Ethical Issues in Modern Medicine

Fifth Edition

John D. Arras
University of Virginia

Bonnie Steinbock
State University of New York–Albany

Mayfield Publishing Company
Mountain View, California
London • Toronto

Library of Congress Cataloging-in-Publication Data
Ethical issues in modern medicine / [edited by] John D. Arras, Bonnie Steinbock.
   —5th ed.
      p.   cm.
   Includes bibliographical references and index.
   ISBN 0-7674-0016-X
   1. Medical ethics.   I. Arras, John.   II. Steinbock, Bonnie.
R724.E788   1998
174' .2—dc21

                                          98-16724
                                          CIP

Manufactured in the United States of America
10 9 8 7 6 5

Mayfield Publishing Company
1280 Villa Street
Mountain View, California 94041

Sponsoring editor, Kenneth King; production,
Publication Services; manuscript editor, Katherine
Coyle; art director, Jeanne M. Schreiber; cover
designer, Diana Coe; manufacturing manager,
Randy Hurst. The text was set in 9/11 Palatino by
Publication Services and printed on 45# Highland
Plus by R. R. Donnelley and Sons Company.

Cover image: Alfred Pasieka/Science Photo
Library. Colored x-ray image of thoracic verte-
brae affected by osteoporosis.

To Daniel Callahan and John Fletcher
with appreciation and gratitude
and
In memory of Benjamin Freedman

PREFACE

As users of *Ethical Issues in Modern Medicine* know, the previous edition represented a complete overhaul of the entire book. It was a job that neither of us was eager to tackle again. Indeed, we expected the new edition to remain relevant for five years, so that we would not have to revise before the year 2000. Enormous technological, legal, and policy developments in several areas, however, made that plan obsolete, and when our editor, Ken King, suggested to me that we needed to do a new edition, we reluctantly conceded that he was right. (John's initial reaction to the idea was something like, "I can't believe we're having this conversation.")

One of those developments concerns the debate over physician-assisted suicide (PAS). The Supreme Court considered, and rejected, a constitutional right to physician-assisted suicide, but its decision in *Vacco* v. *Quill* and *Washington* v. *Glucksberg* has merely returned the debate to the states, not ended it. California and Washington voters rejected measures legalizing PAS, and Oregon is so far the only state to have legalized it, although as of this writing the law has not been implemented. Thus, our expanded section on the moral and policy arguments for and against PAS in Part Two remains timely and urgent.

The field of reproductive medicine continues to grow, and each new development raises moral questions. Since the last edition, the world has seen the birth of a baby to a 63-year-old woman, the development of technology that would permit the freezing of eggs, and the birth of the first surviving set of septuplets. Most dramatic of all, Dr. Ian Wilmut announced the birth of Dolly, a lamb cloned from a cell of an adult sheep. This feat, and the potential for cloning a human being, has given rise to so much debate and speculation that we felt an entire section of Part Four should be devoted to cloning. Although some critics of cloning object to asexual reproduction (or replication) per se, others object to the potential for manipulating the genome, and the creation of children "to spec." Defenders of genetic manipulation respond that we already attempt to make our children healthier and smarter by environmental intervention (from prenatal behavior to diet to piano lessons): the question is, then, whether there is something about genetic intervention that is different and morally problematic.

It must be emphasized that the ability to determine behavior by manipulating genes is greatly exaggerated in the public mind. The belief that genes determine what we are is the "fallacy of genetic determinism," which was strongly criticized in the National Bioethics Advisory Commission Report on Cloning Human Beings. Although many personality traits and susceptibility to many diseases have a genetic component, it does not follow that an individual's behavioral characteristics can be determined through manipulation of his or her genes. Diseases, much less behaviors, are rarely the result of a defect on a single, identifiable gene. Genes interact with each other in complex ways, and genes interact with environmental influences in even more complicated ways. It is simply not the case now or in the foreseeable future that we will be able to determine the level of intelligence, or the degree of compassion or boldness, in an individual by genetic manipulation. Nevertheless, even within the confines of what is scientifically possible, there is room for moral debate about the kinds of traits, if any, it is morally permissible to attempt to control.

The increasing influence of managed care is another development that has required considerable revision, as reflected in two parts in this edition: in "Conflicts of Interest and Informed Consent in Managed Care" in Part One, Sections Three and Four, and in Part Six, Sections Two and Three, on rationing health care. The aim in both places is to give readers a better understanding of the economic forces that have led to the implacable rise of managed care, and of how essential cost-cutting might be accomplished according to just principles and fair procedures.

Despite a firm commitment to the principle "If it ain't broke, don't fix it," we ended up making more changes than we had anticipated. The fifth edition has over 40 new readings—almost as many new readings as the fourth edition. And while some sections remain substantially the same, many are radically changed, and sometimes renamed. Part Six, "Allocation, Social Justice, Health Policy," is a good example of a chapter that required a great deal of rethinking, adding, and subtracting. John did a yeoman's job on this part, with a little help (no, a lot of help, actually) from his friends, especially Len Fleck (Michigan State University) and Peggy Battin (University of Utah). In addition, there are new articles on informed consent, the definition of death, advance directives, abortion, procreative autonomy and responsibility, commodification and the family, and experimentation on human subjects. Some completely new sections have been added, including "Controversies over Contraception," and "'Vulnerable' Populations" in Part Five, "Experimentation on Human Subjects." The book also has 16 case studies, 8 of them new to this edition. We have tried to achieve a balance between application and analysis, because (to paraphrase Kant) analysis without application is empty, while application without analysis is blind.

Two sections were reluctantly deleted: medical futility and maternal-fetal conflicts. As always, adding current material necessitates the sacrifice of something else. We agreed that the debate over medical futility often masked other issues, such as patient self-determination, professional responsibility, and cost, and was best discussed under those headings. As for maternal-fetal conflict, we felt that this topic was cogent only in regard to the legal system's response to pregnant addicts. Within the medical community, there has been a growing consensus that forcing a competent patient to undergo a cesarean section against her will, even when deemed necessary to protect the nearly born fetus, is neither legal nor good medical practice. With such consensus, the issue has become less pressing.

As always, we owe thanks to the many people who have helped us with suggestions, background information, comments, and criticisms. In particular, we would like to single out George Annas, Boston University; Ira Byock, American Academy of Hospice and Palliative Medicine; Jim Childress, Paul Lombardo, Jonathan Moreno, Robert Crouch, and Mark Douglas, University of Virginia; Norman Daniels, Tufts; Rebecca Dresser, Case Western Reserve; Alan Fleischman, New York Academy of Medicine; Norman Fost, University of Wisconsin; Eric T. Juengst, Case Western Reserve; Don Marquis, University of Kansas; Erik Parens, the Hastings Center; Mark Sheldon, Indiana University; Jeffrey Spike, University of Rochester; Benjamin Wilfond, University of Arizona; and the five anonymous reviewers of the fourth edition.

We both owe an enormous debt of gratitude to the members of our "UVa production team," who worked tirelessly and efficiently on all the important and seemingly endless chores involved in the preparation of this book. Carolyn Randolph, the administrative assistant (and heart and soul) of our Bioethics Program, and Sasha Yamshchikov, an outstanding third-year premed and bioethics major, did superlative work on the dreaded job of cutting and pasting the entire manuscript, securing permissions, and updating our lists of contributors and "Resources in Bioethics." Alex John London, a Ph.D. candidate in classical philosophy and bioethics, updated and vastly expanded the bibliographies at the end of each part, wrote an excellent case study for Part Six, and provided timely and sound pedagogical advice on the proposed readings. And Robert Crouch, also a doctoral student in philosophy, helped with both valuable textual suggestions and proofreading. The members of this production crew were unfailingly precise and remarkably good humored from beginning to end. Although their work has taken place behind the scenes, it shows on literally every page. Heartfelt thanks to you all!

In addition, John would like to thank his academic colleagues at the University of Virginia for providing such a welcoming and stimulating intellectual environment. First and foremost, thanks to John Fletcher, who brought John here from New York and has given selflessly of his friendship, time, and knowledge of the field. Now that John Fletcher is in semi-retirement (the equivalent of full-time work for the rest of us), John will cherish their past and future intellectual exchanges, particularly the one that changed John Fletcher's mind on physician-assisted suicide. John also thanks Jim Childress (Religious Studies), Richard Bonnie, Paul Lombardo and Walter Wadlington (Law School), the members of the UVa Philosophy Department, and the Division of Medical Humanities for making his life here in Charlottesville so interesting and challenging.

Bonnie Steinbock owes a debt of gratitude to the members of the working groups on which she has served over the last three years: the National Study Group for Ethics, Genetics, and Alzheimer's Disease, at the Center for Biomedical Ethics, Case Western Reserve University, headed by Stephen Post; the Project on Prenatal Testing for Genetic Disability, at The Hastings Center, headed by Erik Parens; and the Project on Reproductive Choice and Control of Fertility, at the Centre for Social Ethics and Policy, University of Manchester, England, headed by Margot Brazier. From all of these groups, she learned a great deal, enabling her to do a better job updating *Ethical Issues in Modern Medicine*.

We are indebted as well to the following individuals for their thoughtful review of the manuscript for this edition: Ben Bradley, University of Massachusetts at Amherst; Patti L. Brandt, Virginia Commonwealth University; William Harper, University of Alabama; Nelson P. Lande, University of Massachusetts at Boston; Bruce Landesman, University of Utah; Greg Lobean, Center for Bio-ethics at University of Pennsylvania; Cynthia L. Owen, University of Toledo; and William Ruddick, New York University.

For turning the sow's ear of our bulging and tattered manuscript into this silk purse of a book, we are thankful once again to the production staff at Mayfield Publishing Company, this time to April Wells-Hayes and Josh Tepfer. Our friends at Publication Services, ably headed by Dawn Longfellow and Jan Fisher, did what we had hardly thought possible: to bring this book from rough manuscript to finished product within a few short months. Hats off to one and all!

Finally, we wish to thank Ken King, our new editor at Mayfield. He is a fountain of good ideas, good sense, and good humor, and we are immensely grateful for his support, guidance, and gentle *nudzhing*.

Bonnie Steinbock
John D. Arras

CONTENTS

PART TWO
Defining Death, Forgoing Life-Sustaining Treatment, and Euthanasia   131

PART THREE
Contraception, Abortion, and Prenatal Diagnosis   307

PART FOUR
Assisted Reproductive Technologies and Genetics   407

PART SIX
Allocation, Social Justice, and Health Policy   617

THE CONTRIBUTORS

George J. Annas, J.D., M.P.H., is Professor and Chair of the Health Law Department at the Boston University Schools of Medicine and Public Health.

John D. Arras, Ph.D., is the William and Linda Porterfield Professor of Bioethics and Professor of Philosophy at the University of Virginia, Charlottesville.

Adrienne Asch, Ph.D., is the Henry R. Luce Professor in Biology, Ethics, and the Politics of Human Reproduction at Wellesley College.

Margaret Battin, Ph.D., M.F.A., is Professor of Philosophy and Adjunct Professor of Internal Medicine in the Division of Medical Ethics at the University of Utah.

Allan Brandt, Ph.D., is the Amalie Moses Kass Professor of the History of Medicine at the Harvard Medical School, in Boston, Massachusetts.

Dan W. Brock, Ph.D., is the Charles C. Tillinghast, Jr., University Professor and Professor of Philosophy and Biomedical Ethics, and the Director of the Center for Biomedical Ethics at Brown University in Providence, Rhode Island.

Howard Brody, M.D., Ph.D., is Professor and Director of the Center for Ethics and Humanities in the Life Sciences at Michigan State University in East Lansing, Michigan.

Allen Buchanan, Ph.D., is Professor of Philosophy, Affiliate Professor of Medical Ethics at the School of Medicine Program of Medical Ethics, and the Grainger Professor of Business Ethics (School of Business) at the University of Wisconsin, Madison.

Keith Burton is Executive Managing Director and General Manager, Chicago, of Hill and Knowlton, an international public relations and public affairs firm.

William Byne, M.D., is a Lecturer on Brain Sciences and Behavior at the Mount Sinai Medical School in New York.

Daniel Callahan, Ph.D., is Founder and Director of International Programs of the Hastings Center, Briarcliff Manor, New York.

Sidney Callahan, Ph.D., is Professor of Psychology at Mercy College in Dobbs Ferry, New York.

Norman Cantor, J.D., is Professor of Law and Justice Nathan Jacobs Scholar at the Rutgers University School of Law in Newark, New Jersey.

Christine Cassell, M.D., is Professor and Chair of the Department of Geriatrics and Adult Development at Mount Sinai Medical Center in New York.

R. Alta Charo, J.D., is Professor of Law and Medical Ethics at the Law and Medical Schools of the University of Wisconsin. She has served on the NIH Human Embryo Research Panel and the National Bioethics Advisory Commission.

Kate T. Christensen, M.D., F.A.C.P., is an Internist and the Regional Ethics Coordinator at the Department of Ethics of the Kaiser Permanente Medical Group, Inc., in Antioch, California.

Carl Cohen, Ph.D., is Professor of Philosophy at the University of Michigan in Ann Arbor.

Norman Daniels, Ph.D., is the Goldthwaite Professor in the Department of Philosophy at Tufts University in Medford, Massachusetts.

Alan Donagan, Ph.D., was Professor of Philosophy at the University of Chicago and the California Institute of Technology.

Rebecca S. Dresser, J.D., is Professor of Law at Washington University, St. Louis.

Ronald Dworkin, L.L.B., is Professor of Jurisprudence at Oxford University and Professor of Law and Philosophy at New York University.

David Eddy, M.D., Ph.D., is Senior Advisor for Health Policy and Management at Kaiser Permanente of Southern California.

Stuart Eisendrath, Ph.D., is Professor of Clinical Psychiatry at the University of California in San Francisco.

Ezekiel J. Emanuel, M.D., Ph.D., is an oncologist at the Dana-Farber Cancer Institute, a medical ethicist at Harvard Medical School in Boston, Massachusetts, and the Director of the National Institutes of Health Bioethics Program in Bethesda, Maryland.

Linda L. Emanuel, M.D., Ph.D., is Vice President of the Ethics Standards Division at the American Medical Association in Chicago, Illinois.

H. Tristram Engelhardt, Jr., Ph.D., M.D., is Professor of Medicine and Community Medicine at Baylor College of Medicine in Houston, Texas.

Leonard M. Fleck, Ph.D., is Professor of Philosophy and Medical Ethics in the Philosophy Department and the Center for Ethics and Humanities in the Life Sciences, Michigan State University.

Benjamin Freedman, Ph.D., was Professor at the McGill Centre for Medicine, Ethics, and Law, Montreal, Canada, and Clinical Ethicist at the Sir Mortimer B. Davis–Jewish General Hospital, Montreal, until his tragic and untimely death in 1997.

Norman Fost, M.D., is Professor and Vice-Chairman of Pediatrics and the Director of the Program in Medical Ethics at the University of Wisconsin in Madison.

Alan Goldman, Ph.D., is Professor of Philosophy at the University of Miami, Florida.

Mark A. Hall is a Professor of Law and Public Health at Wake Forest University. His recent works include a textbook, *Health Care Law and Ethics* (Aspen, 1998), and *Making Medical Spending Decisions: The Law, Ethics, and Economics of Rationing Mechanisms* (Oxford, 1997).

John Hardwig, Ph.D., is Professor of Philosophy and Medical Ethics in the Department of Philosophy and the Quillen Dishner College of Medicine at East Tennessee State University, Johnson City.

John Harris, Ph.D., is a Reader of Ethics and Medical Ethics at the Victoria University of Manchester, in Manchester, England.

Deborah S. Hellman, M.A., J.D., is Assistant Professor of Law at the University of Maryland, Baltimore.

Samuel Hellman, M.D., is Professor of Radiation and Cellular Oncology at the Cancer Research Center of the University of Chicago School of Medicine.

Albert R. Jonsen, Ph.D., is Professor of Ethics in Medicine and the Chairman of the Department of Medical History and Ethics at the University of Washington School of Medicine in Seattle, Washington.

Leon R. Kass, Ph.D., is the Addie Clark Harding Professor in the Committee on Social Thought at the University of Chicago.

Jay Katz, M.D., is Professor of Law Emeritus at Yale Law School in New Haven, Connecticut.

Jacinta Kerin, Ph.D., teaches medical ethics in the faculty of medicine at Monash University, Melbourne, Australia.

Carol Levine, M.A., is the Director of the Families and Healthcare Project at the United Hospital Fund in New York, New York.

Norman Levinsky, M.D., is Professor and Chair of the Department of Medicine at the Boston University School of Medicine.

Alex John London is a Ph.D. candidate in the Philosophy Department at the University of Virginia. His interests are in ancient philosophy, ethics, and bioethics.

Charles C. Lund, M.D., was in the Department of Surgery at Harvard Medical School and the Surgical Service at Boston City Hospital.

Peter Lurie, M.D., M.P.H., is a Visiting Assistant Research Scientist at the Institute for Social Research at the University of Michigan and an Assistant Professor in the Department of Family and Community Medicine, University of California, San Francisco.

Maurie Markman, M.D., is Director of the Cleveland Clinic Cancer Center, Ohio.

Don Marquis, Ph.D., is Professor of Philosophy at the University of Kansas, Lawrence.

Ron McClamrock, Ph.D., is Associate Professor of Philosophy at the State University of New York at Albany.

Paul T. Menzel, Ph.D., is Professor of Philosophy and Provost at Pacific Lutheran University in Tacoma, Washington.

E. Haavi Morreim, Ph.D., is Professor in the Department of Human Values and Ethics at the University of Tennessee College of Medicine, Memphis.

Alvin H. Moss, M.D., is Professor of Medicine and Director of the Center for Health Ethics and Law at West Virginia University, Morgantown.

Thomas H. Murray, Ph.D., is Professor and Director of the Center for Biomedical Ethics at Case Western Reserve University School of Medicine in Cleveland, Ohio.

Thomas Nagel, Ph.D., is Professor of Law and Professor of Philosophy at New York University.

Robert Nozick, Ph.D., is the Arthur Kingsley Porter Professor of Philosophy at Harvard University.

Timothy E. Quill, M.D., is an internist and Associate Professor of Medicine and Psychiatry at the University of Rochester School of Medicine and Dentistry, New York.

John Rawls, Ph.D., is Professor of Philosophy Emeritus at Harvard University.

Nancy K. Rhoden, J.D., was Professor of Law at the University of North Carolina at Chapel Hill. She was also coeditor of the third edition of *Ethical Issues in Modern Medicine.*

John A. Robertson, J.D., holds the Vinson & Elkins Chair of Law at the University of Texas School of Law, and is the Co-Chair of the Ethics Committee of the American Society of Reproductive Medicine.

Barbara Katz Rothman, Ph.D., is Professor of Sociology at Baruch College and the City University of New York Graduate Center, New York, New York.

James E. Sabin, M.D., Ph.D., is Co-Director of the Center for Ethics in Managed Care at Harvard Pilgrim Healthcare and Harvard Medical School, and Associate Clinical Professor of Psychiatry at Harvard Medical School.

David Satcher, M.D., Ph.D., has been the Director of the Centers for Disease Control and Prevention and an administrator at the Agency for Toxic Substances and Disease Registry in Atlanta, Georgia. He has recently been appointed Surgeon General of the U.S. Public Health Service.

Thomas Scanlon, Ph.D., is Professor of Philosophy at Harvard University.

Udo Schüklenk, Ph.D., is a Lecturer at the Monash University Centre for Human Bioethics, Melbourne, Australia.

Susan Sherwin, Ph.D., is Professor of Philosophy and Women's Studies at Dalhousie University in Halifax, Nova Scotia.

Mark Siegler, M.D., is Director of the Maclean Center for Clinical Medical Ethics at the University of Chicago.

Edward Stein, Ph.D., teaches Philosophy and Lesbian and Gay Science at Yale University in New Haven, Connecticut.

Bonnie Steinbock, Ph.D., is Professor of Philosophy, Public Policy, and Public Health at the State University of New York at Albany.

Stuart Tailor, Jr., is Senior Writer with American Lawyer Media, L.P., and the *American Lawyer* magazine.

Judith Jarvis Thomson, Ph.D., is Professor of Philosophy at the Massachusetts Institute of Technology, Cambridge, Massachusetts.

Robert Truog, M.D., is Director of the Multidisciplinary Intensive Care Unit at Children's Hospital in Boston, and Associate Professor of Anesthesiology and Pediatrics at Harvard Medical School.

Harold Varmus, Ph.D., is the Director of the National Institutes of Health in Bethesda, Maryland.

Robert M. Veatch, Ph.D., is Professor of Medical Ethics at the Kennedy Institute of Ethics at Georgetown University in Washington, D.C.

Mary Anne Warren, Ph.D., is Professor of Philosophy at San Francisco State University.

Robert M. White, M.D., is Professor of Psychiatry at the University of Texas Medical Branch at Galveston.

Benjamin S. Wilfond, M.D., is a physician in the Department of Pediatrics at the University of Arizona Health Sciences Center in Tucson, Arizona.

Sidney Wolfe, M.D., is Director of the Public Citizen Research Group in Washington, D.C.

Robert Wright, B.S., is author of *The Moral Animal: Evolutionary Psychology and Everyday Life* and is a contributing editor at *The New Republic* and at *Slate* magazine.

INTRODUCTION

MORAL REASONING IN THE MEDICAL CONTEXT

John D. Arras
Bonnie Steinbock
Alex John London

BIOETHICS: NATURE AND SCOPE

Doctor Deborah Brody was not looking forward to Jim Lasken's next visit. Jim, a 40-year-old former postman, devoted husband, and father of two teenagers, was at a critical juncture in his treatment for amyotrophic lateral sclerosis, a progressive and ultimately fatal degenerative disease of the nervous system, known to most people as Lou Gehrig's disease. Dr. Brody had been seeing Jim for the past ten years, during which time his condition had been steadily deteriorating. Jim was now in very bad shape. In the past three years he had lost the ability to walk, work, dress himself, and sit up without supports. He was now incontinent, and could only speak a few short words at a time, and only with agonizing difficulty. Jim's psychological state had tracked his physical decline. Although he had kept up a brave front as many of his faculties declined over the first years of his illness, Jim was becoming more and more despondent as his condition worsened. Dr. Brody suspected that Jim was in a deep depression, but, given his life prospects, she could not really blame him.

Dr. Brody dreaded Jim's next visit not simply because he was seriously ill and getting progressively worse, but because Jim had been asking her to help him "end it." As he and his wife, Jane, had explained, Jim's life had become unbearable. He could no longer enjoy his former hobbies, he could no longer communicate with anyone without enduring monumental frustration and fatigue, he knew he was a tremendous burden to his family, and was well aware that things were just going to get worse. It had become

---

EDITORS' NOTE: Although this essay represents a complete reworking and expansion of the introduction from previous editions of this book, the authors gratefully acknowledge the enduring contributions of Robert Hunt, coeditor of the first edition, to these pages.

clear, in fact, that Jim would soon have to be hooked up to a mechanical ventilator to do his breathing for him, or else he would drown in his own secretions.

This was apparently the last straw. Jim was now adamant: he saw no point in either going on the respirator or dying a slow, wasting death without it. He wanted to die now, and he wanted Dr. Brody to help him. "Give me a shot," he implored, "it's all you can do for me now. My life is over."

Dr. Brody now had a serious problem. Should she help her patient commit suicide? Indeed, since Jim could no longer actively do anything to take his own life, the doctor would have to do it herself, engaging in what is called *active euthanasia*. She knew that it was against the law in her state either to assist someone in a suicide or directly to kill another person, but could such an act be ethically permitted if the patient were sufficiently desperate and helpless? Supposing that *someone* might be justified in performing euthanasia, was this the sort of thing that a *doctor* could or should do? As a physician, she empathized with her patient's pain, isolation, and desperation, and would have done just about anything to alleviate his terrible suffering. "A big part of my job is to combat suffering, not just death," she thought. "If my patient's mental and physical suffering can only be ended by death, and if his life is no longer of any use to him, why should I not help him?" On the other hand, she recalled the Hippocratic Oath, a version of which she took upon graduation from medical school, which condemned giving patients "deadly drugs." The message, transmitted from one generation of doctors to the next, was that physicians are supposed to be healers, not killers.

Dr. Brody's dilemma is also society's problem. More and more individuals are claiming that just as they have a right to control what happens to their own bodies during life, so they have a right to control the timing and manner of their deaths. Celebrated cases, like that of Dr. Kevorkian in Michigan, focus public attention on the question of whether the laws that currently constrain Dr. Brody should be changed. Given appropriate circumstances, checks, and balances, should doctors be given legal permission to prescribe deadly drugs for their suicidal patients? Should they be allowed to kill outright? What are the social implications of allowing individuals such a right to die?

Should these practices become widespread, what would be the likelihood of abuse and the "slippery slope" toward killing the mentally infirm, the elderly, and the poor?

Problems of this sort lie at the heart of contemporary bioethics, the field introduced by this anthology. Like its parent disciplines, moral philosophy and religious ethics, bioethics is a study of moral conduct, of right and wrong. As such, it is inescapably *normative*. As opposed to some historical or social scientific approaches to moral conduct that emphasize description of the way the world is, or causal conjectures about why it is the way it is, bioethics inquires about the rightness or wrongness of various actions, character traits, and social policies. Thus, instead of fixing on such issues as the history of physicians' participation in their patients' suicides, or the way in which their attitudes are shaped by age, gender, specialty, and so on, "bioethicists" typically ask whether assisted suicide or euthanasia can be morally justified, whether either practice would be good social policy, and whether these practices are compatible with the character traits of a good physician. (This is not to say, however, that good normative reasoning can or should take place without careful attention to empirical details, which often prove crucial to the careful resolution of practical moral problems.)

In addition to these straightforward normative concerns, bioethicists are also increasingly interested in what philosophers call "metaethical" themes. That is, they are concerned not just with the question, say, of whether assisted suicide is morally justified, but also with broader and more abstract questions bearing on the nature of moral justification and the kind of thinking that supports it. As we shall see near the end of this essay, some bioethicists might claim, for example, that the justifiability of physician-assisted suicide must be sought in the articulation and application of various moral theories or principles, while others might claim that justification must proceed the other way around, beginning with concrete and unmistakable instances of good and bad behavior, and then gradually developing principles that capture and distill our most fundamental moral responses to cases. It is a question, in other words, of whether ethical thought should proceed from the "top down" or from the "bottom up."

SOURCES OF BIOETHICAL PROBLEMS AND CONCERNS

Since its birth in the early 1970s, the contemporary bioethics movement has grown from a mere blip on the radar of public consciousness to a major academic- and service-oriented profession with its own research centers, journals, conferences, and degree programs. Not a week goes by, it seems, without some controversial biomedical case or issue making its way into the nation's headlines and talk shows: "Gene for Homosexuality Discovered!" "Parents Insist on Treatment for Baby Without a Brain!" "Patients Subjected to Radiation Experiments Without Their Consent!" "Dr. Kevorkian Strikes Again!" Why are we beset in this present age with so many fundamental and fascinating questions?

TECHNOLOGICAL INNOVATION

Obviously, much of the ferment in contemporary biomedical ethics is due to the unrelenting pace of technological advance. The story is by now familiar: Clever physicians, researchers, and technicians discover newer and better ways to do things, such as sustaining the lives of terminally ill patients, diagnosing fetal abnormalities in utero, and facilitating conception for infertile couples. Before we know it, however, these new techniques and services begin to take on lives of their own, expanding well beyond the problems and patients for whom they were originally intended.

Cardiopulmonary resuscitation, for example, originally intended for otherwise healthy victims of drowning or electrocution, has gradually and unceremoniously become a violent and final "rite of passage" for many aged, moribund patients in our nation's hospitals. The administration of artificial nutrition and hydration, originally intended as a temporary bridge to the restoration of patients' digestive functioning, now is routinely delivered to thousands of patients who have irretrievably lost all higher brain functions.

Prenatal diagnosis, originally intended for fetuses at high risk of a metabolic or genetic disorder, is now routinely offered to, and sought by, many women in their late twenties or early thirties who are at no special health risk. The availability of this technology has thus expanded choice, while simultaneously imposing new pressures on many women by altering their definition of an "acceptable risk" during pregnancy.

Finally, in vitro fertilization (IVF), originally developed to aid infertile married couples, is now offered to single women, to adult daughters volunteering to serve as surrogate mothers for their own mothers' children (i.e., to be the mothers of their own siblings), and to postmenopausal women in their late forties and fifties. In conjunction with the newly developed techniques of embryo freezing and "embryo splitting," a kind of cloning, IVF might soon make it possible for a woman grown from a split embryo to give birth to her own previously frozen identical twin.

Needless to say, problems such as these, as they spawn new possibilities for remaking ourselves, our families, and our society, call into question the adequacy of our traditional ways of thinking. In some instances, it is clear that scientific and technological developments have brought about a change in values and moral beliefs. As Emmanuel Mesthene has remarked, "By adding new options . . . technology can lead to changes in values in the same way that the appearance of new dishes on the heretofore standard menu of one's favorite restaurant can lead to changes in one's tastes and choices of food."[1] Often, what science and technology make possible soon becomes permissible and, eventually, normal and expected. For example, when the use of anesthesia during childbirth was introduced around 150 years ago, it was condemned as morally wrong. Women were "supposed" to suffer through labor: it was "unnatural" if they did not. But what *could* be done *was* done, and eventually those beliefs were revised.

In the more recent past, we have noted a change in attitude toward heart transplants; at first, many people had moral reservations about this procedure, not because it was new and risky, but because the heart was associated with the soul or personality. Today, although heart transplants continue to raise social policy problems, this particular moral reservation has completely vanished.

Most readers may feel comfortable about the attitudinal changes just mentioned, but in other

1. Emmanuel Mesthene, "The Role of Technology in Society," in *Technology and Man's Future,* edited by A. Teich (New York: St. Martin's Press, 1972), 137.

areas the influence of technology on values and morals has had more controversial results. For example, developments in medical knowledge and techniques have played a major role in reshaping cultural and legal attitudes toward contraception and abortion, and more recent developments— e.g., the "abortion pill," RU 486, and long-acting contraceptives such as Norplant—promise to erode traditional moral qualms even further. Yet not everyone believes that these developments constitute an unalloyed good; some regard them as a profound insult to their conception of the sanctity of life, while others suspect that they will be coercively targeted at vulnerable minority groups. And what about the near future? Already there is widespread concern regarding the ethical implications of techniques and procedures that are still in their developmental stages. Will developments in genetic knowledge made possible by the human genome project and advances in reproductive technologies help usher in a "brave new world"? Is there, perhaps, some knowledge that we ought not try to seek? Or are our reservations about such matters as in vitro fertilization for women old enough to be grandmothers as time-bound and unwarranted as those of the people who opposed anesthesia and heart transplants?

As Nicholas Rescher has pointed out, the phenomenon of value change is a complex one, and technological developments may lead to "value restandardization."[2] The value of good health may not have changed position in our hierarchy of values, but as a result of technology the standard of what constitutes good health may have been revised considerably upward. As technology increases the possibilities in life, as values diversify and expectations rise, abnormalities—and common conditions—that were once taken for granted come to be viewed as pathological conditions requiring treatment and/or prevention. It is, after all, a comparatively recent assumption that medical relief can and should be sought for such conditions as acne, obesity, short stature, crooked teeth, small breasts, and the failure to achieve orgasm.

In addition to curing disease, medicine is now increasingly capable of *optimizing* more or less normal conditions that nevertheless can be improved upon. Drugs like Prozac, for example, promise a future in which individuals might not merely manage clinical depression better, but also alter their personalities in significantly positive ways. Having problems with self-esteem? Having trouble mustering the courage to ask for that promotion? "Cosmetic psychopharmacology" may be able to provide just what you need.[3]

Related to all these issues is, of course, the restandardization of what constitutes adequate health care. Today we expect not only to be cured of ills that were previously incurable, but also to be prevented from experiencing a variety of infirmities and misfortunes that were once the common lot of humankind. And we feel wronged if these expectations go unfulfilled. Driven by the pressure of consumer demand, treatments that many might regard today as "frills," such as in vitro fertilization and cosmetic personality-altering drugs, may well be regarded tomorrow as essential ingredients in the "pursuit of happiness."

The impact of technology on our value systems is also seen in the fact that the development of new knowledge and techniques may blur, rather than sharpen, the very concepts that are central to our norms and values. The advent of organ transplantation and critical-care technologies, for example, has forced physicians and society at large to rethink the very meanings of life and death. The traditional "definition" of life as the presence of respiration and heartbeat has been replaced in every U.S. state over the past twenty years by the notion of whole-brain death, yet few people, even today, can identify a noncontroversial philosophical rationale for the new law's insistence that the entire brain, both "higher" and "lower," must have ceased functioning irreversibly for a patient to be dead. As a result, the moral and legal status of patients with no higher brain functions, those in persistent vegetative states, poses an ongoing challenge to the current approach to brain death. If a patient has permanently lost the capacity for any kind of thought, feeling, and human interaction— if, to put it somewhat crudely, "no one is home"— why not consider him or her to be dead? (Issues such as this also raise methodological questions:

2. Nicholas Rescher, "What Is Value Change? A Framework for Research," in *Values and the Future*, edited by K. Baier and N. Rescher (New York: Free Press, 1969).

3. Peter Kramer, *Listening to Prozac* (New York: Viking, 1993).

e.g., Is the definition of death primarily a matter of discovery, death being some kind of brute fact with contours that merely need better tracing, or is it, rather, something that the citizens of a political community must *invent* for themselves?)

The definition of death is perhaps the most salient conceptual puzzle served up by the new medicine, but it is by no means the only one. Similar issues are posed by the advent of new reproductive technologies (Is a woman who donates an egg to another woman the "mother" of the child born? Is she a mother in any sense that matters?), the human genome project (Is the otherwise healthy 20-year-old carrier of a gene associated with the development of coronary artery disease in later life "diseased" in some sense?), and, of course, abortion (Is the fetus a "person" or full-fledged human being deserving of our respect and protection, is it merely a clump of cells, or is it perhaps something in-between?).

Finally, technology drives the bioethical agenda by virtue of its phenomenal success in addressing medical needs and desires. Hundreds of years ago, when medicine could offer little more than bleeding, blistering, and purging—when the leech represented the cutting edge of biotechnology—there weren't many "tragic choices" to be made. With the advent of technological success, however, has come the need to pay for increasingly expensive curative, diagnostic, and palliative procedures, access to which is increasingly perceived as a matter of right. But as costs skyrocket and as the demand for access spreads, the inevitability of limits and priority-setting gradually comes into focus. Assuming that meeting every conceivable health care need would either break the bank or devour funds earmarked for other important societal needs—such as food, shelter, education, transportation, and the arts—the question of the explicit rationing of health care acquires real seriousness and urgency. Can we afford to pay for a patient's third organ transplant, for his or her experimental bone marrow transplant for advanced cancer, or for the short but otherwise normal child's synthetic growth hormone injections? Can we afford these things when millions of people lack basic health insurance and decent preventive and primary care? Conceived in their broadest framework, these questions ask how our health care system might be reformed so as to provide universal access to a good package of "basic" services, without either bankrupting society or destroying the doctor-patient relationship.

OTHER SOURCES OF BIOETHICAL PROBLEMS

Although the urgency and frequency of bioethical controversies owe much to the magnitude and pace of technological change, there are other factors at work driving the recent explosion of bioethical issues. Some medical-moral problems of long standing, such as the limits of confidentiality, truth-telling, and euthanasia, have more to do with the ethics of human relationships—with what we owe to one another and may (or may not) do to one another—than with the advent of new technologies. More important than technology in reshaping the physician-patient relationship are such widespread social phenomena as the increasing demand, modeled on the civil rights movement, for patients' rights to information and health care; the growing distrust of professional privilege; women's critiques of male dominance within medicine; and the assimilation of medicine to our consumerist and entrepreneurial culture.

Even here, however, it remains true that advances in biology and medicine have often given a characteristically modern spin to some of these traditional problems. Truth-telling, for example, is perhaps now more important and more difficult an obligation than ever before, due in large measure to the vast proliferation of possible treatments and diagnostic interventions available to physicians and their patients. Likewise, our traditional norms governing the confidentiality of medical information are sorely tested when new genetic tests reveal serious abnormalities not only in patients coming for diagnosis and/or treatment, but also, of necessity, in some of their family members as well.

Still, many highly controversial practices require surprisingly little technological assistance in threatening our fundamental values and established customs. Artificial insemination with donated sperm, for example, allows infertile married couples to have children, but it also enables single women and lesbian partners to give birth without the presence of a male spouse; in addition, it makes possible the practice of so-called surrogate motherhood, in which, for example, a woman agrees to be inseminated with the sperm of the husband of a childless marriage. For some, these developments signal serious threats to the welfare of children and to the institution of marriage, the very bedrock of our society; for others, they merely represent the next logical step in the growth of reproductive rights for all individuals, whether they be married or single, straight or gay, fertile or infertile. Ironically, at the heart of this impassioned debate about rights, marriage, and society lies the most ordinary of technological means: the humble turkey baster.

CHALLENGES TO ETHICAL THEORY

The issues raised in the preceding section pose challenging factual, conceptual, and moral problems. People often have strong feelings about some of these issues (for example, abortion and euthanasia). On some issues, many of us do not know what to think (for example, IVF for older women, or using children born without a higher brain as sources of transplantable organs). The assumption in philosophical bioethics is that careful analysis can help us at least make progress on some of these issues, if not resolve all of them. However, some are skeptical about this assumption. They believe, for a variety of reasons, that ethical disputes are, in principle, unresolvable by rational means.

MORAL NIHILISM

Princeton philosopher Gilbert Harman defines *moral nihilism* as "the doctrine that there are no moral facts, no moral truths, and no moral knowledge."[4] Extreme nihilists think that nothing is right or wrong; that morality, like religion, is an illusion that should be abandoned. This implies that torturing, raping, and killing a young child is not wrong—something few people could accept. More moderate nihilists do not recommend abandoning morality, but, rather, offer a theory about the meaning of moral terms that explains why there are no moral facts, truths, or knowledge.

4. Gilbert Harman, *The Nature of Morality: An Introduction to Ethics* (New York: Oxford University Press, 1977), 11.

ETHICS AND FEELINGS

The theory of moral language that is offered by moderate moral nihilists is known as *emotivism*. Emotivists believe that moral utterances do not express facts, or tell us anything about how the world is. Rather, they express our feelings. Therefore, such statements are not—indeed, cannot be—true or false, any more than "Go, Yankees!" is true or false. The sentence, "Abortion is wrong," does not say anything about abortion, but rather expresses someone's negative feelings about abortion.

How plausible is this thesis about moral language? Undoubtedly, moral claims often do express feelings, but it is debatable that that is all they do. Consider Dr. Brody's quandary. She might ask herself, "I wonder if euthanasia is wrong." In an emotivist analysis, this can only mean, "I wonder if I have negative feelings about euthanasia." Is this Dr. Brody's question? It seems rather that she wonders what she *thinks* about euthanasia. Should she be motivated by her empathy for her patient and her desire to alleviate his suffering? Or should she act according to that part of the Hippocratic Oath that requires doctors to be healers, not killers? What would be the larger implications for society if doctors were to engage in terminating their patients' lives? Dr. Brody's internal debate is of a kind familiar to most of us. In other words, when we face a moral dilemma, instead of trying to resolve our puzzlement by an introspective attempt at ascertaining which of our feelings is really the strongest, we tend to look "outward" at various external or objective aspects and implications of the alternatives in order to determine which is right.

We do not deny a relationship between feelings and ethical decisions, for moral issues often, if not always, provoke deep emotional responses. But to assign feelings ultimate authority in these matters is, we think, to put the cart before the horse. Our feelings may provoke us to moral inquiry, but the inquiry does not terminate there.

ETHICS AND CULTURE

Another form of moderate moral nihilism denies the possibility of moral truth *independent of a particular culture*. This view, known as *ethical relativism*, says that morality is relative to the society one lives in and the way one was brought up. The rightness or wrongness of an action or practice cannot be determined apart from the cultural or social context in which it occurs.

Support for ethical relativism comes from three sources. First, it stems from an observation that different cultures have different moral beliefs and practices. However, simply noting moral differences in various cultures does not establish ethical relativism. Ethical relativism goes beyond noting that cultures differ in their moral beliefs and practices; it maintains that when there are moral differences, no one is right (or wrong). According to relativism, right and wrong are always relative to, and determined by, culture.

A reason for thinking that morality is always relative to culture is that there does not seem to be any way to prove that an ethical belief or practice is right (or wrong). Infanticide, for example, is treated as murder in our culture, but is accepted or tolerated in others. Who's to say who's right? The inability to prove an ethical belief is contrasted with the ability to prove factual claims. If we come across people who think that the Earth is flat, we can (in principle) show them that it is round. Note that the difference between ethics and science is not that ethics has a monopoly on disagreement. There are plenty of heated disagreements among scientists. However, scientists agree (in principle) about what kinds of evidence would settle a dispute. There is no such agreement in ethics. In other words, we do not have a decision procedure for resolving ethical disputes. This is the second source of support for ethical relativism.

The above two reasons offered in support of relativism make observations about the world, and then offer a theory about the nature of reality that is consistent with these observations. We might characterize these as intellectual reasons for relativism. The third reason for relativism is quite different. It offers a moral reason for adopting relativism: namely, that relativism promotes tolerance toward people who hold moral beliefs different from one's own. This apparently was the motivation of nineteenth-century anthropologists who wished to prevent Western imperialists from imposing their culture on indigenous peoples.

Assume that we accept the plausible claim that different cultures do in fact differ in their moral beliefs. (Even this statement can be questioned, but let us accept it for the sake of argument.) What about the second support for relativism, that there is no decision procedure in ethics? This claim seems most plausible when we think of controversial issues, such as abortion or euthanasia, about which intelligent people of good will can disagree. Suppose, however, we think instead of a practice that virtually everyone thinks is wrong: for example, slavery. In the eighteenth and nineteenth centuries, slavery was often justified on the grounds that the Africans were inherently inferior to their European masters, incapable of learning or governing themselves. This is a "factual" claim, and it is clearly false. Indeed, had the slaves really been incapable of learning, laws prohibiting the teaching of reading to slaves would have been pointless—there were no laws outlawing the teaching of reading to cows, for example. These and other justifications of slavery are clearly false and self-serving.

Slavery can also be criticized as inconsistent with other fundamental values, such as the equality of all men (or as we would say today, all human beings), as proclaimed in the Declaration of Independence. It seems likely that the discrepancy between the value of equality and the practice of slavery was a motivation for the abolition of slavery, along with its recognition as cruel, exploitative, and unjust. These terms also have considerable factual content, so that it is not "just a matter of opinion" whether a practice is cruel, exploitative, or unjust.

A further point against relativism (parallel to the argument we presented against emotivism) is that it gives an inaccurate account of the meaning of certain moral claims, notably those of moral reformers. According to relativism, right and wrong are always relative to culture. What a culture (or the majority of a culture) thinks is right is right—for them. However, a moral reformer challenges the conventional beliefs of his or her own culture. For example, Martin Luther King, Jr., said that segregation was wrong. According to relativism, this can only mean that segregation is considered wrong by his culture, which was obviously false in the American South in the 1950s. Of course King was not claiming that his culture *regarded* segregation as wrong. He was making the very different claim that segregation *was* wrong.

(Indeed, if his culture already believed that segregation was wrong, he would not have had to demonstrate and go to jail for his beliefs!) Relativism simply cannot make sense of the claims of moral reformers. Since we do understand the claims of moral reformers, and at least sometimes are influenced by them, it seems that relativism cannot be true.

Despite these considerations, ethical relativism holds sway with many people, perhaps because the alternative seems terribly arrogant. One often hears the following sort of argument: "How can anyone say that another person's values are wrong? Who are you to tell me that you're right and I'm wrong? What makes you an authority? Everyone has a right to an opinion." However, we must be careful here. To say that everyone has a right to an opinion is not to say that every opinion is right. One can certainly agree that people have a right to their moral views without being a relativist. Indeed, if we think that everyone has the right to an opinion, we are *not* relativists. For "everyone has the right to an opinion" is itself a moral value. According to relativism, this moral value (like any other) is only true for societies that believe it. But not all cultures accept freedom of thought as a basic value. What if a culture believes in complete conformity of thought, and in brutal suppression of nonconformity? What if they practice conversion by the sword? Can we say that they are wrong to do this, that they ought to be tolerant? Not if we are relativists. Tolerance, then, is not a value that relativists can consistently promote, for tolerance, like all other moral values, is only right in cultures that think it right.

Finally, relativism not only prevents us from criticizing the brutal and intolerant practices of others, it also does not permit us to criticize our own past. We cannot say that slavery or child labor or the oppression of women were mistakes, since this implies an objective moral standard according to which we can evaluate our past practices. There is no moral progress, only moral change. This is another reason for rejecting ethical relativism, at least in its most extreme form.

At the same time, relativism has two things to recommend it, which we believe can be incorporated into a nonrelativist approach. First, the relativist is right to point out that morality occurs in a cultural context. Before presuming to judge another culture's practices and beliefs, we would do well to try to understand them "from the inside." We may still decide ultimately that a practice is wrong, but we are not entitled to make this judgment without understanding the practice in context. Second, relativism encourages multiple perspectives on and solutions to moral problems. Both of these insights are present in "multiculturalism." As we understand it, multiculturalism is *not* an uncritical acceptance of the values and practices of all other cultures. Rather, it is the awareness that there are a range of different ways to live, which offer different solutions to the problems faced by human beings, combined with a recognition that our own solutions—practices, institutions, values, and moral rules—may not be the best ones. Multiculturalism is a welcome corrective to an unfortunate tendency of Western civilization to assume superiority and to dismiss other ways of life as inferior and backward.

One can, however, be a multiculturalist without being a relativist. Indeed, it is only if one *rejects* relativism that one can meaningfully say such things as, "Our culture's attitude toward nature is domineering, exploitative, and wasteful. We could learn something from Native Americans." Multiculturalism requires an open mind toward the customs and beliefs of other cultures, but such open-mindedness need not, and should not, be uncritical. It is entirely consistent with a conception of morality as amenable to rational considerations, and the conviction that there can be better or worse moral justifications.[5]

MORAL THEORIES AND PERSPECTIVES

How are we to assess moral reasons and arguments? Intuitively, most of us can probably recognize good—or especially bad—moral reasoning, but in complicated situations we are often left wondering whether a consideration is pertinent. Is

5. Robert K. Fullinwider, "Ethnocentrism and Education in Judgment," *Report from the Institute for Philosophy & Public Policy* 14 (1994): 6–11. See also Charles Taylor et al., *Multiculturalism and "The Politics of Recognition"* (Princeton, NJ: Princeton University Press, 1992); and Amy Gutmann, "The Challenge of Multiculturalism in Political Ethics," *Philosophy and Public Affairs* 22, no. 3 (Summer 1993): 171–206.

assisted suicide wrong because it helps someone to kill him- or herself, and killing is wrong? Or is it right because it helps someone to do what he or she reasonably wants to do, and thus promotes autonomy? To answer questions of this sort, we need "a framework within which agents can reflect on the acceptability of actions and can evaluate moral judgments and moral character."[6] Such a framework is known as an *ethical theory*.

Traditionally, ethical theories tend to be reductionist; that is, they offer one idea as the key to morality, and attempt to reduce everything to that one idea. For example, classical utilitarians maintain that right actions are those that promote the greatest happiness of the greatest number, while Kantians tell us that right actions are those that can be consistently willed universally. Each theory claims to have discovered the single, overarching standard of morality or right action. In a typical introduction to ethical theory class, each theory is presented and subjected to devastating criticism. The unfortunate result is that students frequently conclude that all of the theories are wrong—or worse, are pretentious nonsense.

In recent years, a number of philosophers have come to doubt that any normative theory can plausibly claim to be *the* correct theory. It may be that moral reality is sufficiently complex that any one theory gives only partial insight. Utilitarians are certainly right that achieving human happiness is an important goal of morality, but nonconsequentialists are also right in insisting, first, that other values such as justice and autonomy are also important, and second, that these values cannot be reduced to happiness. We conclude that it is a mistake to view the various theoretical alternatives as mutually exclusive claims to moral truth. Instead, we should view them as important but partial contributions to a comprehensive, although necessarily fragmented, moral vision.

UTILITARIANISM

Jeremy Bentham (1748–1832) and John Stuart Mill (1806–1873) are generally credited with developing the first detailed and systematic formulation of

the ethical theory known as *utilitarianism*. The heart of utilitarianism is "the greatest happiness principle," which, as Mill puts it, "holds that actions are right in proportion as they tend to promote happiness; wrong as they tend to produce the reverse of happiness."[7] The greatest happiness principle is also known as the principle of utility. The utility of an action is determined by its tendency to produce or promote happiness. Actions that result in happiness have positive utility; those that create misery have negative utility. Clearly, many actions can create both conditions. An act that is pleasurable now (not going to the dentist) can cause considerable suffering later on; and often the happiness of some persons (car thieves) is purchased at the expense of unhappiness for others. The right action is the one that, on balance, promotes the most happiness, or the greatest amount of pleasure over pain.

The first thing to note about utilitarianism is that it is a *consequentialist* theory. That is, it judges the rightness and wrongness of an action by its consequences, or what will happen if the action is or is not performed. Second, utilitarianism's theory of value says that good consequences are those that produce or promote happiness or pleasure, bad consequences those that produce or promote the reverse. As we will see, both consequentialism and utilitarianism's theory of value have lately come under attack.

There are several advantages to utilitarianism. It provides us with a decision procedure for deciding what to do: namely, whichever action produces, on balance, the greatest net amount of happiness. Moreover, happiness is alleged to be something empirical, something both measurable and comparable. In principle, therefore, utilitarianism provides definite answers to the question of how we ought to act.

Features of Utilitarianism As we indicated earlier, utilitarianism is a form of consequentialism, and thus it holds that the results of actions are the *only* relevant feature in assessing actions. Considerations of an agent's intentions, feelings, or convictions are seen as irrelevant to the question, "What is the right thing to do?" Similarly,

6. Tom Beauchamp and James F. Childress, *The Principles of Biomedical Ethics*, 4th ed. (New York: Oxford University Press, 1994), 44.

7. John Stuart Mill, *Utilitarianism* (New York: Liberal Arts Press, 1957), 10.

utilitarianism regards the question of whether a given course of action conforms to established social norms or ethical codes as relevant only to the extent that such conformity has a bearing on the production of happiness or unhappiness. Departing from established social codes typically has adverse consequences for the rule-breaker, and these consequences must be considered in deciding whether departing from the norm is the right thing to do.

Another important feature of utilitarianism is its impartiality. The utilitarian does not say, "The goodness of an action is determined by the amount of happiness it produces *for me*." Rather, the good is determined by the overall net happiness achieved. The utilitarian considers his or her own happiness, but no more and no less than the happiness of others. In weighing the effects of an action, utilitarianism maintains that we must take into consideration all of the parties concerned and that all parties shall be given equal consideration. Thus, utilitarianism is committed to the value of equality.

How far does this equality extend? In the nineteenth century, women were not considered the equals of men. Women were largely under the control of their fathers before marriage, and their husbands after. They could not vote, and their ability to own property was greatly restricted. Mill rejected such inequality. He supported equal rights for women and opposed slavery. Indeed, Mill thought that any creature capable of being happy or miserable—"all sentient creation so far as possible"—was deserving of moral concern. Contemporary utilitarians, like Peter Singer, have argued that nonhuman animals should count equally with humans, and that therefore painful experimentation on animals is wrong.

Utilitarianism has been influential not only in expanding our notion of "who counts" morally, but also in focusing attention on long-term, as well as short-term, results. Many decisions and actions performed today have an impact on the future. Remoteness in time is not, in principle, a reason to ignore a consequence, any more than is remoteness in space (although, of course, our knowledge about the future is less certain than our knowledge of the present). This is particularly important when we think of issues such as genetic engineering and gene therapy, which may have a profound impact on the genetic makeup of people in future generations. Utilitarianism espouses a prudent moral doctrine that requires us to think carefully about what we should do, and to consider not only the immediate effects of our actions, but also their long-term consequences.

To summarize the advantages of utilitarianism, first, it reduces vagueness by providing a single criterion of right action: namely, the promotion of human happiness. Moreover, happiness, whether understood as pleasure or as preference satisfaction, is something that can be empirically measured. Utilitarianism thus provides an objective standard for judging whether an action is right or wrong, and a method for resolving moral disputes. Finally, and more importantly, the principle of utility is derived from the very point of morality, which is to improve the lot of human beings living together. Morality does not relate to the satisfaction of some abstract or arbitrary code; rather, it relates to the improvement of the human condition, which means alleviating suffering and increasing happiness.

That the point of morality is to promote human welfare may seem boringly obvious, but it was regarded as quite radical in the nineteenth century, and not only because of its egalitarian implications. In addition, the focus on human happiness seemed to conflict with Christian teachings; for example, those teachings espousing the value of suffering. As we noted earlier, anesthesia during childbirth was condemned in the nineteenth century as unnatural and contrary to Biblical teachings ("In sorrow shalt thou bring forth children"). Even today the suffering of terminally ill patients is valued by some Catholic theologians, who regard the opportunity to identify with and participate in Christ's suffering on the cross as a positive good. Utilitarians are likely to have little patience with such views. Utilitarianism regards suffering and sacrifice as having moral value only if they promote overall happiness. Suffering and sacrifice have no intrinsic moral worth.

Objections to Utilitarianism Utilitarianism has been subjected to numerous objections, four of which we will consider here. One objection is to utilitarianism's theory of value: namely, the claim that happiness is the greatest good, the ultimate end. Critics have maintained that this theory leaves out many other "goods," such as health, friendship, creativity, intellectual attainment, and so forth. Mill agreed that these things are all valuable, but argued that they are valuable because they contribute to a happy life, one as rich as possible in enjoyment and as free as possible from pain. However, it remains questionable whether all values are commensurable; that is, whether all values can be reduced to happiness, however happiness is interpreted. And even if it were possible to reduce the plurality of values to a single value, happiness, is it possible to compare and weigh the happiness of one person against that of another? What if an action will make one person intensely happy but leave several people somewhat depressed? Exactly how are we to arrive at the right utilitarian solution? Moreover, some people feel things more intensely than others. Should we pay attention to the strength of desires? On the one hand, it seems that we should, since the intensity of an individual's happiness or unhappiness affects the total amount, and utilitarianism tells us to maximize happiness. On the other hand, this gives an advantage to the passionate over the phlegmatic that seems to violate Bentham's dictum that everyone counts for one, nobody for more than one.

A second objection to utilitarianism is that it requires us to calculate the probable consequences of every action, and this task is impossible. The sheer calculations alone would prevent anyone from doing anything. In response, it should be noted that both Bentham and Mill thought of utilitarianism primarily as a guide to legislative policy, rather than as a guide to individual behavior. No one thinks it unreasonable to ask for impact studies on the likely consequences of legislation. These are sometimes called "cost-benefit" analyses, and they are the direct descendants of classical utilitarianism.

Being utilitarians in our private lives does not mean that we must calculate all the consequences of every act, which would be impossible. Instead, we can rely on what Mill calls secondary principles, like "Don't lie," and "Don't harm others." We know from centuries of experience that adherence to these secondary principles promotes the greatest happiness for all, while departure from them causes insecurity and misery.

A more recent criticism of utilitarianism (or consequentialism generally) concerns the theory of responsibility it implies. For nonconsequentialists, it can be very significant whether an outcome occurs because of something *I did*, whereas for consequentialists all that matters ultimately is *what happens*. This has led some consequentialists to reject a time-honored distinction in medicine, the distinction between killing and "letting die." Many doctors believe that it is permissible for them to stop treatment when death is desirable; for example, in the case of a terminally ill patient in a great deal of pain who wants to die. However, they think it would be wrong (as well as illegal) actively to kill a patient in that same situation. Utilitarians, by contrast, are likely to regard killing and letting die as morally equivalent, since the outcome—a desirable death—is achieved in both cases (see Part Two, Section Five).

A final major criticism of utilitarianism is that it is inadequate as a moral theory because it conflicts with some of our most basic moral intuitions.

> Suppose we could greatly increase human happiness and diminish misery by occasionally, and perhaps secretly, abducting derelicts from city streets for use in fatal but urgent medical experiments. If utilitarian considerations were decisive, this practice might well be justifiable, even desirable. Yet it is surely wrong. Such a case suggests that we cannot always explain good and bad simply in terms of increasing or decreasing overall happiness.[8]

A utilitarian might respond by denying the premise that we could in fact promote the greatest happiness by abducting derelicts for medical experiments. He or she might argue that this fails to take into consideration all the negative side effects of such a policy: the impossibility of keeping it secret, the terror of the derelicts not yet abducted, the risk of mistake and abuse, the psychological effect on the doctors performing the experiments, etc. It is precisely because of such long-range negative consequences that policies like informed consent are rational from a utilitarian viewpoint. Still, it seems possible that, in special circumstances, the good effects could outweigh the bad. Some utilitarians will acknowledge that in such circumstances it would be right to use

8. Christina and Fred Sommers, eds., *Vice and Virtue in Everyday Life: Introductory Readings in Ethics*, 2nd ed. (San Diego, CA: Harcourt Brace Jovanovich, 1989), 80.

derelicts in fatal medical experiments (while reminding us that such circumstances are extremely unlikely to obtain, and it is even less likely that we can be sure that they do). However, they maintain that the fact that this practice would conflict with many people's deeply held moral convictions is not a worthwhile criticism of utilitarianism. Many utilitarians are quite skeptical of "deeply held moral convictions," which they regard as often no more than irrational superstitions.

Others, attracted by the virtues of utilitarianism, are nevertheless disturbed by the possibility of conflicts with justice and other basic moral practices, such as telling the truth and keeping promises. Rule-utilitarianism may be seen as one attempt to counter this objection.

RULE-UTILITARIANISM VERSUS ACT-UTILITARIANISM

Mill left unresolved the question whether the greatest happiness principle is to be applied to specific acts or to general kinds of acts. It has been suggested that if we apply the principle to kinds of acts, we can avoid some of the criticisms of utilitarianism. The version of utilitarianism that is primarily concerned with the consequences of specific acts has become known as *act-utilitarianism*, while the version primarily concerned with the consequences of general policies is called *rule-utilitarianism*.

Act-utilitarianism tells us to apply the principle of utility directly to the particular act in question. Suppose a doctor is faced with the question whether it would be morally right to help a terminally ill patient to die. An act-utilitarian would seek to determine which alternative in this particular case would maximize happiness and/or minimize suffering. Relevant considerations would include the possibility of recovery, whether the patient really wanted to die or was in a depression that might be alleviated, the impact on the patient's family, the impact on the doctor, and so forth.

By contrast, rule-utilitarianism uses the principle of utility not to decide which acts to perform or avoid, but rather to formulate and justify moral rules. The correct moral rules are those that promote the greatest happiness of the greatest number. Faced with a decision about how to act, rule-

utilitarianism tells us that we are not to appeal directly to the principle of utility. Rather, we are to consider whether this action falls under a rule that is justified by the principle of utility. Rule-utilitarianism would direct Dr. Brody to ask whether a general rule permitting assisted suicide would maximize happiness. Here, an important consideration would be whether such a practice would start us down a "slippery slope," and threaten the lives of terminally ill patients who do not really want to die, but who, for various reasons, are either afraid of being a burden to their families, or have families that want to get rid of them. Thus, a rule-utilitarian might argue that while helping *this* patient to die might maximize happiness (or minimize misery), it would nevertheless be wrong, because the consequences of a general policy of assisting suicide would be disastrous.

The difference between act- and rule-utilitarianism is *not* that only the latter appeals to moral rules. Both act- and rule-utilitarians use rules to guide their behavior. Rather, the difference lies in the way each group regards moral rules. For the act-utilitarian, rules are *summaries of past experience*. They're what we might call "rules of thumb": handy guides to the future based on past experience. Since it's often difficult to know what will maximize happiness in a particular situation, and since people are likely to be prejudiced by their own self-interest in their calculations, rules help us decide what to do.

Rules are regarded differently by rule-utilitarians. Rules are not just devices to help us figure out what will maximize happiness in a particular case. The rules themselves are justified on the grounds that having these particular rules maximizes happiness. But once we decide what the best rules are (that is, which ones are most likely to maximize happiness over the long run), then those are the rules we should follow, even if following them in a particular situation doesn't maximize happiness.

Thus, the rule-utilitarian can apparently avoid the sorts of situations that make act-utilitarianism unsatisfactory to many. In brief, the rule-utilitarian agrees with the act-utilitarian that the value of just practices resides in their tendency to promote happiness; but he will not agree that it is permissible to perform an unjust act in order to maximize happiness.

Is Rule-Utilitarianism an Improvement over Act-Utilitarianism? Act-utilitarians make this criticism of rule-utilitarianism: It makes no sense for a utilitarian to insist that a rule that will have less than optimal consequences should be followed simply because the rule maximizes happiness *in general*. J. J. C. Smart gives the following example. A good rule of thumb in a chess game is that you shouldn't sacrifice your queen for a pawn. But if, in a particular game of chess, you could checkmate your opponent by sacrificing your queen for a pawn, it would be absurd to stick dogmatically to the "Never sacrifice your queen for a pawn" rule. Smart thinks rule-utilitarianism is guilty of the same absurdity. Just as checkmating your opponent is the whole point of chess, so maximizing happiness is the whole point of utilitarian morality. It would not be rational from the standpoint of utility to refuse to break a moral rule when by doing so you could maximize welfare. For this reason, Smart calls rule-utilitarianism "superstitious rule worship."[9]

A related objection to rule-utilitarianism is that it collapses into act-utilitarianism. For whenever an act-utilitarian would say it was right to *break* a moral rule, it seems that the rule-utilitarian would generally agree, but instead say that the rule should be *modified*. Suppose, for example, that the only way to save someone's life is by telling a lie. An act-utilitarian would say that it was right to lie in such circumstances. But what would a rule-utilitarian say? That it is wrong to lie, knowing that the result will be an avoidable death? Surely not. A rule-utilitarian would say that the original rule, "Don't lie," is too crude. A better rule would be, "Don't lie, except to save a life." Moreover, it is likely that there is more than one exception to the "Don't lie" rule. That is, the rule most likely to maximize happiness probably allows for several situations in which lying is morally right. But now it seems that whatever would lead the act-utilitarian to break the rule would lead the rule-utilitarian to modify the rule. Thus, the two versions give exactly the same advice; they are *extensionally equivalent*, so rule-utilitarianism cannot be an improvement over act-utilitarianism. On the other hand, if the rule-utilitarian holds fast to the original rule, even when modifying it would have better results, he or she deviates from utilitarianism and is guilty of Smart's charge of "rule-worship."

In response, a rule-utilitarian might say that the criticism of extensional equivalence reflects a naive view of the operation of social rules and policies. While the considerations that lead an act-utilitarian to break a rule in a particular case can perhaps be articulated, it is much less easy to formulate a general policy that covers all the relevant exceptions. Consider the case study with which we began. A rule-utilitarian would not only consider whether it would be right for Dr. Brody to help Jim Lasken kill himself, but also whether doctors generally ought to be able to make decisions of this kind. For it is clear that this is not a one-of-a-kind situation; there are lots of Jim Laskens and Dr. Brodys. Should doctors make such decisions on a case-by-case basis? That approach has the advantage of allowing the individual doctor to decide whether the patient's pain outweighs the general rule against killing. The disadvantage of that approach, however, is that most people, including doctors, are not perfect happiness optimizers. There are bound to be mistakes. Some patients who are not terminally ill will be killed, as will some who could have been helped with psychiatric treatment or better pain medicine. Some doctors may be unduly influenced by relatives who want the patient's life to be over when the patient does not. More disturbing, in times of cost-cutting, might there not be a tendency to regard the terminally ill as "expendable" and not worth spending money on, even if a sick individual does not want to die? The problem is not so much that we cannot say when assisted suicide would and would not be justified (though this too is difficult to specify in advance); rather, it is that the practice of this policy on a large scale may result in many unnecessary and undesirable deaths. The question, then, is whether the need for such a policy is outweighed by the risk of mistake and abuse. These rule-utilitarian considerations do not seem to be captured by an act-utilitarian approach, which looks only at the consequences of a specific act. Therefore, rule-utilitarianism does not collapse into act-utilitarianism.

Nevertheless, rule-utilitarianism acknowledges that it is, in principle, possible that a practice we ordinarily think of as completely immoral (such as

9. J. J. C. Smart, "Extreme and Restricted Utilitarianism," in *Theories of Ethics,* edited by Philippa Foot (Oxford: Oxford University Press, 1967), 177.

slavery) might, in unusual circumstances, promote the greatest happiness and would therefore be right. Moreover, the factor that determines whether a practice maximizes happiness (for example, whether the number of people made miserable was sufficiently small) seems morally irrelevant. How can it be right to ride roughshod over the rights of a few people simply to make the majority happy? It is considerations of this kind that lead some people to reject utilitarianism altogether and opt for something completely different.

KANTIAN ETHICS

Utilitarian ethics has a strong appeal. The utilitarian says, "*Surely* consequences are terribly important. Whenever we act, we are trying to bring about certain states of affairs and avoid others. It is right to bring about happiness, and wrong to create misery. How can there be any other criterion of right and wrong? What *makes* lying and cheating wrong, if not that they cause misery?"

At the same time, it seems that there are some things we must not do, even if doing them would accomplish great good. What if we could maximize happiness by deliberately hurting innocent people or by violating their rights? Surely this would be wrong. It seems to matter not just *what* happens, but *how* it comes about.

Kantian ethics, so titled from its most illustrious exponent, Immanuel Kant (1724–1804), captures this intuitive conviction. Whereas Mill said that the right act is the one with the best consequences, Kant argued that consequences can never make an action right or wrong. An action that brings about the greatest amount of happiness might still be wrong. One must never act wrongly in order to bring about good consequences. In other words, the ends do not justify the means.

To understand the Kantian position, consider whether it would be morally right to prevent the deaths of five innocent people, each of whom needs an organ transplant, by killing another innocent person and distributing his or her vital organs. According to utilitarianism this would be right, since it results in a net gain of four lives. Of course, this reasoning fails to take into consideration the side effects we mentioned earlier in the theoretical use of derelicts in urgent medical experiments. For a utilitarian, the moral question turns

on whether the negative side effects outweigh the benefit of saving four net lives. On a Kantian approach, however, killing an innocent person is murder, which is intrinsically wrong. Kant did not claim that we should *ignore* the consequences of actions; that would be absurd. However, consequences are relevant to deciding what to do only if the proposed action is morally permissible. Other things being equal, we should of course try to bring about good consequences, but good consequences can never make a wrong action right.

How then are we to identify wrong or impermissible actions? Most people already have a pretty good idea of the kinds of actions that are wrong. We learn to distinguish right from wrong from our parents, our teachers, and our playmates. We know that lying, breaking promises, cheating, hurting others, and stealing are wrong. But *why* are these things wrong? As we've seen, the utilitarian explanation is that the actions we normally regard as wrong—lying, cheating, stealing, killing—promote unhappiness. The trouble with this explanation is that it seems possible, in a particular case, that no one gets hurt by an act of lying or cheating, or that the negative consequences of such an act are outweighed by the positive. Suppose I can get away with cheating without anyone finding out; would that make it morally acceptable? Kant would say of course not, it's still cheating. The important thing is not the consequences of the act, but the kind of act it is. An action could bring about the best nonmoral consequences—e.g., save the most number of lives, make the most people happy—and still be morally wrong, because it is unjust or dishonest.

Another reason Kant rejects consequentialism is that what happens is often not within our control, and so is not something for which we can be praised, blamed, or held at all responsible. A physician may administer a drug that kills a patient, due to unknown and unforeseeable side effects. Though the outcome is disastrous, surely the physician does not act immorally. Kant holds that if you act rightly, you are not responsible for any bad effects that occur. (Utilitarians distinguish between rightness and moral blameworthiness. They say that what the physician did was *wrong*, though it was not his fault and he should not be *blamed*.)

According to Kant, the fact that an action is likely to promote happiness or human welfare has nothing to do with whether anyone has a moral duty to do it. Duty must be entirely independent of consequences, for if it were otherwise, moral imperatives could only be *hypothetical*. That is, they would tell us only, "If you want to achieve *x*, then do *y*." Thus, if someone is indifferent to *x*, then he or she has no reason to do *y*. Morality, Kant held, is clearly *not* like this. Morality tells us, "Do *y*, whatever you may happen to want or feel." In other words, morality yields *categorical*, rather than mere hypothetical, imperatives.

Imperatives or commands can be either hypothetical or categorical, depending on the implicit principle contained in them. For example, "Treat people with respect" is a hypothetical imperative if the reason for respecting others is to gain their friendship. Interpreted as a hypothetical imperative, this maxim tells us to treat others with respect *if* we want their friendship. However, some people do not care about gaining others' friendship. If "Treat others with respect" were a hypothetical imperative, it would not apply to such people, who are indifferent to others. Since morality is clearly not conditional in this way, however, Kant argued that morality cannot consist of hypothetical imperatives. Instead, morality consists of categorical imperatives: commands that are valid for rational agents as such, independent of their feelings and desires. Moreover, because morality consists of these categorical imperatives devoid of empirical content, it can have necessity; it can tell us what we *must* do.

Because utilitarianism focuses on the prevention of pain and the promotion of pleasure, it regards *sentience,* or the capacity to feel pain and pleasure, as having a great deal of moral significance. As we saw earlier, Mill and Bentham extended moral concern to all sentient beings. By contrast, Kant regarded our capacity to experience pleasure and pain as fairly insignificant in terms of morality. Of far greater importance is our rationality: our ability to think, to plan our lives, to be motivated by abstract considerations. This is allegedly what separates us from the rest of creation, giving us a central and special moral status. As animals, we are subject to the laws of nature, physical and psychological. However, unlike other animals, we are rational beings, or persons. Persons have a special moral status because persons are able to conform their behavior to moral law.

According to Kant, one must treat every person as an end, and never merely as a means. This means that in our dealings with others we are to realize that they have their own goals, aims, and projects. We are never to treat other people as if they do not matter or count, or as if they exist simply to fulfill our purposes. This Kantian idea is reflected in the insistence that patients and research subjects must give informed consent before they can be treated or used in experiments. We also show respect for persons by telling them the truth, even when such knowledge might be painful, and by allowing them to make their own moral choices, even when we think they will choose unwisely. Thus, Kantian ethics has been a strong force against the medical paternalism that held sway until fairly recently.

If we want to know if a proposed action is morally permissible, the right question to ask, Kant says, is not, "What are the likely consequences of doing (or not doing) this action?" but rather, *"Can I, as a rational agent, consistently will that everyone in a similar situation should act this way?"* If we convert this question into an imperative, we get "Act always on that maxim (or principle) that you can consistently will as a principle of action for everyone similarly situated." Kant calls this rule the Categorical Imperative, and it is the foundation of his ethical system. The intuitive idea here is that morality requires us not to make exceptions of ourselves. If the proposed action is one that would be wrong if done generally, then the particular action is wrong, too—even if it would not, in the case at hand, have harmful consequences. For Kant, it is *irrelevant* that a particular act of cheating might not have, on balance, harmful consequences. What matters is that you cannot consistently will that people should cheat on exams. (Kant's own example was making a lying promise, which we adapt here to the analogous case of cheating on an exam.)

It is important at this point to clarify precisely what Kant means by "cannot consistently will." According to Mill, you can consistently will *anything:* it's just that the consequences of universal adoption of the principle of your action would be undesirable. That is, if people invariably cheated on exams, exams wouldn't test anything and there would be no point in administering them. That is a utilitarian reason against cheating.

Kant's argument is quite different. He does not say that cheating is wrong because the consequences of cheating (the destruction of an examination system) are undesirable. Kant's point is this: When you cheat, you are operating on a certain principle or maxim; in this case, I will cheat whenever cheating will help me improve my grade. To see if that is morally permissible, *universalize* it: Everyone cheats whenever cheating will improve his or her grade. However, this universalized principle contains an inconsistency. You are willing, first, *that examinations exist* because they are necessary for you to achieve your aim of improving your grade. But you are at the same time willing *that examinations cease to exist*, because if everyone always cheats, the system of examinations will have no point and will self-destruct. This inconsistency has nothing to do with finding the consequences of cheating undesirable.

Kant thought that consistency and universality are clearly part of our concept of morality and duty. In trying to explain why we ought to do certain things (like voting) or refrain from doing others (like cheating on exams) we ask things like, "What would happen if everyone acted that way?" But note that we do not regard it as a rebuttal if it is pointed out that not everyone *will* act that way. Universalization requires us to abstract from the actual circumstances, and to refrain from making exceptions of ourselves. This test of right action is considered so important that many moral philosophers hold that a person "has a morality" only if that person is willing to universalize his or her moral judgments.[10]

How would a Kantian resolve Dr. Brody's dilemma? Kant himself thought that suicide was as self-contradictory (and therefore morally wrong) as cheating. His argument is as follows: Suicides kill themselves to spare themselves the pain of living. However, the desire to avoid pain is intrinsic to self-preservation. Committing suicide is thus acting from both self-preservation and self-destruction at the same time, and so is self-contradictory. Kant's argument here seems extremely murky. It is far from clear why it is self-contradictory to prefer death to life under horrible conditions. Kant's absolute opposition to suicide seems more a prod-

uct of the conventional morality of his time than a requirement of the categorical imperative.

Kant's difficulty in demonstrating the self-contradiction in suicide brings out an important feature of Kantian ethics. Often in deciding what to do, I am faced with a range of alternatives, none of which conflict with the categorical imperative. They are all therefore permissible. How, then, am I to decide which alternative to choose? Kantian ethics gives the individual a great deal more latitude than does utilitarianism, which commands us to choose the act that has the *best* consequences. However, while allowing for more individual autonomy, Kantian ethics gives proportionately less guidance. Indeed, it seems that the categorical imperative functions only as a kind of *necessary condition* of the morality of actions, telling us what we *cannot* do, and not as a *sufficient condition* that would specify, from a list of permissible acts, what we *should* do. Does this ethical perspective give any guidance at all to Dr. Brody?

To see if it does, we need to remember that the ability to universalize is only one value in Kantian ethics; the other is respect for persons. Does a policy of assisted suicide or voluntary euthanasia promote respect for persons? Someone like Jim wishes to end his life not simply to avoid pain, but also to avoid the certain deterioration of his mental powers, the subsequent loss of rationality, and the gradual erosion of his own sense of dignity and meaning. This reasoning should have considerable weight from a Kantian perspective. Thus a Kantian (though not the historical Kant) might support assisted suicide and voluntary euthanasia as promoting autonomy and self-determination. On the other hand, it is possible that a policy of voluntary euthanasia would lead to the devaluing of human life, and ultimately the nonvoluntary killing of the weak, the vulnerable, and the poor. If so, this would violate the values of autonomy and respect for persons, which would lead Kantians to oppose euthanasia. (Remember that Kantians do not ignore consequences; they simply do not regard consequences themselves as determinative of right and wrong.)

Thus, we may expect to find Kantians—as well as utilitarians—on both sides of the euthanasia issue, depending on their factual predictions and their conceptions of basic moral concepts such as autonomy and personhood. This conclusion will

10. See, for example, William Frankena, *Ethics*, 2nd ed. (Englewood Cliffs, NJ: Prentice-Hall, 1973), 113–114.

be discouraging for anyone who expects ethical theories to provide handy-dandy formulas for resolving moral issues. But ethical theories are not meant to provide formulas; instead, they provide frameworks for trying to reach workable solutions to complex and difficult questions.

SOCIAL CONTRACT THEORY

Any ethical theory must answer two fundamental questions. The first is about the content of our moral obligations: What are we required to do? The second is about our motivation for acting: Why are we required to do it? The social contract approach to ethics gives related answers to these questions. Our obligations are determined by the agreements we have made, and we ought to fulfill our obligations because we have agreed to them.[11]

There are two basic forms of contemporary social contract theory. Philosopher Will Kymlicka explains their difference this way:

> One approach stresses a natural equality of physical power, which makes it mutually advantageous for people to accept conventions that recognize and protect each other's interests and possessions. The other approach stresses a natural equality of moral status, which makes each person's interests a matter of common or impartial concern. This impartial concern is expressed in agreements that recognize each person's interests and moral status.[12]

Kymlicka calls proponents of the mutual advantage theory "Hobbesian contractarians," and proponents of the impartial theory "Kantian contractarians," because Hobbes and Kant inspired and foreshadowed these two forms of contract theory.

Hobbesian Contractarianism Hobbesian contractarianism is a form of moral nihilism in its rejection of objective (or real) moral values. There is nothing inherently right or wrong about the goals one chooses to pursue, or the means one uses to pursue these goals. However, unless there are restrictions on the goals people pursue and the means by which they pursue them, the world is a threatening, dangerous place. Everyone is better-off restricting his or her own liberty to injure others, so long as the others do likewise. Harming others is not inherently wrong in this view, but it is to our mutual advantage to accept conventions that define such harm as wrong.[13]

Hobbesian contractarianism replicates a good deal of ordinary morality, but not all of it. For one thing, it is clear that there is no mutual advantage in bargaining with those who are too weak to pose a threat of retaliation. Thus, Hobbesian contractarianism leaves out defenseless human beings, such as babies and the disabled.[14] This departure from everyday morality is no argument against Hobbesian contractarianism since, as Kymlicka points out, the theory denies that we have any natural duties to others; it is, as we said, a form of moral nihilism. Hobbesian contractarianism may be the best we can do in a world without natural duties or objective values.[15]

How would a Hobbesian contractarian approach the problem of doctor-assisted suicide? The question is whether it is to everyone's mutual advantage to allow doctors to kill (or help to die) their terminally ill patients who request such help. On the one hand, it would appear irrational to rule out an option that a great many people apparently wish to have at the end of life. On the other hand, when we become terminally ill, we do not want doctors killing us for cost-control, to convenience our relatives, etc. Thus, the Hobbesian contractarian analysis looks a great deal like a rule-utilitarian analysis.

Kantian Contractarianism The best-known exponent of Kantian contractarianism is John Rawls. According to Rawls, people matter not because they can harm or benefit others (as in the Hobbesian view), but because they are ends in themselves (as Kant held). Everyone is entitled to equal consideration, and this basic notion of equality gives rise to a natural duty to promote a just society. A just society is one based on fair principles. However, the social contract approach creates a problem in attempting to derive fair principles. The problem is that, in a bargaining situation, the

---

11. Will Kymlicka, "The Social Contract Tradition," in *A Companion to Ethics*, edited by Peter Singer (Oxford: Basil Blackwell, 1993), 186.

12. Ibid., 188.

13. Ibid., 189.

14. David Gauthier, *Morals by Agreement* (Oxford: Oxford University Press, 1986), 286.

15. Kymlicka, 191 (see note 11).

strong have a clear advantage over the weak, which is intuitively unfair. Rawls's solution to the problem of natural inequality is a hypothetical social contract whereby a society chooses its basic social principles from the standpoint of "the original position."

In the original position, all parties are under a "veil of ignorance." That is, while they know that they are human and have basic human needs, they are deprived of all knowledge of their special characteristics. No one knows if he or she is rich or poor, black or white, male or female, or politically liberal or conservative. This ignorance prevents people from tailoring social principles to their own advantage.

In the original position, each contractor is motivated by self-interest; that is, each is trying to do the best for him- or herself. But since no one knows what his or her position in society eventually will be, this self-interest amounts to acting impartially. To promote my own good, I must put myself in the shoes of every member of society and see what promotes his or her good, since I may end up being any one of these members.[16] It would be contrary to my own self-interest to choose a society that permitted slavery, since I might be a slave. Of course, it might turn out that I get to be a master, in which case I would be better-off living in a slave-owning society. However, one cannot know one's place in advance. Rawls thinks that it would be irrational to opt for a slave-owning society, since being a slave in a slave-owning society is much worse than living as a free person in a society that prohibits slavery. Similarly, individuals in the original position could not choose a caste system, since they might turn out to be untouchables; they could not choose a male-dominated society, since they might turn out to be women. The very arrangements we intuitively reject as unfair turn out to be irrational from the perspective of the original position.

Rawls goes on to argue that rational people in the original position would choose two basic principles to guide and determine the institutions of their society. The first principle is a principle of liberty. It maintains that everyone is to have as much liberty as possible, consonant with everyone else's having the same amount of liberty. This principle would be chosen from the standpoint of the original position because it would be irrational to choose a principle that gives some people more liberty than others. After all, you might end up being one of the people with less liberty.

The second principle is a principle of equality. It has two parts. The first part is a principle of distribution, often referred to as the "difference principle." It says that all goods should be equally distributed, except where an unequal distribution makes everyone, especially the worst-off, better-off. Why would choosers in the original position opt for equal distribution? Because if you don't know your position in society, it would be irrational to choose a distribution in which some have enormous wealth and others are impoverished. True, you might be Donald Trump, but it's better to forgo the chance for great wealth than to risk being impoverished. At the same time, it would be irrational to insist on absolute equal distribution if an unequal distribution would make everyone better-off. (For example, it is in the best interests of the worst-off to have an adequate supply of well-trained brain surgeons who are paid much more than the average person, if this inequality is the necessary incentive for them to set aside so many years for training.)

The second part of the principle of equality is a principle of equality of opportunity. Everyone is to have equal opportunity in achieving the various offices and roles in society; they are all to be open to everyone. Rawls's principle of fair equality of opportunity has been used by Norman Daniels as the basis for a universal right to health care.[17] The basic idea is that sickness and disability prevent us from functioning normally, and deprive us of the opportunity to compete on an equal basis with others for the goods in society. While we can strive to keep ourselves healthy through various means (e.g., abstaining from smoking, following a low-fat diet, exercising regularly), for the most part, we have no control over becoming sick or disabled. The sick and the disabled are therefore at a considerable and unfair disadvantage. Those who do not get the medical attention that can restore "normal species-functioning" are thus doubly disadvantaged, first by "nature's lottery," and second by

---

16. Kymlicka, 192 (see note 11).

17. See Norman Daniels, *Just Health Care* (Cambridge: Cambridge University Press, 1985).

social arrangements that give some, but not others, access to health care. If equal opportunity is to be a reality, we must guarantee universal access to health care. Moreover, the concept of "normal species-functioning" is a guide for what kinds of treatment should be provided. Vaccination and eyeglasses are obvious candidates, while cosmetic surgery is not.

Rawls requires that his principle of liberty take precedence over his principle of equality. He states that the claims of liberty must be satisfied before social and economic inequalities can be contemplated, and that departures from the principle of equal liberty cannot be justified or made good by greater social and economic advantages.[18] The elements of the principle of equality are similarly ordered: Rawls sees that genuinely fair equality of opportunity (as opposed to merely formal access) must be guaranteed before we can address ourselves to social or economic inequalities.

If we compare Rawls's vision of "justice as fairness" with utilitarianism, we see some striking differences. The most dramatic difference concerns the respective theories of the "good" and the "right," and the way these important moral concepts are related. Utilitarian theories define the good independently of the right; first the good is defined as happiness, then the right is defined as that which maximizes happiness. Because justice is defined as a function of utility, it cannot limit the claims of utility. By contrast, Rawls sees the concepts of right and justice as preceding the concept of the good.[19] He states that for desires to have any value or to play any role in ethical calculations, they must accord with the principles of justice.

Rawls's theory of justice has been criticized as embodying problematic notions of rationality—in particular, a fundamental aversion to risk. Why assume that a rational person behind the veil of ignorance would opt for the equality of the difference principle? A gambler might be willing to take a relatively small risk of being impoverished for the chance of becoming very wealthy. Is this obviously irrational? A related criticism is that the contract does no real work. As we have seen, and as Rawls acknowledges, there can be different interpretations of the original position. A risk-aversive interpretation, which yields the difference principle, is not the only possible one. According to Rawls, we decide which interpretation of the original position is most suitable by determining which interpretation yields principles that match our convictions of justice. But, as Kymlicka points out, "if each theory of justice has its own account of the contracting situation, then we have to decide *beforehand* which theory of justice we accept, in order to know which description of the original position is suitable."[20] If this is so, then the contract cannot be used to establish the correct theory of justice. Nevertheless, contracting from an original position has some useful purposes. The veil of ignorance is a vivid expression of the moral requirement of our commitment to others, and of putting ourselves in their shoes. It dramatizes the claim that we would accept a certain principle, however it affected us. As Kymlicka says, "In these and other ways, the contract device illuminates the basic ideas of morality as impartiality, even if it cannot help defend those ideas."[21]

So how would a Kantian contractarian, or Rawlsian, approach Dr. Brody's dilemma? The principle of liberty requires that each individual have the maximum liberty possible, consistent with equal liberty for others. That requirement seems to argue in favor of allowing people to choose the time and manner of their death at the end of their life, in order to avoid great suffering, as well as financial loss for their families. At the same time, Rawls is concerned to protect the weak and vulnerable who cannot bargain on their own behalf. That would militate against a policy that could have a discriminatory impact on the elderly, the disabled, and the poor. Thus, a Rawlsian would be likely to approve of a policy of doctor-assisted suicide if it promoted the value of individual autonomy, but not if it violated equal respect for persons.

RELIGIOUS ETHICS

We noted above that religious ethics is one of the parent disciplines of bioethics. We are not suggesting that "religious ethics" is an ethical theory in

18. John Rawls, *A Theory of Justice* (Cambridge, MA: Harvard University Press, 1971), 61.

19. Ibid., 31.

20. Kymlicka, 193 (see note 11).

21. Ibid.

the same sense as utilitarianism and Kantian ethics; religious beliefs do not, in general, imply any one particular ethical orientation. Some Christians take a utilitarian approach, while others have views closer to Kantianism. Although there are certainly ethical directives inherent in religious belief (e.g., "Do unto others as you would be done by"), each of these directives can be compatible with very different ethical theories.

Some religious traditions have been more influential than others in bioethics; for example, Roman Catholic moral thought. One reason for this influence is that the Roman Catholic church is characterized by considerable unanimity. There is, on a number of issues, an official Church doctrine—this is not generally true of Protestantism, which has a great many denominations, or Judaism, which is divided into Orthodox, Conservative, and Reform. Another reason for the more powerful influence of Roman Catholicism is that it includes a well-developed, written body of thought on medical-moral issues, which has had considerable influence on prevailing attitudes (even among many non-Catholics), as well as on legal doctrine regarding a wide range of biomedical ethical issues. Lastly, the Catholic tradition includes an alternative ethical theory—known as natural law ethics—that provides principles for interpreting the general ethical directives of the Christian faith.

NATURAL LAW THEORIES

Natural law theorists offer an account of the human good and ethical duty that contrasts sharply with the views of both utilitarianism and Kantianism on these issues. Utilitarianism defines the good in terms of happiness or the satisfaction of desire, while Kant repudiated all ethical theories based in any way upon desire or inclination. In contrast to utilitarianism, natural law ethicists insist that the human good cannot be reduced to a mere function of what people happen to desire. In this view, things are not good because we desire them; rather, we desire them, or should desire them, because they are good.

But natural law ethics is also opposed to Kantian ethics, in that it is based on a conception of human nature. Kant insists that the categorical imperative must be empty of all empirical content;

otherwise it could not have the necessity characteristic of the moral law. But what else, if not a concern for human welfare, can ethics possibly be founded upon, and how can it have any motivational force? Why, asks the natural law theorist, should we desire to be moral in the first place and follow the dictates of morality, unless such behavior holds out some prospect of promoting human well-being and happiness?

Natural law theorists thus agree with utilitarians that ethics must be grounded in a concern for the human good. But they agree with Kantians that the good cannot be defined simply in terms of what people "happen" to want. Instead, there is a good for human beings that, based on their nature, is objectively desirable.

Catholic theologians conceive of natural law as the law inscribed by God into the nature of things—as a species of divine law. According to this conception, the Creator endows all things with certain potentialities or tendencies that serve to define their natural end; the fulfillment of a thing's natural tendencies constitutes the specific "good" of that thing. The natural potential of an acorn is to become an oak. But what is the natural potential of human beings? Like Kant, the natural law theorist focuses on what makes human beings distinctive, what separates us from the rest of the natural world—namely, the ability to reason. Through our ability to reason, we can participate actively in God's plan. However, natural law ethics is distinct from Kantian ethics in that natural law ethicists do not attempt to empty their theories of all empirical content. On the contrary, our moral obligations are derived from a conception of the good life for human beings. For example, the Church opposes both abortion and birth control because these are inconsistent with a conception of sexuality as expressed within monogamous marriage only, and primarily oriented toward its natural end or purpose, procreation.

The most general moral precept of the natural law is "do good and avoid evil." Evil must always be avoided, even if avoiding evil will bring about great harm. As St. Paul put it, "Do not evil that good may come." The commission of an evil deed, such as the murder of an innocent person, can never be condoned, even if it is intended to advance the noblest of ends.

THE DOCTRINE OF THE DOUBLE EFFECT

The doctrine of the double effect (DDE) was formulated in response to the recognition that an act may have both a good and a bad effect. Are we to shun such an action because of its bad effect? For example, administering morphine to a dying cancer patient may be necessary to ease his or her pain, but it may also depress respiration and hasten death. Must a doctor refrain from using the most effective pain medication because it might also kill the patient? Would this count as "doing evil (causing death) that good (relieving pain) may come"?

According to Catholic doctrine, the permissibility of the action depends largely on whether the bad effect is intended, or merely foreseen and permitted to happen. In addition, it must also be the case that

1. The act itself is not intrinsically wrong.
2. The good effect is produced directly by the action and not by the bad effect.
3. The good effect is sufficiently desirable to compensate for allowing the bad effect.[22]

Applying these conditions, the use of pain-relieving drugs that may also shorten life can be justified. The physician's purpose is not to kill, but rather to ease pain, although he or she foresees that death is a possible, or even likely, result. Giving drugs for pain relief is not intrinsically wrong; indeed, it is a central function of the physician. The good effect—the relief of pain—is produced directly by the administering of the drug, and not by the bad effect: namely, the patient's death. And lastly, when a patient is both terminally ill and suffering, the desirability of relieving suffering compensates for the shortening of his or her life. Thus, the DDE can be a useful tool for justifying an action that has a bad effect.

Double-effect reasoning has sometimes been incorrectly and speciously used. Someone who shoots a person at point-blank range cannot use the DDE to mitigate his or her responsibility, saying, "I didn't mean to kill him, only to get him out of the way." One is guilty of killing a person even if death is not desired in itself, but only as a means to achieve an end. Recently, a Michigan jury used

22. "Double Effect," *New Catholic Encyclopedia.*

such specious reasoning in their acquittal of Dr. Jack Kevorkian, who was accused of violating the state's assisted-suicide law when he helped a terminally ill man to die by carbon monoxide poisoning. The law made an exception for physicians who administer pain relieving drugs that may cause death. The jury accepted Kevorkian's argument that he did not intend to cause the man's death, but only to relieve his suffering. This reasoning, however, is a perversion of the DDE. Carbon monoxide, unlike morphine, is never offered as a means of pain relief. It has no medical use at all. It causes death, and death causes cessation of pain, but this is bringing about the good effect by means of the bad effect, which violates the second condition of the DDE. Thus, the DDE cannot be used to justify Dr. Kevorkian's act or to sustain his claim that he did not intend to cause the man's death. After the acquittal, law professor Yale Kamisar characterized the jury's decision as "confused." However, it seems likely that the decision was less the result of confusion about the appropriate application of double-effect reasoning, and more the result of their belief that Dr. Kevorkian was *right* in doing what he did, and should not be punished.

Critics of the DDE argue that the principle is confusing and difficult to apply. It is not always easy to know whether a result is intended or merely foreseen, or whether it is brought about (impermissibly) by means of the bad effect or (permissibly) by the morally neutral action. The concepts of "means" and "intention" need to be made clearer before the DDE can give clear guidance.

Some theorists doubt that the DDE has moral significance even if it can be clearly and correctly applied. They note that the whole point of the doctrine is to avoid the counterintuitive implications of an absolutist ethic that insists that some acts (like directly causing the death of an innocent person) are absolutely wrong, regardless of reason or context. However, why should we assimilate garden-variety murder with causing the death of a terminally ill patient who wants to die? The solution, these critics say, is to recognize that causing death is not always wrong. If death is desirable, why should it make any difference *how* death is brought about—whether indirectly, by pain relief, or directly, by carbon monoxide?

ORDINARY VERSUS EXTRAORDINARY TREATMENT

Another influential distinction devised by Catholic medical ethicists is the distinction between "ordinary" and "extraordinary" treatment. Ordinary treatment is considered obligatory, while there is no obligation to provide extraordinary treatment. How are these two types of treatment to be best defined?

This question is complicated because there are various different grounds that have been used to distinguish ordinary and extraordinary treatments. For example, "ordinary" treatment may be viewed as routine or standard care, while "extraordinary" treatment is considered unusual. This distinction has the advantage of providing an empirical definition, based on current medical practice. However, it is not clear that this basis has moral significance. If a treatment is helpful to a patient, what difference does it make that it is unusual, or even unique? For this reason, some people prefer to think of the distinction between ordinary and extraordinary treatment as being a distinction between "beneficial" and "nonbeneficial" treatment.

Understood this way, the ordinary/extraordinary distinction is context dependent. Treatment such as a respirator may be ordinary in one context (e.g., to sustain a patient through a severe bout with a respiratory disease), but extraordinary in another (e.g., to sustain the life of a severely brain-damaged patient in a persistent vegetative state [PVS]). This makes the normative assumption that a PVS individual is not benefited by continued existence with no hope of recovery to consciousness. Someone who regards biological life itself as valuable will not agree that the use of a respirator to sustain the life of a PVS patient is "nonbeneficial," and so will not classify the treatment as extraordinary. However, this reasoning raises serious doubts about the usefulness of the distinction. If our moral views determine whether a treatment is to be classified as ordinary or extraordinary, the distinction itself cannot provide moral guidance.

Despite this difficulty, doctors and laypeople alike often use terms like "extraordinary" and "heroic" to characterize treatment they regard as inappropriate. Rather than regarding these classifications as morally significant in themselves, it is important to understand the moral presuppositions lying behind them. It is these presuppositions—not the shorthand labels that stand for them—that need discussion and debate (see "In the Matter of Claire C. Conroy," Part Two, Section Four).

"RIGHTS-BASED" APPROACHES

The idea that, simply by virtue of being human, people can have rights regardless of the legal system under which they live, has ancient roots. The Stoic philosophers recognized the possibility that actual human laws might be unjust. They contrasted conventional laws with an unvarying natural law, to which everyone had access through individual conscience, and by which actual laws could be judged.[23] Later, the spread of the Roman Empire provided a system of law that applied to all people, whatever their tribe, race, or nationality. Christianity also incorporated the idea of natural law as the paramount standard by which all social institutions and laws should be judged.

However, neither the ancient Greeks, nor the Romans, nor the medieval Christians made the transition to natural rights. The notion of natural rights had its heyday in the seventeenth century, with writers like Grotius, Pufendorf, and Locke. Rights also played a crucial role in the American and French revolutions in the late eighteenth century. However, states Brenda Almond, "In the nineteenth and early twentieth centuries, . . . appeal to rights was eclipsed by movements such as utilitarianism and Marxism, which could not, or would not, accommodate them."[24]

Appeal to natural rights revived in the aftermath of World War II, during the Nuremberg trials. Some theorists argued that since the actions of the accused were not contrary to German law (indeed, were required by it), the trials had no legal basis, but were merely a cynical attempt by the victors to punish the losers. Others maintained that the trials were a return to principles of legality and justice in the aftermath of Nazi barbarism, and that these principles have their foundation in both international and natural law.

23. Brenda Almond, "Rights," in *A Companion to Ethics*, edited by Peter Singer (Basil Blackwell, 1993), 259.
24. Ibid.

Natural or human rights unquestionably occupy an important role in contemporary international moral and political debate. Apartheid, the death penalty, and female genital mutilation, to take just a few examples, have all been condemned as violations of human rights. Discussions of abortion, euthanasia, access to health care, the treatment of animals and the environment, and our obligations to future generations are typically framed in terms of conflicting moral rights.

Some see "rights talk" as unnecessary and vague. Bentham regarded the notion of moral—as opposed to legal—rights as "nonsense," and the notion of natural rights as "nonsense on stilts."[25] According to Bentham and other legal positivists, legal rights can be explained as claims that will be upheld by the power of the state. Legal rights can be identified because they stem from legislative acts or judicial decisions. So-called moral rights have no such legitimation, and it is partly for this reason that positivists regard them as empty rhetoric. According to utilitarianism, to say that someone has a moral right to something is only a shorthand way of saying that he or she *ought* to have it, and ought to be protected in his or her possession of it. There is, then, a role for moral rights in utilitarianism, but it is completely derivative from the principle of utility. To some extent, rights can serve as barriers against the application of overall utility. For example, utilitarians might, on grounds of utility, take property rights very seriously. They will agree that individuals should not be deprived of their property, unless this is essential to the general welfare, and even then there should be compensation. In other words, while utilitarians reject the Lockean idea of a "natural right to property," they are likely to agree that there are good utilitarian reasons to create something very like our existing system of property rights.

Rights-based critics of utilitarianism maintain that its conception of rights gives insufficient protection to individuals, whose happiness may be sacrificed for the benefit of the many. In *Taking Rights Seriously*, Ronald Dworkin offers a penetrating critique of the positivist analysis of law, as well as the utilitarian morality intimately linked to it. Rather than seeing rights as a device to achieve net utility, Dworkin sees rights as "trumps," as claims that supersede other kinds of claims. Similarly, Robert Nozick conceives of rights as "side constraints," which place limits on the things we may do to achieve goals.

In *Anarchy, State, and Utopia*, Nozick presents a libertarian view that is fundamentally opposed to utilitarianism.[26] He thus joins Kant, Rawls, and Dworkin in this opposition, holding that an action that is unfair or that violates someone's rights cannot be right, even if it does achieve the greatest net happiness. Happiness might be maximized by forcing people to volunteer their time to work in hospitals, or by making them donate blood or spare kidneys, but they have no obligation to do so according to Nozick; indeed, they have a right not to do so.

Nozick is equally opposed to Rawls's contractarianism. The central question of distributive justice is, "How should the goods of society be distributed?" According to Nozick, this question misconceives the issue because it implies that the goods of society—money, property, services—are there simply to be distributed, like manna fallen from the heavens. Instead, these goods already belong to people who have invested their labor in them, been given them, or traded something for them. Taking goods away from those who are entitled to them violates their rights, and so is fundamentally unfair.

Another important feature of libertarianism is the distinction between negative and positive rights. Libertarians maintain that the only rights are negative rights: rights to be left alone, rights not to be interfered with. They reject positive rights—rights to be helped—because recognition of such rights would infringe on the freedom of individuals to spend their time and money as they choose. An example of a positive right is a right to an education. Libertarians oppose taxation generally on the grounds that it deprives individuals of their legitimate property; thus, they oppose taxation for the creation and support of public schools. However, they recognize the need for an army to

---

25. From *Anarchical Fallacies: Being an Examination of the Declaration of Rights Issued During the French Revolution*. Cited in Ronald Dworkin, *Taking Rights Seriously* (Cambridge, MA: Harvard University Press, 1977), 184.

26. Robert Nozick, *Anarchy, State, and Utopia* (New York: Basic Books, 1974).

defend a country from foreign enemies, for a police force to protect citizens against aggression and attack, and for a legal system to uphold contractual agreements. Taxation to support these purposes is regarded as legitimate.

Libertarians reject the idea of a right to health care, since health care is regarded as a positive right—a right to be given certain treatment. However, it is not clear why they assume this distinction to have such moral significance. If it is legitimate to tax people for a police force that will protect their lives, why isn't it equally legitimate to tax people to provide them with health care, which is also often necessary for survival?

Perhaps the biggest objection to libertarianism is that it works to the disadvantage of those who, through no fault of their own, are born into poverty. Poverty limits people's life chances. The poor typically get substandard health care, inferior schools, and inadequate housing. These disadvantages make it unlikely that they will have an equal opportunity to obtain the goods of society: jobs, money, and material goods. Rawls attempts to compensate for life's initial unfairness, but libertarianism reinforces it.

In a rights-based approach, the fundamental question in our opening case study would be whether Jim Lasken has a right to end his life, and to ask his doctor for help in doing so. Those who oppose voluntary euthanasia and physician-assisted suicide maintain that Lasken has no such right. They see a distinction between the established right to refuse medical treatment, and an affirmative right to seek help in dying. However, this interpretation was disputed for the first time by a federal judge on May 3, 1994, when Judge Barbara F. Rothstein found Washington state's assisted-suicide law unconstitutional. Rothstein held that the law places an undue burden on the Fourteenth Amendment interests of terminally ill, mentally competent patients. Moreover, she found that the law "unconstitutionally distinguishes between two similarly situated groups," namely, those on life-support and those not on life-support. Washington permits terminally ill patients to hasten their deaths by allowing removal of life-support systems, yet bars physicians from giving medication that would bring about the same results. Rothstein wrote that from "a constitutional perspective, the court does not believe that a distinction can be drawn between

refusing life-sustaining medical treatment, and physician-assisted suicide by an uncoerced, mentally competent, terminally ill adult."[27]

Rights play an important role in moral discourse. Without the notion of individual rights, it would be difficult—if not impossible—to express our convictions about informed consent, protections for research subjects, and other such issues. However, this should not lead us to conclude that the application of individual rights is always appropriate, or that such rights are the only relevant factors.

The area of treatment refusal presents an obviously inappropriate instance of invoking the right to self-determination. Suppose that a patient enters an emergency room screaming from the pain of severe burns. The attending physicians conclude that, although her burns are serious, she will recover if given immediate and sustained treatment. Suddenly the patient, on the verge of shock, rebuffs the efforts of the medical staff on the grounds that she has a right to "die with dignity." Clearly, in this sort of case it would be wrong for the medical staff to honor the claimed right to refuse treatment. Not only is the woman mistaken in her belief that she is about to die, regardless of treatment, but her capacity for self-determination has itself been substantially impaired or temporarily eclipsed by her recent trauma. To honor her refusal would be tantamount to treating this incompetent person as though she were competent, with morally disastrous results.

The above example demonstrates limits to the scope of the right of self-determination, namely, that it should be restricted to competent individuals. Conflicts between individual rights and the welfare of other persons—including, on occasion, the welfare of the entire community—constitute another set of problematic issues of libertarianism. For example, some libertarians argue that people should have the right to do whatever they please, so long as they do not violate anyone's rights. On a small-scale, interpersonal level, this principle is extremely problematic. Imagine a jilted lover who decides on impulse to marry another woman, not because he loves her, but merely to spite the woman who rejected him. We might all agree that this man has a right to marry whomever he chooses, but is "having a right" the same as "doing the

27. *National Law Journal* (May 16, 1994): A6.

right thing"? Obviously not, since the decision to marry out of spite will predictably inflict great suffering upon his unsuspecting bride.

On a broader social scale, libertarians often assert that individual freedom should include the right to shoot heroin, smoke crack cocaine, and take any other accurately labeled drug, so long as an individual freely chooses to do so. If our liberty is to mean anything, so the argument goes, it must encompass the right to take risks. To allow the government to decide what we may or may not put into our own bodies is to give up control over them. It is analogous to slavery.[28]

The trouble with a libertarian approach to the drug problem is that it ignores social consequences, and focuses only on individual rights. Drugs have destroyed many inner-city neighborhoods. Some of the related problems—such as crime due to illegal trafficking—might be solved by legalization, but not all of them would. Drug addiction has contributed to a skyrocketing rate of child abuse and neglect, because addicts—especially crack addicts—make notoriously poor parents. In addition, drug abuse by pregnant women is connected with dramatic increases in infant mortality, congenital syphilis, and HIV-positive infants. Serious students of the drug problem realize that hard questions remain even after the right of the individual to go to the devil has been invoked. What, for example, is the causal connection, if any, between unemployment, poverty, and ghetto conditions on the one hand, and hard drug addiction on the other? Would not an important consideration be if widespread use of drugs could be shown to reinforce racism and poverty? When unthinkingly waved as a trump, the right to self-determination can mask injustice and justify inequity.

We also need to ask what the effect of legalization on access and consumption would be. Some say that it would have little effect, since it is already so easy to obtain drugs in certain areas. At the same time, it should be remembered that three times as many Americans abuse alcohol as use illegal drugs, largely because of availability. From a public health perspective, if the end result of legalization is high-er addiction rates, this is a serious argument against it. Astonishingly, this consideration has no bearing at all on a libertarian view. For the libertarian, the level of addiction in society is irrelevant; the only thing that matters is whether the individual has made a free and voluntary decision to use drugs. Once again, the individual's freedom is everything, and the impact on society is ignored.[29]

Rights are important, for they protect individuals from—as Mill called it—"the tyranny of the majority." Nevertheless, an overemphasis on rights can sometimes exacerbate conflict. For example, to justify criminal punishment of women who use drugs during pregnancy, conservatives appeal to fetal rights. At the other extreme, some feminists and civil libertarians insist that a woman has a right to control her own body during pregnancy, regardless of the harm she causes to her future child. A recognition that mother and fetus are a unit, whose interests are generally promoted together, might be preferable to a rigid rights-based approach.

COMMUNITARIAN ETHICS

For all their differences, Hobbes, Mill, Kant, Rawls, Gauthier, and Nozick share the belief, bequeathed to us by the Enlightenment philosophers of the eighteenth century, that people should find moral rules in the application of reason to practical conduct. For this tradition, which we shall call "liberal individualism," ethical truth must be sought not in the vagaries of history, tradition, and religious faith, but rather in the universal tenets of rationality. Whether ethical norms are conceived in terms of enlightened self-interest, maximized utility, or the recognition of autonomy and human rights, they are viewed by this tradition as objective and universal, applicable to all times and places.

Another important theoretical strand connecting these theorists is their commitment to the individual as the unique focal point of moral concern. In utilitarianism, the collective preferences of each individual determine right and wrong. Everyone is to count as one, and nobody for more than one. However, the interest of the community as a

28. Walter Block, "Drug Prohibition: A Legal and Economic Analysis," in *Drugs, Morality, and the Law*, edited by Steven Luper-Foy and Curtis Brown (New York: Garland Publishing, Inc.), 199–216.

29. Bonnie Steinbock, "Drug Prohibition: A Public-Health Perspective," in *Drugs, Morality, and the Law*, 233–234.

whole may conflict with any particular individual's interest. Thus, a perennial problem for utilitarianism is the conflict between individual rights and the welfare of society as a whole. By contrast, "rights-based" Kantian and contractarian moral theory, as well as Nozick's brand of libertarianism, are committed to the notion that the rights and dignity of the individual should never (or rarely) be sacrificed to the interests of the larger society. Indeed, the whole point of social organization, of the "social contract," according to this tradition is the advancement of the *individual's* interests, rights, and happiness.

An important corollary of this view is the claim that, since different individuals will naturally have different values and conflicting visions of the good life, a truly liberal society will not—indeed cannot justifiably—adopt any particular conception of the good life to the exclusion or diminution of others.[30] Thus, a liberal society must remain "neutral" with regard to these competing conceptions of value and the good. To do otherwise—for example, by imposing a religion-based test on what kind of literature people should be allowed to read— amounts to a serious form of tyranny.

This ethical consensus on rationalism and individualism has had a profound impact on the development of contemporary biomedical ethics. Recently, however, the consensus has been challenged by a number of critics who can usefully, if somewhat uneasily, be lumped under the common banner of "communitarianism."[31] According to communitarian ethical theorists, all of our guiding ethical norms, rules, principles, theories, and virtues can be traced to distinct ethical traditions

and ways of life. They argue that it is impossible for us to "bootstrap" ourselves outside of time and space in order to discover some eternal realm of ethical insight. Rather, they claim, history, tradition, and concrete moral communities are the real wellsprings of our moral thought, judgment, and action. As Aristotle put it, we are social beings; our values, our conceptual schemes, our very identities are engendered, shaped, and nurtured within the confines of community.

Within this countertradition, ethical truth is thus particular, not universal. In contrast to the liberal claim that society must remain neutral vis-à-vis competing conceptions of the good life, communitarians argue that if any progress is to be made on a host of public controversies, ranging from pornography to the treatment of dying patients, we will have to begin not with abstract statements of rights, nor with an attempt to promote the good of all by promoting the good of each, but rather with some conception of common meanings, with a vision of what we take to be a "good society." Necessarily, our conception of this good society will crucially depend upon our own history, traditions, institutions, and customs.

Communitarians reject both the rationalism of liberalism's approach to method and their claim to value neutrality. In opposition to individualistic utilitarianism, they offer the idea of a *common good.* That is, where utilitarianism looks to the welfare of all individuals taken together, communitarianism looks to the *shared* values, ideals, and goals of a community. Where utilitarianism asks, "Which policies will produce the greatest happiness, on balance, of all of the individuals in society?" communitarianism asks, "Which policies will promote the kind of community in which we want to live?" The difference is subtle, but real. Against rights-based approaches, communitarians reject the penchant for elevating the individual above the social group or community. According to communitarians, the tendency of liberalism to focus so insistently on individual rights—to the exclusion of other social interests—can give rise to circumstances that a good society would not, and should not, tolerate.[32] Take, for example, the practice of

30. Ronald Dworkin, "Liberalism," in *A Matter of Principle* (Cambridge, MA: Harvard University Press, 1985), 181–204.

31. See, for example, Alasdair MacIntyre, *After Virtue* (Notre Dame, IN: University of Notre Dame Press, 1981). Reprinted in *Contemporary Moral Problems,* 4th ed., edited by James E. White (St. Paul, MN: West Publishing Company, 1994). See also Michael Sandel, *Liberalism and the Limits of Justice* (Cambridge: Cambridge University Press, 1982); Charles Taylor, "Atomism," in *Philosophical Papers,* vol. 2 (Cambridge: Cambridge University Press, 1982); Michael Walzer, *Spheres of Justice* (New York: Basic Books, 1983); Shlomo Avineri and Avner de-Shalit, eds., *Communitarianism and Individualism* (Oxford: Oxford University Press, 1992); and, for a good general overview, Stephen Mulhall and Adam Swift, *Liberals and Communitarians* (Oxford: Basil Blackwell, 1992).

32. See, e.g., Mary Ann Glendon, *Rights Talk: The Impoverishment of Political Discourse* (New York: Free Press, 1991).

some very large corporations with deep community roots—firms employing thousands of workers in relatively small cities—of simply pulling up stakes to search for cheaper labor markets in Mexico. In a society that gives pride of place to rights of ownership, such companies are given total freedom of movement; but the social costs of such rights and freedom can be enormous and often devastating to the affected communities, adding to unemployment, poverty, and the disintegration of neighborhoods and families. A good society, it is argued, would focus not only on individual rights, but also on the good of the larger community.

The dominance of liberal individualism within bioethics has recently been challenged on a number of fronts. Daniel Callahan has brought a communitarian perspective to debates over health care issues, such as rationing and reform (see Part Six, Section Two). According to Callahan, the combination of our desire to provide universal access to care, the burgeoning cost of high-tech medicine, and the sharp rise in the population of the elderly force some very hard choices that may decide who will live. Instead of starting, in standard liberal fashion, with individual wants, needs, interests, and rights, Callahan urges us to begin by asking what kind of society we wish to have—or as one of his book titles puts it, "What kind of life?"[33] To get at this big question, Callahan must confront some other very difficult and controversial questions, such as, What ought to be the goals and virtues of elderly persons? Should they seek individual happiness, or devote themselves to the education and welfare of future generations? And what ought to be the goals of medicine at various stages of the life cycle? Should medicine seek, at great expense, to forestall death for the very old with the latest high-tech devices, or should it merely try to provide dignified terminal *care?* Clearly, all this talk about goals and virtues necessarily implicates us in a quest for common meanings and values. Rather than ruling such questions off-limits due to

the strictures of liberal neutrality, Callahan claims simply that we *must* address them as a community if we are to act responsibly. Failure to do so, thus allowing each person to chart his or her own course, could well vindicate individual freedom of the elderly at the expense of the young.

How might a communitarian interpret our case of physician-assisted suicide? This is a difficult question to answer in light of the remarkable diversity among communitarian thinkers. For communitarians such as Alasdair MacIntyre, the emphasis upon history, traditional practices, and virtues leads to the wholesale abandonment of liberal individualism and the embrace of a rather "conservative" political agenda. More moderate communitarians, on the other hand, some of whom are politically quite "progressive," stress the importance of social meanings and communal values while attempting to preserve a more modest role for the language of individual rights.

Some communitarians, then, might approach the case of Dr. Brody and Jim Lasken by stressing the customary and time-honored prohibition of assisted suicide and euthanasia in all Western societies. They might argue that, in spite of individuals' strong claims to liberty in this area, the claims of society are stronger. The needs of many suicidal patients might well be met in ways other than by killing them, and society will be a better place if it acknowledges the sanctity and inviolability of human life. A similar argument might be mounted by physicians who could point to their own traditional professional commitments and values: "We heal; we don't kill. That's who we are as doctors; that's how we have always been."

An alternative communitarian reading of the case might reach the same conclusion, but for very different reasons. One could argue, for example, that even though individuals have a powerful claim of self-determination in this matter, the social costs of allowing a right of assisted suicide in a society distinguished by widespread poverty, lack of access to health care, and discrimination against vulnerable minority groups would be prohibitive. While the first communitarian response to our case has a distinctly conservative political flavor, the second might issue from a highly progressive, even Marxist, critique of existing social relationships.

An overall evaluation of communitarianism is an exceedingly complicated matter, due to the

33. Daniel Callahan, *What Kind of Life?* (New York: Simon and Schuster, 1990). See also his *Setting Limits* (New York: Simon and Schuster, 1987). For a recent attempt to develop a comprehensive communitarian theory of bioethics, focusing specifically on end-of-life and access to health care issues, see Ezekiel Emanuel, *The Ends of Human Life: Medical Ethics in a Liberal Polity* (Cambridge, MA: Harvard University Press, 1991).

disparate character of the theorists and theories lumped under its banner. For the purposes of this brief introduction, however, we venture the following conclusions and recommendations. (1) We agree with the claim that all ethical principles, rules, and virtues grow out of concrete historical traditions and derive their meaning and weight from those traditions. Thus, although our moral principles might extend very far indeed in both space and time, they are not the products of disembodied "reason." (2) The emphasis upon the communal dimension of our moral lives should be viewed as a welcome corrective to the largely asocial invocation of individual rights. We should worry a lot more about the "ecology of rights,"[34] the kind of society, neighborhood, and family life within which rights are developed and claimed.

On the negative side, (3) the more hardcore communitarians' wholesale rejection of liberal rights in favor of traditional practices and virtues is especially problematic. Curbing the socially destructive invocation of property rights is one thing, but limiting the freedom of individuals, in the name of communal values, to read pornography, obtain contraceptives, have abortions, or engage in homosexual relationships is, to us, a more disturbing prospect.[35] Finally, (4) it must be noted that an emphasis upon community, neighborhood, family, and traditional values will always express a preference for some *particular conception* of family, neighborhood, and community. For minority groups and women struggling to assert their own, quite varied, conceptions of individual and cultural identity, the communitarian impulse must learn to appreciate and respect such differences within our increasingly cosmopolitan societies.[36]

FEMINIST ETHICS

Just as communitarianism started as a critique of certain assumptions in liberal theory, so too the idea of a feminist ethic stems, in part, from a critique of traditional ethical theories as representing the experiences of men, not women. Feminist approaches to morality seek to correct this underlying bias.

Feminism is not a monolithic theory; thus, there is no one definition of "feminist ethics." Rather, feminism incorporates a variety of social and political beliefs, and there are even differing conceptions of feminism itself. All varieties of feminism are characterized by a concern for the welfare of all women, and a belief that women have historically been—and continue to be—oppressed by patriarchal societies. As Alison Jaggar writes, "Feminist approaches to ethics are distinguished by their explicit commitment to rethinking ethics with a view to correcting whatever forms of male bias it may contain."[37] They all seek to unmask and challenge the oppression, discrimination, and exclusion that women have faced. Feminist approaches to ethics are political, in the sense that they are keenly aware of imbalances of power between women and men, rich and poor, healthy and disabled, white people and people of color, and first world and third world peoples.

Feminist approaches to ethics are also marked by attention to the so-called "private sphere," including reflection on intimate relations, such as affection and sexuality, which were ignored by modern moral theory until quite recently. Finally, feminist ethics, rather than seeing women as less fully developed versions of men, insists on taking the moral experience of all women seriously. Modern feminists also warn against the tendency to make generalizations about "women" based on the experience of the relatively small group of middle-class white women. Many feminists today emphasize that sexual oppression is only one form of oppression, and that all forms—whether based on gender, class, race, or disability—must be acknowledged and fought.

Some issues, such as abortion and reproductive technology, are traditionally conceived as "women's issues," and many feminists have written on these topics. However, feminist approaches

---

34. Mary Ann Glendon, *Rights Talk*, 136–144 (see note 32).

35. See Amy Gutmann, "Communitarian Critics of Liberalism," *Philosophy and Public Affairs* 14 (1985): 308–322.

36. See Iris Marion Young, *Justice and the Politics of Difference* (Princeton, NJ: Princeton University Press, 1990); and Marilyn Friedman, "Feminism and Modern Friendship: Dislocating the Community," *Ethics* 99 (1989): 275–290.

37. Alison M. Jaggar, "Feminist Ethics: Some Issues for the Nineties," in *Contemporary Moral Problems*, 4th ed., edited by James E. White (St. Paul, MN: West Publishing Company, 1994), 61.

to bioethics are not limited to this sphere; feminist thought has influenced thinking about the health professional–patient relationship, informed consent, experimental trials, disability, access to health care, and other issues.[38]

One issue that divides feminists is whether virtue is "gendered"; that is, whether there are virtues that are specifically female and male. Many feminists reject this approach, as the idea of "feminine virtues"—including selflessness, devotion to family needs, and submissiveness to men—has long been linked with the oppression of women. Nevertheless, many nineteenth-century women, including many who were concerned with women's emancipation, believed not only that there were specifically female virtues, but also that women were morally superior to men and that society could be transformed through the influence of women. Today, some feminists regard many of the evils of society—war, violence, racism, the destruction of the environment—as the result of specifically male faults, such as aggression.[39] They believe that the "feminine" virtues of kindness, generosity, helpfulness, and sympathy can serve as a corrective to these evils.

A related issue on which feminists divide is the meaning of sexual equality. Are men and women treated equally when they are treated the same? Jaggar states that "By the end of the 1960s, most feminists in the United States had come to believe that the legal system should be sex-blind, that it should not differentiate in any way between women and men."[40] However, this version of equality does not always promote women's interests. A notorious example is "no-fault" divorce settlements that divide family property equally between husband and wife. Here, equal distribution leaves many women much worse-off financially, because women—who often shoulder most of the family responsibilities, such as housework and caring for children—typically have much

lower job qualifications and less work experience than men. Divorce settlements that do not take social realities into account are egregiously unfair, and moreover reinforce sexual inequality. At the same time, the alternative way of seeking equality, by providing women with special legal protection, appears to promote sexual stereotypes.

Feminists continue to debate the correct interpretation of equality, even while some feminists reject the entire concept of equality as part of an "ethic of justice" that is characteristically masculine, relying on rules and abstracting from particular, concrete situations, instead of responding to immediately perceived needs.[41] Such feminists suggest an alternative "ethic of care,"[42] stressing connectedness, the importance of human relationships, empathy, and an acknowledgement of dependency. It shares with virtue ethics the conviction that undue emphasis on moral rules obscures the crucial role of moral insight, virtue, and character in determining how to deal with ethical issues.

Some feminists have claimed that the ethic of caring fails to give enough attention to moral principles. Virginia Held reminds us that "an absence of principles can be an invitation to capriciousness."[43] Moreover, issues such as economic justice "cry out for relevant principles. Although caring may be needed to motivate us to act on such principles, the principles are not dispensable."[44] Without such principles, the claims of those unrelated to us, or different from us, may go unheeded. Moreover, it is not clear that an ethic of care would ensure the rights of women to equality and fair treatment.[45]

The emphasis on the importance of emotions is seen by many (and not just feminists) as a welcome

38. See Susan Wolf, ed., *Feminism and Bioethics: Beyond Reproduction* (New York: Oxford University Press, 1995); Helen B. Holmes and Laura Purdy, eds., *Feminist Perspectives in Medical Ethics* (Bloomington: Indiana University Press, 1992); and Susan Sherwin, *No Longer Patient* (Philadelphia, PA: Temple University Press, 1992).

39. Mary Daly, *Gyn/Ecology: The Metaethics of Radical Feminism* (Boston, MA: Beacon Press, 1978).

40. Jaggar, "Feminist Ethics," 63 (see note 37).

41. Ibid., 64.

42. Carol Gilligan, *In a Different Voice: Psychological Theory and Women's Development* (Cambridge, MA: Harvard University Press, 1982); Nell Noddings, *Caring: A Feminine Approach to Ethics and Moral Education* (Berkeley: University of California Press, 1984).

43. Virginia Held, "Feminism and Moral Theory," in *Contemporary Moral Problems*, 4th ed., edited by James E. White (St. Paul, MN: West Publishing Company, 1994), 75.

44. Ibid.

45. Ibid., 76. See also Joan Tronto, *Moral Boundaries: A Political Argument for an Ethic of Care* (New York: Routledge, 1993).

balance to the sort of moral theory that completely ignores feeling. At the same time, taking emotion as a guide can often degenerate into a "do what feels good" kind of subjective relativism.[46] The problem of relativism remains a difficult one for feminism. On the one hand, many feminists join with postmodernists and communitarians in rejecting the Enlightenment notion of a universal morality, valid for all people at all times and places. This notion ignores the particularity most feminists regard as essential and too long ignored by Western ethics. On the other hand, however, feminists are understandably concerned that their critique of the oppression of women not be dismissed as a single point of view.[47]

The problem of relativism for feminists is poignantly posed by the practice of clitoridectomy, or female "circumcision." This practice, common among certain groups in Africa, involves the excision of the clitoris. Sometimes the vulva is sewn up as well. The clitoris is removed to reduce sexual pleasure and remove temptation to sexual activity; the lips of the vulva are sewn up to ensure that the young woman will remain a virgin until her marriage. The circumcision is usually done when a girl reaches puberty, although it is also often performed on very young children. It is performed without anesthesia, using unsterilized razor blades, while the girl is held down by older women. It frequently causes life-threatening blood loss and infection. It can lead to painful intercourse, infertility, and difficult childbirth.

> Ironically, the frigidity or infertility caused by the mutilation leads many husbands to shun their brides. . . . Doctors throughout Africa recognize the harmful effects of female circumcision but feel powerless to stop a practice so entrenched in custom and tradition. Many organizations are campaigning against it, and the new African Charter on the Rights of Children includes items condemning circumcision. Governments in Sudan and elsewhere have passed laws against it, but they are seldom enforced.[48]

46. Jaggar, 68 (see note 37).
47. Ibid., 67.
48. *Time* (Fall 1990), 39. Cited in Joel Feinberg, *Freedom and Fulfillment: Philosophical Essays* (Princeton, NJ: Princeton University Press, 1992), 199.

Despite this opposition, many Africans continue to regard female circumcision as an important cultural and religious ritual.

The practice of female circumcision poses a dilemma for feminists. On the one hand, feminism is committed to multiculturalism, that is, to the view that no culture has a monopoly on the right way to live, and that the voices of all people must be heard. On the other hand, feminists must reject a practice they regard as patently contrary to the interests of women. Not only is clitoridectomy painful and dangerous, but its justification stems from suppositions antithetical to feminist thought: that women are male property, that female virginity must be preserved, that women ought not to have sexual feelings, that adultery is a male prerogative, and so forth. Is there a way out of the dilemma, a way to remain faithful to feminist ideals without rejecting multiculturalism?

We think that there is a way out. As suggested earlier, we need to develop an interpretation of multiculturalism that does not imply relativism. Keeping an open mind about the practices of other cultures, and attempting to understand them "from within," does not commit us to unqualified acceptance of these practices, particularly when they conflict with our deepest values and principles. For feminists, a core value is the conviction that women are full human persons, entitled to equality and justice. Clitoridectomy is not compatible with the recognition of women as free and equal members of society; indeed, it contributes to women's oppression, and is thus opposed by many African women and men. Western feminists can support these Africans in this struggle, and not be guilty of arrogance, smugness, or cultural imperialism.

VIRTUE ETHICS

In light of the problems facing consequentialist and deontological moral theories, the last fifty years or so have witnessed a growing interest in what is called "virtue ethics." Virtue ethics does not represent a single distinctive moral theory. Rather, it is a label for a family of moral theories that are specially concerned with or that give special priority to the role of the virtues in the moral life. In fact, one of the main challenges facing theories of this kind is to differentiate themselves from the moral theories we have already discussed. After all, a utilitarian like Mill will value the moral virtues on the grounds that they motivate those who possess them to reliably perform actions that maximize the overall good. Contractarians like Hobbes will value them because of the way they contribute to our ability to cooperate with one another and to form a stable community.[49] In fact, virtue plays a central role in Kant's moral philosophy. For Kant, the good will is the only thing unconditionally good, and virtue is what makes the good will good. Virtue is the strength of the will's commitment to performing actions from the motive of duty, and it is, therefore, the condition for the goodness of anything the will does. To begin with, then, it will be useful to mark a very general contrast between the role the virtues play in these moral theories and the more central place they occupy in virtue ethics.

According to an act-consequentialist moral theory, the right action is the one that produces the best consequences. In order to be practically useful, such theories must provide us with a meaningful account of the relevant consequences and how they are to be calculated or measured. Similarly, according to a deontological moral theory, the right action is the one specified by a particular rule of some sort. In order to be of any practical benefit, such theories must supply us with the appropriate set of rules or with some procedure or criteria by which we can generate the relevant rules. In contrast, the right action in a virtue-theoretic account is the one that the virtuous person would perform. In order to be practically useful, this sort of theory must tell us who the virtuous people are and it must give us an account of the nature and number of whatever virtues it recognizes.[50] Unlike consequentialist or rule-based theories, then, virtue ethics begins with an account of the moral virtues and then links the possession of these traits to the

ability to reliably perform certain kinds of actions and, importantly, to an inability to perform certain others. As a result, moral theories in this family may differ in the kinds of things they count as virtues and vices, the number of virtues and vices they recognize, their reasons why the virtues are valuable, and the relationship of the virtues to right actions.

Contemporary virtue ethicists tend to see themselves as carrying on or working within a tradition of moral philosophy that begins with Aristotle. According to Aristotle, the priorities reflected in the choices we make in our lives reveal our conception of the good life, or human flourishing—what Aristotle calls *eudaimonia*. We may disagree about the nature of the good life, but we can all agree that it is around some conception of happiness or doing well that we structure our various activities and give a distinctive shape to our lives. As a result, a central question for Aristotle is, What is the best life for a person to lead?

For Aristotle, a candidate for this highest good must not be something that others bestow upon us. Rather, it must be proper to its possessor and not easily taken away (1095b26-27).[51] Because honor or fame fail both of these tests, the life dedicated to their pursuit is ruled out as a candidate for the good life. Similarly, any candidate for the highest good must be a final good in the sense that we choose other things for the sake of it, but we don't choose it for the sake of anything else (1097a30). As a result, the life of money making is ruled out. In addition, the candidate must be self-sufficient in the sense that the presence of it alone makes life desirable and worth living (1097b ff). In Aristotle's view, the virtues of temperance, courage, justice, wisdom, and practical reason represent the excellent states of our emotional and intellectual faculties. Because each of these traits represents the proper development of some human faculty, they are valuable for themselves (1097b2-5, 1144a1-7). But Aristotle believes that the virtues are also valuable for the activities that they produce and that happiness, or the highest human good, is a life of activity that consists in

49. For an analysis of the role of moral virtues in Hobbes' moral philosophy and a contrast of this view with those of Plato and Aristotle, see Alex John London, "Virtue and Consequences: Hobbes on the Value of the Moral Virtues," *Social Theory and Practice* (Spring 1998)

50. This way of contrasting virtue ethics with consequentialist and deontological moral theories is explained at length by Rosalind Hursthouse in "Normative Virtue Ethics," *How Should One Live One's Life?* edited by Roger Crisp (New York: Oxford University Press, 1996), 19–36.

51. These numbers refer to the page and line numbers of Bekker's edition of Aristotle's works. They are the standard method of citing particular passages in the works of Aristotle and can be found in the margins of the text of most translations.

the exercise of such well-developed emotional and intellectual faculties under the guidance of our distinctly human capacity for rationality.

To cultivate the virtues, however, one must first perform actions that are noble and good. Noble and just actions have a kind of symmetry or balance about them—they are a mean between unacceptable extremes—and the only way to cultivate character states that share this symmetry is to repeatedly perform virtuous actions. To understand what is right, noble, and just, however, one must have received a proper upbringing. One must have cultivated good habits, such as consideration for others, truthfulness, and self-control, because one becomes just and temperate by first doing just and temperate things. But virtue isn't simply a matter of practice or mere habit. Rather, it is only by acting in certain ways that we can come to understand what is noble and just and why this is so. Those who lack appropriate role models or guardians to instruct them will be unable to appreciate these things. Furthermore, Aristotle thinks that right, noble, and just actions are of such a diverse nature that they cannot be adequately captured by a set of rules or decision procedures. As a result, one cannot rely solely on some external theory or decision principle to determine which actions one ought to perform. To reliably perform the right action, one must cultivate the virtues for oneself and rely on one's experience and ability to appreciate and judge such things for oneself.

This does not mean that one will not be able to explain why something was the right thing to do given a particular situation. To the contrary, the virtuous person will be able to bring out the salient features of a situation and to say why some action is morally acceptable. This ability to appreciate the facts of a situation and to justify acting in one way rather than another, however, is quite different from the ability to give a general and practically useful account of the features that are morally important to situations in general and of what makes an action right and noble such that nonvirtuous people could use this account as a guide to action. For Aristotle, the only reliable way to understand what must be done, and to ensure that one is sufficiently willing to act on this understanding, is to become a just person oneself.

In this reading of Aristotle, the virtues play a central role in his ethical theory for several reasons. First, because they represent the excellent states of important human emotional and intellectual capacities, they are valuable in their own right. Second, the virtues play an important role in human flourishing, since the exercise of these well-developed states of our faculties is what Aristotle regards as happiness, or *eudaimonia*. Third, the virtues play an important epistemological role in the good life—namely, without the virtues, one will not fully understand what makes an action noble and just, or be able to appreciate the morally relevant factors of complicated situations. Fourth, the moral virtues provide the motivation for consistently performing the right actions since the person who possesses them will not only understand what makes them noble and just, but will also take pleasure in acting will and will do so for its own sake and not for the sake of some external consideration. Those who lack the proper upbringing will regard such actions as painful, to be done only to avoid punishment or to gain some advantage, such as obtaining money, power, or friends.

Some contemporary versions of virtue ethics differ from Aristotle on one or more of these points. For example, Aristotle says that the right action is the one that the virtuous person would perform because the virtuous person "judges each thing rightly" and "things appear to him as they truly are," so that what sets the virtuous person apart from others is that "he sees the truth in each thing, being himself the norm and measure of the noble and the pleasant" (1113a26-35 cf. 1176a12-19). We can use the virtuous person as a standard or measure of what is right because she understands why some action is right and just and can be counted on to reliably perform such actions. The virtuous person is thus an epistemological guide to determining which actions are right. But the rightness of those actions is not a product of the fact that they are the actions virtuous people would perform, although some contemporary virtue theorists embrace this view.

According to these theorists, the virtues are of primary importance to the moral life because they are the primary locus of moral value. As such, the virtuous are the norm and measure of what is right and good precisely because actions derive whatever moral value they possess from their relationship to the virtues. If an action is one that the virtuous person would perform, then this makes the action right and just.[52] The value of the action is therefore determined by the judgment of the virtuous person. One major problem for a view of this sort lies in explaining the grounds on which virtuous agents make their initial judgment. On what grounds do they decide whether an action is the right one? Certainly it cannot be simply because it is the action they did in fact choose. This would make their judgment seem arbitrary and capricious. But if it is because it is the action they *should* choose, then we want to know what it is about the action that makes it worthy of choice. In either case it looks like such a theory will either turn out to be arbitrary and unhelpful or it will have to advert to some explanation of the value of an action that reaches beyond its relation to the judgment of the virtuous themselves.

Similarly, many contemporary virtue ethicists differ from Aristotle in rejecting the view that the virtues are excellent states of our cognitive and affective faculties. For example, Alasdair MacIntyre argues that the virtues should not be thought of as timeless, human excellences. Rather, they are acquired human qualities that allow us to achieve goods internal to those cultural roles and practices that can be shaped into a coherent vision of the good life within a particular community.[53] As such, cultural traditions, community membership, and role obligations play a crucial part in determining which kinds of human qualities are virtues and what kinds of activities count as virtuous activities.

In MacIntyre's view, Dr. Brody has to ask herself whether assisting in suicide is consistent with the goods that are internal to the practice of medicine in late twentieth-century America and the obligations that she has taken on in her role as physician. On the one hand, Dr. Brody is committed to ameliorating pain and suffering, but she is also aware that doctors have traditionally conceived of themselves as the agents of health, not death. She also knows that there may be considerable consequences to a choice to assist Jim's suicide, and she has to weigh these consequences against her own well-being and self-interest. Is it

fair that Jim cannot receive help in ending his suffering until his condition degenerates to the point that his life is being sustained by machines, the support of which it might then be permissible to withdraw? Is it acceptable for her to lie or dissemble in order to help Jim and avoid going to jail, or to comfort or assuage Jim if she decides not to come to his aid?

These are difficult questions, and the fact that virtue ethics does not provide us with easy answers to them is not peculiar to this ethical theory. Even so, critics are generally nonplussed by the advice to do whatever the virtuous person would do, especially in situations where compassion, fidelity, courage, prudence, and self-interest seem to be at odds with one another. What critics demand is some way of ranking the virtues and their hold on us so that people like Dr. Brody will know how to negotiate such conflicts. In the eyes of critics, without such a ranking, virtue ethics will never entirely substitute for a more principled approach.

Yet the fact that the virtue ethicist relies on the good judgment of the virtuous person to negotiate such apparent conflicts should not detract from the fact that the consequentialist and the deontologist face very similar problems. The consequentialist must provide Dr. Brody with an account of the relevant consequences and with a procedure by which to weigh or measure them without running afoul of our deepest intuitions about this case. Similarly, the deontologist must produce a set of rules or decision procedures flexible enough to accommodate the nuances of the situation. So it appears that with each of these theories as well, Dr. Brody is going to have to exercise her deliberative skills to do what is right for Jim and for herself.

Nevertheless, the virtue-based approach to cases like this does have certain advantages. For example, it brings out a variety of *prima facie* concerns, each of which makes a serious claim on us and demands that we apply ourselves to finding a judicious way to address each of them as best we can. It also brings out the way in which a physician must be committed to her patients and to her craft. The goal and goods of medicine require physicians to take chances for their patients—to have the courage to attend to them even when this may conflict with their own self-interest. Willingness to expose oneself to risk, including

52. A version of this view can be found in Rosalind Hursthouse, "Virtue Theory and Abortion,"*Philosophy & Public Affairs* 20 (1991): 223–246.

53. Alasdair MacIntyre, *After Virtue*, 2nd ed. (Notre Dame, IN: University of Notre Dame Press, 1984), 191.

disease and sickness, is part of what it means to be a physician. As Arnold Relman puts it, "the risk of contracting the patient's disease is one of the risks that is inherent in the profession of medicine. Physicians who are not willing to accept that risk . . . ought not to be in the practice of medicine."[54] Although there are limits to the duty to put oneself at risk, a virtue-based approach establishes a strong presumption in favor of the duty to treat over doctors' rights to decide whom to treat and what risks to take.[55] Indeed, one of the shortcomings of a narrowly contractualist approach to the doctor-patient relationship, an approach that specifies numerous duties *within* that relationship, is its silence on the question of whether doctors have moral and professional obligations to *establish* relationships with needy, dangerous, or HIV-infected patients.

NONMORAL CONSIDERATIONS

The dizzying array of moral theories and perspectives presented above make it hard enough to decide how to act in a given situation. We suggested that it is not a question of determining which moral theory is correct; all of them contribute to an extraordinarily complex moral reality. Still, in deciding what to do, one must decide when utilitarian considerations should prevail, or when one ought to adhere to absolutist principles; when to appeal to principles and when to seek guidance in virtues; when to abide by universal, impartial considerations and when to concentrate on personal relationships and feelings.

As if the moral dimension of decision making were not complicated enough, there is another dimension we have not so far discussed: the "nonmoral" dimension. How should we think about the political, personal, prudential, economic, or legal implications of our actions? According to one school of thought, moral reasons are the "best" reasons; they always "trump" other considerations. Thus, if it would be morally right to do something, then one ought to do it, even if it would have adverse nonmoral consequences. More recently, philosophers like Bernard Williams[56] and Susan Wolf[57] have argued that one is sometimes entirely justified in overriding impartial moral reasons to pursue a significant personal goal or defining relationship. Conceivably, many of the considerations left out of traditional ethics can be recovered if we take seriously the idea, advocated by feminists and others, that personal relations and feelings are as important to ethics as universal and impartial principles. Nevertheless, however broadly ethics is conceived, there will always be the possibility of conflict between moral and nonmoral considerations. In such cases, how are we to decide what to do?

Consider, once again, Dr. Brody. Suppose she decides that the morally right thing to do is to help Jim Lasken. Helping him is breaking the law. She could be prosecuted and go to jail; even if she is not convicted, she could lose her license to practice medicine. It seems clear that these are important considerations and that it would be absurd (as opposed to noble) for Dr. Brody to completely ignore them. Whether her personal risk should override her view of the morally right action depends, in part, on the degree of the risk. If the risks of discovery, prosecution, and punishment are sufficiently low, and if she believes that it is morally right to help Jim, Dr. Brody should perhaps be willing to risk legal and professional repercussions. In other situations, doing the morally right thing might ask too much of a person. The hard thing in life is having the wisdom to figure out when nonmoral actions are justified.

MODES OF MORAL REASONING

The above survey of moral theories suggests the richness and diversity of our repertoire of ethical language and concepts. The task for this section is to show how these disparate and sometimes conflicting elements of morality figure into the moral judgments that we make. What should we *do* with all this ethical "raw material"?

54. *Cardiovascular News* (August 1987): 7.

55. Norman Daniels argues that a virtue-based approach to the question of the duty to treat implies a contractualist theory. See "Duty to Treat or Right to Refuse?" *Hasting Center Report* 21, no. 2 (1991): 36–46.

56. Bernard Williams, *Ethics and the Limits of Philosophy* (Cambridge, MA: Harvard University Press, 1985).

57. Susan Wolf, "Moral Saints," *Journal of Philosophy* (August 1982): 419–439.

Many of the enumerated theoretical perspectives—such as utilitarianism, Kantianism, and rights-based theories—articulate basic moral values, principles, and rules at a fairly high level of abstraction. We are told, for example, to maximize happiness, respect persons, honor patients' rights to confidentiality, and so on. But we are also told—for example, by the partisans of an ethic of care—to de-emphasize such abstractions in favor of a heightened caring responsiveness to individual people and situations. An important question arises, then, about precisely how these generalities are, or should be, brought to bear in specific cases. In the language of the philosophical tradition, it is a question about the relationship between the universal and the particular.

This is also a question about the nature of moral justification. In pointing out the importance of happiness, personhood, rights, virtues, caring, etc., each of the above theories contributes to our search for ethical *warrants* or reasons that tend to *justify* our actions. When called upon to justify or defend individual actions or social policies, how do—or how should—we respond? Insofar as it makes sense to pursue ethical certitude about our actions, where does such certitude lie: in our philosophical or religious theories, in our pre-theoretical convictions of right and wrong generated by our history and culture, or perhaps in some combination of these two areas?

THE PRINCIPLES APPROACH

One tempting response to these questions is to hold that justification in ethics is a matter of deducing the best and most comprehensive ethical theory from the foregoing list, and deriving this theory's correct conclusions. Thus, one should throw in his or her lot with, say, utilitarianism or Kantianism and then "apply" this theoretical framework to the facts at hand. Understood in this way, bioethics has been described as a kind of "applied ethics," as though philosophers and theologians do all the ethical heavy lifting, while others simply apply their findings to this or that set of factual circumstances. Tempting as it is in its simplicity, this conception of bioethics must nevertheless be rejected.

First, although this approach identifies philosophical theory as the ultimate locus of moral certitude, it is far from clear what the "best and most comprehensive" ethical theory is. Indeed, after centuries of moral debates, we still disagree, sometimes vehemently, about justice and the nature of the good life. Second, as we have seen in the application of various theories to our case of physician-assisted suicide, theories are often stated at such a high level of generality (e.g., "Maximize happiness," "Respect persons") that they are capable of generating contradictory answers to the same moral questions. Third, this way of understanding "theory"—i.e., as an abstract construction built upon one or two overarching values—tends to obscure the extraordinary richness and diversity of the moral life. So, even if one of the enumerated "standard" theories were miraculously to attract a consensus, the result would be more impoverishing than liberating. To repeat, ethical theories as we understand them are best viewed as partial perspectives on a complex moral reality.

A powerful alternative to theory-driven approaches to bioethics emphasizes the role in moral reasoning of a small cluster of middle-level ethical principles. Instead of pursuing difficult and highly divisive foundational issues, the partisans of the "principles approach" (or "principlism") begin with our common moral experience and the manifest importance of keeping a short list of moral duties. Originally developed by Professors Tom Beauchamp and James Childress in their justly influential book, *The Principles of Bioethics*,[58] and later endorsed by prestigious governmental ethics commissions,[59] the method of principlism rapidly became the dominant mode of "doing bioethics" in the United States.

Stated in their popular tongue-twisting, Latinate formulations, these norms include the principles of autonomy, beneficence, nonmaleficence, and justice. In simpler terms, the core principles of bioethics bid us to (1) respect the capacity of individuals to choose their own vision of the good life and act accordingly; (2) foster the interests and happiness of other persons and of society at large;

58. Beauchamp and Childress, *The Principles of Bioethics* (see note 6).

59. National Commission for the Protection of Human Subjects of Biomedical and Behavioral Research, *The Belmont Report: Ethical Principles and Guidelines for the Protection of Human Subjects of Research* (Washington, D.C.: U.S. Government Printing Office, 1978).

(3) refrain from harming other persons; and (4) act fairly, distribute benefits and burdens in an equitable fashion, and resolve disputes by means of fair procedures.

In contrast to the partisans of applied moral theory, who tend to reduce the sources of normative guidance and criticism to a single overarching value (for example, Kantian respect for persons or the maximization of utility), the principlists settle for a small cluster of "middle level" norms, each one consistent with a number of ethical theories, no one of which enjoys automatic supremacy over the others. They reject the notion that serious moral conflict can always be resolved by appeal to a higher moral standard provided by some ultimate theory. Instead, they frankly admit the necessity of "weighing and balancing" the various principles against one another in each concrete moral situation.

While each principle articulates a serious moral duty, these duties are not absolute. They are, in the words of the late philosopher W. D. Ross, *prima facie* obligations.[60] This means that the ethical principles are indeed binding, but on any given occasion one principle may eclipse another with which it conflicts. So we say that a given principle is binding *prima facie,* or "at first blush," but that in the final analysis, all things having been considered, the pull of another principle might turn out to be even stronger. Importantly, however, even when a principle is outweighed, it usually continues to exert a strong moral pull on our behavior; it does not simply become irrelevant.

The conflict between the demands of confidentiality and the protection of public health in the context of AIDS provides a useful example of how principlism could be applied. On the one hand, physicians swear an oath to uphold the confidentiality of their patients. Since Hippocrates, this duty has been utterly central to the vocation of physicians. Without assurances that their often embarrassing secrets are safe with the doctor, patients will be reluctant to speak frankly about their symptoms or medical history, and in some cases may avoid seeking medical attention to the detriment of their condition. A doctor's violations of confidentiality thus might be seen as violating the principles of beneficence and nonmaleficence.

60. W. D. Ross, *The Right and the Good* (Oxford: Clarendon Press, 1930).

The principle of autonomy provides further warrant for a doctor's confidentiality. Patients have a right to determine who knows what about their medical history. When physicians or nurses share this information with others who do not have a legitimate medical need to know, they rob their patients of control over information that is rightfully theirs. Combined, then, the principles of autonomy, beneficence, and nonmaleficence make an exceedingly strong case for respecting patient confidentiality.

But now suppose that you are a physician caring for a bisexual male infected with the AIDS virus. Your patient admits to having regular unprotected sex with his fiancée, who does not suspect his HIV status, yet he insists upon absolute confidentiality out of a (well-founded) fear of losing her. On one hand, you feel the pull of your duty to respect confidentiality; but, on the other hand, your patient's behavior is placing another human being in mortal peril and you are in a unique position to protect this unsuspecting, vulnerable person.

This ethical dilemma, discussed at greater length in Part One, Section Three, effectively illustrates the *prima facie* character of the principles approach. As a physician, you are clearly bound by your duty of confidentiality, but you are also bound to prevent grave harm to highly vulnerable people, especially when you are in a unique position to do so. According to principlism, you cannot simply invoke a supreme value that always wins; you must instead undertake the difficult task of weighing and balancing conflicting values. In this case, you might decide that the principle of autonomy is outweighed by the prevention of harm to others. The risk is great, the projected harm exceedingly grave, and your patient's insistence upon his autonomy might be discounted as self-contradictory and hypocritical in light of his irresponsible disregard of his fiancée's autonomy, as well as her life.

On balance, then, your *prima facie* duty to respect your patient's confidentiality might fall short as a duty *all things considered* in this particular situation. But this does not mean either that these rival concerns will always prevail in similar circumstances or that confidentiality simply becomes irrelevant once it is outweighed. If your patient is an HIV-infected woman who (credibly) claims that her abusive, drug-taking, and possibly

HIV-infected boyfriend will kill her should he discover her secret, you will most likely find another way to solve the problem than by violating your patient's confidentiality. And even when you decide that, all things considered, confidentiality must yield to another principle, such as the prevention of harm, confidentiality continues to exert moral influence by setting the terms of legitimate disclosure. Even though the bisexual's fiancée has a right to know the truth, the same cannot be said of his employer, the other patients in your waiting room, or the members of your weekly poker game.

OBJECTIONS TO THE PRINCIPLES APPROACH

In spite of its enormous success, the method of principlism has recently been criticized on a number of fronts. Although some of these objections lack merit, others pose important challenges to principlism. As we shall see, principlism has nevertheless proved itself remarkably adaptive in responding to many of these complaints.[61]

1. Principlism Is Mechanistic and Vacuous. Although astute commentators like Beauchamp and Childress have wielded principlism in a thoughtful, carefully nuanced, and fruitful manner, in less skilled hands this method has tended to degenerate into a ritualistic incantation of empty abstractions. Bioethical literature abounds with superficial claims that "the principle of autonomy (or of beneficence, or of the 'best interests' of the patient) *requires* that we do such and such." The problem with this common locution is that it ignores the difficulty (or the vacuousness) of passing immediately from very abstract statements of principle to very concrete conclusions about what to do here and now. Quite apart from the vexing problem of rank ordering *competing* principles in morally complex situations, we first have to determine what these abstract formulations of principle actually mean.

What does it mean, for example, to invoke the moral principle that caregivers should always seek

the "best interests" of all patients, including severely impaired newborns? How are the interests of such a child to be assessed, and according to which conception of the good? Some argue that life is sacred and that continued life is always in the child's interest; others contend that a life of constant suffering is not a life worth living; while still others advance a conception of the good based on more complex notions of human flourishing and dignity, which might sanction nontreatment decisions even given the absence of pain and suffering.[62]

Whatever the merit of these individual suggestions, the point is that unless we *interpret* "the principles of bioethics," they will merely play the role of empty "chapter headings,"[63] doing little, if any, actual work in moral analysis. Unless we furnish principles with a definite shape and content— *Which* principle of justice? *Which* conception of autonomy?—they will merely lend a patina of objectivity to bioethical debates while masking the need to pin down arguments and choices defining the substance of those principles.

2. Principlism Founders on the Problem of Moral Conflict. Other critics call attention to principlism's inability or unwillingness to provide a rationally defensible framework for settling conflicts between competing principles. Clearly, such critics have a point here. Unlike utilitarians or Rawlsians who could settle, at least to their own satisfaction, the inevitable conflicts of the moral life using some overarching principle of "lexical ordering," the principlists forthrightly admit that their moral principles do not come with pre-established theoretical weights; consequently, conflicts have to be settled through a subtle process of weighing and balancing of principles in the midst of real cases, an approach to conflict resolution that some philosophers regard as excessively subjective. We believe, however, that there is wisdom in the principlists' modesty. Their critics have neither established the clear superiority of any monistic theory, such as utilitarianism, nor have they produced a convincing account of why, within

---

61. The following account of the role of principles and cases in moral argument is based upon John Arras's more extensive discussion in "Principles and Particularity: The Roles of Cases in Bioethics," *Indiana Law Journal* 69, no. 4 (Symposium on Emerging Paradigms in Bioethics, Fall 1994): 983–1014.

62. See Ezekiel Emanuel, *The Ends of Human Life,* 70–87 (see note 33).

63. K. Danner Clouser and Bernard Gert, "A Critique of Principlism," *Journal of Medicine and Philosophy* 15 (1990): 227.

more pluralistic systems, certain favored values such as utility or liberty should *always* prevail over all other competing values in a myriad of convoluted real world situations.

3. Principlism Is Deductivistic. Another group of critics, the partisans of a more "case-driven" mode of analysis, object to the apparently unidirectional movement from principles to cases within principlism. Although a careful analysis of Beauchamp and Childress's early editions of *The Principles of Bioethics* might well suggest a more complicated relationship between principles and cases in the process of moral justification, earlier editions of their book gave the distinct impression that theory justifies principles, that principles justify moral rules, and that rules justify moral judgments in particular cases.[64]

This "top down" conception of moral reasoning has been faulted for ignoring the pivotal role of intuitive, case-based judgments of right and wrong. To be sure, the judgments in question are not to be confused with just any responses to cases, no matter how prejudiced, ill-considered, or subject to coercion they might be. Rather, the critics have in mind something more akin to John Rawls's notion of "considered" moral judgments;[65] i.e., those judgments about whose genesis and moral rectitude we feel most confident, such as that slavery is wrong. It is precisely these judgments, they claim, that give concrete meaning, definition, and scope to our moral principles, thus providing us with critical leverage in refining their articulation.

The ultimate point of this criticism is that the relationship between principles and cases is dialectical or reciprocal: the principles provide normative guidance and the cases provide considered judgments that, in turn, help shape the principles, which then provide more precise guidance. Another way of putting this, following Rawls's terminology, is that principles and cases exist together in creative tension or "reflective equilibrium."[66] One can thus insist on a robust role for principles

in moral reasoning without being committed to a "top down" or deductivistic approach.[67]

CASUISTRY OR "CASE-BASED" REASONING

The renaissance of casuistry, or "case-based" reasoning, in practical ethics has stressed the pivotal role of the particularity of cases while de-emphasizing the role of theory and routinized appeals to "the principles of bioethics."[68] According to its leading proponents, a casuistical method must begin with a typology or grouping of cases around paradigmatic instances of a moral rule or principle. In the area of research ethics, for example, the atrocities of Nazi medicine still serve to exemplify unethical dealing with human subjects. From this signal case, one then branches out to analogous cases of greater complexity and difficulty, such as research on children or the demented elderly, proceeding by a method akin to "moral triangulation." As one goes from case to case, responding to the particularities of different settings, treatments, and categories of research subjects, principles emerge and become increasingly refined and complex.

Crucially, the casuists contend that whatever "weight" a principle might have vis-à-vis competing principles must be determined not in the abstract, but rather in response to the particularities of individual cases.[69] Suppose, for example, that physicians and nurses at a nursing home wish to study the refusal to eat of many elderly patients with Alzheimer's disease. Further suppose that informed consent to participate in the study can-

---

64. Beauchamp and Childress, *The Principles of Biomedical Ethics,* 1st edition (1979), 5.

65. Rawls, 47 (see note 18).

66. Rawls, 20ff, 48–50.

67. The principlists' response to this line of criticism has been to embrace it, over time, with increasing forthrightness and enthusiasm. Although they may have been slower than others to discern the formative and critical roles of case analysis with regard to principles and theories, Beauchamp and Childress (4th ed.) now embrace reflective equilibrium as *the* methodology of principlism, and emphatically denounce deductivism for precisely the same reasons given by their critics. See chapters 1–2 (see note 6).

68. See, e.g., Albert Jonsen and Stephen Toulmin, *The Abuse of Casuistry* (Berkeley: University of California Press, 1988); John D. Arras, "Getting Down to Cases: The Revival of Casuistry in Bioethics," *Journal of Medicine and Philosophy* 16 (1991): 29–51; and Baruch Brody, *Life and Death Decision Making* (New York: Oxford University Press, 1988).

69. Albert Jonsen, "Of Balloons and Bicycles, or the Relationship between Ethical Theory and Practical Judgment," *Hastings Center Report* 21 (1991): 14–16.

not be expected from this impaired patient population. According to the dictates of our paradigm case—e.g., the infamous and lethal experiments of the Nazi doctors—the principle of respect for persons always requires the free and informed consent of the research subject. But according to the casuists, whether the principle of autonomy should prevail over the principle of beneficence in nursing home research—a result that many consider the primary lesson of Nazi research atrocities—will be determined in the context of a nuanced investigation into the "who" (enslaved ethnic populations versus patients with Alzheimer's disease); the "what" (experiments designed to kill versus studying and filming patients' eating behaviors); the "where" (death camps versus a regulated nursing home with a competent research review board); and the "when" (after capture and before execution versus after the consent of family, the loss of decision-making capacity, and the approval and ongoing oversight of an ethics committee). Rather than assigning a timeless relative weight to a certain principle, casuistry holds that the weight lies in the details. In this hypothetical situation, a proposed protocol might be so far removed from our paradigm of unethical research, and the potential benefits to future patients might be so great, that our moral approval may be justified even without the patient's consent.

Presented in this way, the casuistical method obviously has much in common with the method of the common law. Indeed, given the pivotal and ubiquitous role of legal cases in the recent history of bioethics—a history punctuated by such names as Karen Quinlan, Claire Conroy (see Part Two, Section Four), Nancy Cruzan, and Baby M (Part Four, Section Two)—it was entirely natural for bioethicists to begin drawing parallels between case-based reasoning in ethics and in law. In both casuistry and law, we seem to reason from the "bottom up" (from specific cases to fleshed-out principles) rather than from the "top down" (as in most versions of applied ethics); the principles themselves are consequently "open textured," always subject to further revision and specification; and our final judgments usually turn on a fine-grained analysis of the particularities of the case.

To many ethicists, this account of reasoning in both ethics and law accurately describes how we actually think, both in clinical situations and in the classroom; that is, we tend to see cases, which serve as a kind of shorthand, as exemplars for moral analysis and assessment. "This is a Quinlan-type case, except instead of a ventilator the issue is a feeding tube (or antibiotics, or the sustainment of minimal conscious awareness, or a family insisting that everything be done, etc.). How does each different variable alter the case? Is it so different that it should dictate an alternative result?" Instead of ritualistically invoking the mantra of principles, casuistic ethicists thus urge us all to conform our rhetoric to our actual practice.

Just as the casuists insist that the weight of principles resides in the details, they also insist that moral certainty resides in our responses to paradigmatic cases, rather than in abstractions of theory or principle. We are much more confident in our knowledge that torturing and killing Jews to learn about hypothermia is wrong than we are in our assessment of which moral theory or constellation of moral principles best explains why. We would, in fact, be much more likely to switch our allegiance to a different moral theory or set of principles than to change our judgment on what the Nazi doctors did. Indeed, were a moral theory to approve of the Nazis' experiments, we would most likely take that specific judgment as sufficient reason to reject the theory.

Although some extreme casuists reject principles entirely, more moderate versions of casuistry make room for principles, theories, and cultural norms, while still insisting on the priority of the particular. Instead of imposing a false choice between principles and responses to cases, these ethicists envision, in the words of Martha Nussbaum, a "process of loving conversation between rules and concrete responses, general conceptions and unique cases, in which the general articulates the particular and is in turn further articulated by it."[70] Principles play a role, then, but rarely—if ever—as mere axioms from which to deduce moral conclusions. Indeed, whatever validity or usefulness general principles might have depends upon the insight, moral sensitivity, and casuistical

70. Martha Nussbaum, "The Discernment of Perception: An Aristotelian Conception of Private and Public Rationality," in *Love's Knowledge: Essays on Philosophy and Literature* (New York: Oxford University Press, 1990), 95.

skill that mediate their "application" to the particulars of a case.

At this point it should be clear that principlism and the emerging paradigm of casuistry are not necessarily as antithetical as their respective partisans often suggest. On the contrary, chastened principlists who have abandoned deductivism, and moderate casuists who admit a role for principles and general norms, could endorse Martha Nussbaum's dictum with equal enthusiasm; it is, after all, just another way of calling for reflective equilibrium between principles and cases.

According to this emerging consensus, then, moral justification lies not in the correspondence between our moral theories and some sort of moral bedrock, such as nature or God's will; rather, justification resides in the coherence or "fit" among the whole network of our considered judgments and the principles and rules that emanate from them. Insofar as our most confident moral judgments cohere with the system of norms built upon them, they can be considered justified. Contrary to deductivism, moral certainty does not lie in either principles or theory; and contrary to extreme casuistry, certainty does not lie only in our responses to paradigmatic cases. Instead, we believe that any moral certitude lies at the intersection between our abstract norms and our responses to cases.

Judgments that conflict with well-established moral norms, even judgments that might have once seemed unassailable, should be subjected to further scrutiny. Even though it might have once been "plain as day" that African-Americans deserve second-class status or that doctors should never assist patients to commit suicide, the principles of respect for persons or individual autonomy might well prompt us to rethink—and in some cases reject—what was once thought to be our moral bedrock. By the same token, as we have seen, principles develop out of reflection on our considered judgments and acquire their precise meaning and weight within the crucible of contextualized judgments.

It should be noted, however, that even though we speak of reflective "equilibrium" and the "system" of coherent judgments and general norms, the moral life will always be more dynamic and less tidy than these terms imply. The uneasy balance between particular judgments and general norms will most likely never reach equilibrium. Our considered judgments are in a state of constant, if glacially slow, flux, and our concepts, principles, and rules are always merely provisional—always subject to further expansion in scope, specification of meaning, and fluctuation in importance vis-à-vis other general norms. The best we can hope for, then, is a constant striving for greater and greater coherence. Complete coherence—a total seamless system of morality—is most likely beyond our grasp, kept out of reach by both the limitations of our mental capacities and the inherent fragmentation among the values that constitute our complicated moral lives.

PART ONE

FOUNDATIONS OF THE HEALTH PROFESSIONAL–PATIENT RELATIONSHIP

The success of scientific medicine, the growing impersonality of the medical setting, and the rise of consumerism—together with the recent emergence of managed care—have combined to shake the foundations of the traditional doctor-nurse-patient relationship. The burgeoning number of medical mal-practice suits alone provides eloquent testimony of profound changes taking place both in our expectations of medical science and in our awareness of patients' rights. What responsibilities and rights *should* attach to the roles of nurse, doctor, and patient? And how should health professionals think about the inevitable conflicts of duty that arise from the intersection of their specific roles? Part One is devoted to the exploration of these questions. Although clarifying the moral foundations of the health professional–patient relation-ship is an interesting and important task in its own right, the resolution of these basic issues will also shed welcome light on the bioethical problems raised in subsequent parts of the text.

AUTONOMY, PATERNALISM, AND MEDICAL MODELS

How should we think of the bond uniting health care providers and patients? The disparate ways of viewing this relationship emerge from the metaphors used to describe it: parent/child, teacher/student, seller/buyer, priest/peni-tent, oppressor/victim, friends, contractors. Clearly, our choice of an ethical "model" of the provider-patient relationship will profoundly shape both our outlook on medical ethics generally and our views on particular controversies. In order to give content to our deliberations on this important question, we begin Section One with a case study selected to elicit very different responses from the partisans of competing ethical models. In "The Dying Cancer

Patient," Robert Veatch portrays the plight of a 54-year-old woman who has just undergone exploratory surgery to assess a painful mass. The diagnosis is advanced cancer of the cervix; the prognosis is grim. Should she be told the truth about her condition?

If we turn to one of the most venerable sources of medical ethics, the Hippocratic Oath, we find little specific guidance. The Oath is, in fact, entirely silent on the question of truth-telling. The doctor pledges to "apply dietetic measures for the benefit of the sick according to [his] ability and judgment," and he promises to keep patients from "harm and injustice." Although this "moral core" of the Oath admirably commits the physician above all else to the health and well-being of his patients—as opposed, for example, to the advancement of medical science, profits, or cost-containment—it does not say that he must not lie to them. Indeed, the medical tradition based on this Oath has hardly considered lying or shielding the patient from the truth to be a form of "injustice," as the following passage from the "Decorum," another Hippocratic text, strikingly shows: "Perform [these duties] calmly and adroitly, concealing most things from the patient while you are attending to him. Give necessary orders with cheerfulness and serenity, turning his attention away from what is being done to him; sometimes reprove sharply and emphatically, and sometimes comfort with solicitude and attention, revealing nothing of the patient's future or present condition."

Traditionally, physicians have resisted giving a categorical answer to the problem of truth-telling, preferring instead to apply the Hippocratic injunction to "do no harm" on a case-by-case basis. This consequentialist approach is well illustrated in Charles C. Lund's essay, "The Doctor, the Patient, and the Truth." According to Dr. Lund, the physician's duty to tell the truth to the cancer patient in our case study would always be subordinate to (and derivative from) his or her primary duty never to harm the patient. If telling her the truth would predictably depress her or impact adversely upon her care, then the doctor is duty-bound to withhold the truth; conversely, if telling the truth would advance important treatment goals, then she should be told. Within the Hippocratic tradition, then, the dominant value is securing the

health and well-being of the patient, as determined by the physician. Truth, like any other implement in the physician's black bag, should be used sparingly and only to advance therapeutic goals.

Some critics of this paternalistic approach to truth-telling have attempted to refute it on its own terms. Instead of arguing that lying violates a patient's right to be told the truth, a strategy that would eventually have to invoke a full-blown theory of rights, they have tried to refute Dr. Lund's case exclusively on empirical grounds. Thus, whereas Lund assumes that most patients do not want to be told bad news, these critics have countered with studies showing that, in fact, most patients want the unvarnished truth. Contrary to Lund's assumption that physicians are well qualified to assess the risks and benefits of withholding the truth, it has been tellingly argued that doctors rarely possess good evidence for their customary refusal to disclose the truth and that they have no special training to make such difficult value-laden decisions regarding what is really best for patients and their families.

The argument for truth-telling is cogently made by Alan Goldman in "The Refutation of Medical Paternalism." Goldman first points out that doctors and patients do not always share the same values or aim at the same treatment goals. Whereas many physicians tend to regard the extension of life as the predominant value, their patients might well value the quality of future life more than its mere quantity. Secondly, Goldman suggests that even if doctors excelled at making value-laden judgments for their patients, they would still have no right to do so. According to Goldman, the duty to tell the truth is subordinated not to the physician's duty to avoid harm, but rather to the patient's moral and legal rights to self-determination. It stands to reason that, unless the patient has sufficient information upon which to base a judgment, his or her consent will not be informed; and in the absence of informed consent, the patient's self-determination is effectively thwarted. From this perspective, the physician always has a strong duty to be truthful with patients—a duty that is grounded ultimately on the patient's dignity as a choosing being. All the various tried and true forms of deceit—from outright lying, to withholding information, to using medical jargon ("No need to worry; it's just a little carcinoma")—undermine the status of the patient as an autonomous agent. Therefore, according to Goldman and advocates of the contractual model, patients should be told the truth (in most cases) out of respect for them as persons.

Goldman's vindication of patient autonomy against traditional physician paternalism provides a strong foundation for an alternative vision or model of the doctor-patient relationship, one based on the metaphor of a contract or covenant. According to this "contractual model," both the patient and the physician are conceived as responsible moral agents capable of making important decisions that will have bearing on their lives. Contrary to the paternalistic or Hippocratic model, the patient within a "contractual" relationship is charged with making important value-laden decisions that will affect the overall direction of treatment, while the physician is responsible for presenting the available treatment options to the patient and carrying out the details of the agreed-upon plan of care with professional expertise. Importantly, the physician retains his or her moral integrity within the contractual model and is not reduced to the status of a mere "body mechanic" or "engineer" doing the bidding of patients. Since a contractual relationship is a two-way street, the physician may decide to terminate the relationship if, for example, the patient makes unreasonable demands or is flagrantly noncompliant with treatment (Veatch 1972).* This contractual understanding of the physician-patient relationship has proven to be a powerful counterpoint to traditional physician ethics.

Both the paternalistic and contractual models receive closer scrutiny in "Four Models of the Physician-Patient Relationship" by Ezekiel and Linda Emanuel. The Emanuels present a typology of various models of the physician-patient relationship, including (1) the paternalistic model, (2) the informative model, (3) the interpretive model, and (4) the deliberative model. The first is the familiar Hippocratic approach, while the second and third together constitute what others

would call the contractual approach. Their version of the informative model makes a sharp distinction between facts and values, assigning the patient the role of decision maker concerning values, while relegating the physician to the role of providing expert factual information to the patient. Thus, the informative model in the Emanuels' schema tends to reduce the physician to a mere "tool" of the patient's wishes; in this respect it deviates from standard conceptions of the contractual model.

The interpretive model, like the standard contractual approach, lodges final decision-making authority in the patient, but it emphasizes the problematic nature of discovering what the patient's values and preferences really are. Advocates of the contractual model often seem to assume, quite erroneously, that patients always know exactly how they feel and what they want in enormously complex and emotionally trying circumstances. In this interpretive model, by contrast, the doctor's role is analogous to that of a counselor who engages the patient in a mutual effort to understand what the patient's values really are and to discern which medical interventions will best advance those values.

The Emanuels' deliberative model encompasses the information-sharing and interpretive efforts of previous models, but goes one controversial step further in recommending that the patient choose the "best" or "most admirable" course involving health-related values. Here the doctor's role is that of a teacher or moral guide who, though shunning coercive methods, recommends to the patient the medically best choice. For example, instead of simply laying out all the pros and cons of gluttony and smoking, a "deliberative" physician will directly recommend that the patient eat in moderation and stop smoking altogether.

The Emanuels' schema is instructive because it presents a much richer and more complicated picture of patient autonomy than we usually get from overly simplistic juxtapositions of "autonomy versus paternalism." They note that all of the above models, excluding, of course, all frankly coercive approaches, accept some notion of autonomy, ranging from the mere acceptance of the doctor's recommendations to the more robust notion of moral learning and development in the deliberative model. The directive aspect of their favored

*EDITORS' NOTE: See "Recommended Supplementary Reading" at the end of Part One. All subsequent parenthetical references in the Part introductions refer to their respective Recommended Reading lists.

deliberative model, however, remains a point of controversy. Many readers might well wonder how physicians are to distinguish in-practice recommendations based upon "health-related values," which are permitted in this model, from those recommendations based on the physician's personal moral code, which are not permitted.

INFORMED CONSENT

The ethical cornerstone of the contractual and interpretive models is their insistence that the patient should make value-laden decisions bearing on his or her body and future life. The philosophical basis for this position is based on two distinct values: advancement of the patient's well-being and respect for the patient's autonomy. Partisans of the contractual and interpretive models contend that the patient, if adequately informed, is usually the best judge of his or her own best interests and should therefore possess the ultimate decision-making authority. Moreover, as Goldman points out, most of us value the ability to make decisions on our own behalf, quite apart from the consequences.

This ethical ideal of self-determination has received legal sanction in the doctrine of informed consent. As articulated by Justice Cardozo in a justly celebrated formulation in the case of *Schloendorff* v. *Society of New York Hospital* (1914), "Every adult human being of adult years and sound mind has a right to determine what shall be done with his own body. . . ." In order to consent freely, the patient must not be subject to any coercion or undue influence; and in order that the patient's consent be *informed*, the patient must, as we shall see in the readings, receive adequate information on which to base his or her choice. A final threshold condition for informed consent, in the words of Cardozo, is that the patient have a "sound mind" (a requirement that is addressed in Part Two, Section Two).

How much information is required in order to render the patient's consent truly informed? The law's attempt to answer this difficult question can be found in the 1972 California Supreme Court case of *Cobbs* v. *Grant*.

Mr. Cobbs, the plaintiff, had the misfortune of experiencing a number of remote "maloccurrences" incidental to his original surgery for a peptic ulcer. Since none of his physicians had warned him of any of these risks, Mr. Cobbs sued on the ground that his right to informed consent had been violated.

At the time he brought suit, however, the hapless Cobbs had little reason to think that his claim would hold up in court. In determining the scope of a physician's duty to inform patients, most American jurisdictions had adopted a "professional standard" approach that placed lay claimants at a severe disadvantage. Under this rule, a physician's conduct in disclosing information was to be judged by the standards actually observed by members of the local medical community. If it was not common practice to disclose a given risk, then the patient could not recover damages for breach of informed consent. Under this legal doctrine, good medical practice (as defined by the local medical community) made good law.

Cobbs sued nonetheless, arguing that the "professional standard" approach placed too much discretion in the hands of physicians. Happily for Cobbs, he again found himself on the cutting edge, but this time of a revolution in the law of informed consent. His case, *Cobbs* v. *Grant*, along with several others decided in the early 1970s, made the patient's right of self-determination the measure of the doctor's duty to reveal. Doctors were found to have a duty to disclose "all information relevant to a meaningful decisional process." Instead of asking, "What do physicians ordinarily disclose around here?" the *Cobbs* court asked, "What information would a competent patient need to make a reasonable decision?"

In response to those critics who debunk the informed consent requirement as a sheer impossibility, presiding Judge Mosk noted that a "minicourse" in medicine is not required, nor is a useless list of remote minor risks. Simply put, the patient must be told what a reasonable person would need to know about the procedure and its attendant risks in order to make a rational decision on the basis of his or her own values. In a passage strongly influenced by the contractual model, Mosk noted that the physician's expert *medical function* is limited to describing the nature of the procedure and its risks; the actual decision must incorporate those risks, must weigh them against a patient's values, hopes, and fears, and must therefore be left to the patient.

Against this historical background, in Section Two we present two case studies designed both to probe the moral dimensions of informed consent law and to update the legal standard as enunciated in *Cobbs*. In the 1993 legal case *Arato* v. *Avedon*, the plaintiffs attempted to extend the law as articulated in *Cobbs* by charging that physicians had a duty to disclose not merely the risks of a certain medical procedure, but also the statistical likelihood of the patient's survival. Miklos Arato was a successful electrical contractor and real estate developer who was diagnosed at the age of 42 with pancreatic cancer. Acting on the advice of his physicians, Mr. Arato consented to an aggressive experimental course of surgery with combined chemotherapy and radiation. His doctors had informed him of the grave nature of this particular disease; the experimental nature of the treatment, including its risks and benefits; the incurable nature of the illness should it recur after surgery; and the option of doing nothing. However, they did not inform him of the very low statistical probability (approximately 1–5 percent) of patients with his diagnosis living another five years. Unfortunately, Mr. Arato died about one year after his surgery.

Mr. Arato's wife and family sued the physicians on the ground that their failure to reveal such a low statistical probability gave the patient false hopes of survival and prevented him from properly ordering his financial affairs to avoid the failure of his business enterprises. They claimed that, had he been properly informed, Mr. Arato would not have consented to such a rigorous and painful course of experimental treatment and would have had time to put his affairs in order. This lawsuit thus attempted to push the established boundaries of informed consent law in two ways. First, it attempted to expand physicians' duty of disclosure to include relevant prognostic information, preferably in the form of statistical odds of survival; second, it would have expanded the range of information deemed "material" to the patient's decision to include data concerning the relevance of his medical condition to his *nonmedical* interests, including his financial affairs. Although the California Court of Appeal sided with Mr. Arato's family, arguing that his consent was meaningless in the absence of some statistical information on the virulence of his particular cancer, the state

Supreme Court reversed the decision and sided with the jury in refusing to impose these additional informational requirements on physicians. Students should ask themselves as they read this excerpt from the Supreme Court's decision whether this result is consistent with the spirit of an autonomy-inspired legal doctrine of informed consent.

In our second case study, "Antihypertensives and the Risk of Temporary Impotence," John D. Arras shows how difficult problems of information sharing arise not merely in high-profile surgical cases such as *Cobbs* and *Arato,* but also in the course of the undramatic and mundane practice of primary-care medicine. This case asks whether a physician should inform a patient with high blood pressure that a cheap and effective medication also poses a very small risk of inducing temporary impotence, a risk that would be magnified by the very act of informing the patient.

The ethical and legal challenges posed by cases such as these have elicited a wide range of critical responses. Here we present two especially thoughtful but diverging critical responses from Jay Katz and Howard Brody. In his article "Informed Consent—Must It Remain Fairy Tale?" Katz contends that the ethical ideal of self-determination at the core of informed consent has been resisted by medicine and distorted by the law. Contrary to those who view the advent of informed consent as the triumph of patient autonomy over medical paternalism, Katz shows how the framework of malpractice law has systematically betrayed the ethical ideal of self-determination out of deference to medical professionalism. Notwithstanding a brief flirtation with autonomy in cases like *Cobbs*, Katz argues that the law has fallen far short of its promise in reshaping the doctor-patient relationship. At most, he says, the law has created an expanded *duty to warn* rather than a more supportive context for patient decision making.

Although Katz would agree with critics who charge that the law's capacity for fundamental reform of the doctor-patient relationship is quite limited, and that real progress will most likely come (if at all) from a different kind of medical education, he nevertheless claims that the doctrine of informed consent has posed some very powerful and disturbing questions for the medical profession. In particular, he asks doctors to question whether their opposition to informed consent stems not merely from patients' alleged incompetence to handle harsh truths, but also perhaps from their own deep-seated reluctance to admit the widespread existence of medical uncertainty both to their patients and to themselves. For Katz, the ethical ideal of informed consent, as opposed to its legalistic trappings, is an appeal to the medical profession to discover new ways of relating to patients, new modes of communication that might foster hope on the basis of mutual respect rather than deceit.

Two points are particularly noteworthy about Katz's article. First, in stark contrast to courts and physicians, who tend to view informed consent either as a mere recitation of potential risks or, worse yet, as the signing of a form, Katz envisions true informed consent as a kind of searching conversation between patient and physician. Second, as to whether physicians ought to be required to converse with their patients about statistical probabilities, Katz sides with the lower court in *Arato* in holding that physicians should be required to inform patients of their dire prognosis and that patients have a right to make decisions not only about their bodies, but also about their lives.

In "Transparency: Informed Consent in Primary Care," physician-ethicist Howard Brody concurs with Katz that the courts' emphasis on a mere duty to warn patients of possible maloccurrences sends the wrong message to practicing physicians, prompting them only to ask, "Have I *told* the patient of everything that could possibly go wrong?" Moreover, Brody agrees with Katz that the notion of a conversation between doctor and patient nicely captures the ethical essence of the informed consent requirement. Brody worries, however, that this conversational norm is notoriously vague and slippery, thus making it difficult for physicians to determine just when they have properly discharged their legal duty to disclose. Although as an ethical matter it might be clear to a physician when any particular conversation has lasted sufficiently long and covered a sufficient number of topics for a patient to make a responsible decision, as a legal matter, Brody contends, such a subjective standard does not set for physicians a sufficiently determinate standard. So, without abandoning Katz's commitment to conversation, Brody suggests an alternative legal norm

based on the notion of "transparency," which, he claims, should be especially useful in the context of primary-care medicine, the field of Arras' case study. Brody contends that disclosure should be considered adequate when the physician's basic thinking about a decision and recommendation has been made clear or transparent to the patient. Thus, the doctor's duty is not merely to disclose what other reasonable practitioners would disclose, nor what a putative "reasonable patient" would want to know. Instead, the doctor must make her own reasoning clear to the patient, and then invite the patient to ask questions. The physician should facilitate the level of conversational participation desired by the patient. Although Brody's proposal has a number of virtues, including a somewhat more determinate legal standard than the one advocated by Katz, in practice it could conceivably reintroduce medical paternalism through the back door. While it would clearly obligate physicians to reveal the nature, gravity, and likelihood of any risks they considered in making up their own minds about any particular recommendations, Brody's standard could lead some physicians, such as Dr. Black in Arras' case study, to remain silent on aspects of a decision that they might dismiss as insignificant—such as the remote possibility of temporary, reversible impotence—but that any given patient might consider to be very important indeed.

PROFESSIONAL RESPONSIBILITIES: CONFLICTS OF INTEREST IN MANAGED CARE

After making their way through the foregoing controversies, some readers might well be led to conclude that the important issues in bioethics can be discussed without reference to the special functions and roles played by health professionals. Indeed, much of the best bioethical literature seems devoted to establishing the proposition that the doctor's role as healer supplies no special warrant for violating the rights of persons that would normally obtain in other settings. Medical ethics, it is said, is simply a subset of general ethics.

This impression that the roles of health professionals are irrelevant to bioethical disputes is strengthened by exposure to the literature on such subjects as abortion, euthanasia, behavior control, and health care delivery. With rare exceptions, these issues are usually discussed in the language of utility and individual rights—that is, in the language of general ethics. Abstract ethical principles of a quite general nature—such as that persons have a right to be told the truth—are thus applied in a straightforward way to the facts of medical situations. In spite of these appearances, however, such an impression would be seriously mistaken.

Although the Hippocratic tradition would have us believe that the physician's only obligation is to his or her patient, it is a fact of professional life that this duty often conflicts with duties to other parties—such as the patient's family, other patients, other members of the health care team, or persons who might be harmed in some way by the patient. In addition, physicians and other health professionals are increasingly employed by large institutions—such as the armed forces, prisons, insurance companies, and corporations—whose goals have more to do with killing, retribution, and profits than with healing. When health workers act as "double agents" on behalf of both patients and agencies of social control, how should they resolve the inevitable conflicts of loyalty stemming from their conflicting roles? While we might think it appropriate for company physicians to report workers who pose a health hazard to other employees or to the public at large, what are we to think when psychiatrists are required to warn third parties about the violent tendencies of their patients, or when physicians are asked to administer capital punishment by means of lethal injections?

In Section Three, we restrict our attention to some of the most important role conflicts encountered by physicians today, those engendered by the recently emerged phenomenon of "managed care." It is often claimed that managed care threatens to undermine the ethical foundations of the patient-physician relationship and sacrifices the legitimate interests of patients at the altar of cost containment and, worse yet, corporate profits. In order to understand and critically assess these charges, especially as they apply to the physician-patient relationship, we must first lay down an adequate factual basis, determining (a) what exactly constitutes the ethical core of the patient-physician relationship, (b) the basic structures and

varieties of managed care organizations (MCOs), and (c) the respective implications of these structures and types of managed care for the patient-physician relationship.

The traditional doctor-patient relationship has been well described as resting on an ethic of "personal care" (Fried 1974). According to this conception, the patient's vulnerability combines with the doctor's expertise to yield a *fiduciary* relationship; that is, a relationship based not upon mere self-interest but rather on loyalty and concern for those in need. According to this ethic, well articulated by Norman Levinsky in "The Doctor's Master," the physician's primary loyalty is to the individual patient, not to the population at large or to other utilitarian abstractions such as "future patients" or "the future of medical science." When physicians have strayed from this ethic of personal care—as they did in Nazi Germany by forcing Jews and Gypsies to serve as subjects in lethal medical experiments (see Part Five, Section One)—the results have tended to be scandalous and morally disastrous.

Today, serious threats to this ethic of personal care loom on the horizon, and they stem not so much from the errant motives of unethical researchers as from changes in the very organization and financing of health care. Gone are the days of unfettered "fee for service" medicine when doctors would be generously reimbursed for just about any kind of medical care they ordered for patients. While this system encouraged doctors always to do more for their patients, it was also a horribly wasteful and expensive system, full of incentives to overtreat. In its place, we are now witnessing the birth and development of alternative financing arrangements, such as "managed care," in which public and private insurers exercise strict control over doctors' medical choices, and "health maintenance organizations" (HMOs), in which doctors are given incentives to contain costs by the prudent shepherding of medical resources.

In addition to merely saving money, there is an ethical rationale for such efforts at cost containment. As we shall see in Part Six, the demand for universal access to health care, together with the high cost of new medicines and technologies, gives rise to an ethical imperative to control costs. Continued profligate spending on marginal or worthless medical care will seriously undermine efforts to extend needed care to those who cannot presently gain access to it. Doctors must worry, then, not merely about their obligations to patients in their waiting rooms, but also, to some extent, about the effects of their treatment decisions on those who might lack access to health care, now or in the future.

But what exactly is managed care, and how does it impact this ethical core of the patient-physician relationship? It is often said by defenders of managed care that if you've seen one MCO, you've seen one MCO. In other words, managed care organizations do not uniformly exhibit a common set of features; rather, what we call "managed care" actually represents a broad umbrella encompassing a wide variety of methods for delivering health care, a variety of incentives for providers to cut costs and provide quality care, and a variety of relationships between physicians and patients. In spite of this confusing diversity—nicely articulated in Kate T. Christensen's article, "Ethically Important Distinctions Among Managed Care Organizations"—we might still venture an extremely broad and loose definition of managed care as consisting of the following four basic elements: (1) arrangements with selected health care providers, such as a group of physicians, to provide a comprehensive package of benefits to members; (2) the use of explicit standards for the selection and retention of participating physicians; (3) carefully formulated programs for ongoing review of costs and quality of care; and (4) significant financial incentives for consumer-members (formerly called patients) to utilize providers and procedures associated with the plan, coupled with significant incentives for physicians to cut out wasteful and marginally beneficial care (Hoy 1991).

After providing us with a serviceable map of the territory, carefully demarcating the most important varieties of MCOs, their financial structures, and their methods for cost containment, Christensen proceeds to suggest ways in which the traditional values of the patient-physician relationship might best be preserved within the ambit of this new system. She recommends, contrary to existing trends, that MCOs should be nonprofit, that physicians should be salaried instead of tempted by financial incentives to undertreat their patients, and that techniques of cost containment such as "capitation" (the set amount of money per patient paid out by an MCO to physician-

providers to cover all the health care needs of their patients) should focus not on individual physicians, thereby placing them in a direct financial conflict of interest with their patients' well-being, but rather on broad *groups* of physicians, thereby diluting the possibilities for conflicts of interest.

As helpful as Christensen's suggestions may be for the ethical deployment of managed care, they do not altogether resolve the fundamental ethical question formulated by Levinsky: Should doctors attempt to serve two "masters"—their patients and the requirements of cost containment? The existence of financial incentives to contain costs introduces an additional "master," or source of moral tension, for physicians. In addition to their conflicting ethical roles as financial gatekeepers and patient advocates, such incentives tend to involve physicians in potential conflicts of interest between their duties (e.g., to patients) and their own financial well-being. So a further question arises: When, if ever, may physicians allow their financial self-interest to eclipse their duties to patients? Even if we can agree with the macro-level question posed in Sections Two and Three of Part Six on the ethical acceptability of rationing health care, the question remains whether *physicians* ought to be the agents of cost containment, rationing care to patients literally at the bedside.

Suppose, then, that you are a physician confronted by the dilemma sketched in the case study, "The HMO Physician's Duty to Cut Costs." You have concluded that an entirely patient-centered ethic of personal care would dictate prescribing two drugs for your patient, one very cheap and the other very expensive. On the other hand, the HMO's physicians are under constant pressure to rein in costs by prescribing cheaper drugs whenever possible. You think your patient would be better-off with the more expensive drug, but only marginally so. As a physician, you ask, "Is the small extra benefit worth the $400 cost differential per year? Would it be worth, say, an additional $16,000 spread out over the next 40 years?"

According to Norman Levinsky, the doctor can and should serve only one "master," and that is the patient. Others might worry about cost containment and the percentage of the national budget spent on health care, but for Levinsky the doctor's entire loyalty belongs to the individual patient. E. Haavi Morreim, on the other hand, contends that the social and economic system that once supported Levinsky's ideal no longer exists, and that the doctor's traditional aloofness from the grubby realities of cost is no longer a tenable attitude. She argues that "fiscal scarcity"—i.e., the fact that there isn't enough money to pay for everything that medical science might provide for everyone—necessitates serious cost constraints, and that meaningful constraints will require some compromises with patient care at the bedside. Morreim concludes that the moral question for physicians today "is no longer whether to participate in cost containment, . . . but how to do so in morally credible ways."

MANAGED CARE AND INFORMED CONSENT

As Christensen notes in her survey, MCOs use a variety of means to induce physicians to observe the imperative to cut medical costs. As we have just seen, one method is to establish links of varying strength and directness between physicians' financial well-being and their clinical decisions. Another method of saving money is to tightly control the flow of information from MCOs and their physicians to patient-members. This might take place on two different levels. First, MCOs might advertise their services to the general public in a way that falsely emphasizes desirable features, such as personal attention and choice of physicians, while downplaying the often unsavory methods actually used to control costs (e.g., making care more impersonal and routinized, and reducing choice of physicians and access to the services of specialists). Second, MCOs might attempt to limit the amount of information physicians are permitted to disclose to patients as a part of their informed consent conversations. On the one hand, many MCOs have imposed so-called gag rules forbidding physicians from disclosing to patients the ways they control costs in order to maximize savings and/or profits. These rules have proven to be immensely unpopular among physicians, patients, and, most recently, state and federal legislatures, which have moved to ban them by law. A closely related strategy is for MCOs to prohibit physicians from disclosing to patient-members the existence of noncovered services.

Suppose, for example, that a particular patient, a long-time smoker, suffers from terminal emphysema, and that at the rate his disease is progressing, he will die in a matter of months. Suppose further that his managed care physician knows of an experimental treatment, called lung reduction surgery, that might possibly buy her patient several additional years of life with acceptable quality. This treatment, let us suppose, is still in an early investigational stage; its various risks and benefits have not yet been scientifically determined in a trustworthy clinical trial. For this reason, the patient's MCO has decided not to fund any lung reduction surgeries. Suppose further that the physician knows of another reputable hospital across town where a surgical team seems to be achieving significant results through this experimental procedure.

A crucial question arises: What exactly does "informed consent" mean in this situation? Does the physician have a duty to disclose the existence of a possibly beneficial treatment to her patient, even though the MCO has already determined that, for the time being at least, this treatment will not be made available to him within the health plan? Traditionally, physicians have only been held accountable for disclosing the risks and benefits of various potential treatment options. Apart from the option of doing nothing, physicians' traditional duty of information disclosure has thus far centered on what they proposed to do for a patient. In the present case, however, the question is whether the physician has a duty to disclose what neither she nor the MCO is prepared to do for the patient. Does the physician, in short, have a moral and legal duty to inform this patient of what she *won't* be doing for him? That is, does she have a duty to disclose the fact that even though this potentially beneficial, albeit experimental, treatment is unavailable within the plan, it is being performed by others across town and could possibly extend the patient's life?

Section Four begins with an article by law professor Mark A. Hall. In "Informed Consent to Rationing Decisions," Hall contends that, under a certain set of presuppositions, there is no such legal duty. Hall notes that at the time they enroll in a health plan, individuals in effect give a kind of "bundled" consent to have their treatment rationed according to the rules of the plan. Assuming that they have been adequately informed from the start about what the plan will and will not cover, Hall contends that it is neither legally nor ethically necessary to remind them again at the bedside, for example, that "experimental" treatments such as lung reduction surgery will not be covered. It could be said in Hall's defense that requiring physicians to inform patients of expensive treatments that will not be available to them within their plan will only serve to frustrate and anger patients. It is bad enough, one might think, to be denied access; but to have that denial rubbed in one's face can be downright humiliating. (Imagine the worst: "There is indeed a treatment that might save your life, Mr. Jones, but you can't have it because we're trying, you see, to save money.")

Psychiatrist-ethicist Paul S. Appelbaum disagrees with this assessment. In a direct rebuttal to Mark Hall, Appelbaum challenges the assumption that consumer ignorance is a necessary prerequisite of cost containment. He argues, first, that prior disclosure of treatment limits at the time of enrollment in a plan is likely to be poorly understood and immediately forgotten by most patients. Second, he observes that even if a plan intends to deny a certain treatment, the knowledge of that treatment's existence and availability elsewhere could prove highly useful to patients who could, for example, attempt to raise the money separately or lobby their own plan for an exception to the rule or a change of policy. Appelbaum worries that the widespread practice of witholding such information could seriously undermine the traditional ethic of "personal care" and destroy patients' trust in the medical profession. That would indeed be a high price to pay for health care reform. Still, Hall might well wonder what sense it makes for our society to abandon a standard of care based on profligate spending, as we have done through the managed care revolution, while still adhering to a set of informational requirements and consumer expectations based on that abandoned system.

SECTION 1

Autonomy, Paternalism, and Medical Models

The Dying Cancer Patient

Robert M. Veatch

This was the first hospitalization for the 54-year-old patient. She was born in Puerto Rico but had lived in the States for the last ten years. She had come to the emergency room two weeks before with a severe pain and a mass in the right lower quadrant. The previous December the patient had had a severe attack in the same area. Her history revealed that she was past menopause. She had worked in a nursing home and so was familiar with medical procedure. A third-year medical student obtained the pertinent material in her medical history and engaged in a brief conversation with her. The patient explained that she was afraid she had cancer. The student assured her that she would have a complete work-up. She replied in a sad manner that she knew, "If it was cancer, you doctors wouldn't tell me." The student did not comment on this statement but said that the lab tests and examinations would tell them much more about the possible causes of the trouble.

Two days later, after the patient had been examined by the medical students, the resident, the chief resident, and the attending physician, the diagnosis was made of a degenerating fibroid. This diagnosis would explain the severe pain and the mass, although it was pointed out that after menopause the most common cause of a painful mass is cancer.

The patient went to surgery Wednesday morning. The medical student spoke to the resident the same day. He reported that she had stage IV cancer of the cervix, the most advanced stage. They cleaned out all the tumor they could see, but since the tumor had spread to the pelvic wall, all they could now do was to try chemotherapy and radiation. The five-year survival rate of stage IV cancer is 0 to 20 percent.

When the patient awoke from surgery, the medical student's first reaction was to go to her and explain the findings. He felt that he should speak frankly with her, attempt to share the grief, and be there for support. However, since he had not had much experience with cancer and this was the first patient of his "who had been given a death notice," he decided to speak first to the chief resident about how best to approach telling this woman.

The chief resident was sitting in the lounge. The medical student explained that he wanted to tell the patient she had cancer, and that he felt close enough to her to share some of the process. The chief resident's reaction was agitated. "Never use the word 'cancer' with a patient," he said, "because then they give up hope." He suggested using other words or medical jargon.

The student's mind was in a turmoil. He felt that it was important to convey to the patient what he knew himself. According to their best medical understanding of her condition, she had a limited time to live. New biomedical technology and medical discoveries had resulted in several possible treatments, and these would be tried. New discoveries were also being made which might help. But somehow he wanted to convey to her that, knowing what they did, the chances were not good that she would live out her normal life span. In fact, the chances were that she would not survive more than a few years.

The discussion got more heated. The resident angrily asked, "I'd like to know how you'll feel when the patient jumps out the window?" The student's response was that he felt he had to evaluate the patient's desire to know and that this woman had given a clear message that she wished to know.

The resident told the young student a story about the senior attending physician on their service, an internist and an internationally known author of a major medical textbook, who on rounds one day had asked if there was anyone present who would tell the patient they had just seen that he had cancer. When one medical student raised his hand, the internist, who was the awesome patriarch of the medical school, said, "You march down to the Dean's office and tell him that I said you are to be kicked out of medical school." Since an authoritarian and often hostile relation between master and student is not unusual in the clinical teaching setting, the student took him very seriously and turned toward the door. At that point the internist said, "Now you know what it's like to be told you have cancer. Tell a patient that, and it will destroy the last years of his life."

The student left the meeting with the chief resident wondering what should be told to the patient and who should do the telling. He had a good idea what would be said by the senior attending, by the resident, and by himself.[1]

This case raises all of the classical issues in the morality of what the patient should be told. The issues divide into three separate problems of ethics: whether the consequences have been accurately determined (value theory); whether consequences are definitive or moral principles indicate right and wrong in a particular situation independent of consequences (normative ethics); and whether situations should be evaluated individually or general moral rules should apply.

The physician chooses in this case to withhold the terminal cancer diagnosis from the patient because of what he thinks would be the consequences of telling it. Cost-benefit analysis is one of the classical methods for resolving ethical dilemmas and is particularly favored by the physician. The Hippocratic oath pledges the physician to do

that which, according to his judgment and ability, will benefit the patient and protect him from harm. In this case the costs and benefits are clearly not thought of primarily in economic terms. The focus is on the psychological impact of the disclosure of the ultimate bad news. Concern is expressed over the possibility of suicide following the disclosure and more generally over the needless suffering, anxiety, and depression upon learning of her fate.

Yet there are dangers in leaping quickly to the conclusion that these possible consequences imply that the patient should not be told of the diagnosis or even that they create a predisposition not to tell. In ethical theory the position that rightness or wrongness of an action is determined by the consequences, called utilitarianism or consequentialism, is hotly debated, but even if consequences are accepted as the sole determinant, there are reasons to argue for telling the patient of her cancer diagnosis.

Some of those consequences are apparent to the medical student and probably even to the chief resident who is so vehemently opposed to the disclosure. The uncertainty of not knowing can produce anxiety. With knowledge, financial budgeting can take place more accurately. Two other problems derive from depending on the medical professional's calculation of the consequences. First, he may not have included some values that are important to the patient. This woman may have grandchildren in Puerto Rico whom she would want to see more than anything in the world before she dies. She may value conversation with her priest or the Catholic last rite. Some patients may value human freedom and self-determination very highly. The consequences to the patient of being told or not being told can be accurately determined only if the proper values are included in the calculation and if they are given the proper weighting.

The second problem is that even if the proper values have been included, there may be differences between the physician and the patient which lead to serious errors in calculating the consequences. Suppose both patient and physician agree that psychological consequences are crucial and that serious anxiety and mental suffering are to be avoided. Suppose also, however, that the thought of death produces high anxiety in the mind of the physician, whereas the patient can handle the thought with comparatively little psychological trauma. Some patients reportedly are able to adjust to the thought of their own death because of particular religious convictions, because they have worked through their feelings, or because they can come to grips with the psychological impact rapidly once given the news. In fact, one psychological study of physicians suggests they have a uniquely high anxiety when confronted with the subject of death.[2] If this is so, then one can anticipate systematic errors in estimating the psychological harm done by telling the patient of the fatal diagnosis. The same would be true in the opposite case, if the physician is eager to tell while the patient shows a uniquely high anxiety on the subject of death.

Even if the physician uses the same values as the patient, weighs them properly, and quantifies the benefit or harm in the correct way, there still are moral problems in deciding whether to tell something to the patient on the basis of estimating the consequences. The patient may make moral judgments using considerations other than consequences.

Many systems of ethical reasoning emphasize factors other than the consequences in deciding which actions are right and which are wrong. In fact, the utilitarian or consequentialist position has been treated rather harshly in discussions of normative philosophical theory.[3] Those who are not satisfied with the utilitarian position claim that there are right-making characteristics inherent in actions independent of their consequences. Holders of this position, called the formalist or deontological position, claim that the utilitarians cannot adequately account for intuitive moral judgments and that honesty, promise-keeping, justice, and similar characteristics are important even if they do not necessarily lead to the best consequences. One need not be personally convinced of the formalist position to recognize the problems it raises for the decision about whether to tell the dying cancer patient of the diagnosis. One need only recognize the undisputable fact that some patients do hold such a position. Certain sophisticated forms of the formalist position do not deny the importance of consequences but claim that there are other important considerations as well.

Kant was a representative of the formalist tradition. On the subject of truth-telling he argued:

> The duty of being truthful . . . is unconditional. . . . Although in telling a certain lie I do not actually do anyone a wrong, I formally but not materially violate the principle of right. . . . To be truthful (honest) in all declarations, therefore, is a sacred and absolutely commanding decree of reason, limited by no expediency.
>
> Thus, the definition of a lie as merely an intentional untruthful declaration to another person does not require the additional condition that it must harm another. . . . For a lie always harms another; if not some other particular man, still it harms mankind generally, for it vitiates the source of law itself.[4]

Kant may have stated the matter more strongly than the typical twentieth-century patient, but it seems clear that some of those patients give importance to truth-telling independent of or in addition to the consequences. For those patients, the argument that the deception is justified by the harmful consequences of the disclosure is not necessarily sufficient.

Some who feel that withholding of information is the right course may reply that withholding the information is not the same as lying. They grant the duty to tell the truth, but not the duty to tell the whole truth. The distinction is between actions and omissions, and it is one that troubles medical ethics at many points, not only in comparing lying with withholding information but also in comparing the killing of a dying patient with not starting a respirator or abandoning a patient with failing to take him on in the first place.

Whether the distinction is valid is debatable. But even if one concludes that it is valid, the issue is not resolved. The question is still open whether inherently it is morally acceptable to withhold information which is potentially meaningful to a patient even if that action is different from lying. The formalist may well take the position that in addition to the moral duty to avoid lying, there is another moral duty to disclose information which is potentially meaningful when one is in a position to do so conveniently.

The duty to disclose information that is potentially meaningful is not the only formalist or nonconsequentialist factor in deciding whether the woman should be told about her diagnosis. Some would hold that the patient has the right and the duty to give informed consent for medical treatment, and that right and duty exist independent of the consequences of giving that consent. Not only may failure to disclose the diagnosis make it difficult to get patient cooperation in therapy, but continued treatment of the patient may also violate the requirements of reasonably informed consent and thus be assault and battery.

The conclusion seems clear, that one reason the issue of what to tell a dying patient is so controversial is that different people in the debate have widely differing ethical norms which they bring to bear on the decision. If one person has the objective of doing what will have the best consequences and another has the objective of disclosing potentially meaningful information or of obtaining informed consent or of protecting patient dignity, the moral conclusions may be quite different, even if the two can agree on what values are important and what the consequences will be.

The third major issue in ethics raised by this case is the conflict between those who insist that moral rules must be followed in specific cases and those who argue that each situation, each case, is unique and must be evaluated anew. The formalists are often accused of being legalistic, of insisting on the rules of truth-telling or promise-keeping or consent-getting. But the rules-situation debate is really independent of the utilitarian-formalist debate. It is quite possible to argue that a rule to tell the truth should be followed even if in a particular case it appears that the consequences would be better if the rule were not followed, and to argue this on the grounds that following the rule will produce the best consequences in the long run. It is also possible, even for the formalist, to argue that on the question of what to tell the patient every case must be treated as a unique entity in which no general rules can be followed. In every case the situation would therefore have to be examined to determine what formal right-making characteristics are present and how they can be balanced, independent of the consequences or with the consequences being only one consideration.

The case of the woman who has cancer and does not yet know it is a good case to test the value of the rule. The evidence from surveys indicates that the overwhelming percentage of physicians would tend not to tell patients of a cancer diagnosis.

According to Donald Oken, the figure is 88 percent.[5] In contrast, an overwhelming percentage of laypeople, between 82 and 98 percent, say they would like to be told of such a diagnosis.[6] Of course, some might argue that they say they want to be told when they really do not want to, but such judgment requires a paternalistic second-guessing of the layperson's judgment, which has moral implications of its own. In any case it would appear that the gap in judgment between the professional and the layperson is extremely great. If every physician considered each case as a special situation and did what he thought best, then it seems very likely that in many cases he would make a judgment in which the layperson would not concur. He may do so because he is a consequentialist while his patient is a formalist; he may do so because he is considering some consequences while his patient would have considered others; or he may do so because he evaluates some consequences, such as anxiety in the face of death, as much more serious than his patient would. There are good and predictable reasons why the problem of the medical student and his mentors about what to tell the woman with cancer creates heated ethical disputes in the hospital as well as in the classroom.

One kind of difference in the consequences considered is between those that are long-range and those that are short-range. When the woman with cancer says, "if it was cancer, you doctors wouldn't tell me," she is making a statement based on prior experience or beliefs. If many years ago her dying mother was not told of a cancer, she may have learned that in some cases the physician will not disclose the true diagnosis and prognosis to the patient. It is unlikely that the physician caring for her mother would have included in his calculation of consequences the impact on this patient who is now in the miserable condition of not being able to depend on the word of the medical profession. It may be that some people, including physicians, are uniquely committed to considering short-range consequences. If the physician's duty is to his patient and not to others, it might even be considered immoral to include such consequences. On the contrary, the classical utilitarian may

*EDITORS' NOTE: The study Veach refers to was published in 1961 and is thus outdated.

well be very interested in such long-term consequences.

NOTES

1. Based on a case provided by Keith Sedlacek, M.D.
2. Herman Feifel et al., "Physicians Consider Death," *Proceedings, American Psychological Association*, 1967, pp. 201–202.
3. For this classical ethical debate, see Richard B. Brandt, *Ethical Theory: The Problems of Normative and Critical Ethics* (Englewood Cliffs, N.J.: Prentice-Hall, 1959), pp. 380–432; William Frankena, *Ethics* (Englewood Cliffs, N.J.: Prentice-Hall, 1963), pp. 11–46. For utilitarian ethics, see David Lyons, *Forms and Limits of Utilitarianism* (Oxford: Oxford University Press, 1965; W. D. Ross, *The Right and the Good* (Oxford: Oxford University Press, 1939).
4. Immanuel Kant, "On the Supposed Right to Tell Lies from Benevolent Motives," in *Kant's Critique of Practical Reason and Other Works on the Theory of Ethics*, trans. Thomas Kingsmill Abbott (London: Longmans, 1909), pp. 361–365.
5. Donald Oken, "What to Tell Cancer Patients," *Journal of the American Medical Association* 175 (Apr. 1, 1961): 1120–1128.
6. W. D. Kelly and S. R. Friesen, "Do Cancer Patients Want to Be Told?" *Surgery* 27 (June 1950): 822–826.

The Hippocratic Oath

I swear by Apollo Physician and Asclepius and Hygieia and Panaceia and all the gods and goddesses, making them my witness, that I will fulfil according to my ability and judgment this oath and this covenant:

To hold him who has taught me this art as equal to my parents and to live my life in partnership with him, and if he is in need of money to give him a share of mine, and to regard his offspring as equal to my brothers in male lineage and to teach them this art—if they desire to learn it—without fee and covenant; to give a share of precepts and oral instruction and all the other learning to my sons and to the sons of him who has instructed me and to pupils who have signed the covenant and have taken an oath according to the medical law, but to no one else.

I will apply dietetic measures for the benefit of the sick according to my ability and judgment; I will keep them from harm and injustice.

I will neither give a deadly drug to anybody if asked for it, nor will I make a suggestion to this effect. Similarly I will not give to a woman an abortive remedy. In purity and holiness I will guard my life and my art.

I will not use the knife, not even on sufferers from stone, but will withdraw in favor of such men as are engaged in this work.

Whatever houses I may visit, I will come for the benefit of the sick, remaining free of all intentional injustice, of all mischief and in particular of sexual relations with both female and male persons, be they free or slaves.

What I may see or hear in the course of the treatment or even outside of the treatment in regard to the life of men, which on no account one must spread abroad, I will keep to myself holding such things shameful to be spoken about.

If I fulfil this oath and do not violate it, may it be granted to me to enjoy life and art, being honored with fame among all men for all time to come; if I transgress it and swear falsely, may the opposite of all this be my lot.

From Ludwig Edelstein, *Ancient Medicine: Selected Papers of Ludwig Edelstein*. Owsei Temkin and C. Lillian Temkin, eds., Baltimore, MD: Johns Hopkins University Press, 1967.

The Doctor, the Patient, and the Truth*

Charles C. Lund

When Pilate asked Jesus, "What is the truth?", He did not answer. After a doctor has completed a careful examination he will frequently be in possession of information about a patient that will indicate to him quite definitely that the patient is suffering from a serious disease which is in a probably or possibly curable condition if a certain course of treatment or of surgery is carried out promptly. Should he then and there tell the patient "the truth, the whole truth, and nothing but the truth" and then ask the patient to let him arrange for the treatment? Is it *possible* to convey the "truth" about a serious matter to a patient? Henderson has discussed this subject in an article that should be read by every one interested, and gives the following example:

> Consider the statement, "This is a carcinoma." . . . Let us assume . . . that the statement has nearly the same validity as the assertions in the nautical almanac. If we now look at things not from the standpoint of philosophers, moralists or lawyers, but from the standpoint of biologists, we may regard the statement as a stimulus applied to the patient. This stimulus will produce a response and the response, together with the mechanism that is involved in its production, is an extremely complex one, at least in those cases where a not too vague cognition of the meaning of the four words is involved in the process. . . . With the cognition there is a correlated fear. There will be a concern for the economic interests of others for example, of wife and children. I suggest, in view of these obvious facts, that if you recognize the duty of telling the truth to the patient, you range yourself outside the class of biologists, with lawyers and philosophers. The idea that the truth, the whole truth,

and nothing but the truth can be conveyed to the patient is an example of false abstraction, of that fallacy called by Whitehead, "The fallacy of misplaced concreteness." It results from neglecting factors that cannot be excluded from the concrete situation and that have an effect that cannot be neglected. Another fallacy also is involved, the belief that it is not too difficult to know the truth; but of this I will not speak further.

I beg that you will not suppose that I am recommending, for this reason, that you should always lie to your patients. Such a conclusion from what I have said would correspond roughly to a class of fallacies that I have already referred to above. Since telling the truth is impossible, there can be no sharp distinction between what is true and what is false. But surely that does not relieve the physician of his moral responsibility. On the contrary the difficulties that arise from the immense complexity of the phenomena do not diminish, but rather increase, the moral responsibility of the physician, and one of my objects has been to describe the facts through which the nature of that moral responsibility is determined.

Far older than the precept, "the truth, the whole truth, and nothing but the truth," is another that originates within our profession, that has always been the guide of the best physicians, and, if I may venture a prophecy, will always remain so: So far as possible, "Do no harm." You can do harm by the process that is quaintly called telling the truth. You can do harm by lying. In your relations with your patients you will inevitably do much harm, and this will be by no means confined to your strictly medical blunders. It will also arise from what you say and what you fail to say. But try to do as little harm as possible, not only in treatment with drugs, or with the knife, but also in treatment with words, with the expression of your sentiments and emotions. Try at all times to act upon the patient so as to modify his sentiments to his own advantage, and remember that, to this end, nothing is more effective than arousing in him the belief that you are concerned wholeheartedly and exclusively for his welfare.

From Charles C. Lund, "The Doctor, the Patient, and the Truth," *Annals of Internal Medicine* 1946; 24:955–959. Used with permission of the publisher.

*Editors' Note: Author's notes have been deleted. Students who wish to follow up on sources should consult the original article.

In any group of patients with identical surgical or medical conditions there will be a very wide variation in their mental states, physical states, social circumstances, and in the amount of information or misinformation concerning disease in their possession. Let us assume that a group of patients has gone to a man who is their final authority because they believe him to be an expert in the care of such cases. The doctor considers himself equipped by knowledge and training to assume this responsibility. All examinations have been completed and the doctor knows that the patients have carcinoma of the breast. If he operates on them there is essentially no danger of immediate death and after operation, according to known average results in cases at this particular stage of the disease, one half the group will survive five years without recurrence of the disease. But he does not know at this time and has no further tests to use to differentiate the potentially cured patients from the potential failures. Also let us assume that if operation is not done promptly but is done later, the chance of cure declines progressively. Also that treatment by other means, such as radiation, would result in only one cure out of the group and again that there is no way to predict which case would receive this fortunate result. Also let us assume that all patients want very earnestly to live but that all of them would prefer to have any reasonable treatment short of surgery. It is clear that in these situations the most important accomplishment for the benefit of the patients is to secure their prompt consent to operations.

Now suppose a blunt doctor starts his conversations with the statement, "This is a cancer," and follows up by outlining all the facts in the assumptions given above. This statement will be given a very different interpretation by each of 10 different patients and none of them will interpret from it exactly what is going on in the doctor's mind. Many will interpret "cancer" as identical in meaning with "hopeless cancer." Perhaps eight of the patients might consent to proper operations but of these half might never forgive the doctor for his brutality. One of the remaining two might be among the number of people who believe erroneously that cancer is never cured and therefore decide to have no treatment. The other might be so upset mentally that she leaves the doctor and goes to a charlatan in whose hands all hope of cure will be lost.

On the other hand, suppose the doctor avoids the word cancer and minimizes the seriousness of the situation. Again eight patients consent. However, of these eight the one who recurred the earliest will blame the doctor by stating that the operation was not worth while and if she had known how serious the condition was she would not have consented. The other two refuse operation by telling the doctor they need time to make arrangements but in reality because they have not taken in the urgency of the situation, and as a result they delay so long they lose their chance of cure.

It is seen then that blunt "truth" is not good and that avoidance of truth may be as bad. How then should the doctor proceed with such an interview with some hope of doing no harm or at least of doing less harm to his patients?

Certainly at the start of the interview he should avoid the words carcinoma or cancer. He should use cyst, nodule, tumor, lesion, or some other loosely descriptive word that has not so many frightening connotations. He should then suggest that operation is indicated and give some rough idea of the extent of the operation. If consent is given at this stage, this is enough. But he should inform the most interested relative that there is only a 50 per cent chance of a successful outcome. Again, however, two patients in the group that are handled in this way are also resistive to the idea of operation. Now, however, no bridges have been crossed and many resources are still open to the doctor to secure consent for proper treatment. In one case the matter may be presented to the family and the family doctor who can take over at this point and who can frequently present the situation in such a light that the patient will consent. The other patient, however, is in a situation not infrequently encountered and has no family or family doctor who can be asked to assist. For instance, a patient who has warned you in advance that she does not want her husband to be told anything because he is not well himself. In this situation, it seems clear that the doctor can only fully meet his obligations to the patient if she makes her final decision after being put in possession of as close approximation to the truth as can fairly be conveyed to her. One should, at least, state that the lesion is in imminent danger of becoming a cancer and that a good chance of cure still remains if action is immediate. If the patient asks directly, "Is this cancer?" the doctor is forced to answer, "Yes," but can always go on to explain in the same sentence, "but it probably is not as serious as you fear because you have a good chance of cure." In this way he can reduce greatly the shock that always is associated with the bald assertion.

After operation, the first things many patients want to know are what was found, what was done, and what is the expected result? What should the doctor tell the patient at this time? When the patient is still under the influence of opiates or sedatives, he must be told nothing because of great danger that the simplest statement will be misunderstood. Later, however, at a more opportune time, the doctor must be frank. In spite of the frequent requests by relatives not to do so, the patient should almost always be told exactly what was found at operation and exactly what was done. Harsh words and bald facts should be tempered to a reasonable degree. If the outlook is probably but not surely favorable, this statement must be made so that the patient will coöperate properly in follow up examinations or treatments necessary to prompt recognition and care of any sequelae. If the outlook is thoroughly bad and the doctor is quite sure the patient will die shortly, what should he do? Of course, tell the responsible relative at once. His procedure with regard to the patient must vary with different patients. Usually the variations in procedure should be according to the patient's expressed desires. Almost always it does more good than harm to tell the patient who is in a hopeless situation the truth about his prospects. This must always be done gently, and perhaps, indirectly. A question as to whether the patient would like to see his clergyman or to make his will would mean much to some patients. Following such a suggestion the patient will often ask a direct question and should be given a direct answer. It was the author's duty as an intern to break the news to an old man from another state that the surgeons could do nothing further for his bladder carcinoma and that he might go home. While I was "beating around the bush" in a clumsy way, the man understood what was meant and said "You should not be afraid to tell me that I am going to die. I thought I was, but came down here to make sure. I will go home perfectly happy."

One reason it usually does good to patients to tell them their outlook is hopeless is that dying patients usually have a fairly good insight into their condition and the shock of confirming this belief is not great. Another reason is that they can relax and stop struggling to do all the things they have previously been doing to try to get well and to keep up their own or their family's morale. On the other hand, there are unusual patients suffering from fatal illnesses who ask the doctor not to tell them anything. Such a request is in quite a different category from a request of the relatives. Usually it means that they have decided themselves that the situation is hopeless but they cannot bear to be told about it. If this is true, and if the patient is allowing all measures important to her comfort to be carried out, everything is to be gained by acceding to her request. Such a patient frequently shows great courage in facing the unpleasant facts of her disease during the process of dying.

SUMMARY

The doctor is bound in his duty to his patient to do whatever is best for his patient and to avoid doing him harm.

In discussing his patient's condition, the doctor realizes that there are some circumstances when he cannot, for the patient's own good, tell him the "whole truth."

However, there are other frequent circumstances in which friends and relatives want the "whole truth" (unpleasant) kept from the patient when it is much better for the patient for the doctor to be quite frank.

The Refutation of Medical Paternalism

Alan Goldman

In the case of doctors the question is whether they have the authority to make decisions for others that they would lack as nonprofessionals. The goal of providing optimal health treatment may be seen to conflict in some circumstances with the otherwise overriding duties to tell the patient the truth about his condition or to allow him to make decisions vitally affecting his own interests. Again the assumption of the profession itself appears to be that the doctor's role is strongly differentiated in this sense. The Principles of Medical Ethics of the American Medical Association leaves the question of informing the patient of his own condition up to the professional judgment of the physician, presumably in relation to the objective of maintaining or improving the health or well-being of the patient.[1] I shall concentrate upon these issues of truth telling and informed consent to treatment in the remainder of this chapter. They exemplify our fundamental issue because the initially obvious answer to the question of who should make decisions or have access to information vital to the interests of primarily one person is that person himself.[2]

Rights are recognized, we have said, partially to permit individuals control over their own futures. Regarding decisions vital to the interests of only particular individuals, there are three main reasons why such decisions should normally be left to the individuals themselves, two want-regarding and one ideal-regarding. First is the presumption of their being the best judges of their own interests, which may depend upon personal value orderings known only to them. There is often a temptation for others to impose their own values and preferences, but this would be less likely to produce satisfaction for the individuals concerned.

The second reason is the independent value of self-determination, at least in regard to important decisions (in medical contexts decisions may involve life and death alternatives, affect the completion of major life projects, or affect bodily integrity). Persons desire the right or freedom to make their own choices, and satisfaction of this desire is important in itself. In addition, maximal freedom for individuals to develop their own projects, to make the pivotal choices that define them and to act to realize them, allows for the development of unique creative personalities, who become sources of new value in the goods they create and that they and others enjoy.

Resentment as well as overall harm is therefore generally greater when caused by a wrong, even if well-meaning, decision of another than when caused to oneself. There is greater chance that the other person will fail to realize one's own values in making the decision, and, when this happens, additional resentment that one was not permitted the freedom to decide. Thus, since individuals normally have rights to make decisions affecting the course of their lives and their lives alone, doctors who claim authority to make medical decisions for them that fall into this self-regarding category are claiming special authority. The normally existing right to self-determination implies several more specific rights in the medical context. These include the right to be told the truth about one's condition, and the right to accept or refuse or withdraw from treatment on the basis of adequate information regarding alternatives, risks and uncertainties. If doctors are permitted or required by the principle of providing optimal treatment, cure or health maintenance for patients sometimes to withhold truth or decide on their own what therapeutic measures to employ, then the Hippocratic principle overrides important rights to self-determination that would otherwise obtain, and the practice of medicine is strongly role differentiated.

This is clear enough in the case of informed consent to therapy; it should be equally clear in the

From *The Moral Foundations of Professional Ethics* by Alan Goldman, Rowman and Littlefield, 1980. Reprinted by permission of the publisher.

EDITORS' NOTE: Sections of this essay have been omitted, and the notes have been renumbered.

case of withholding truth, from terminally ill patients for example. The right violated or overridden when truth is withheld in medical contexts is not some claim to the truth per se, but this same right to self-determination, to control over decisions vital to the course of one's life. In fact, it seems on the face of it that there is a continuum of medical issues in which this right figures prominently. These range from the question of consent to being used as a subject in an experiment designed primarily to benefit others, to consent to treatment intended as benefit to the patient himself, to disclosure of information about the patient's condition. In the first case, that of medical experimentation, if the consent of subjects is required (as everyone these days admits it is), this is partly because the duty not to harm is stronger than the duty to provide benefits. Hence if there is any risk of harm at all to subjects, they cannot be used without consent, even if potential benefits to others is great. But consent is required also because the right to self-determination figures independently of calculations of harms and benefits. Thus a person normally ought not to be used without his consent to benefit others even if he is not materially harmed. This same right clearly opposes administration of treatment to patients without their consent for their own benefit. It opposes as well lying to patients about their illnesses in order to save them distress.

What is at least prima facie wrong with lying in such cases is that it shifts power to decide future courses of action away from the person to whom the lie is told.[3] A person who is misinformed about his own physical condition may not complete certain projects or perform certain actions that he would choose to perform in full knowledge. If a person is terminally ill and does not know it, for example, he may fail to arrange his affairs, prepare himself for death, or may miss opportunities to complete projects or seek certain experiences always put off before. Being lied to can reduce or prevent from coming into view options that would otherwise be live. Hence it is analogous to the use of force, perhaps more coercive than the use of force in that there is not the same chance to resist when the barrier is ignorance. The right to know the truth in this context then derives from the right to make for oneself important decisions relating primarily to one's own welfare and to the course

of one's life. If the doctor's authority is to be augmented beyond that of any nonprofessional, allowing him to override these important rights in contexts in which this is necessary to prevent serious harm to the patient's health, then his position appears to meet in a dramatic way our criteria for strong role differentiation.

THE CASE FOR MEDICAL PATERNALISM

Since the primary rights in potential conflict with the presumed fundamental norm of medical ethics are rights of patients themselves, and since the norm seeks to serve the health needs of patients themselves, arguments in favor of strong role differentiation in this context are clearly paternalistic. We may define paternalism as the overriding or restricting of rights or freedoms of individuals for their own good. It can be justified even for competent adults in contexts in which they can be assumed to act otherwise against their own interests, values, or true preferences. Individuals might act in such self-defeating ways from ignorance of the consequences of their actions, from failure to weigh the probabilities of various consequences correctly, or from irrational barriers to the operation of normal short-term motivations. Paternalistic measures may be invoked when either the individual in question, or any rational person with adequate knowledge of the situation, would choose a certain course of conduct, and yet this course is not taken by the individual solely because of ignorance, carelessness, fear, depression, or other uncontroversially irrational motives.[4]

PARADIGM CASES

It will be useful in evaluating arguments for strong role differentiation for doctors to look first at criteria for justified paternalism in nonmedical cases, in order to see then if they are met in the medical context. In approaching the controversial case of withholding truth from patients, we may begin with simpler paradigm cases in which paternalistic behavior is uncontroversially permissible or required. We can derive a rule from these cases for the justification of such conduct and then apply the rule to decide this fundamental question of medical ethics.

The easiest cases to justify are those in which a person is acting against even his immediate desires out of ignorance: Dick desires to take a train to New York, is about to board the train for Boston on the other side of the platform, and, without time to warn him, he can only be grabbed and shoved in the other direction. Coercing him in this way is paternalistic, since it overrides his right of free movement for his own good. "His own good" is uncontroversial in interpretation in this easiest case. It is defined by his own clearly stated immediate and long-range preferences (the two are not in conflict here). Somewhat more difficult are cases in which persons voluntarily act in ways inconsistent with their long-range preferences: Jane does not desire to be seriously injured or to increase greatly her chances of serious injury for trivial reasons; yet, out of carelessness, or just because she considers it a nuisance and fails to apply statistical probabilities to her own case, she does not wear a helmet when riding a motorcycle. Here it might be claimed that, while her action is voluntary in relation to trivial short-term desires, it is nevertheless not fully voluntary in a deeper sense. But to make this claim we must be certain of the person's long-range preferences, of the fact that her action is inconsistent with these preferences (or else uncontroversially inconsistent with the preferences of any rational person). We must predict that the person herself is likely to be grateful in the long run for the additional coercive motivation. In this example we may assume these criteria to be met. For rational people, not wearing a helmet is not an essential feature in the enjoyment of riding a motorcycle, even if people ride them primarily for the thrill rather than for the transportation. The chances are far greater that a rider will at some time fall or be knocked off the cycle and be thankful for having a helmet than that one will prefer serious head injury to the inconvenience of wearing protection that can prevent such injury. Therefore we may justifiably assume that a person not wearing a helmet is not acting in light of her own true long-range values and preferences.

As the claim that the individual's action is not truly voluntary or consistent with his preferences or values becomes more controversial, additional criteria for justified paternalism must come into play. They become necessary to outweigh the two considerations mentioned earlier: the presumption that individuals know their own preferences best (that interference will be more often mistaken than not), and that there is an important independent value to self-determination or individual freedom and control (the latter being true both because persons value freedom and because such freedom is necessary to the development of genuinely individual persons). The additional criteria necessary for justifying paternalism in more controversial cases relate to the potential harm to the person from the action in question: it must be relatively certain, severe, and irreversible (relative to the degree of coercion contemplated). These further criteria are satisfied as well in the case of motorcycle helmets, because the action coerced is only a minor nuisance in comparison to the severity of potential harm and the degree of risk.

It is important for the course of the later argument to point out that these additional criteria relating to the harm that may result from self-regarding actions need not be viewed in terms of a simple opposition between allowing freedom of action and preventing harm. It is not simply that we can override a person's autonomy when in our opinion the potential harm to him from allowing autonomous decision outweighs the value of his freedom. His right to self-determination, fundamental to individuality itself, bars such offsetting calculations. The magnitude of harm is rather to be conceived as *evidence* that the person is not acting in accord with *his own* values and preferences, that he is not acting autonomously in the deepest sense. A rights-based moral theory of the type I am assuming as the framework for this study will view the autonomy of the individual as more fundamental than the particular goods he enjoys or harms he may suffer. The autonomous individual is the source of value for those other goods he enjoys and so not to be sacrificed for the sake of them. The point here is that cases of justified paternalism, even where the agent's immediate or short-term preferences are overridden, need not be viewed as reversing that order of priority.

Criteria for justified paternalism are also clearly satisfied in certain medical contexts, to return to the immediate issue at hand. State control over physician licensing and the requirement that prescriptions be obtained for many kinds of drugs are medical cases in point. Licensing physicians prevents some quacks from harming other persons, but also limits these persons' freedom of choice for their own good. Hence it is paternalistic. We may assume that no rational person would want to be treated by a quack or to take drugs that are merely harmful, but that many people would do so in the absence of controls out of ignorance or irrational hopes or fears. While controls impose costs and bother upon people that may be considerable in the case of having to see a doctor to obtain medication, these are relatively minimal in comparison to the certainty, severity and irreversibility of the harm that would result from drugs chosen by laymen without medical assistance. Such controls are therefore justified, despite the fact that in some cases persons might benefit from seeing those who could not obtain licenses or from choosing drugs themselves. We can assume that without controls mistakes would be made more often than not, that serious harm would almost certainly result, and that people really desire to avoid such harm even given additional costs.

There is another sense too in which paternalistic measures here should not be viewed as prevention of exclusively self-regarding harm by restriction of truly autonomous actions. The harm against which laymen are to be protected in these cases, while deriving partly from their own actions in choosing physicians or drugs, can be seen also as imposed by others in the absence of controls. It results from the deception practiced by unqualified physicians and unscrupulous drug manufacturers. Hence controls, rather than interfering with autonomous choice by laymen, help to prevent deceptive acts of others that block truly free choice.[5] This is not to say that some drugs now requiring prescriptions could not be safely sold over the counter at reduced cost, or that doctors have not abused their effective control over entrance to the profession by restraining supply in relation to demand, maintaining support for exorbitant prices. Perhaps controls could be imposed in some other way than by licensing under professional supervision. This issue is beyond our scope here. The point for us is that some such restraints appear to be necessary. Whichever form they take, they will be paternalistic, justifiably so, in their relation to free patient choice.

We have now defined criteria for justified paternalism from considering certain relatively easy examples or paradigm cases. The principal criterion is that an individual be acting against *his own*

predominant long-range value preferences, or that a strong likelihood exist that he will so act if not prevented. Where either clause is controversial, we judge their truth by the likelihood and seriousness of the harm to the person risked by his probable action. It must be the case that this harm would be judged clearly worse from the point of view of the person himself than not being able to do what we prevent him from doing by interfering. Only if the interference is in accord with the person's real desires in this way is it justified. Our question now is whether these criteria are met in the more controversial medical cases we are considering, those of doctors' withholding truth or deciding upon courses of treatment on their own to prevent serious harm to the health of their patients.

APPLICATION OF THE CRITERIA TO MEDICAL PRACTICE

The argument that the criteria for justified paternalism are satisfied in these more controversial medical cases begins from the premise that the doctor is more likely to know the course of treatment optimal for improving overall health or prolonging life than is his patient. The patient will be comparatively ignorant of his present condition, alternative treatments, and risks, even when the doctor makes a reasonable attempt to educate him on these matters. More important, he is apt to be emotional and fearful, inclined to hold out false hope for less painful treatments with little real chance of cure, or to despair of the chance for cure when that might still be real. In such situations it again could be claimed, as in the examples from the previous subsection, that patient choice in any event would not be truly voluntary. A person is likely to act according to his true long-range values only when his decision is calm, unpressured, and informed or knowledgeable. A seriously ill person is unlikely to satisfy these conditions for free choice. Choice unhindered by others is nevertheless not truly free when determined by internal factors, among them fear, ignorance, or other irrational motivation, which result in choice at variance with the individual's deeper preferences. In such circumstances interference is not to be criticized as restrictive of freedom.

The second premise states that those who consult doctors really desire to be cured above all else.

Health and the prolonging of life may be assumed (according to this argument) to have priority among values for any rational person, since they are necessary conditions for the realization of almost every other personal value. While such universally necessary means ought to have priority in personal value orderings, persons may again fail to act on such orderings out of despair or false hope, or simply lack of knowledge, all irrational barriers to genuinely voluntary choice. When they fail to act rationally in medical contexts, the harm may well be serious, probable and irreversible. Hence another criterion for justified paternalism appears to be met; we have another sign that the probable outcome in these circumstances of unhindered choice is not truly desired, hence the choice not truly voluntary.

While it is possible that a doctor's prognosis might be mistaken, this can be argued to support further rather than weaken the argument for paternalism. For if the doctor is mistaken, this will infect the patient's decision-making process as well, since his appreciation of the situation can only fall short of that of his source of information. Furthermore, bad prognoses may tend to be self-fulfilling when revealed, even if their initial probability of realization is slight. A positive psychological attitude on the part of the patient often enhances chances for cure even when they are slight; and a negative attitude, which might be incurred from a mistaken prognosis or from fear of an outcome with otherwise low probability, might increase that probability. In any case it can be argued that a bad prognosis is more likely to depress the patient needlessly than to serve a positive medical purpose if revealed. The doctor will most likely be able to convince the patient to accept the treatment deemed best by the doctor even after all risks are revealed. The ability to so convince might well be conceived as part of medical competence to provide optimal treatment. If the doctor knows that he can do so in any case, why needlessly worry or depress the patient with discussion of risks that are remote, or at least more remote or less serious than those connected with alternative treatments? Their revelation is unlikely to affect the final decision, but far more likely to harm the patient. It therefore would appear cruel for the doctor not to assume responsibility for the decision or for remaining silent on certain of its determining factors.

Thus all the criteria for justified paternalism might appear to be met in the more controversial cases as well. The analogies with our earlier examples appear to support overriding the patient's right to decide on the basis of the truth by the fundamental medical principle of providing optimal care and treatment. Let us apply this argument more specifically to . . . the case of withholding truth when no other medical decisions remain to be made, when the question is what to tell the terminally ill patient for example. Here recognition of an absolute right of the patient is likely to result in needless mental suffering and even in some cases hasten death. The dying patient is likely to realize at a certain point that he is dying without having to be informed. If he does realize it, blunt and open discussion of the fact may nevertheless be depressing. What appear to be pointless deceptive games played out between patients and relatives in avoiding such discussion may actually express delicate defense mechanisms whose solace may be destroyed by the doctor's intrusion. When the doctor has no reason to predict such detrimental effects, then perhaps he ought to inform. But why do so when this is certain to cause needless additional suffering or harm? To do so appears not only wrong, but cruel.

We certainly are justified in lying to a person in order to prevent serious harm to another. If I must lie to someone in order to save the life of another whom the first person might kill if told the truth (even if the killing would be nonintentional), there is no doubt at all that I should tell the lie or withhold the information. Rights to be told the truth are not absolute, but, like all rights, must be ordered in relation to others. If I may lie to one person to save another from harm, why not then when the life of the person himself might be threatened or seriously worsened by the truth, as it might be in the medical contexts we are considering? Why should the fact that only one person is involved, that only the person himself is likely to be harmed by the truth, alter the duty to deceive or withhold information in order to prevent the more serious harm? If it is replied that when only one person is involved, that person is likely to know the best course of action for himself, the answer is that in medical contexts this claim appears to be false. The doctor is likely to be better informed than the patient about his condition and the optimal treatments for it.

Thus there are two situations in which the doctor's duty not to harm his patient's health or shorten his life might appear to override otherwise obtaining rights of the patients to the full truth. One is where the truth will cause direct harm—depression or loss of continued will to live. The other is where informing may be instrumentally harmful in leading to the choice of the wrong treatment or none at all. Given that information divulged to the patient may be harmful or damaging to his health, may interfere with other aspects of optimal or successful treatment, it is natural to construe what the doctor tells the patient as an aspect of the treatment itself. As such it would be subject to the same risk-benefit analysis as other aspects. Doctors must constantly balance uncertain benefits and risks in trying to provide treatment that will maximize the probability of cure with least damaging side effects. Questions regarding optimal treatment are questions for medical expertise. Since psychological harm must figure in the doctor's calculations if he is properly sensitive, since it may contribute as well to physical deterioration, and since what he says to a patient may cause such harm, it seems that the doctor must construe what he *says* to a patient as on a par with what he *does* to him, assuming full responsibility for any harm that may result. Certainly many doctors do so conceive of questions of disclosure. A clear example of this assimilation to questions regarding treatment is the following:

> From the foregoing it should be self-evident that what is imparted to a patient about his illness should be planned with the same care and executed with the same skill that are demanded by any potentially therapeutic measure. Like the transfusion of blood, the dispensing of certain information must be distinctly indicated, the amount given consonant with the needs of the recipient, and the type chosen with the view of avoiding untoward reactions.[6]

When the patient places himself in the care of a physician, he expects the best and least harmful treatment, and the physician's fundamental duty, seemingly overriding all others in the medical context, must be to provide such treatment. Indeed the terminology itself, "under a physician's care," suggests acceptance of the paternalistic model of strong role differentiation. To care for someone is to provide first and foremost for that person's welfare.[7] The doctor ministers to his patient's needs, not to his immediate preferences. If this were not the case, doctors would be justified in prescribing whatever drugs their patients requested. That a person needs care suggests that, at least for the time being, he is not capable of being physically autonomous; and given the close connection of physical with mental state, the emotional stress that accompanies serious illness, it is natural to view the patient as relinquishing autonomy over medical decisions to the expert for his own good. Being under a physician's care entails a different relationship from that involved in merely seeking another person's advice.

THE REFUTATION OF MEDICAL PATERNALISM

In order to refute an argument, we of course need to refute only one of its premises. The argument for medical paternalism, stripped to its barest outline, was:

1. Disclosure of information to the patient will sometimes increase the likelihood of depression and physical deterioration, or result in choice of medically inoptimal treatment.
2. Disclosure of information is therefore sometimes likely to be detrimental to the patient's health, perhaps even to hasten his death.
3. Health and prolonged life can be assumed to have priority among preferences for patients who place themselves under physicians' care.
4. Worsening health or hastening death can therefore be assumed to be contrary to patients' own true value orderings.
5. Paternalism is therefore justified: doctors may sometimes override patients' prima facie rights to information about risks and treatments or about their own conditions in order to prevent harm to their health.

THE RELATIVITY OF VALUES: HEALTH AND LIFE

The fundamentally faulty premise in the argument for paternalistic role differentiation for doctors is that which assumes that health or prolonged life must take absolute priority in the patient's value orderings. In order for paternalistic interference to be justified, a person must be acting irrationally or inconsistently with his own long-range preferences. The value ordering violated by the action to be prevented must either be known to be that of the person himself, as in the train example, or else be uncontroversially that of any rational person, as in the motorcycle helmet case. But can we assume that health and prolonged life have top priority in any rational ordering? *If* these values could be safely assumed to be always overriding for those who seek medical assistance, then medical expertise would become paramount in decisions regarding treatment, and decisions on disclosure would become assimilated to those within the treatment context. But in fact very few of us act according to such an assumed value ordering. In designing social policy we do not devote all funds or efforts toward minimizing loss of life, on the highways or in hospitals for example.

If our primary goal were always to minimize risk to health and life, we should spend our entire federal budget in health-related areas. Certainly such a suggestion would be ludicrous. We do not in fact grant to individuals rights to minimal risk in their activities or to absolutely optimal health care. From another perspective, if life itself, rather than life of a certain quality with autonomy and dignity, were of ultimate value, then even defensive wars could never be justified. But when the quality of life and the autonomy of an entire nation is threatened from without, defensive war in which many lives are risked and lost is a rational posture. To paraphrase Camus, anything worth living for is worth dying for. To realize or preserve those values that give meaning to life is worth the risk of life itself. Such fundamental values (and autonomy for individuals is certainly among them), necessary within a framework in which life of a certain quality becomes possible, appear to take precedence over the value of mere biological existence.

In personal life too we often engage in risky activities for far less exalted reasons, in fact just for the pleasure or convenience. We work too hard, smoke, exercise too little or too much, eat what we know is bad for us, and continue to do all these things even when informed of their possibly fatal effects. To doctors in their roles as doctors all this may appear irrational, although they no more act

always to preserve their own health than do the rest of us. If certain risks to life and health are irrational, others are not. Once more the quality and significance of one's life may take precedence over maximal longevity. Many people when they are sick think of nothing above getting better; but this is not true of all. A person with a heart condition may decide that important unfinished work or projects must take priority over increased risk to his health; and his priority is not uncontroversially irrational. Since people's lives derive meaning and fulfillment from their projects and accomplishments, a person's risking a shortened life for one more fulfilled might well justify actions detrimental to his health. . . .

To doctors in their roles as professionals whose ultimate concern is the health or continued lives of patients, it is natural to elevate these values to ultimate prominence. The death of a patient, inevitable as it is in many cases, may appear as an ultimate defeat to the medical art, as something to be fought by any means, even after life has lost all value and meaning for the patient himself. The argument in the previous section for assuming this value ordering was that health, and certainly life, seem to be necessary conditions for the realization of all other goods or values. But this point, even if true, leaves open the question of whether health and life are of ultimate, or indeed any, intrinsic value, or whether they are valuable *merely* as means. It is plausible to maintain that life itself is not of intrinsic value, since surviving in an irreversible coma seems no better than death. It therefore again appears that it is the quality of life that counts, not simply being alive. Although almost any quality might be preferable to none, it is not irrational to trade off quantity for quality, as in any other good.

Even life with physical health and consciousness may not be of intrinsic value. Consciousness and health may not be sufficient in themselves to make the life worth living, since some states of consciousness are intrinsically good and others bad. Furthermore, if a person has nothing before him but pain and depression, then the instrumental worth of being alive may be reversed. And if prolonging one's life can be accomplished only at the expense of incapacitation or ignorance, perhaps preventing lifelong projects from being completed, then the instrumental value of longer life again seems overbalanced. It is certainly true that normally life itself is of utmost value as necessary for all else of value, and that living longer usually enables one to complete more projects and plans, to satisfy more desires and derive more enjoyments. But this cannot be assumed in the extreme circumstances of severe or terminal illness. Ignorance of how long one has left may block realization of such values, as may treatment with the best chance for cure, if it also risks incapacitation or immediate death.

Nor is avoidance of depression the most important consideration in such circumstances, as a shallow hedonism might assume. Hedonistic theories of value, which seek only to produce pleasure or avoid pain and depression, are easily disproven by our abhorrence at the prospect of a "brave new world," or our unwillingness, were it possible, to be plugged indefinitely into a "pleasure machine." The latter prospect is abhorrent not only from an ideal-regarding viewpoint, but, less obviously, for want-regarding reasons (for most persons) as well. Most people would in fact be unwilling to trade important freedoms and accomplishments for sensuous pleasures, or even for the illusion of greater freedoms and accomplishments. As many philosophers have pointed out, while satisfaction of wants may bring pleasurable sensations, wants are not primarily *for* pleasurable sensations, or even for happiness more broadly construed, per se. Conversely, the avoidance of negative feelings or depression is not uppermost among primary motives. Many people are willing to endure frustration, suffering, and even depression in pursuit of accomplishment, or in order to complete projects once begun. Thus information relevant to such matters, such as medical information about one's own condition or possible adverse effects of various treatments, may well be worth having at the cost of psychological pain or depression.

THE VALUE OF SELF-DETERMINATION

We have so far focused on the inability of the doctor to assume a particular value ordering for his patient in which health, the prolonging of life, or the avoidance of depression is uppermost. The likelihood of error in this regard makes it probable that the doctor will not know the true interests of his patient as well as the patient himself. He is therefore less likely than the patient himself to make choices in accord with that overall interest, and paternalistic assumption of authority to do so is therefore unjustified. There is in addition another decisive consideration mentioned earlier, namely the independent value of self-determination or freedom of choice. Personal autonomy over important decisions in one's life, the ability to attempt to realize one's own value ordering, is indeed so important that normally no amount of other goods, pleasures or avoidance of personal evils can take precedence. This is why it is wrong to contract oneself into slavery, and another reason why pleasure machines do not seem attractive. Regarding the latter, even if people were willing to forgo other goods for a life of constant pleasure, the loss in variety of other values, and in the creativity that can generate new sources of value, would be morally regrettable. The value of self-determination explains also why there is such a strong burden of proof upon those who advocate paternalistic measures, why they must show that the person would otherwise act in a way inconsistent with his own value ordering, that is irrationally. A person's desires are not simply evidence of what is in his interest—they have extra weight.

Especially when decisions are important to the course of our lives, we are unwilling to relinquish them to others, even in exchange for a higher probability of happiness or less risk of suffering. Even if it could be proven, for example, that some scientific method of matching spouses greatly increased chances of compatibility and happiness, we would insist upon retaining our rights over marriage decisions. Given the present rate of success in marriages, it is probable that we could in fact find some better method of matching partners in terms of increasing that success rate. Yet we are willing to forgo increased chances of success in order to make our own choices, choices that tend to make us miserable in the long run. The same might be true of career choices, choices of schools, and others central to the course of our lives. Our unwillingness to delegate these crucial decisions to experts or computers, who might stand a better chance of making them correctly (in terms of later satisfactions), is not to be explained simply in terms of our (sometimes mistaken) assumptions that we know best how to satisfy our own interests, or that we personally will choose correctly, even though most other people do not. If our retaining such authority for ourselves is not simply irrational, and I do not believe it is, this can only be because of the great independent value of self-determination. We value the exercise of free choice itself in personally important decisions, no matter what the effects of those decisions upon other satisfactions. The independent value of self-determination in decisions of great personal importance adds also to our reluctance to relinquish medical decisions with crucial effects on our lives to doctors, despite their medical expertise.

Autonomy or self-determination is independently valuable, as argued before, first of all because we value it in itself. But we may again add to this want-regarding or utilitarian reason a second ideal-regarding or perfectionist reason. What has value does so because it is valued by a rational and autonomous person. But autonomy itself is necessary to the development of such valuing individual persons or agents. It is therefore not to be sacrificed to other derivative values. To do so as a rule is to destroy the ground for the latter. Rights in general not only express and protect the central interests of individuals (the raison d'être usually emphasized in their exposition); they also express the dignity and inviolability of individuality itself. For this reason the most fundamental right is the right to control the course of one's life, to make decisions crucial to it, including decisions in life-or-death medical contexts. The other side of the independent value of self-determination from the point of view of the individual is the recognition of him by others, including doctors, as an individual with his own possibly unique set of values and priorities. His dignity demands a right to make personal decisions that express those values. . . .

NOTES

1. American Medical Association, *Principles of Medical Ethics*.
2. I restrict discussion for the time being to competent adults. I assume for now that if they have rights to information or to make their own decisions in medical contexts, then parents or guardians, not doctors, have these same rights in relation to children or the mentally incapacitated.
3. Compare Sissela Bok, *Lying* (New York: Pantheon, 1978), pp. 18–19.
4. See Gerald Dworkin, "Paternalism," in R. Wasserstrom, ed., *Morality and the Law* (Belmont, Cal.: Wadsworth, 1971).
5. Compare Norman Cantor, "A Patient's Decision to Decline Life-Saving Medical Treatment: Bodily Integrity Versus the Preservation of Life," in T. Beauchamp and S. Perlin, eds., *Ethical Issues in Death and Dying* (Englewood Cliffs, N.J.: Prentice-Hall, 1978), pp. 208–209.
6. Bernard Meyer, "Truth and the Physician," in Beauchamp and Perlin ed., op. cit., p. 160.
7. Compare A. R. Jonsen, "Do No Harm: Axiom of Medical Ethics," *Philosophy and Medicine* 3 (1977): 27–41, p. 30.

Four Models of the Physician-Patient Relationship

Ezekiel J. Emanuel and Linda L. Emanuel

During the last two decades or so, there has been a struggle over the patient's role in medical decision making that is often characterized as a conflict between autonomy and health, between the

From *Journal of the American Medical Association* 267, no. 16, April 22/29, 1992: 2221–2226. Copyright © 1992 American Medical Association.

*EDITORS' NOTE: Author's notes have been deleted. Students who wish to follow up on sources should consult the original article.

values of the patient and the values of the physician. Seeking to curtail physician dominance, many have advocated an ideal of greater patient control. Others question this ideal because it fails to acknowledge the potentially imbalanced nature of this interaction when one party is sick and searching for security, and when judgments entail the interpretation of technical information. Still others are trying to delineate a more mutual relationship. This struggle shapes the expectations of physicians and patients as well as the ethical and legal standards for the physician's duties, informed consent, and medical malpractice. This struggle forces us to ask, What should be the ideal physician-patient relationship?

We shall outline four models of the physician-patient interaction, emphasizing the different understandings of (1) the goals of the physician-patient interaction, (2) the physician's obligations, (3) the role of patient values, and (4) the conception of patient autonomy. To elaborate the abstract description of these four models, we shall indicate the types of response the models might suggest in a clinical situation. Third, we shall also indicate how these models inform the current debate about the ideal physician-patient relationship. Finally, we shall evaluate these models and recommend one as the preferred model.

As outlined, the models are Weberian ideal types. They may not describe any particular physician-patient interactions but they highlight, free from complicating details, different visions of the essential characteristics of the physician-patient interaction. Consequently, they do not embody minimum ethical or legal standards, but rather constitute regulative ideals that are "higher than the law" but not "above the law."

THE PATERNALISTIC MODEL

First is the *paternalistic* model, sometimes called the parental or priestly model. In this model, the physician-patient interaction ensures that patients receive the interventions that best promote their health and well-being. To this end, physicians use their skills to determine the patient's medical condition and his or her stage in the disease process and to identify the medical tests and treatments most likely to restore the patient's health or ameliorate pain. Then the physician presents the patient with selected information that will encourage the patient to consent to the intervention the physician considers best. At the extreme, the physician authoritatively informs the patient when the intervention will be initiated.

The paternalistic model assumes that there are shared objective criteria for determining what is best. Hence the physician can discern what is in the patient's best interest with limited patient participation. Ultimately, it is assumed that the patient will be thankful for decisions made by the physician even if he or she would not agree to them at the time. In the tension between the patient's autonomy and well-being, between choice and health, the paternalistic physician's main emphasis is toward the latter.

In the paternalistic model, the physician acts as the patient's guardian, articulating and implementing what is best for the patient. As such, the physician has obligations, including that of placing the patient's interest above his or her own and soliciting the views of others when lacking adequate knowledge. The conception of patient autonomy is patient assent, either at the time or later, to the physician's determinations of what is best.

THE INFORMATIVE MODEL

Second is the *informative* model, sometimes called the scientific, engineering, or consumer model. In this model, the objective of the physician-patient interaction is for the physician to provide the patient with all relevant information, for the patient to select the medical interventions he or she wants, and for the physician to execute the selected interventions. To this end, the physician informs the patient of his or her disease state, the nature of possible diagnostic and therapeutic interventions, the nature and probability of risks and benefits associated with the interventions, and any uncertainties of knowledge. At the extreme, patients could come to know all medical information relevant to their disease and available interventions and select the interventions that best realize their values.

The informative model assumes a fairly clear distinction between facts and values. The patient's values are well defined and known; what the patient lacks is facts. It is the physician's obligation to provide all the available facts, and the patient's values then determine what treatments are to be given. There is no role for the physician's values, the physician's understanding of the patient's values, or his or her judgment of the worth of the patient's values. In the informative model, the physician is a purveyor of technical expertise, providing the patient with the means to exercise control. As technical experts, physicians have important obligations to provide truthful information, to maintain competence in their area of expertise, and to consult others when their knowledge or skills are lacking. The conception of patient autonomy is patient control over medical decision making.

THE INTERPRETIVE MODEL

The third model is the *interpretive* model. The aim of the physician-patient interaction is to elucidate the patient's values and what he or she actually wants, and to help the patient select the available medical interventions that realize these values. Like the informative physician, the interpretive physician provides the patient with information on the nature of the condition and the risks and benefits of possible interventions. Beyond this, however, the interpretive physician assists the patient in elucidating and articulating his or her values and in determining what medical interventions best realize the specified values, thus helping to interpret the patient's values for the patient.

According to the interpretive model, the patient's values are not necessarily fixed and known to the patient. They are often inchoate, and the patient may only partially understand them; they may conflict when applied to specific situations. Consequently, the physician working with the patient must elucidate and make coherent these values. To do this, the physician works with the patient to reconstruct the patient's goals and aspirations, commitments and character. At the extreme, the physician must conceive of the patient's life as a narrative whole, and from this specify the patient's values and their priorities. Then the physician determines which tests and treatments best realize these values. Importantly, the physician does not dictate to the patient; it is the patient who ultimately decides which values and course of action best fit who he or she is. Neither is the physician judging the patient's values; he or she helps the patient to understand and use them in the medical situation.

In the interpretive model, the physician is a counselor, analogous to a cabinet minister's advisory role to a head of state, supplying relevant information, helping to elucidate values, and suggesting what medical interventions realize these values. Thus the physician's obligations include those enumerated in the informative model but

also require engaging the patient in a joint process of understanding. Accordingly, the conception of patient autonomy is self-understanding; the patient comes to know more clearly who he or she is and how the various medical options bear on his or her identity.

THE DELIBERATIVE MODEL

Fourth is the *deliberative* model. The aim of the physician-patient interaction is to help the patient determine and choose the best health-related values that can be realized in the clinical situation. To this end, the physician must delineate information on the patient's clinical situation and then help elucidate the types of values embodied in the available options. The physician's objectives include suggesting why certain health-related values are more worthy and should be aspired to. At the extreme, the physician and patient engage in deliberation about what kind of health-related values the patient could and ultimately should pursue. The physician discusses only health-related values, that is, values that affect or are affected by the patient's disease and treatments; he or she recognizes that many elements of morality are unrelated to the patient's disease or treatment and beyond the scope of their professional relationship. Further, the physician aims at no more than moral persuasion; ultimately, coercion is avoided, and the patient must define his or her life and select the ordering of values to be espoused. By engaging in moral deliberation, the physician and patient judge the worthiness and importance of the health-related values.

In the deliberative model, the physician acts as a teacher or friend, engaging the patient in dialogue on what course of action would be best. Not only does the physician indicate what the patient could do, but, knowing the patient and wishing what is best, the physician indicates what the patient should do—what decision regarding medical therapy would be admirable. The conception of patient autonomy is moral self-development; the patient is empowered not simply to follow unexamined preferences or examined values, but to consider, through dialogue, alternative health-related values, their worthiness, and their implications for treatment.

COMPARING THE FOUR MODELS

Importantly, all models have a role for patient autonomy; a main factor that differentiates the models is their particular conceptions of patient autonomy. Therefore, no single model can be endorsed because it alone promotes patient autonomy. Instead the models must be compared and evaluated, at least in part, by evaluating the adequacy of their particular conceptions of patient autonomy.

The four models are not exhaustive. At a minimum, there might be added a fifth: the *instrumental* model. In this model, the patient's values are irrelevant; the physician aims for some goal independent of the patient, such as the good of society or the furtherance of scientific knowledge. The Tuskegee syphilis experiment and the Willowbrook hepatitis study (see Part Five, Section One) are examples of this model. As the moral condemnation of these cases reveals, this model is not an ideal, but an aberration. Thus we have not elaborated it herein.

A CLINICAL CASE

To make tangible these abstract descriptions and to crystallize essential differences among the models, we will illustrate the responses they suggest in a clinical situation, that of a 43-year-old premenopausal woman who has recently discovered a breast mass. Surgery reveals a 3.5-cm ductal carcinoma with no lymph node involvement that is estrogen receptor positive. Chest roentgenogram, bone scan, and liver function tests reveal no evidence of metastatic disease. The patient was recently divorced and has gone back to work as a legal aide to support herself. What should the physician say to this patient?

In the paternalistic model a physician might say, "There are two alternative therapies to protect against recurrence of cancer in your breast: mastectomy or radiation. We now know that the survival with lumpectomy combined with radiation therapy is equal to that with mastectomy. Because lumpectomy and radiation offers the best survival and the best cosmetic result, it is to be preferred. I have asked the radiation therapist to come and discuss radiation treatment with you. We also need to

protect you against the spread of the cancer to other parts of your body. Even though the chance of recurrence is low, you are young, and we should not leave any therapeutic possibilities untried. Recent studies involving chemotherapy suggest improvements in survival without recurrence of breast cancer. Indeed, the National Cancer Institute (NCI) recommends chemotherapy for women with your type of breast cancer. Chemotherapy has side effects. Nevertheless, a few months of hardship now are worth the potential added years of life without cancer."

In the informative model, a physician might say, "With node-negative breast cancer there are two issues before you: local control and systemic control. For local control, the options are mastectomy or lumpectomy with or without radiation. From many studies we know that mastectomy and lumpectomy with radiation result in identical overall survival, about 80 percent 10-year survival. Lumpectomy without radiation results in a 30 percent to 40 percent chance of tumor recurrence in the breast. The second issue relates to systemic control. We know that chemotherapy prolongs survival for premenopausal women who have axillary nodes involved with tumor. The role for women with node-negative breast cancer is less clear. Individual studies suggest that chemotherapy is of no benefit in terms of improving overall survival, but a comprehensive review of all studies suggests that there is a survival benefit. Several years ago, the NCI suggested that for women like yourself, chemotherapy can have a positive therapeutic impact. Finally, let me inform you that there are clinical trials, for which you are eligible, to evaluate the benefits of chemotherapy for patients with node-negative breast cancer. I can enroll you in a study if you want. I will be happy to give you any further information you feel you need."

The interpretive physician might outline much of the same information as the informative physician, then engage in discussion to elucidate the patient's wishes, and conclude, "It sounds to me as if you have conflicting wishes. Understandably, you seem uncertain how to balance the demands required for receiving additional treatment, rejuvenating your personal affairs, and maintaining your psychological equilibrium. Let me try to express a perspective that fits your position. Fighting your cancer is important, but it must leave you with a healthy self-image and quality time outside the hospital. This view seems compatible with undergoing radiation therapy but not chemotherapy. A lumpectomy with radiation maximizes your chance of surviving while preserving your breast. Radiotherapy fights your breast cancer without disfigurement. Conversely, chemotherapy would prolong the duration of therapy by many months. Further, the benefits of chemotherapy in terms of survival are smaller and more controversial. Given the recent changes in your life, you have too many new preoccupations to undergo months of chemotherapy for a questionable benefit. Do I understand you? We can talk again in a few days."

The deliberative physician might begin by outlining the same factual information, then engage in a conversation to elucidate the patient's values, but continue, "It seems clear that you should undergo radiation therapy. It offers maximal survival with minimal risk, disfigurement, and disruption of your life. The issue of chemotherapy is different, fraught with conflicting data. Balancing all the options, I think the best one for you is to enter a trial that is investigating the potential benefit of chemotherapy for women with node-negative breast cancer. First, it ensures that you receive excellent medical care. At this point, we do not know which therapy maximizes survival. In a clinical study the schedule of follow-up visits, tests, and decisions is specified by leading breast cancer experts to ensure that all the women receive care that is the best available anywhere. A second reason to participate in a trial is altruistic; it allows you to contribute something to women with breast cancer in the future who will face difficult choices. Over decades, thousands of women have participated in studies that inform our current treatment practices. Without those women, and the knowledge they made possible, we would probably still be giving you and all other women with breast cancer mastectomies. By enrolling in a trial you participate in a tradition in which women of one generation receive the highest standard of care available but also enhance the care of women in future generations because medicine has learned something about which interventions are better. I must tell you that I am not involved in the study; if you elect to enroll in this trial, you will initially see another breast cancer expert to plan your ther-

apy. I have sought to explain our current knowledge and offer my recommendation so you can make the best possible decision."

Lacking the normal interchange with patients, these statements may seem contrived, even caricatures. Nevertheless, they highlight the essence of each model and suggest how the objectives and assumptions of each inform a physician's approach to his or her patients. Similar statements can be imagined for other clinical situations such as an obstetrician discussing prenatal testing or a cardiologist discussing cholesterol-reducing interventions.

THE CURRENT DEBATE AND THE FOUR MODELS

In recent decades there has been a call for greater patient autonomy or, as some have called it, "patient sovereignty," conceived as patient *choice* and *control* over medical decisions. This shift toward the informative model is embodied in the adoption of business terms for medicine, as when physicians are described as health care providers and patients as consumers. It can also be found in the propagation of patient rights statements, in the promotion of living-will laws, and in rules regarding human experimentation. For instance, the opening sentences of one law state: "The Rights of the Terminally Ill Act authorizes an adult person to *control* decisions regarding administration of life-sustaining treatment. . . . The Act merely provides one way by which a terminally-ill patient's *desires* regarding the use of life-sustaining procedures can be legally implemented" (emphasis added). Indeed, living-will laws do not require or encourage patients to discuss the issue of terminating care with their physicians before signing such documents. Similarly, decisions in "right-to-die" cases emphasize patient control over medical decisions. As one court put it:

> The right to refuse medical treatment is basic and fundamental. . . . Its exercise requires no one's approval. . . . [T]he controlling decision belongs to a competent informed patient. . . . It is not a medical decision for her physicians to make. . . . It is a moral and philosophical decision that, being a competent adult, is [the patient's] alone.[1] (emphasis added)

Probably the most forceful endorsement of the informative model as the ideal inheres in informed consent standards. Prior to the 1970s, the standard for informed consent was "physician based." Since 1972 and the *Canterbury* case, however, the emphasis has been on a "patient-oriented" standard of informed consent in which the physician has a "duty" to provide appropriate medical facts to empower the patient to use his or her values to determine what interventions should be implemented.

> True consent to what happens to one's self is the informed exercise of a choice, and that entails an opportunity to evaluate knowledgeably the options available and the risks attendant upon each. . . . *[I]t is the prerogative of the patient, not the physician, to determine for himself the direction in which his interests seem to lie.* To enable the patient to chart his course understandably, some familiarity with the therapeutic alternatives and their hazards becomes essential.[2] (emphasis added)

SHARED DECISION MAKING

Despite its dominance, many have found the informative model somewhat "arid." The President's Commission and others contend that the ideal relationship does not vest moral authority and medical decision-making power exclusively in the patient but must be a process of shared decision making constructed around "mutual participation and respect." The President's Commission argues that the physician's role is "to help the patient understand the medical situation and available courses of action, and the patient conveys his or her concerns and wishes." Brock and Wartman[3] stress this fact-value "division of labor"—having the physician provide information while the patient makes value decisions—by describing "shared decision making" as a collaborative process

> in which both physicians and patients make active and essential contributions. Physicians bring their medical training, knowledge, and expertise—including an understanding of the available treatment alternatives—to the diagnosis and management of patients' conditions. Patients bring knowledge of their own subjective aims and values, through which risks and

benefits of various treatment options can be evaluated. With this approach, selecting the best treatment for a particular patient requires the contribution of both parties.

Similarly, in discussing ideal medical decision making, Eddy[4] argues for this fact-value division of labor between the physician and patient as the ideal:

> It is important to separate the decision process into these two steps. . . . The first step is a question of facts. The anchor is empirical evidence. . . . [T]he second step is a question not of facts but of personal values or preferences. The thought process is not analytic but personal and subjective. . . . [I]t is the patient's preferences that should determine the decision. . . . Ideally, you and I [the physicians] are not in the picture. What matters is what Mrs. Smith thinks.

This view of shared decision making seems to vest the medical decision-making authority with the patient while relegating physicians to technicians "transmitting medical information and using their technical skills as the patient directs." Thus, while the advocates of "shared decision making" may aspire toward a mutual dialogue between physician and patient, the substantive view informing their ideal reembodies the informative model under a different label.

Other commentators have articulated more mutual models of the physician-patient interaction. Prominent among these efforts is Katz's *The Silent World of the Doctor and Patient*. Relying on a Freudian view in which self-knowledge and self-determination are inherently limited because of unconscious influences, Katz views dialogue as a mechanism for greater self-understanding of one's values and objectives. According to Katz, this view places a duty on physicians and patients to reflect and communicate so that patients can gain a greater self-understanding and self-determination. Katz's insight is also available on grounds other than Freudian psychological theory and is consistent with the interpretive model.

OBJECTIONS TO THE PATERNALISTIC MODEL

It is widely recognized that the paternalistic model is justified during emergencies when the time taken to obtain informed consent might irreversibly harm the patient. Beyond such limited circumstances, however, it is no longer tenable to assume that the physician and patient espouse similar values and views of what constitutes a benefit. Consequently, even physicians rarely advocate the paternalistic model as an ideal for routine physician-patient interactions.

OBJECTIONS TO THE INFORMATIVE MODEL

The informative model seems both descriptively and prescriptively inaccurate. First, this model seems to have no place for essential qualities of the ideal physician-patient relationship. The informative physician cares for the patient in the sense of competently implementing the patient's selected interventions. However, the informative physician lacks a caring approach that requires understanding what the patient values or should value and how his or her illness impinges on these values. Patients seem to expect their physician to have a caring approach; they deem a technically proficient but detached physician as deficient, and properly condemned. Further, the informative physician is proscribed from giving a recommendation for fear of imposing his or her will on the patient and thereby competing for the decision-making control that has been given to the patient. Yet, if one of the essential qualities of the ideal physician is the ability to assimilate medical facts, prior experience of similar situations, and intimate knowledge of the patient's view into a recommendation designed for the patient's specific medical and personal condition, then the informative physician cannot be ideal.

Second, in the informative model, the ideal physician is a highly trained subspecialist who provides detailed factual information and competently implements the patient's preferred medical intervention. Hence, the informative model perpetuates and accentuates the trend toward specialization and impersonalization within the medical profession.

Most importantly, the informative model's conception of patient autonomy seems philosophically untenable. The informative model presupposes that persons possess known and fixed values, but

this is inaccurate. People are often uncertain about what they actually want. Further, unlike animals, people have what philosophers call "second-order desires," that is, the capacity to reflect on their wishes and to revise their own desires and preferences. In fact, freedom of the will and autonomy inhere in having "second order desires" and being able to change our preferences and modify our identities. Self-reflection and the capacity to change what we want often require a "process" of moral deliberation in which we assess the value of what we want. And this is a process that occurs with other people who know us well and can articulate a vision of who we ought to be that we can assent to. Even though changes in health or implementation of alternative interventions can have profound effects on what we desire and how we realize our desires, self-reflection and deliberation play no essential role in the informative physician-patient interaction. The informative model's conception of autonomy is incompatible with a vision of autonomy that incorporates second-order desires.

OBJECTIONS TO THE INTERPRETIVE MODEL

The interpretive model rectifies this deficiency by recognizing that persons have second-order desires and dynamic value structures and placing the elucidation of values in the context of the patient's medical condition at the center of the physician-patient interaction. Nevertheless, there are objections to the interpretive model.

Technical specialization militates against physicians cultivating the skills necessary to the interpretive model. With limited interpretive talents and limited time, physicians may unwittingly impose their own values under the guise of articulating the patient's values. And patients, overwhelmed by their medical condition and uncertain of their own views, may too easily accept this imposition. Such circumstances may push the interpretive model toward the paternalistic model in actual practice.

Further, autonomy viewed as self-understanding excludes evaluative judgment of the patient's values or attempts to persuade the patient to adopt other values. This constrains the guidance and recommendations the physician can offer. Yet in practice, especially in preventive medicine and risk-reduction interventions, physicians often attempt to persuade patients to adopt particular health-related values. Physicians frequently urge patients with high cholesterol levels who smoke to change their dietary habits, quit smoking, and begin exercise programs before initiating drug therapy. The justification given for these changes is that patients should value their health more than they do. Similarly, physicians are encouraged to persuade their human immunodeficiency virus (HIV)–infected patients who might be engaging in unsafe sexual practices either to abstain or, realistically, to adopt "safer sex" practices. Such appeals are not made to promote the HIV–infected patient's own health, but are grounded on an appeal for the patient to assume responsibility for the good of others. Consequently, by excluding evaluative judgments, the interpretive model seems to characterize inaccurately ideal physician-patient interactions.

OBJECTIONS TO THE DELIBERATIVE MODEL

The fundamental objections to the deliberative model focus on whether it is proper for physicians to judge patients' values and promote particular health-related values. First, physicians do not possess privileged knowledge of the priority of health-related values relative to other values. Indeed, since ours is a pluralistic society in which people espouse incommensurable values, it is likely that a physician's values and view of which values are higher will conflict with those of other physicians and those of his or her patients.

Second, the nature of the moral deliberation between physician and patient, the physician's recommended interventions, and the actual treatments used will depend on the values of the particular physician treating the patient. However, recommendations and care provided to patients should not depend on the physician's judgment of the worthiness of the patient's values or on the physician's particular values. As one bioethicist put it:

> The hand is broken; the physician can repair the hand; therefore the physician must repair the

hand—as well as possible—without regard to personal values that might lead the physician to think ill of the patient or of the patient's values. . . . [A]t the level of clinical practice, medicine should be value-free in the sense that the personal values of the physician should not distort the making of medical decisions.[5]

Third, it may be argued that the deliberative model misconstrues the purpose of the physician-patient interaction. Patients see their physicians to receive health care, not to engage in moral deliberation or to revise their values. Finally, like the interpretive model, the deliberative model may easily metamorphose into unintended paternalism, the very practice that generated the public debate over proper physician-patient interaction.

THE PREFERRED MODEL AND THE PRACTICAL IMPLICATIONS

Clearly, under different clinical circumstances, different models may be appropriate. Indeed, at different times, all four models may justifiably guide physicians and patients. Nevertheless, it is important to specify one model as the shared, paradigmatic reference; exceptions to use other models would not be automatically condemned, but would require justification based on the circumstances of a particular situation. Thus, it is widely agreed that in an emergency where delays in treatment to obtain informed consent might irreversibly harm the patient, the paternalistic model correctly guides physician-patient interactions. Conversely, for patients who have clear but conflicting values, the interpretive model is probably justified. For instance, a 65-year-old woman who has been treated for acute leukemia may have clearly decided against reinduction chemotherapy if she relapses. Several months before the anticipated birth of her first grandchild, the patient relapses. The patient becomes torn about whether to endure the risks of reinduction chemotherapy in order to live to see her first grandchild or whether to refuse therapy, resigning herself to not seeing her grandchild. In such cases, the physician may justifiably adopt the interpretive approach. In other circumstances, where there is only a one-time physician-patient interaction without an ongoing relationship in which the patient's values can be elucidated and compared with ideals, such as in a walk-in center, the informative model may be justified.

Descriptively and prescriptively, we claim that the ideal physician-patient relationship is the deliberative model. We will adduce six points to justify this claim. First, the deliberative model more nearly embodies our ideal of autonomy. It is an oversimplification and distortion of the Western tradition to view respecting autonomy as simply permitting a person to select, unrestricted by coercion, ignorance, physical interference, and the like, his or her preferred course of action from a comprehensive list of available options. Freedom and control over medical decisions alone do not constitute patient autonomy. Autonomy requires that individuals critically assess their own values and preferences; determine whether they are desirable; affirm, upon reflection, these values as ones that should justify their actions; and then be free to initiate action to realize the values. The process of deliberation integral to the deliberative model is essential for realizing patient autonomy understood in this way.

Second, our society's image of an ideal physician is not limited to one who knows and communicates to the patient relevant factual information and competently implements medical interventions. The ideal physician—often embodied in literature, art, and popular culture—is a caring physician who integrates the information and relevant values to make a recommendation and, through discussion, attempts to persuade the patient to accept this recommendation as the intervention that best promotes his or her overall well-being. Thus, we expect the best physicians to engage their patients in evaluative discussions of health issues and related values. The physician's discussion does not invoke values that are unrelated or tangentially related to the patient's illness and potential therapies. Importantly, these efforts are not restricted to situations in which patients might make "irrational and harmful" choices but extend to all health care decisions.

Third, the deliberative model is not a disguised form of paternalism. Previously there may have been category mistakes in which instances of the deliberative model have been erroneously identified as physician paternalism. And no doubt, in practice, the deliberative physician may occasionally lapse into paternalism. However, like the ideal teacher, the deliberative physician attempts to *persuade* the patient of the worthiness of certain values, not to *impose* those values paternalistically; the physician's aim is not to subject the patient to his or her will, but to persuade the patient of a course of action as desirable. In the *Laws*, Plato[6] characterizes this fundamental distinction between persuasion and imposition for medical practice that distinguishes the deliberative from the paternalistic model:

> A physician to slaves never gives his patient any account of his illness. . . . [T]he physician offers some orders gleaned from experience with an air of infallible knowledge, in the brusque fashion of a dictator. . . . The free physician, who usually cares for free men, treats their disease first by thoroughly discussing with the patient and his friends his ailment. This way he learns something from the sufferer and simultaneously instructs him. Then the physician does not give his medications until he has persuaded the patient; the physician aims at complete restoration of health by persuading the patient to comply with his therapy.

Fourth, physician values are relevant to patients and do inform their choice of a physician. When a pregnant woman chooses an obstetrician who does not routinely perform a battery of prenatal tests or, alternatively, one who strongly favors them; and when patients seek an aggressive cardiologist who favors procedural interventions or one who concentrates therapy on dietary changes, stress reduction, and life-style modifications, they are, consciously or not, selecting a physician based on the values that guide their medical decisions. And, when disagreements between physicians and patients arise, there are discussions over which values are more important and should be realized in medical care. Occasionally, when such disagreements undermine the physician-patient relationship and a caring attitude, a patient's care is transferred to another physician. Indeed, in the informative model the grounds for transferring care to a new physician is either the physician's ignorance or incompetence. But patients seem to switch physicians because they do not "like" a particular physician or that physician's attitude or approach.

Fifth, we seem to believe that physicians should not only help fit therapies to the patients' elucidated values, but should also promote health-related values. As noted, we expect physicians to promote certain values, such as "safer sex" for patients with HIV or abstaining from or limiting alcohol use. Similarly, patients are willing to adjust their values and actions to be more compatible with health-promoting values. This is in the nature of seeking a caring medical recommendation.

Finally, it may well be that many physicians currently lack the training and capacity to articulate the values underlying their recommendations and persuade patients that these values are worthy. But, in part, this deficiency is a consequence of the tendencies toward specialization and the avoidance of discussions of values by physicians that are perpetuated and justified by the dominant informative model. Therefore, if the deliberative model seems most appropriate, then we need to implement changes in medical care and education to encourage a more caring approach. We must stress understanding rather than mere provisions of factual information in keeping with the legal standards of informed consent and medical malpractice; we must educate physicians not just to spend more time in physician-patient communication but to elucidate and articulate the values underlying their medical care decisions, including routine ones; we must shift the publicly assumed conception of patient autonomy that shapes both the physician's and the patient's expectations from patient control to moral development. Most important, we must recognize that developing a deliberative physician-patient relationship requires a considerable amount of time. We must develop a health care financing system that properly reimburses—rather than penalizes—physicians for taking the time to discuss values with their patients.

CONCLUSION

Over the last few decades, the discourse regarding the physician-patient relationship has focused on two extremes: autonomy and paternalism. Many have attacked physicians as paternalistic, urging the empowerment of patients to control their own care. This view, the informative model, has become dominant in bioethics and legal standards. This model embodies a defective conception of patient autonomy, and it reduces the physician's role to that of a technologist. The essence of doctoring is a fabric of knowledge, understanding, teaching, and action, in which the caring physician integrates the patient's medical condition and health-related values, makes a recommendation on the appropriate course of action, and tries to persuade the patient of the worthiness of this approach and the values it realizes. The physician with a caring attitude is the ideal embodied in the deliberative model, the ideal that should inform laws and policies that regulate the physician-patient interaction.

Finally, it may be worth noting that the four models outlined herein are not limited to the medical realm; they may inform the public conception of other professional interactions as well. We suggest that the ideal relationships between lawyer and client, religious mentor and laity, and educator and student are well described by the deliberative model, at least in some of their essential aspects.

NOTES

1. *Bouvia v. Superior Court*, 225 Cal Rptr 297 (1986).
2. *Canterbury v. Spence*, 464 F2d 772 (D.C. Cir 1972).
3. Brock DW, Wartman SA. When competent patients make irrational choices. *N Engl J Med*. 1990;322: 1595–1599.
4. Eddy DM. Anatomy of a decision. *JAMA*. 1990; 263:441–443.
5. Gorovitz S. *Doctors' Dilemmas: Moral Conflict and Medical Care*. New York, NY: Oxford University Press Inc; 1982:chap 6.
6. Plato; Hamilton E, Cairns H, eds; Emanuel EJ, trans. *Plato: The Collected Dialogues*. Princeton, NJ: Princeton University Press; 1961:720 c–e.

SECTION 2

Informed Consent

Arato v. *Avedon*

Supreme Court of California, En Banc, 1993
5 Cal. 4th 1172, 23 Cal. Rptr. 2d 131, 858 P. 2d 589

ARABIAN, Justice.

A physician's duty to disclose to a patient information material to the decision whether to undergo treatment is the central constituent of the legal doctrine known as "informed consent." In this case, we review the ruling of a divided Court of Appeal that, in recommending a course of chemotherapy and radiation treatment to a patient suffering from a virulent form of cancer, the treating physicians breached their duty to obtain the patient's informed consent by failing to disclose his statistical life expectancy. . . .

I., A

Miklos Arato was a successful 42-year-old electrical contractor and part-time real estate developer when, early in 1980, his internist diagnosed a failing kidney. On July 21, 1980, in the course of surgery to remove the kidney, the operating surgeon detected a tumor on the "tail" or distal portion of Mr. Arato's pancreas. After Mrs. Arato gave her consent, portions of the pancreas were resected, or removed, along with the spleen and the diseased kidney. A follow-up pathological examination of the resected pancreatic tissue confirmed a malignancy. Concerned that the cancer could recur and might have infiltrated adjacent organs, Mr. Arato's surgeon referred him to a group of oncology practitioners for follow-up treatment.

During his initial visit to the oncologists, Mr. Arato filled out a multipage questionnaire routinely given new patients. Among the some 150 questions asked was whether patients "wish[ed] to be told the truth about [their] condition" or whether they wanted the physician to "bear the burden" for them. Mr. Arato checked the box indicating that he wished to be told the truth.

The oncologists discussed with Mr. and Mrs. Arato the advisability of a course of chemotherapy known as "F.A.M.," a treatment employing a combination of drugs which, when used in conjunction with radiation therapy, had shown promise in treating pancreatic cancer in experimental trials. The nature of the discussions between Mr. and Mrs. Arato and the treating physicians, and in particular the scope of the disclosures made to the patient by his doctors, was the subject of conflicting testimony at trial. By their own admission, however, neither the operating surgeon nor the treating oncologists specifically disclosed to the patient or his wife the high statistical mortality rate associated with pancreatic cancer.

Mr. Arato's oncologists determined that a course of F.A.M. chemotherapy was indicated for several reasons. According to their testimony, the high statistical mortality of pancreatic cancer is in part a function of what is by far the most common diagnostic scenario—the discovery of the malignancy well after it has metastasized to distant sites, spreading throughout the patient's body. As noted, in Mr. Arato's case, the tumor was comparatively localized, having been discovered in the tail of the pancreas by chance in the course of surgery to remove the diseased kidney.

Related to the "silent" character of pancreatic cancer is the fact that detection in such an advanced state usually means that the tumor cannot as a practical matter be removed, contributing to the high mortality rate. In Mr. Arato's case, however, the operating surgeon determined that it was possible to excise cleanly the tumorous portion of the pancreas and to leave a margin of about one-half centimeter around the surgical site, a margin that appeared clinically to be clear of cancer cells. Third, the mortality rate is somewhat lower, according to defense testimony, for pancreatic tumors located in the distal part of the organ than for those found in the main body. Finally, then-recent experimental studies on the use of F.A.M. chemotherapy in conjunction with therapeutic radiation treatments had shown promising response rates—on the order of several months of extended life—among pancreatic cancer patients.

Mr. Arato's treating physicians justified not disclosing statistical life expectancy data to their patient on disparate grounds. According to the testimony of his surgeon, Mr. Arato had exhibited great anxiety over his condition, so much so that his surgeon determined that it would have been medically inappropriate to disclose specific mortality rates. The patient's oncologists had a somewhat different explanation. As Dr. Melvin Avedon, his chief oncologist, put it, he believed that cancer patients in Mr. Arato's position "wanted to be told the truth, but did not want a cold shower." Along with the other treating physicians, Dr. Avedon testified that in his opinion the direct and specific disclosure of extremely high mortality rates for malignancies such as pancreatic cancer might effectively deprive a patient of any hope of cure, a medically inadvisable state. Moreover, all of the treating physicians testified that statistical life expectancy data had little predictive value when applied to a particular patient with individualized symptoms, medical history, character traits and other variables.

According to the physicians' testimony, Mr. and Mrs. Arato were told at the outset of the treatment that most victims of pancreatic cancer die of the disease, that Mr. Arato was at "serious" or "great" risk of a recurrence and that, should the cancer return, his condition would be judged incurable. This information was given to the patient and his wife in the context of a series of verbal and behavioral cues designed to invite the patient or family member to follow up with more direct and diffi-

cult questions. Such follow-up questions, on the order of "how long do I have to live?," would have signaled to his doctors, according Dr. Avedon's testimony, the patient's desire and ability to confront the fact of imminent mortality. In the judgment of his chief oncologist, Mr. Arato, although keenly interested in the clinical significance of the most minute symptom, studiously avoided confronting these ultimate issues; according to his doctors, neither Mr. Arato nor his wife ever asked for information concerning his life expectancy in more than 70 visits over a period of a year. Believing that they had disclosed information sufficient to enable him to make an informed decision whether to undergo chemotherapy, Mr. Arato's doctors concluded that their patient had as much information regarding his condition and prognosis as he wished.

Dr. Avedon also testified that he told Mr. Arato that the effectiveness of F.A.M. therapy was unproven in cases such as his, described its principal adverse side effects, and noted that one of the patient's options was not to undergo the treatment. In the event, Mr. Arato consented to the proposed course of chemotherapy and radiation, treatments that are prolonged, difficult and painful for cancer patients. Unfortunately, the treatment proved ineffective in arresting the spread of the malignancy. Although clinical tests showed him to be free of cancer in the several months following the beginning of the F.A.M. treatments, beginning in late March and into April of 1981, the clinical signs took an adverse turn.[1] By late April, the doctors were convinced by the results of additional tests that the cancer had returned and was spreading. They advised the patient of their suspicions and discontinued chemotherapy. On July 25, 1981, a year and four days following surgery, Mr. Arato succumbed to the effects of pancreatic cancer.

B

Not long after his death, Mr. Arato's wife and two children brought this suit against the physicians who had treated their husband and father in his last days, including the surgeon who performed the pancreas resection and the oncologists who had recommended and administered the chemotherapy/radiation treatment. As presented to the jury, the gist of the lawsuit was the claim that in discussing with their patient the advisability of undergoing a course of chemotherapy and radiation, Mr. Arato's doctors had failed to disclose adequately the shortcomings of the proposed treatment in light of the diagnosis, and thus had failed to obtain the patient's informed consent. Specifically, plaintiffs contended that the doctors were aware that, because early detection is difficult and rare, pancreatic cancer is an especially virulent malignancy, one in which only 5 to 10 percent of those afflicted live for as long as five years, and that given the practically incurable nature of the disease, there was little chance Mr. Arato would live more than a short while, even if the proposed treatment proved effective.

Such mortality information, the complaint alleged—especially the statistical morbidity rate of pancreatic cancer—was material to Mr. Arato's decision whether to undergo postoperative treatment; had he known the bleak truth concerning his life expectancy, he would not have undergone the rigors of an unproven therapy, but would have chosen to live out his last days at peace with his wife and children, and arranging his business affairs. Instead, the complaint asserted, in the false hope that radiation and chemotherapy treatments could effect a cure—a hope born of the negligent failure of his physicians to disclose the probability of an early death—Mr. Arato failed to order his affairs in contemplation of his death, an omission that, according to the complaint, led eventually to the failure of his contracting business and to substantial real estate and tax losses following his death.

As the trial neared its conclusion and the court prepared to charge the jury, plaintiffs requested that several special instructions be given relating to the nature and scope of the physician's duty of disclosure. Two proffered instructions in particular are pertinent to this appeal. In the first, plaintiffs asked the trial court to instruct the jury that "A physician has a fiduciary duty to a patient to make a full and fair disclosure to the patient of all facts which materially affect the patient's rights and interests." The second instruction sought by plaintiffs stated that "The scope of the physician's duty to disclose is measured by the amount of knowledge a patient needs in order to make an

informed choice. All information material to the patient's decision should be given."

The trial judge declined to give the jury either of the two instructions sought by the plaintiffs. Instead, the court read to the jury a modified version of BAJI No. 6.11, the so-called "reality of consent" instruction drawn from our opinion in *Cobbs v. Grant* (1972). . . . As can be seen by a comparison of the two instructions, the texts of which are set out in the margin,[2] the instruction actually given the jury by the trial court substantially recapitulated the wording of BAJI No. 6.11, except for the omission of two brief paragraphs dealing with exceptions to the duty of disclosure and a third paragraph that appears on its face not to have been relevant to the case as it developed at trial.

In addition to the modified version of BAJI No. 6.11, the trial court supplemented its informed consent instruction to the jury with the three special instructions, two requested by plaintiffs and a third offered by defendants, set out below.[3] Finally, with plaintiffs' approval, the trial court gave the jury several generic BAJI instructions dealing with such topics as the general legal duties of physicians and specialists (BAJI Nos. 6.00 & 6.11), the negligence standard of care in medical cases (BAJI Nos. 6.02 & 6.30) and when patient consent is necessary (BAJI No. 6.10).

After concluding its deliberations, the jury returned two special verdicts—on a form approved by plaintiffs' counsel—finding that none of the defendants was negligent in the "medical management" of Mr. Arato, and that defendants "disclosed to Mr. Arato all relevant information which would have enabled him to make an informed decision regarding the proposed treatment to be rendered him." Plaintiffs appealed from the judgment entered on the defense verdict, contending that the trial court erred in refusing to give the jury the special instructions requested by them. As noted, a divided Court of Appeal reversed the judgment of the trial court, and ordered a new trial. We granted defendants' ensuing petition for review and now reverse the judgment of the Court of Appeal.

C

In the Court of Appeal's view, Mr. Arato's doctors had breached the duty to disclose to their patient information material to the decision whether to undergo the radiation and drug therapy. According to the Court of Appeal, because there are so many different cancers, the lethality of which varies dramatically, telling a patient that cancer might recur and would then be incurable, without providing at least some general information concerning the virulence of the particular cancer at issue as reflected in mortality tables, was "meaningless." In addition, the Court of Appeal reasoned that his physicians were under a duty to disclose numerical life expectancy information to Mr. Arato so that he and his wife might take timely measures to minimize or avoid the risks of financial loss resulting from his death. . . .

The fount of the doctrine of informed consent in California is our decision of some 20 years ago in *Cobbs v. Grant, supra,* 8 Cal.3d 229, 104 Cal.Rptr. 505, 502 P.2d 1, an opinion by a unanimous court that built on several out-of-state decisions significantly broadening the scope and character of the physician's duty of disclosure in obtaining the patient's consent to treatment.[4] In *Cobbs v. Grant,* we not only anchored much of the doctrine of informed consent in a theory of negligence liability, but also laid down four "postulates" as the foundation on which the physician's duty of disclosure rests.

"The first [of these postulates,]" we wrote, "is that patients are generally persons unlearned in the medical sciences and therefore, except in rare cases, courts may safely assume the knowledge of patient and physician are not in parity. The second is that a person of adult years and in sound mind has the right, in the exercise of control over his own body, to determine whether or not to submit to lawful medical treatment." . . .

"The third [postulate,]" we continued, "is that the patient's consent to treatment, to be effective, must be an informed consent. And the fourth is that the patient, being unlearned in medical sciences, has an abject dependence upon and trust in his physician for the information upon which he relies during the decisional process, thus raising an obligation in the physician that transcends arms-length transactions." . . . From these ethical imperatives, we derived the obligation of a treating physician "of reasonable disclosure of the available choices with respect to proposed therapy and of the dangers inherently and potentially involved in each." . . .

II., B

Together with companion decisions in other jurisdictions, *Cobbs v. Grant, supra,* . . . is one of the epochal opinions in the legal recognition of the medical patient's protectible interest in autonomous decisionmaking. After more than a generation of experience with the judicially broadened duty of physician disclosure, the accumulated medicolegal comment on the subject of informed consent is both large and discordant. Those critics writing under the banner of "patient autonomy" insist that the practical administration of the doctrine has been thwarted by a failure of judicial nerve and an unremitting hostility to its underlying spirit by the medical profession. Others, equally earnest, assert that the doctrine misapprehends the realities of patient care and enshrines moral ideals in the place of workable rules.

Despite the critical standoff between these extremes of "patient sovereignty" and "medical paternalism," indications are that the *Cobbs*-era decisions helped effect a revolution in attitudes among patients and physicians alike regarding the desirability of frank and open disclosure of relevant medical information.[5] The principle question we must address is whether our holding in *Cobbs v. Grant, supra,* . . . as embodied in BAJI No. 6.11, accurately conveys to juries the legal standard under which they assess the evidence in determining the adequacy of the disclosures made by physician to patient in a particular case or whether, as the Court of Appeal here appeared to conclude, the standard instruction should be revised to mandate specific disclosures such as patient life expectancy as revealed by mortality statistics.

In our view, one of the merits of the somewhat abstract formulation of BAJI No. 6.11 is its recognition of the importance of the overall medical context that juries ought to take into account in deciding whether a challenged disclosure was reasonably sufficient to convey to the patient information material to an informed treatment decision. The contexts and clinical settings in which physician and patient interact and exchange information material to therapeutic decisions are so multifarious, the informational needs and degree of dependency of individual patients so various, and the professional relationship itself such an intimate and irreducibly judgment-laden one, that we believe it is unwise to require *as a matter of law* that a particular species of information be disclosed. We agree with the insight in *Salgo, supra,* 154 Cal. App.2d at page 578, 317 P.2d 170, that in administering the doctrine of informed consent, "each patient presents a separate problem, that the patient's mental and emotional condition is important and in certain cases may be crucial, and that in discussing the element of risk a certain amount of discretion must be employed consistent with the full disclosure of facts necessary to an informed consent."

Our opinion in *Cobbs v. Grant, supra,* . . . recognized these "common practicalities" of medical treatment which, we said, make the ideal of "full disclosure" a "facile expression[ ]." . . . Eschewing both a "mini-course in medical science" and a duty to discuss "the relatively minor risks inherent in common procedures," we identified the touchstone of the physician's duty of disclosure in the patient's need for "adequate information to enable an intelligent choice," a peculiarly fact-bound assessment which juries are especially well-suited to make. . . .

This sensitivity to context seems all the more appropriate in the case of life expectancy projections for cancer patients based on statistical samples. Without exception, the testimony of every physician-witness at trial confirmed what is evident even to a nonprofessional: statistical morbidity values derived from the experience of population groups are inherently unreliable and offer little assurance regarding the fate of the individual patient; indeed, to assume that such data are conclusive in themselves smacks of a refusal to explore treatment alternatives and the medical abdication of the patient's well-being. Certainly the jury here heard evidence of articulable grounds for the conclusion that the particular features of Mr. Arato's case distinguished it from the typical population of pancreatic cancer sufferers and their dismal statistical probabilities—a fact plaintiffs [implicitly] acknowledged at trial in conceding that the oncologic referral of Mr. Arato and ensuing chemotherapy were not in themselves medically negligent.

In declining to endorse the mandatory disclosure of life expectancy probabilities, we do not mean to signal a retreat from the patient-based standard of disclosure explicitly adopted in *Cobbs v. Grant.* . . . We reaffirm the view taken in *Cobbs*

that, because the "weighing of these risks [i.e., those inherent in a proposed procedure] against the individual subjective fears and hopes of the patient is not an expert skill," the test "for determining whether a potential peril must be divulged is its materiality to the patient's decision." . . . In reaffirming the appropriateness of that standard, we can conceive of no trier of fact more suitable than lay jurors to pronounce judgment on those uniquely human and necessarily situational ingredients that contribute to a specific doctor-patient exchange of information relevant to treatment decisions; certainly this is not territory in which appellate courts can usefully issue "bright line" guides.

Rather than mandate the disclosure of specific information as a matter of law, the better rule is to instruct the jury that a physician is under a legal duty to disclose to the patient all material information—that is, "information which the physician knows or should know would be regarded as significant by a reasonable person in the patient's position when deciding to accept or reject a recommended medical procedure"—needed to make an informed decision regarding a proposed treatment. That, of course, is the formulation embodied in BAJI No. 6.11 and the instruction given in this case. Having been properly instructed, the jury returned a defense verdict—on a form approved by plaintiffs' counsel—specifically finding that defendants had "disclosed to Mr. Arato all relevant information which would have enabled him to make an informed decision regarding the proposed treatment to be rendered him."

We decline to intrude further, either on the subtleties of the physician-patient relationship or in the resolution of claims that the physician's duty of disclosure was breached, by requiring the disclosure of information that may or may not be indicated in a given treatment context. Instead, we leave the ultimate judgment as to the factual adequacy of a challenged disclosure to the venerable American jury, operating under legal instructions such as those given here and subject to the persuasive force of trial advocacy.

Here, the evidence was more than sufficient to support the jury's finding that defendants had reasonably disclosed to Mr. Arato information material to his decision whether to undergo the proposed chemotherapy/radiation treatment. There was testimony that Mr. and Mrs. Arato were informed that cancer of the pancreas is usually fatal; of the substantial risk of recurrence, an event that would mean his illness was incurable; of the unproven nature of the F.A.M. treatments and their principal side effects; and of the option of forgoing such treatments. Mr. Arato's doctors also testified that they could not with confidence predict how long the patient might live, notwithstanding statistical mortality tables.

In addition, the jury heard testimony regarding the patient's apparent avoidance of issues bearing upon mortality; Mrs. Arato's testimony that his physicians had assured her husband that he was "clear" of cancer; and the couple's common expectation that he had been "cured," only to learn, suddenly and unexpectedly, that the case was hopeless and life measurable in weeks. The informed consent instructions given the jury to assess this evidence were an accurate statement of the law, and the Court of Appeal in effect invaded the province of the trier of fact in overturning a fairly litigated verdict.

C

In addition to their claim that his physicians were required to disclose statistical life expectancy data to Mr. Arato to enable him to reach an informed treatment decision, plaintiffs also contend that defendants should have disclosed such data because it was material to the patient's *nonmedical* interests, that is, Mr. Arato's business and investment affairs and the potential adverse impact of his death upon them. . . . Plaintiffs contend that since Mr. Arato's contracting and real estate affairs would suffer if he failed to make timely changes in estate planning in contemplation of imminent death, and since these matters are among "his rights and interests," his physicians were under a legal duty to disclose all material facts that might affect them, including statistical life expectancy information. We reject the claim as one founded on a premise that is not recognized in California.

The short answer to plaintiffs' claim is our statement in *Moore, supra,* . . . that a "physician is not the patient's financial adviser." . . . From its inception, the rationale behind the disclosure requirement implementing the doctrine of informed con-

sent has been to protect the patient's freedom to "exercise . . . control over [one's] own body" by directing the course of *medical treatment*. . . . Although an aspect of personal autonomy, the conditions for the exercise of the patient's right of self-decision presuppose a therapeutic focus, a supposition reflected in the text of BAJI No. 6.11 itself. The fact that a physician has "fiducial" obligations which, as the result in *Bowman* illustrates, prohibit misrepresenting the nature of the patient's medical condition, does not mean that he or she is under a duty, the scope of which is undefined, to desclose every contingency that might affect the patient's *nonmedical* "rights and interests." Because plaintiffs' open-ended proposed instruction—that the physician's duty embraces the "disclosure . . . of all facts which materially affect the patient's rights and interests"—failed to reflect the therapeutic limitation inherent in the doctrine of informed consent, it would have been error for the trial judge to give it to the jury.

Finally, plaintiffs make much of the fact that in his initial visit to Dr. Avedon's office, Mr. Arato indicated in a lengthy form he was requested to complete that he "wish[ed] to be told the truth about [his] condition." In effect, they contend that as a result of Mr. Arato's affirmative answer, defendants had an absolute duty to make specific life expectancy disclosures to him. Whether the patient has filled out a questionnaire indicating that he or she wishes to be told the "truth" about his or her condition or not, however, a physician is under a legal duty to obtain the patient's informed consent to any recommended treatment. Although a patient may validly waive the right to be informed, we do not see how a request to be told the "truth" in itself heightens the duty of disclosure imposed on physicians as a matter of law.

III.

The final issue we must resolve concerns the use of expert testimony at trial. As noted, the Court of Appeal concluded that expert testimony offered on behalf of defendants went beyond what was appropriate in support of the so-called "therapeutic exception" to the physician's duty of disclosure, misleading the jury and prejudicing plaintiffs' case. Resolution of this issue requires an understanding of the proper, albeit limited, role of expert testimony in informed consent cases.

Over plaintiffs' objection, the trial court admitted the testimony of two medical experts, Drs. Plotkin and Wellisch, the former a professor of clinical medicine and the latter and expert in the psychological management of cancer patients. Both testified that the standard of medical practice cautioned against disclosing to pancreatic cancer patients specific life expectancy data unless the patient directly requested such information and that, in effect, defendants complied with that standard in not disclosing such information to Mr. Arato under the circumstances. Plaintiffs offered expert medical testimony of their own to counter this evidence; their expert testified that there are a number of indirect and compassionate ways to approach the issue of imminent mortality in dealing with patients with terminal cancer and that the standard of professional practice required that a patient in Mr. Arato's circumstances be given specific numerical life expectancy information.

Plaintiffs now complain that it was error for the trial court to admit expert defense testimony, relying on our statement in *Cobbs v. Grant, supra,* . . . that the weighing of the risks accompanying a given therapy "against the individual subjective fears and hopes of the patient is not an expert skill." Plaintiffs fail to distinguish between the two kinds of physician disclosure discussed in *Cobbs.* Our formulation of the scope of the duty of disclosure encompassed "the potential of death or serious harm" known to be inherent in a given procedure and an explanation "in lay terms [of] the complications that might possibly occur." . . . In addition to these disclosures, which we termed the "minimal" ones required of a physician to ensure the patient's informed decisionmaking, we said that the physician must also reveal to the patient "such additional information as a skilled practitioner of good standing would provide under similar circumstances." . . .

As its verbatim presence in BAJI No. 6.11 testifies, the quoted language, including the reference to the standard of professional practice as the benchmark for measuring the scope of disclosure beyond that implicated by the risks of death or serious harm and the potential for complications, has become an integral part of the legal standard in California for measuring the adequacy of a physician's disclosure in informed consent cases.

In reckoning the scope of disclosure, the physician will for the most part be guided by the patient's decisional needs—or, as we said in *Cobbs v. Grant, supra,* "the test for determining whether a potential peril must be divulged is its materiality to the patient's decision." . . . A physician, however, evaluates the patient's decisional needs against a background of professional understanding that includes a knowledge of what information beyond the significant risks associated with a given treatment would be regarded by the medical community as appropriate for disclosure under the circumstances.

It is thus evident that under the formulation we adopted in *Cobbs v. Grant, supra,* . . . situations will sometimes arise in which the trier of fact is unable to decide the ultimate issue of the adequacy of a particular disclosure without an understanding of the standard of practice within the relevant medical community. For that reason, in an appropriate case, the testimony of medical experts qualified to offer an opinion regarding what, if any, disclosures—in addition to those relating to *the risk of death or serious injury and significant potential complications posed by consenting to or declining a proposed treatment*—would be made to the patient by a skilled practitioner in the relevant medical community under the circumstances is relevant and admissible. . . .

Because statistical life expectancy data is information that lies outside the significant risks associated with a given treatment, the disclosure of which is mandated by *Cobbs v. Grant, supra,* . . . it falls within the scope of the "additional information . . . a skilled practitioner . . . would provide" language of *Cobbs.* . . . And since the question of whether a physician should disclose such information turns on the standard of practice within the medical community, the trial court did not err in permitting expert testimony directed at that issue.

CONCLUSION

The judgment of the Court of Appeal is reversed and the cause is remanded with directions to affirm the judgment of the trial court.

LUCAS, C.J., and MOSK, PANELLI, KENNARD, BAXTER and GEORGE, JJ., concur.

NOTES

1. Around this time—on March 12, 1981, according to the record— an article appeared in the Los Angeles Times stating that only 1 percent of males and 2 percent of females diagnosed as having pancreatic cancer live for five years. According to his wife's testimony, Mr. Arato read the Times article and brought it to the attention of his oncologists. One of his oncologists confirmed such a discussion but denied that he told Mr. Arato that the statistics did not apply to his case, as Mrs. Arato testified. Mr. Arato continued to undergo chemotherapy treatment after reading the article and evidently made no changes in his estate planning or business and real estate affairs.

2. The trial judge read to the jury the following instruction:

"Except as hereinafter explained, it is the duty of the physician to disclose to the patient all material information to enable the patient to make an informed decision regarding proposed treatment. [¶] Material information is information which the physician knows or should know would be regarded as significant by a reasonable person in the patient's position when deciding to accept or reject a recommended medical procedure. To be material a fact must also be one which is not commonly appreciated. [¶] A physician has no duty of disclosure beyond that required of physician of good standing in the same or similar locality when he or she relied upon facts which would demonstrate to a reasonable person that the disclosure would so seriously upset the patient that the patient would not have been able to rationally weigh the risks of refusing to undergo the recommended treatment. [¶] Even though the patient has consented to a proposed treatment or operation, the failure of the physician to inform the patient as stated in this instruction before obtaining such consent is negligence and renders the physician subject to liability for any damage legally resulting from the failure to disclose or for any injury legally resulting from the treatment if a reasonably prudent person in the patient's position would not have con-

sented to the treatment if he or she had been adequately informed of the likelihood of his [sic] premature death."

3. As modified, the following two instructions requested by plaintiffs were read to the jury:

"The law recognizes that patients are generally persons unlearned in the medical sciences and that the knowledge of the patient and physician are not in parity.

"The law recognizes that a person of adult years and in sound mind has the right, in the exercise of control over his own body, to determine whether or not to submit to lawful medical treatment."

The following instruction, modified by the trial court, was given at defendants' request:

"The doctrine of informed consent imposes upon a physician a duty to disclose relevant information concerning a proposed treatment. However, the doctrine recognizes that the primary duty of a physician is to do what is best for his patient."

4. Influential contemporaneous decisions of other courts include *Canterbury v. Spence* (D.C.Cir. 1972) 464 F.2d 772 and *Natanson v. Kline* (1960) 186 Kan. 393, 350 P.2d 1093, as well as the much earlier but still powerful opinion by Judge Cardozo in *Schloendorff v. Society of New York Hospital* (1914) 211 N.Y. 125, 105 N.E. 92. The origin of the phrase "informed consent" is often attributed to the opinion by Justice Bray in *Salgo v. Leland Stanford etc. Bd. Trustees* (1957) 154 Cal.App.2d 560, 578, 317 P.2d 170 (*Salgo*). (See, e.g., Katz, *Informed Consent—A Fairy Tale? Law's Vision* (1977) 39 U.Pitt.L.Rev. 137.) We recently traced the origin and development of the doctrine in American law in *Thor v. Superior Court* (1993) 5 Cal.4th 725, 21 Cal. Rptr.2d 357, 855 P.2d 375.

5. According to the report of the Presidential Commission (see, *ante,* fn. 6) a survey conducted in 1961 by the Journal of the American Medical Association found that 90 percent of physicians preferred not to inform patients of a diagnosis of cancer; in a follow-up study conducted in 1977, 97 percent of the physicians surveyed said they routinely disclosed cancer diagnoses to patients. (1 Making Health Care Decisions, supra, p. 76, fn. 14.)

Antihypertensives and the Risk of Temporary Impotence: A Case Study in Informed Consent

John D. Arras

Dr. Sylvia Kramer pondered what she would tell Robert Williams on his next visit to her primary care clinic. Mr. Williams was an affable 40-year-old African-American, and one of Dr. Kramer's favorite patients. He had recently remarried, and enjoyed telling his doctor about his two young stepdaughters. The problem that brought him to this inner-city clinic was high blood pressure, which was first diagnosed by Dr. Kramer a year ago, during her first year as a resident in family medicine. Mr. Williams's blood pressure had then measured 180/103: not frightening numbers, to be sure, but still very much on the high side of "mild hypertension." If his blood pressure were not lowered, Mr. Williams could anticipate some serious related health problems, such as an increased risk of stroke.

Dr. Kramer's initial recommendation to Mr. Williams was that he attempt to control his weight and blood pressure through a regimen of regular exercise and a sensible diet low in salt and fat. She had recalled one of her mentor's lectures on hypertension: "No need to burden your patients with expensive drugs with side effects when they can solve the problem on their own through good behavior." Although Mr. Williams had achieved some lowering of his blood pressure during the ensuing months, down to 160/95, this improvement still left him in the marginal zone and was, in any case, short-lived. His blood-pressure readings were now consistently elevated. On his last visit, he had expressed some frustration to Dr. Kramer that, try as he might, no amount of exercise or diet seemed to be working.

Given Mr. Williams's lack of progress, Dr. Kramer was considering prescribing a common diuretic, hydrochlorothiazide, as the second line of defense against his hypertension. This particular drug, she knew, has a long history as a cheap and highly effective remedy. The price tag, 5 cents per pill, was particularly attractive to Dr. Kramer, who realized that her clinic

patients often had a hard time paying for some of the more "high-tech" and high-priced hypertension medications that had been flooding the market in recent years.

Notwithstanding its relative safety, efficacy, and affordability, this particular drug still posed problems. First, it had a tendency to leech potassium from the body. She could address that problem by prescribing bananas. The second problem, a more serious matter, was a risk of causing impotence in males. The risk was small, however: only about 3 to 5 percent of men who took the pill were likely to be affected, and the impotence was easily reversible. One simply had to stop taking the drug for this side effect to disappear.

Dr. Kramer pondered the question of what "informed consent" should mean in this situation. In particular, she wondered whether she had an obligation to inform Mr. Williams of the risk of temporary impotence when recommending that he start with this diuretic. While this risk was certainly a lot less worrisome than the remote possibility of death attendant upon many medical and surgical procedures, it was still significant. If Mr. Williams, a newlywed, were to experience an unexpected and unexplained episode of sexual dysfunction, he would no doubt be extremely upset and anxious about it. Dr. Kramer, the product of a family-medicine training program committed to the value of patient self-determination, initially felt that she should share all the risks that Mr. Williams would likely consider relevant to his decision. Cost was certainly a factor, but so was his sex life. He should have the right, she reasoned, to make his own trade-offs among competing values. If sexual dysfunction is high on his list of things to avoid, especially at this time in his marriage, he might be willing to pay extra for another drug.

Still somewhat uncomfortable with her conclusion, Dr. Kramer asked the advice of Dr. Robert Black, a senior physician in her program. Dr. Black registered total disbelief upon hearing the resident's plan of action. "Look," he said, "I'm a staunch supporter of patients' rights, autonomy, and all that, but this is just ridiculous. The risk is quite low, entirely reversible, and consider this: if you share this possible side effect with your patient, this

This case study has benefited from helpful discussions with my brother, Ernest Arras, M.D., and from the careful scrutiny of several physician-colleagues at Montefiore Medical Center, including Michael Alderman, Ellen Cohen, Tom McGinn, and Doug Shenson.

little bit of truth is likely to make him extremely anxious about what could happen. You've heard of the Hawthorne effect, haven't you? Telling him about the risk of impotence could actually make Mr. Williams so worried that he would become impotent at your suggestion. I've been practicing medicine for fifteen years, and I've never told a patient about this sort of thing beforehand. If Mr. Williams comes back to you in a couple of weeks complaining about his sex life, you can deal with it then. But in the meantime, don't make a counterproductive fetish of informed consent. Lighten up!"

At this point, Dr. Kramer was truly puzzled. If she were to be entirely honest with her patient, she might end up doing him harm, and all for a very remote and reversible risk. On the other hand, it still bothered her to hide a fact from her patient that she suspected he would consider sig-

nificant. He was, moreover, a rather shy man, especially about sexual matters. Dr. Kramer was not entirely confident that, should a problem develop, Mr. Williams would feel comfortable talking with a young female physician about his sexual "failure." He might just conclude that it was his or his new wife's fault, not the result of the drug, and live with impaired sexual function for some time.

How should Dr. Kramer resolve her ethical conflict? Should she (a) have a serious discussion with Mr. Williams about the small risk of temporary impotence, (b) casually mention the risk, perhaps using medical jargon, but only in passing along with many other minor risks, (c) withhold information about this particular risk until the patient complained of sexual dysfunction, or (d) withhold the information at first, but inquire specifically at a later date about the patient's sex life?

Informed Consent — Must It Remain a Fairy Tale?*

Jay Katz

I. THE PRE-HISTORY OF INFORMED CONSENT IN MEDICINE

The idea that, prior to any medical intervention, physicians must seek their patients' informed consent was introduced into American law in a brief paragraph in a 1957 state court decision,[1] and then elaborated on in a lengthier opinion in 1960.[2] The emerging legal idea that physicians were from now on obligated to share decisionmaking authority with their patients shocked the medical community, for it constituted a radical break with the silence that had been the hallmark of physician-patient interactions throughout the ages. Thirty-five years are perhaps not long enough for either law or medicine to resolve the tension between legal theory and medical practice, particularly since judges were reluctant to face up to implications of their novel doctrine, preferring instead to remain quite deferential to the practices of the medical profession.

Viewed from the perspective of medical history, the doctrine of informed consent, if taken seriously, constitutes a revolutionary break with customary practice. Thus, I must review, albeit all too briefly, the history of doctor-patient communication. Only then can one appreciate how unprepared the medical profession was to heed these new legal commands. But there is more: Physicians could not easily reject what law had begun to impose on them, because they recognized intuitively that the radical transformation of medicine since the age of medical science made it possible, indeed imperative, for a doctrine of informed consent to emerge. Yet, bowing to the doctrine did not mean accepting it. Indeed, physicians could not accept it because, for reasons I shall soon explore, the nature of informed consent has remained in the words of Churchill, "an enigma wrapped in a mystery."

Throughout the ages physicians believed that they should make treatment decisions for their patients. This conviction inheres in the Hippocratic

From *Journal of Contemporary Health Law and Policy*, Vol. 10–67. Used with permission. Deletions approved by the author.

*EDITORS' NOTE: Space limitations have forced us to cut several sections of this article. Many footnotes have been deleted, and the remainder have been renumbered.

Oath: "I swear by Apollo and Aesculepius [that] I will follow that system of regimen which according to *my* ability and judgment *I* consider for the benefit of *my* patients. . . ."[3] The patient is not mentioned as a person whose ability and judgment deserve consideration. Indeed, in one of the few references to disclosure in the Hippocratic Corpus, physicians are admonished "to [conceal] most things from the patient while attending to him; [to] give necessary orders with cheerfulness and serenity, . . . revealing nothing of the patient's future or present condition."[4] When twenty-five centuries later, in 1847, the American Medical Association promulgated its first Code of Ethics, it equally admonished patients that their "obedience . . . to the prescriptions of [their] physician should be prompt and implicit. [They] should never permit (their) own crude opinions . . . to influence [their] attention to [their physicians]."[5]

The gulf separating doctors from patients seemed unbridgeable both medically and socially. Thus, whenever the Code did not refer to physicians and patients as such, the former were addressed as "gentlemen" and the latter as "fellow creatures." To be sure, caring for patients' medical needs and "abstain[ing] from whatever is deleterious and mischievous"[6] was deeply imbedded in the ethos of Hippocratic medicine. The idea that patients were also "autonomous" human beings, entitled to being partners in decisionmaking, was, until recently, rarely given recognition in the lexicon of medical ethics. The notion that human beings possess individual human rights, deserving of respect, of course, is of recent origin. Yet, it antedates the twentieth century and therefore could have had an impact on the nature and quality of the physician-patient relationship.

It did not. Instead, the conviction that physicians should decide what is best for their patients, and, therefore, that the authority and power to do so should remain vested in them, continued to have a deep hold on the practices of the medical profession. For example, in the early 1950s the influential Harvard sociologist Talcott Parsons, who echoed physicians' views, stated that the physician is a technically competent person whose competence and specific judgments and measures cannot be competently judged by the layman and that the latter must take doctors' judgments and measures on 'authority.'[7] The

necessity for such authority was supported by three claims:

First, *physicians' esoteric knowledge, acquired in the course of arduous training and practical experience, cannot be comprehended by patients.* While it is true that this knowledge, in its totality, is difficult to learn, understand and master, it does not necessarily follow that physicians cannot translate their esoteric knowledge into language that comports with patients' experiences and life goals (i.e., into language that speaks to quality of future life, expressed in words of risks, benefits, alternatives and uncertainties). Perhaps patients can understand this, but physicians have had too little training and experience with, or even more importantly, a commitment to, communicating their "esoteric knowledge" to patients in plain language to permit a conclusive answer as to what patients may comprehend.

Second, *patients, because of their anxieties over being ill and consequent regression to childlike thinking, are incapable of making decisions on their own behalf.* We do not know whether the childlike behavior often displayed by patients is triggered by pain, fear, and illness, or by physicians' authoritarian insistence that good patients comply with doctors' orders, or by doctors' unwillingness to share information with patients. Without providing such information, patients are groping in the dark and their stumbling attempts to ask questions, if made at all, makes them appear more incapable of understanding than they truly are.

We know all too little about the relative contributions which being ill, being kept ignorant, or being considered incompetent make to these regressive manifestations. Thus, physicians' unexamined convictions easily become self-fulfilling prophesies. For example, Eric Cassell has consistently argued that illness robs patients of autonomy and that only subsequent to the act of healing is autonomy restored.[8] While there is some truth to these contentions, they overlook the extent to which doctors can restore autonomy prior to the act of healing by not treating patients as children but as adults whose capacity for remaining authors of their own fate can be sustained and nourished. Cassell's views are reminiscent of Dostoyevsky's Grand Inquisitor who proclaimed that "at the most fearful moments of life," mankind is in need of "miracle, mystery and authority."[9] While, in this modern age, a person's capacity and right to take responsibility for his or her conduct has been given greater recognition than the Grand Inquisitor was inclined to grant, it still does not extend to patients. In the context of illness, physicians are apt to join the Grand Inquisitor at least to the extent of asserting that, while patients, they can only be comforted through subjugation to miracle, mystery and authority.

Third, *physicians' commitment to altruism is a sufficient safeguard for preventing abuses of their professional authority.* While altruism, as a general professional commitment, has served patients well in their encounters with physicians, the kind of protection it does and does not provide has not been examined in any depth. I shall have more to say about this later on. For now, let me only mention one problem: Altruism can only promise that doctors will try to place their patients' medical needs over their own personal needs. Altruism cannot promise that physicians will know, without inquiry, patients' needs. Put another way, patients and doctors do not necessarily have an identity of interest about matters of health and illness. Of course, both seek restoration of health and cure, and whenever such ends are readily attainable by only one route, their interests indeed may coincide.

In many physician-patient encounters, however, cure has many faces and the means selected affect the nature of cure in decisive ways. Thus, since quality of life is shaped decisively by available treatment options (including no treatment), the objectives of health and cure can be pursued in a variety of ways. Consider, for example, differences in value preferences between doctors and patients about longevity versus quality of remaining life. Without inquiry, one cannot presume identity of interest. As the surgeon Nuland cogently observed: "A doctor's altruism notwithstanding, his agenda and value system are not the same as those of the patient. That is the fallacy in the concept of beneficence so cherished by many physicians."[10]

II. THE AGE OF MEDICAL SCIENCE AND INFORMED CONSENT

During the millennia of medical history, and until the beginning of the twentieth century, physicians could not explain to their patients, or—from the perspective of hindsight—to themselves, which of their treatment recommendations were curative and which were not. To be sure, doctors, by careful bedside observation, tried their level best "to abstain from what is deleterious and mischievous," to help if they could, and to be available for comfort during the hours, days or months of suffering. Doing more curatively, however, only became possible with the advent of the age of medical science. The introduction of scientific reasoning into medicine, aided by the results of carefully conducted research, permitted doctors for the first time to discriminate more aptly between knowledge, ignorance and conjecture in their recommendations for or against treatment. Moreover, the spectacular technological advances in the diagnosis and treatment of disease, spawned by medical science, provided patients and doctors with ever-increasing therapeutic options, each having its own particular benefits and risks.

Thus, for the first time in medical history it is possible, even medically and morally imperative, to give patients a voice in medical decisionmaking. It is possible because knowledge and ignorance can be better specified; it is medically imperative because a variety of treatments are available, each of which can bestow great benefits or inflict grievous harm; it is morally imperative because patients, depending on the lifestyle they wish to lead during and after treatment, must be given a choice.

All this seems self-evident. Yet, the physician-patient relationship—the conversations between the two parties—was not altered with the transformation of medical practice during the twentieth century. Indeed, the silence only deepened once laboratory data were inscribed in charts and not in patients' minds, once machines allowed physicians' eyes to gaze not at patients' faces but at the numbers they displayed, once x-rays and electrocardiograms began to speak for patients' suffering rather than their suffering voices.

What captured the medical imagination and found expression in the education of future physicians, was the promise that before too long the diagnosis of patients' diseases would yield objective, scientific data to the point of becoming algorithms. *Treatment,* however, required subjective data from patients and would be influenced by doctors' subjective judgments. This fact was overlooked in the quest for objectivity. Also overlooked was the possibility that greater scientific understanding of the nature of disease and its treatment facilitated better communication with patients. In that respect contemporary Hippocratic practices remained rooted in the past.

III. THE IMPACT OF LAW

The impetus for change in traditional patterns of communication between doctors and patients came not from medicine but from law. In a 1957 California case,[11] and a 1960 Kansas case,[12] judges were astounded and troubled by these undisputed facts: That without any disclosure of risks, new technologies had been employed which promised great benefits but also exposed patients to formidable and uncontrollable harm. In the California case, a patient suffered a permanent paralysis of his lower extremities subsequent to the injection of a dye, sodium urokan, to locate a block in the abdominal aorta. In the Kansas case, a patient suffered severe injuries from cobalt radiation, administered, instead of conventional x-ray treatment, subsequent to a mastectomy for breast cancer. In the latter case, Justice Schroeder attempted to give greater specifications to the informed consent doctrine, first promulgated in the California decision: "To disclose and explain to the patient, in language as simple as necessary, the nature of the ailment, the nature of the proposed treatment, the probability of success or of alternatives, and perhaps the risks of unfortunate results and unforeseen conditions within the body."[13]

From the perspective of improved doctor-patient communication, or better, shared decision-making, the fault lines inherent in this American legal doctrine are many:

One: The common law judges who promulgated the doctrine restricted their task to articulating new and more stringent standards of liability whenever physicians withheld material information that patients should know, particularly in light of the harm that the spectacular advances in medical technology could inflict. Thus, the doctrine was limited in scope, designed to specify those minimal disclosure obligations that physicians must fulfill to escape *legal* liability for alleged non-disclosures. Moreover, it was shaped and confined by legal assumptions about the objectives of the laws of evidence and negligence, and by economic philosophies as to who should assume the financial burdens for medical injuries sustained by patients.

Even though the judges based the doctrine on "Anglo-American law['s] . . . premise of thorough-going self-determination,"[14] as the Kansas court put it, or on "the root premise . . . fundamental in American jurisprudence that 'every human being of adult years and sound mind has a right to determine what shall be done with his own body,'"[15] as the Circuit Court for the District of Columbia put it in a subsequent opinion, the doctrine was grounded not in battery law (trespass), but in negligence law. The reasons are many. I shall only mention a compelling one: Battery law, based on unauthorized trespass, gives doctors only one defense—that they have made adequate disclosure. Negligence law, on the other hand, permits doctors to invoke many defenses, including "the therapeutic privilege" not to disclose when in their judgment, disclosure may prove harmful to patients' welfare.

[A] recent opinion illustrate[s] the problems identified here.* . . . [T]he Court of Appeals of California, in a ground-breaking opinion, significantly reduced the scope of the therapeutic privilege by requiring that in instances of hopeless prognosis (the most common situation in which the privilege has generally been invoked) the patient be provided with such information by asking, "If not the physician's duty to disclose a terminal illness, then whose?"[16] The duty to disclose prognosis had never before been identified specifically as one of the disclosure obligations in an informed consent opinion.

Thus, the appellate court's ruling constituted an important advance. It established that patients have a right to make decisions not only about the fate of their bodies but about the fate of their lives as well. The California Supreme Court, however, reversed. In doing so, the court made too much of an issue raised by the plaintiffs that led the appellate court to hold that doctors must disclose "statistical life expectancy information."[17] To be sure, disclosure of statistical information is a complex problem, but in focusing on that issue, the supreme court's attention was diverted from a more important new disclosure obligation promulgated by the appellate court: the duty to inform

*EDITOR'S NOTE: The case is Arato v. Avedon, reprinted on p.p. 77–85 of this volume.

patients of their dire prognosis. The supreme court did not comment on that obligation. Indeed, it seemed to reverse the appellate court on this crucial issue by reinforcing the considerable leeway granted physicians to invoke the therapeutic privilege exception to full disclosure: "We decline to intrude further, either on the subtleties of the physician-patient relationship or in the resolution of claims that the physician's duty of disclosure was breached, by requiring the disclosure of information that may or may not be indicated in a given treatment context."[18]

Two: The doctrine of informed consent was not designed to serve as a *medical* blueprint for interactions between physicians and patients. The medical profession still faces the task of fashioning a "doctrine" that comports with its own vision of doctor-patient communication and that is responsive both to the realities of medical practices in an age of science and to the commands of law. . . . Thus, disclosure practices only changed to the extent of physicians disclosing more about the risks of a proposed intervention in order to escape legal liability.

Three: Underlying the legal doctrine there lurks a broader assumption which has neither been given full recognition by judges nor embraced by physicians. The underlying idea is this: That from now on patients and physicians must make decisions jointly, with patients ultimately deciding whether to accede to doctors' recommendations. In *The Cancer Ward*, Solzhenitsyn captured, as only a novelist can, the fears that such an idea engenders. When doctor Ludmilla Afanasyevna was challenged by her patient, Oleg Kostoglotov, about physicians' rights to make unilateral decisions on behalf of patients, Afanasyevna gave a troubled, though unequivocal, answer: "But doctors *are* entitled to the right—doctors above all. Without that right, there'd be no such thing as medicine."[19]

If Afanasyevna is correct, then patients must continue to trust doctors silently. Conversation, to comport with the idea of informed consent, ultimately requires that both parties make decisions jointly and that their views and preferences be treated with respect. Trust, based on blind faith—on passive surrender to oneself or to another—must be distinguished from trust that is earned after having first acknowledged to oneself and

then shared with the other what one knows and does not know about the decision to be made. If all of that had been considered by physicians, they would have appreciated that a new model of doctor-patient communication, that takes informed consent seriously required a radical break with current medical disclosure practice.

Four: The idea of joint decisionmaking is one thing, and its application in practice another. . . . To translate social policy into *medical* policy is an inordinately difficult task. It requires a reassessment of the limits of medical knowledge in the light of medical uncertainty, a reassessment of professional authority to make decisions for patients in light of the consequences of such conduct for the well-being of patients, and a reassessment of the limits of patients' capacities to assume responsibility for choice in the light of their ignorance about medical matters and their anxieties when ill. Turning now to these problems, I wish to highlight that, in the absence of such reassessments, informed consent will remain a charade, and joint decisionmaking will elude us.

IV. BARRIERS TO JOINT DECISIONMAKING

A. MEDICAL UNCERTAINTY

The longer I reflect about doctor-patient decisionmaking, the more convinced I am that in this modern age of medical science, which for the first time permits sharing with patients the uncertainties of diagnosis, treatment, and prognosis, the problem of uncertainty poses the most formidable obstacle to disclosure and consent. By medical uncertainty I mean to convey what the physician Lewis Thomas observed so eloquently, albeit disturbingly:

The only valid piece of scientific truth about which I feel totally confident is that we are profoundly ignorant about nature . . . It is this sudden confrontation with the depth and scope of ignorance that represents the most significant contribution of twentieth-century science to the human intellect. *We are, at last facing up to it.* In earlier times, we either pretended to understand . . . or ignored the problem, or simply made up stories to fill the gap.[20]

Alvan Feinstein put this in more concrete language: "Clinicians are still uncertain about the best means of treatment for even such routine problems as . . . a fractured hip, a peptic ulcer, a stroke, a myocardial infarction. . . . At a time of potent drugs and formidable surgery, the exact effects of many therapeutic procedures are dubious or shrouded in dissension."[21]

Medical uncertainty constitutes a formidable obstacle to joint decisionmaking for a number of reasons: Sharing uncertainties requires physicians to be more aware of them than they commonly are. They must learn how to communicate them to patients and they must shed their embarrassment over acknowledging the true state of their own and of medicine's art and science. Thus, sharing uncertainties requires a willingness to admit ignorance about benefits and risks; to acknowledge the existence of alternatives, each with its own known and unknown consequences; to eschew one single authoritative recommendation; to consider carefully how to present uncertainty so that patients will not be overwhelmed by the information they will receive; and to explore the crucial question of how much uncertainty physicians themselves can tolerate without compromising their effectiveness as healers. . . .

Moreover, acknowledgement of uncertainty is undermined by the threat that it will undermine doctors' authority and sense of superiority. As Nuland put it, to feel superior to those dependent persons who are the sick, is after all a motivating factor that often influences their choice of medicine as a profession.[22] All of this suggests that implementation of the idea of informed consent is, to begin with, not a patient problem but a physician problem.

B. PATIENT INCOMPETENCE

Earlier, I touched on physicians' convictions that illness and medicine's esoteric knowledge rob patients of the capacity to participate in decisionmaking. Yet we do not know whether this is true. The evidence is compromised by the groping, halfhearted, and misleading attempts to inform patients about uncertainty and other matters which can make doctors' communications so confusing and incomprehensible. If patients then appear stupid and ignorant this should come as no surprise; nor should patients' resigned surrender to this dilemma: "You are the doctor, you decide."

It is equally debatable, as Thomas Duffy has contended, that "[p]aternalism exists in medicine . . . to

fulfill a need created by illness."[23] It led him to argue, echoing Cassell, that "obviously autonomy cannot function as the cornerstone of the doctor-patient relationship [since] the impact of disease on personal integrity results in the patient's loss of autonomy. . . . In the doctor-patient relationship, the medical profession should always err on the side of beneficence."[24] If Duffy is correct, however, then informed consent is *ab initio* fatally compromised.

C. PATIENT AUTONOMY

Duffy's invocation of beneficence as the guiding principle is deeply rooted in the history of Hippocratic medicine. It finds expression in the ancient maxim: *primum non nocere*, above all do no harm, with "harm" remaining undefined but in practice being defined only as physical harm. Before presenting my views on the controversy over the primacy of autonomy or beneficence, let me briefly define their meaning.

In their authoritative book *Principles of Biomedical Ethics*, Thomas Beauchamp and James Childress defined these principles:

> Autonomy is a form of personal liberty of action where the individual determines his or her own course of action in accordance with a plan chosen by himself or herself. [Respect for individuals as autonomous agents entitles them] to such autonomous determinations without limitation on their liberty being imposed by others.[25]

Beneficence, on the other hand,

> [r]equires not only that we treat persons autonomously and that we refrain from harming them, but also that we contribute to their welfare including their health. [Thus the principle asserts] the duty to help others further their important and legitimate interests . . . to *confer* benefits and actively to prevent and remove harms . . . [and] to *balance* possible goods against the possible harms of an action.[26]

Beauchamp and Childress' unequivocal and strong postulate on autonomy contrasts with the ambiguities contained in their postulate on beneficence. What do they mean by "benefits" and "harms" that allow invocation of beneficence? Do they mean only benefits and harms to patients' physical integrity, or to their dignitary integrity as choice-making individuals as well? Furthermore, what degree of discretion and license is permissible in the duty "to balance?" I have problems with balancing unless it is resorted to only as a *rare* exception to respect for autonomy. While human life is, and human interactions are, too complex to make any principle rule absolute, any exceptions must be rigorously justified.

I appreciate that mine is a radical proposal and constitutes a sharp break with Hippocratic practices. If informed consent, however, is ever to be based on the postulate of joint decisionmaking, the obligation "to respect the autonomous choices and actions of others,"[27] as Childress has put it, must be honored. Otherwise, informed consent is reduced to doctors providing more information but leaving decision-making itself to the authority of physicians. . . .

VI. THE CURRENT STATE OF PHYSICIAN-PATIENT DECISION-MAKING

In his recent book, entitled *How We Die*, Sherwin Nuland, a distinguished surgeon, reflects with profundity and insight on his lifelong interactions with patients. In a chapter on cancer and its treatment he speaks movingly about "death belong-[ing] to the dying and to those who love them."[28] Yet, that privilege is often wrested from them when,

> [d]ecisions about continuation of treatment are influenced by the enthusiasm of the doctors who propose them. Commonly, the most accomplished of the specialists are also the most convinced and unyielding believers in biomedicine's ability to overcome the challenge presented by a pathological process. . . . [W]hat is offered as objective clinical reality is often the subjectivity of a devout disciple of the philosophy that death is an implacable enemy. To such warriors, even a temporary victory justifies the laying waste of the fields in which a dying man has cultivated his life.[29]

Looking back at his work, he concludes that "more than a few of my victories have been Pyrrhic. The suffering was sometimes not worth the success. . . . [H]ad I been able to project myself into the place of the family and the patient, I would have been less often certain that the desperate struggle should be undertaken."[30]

In his view, a surgeon,

> [t]hough he be kind and considerate of the patient he treats . . . allows himself to push his kindness aside because the seduction of The Riddle [the quest for diagnosis and cure] is so strong and the failure to solve it renders him so weak. [Thus, at times he convinces] patients to undergo diagnostic or therapeutic measures at a point in illness so far beyond reason that The Riddle might better have remained unsolved.[31]

Speaking then about the kind of doctor he will seek out when afflicted with a major illness, Nuland does not expect him to "understand my values, my expectations for myself . . . my philosophy of life. *That is not what he is trained for and that is not what he will be good at.*"[32] Doctors can impart information, but "[i]t behooves every patient to study his or her own disease and learn enough about it. [Patients] should no longer expect from so many of our doctors what they cannot give."[33]

Nuland's views, supported by a great many poignant clinical vignettes, sensitively and forthrightly describe the current state of physician-patient decisionmaking, so dominated by physicians' judgments as to what is best. He presents many reasons for this state of affairs. One is based on doctors' "fear of failure:"

> A need to control that exceeds in magnitude what most people would find reasonable. When control is lost, he who requires it is also a bit lost and so deals badly with the consequences of his impotence. In an attempt to maintain control, a doctor, usually without being aware of it, convinces himself that he knows better than the patient what course is proper. He dispenses only as much information as he deems fit, thereby influencing a patient's decision-making in ways he does not recognize as self-serving. [34]

I have presented Nuland's observations at some length because they illustrate and support my contentions that joint decisionmaking between doctors and patients still eludes us. My critics had claimed earlier that my work on informed consent was dated because informed consent had become an integral aspect of the practice of medicine. In the paperback edition of *The Silent World of Doctor and Patient*, I argued that they have dismissed too lightly my central arguments:

[T]hat meaningful collaboration between physicians and patients cannot become a reality until physicians have learned (1) how to treat their patients not as children but as the adults they are; (2) how to distinguish between their ideas of the best treatment and their patients' ideas of what is best; (3) how to acknowledge to their patients (and often to themselves as well) their ignorance and uncertainties about diagnosis, treatment, and prognosis; [and to all this, I now want to add, (4) how to explain to patients the uncertainties inherent in the state of the art and science of medicine which otherwise permits doctors on the basis of their clinical experience to leave unacknowledged that their colleagues on the basis of their clinical experience have different beliefs as to which treatment is best].[35] . . .

The moral authority of physicians will not be undermined by this caring view of interacting with patients. Doctors' authority resides in the medical knowledge they possess, in their capacity to diagnose and treat, in their ability to evaluate what can be diagnosed and what cannot, what is treatable and what is not, and what treatment alternatives to recommend, each with its own risks and benefits and each with its own prognostic implications as to cure, control, morbidity, exacerbation or even death.

The moral authority of physicians resides in knowing better than others the certainties and the uncertainties that accompany diagnosis, treatment, prognosis, health and disease, as well the extent and the limits of their *scientific* knowledge and *scientific* ignorance. Physicians must learn to face up to and acknowledge the tragic limitations of their own professional knowledge, their inability to impart all their insights to all patients, and their own personal incapacities—at times more pronounced than others—to devote themselves fully to the needs of their patients. They must learn not to be unduly embarrassed by their personal and professional ignorance and to trust their patients to react appropriately to such acknowledgment. From all this it follows that ultimately the moral authority of physicians resides in their capacity to sort out *with* patients the choices to be made.

It is in this spirit that duty and caring become interwoven. Bringing these strands together imposes upon physicians the duty to respect patients as persons so that care will encompass allowing patients to live their lives in their own self-willed ways. To let patients follow their own lights is not an abandonment of them. It is a professional duty that, however painful, doctors must obey.

Without fidelity to these new professional duties, true caring will elude physicians. There is much new to be learned about caring that in decades to come will constitute the kind of caring that doctors in the past have wished for but have been unable to dispense, and that patients may have always yearned for. . . .

NOTES

1. Salgo v. Leland Stanford Jr. Univ. Bd. of Trustees, 317 P.2d 170, 181 (Cal. Dist. Ct. App. 1957).

2. Natanson v. Kline, 350 P.2d 1093 (Kan. 1960).

3. Hippocrates, *Oath of Hippocrates, in* 1 HIPPOCRATES 299-301 (W.H.S. Jones trans., 1962).

4. 2 Hippocrates 297 (W.H.S. Jones trans., 1962).

5. American Medical Association: Code of Ethics (1847), reprinted in Katz, The Silent World of Doctor and Patient 232 (1986).

6. Hippocrates, *supra* note 3, at 301.

7. Talcott Parsons, The Social System 464-65 (1951).

8. Eric Cassell, *The Function of Medicine,* Hastings Center Rep., Dec. 1977, at 16, 18.

9. Fyodor Dostoyevsky, The Brothers Karamazov 307 (A.P. MacAndrew trans., 1970).

10. Interview with Sherwin Nuland (1993).

11. Salgo v. Leland Stanford Jr. Univ. Bd. of Trustees, 317 P.2d 170 (Cal. Dist. Ct. App. 1957).

12. Natanson v. Kline, 350 P.2d 1093 (Kan. 1960).

13. *Id.* at 1106.

14. *Id.* at 1104.

15. Canterbury v. Spence, 464 F.2d 772, 780 (D.C. Cir. 1972).

16. Arato v. Avedon, 11 Cal. Rptr. 2d 169, 181 n.19 (Cal. Ct. App. 1992), *vacated,* 858 P.2d 598 (Cal. 1993).

17. *Arato,* 11 Cal. Rptr. 2d at 177.

18. *Arato,* 858 P.2d at 607.

19. Alexander Solzhenitsyn, The Cancer Ward 77 (N. Bethell & D. Burg trans., 1969).

20. Lewis Thomas, The Medusa and the Snail 73-74 (1979).

21. Alvan R. Feinstein, Clinical Judgment 23-24 (1967). Even though written 27 years ago, he has not changed his views. Interview with Alvan R. Feinstein (1994).

22. Interview with Sherwin B. Nuland (1994).

23. Thomas P. Duffy, *Agamemnon's Fate and the Medical Profession,* 9 W. New Eng. L. Rev. 21, 27 (1987).

24. *Id.* at 30.

25. Thomas L. Beauchamp & James F. Childress, Principles of Biomedical Ethics 56, 58 (1st ed. 1979).
26. Thomas L. Beauchamp & James F. Childress, Principles of Biomedical Ethics 148-49 (2d ed. 1983).
27. James F. Childress, *The Place of Autonomy in Bioethics*, Hastings Center Rep., Jan.-Feb. 1990, at 12, 12-13.
28. Sherwin B. Nuland, How We Die 265 (1994).

29. *Id.*
30. *Id.* at 266.
31. *Id.* at 249.
32. *Id.* at 266 (emphasis added).
33. *Id.* at 260.
34. *Id.* at 258.
35. Jay Katz, *supra* note 5, at xi (1986).

Transparency: Informed Consent in Primary Care

Howard Brody

While the patient's right to give informed consent to medical treatment is now well-established both in U.S. law and in biomedical ethics, evidence continues to suggest that the concept has been poorly integrated into American medical practice, and that in many instances the needs and desires of patients are not being well met by current policies.[1] It appears that the theory and the practice of informed consent are out of joint in some crucial ways. This is particularly true for primary care settings, a context typically ignored by medical ethics literature, but where the majority of doctor-patient encounters occur. Indeed, some have suggested that the concept of informed consent is virtually foreign to primary care medicine where benign paternalism appropriately reigns and where respect for patient autonomy is almost completely absent.[2]

It is worth asking whether current legal standards for informed consent tend to resolve the problem or to exacerbate it. I will maintain that accepted legal standards, at least in the form commonly employed by courts, send physicians the wrong message about what is expected of them. An alternative standard that would send physicians the correct message, a conversation standard, is probably unworkable legally. As an alternative, I will propose a transparency standard as a compromise that gives physicians a doable task and allows courts to review appro-priately. I must begin, however, by briefly identifying some assumptions crucial to the development of this position even though space precludes complete argumentation and documentation.

CRUCIAL ASSUMPTIONS

Informed consent is a meaningful ethical concept only to the extent that it can be realized and promoted within the ongoing practice of good medicine. This need not imply diminished respect for patient autonomy, for there are excellent reasons to regard respect for patient autonomy as a central feature of good medical care. Informed consent, properly understood, must be considered an essential ingredient of good patient care, and a physician who lacks the skills to inform patients appropriately and obtain proper consent should be viewed as lacking essential medical skills necessary for practice. It is not enough to see informed consent as a nonmedical, legalistic exercise designed to promote patient autonomy, one that interrupts the process of medical care.

However, available empirical evidence strongly suggests that this is precisely how physicians currently view informed consent practices. Informed consent is still seen as bureaucratic legalism rather than as part of patient care. Physicians often deny the existence of realistic treatment alternatives, thereby attenuating the perceived need to inform the patient of meaningful options. While patients may be informed, efforts are seldom made to assess

The Hastings Center Report, Vol. 19, No. 5, Sept/Oct 1989, 5–9. Reprinted with permission.

accurately the patient's actual need or desire for information, or what the patient then proceeds to do with the information provided. Physicians typically underestimate patients' desire to be informed and overestimate their desire to be involved in decisionmaking. Physicians may also view informed consent as an empty charade, since they are confident in their abilities to manipulate consent by how they discuss or divulge information.[3]

A third assumption is that there are important differences between the practice of primary care medicine and the tertiary care settings that have been most frequently discussed in the literature on informed consent. The models of informed consent discussed below typically take as the paradigm case something like surgery for breast cancer or the performance of an invasive and risky radiologic procedure. It is assumed that the risks to the patient are significant, and the values placed on alternative forms of treatment are quite weighty. Moreover, it is assumed that the specialist physician performing the procedure probably does a fairly limited number of procedures and thus could be expected to know exhaustively the precise risks, benefits, and alternatives for each.

Primary care medicine, however, fails to fit this model. The primary care physician, instead of performing five or six complicated and risky procedures frequently, may engage in several hundred treatment modalities during an average week of practice. In many cases, risks to the patient are negligible and conflicts over patient values and the goals of treatment or nontreatment are of little consequence. Moreover, in contrast to the tertiary care patient, the typical ambulatory patient is much better able to exercise freedom of choice and somewhat less likely to be intimidated by either the severity of the disease or the expertise of the physician; the opportunities for changing one's mind once treatment has begun are also much greater. Indeed, in primary care, it is much more likely for the full process of informed consent to treatment (such as the beginning and the dose adjustment of an antihypertensive medication) to occur over several office visits rather than at one single point in time.

It might be argued that for all these reasons, the stakes are so low in primary care that it is fully appropriate for informed consent to be interpreted only with regard to the specialized or tertiary care setting. I believe that this is quite incorrect for three reasons. First, good primary care medicine ought to embrace respect for patient autonomy, and if patient autonomy is operationalized in informed consent, properly understood, then it ought to be part and parcel of good primary care. Second, the claim that the primary care physician cannot be expected to obtain the patient's informed consent seems to undermine the idea that informed consent could or ought to be part of the daily practice of medicine. Third, primary care encounters are statistically more common than the highly specialized encounters previously used as models for the concept of informed consent.[4]

ACCEPTED LEGAL STANDARDS

Most of the literature on legal approaches to informed consent addresses the tension between the community practice standard and the reasonable patient standard, with the latter seen as the more satisfactory, emerging legal standard.[5] However, neither standard sends the proper message to the physician about what is expected of her to promote patient autonomy effectively and to serve the informational needs of patients in daily practice.

The community practice standard sends the wrong message because it leaves the door open too wide for physician paternalism. The physician is instructed to behave as other physicians in that specialty behave, regardless of how well or how poorly that behavior serves patients' needs. Certainly, behaving the way other physicians behave is a task we might expect physicians to readily accomplish; unfortunately, the standard fails to inform them of the end toward which the task is aimed.

The reasonable patient standard does a much better job of indicating the centrality of respect for patient autonomy and the desired outcome of the informed consent process, which is revealing the information that a reasonable person would need to make an informed and rational decision. This standard is particularly valuable when modified to include the specific informational and decisional needs of a particular patient.

If certain things were true about the relationship between medicine and law in today's society, the reasonable patient standard would provide acceptable guidance to physicians. One feature would be that physicians esteem the law as a positive force in guiding their practice, rather than as a threat to their well-being that must be handled defensively. Another element would be a prospective consideration by the law of what the physician could reasonably have been expected to do in practice, rather than a retrospective review armed with the foreknowledge that some significant patient harm has already occurred.

Unfortunately, given the present legal climate, the physician is much more likely to get a mixed or an undesirable message from the reasonable patient standard. The message the physician hears from the reasonable patient standard is that one must exhaustively lay out all possible risks as well as benefits and alternatives of the proposed procedure. If one remembers to discuss fifty possible risks, and the patient in a particular case suffers the fifty-first, the physician might subsequently be found liable for incomplete disclosure. Since lawsuits are triggered when patients suffer harm, disclosure of risk becomes relatively more important than disclosure of benefits. Moreover, disclosure of information becomes much more critical than effective patient participation in decisionmaking. Physicians consider it more important to document what they said to the patient than to document how the patient used or thought about that information subsequently.

In specialty practice, many of these concerns can be nicely met by detailed written or videotaped consent documents, which can provide the depth of information required while still putting the benefits and alternatives in proper context. This is workable when one engages in a limited number of procedures and can have a complete document or videotape for each.[6] However, this approach is not feasible for primary care, when the number of procedures may be much more numerous and the time available with each patient may be considerably less. Moreover, it is simply not realistic to expect even the best educated of primary care physicians to rattle off at a moment's notice a detailed list of significant risks attached to any of the many drugs and therapeutic modalities they recommend.

This sets informed consent apart from all other aspects of medical practice in a way that I believe is widely perceived by nonpaternalistic primary care physicians, but which is almost never commented upon in the medical ethics literature. To the physician obtaining informed consent, *you never know when you are finished.* When a primary care physician is told to treat a patient for strep throat or to counsel a person suffering a normal grief reaction from the recent death of a relative, the physician has a good sense of what it means to complete the task at hand. When a physician is told to obtain the patient's informed consent for a medical intervention, the impression is quite different. A list of as many possible risks as can be thought of may still omit some significant ones. A list of all the risks that actually have occurred may still not have dealt with the patient's need to know risks in relation to benefits and alternatives. A description of all benefits, risks, and alternatives may not establish whether the patient has understood the information. If the patient says he understands, the physician has to wonder whether he really understands or whether he is simply saying this to be accommodating. As the law currently *appears* to operate (in the perception of the defensively minded physician), there never comes a point at which you can be certain that you have adequately completed your legal as well as your ethical task.

The point is not simply that physicians are paranoid about the law; more fundamentally, physicians are getting a message that informed consent is very different from any other task they are asked to perform in medicine. If physicians conclude that informed consent is therefore not properly part of medicine at all, but is rather a legalistic and bureaucratic hurdle they must overcome at their own peril, blame cannot be attributed to paternalistic attitudes or lack of respect for patient autonomy.

THE CONVERSATION MODEL

A metaphor employed by Jay Katz, informed consent as conversation, provides an approach to respect for patient autonomy that can be readily integrated within primary care practice.[7] Just as the specific needs of an individual patient for information, or the meaning that patient will attach to the information as it is presented, cannot be known in advance, one cannot always tell in advance how a conversation is going to turn out.

One must follow the process along and take one's cues from the unfolding conversation itself. Despite the absence of any formal rules for carrying out or completing a conversation on a specific subject, most people have a good intuitive grasp of what it means for a conversation to be finished, what it means to change the subject in the middle of a conversation, and what it means to later reopen a conversation one had thought was completed when something new has just arisen. Thus, the metaphor suggests that informed consent consists not in a formal process carried out strictly by protocol but in a conversation designed to encourage patient participation in all medical decisions to the extent that the patient wishes to be included. The idea of informed consent as physician-patient conversation could, when properly developed, be a useful analytic tool for ethical issues in informed consent, and could also be a powerful educational tool for highlighting the skills and attitudes that a physician needs to successfully integrate this process within patient care.

If primary care physicians understand informed consent as this sort of conversation process, the idea that exact rules cannot be given for its successful management could cease to be a mystery. Physicians would instead be guided to rely on their own intuitions and communication skills, with careful attention to information received from the patient, to determine when an adequate job had been done in the informed consent process. Moreover, physicians would be encouraged to see informed consent as a genuinely mutual and participatory process, instead of being reduced to the one-way disclosure of information. In effect, informed consent could be demystified, and located within the context of the everyday relationships between physician and patient, albeit with a renewed emphasis on patient participation.[8]

Unfortunately, the conversation metaphor does not lend itself to ready translation into a legal standard for determining whether or not the physician has satisfied her basic responsibilities to the patient. There seems to be an inherently subjective element to conversation that makes it ill-suited as a legal standard for review of controversial cases. A conversation in which one participates is by its nature a very different thing from the same conversation described to an outsider. It is hard to imagine how a jury could be instructed to determine in retrospect whether or not a particular conversation was adequate for its purposes. However, without the possibility for legal review, the message that patient autonomy is an important value and that patients have important rights within primary care would seem to be severely undermined. The question then is whether some of the important strengths of the conversation model can be retained in another model that does allow better guidance.

THE TRANSPARENCY STANDARD

I propose the transparency standard as a means to operationalize the best features of the conversation model in medical practice. According to this standard, adequate informed consent is obtained when a reasonably informed patient is allowed to participate in the medical decision to the extent that patient wishes. In turn, "reasonably informed" consists of two features: (1) the physician discloses the basis on which the proposed treatment, or alternative possible treatments, have been chosen; and (2) the patient is allowed to ask questions suggested by the disclosure of the physician's reasoning, and those questions are answered to the patient's satisfaction.

According to the transparency model, the key to reasonable disclosure is not adherence to existing standards of other practitioners, nor is it adherence to a list of risks that a hypothetical reasonable patient would want to know. Instead, disclosure is adequate when the physician's basic thinking has been rendered transparent to the patient. If the physician arrives at a recommended therapeutic or diagnostic intervention only after carefully examining a list of risks and benefits, then rendering the physician's thinking transparent requires that those risks and benefits be detailed for the patient. If the physician's thinking has not followed that route but has reached its conclusion by other considerations, then what needs to be disclosed to the patient is accordingly different. Essentially, the transparency standard requires the physician to engage in the typical patient-management thought process, only to *do it out loud in language understandable to the patient.*[9]

To see how this might work in practice, consider the following as possible general decision-making strategies that might be used by a primary physician:

1. The intervention, in addition to being presumably low-risk, is also routine and automatic. The physician, faced with a case like that presented by the patient, almost always chooses this treatment.
2. The decision is not routine but seems to offer clear benefit with minimal risk.
3. The proposed procedure offers substantial chances for benefit, but also very substantial risks.
4. The proposed intervention offers substantial risks and extremely questionable benefits. Unfortunately, possible alternative courses of action also have high risk and uncertain benefit.

The exact risks entailed by treatment loom much larger in the physician's own thinking in cases 3 and 4 than in cases 1 and 2. The transparency standard would require that physicians at least mention the various risks to patients in scenarios 3 and 4, but would not necessarily require physicians exhaustively to describe risks, unless the patient asked, in scenarios 1 and 2.

The transparency standard seems to offer some considerable advantages for informing physicians what can legitimately be expected of them in the promotion of patient autonomy while carrying out the activities of primary care medicine. We would hope that the well-trained primary care physician generally thinks before acting. On that assumption, the physician can be told exactly when she is finished obtaining informed consent—first, she has to share her thinking with the patient; secondly, she has to encourage and answer questions; and third, she has to discover how participatory he wishes to be and facilitate that level of participation. This seems a much more reasonable task within primary care than an exhaustive listing of often irrelevant risk factors.

There are also considerable advantages for the patient in this approach. The patient retains the right to ask for an exhaustive recital of risks and alternatives. However, the vast majority of patients, in a primary care setting particularly, would wish to supplement a standardized recital of risks and benefits of treatment with some ques-

tions like, "Yes, doctor, but what does this really mean for me? What meaning am I supposed to attach to the information that you've just given?" For example, in scenarios 1 and 2, the precise and specific risk probabilities and possibilities are very small considerations in the thinking of the physician, and reciting an exhaustive list of risks would seriously misstate just what the physician was thinking. If the physician did detail a laundry list of risk factors, the patient might very well ask, "Well, doctor, just what should I think about what you have just told me?" and the thoughtful and concerned physician might well reply, "There's certainly a small possibility that one of these bad things will happen to you; but I think the chance is extremely remote and in my own practice I have never seen anything like that occur." The patient is very likely to give much more weight to that statement, putting the risks in perspective, than he is to the listing of risks. And that emphasis corresponds with an understanding of how the physician herself has reached the decision.

The transparency standard should further facilitate and encourage useful questions from patients. If a patient is given a routine list of risks and benefits and then is asked "Do you have any questions?" the response may well be perfunctory and automatic. If the patient is told precisely the grounds on which the physician has made her recommendation, and then asked the same question, the response is much more likely to be individualized and meaningful.

There certainly would be problems in applying the transparency standard in the courtroom, but these do not appear to be materially more difficult than those encountered in applying other standards; moreover, this standard could call attention to more important features in the ethical relationship between physician and patient. Consider the fairly typical case, in which a patient suffers harm from the occurrence of a rare but predictable complication of a procedure, and then claims that he would not have consented had he known about that risk. Under the present "enlightened" court standards, the jury would examine whether a reasonable patient would have needed to know about that risk factor prior to making a decision on the proposed intervention. Under the transparency standard, the question would instead be whether the physician thought about that risk factor as a relevant consideration prior to recommending the course of action to the patient. If the physician did seriously consider that risk factor, but failed to reveal that to the patient, he was in effect making up the patient's mind in advance about what risks were worth accepting. In that situation, the physician could easily be held liable. If, on the other hand, that risk was considered too insignificant to play a role in determining which intervention ought to be performed, the physician may still have rendered his thinking completely transparent to the patient even though that specific risk factor was not mentioned. In this circumstance, the physician would be held to have done an adequate job of disclosing information.[10] A question would still exist as to whether a competent physician ought to have known about that risk factor and ought to have considered it more carefully prior to doing the procedure. But that question raises the issue of negligence, which is where such considerations properly belong, and removes the problem from the context of informed consent. Obviously, the standard of informed consent is misapplied if it is intended by itself to prevent the practice of negligent medicine.

TRANSPARENCY IN MEDICAL PRACTICE

Will adopting a legal standard like transparency change medical practice for the better? Ultimately only empirical research will answer this question. We know almost nothing about the sorts of conversations primary care physicians now have with their patients, or what would happen if these physicians routinely tried harder to share their basic thinking about therapeutic choices. In this setting it is possible to argue that the transparency standard will have deleterious effects. Perhaps the physician's basic thinking will fail to include risk issues that patients, from their perspective, would regard as substantial. Perhaps how physicians think about therapeutic choice will prove to be too idiosyncratic and variable to serve as any sort of standard. Perhaps disclosing basic thinking processes will impede rather than promote optimal patient participation in decisions.

But the transparency standard must be judged, not only against ideal medical practice, but also against the present-day standard and the message it sends to practitioners. I have argued that that message is, "You can protect yourself legally only by guessing all bad outcomes that might occur and warning each patient explicitly that he might suffer any of them." The transparency standard is an attempt to send the message, "You can protect yourself legally by conversing with your patients in a way that promotes their participation in medical decisions, and more specifically by making sure that they see the basic reasoning you used to arrive at the recommended treatment." It seems at least plausible to me that the attempt is worth making.

The reasonable person standard may still be the best way to view informed consent in highly specialized settings where a relatively small number of discrete and potentially risky procedures are the daily order of business. In primary settings, the best ethical advice we can give physicians is to view informed consent as an ongoing process of conversation designed to maximize patient participation after adequately revealing the key facts. Because the conversation metaphor does not by itself suggest measures for later judicial review, a transparency standard, or something like it, may be a reasonable way to operationalize that concept in primary care practice. Some positive side-effects of this might be more focus on good diagnostic and therapeutic decisionmaking on the physician's part, since it will be understood that the patient will be made aware of what the physician's reasoning process has been like, and better documentation of management decisions in the patient record. If these occur, then it will be clearer that the standard of informed consent has promoted rather than impeded high quality patient care.

REFERENCES

1. Charles W. Lidz *et al.*, "Barriers to Informed Consent," *Annals of Internal Medicine* 99:4 (1983), 539-43.

2. Tom L. Beauchamp and Laurence McCullough, *Medical Ethics: The Moral Responsibilities of Physicians* (Englewood Cliffs, NJ: Prentice-Hall, 1984).

3. For a concise overview of empirical data about contemporary informed consent practices see Ruth R. Faden and Tom L. Beauchamp, *A History and Theory of Informed Consent* (New York: Oxford University Press, 1986), 98-99 and associated footnotes.

4. For efforts to address ethical aspects of primary care practice, see Ronald J. Christie and Barry Hoffmaster, *Ethical Issues in Family Medicine* (New York: Oxford University Press, 1986); and Harmon L. Smith and Larry R. Churchill, *Professional Ethics and Primary Care Medicine* (Durham, NC: Duke University Press, 1986).

5. Faden and Beauchamp, *A History and Theory of Informed Consent*, 23-49 and 114-50. I have also greatly benefited from an unpublished paper by Margaret Wallace.

6. For a specialty opinion to the contrary, see W. H. Coles *et al.,* "Teaching Informed Consent," in *Further Developments in Assessing Clinical Competence,* Ian R. Hart and Ronald M. Harden, eds. (Montreal: Can-Heal Publications, 1987), 241-70. This paper is interesting in applying to special-ty care a model very much like the one I propose for primary care.

7. Jay Katz, *The Silent World of Doctor and Patient* (New York: Free Press, 1984).

8. Howard Brody, *Stories of Sickness* (New Haven: Yale University Press, 1987), 171-181.

9. For an interesting study of physicians' practices on this point, see William C. Wu and Robert A. Pearlman, "Consent in Medical Decisionmaking: The Role of Communication," *Journal of General Internal Medicine* 3:1 (1988), 9-14.

10. A court case that might point the way toward this line of reasoning is *Precourt v. Frederick,* 395 Mass. 689 (1985). See William J. Curran, "Informed Consent in Malpractice Cases: A Turn Toward Reality," *New England Journal of Medicine* 314:7 (1986), 429-31.

SECTION 3

Professional Responsibilities: Conflicts of Interest in Managed Care

The Doctor's Master

Norman Levinsky

There is increasing pressure on doctors to serve two masters. Physicians in practice are being enjoined to consider society's needs, as well as each patient's needs, in deciding what type and amount of medical care to deliver. Not surprisingly, many government leaders and health planners take this position. More remarkably, important elements of the medical profession are promoting this view.

I would argue the contrary, that physicians are required to do everything that they believe may benefit each patient without regard to costs or other societal considerations. In caring for an individual patient, the doctor must act solely as that patient's advocate, against the apparent interests of society as a whole, if necessary. An analogy can be drawn with the role of a lawyer defending a client against a criminal charge. The attorney is obligated to use all ethical means to defend the client, regardless of the cost of prolonged legal proceedings or even of the possibility that a guilty person may be acquitted through skillful advocacy. Similarly, in the practice of medicine, physicians are obligated to do all that they can for their patients without regard to any costs to society.

Society benefits if it expects its medical practitioners to follow this principle. As Fried[1] has elo-

From *New England Journal of Medicine* 311, no. 24, December 13, 1984: 1573–1575. Reprinted by permission of the publisher. Copyright © 1984 Massachusetts Medical Society.

quently argued, in any decent, advanced society there are rights in health care, in that "one is entitled to be treated decently, humanely, personally and honestly in the course of medical care. . . ." In such a just society, "the physician who withholds care that it is in his power to give because he judges it is wasteful to provide it to a particular person breaks faith with his patient." A similar position has been stated by Hiatt[2]: "A physician or other provider must do all that is permitted on behalf of his patient. . . . The patient and the physician want no less, and society should settle for no less." A just society must have a group of professionals whose sole responsibility as health-care practitioners is to their patients as individuals.

The issue is not whether physicians must do everything technically possible for each patient. Rather it is that they should decide how much to do according to what they believe best for that patient, without regard for what is best for society or what it costs. I do not argue, as some have[3], that doctors are obligated to prolong life under all circumstances or that they are required to use their expertise to confer technological immortality on dehumanized bodies. Actual practice is infinitely complex and varied. Caring and experienced doctors will differ about what to do in individual cases. In my opinion, ethical physicians may discontinue life-extending treatment if their decisions are based solely on what they and the patient or his or her surrogate believe to be the patient's best interests. (The legal issues surrounding such decisions are beyond the scope of this paper.) They are not entitled to discontinue treatment on the basis of other considerations, such as cost. This distinction may become blurred if physicians are pressed to balance the needs of their patients with societal needs. The practitioner may make decisions for economic reasons but rationalize them as in the best interests of the individual patient. This phenomenon may be occurring in Britain, where physicians "seem to seek medical justification for decisions forced on them by resource limits. Doctors gradually redefine standards of care so that they can escape the constant recognition that financial limits compel them to do less than their best."[4]

A similar danger lurks if physicians attempt to conserve resources by using probabilities of success or failure to make decisions about the care of individual patients. Estimates of the probable outcome of a clinical condition in a given patient are almost invariably based on "soft data": uncontrolled studies, reports of cases of dubious comparability, or the physician's anecdotal clinical experience—all further devalued by rapidly changing diagnostic and therapeutic techniques. The standard errors of such estimates are undefined but undoubtedly large. Yet leading physicians[5,6] advise doctors to practice probabilistic medicine—i.e., to withhold expensive treatment if the probability of success is low. How is the practitioner to define "low" in everyday practice—2, 5, 10, or 20 percent likelihood of survival with a good quality of life? Even if the dividing line were defined and the requisite precision in estimating outcome could be achieved, the role of the doctor as patient advocate would be subverted by probabilistic practice. This point should not be blurred by using the phrase "hopelessly ill."[5] If there is no hope for a patient, then there is no problem for the doctor in discontinuing treatment. In practice, doctors can rarely be certain who is hopelessly ill. This problem is not resolved by redefining the phrase to exclude consideration of the "rare report of a patient with a similar condition who survived"[5] in deciding whether to continue aggressive treatment. Physicians cannot discharge their responsibility to their individual patients if they try to conserve societal resources by discontinuing treatment on statistical grounds.

An example may indicate the possibilities for disregarding the best interests of a patient in an attempt to conserve societal resources by probabilistic practice. A gerontologist has suggested that we may rapidly be approaching a time when the majority of people will live until the end of a maximal life span to the point of "natural death" at about 85 years of age.[7] Even if the argument is correct as applied to populations, what is the individual doctor to do when caring for a desperately ill 85-year-old patient? Should advanced treatment be withheld, because "high-level medical technology applied at the end of a natural life span epitomizes the absurd"[7]? In terms of probability, the practitioner may be correct in predicting that the patient will not respond to treatment, but how is the physician to know that this person was not destined for a life span of 90 years? On what grounds can the physician withhold maximal treatment?

Another consideration weighs against any dilution of the mandate to doctors to consider solely the needs of their individual patients. Societal decisions about the proper allocation of resources are highly subjective and open to bias. For example, Avorn[8] has argued that cost-benefit analyses in geriatric care tend to turn age discrimination into health policy, because they depend on techniques for quantifying benefits that have a built-in bias against expenditures on health care for the elderly. A large part of the recent increase in overall health-care costs is due to the growing expense of care for older people. Negative attitudes toward aging and the elderly may influence our willingness to meet these costs. Society may encourage physicians to withhold expensive care on the basis of age, even if such care is likely to benefit the individual patient greatly. In Great Britain, persons over age 55 who have end-stage renal disease are steered away from long-term dialysis.[4]

None of the foregoing implies that in caring for individual patients doctors should disregard the escalating cost of medical care. Physicians can help control costs by choosing the most economical ways to deliver optimal care to their patients. They can use the least expensive setting, ambulatory or inpatient, in which first-class care can be given. They can eliminate redundant or useless diagnostic procedures ordered because of habit, deficient knowledge, personal financial gain, or the practice of "defensive medicine" to avoid malpractice judgments.

However, it is society, not the individual practitioner, that must make the decision to limit the availability of effective but expensive types of medical care. Heart and liver transplantation are current cases in point. These are extraordinarily expensive procedures that may prolong a life of "good quality" for some people. Society, through its elected officials, is entitled to decide that the resources required for such programs are better used for other purposes. However, a physician who thinks that his or her patient may benefit from a transplant must make that patient aware of this opinion and assist the patient in obtaining the organ.

The continuous increase in the costs of medical care is a difficult social issue. However, it is not self-evident that expenditures for health care should be limited to any arbitrary percentage of the gross national product, such as the current 11 percent figure. Moreover, if physicians and others make concerted and effective attempts to eliminate health-care expenditures that do not truly benefit patients, it is not a given fact that the proportion of the national wealth devoted to health care will increase indefinitely. It certainly is not self-evident that resources saved by limiting health care will be allocated to other equally worthy programs, such as preventive medicine, health maintenance, or improved nutrition and housing for the needy. In the United States, the societal decision to limit potentially lifesaving health care will not easily be made or enforced—nor should it be, in my opinion. Officials who press for the rationing of medical resources must be prepared for a public outcry, since unlimited availability of useful medical care has been perceived as a right in American society. Governor Lamm of Colorado was recently the target of such a response. Concerned that society cannot afford technological advances such as heart transplants, he quoted favorably a philosopher who believes that it is our societal duty to die. If society decides to ration health care, political leaders must accept responsibility. David Owen, who is both a political leader in Britain and a physician, believes that "it is right for doctors to demand that politicians openly acknowledge the limitations within which medical practice has to operate."[9] I agree and would add that doctors are entitled to lobby vigorously in the political arena for the resources needed for high-quality health care.

Through its democratic processes, American society may well choose to ration medical resources. In that event, physicians as citizens and experts will have a key role in implementing the decision. Their advice will be needed in allocating limited resources to provide the greatest good for the greatest number. As experience in other countries has shown[4], it may be difficult for doctors to separate their role as citizens and expert advisors from their role in the practice of medicine as unyielding advocates for the health needs of their individual patients. They must strive relentlessly to do so. When practicing medicine, doctors cannot serve two masters. It is to the advantage both of our society and of the individuals it comprises that physicians retain their historic single-mindedness. The doctor's master must be the patient.

NOTES

1. Fried C. Rights and health care—beyond equity and efficiency. *N Engl J Med* 1975; 293:241–5.
2. Hiatt HH. Protecting the medical commons: who is responsible? *N Engl J Med* 1975; 293:235–41.
3. Epstein FH. The role of the physician in the prolongation of life. In: Ingelfinger FJ, Ebert RV, Finland M, Relman AS, eds. *Controversy in internal medicine II.* Philadelphia: WB Saunders, 1974:103–9.
4. Aaron HJ, Schwartz WB. *The painful prescription: rationing hospital care.* Washington, D.C.: Brookings Institution, 1984.

5. Wanzer SH, Adelstein SJ, Cranford RE, et al. The physician's responsibility toward hopelessly ill patients. *N Engl J Med* 1984; 310:955–9.
6. Leaf A. The doctor's dilemma—and society's too. *N Engl J Med* 1984; 310:718–21.
7. Fries JF. Aging, natural death, and the compression of morbidity. *N Engl J Med* 1980; 303:130–5.
8. Avorn J. Benefit and cost analysis in geriatric care: turning age discrimination into health policy. *N Engl J Med* 1984; 310:1294–301.
9. Owen D. Medicine, morality and the market. *Can Med Assoc J* 1984; 130:1341–5.

Ethically Important Distinctions Among Managed Care Organizations*

Kate T. Christensen

Due to society's need to control health care costs and to the failure of legislated health care reform, managed care is expanding at a rapid rate and will soon be the predominant form of health care delivery. Plans by Congress to bring Medicare and Medicaid under managed care will further consolidate this trend. Barring some legislative fiat, managed care is here to stay.

The term *managed care* describes a diverse set of organizational forms. Wide variations in approach, financing, physician involvement, and philosophy exist among the different types of managed care organizations (MCOs). While many articles on the ethics of managed care acknowledge this variety, most analyses focus on the for-profit entities, paying less attention to the ethical distinctions among the different forms of managed care. This paper discusses the key distinctions among MCO types, in particular the difference between for-profit and non-profit plans; the relationship of the physician to the MCO; the incentives used to control costs; the incentives that improve patient care; and the organizational features that nurture the principled practice of medicine.

KEY DISTINCTIONS AMONG MCOS

FOR-PROFIT VERSUS NON-PROFIT MANAGED CARE

Although MCOs come in a bewildering array of structures, three crucial distinctions can be made among them: profit status, the relationship of physicians to the organization, and the nature of the capitation arrangement. The most important difference is between for-profit and non-profit health plans. For-profit plans make up the fastest growing segment of the managed care market, are growing at a much faster rate than the non-profits, and receive most of the business news attention. Although all MCOs must generate surplus revenue to continue to operate, for-profit plans differ from non-profit in that they trade their

Journal of Law, Medicine & Ethics, 23 (1996): 223–29. Reprinted with the permission of the American Society of Law, Medicine & Ethics.

*EDITORS' NOTE: Author's notes have been deleted. Students who wish to follow up on sources should consult the original article.

shares publicly and are not governed by the rules of charitable organizations. As a result, their administrative costs as a percentage of total income tend to be much higher. For-profit administrative costs often include extraordinarily large CEO salaries and bonuses, dividends to shareholders, and cash reserves for acquisition of competitors. A recent survey in California revealed a wide range between the total administrative expenses of for-profit organizations, which run as high as 30.9 percent of total revenue, and non-profit organizations, like Kaiser Foundation Health Plan, Inc. in California, which run at 3.1 percent. Other non-profit health plans also tend to have a larger share of income devoted to health services and a smaller profit/income ratio. This difference becomes ethically relevant when we consider the pressure on physicians to limit health care costs. Subscriber premiums or dues are set by the marketplace, and, because of direct competition between plans, the costs of the different plans tend to be very close. Therefore, in order to create more profit, the surplus is generated elsewhere. Part of it comes from reducing the amount spent on doctors, tests, treatments, and hospitalization. It stands to reason then that physicians in an MCO that has both less to spend on patient care and stockholders to please will be under more pressure to cut corners. Corner-cutting, or erring on the side of doing less instead of more, is a reality now. Only future research will tell us whether such practices are having a negative impact on patient care.

PHYSICIANS AND THE MCO

The second relevant distinction between MCO types is the relationship of the physician to the organization, which manifests itself in the various incentives to control patient care costs. For physicians, incentives can influence their professional autonomy as well as their practice stability and quality of professional work life, which in turn impact the quality of patient care in a variety of ways.

All health care delivery systems have financial incentives that can influence physician behavior. Under the traditional fee-for-service (FFS) model, physicians are rewarded financially for overtreating patients. And, because many patients believe that more health care is better health care, physi-

cians have a further incentive to keep patients happy by doing more. This system (along with technological advances and increased public expectations) has led to spiraling health care costs and, at times, iatrogenic harm to patients. Few tests or procedures are entirely risk free, and incidental findings can cause unnecessary anxiety as well as further tests or procedures. Although FFS allows physicians more practice and administrative autonomy than any other system, this system is rapidly withering in the face of the massive growth and consolidation of MCOs, as well as the cost-containment measures to limit Medicare and Medicaid reimbursements. Many FFS physicians are now contracting with a variety of MCOs.

For many years, Kaiser Permanente was the only large-scale alternative to FFS in the United States. Now MCOs include a growing array of reimbursement and health care delivery systems. Many MCOs offer a number of different products to enrollees and employers, giving each a choice from a menu of managed care and traditional indemnity plans. The basic forms currently are the independent practice associations (IPAs), preferred provider organizations (PPOs), the group model HMOs (like Kaiser Permanente), and the staff model HMOs.

PPO physicians contract with the MCO, and are paid on an FFS basis (see Table 1). Fees are usually discounted deeply by the health plan, and, as a result, many FFS physicians have experienced declining incomes in the last five years. Physicians in PPOs typically have contracts with a number of different MCOs and some indemnity plans. Because these physicians are still paid per service rendered, an inherent incentive arises to generate more health care costs by seeing patients more often and/or by ordering more tests and interventions (see Table 2). These physicians also are exposed to sudden changes in their relationship with the health plan, such as contract termination and the subsequent loss of covered patients. Therefore, income security is lowest for this group of physicians, in particular for the subspecialists. Physicians in IPAs also contract with one or more MCOs, but are given organizational coherence and negotiating power by the practice association. They are usually reimbursed on a capitated basis.

In the group model HMO, the physician is part of a group that contracts with the HMO. Instead of

Table 1. The Financial Relationship of the Physician to the MCO.

Practice Type	Relationship of Physician to MCO	Physician Payment	Physician Involvement in QA/UR
PPO	Physicians contract with MCO	Discounted FFS	High
IPA/Network	Physicians contract with MCOs through IPA	Usually capitation	High
Group Model	Group contracts with MCO	Capitation to group; salary with various incentives	High
Staff Model	Physician is employee of MCO	Salary with various incentives	Low

Table 2. Spectrum of Physician Incentives.*

	Traditional FFS	Managed Care
Compensation:	Fee per service rendered	Fee per person enrolled (capitation)
General Incentive:	Do more, get more	Do less, get more
Examples of Specific Financial Incentives:	Direct reimbursement for patient care; income from laboratory or radiology services; partnership in hospital	Withhold part of income; capitation, direct or diffused; bonuses; threat of deselection

*This chart is abstract, in that it does not take into account the many variations on these basic themes among MCOs.

receiving a fee for each service rendered, the group is paid a capitated amount by the health plan in advance of providing patient care services. The physicians are typically paid a basic salary plus a variety of financial incentives, such as bonuses. In contrast, physicians in staff model HMOs are employees of the MCO. They are salaried, and are also paid a variety of incentives—similar to group model physicians—designed to promote cost-effective medical care. Job security is often low in this group, because of the employee status of the physicians. Some predict that the majority of physicians will be working for staff model HMOs in the future.

Financial incentives common to many MCOs are the payment of bonuses from any unspent funds and withholding of portions of income, which may be paid out at the end of the year if certain cost-containment targets are met. Such targets may include keeping hospital utilization below a certain rate or limiting referrals to specialists. The larger the amount of the withheld income, the stronger the incentive to toe the line. Laboratory and radiology costs are frequently deducted from the pooled funds as well. In all but the group model HMOs, the threat of job loss or loss of one's patients also serves as a potent incentive to adhere to the MCO's rules.

Another significant aspect of the relationship of physicians to MCOs is the degree of control physicians have over the administrative and clinical aspects of their practices. In IPAs and PPOs, income security may be low but physician autonomy over medical practice is high, because physicians retain much of the traditional FFS prerogatives and practice format. Although practice autonomy is more restricted in group model HMOs than in IPAs or PPOs, physicians in IPAs, PPOs, and group model HMOs typically manage their own utilization review, quality assurance, and cost controls. Practice autonomy is usually lowest in the staff model HMOs, where utilization review and cost controls are usually managed and implemented by health plan administrators. Experience to date indicates that when control over the clinical aspects of practice rests with nonphysician administrators, the quality of patient care is threatened and physician morale plummets.

Many physicians are happy to relinquish administrative responsibility for their medical practices, but are uncomfortable with losing control over the clinical aspects, such as utilization and quality management. Physicians in MCOs know that utilization review can be benign or malignant, depending on who is doing it and to what end. This is the nightmare of utilization review: a stranger in another city, who has no clinical experience, calls the doctor and tells her to discharge a patient, or denies approval for a test the physician deems necessary. When used in this way, utilization review can function as a barrier to patient care. Physicians' job stress can be significantly increased by having to negotiate these hurdles on behalf of their patients. That situation also raises a direct conflict of interest between physicians' duty to provide good patient care and their own financial health.

However, when managed and implemented by physicians, utilization review can both promote better patient care (by minimizing unnecessary treatments or hospital stays) and save money. Utilization review should not put up barriers to good patient care, and, in the hands of physicians, it is less likely to do so.

Similarly, practice guidelines can be imposed on physicians, as in many staff model MCOs, or developed and implemented by physicians, as in the group model MCOs. When used inappropriately, such guidelines are applied as standards to measure, reward, and punish physician behavior. But with physician involvement, this process serves as a useful extension of peer review, and helps to maintain a high quality of care. When physicians are involved in the development and implementation of practice guidelines, it is less likely that they will mistake guidelines for standards (which require more stringent outcomes studies and stricter enforcement) and inappropriately use the guidelines to reward and punish.

CAPITATION

Another useful distinction among MCOs is the way members' premiums are distributed to the physicians. Capitation forms the core financial process in all of the systems discussed above. In a capitated system, the pool of funds for the provision of services is collected by the health plan and then distributed in various ways, often called *risk sharing*. Some plans give a physician group the money (less administrative costs and, if applicable, profit), and the money is kept in a central pool to pay for health care services. Other plans give the funds to the physicians, or to small physician groups, and the physicians then keep whatever is left at the end of the period (monthly, quarterly, or yearly). The more individualized the capitation arrangement is in relation to the physician, the greater the ethical strain on his or her relationship with the patient. For example, if a physician in a large group with a centralized fund orders an MRI to evaluate a young woman for multiple sclerosis, cost will not be a primary concern, because it is spread out over the group. If that same physician orders the MRI and the money comes out of his or her own capitated fund, it directly impacts that physician's income. The temptation to assign a heart murmur a benign status or to forgo a cardiology consult is greater if every penny spent comes out of the physician's own pocket. Most conscientious physicians will resist this temptation, but it injects an unnecessary "ethical stress" into the clinical encounter, and may in some cases influence treatment decisions to the detriment of good patient care. Many HMOs now shy away from such direct capitation, and instead capitate physicians as a group.

CONSEQUENCES OF MANAGED CARE FINANCIAL INCENTIVES

What are the possible consequences of capitation and other financial inducements to physicians to control costs? The most widely discussed is the temptation to withhold needed services. Whether this really happens is hard to prove, and has not been supported in the few studies that have examined the question. However, anecdotes about harm to patients from undertreatment abound, and this issue remains a primary concern of those who study managed care. It may also be that a disincentive arises to retain ill patients in one's health plan or patient panel, as they will tend to cost more than they (or their employers) pay into the plan. This could endanger the care of patients with complex chronic illnesses, such as AIDS.

The beneficial impact of managed care incentives includes the reduction of wasteful treatments, less iatrogenic harm to patients by the avoidance of unnecessary tests and procedures, more emphasis on preventive care, the potential for better case management of very ill patients in an integrated setting, and cost savings. All of these benefits result in improvements in the quality of the care provided under managed care. Although the degree of cost savings under managed care also has been contested, this is the aspect of managed care that has propelled it to the forefront of health care delivery systems.

BALANCING THE INCENTIVE TO UNDERTREAT

So far, I have focused primarily on the financial relationships that are intended to influence physician behavior and to decrease health care costs. But physicians are influenced by nonfinancial considerations as well. What kinds of incentives exist that may balance or buffer the temptation to limit treatment for the physician's own pecuniary benefit?

The strongest forces that balance the temptation to undertreat are the principles most physicians acquired in medical school. The most important and pervasive principle is the professional duty to benefit, or at least not harm, their patients. Applying this principle in traditional FFS would counteract the temptation to overtreat. Under managed care, physicians will be less likely to withhold necessary treatments if their primary allegiance is to the patient's well-being. Next in importance is the maintenance of the physician's professional and personal integrity, which again requires that they prevent harm to their patients.

The approval of one's colleagues also exerts a strong effect on the behavior of many physicians, and is why peer review is such a powerful tool to change physician behavior. If the philosophy and practice of the physician group reflect the primacy of good patient care over all other considerations, it is less likely that patients will suffer under managed care. Reinforcing these principles in medical school and residency will be an important factor in maintaining good patient care as practiced in the managed care setting.

Health systems have mechanisms for reinforcing the principle of beneficence and for maintaining high-quality patient care, such as peer review and practice guidelines. These mechanisms, for example, give the physician feedback if he or she is not providing the quality for care that colleagues expect, or let a physician know, for example, if he or she is not ordering enough mammograms or vaccinations. The threat of malpractice is a reality in all treatment settings, and it can both promote overtreatment in FFS and deter undertreatment in managed care (see Table 3). State and federal regulations, and future legislation, will also impact MCOs. Finally, if health plan subscribers are educated and involved in their health care, they may be less likely to accept inadequate care, and more likely to understand the financial trade-offs involved in every health care decision.

THE ETHICAL HMO

Enumerating ethical principles and good practices is not enough to help us identify those organizations that are best suited to promote the provision of health care in an atmosphere relatively untainted by financial conflicts of interest. Many authors have developed important and useful

Table 3. Forces Balancing the Negative Consequences of Managed Care Incentives

Principles of Practice	External Forces
Desire to prevent harm from undertreatment (beneficence)	Treatment guidelines
Professionalism/self-respect (integrity)	Peer review
Desire for the respect of one's peers	Fear of malpractice
	Patient/member involvement
	Regulation and legislation

guidelines and principles for MCOs, but I would like to summarize from the above discussion the structural features of health care organizations that nurture and reinforce the best principles of medical practice. MCO structure determines in large part the nature of the conflicts providers within it have to face, and it can also impact the quality of the care delivered. For example, having pre-approval admission requirements for hospitalization is a structural barrier to good patient care. A direct financial incentive to reduce hospital admissions is an ethical hurdle the physician must overcome to keep the patient's welfare foremost.

What would an MCO look like were it structured to buffer or neutralize the incentives to undertreat patients and to maximize the incentives to provide quality medical care? What features should we look for in evaluating the degree of ethical stress a physician experiences in providing health care in different practice settings?

• The organization should be non-profit. This removes shareholders and profit maximization as the bottom line, which theoretically puts less pressure on the physician to meet financial goals (as opposed to patient outcome goals).

• To remove the cash register from the examination room, physicians should be salaried. Divorcing the individual patient encounter from the physician's immediate income helps to focus the encounter on meeting the patient's needs, and frees the physician to practice according to his or her professional principles. Group model and staff model HMOs both meet this ideal.

• Sharing the risk of capitation across a large group of physicians dilutes the temptation to cut corners inappropriately. The manner in which capitated funds are distributed varies and influences the degree of conflict of interest the physician experiences. Direct or individual capitation and linking financial incentives directly to cost-containment targets should be avoided.

• Clinical practice should be managed by physicians. Physicians should be heavily involved with utilization review, quality management, and the development and implementation of practice guidelines. Utilization review should not serve as a barrier to providing health care services.

• The patients or members of the MCO should have a role in the operations of the organization, at a number of levels. First, subscribers should receive full disclosure from the health plan about any incentives to limit treatment and any restrictions on coverage. Second, MCOs need to find a mechanism to include health plan members in discussions of benefit coverage and conflict resolution procedures. Third, community members should be involved in the ethics committees of managed care hospitals and in the organizational ethics committees of health plans, where these committees exist. Fourth, vigorous efforts at patient/member health education should be fundamental, both to improve the health of members, and to improve their understanding of the financial trade-offs involved in treatment and benefit decisions. An educated member may be more likely to challenge unfair limits to treatment.

CONCLUSION

Managed care is not one entity; it is a broad umbrella that includes a variety of health care delivery structures, relationships with physicians, and physician incentives. While all managed care forms face the challenge of avoiding undertreatment, some are more challenged than others. Whether an MCO minimizes conflicts of interest for physicians depends on the way it is organized and financed, the degree of physician involvement in managing patient care quality, and the nature of the incentives used to control costs. The form of managed care which currently works best to prevent undertreatment is one that is non-profit and has a large salaried physician group that manages the clinical aspects of the provision of health care services.

Having drawn these distinctions, it is clear that managed care as a subject of study is a rapidly moving target. Non-profit HMOs themselves are sorely challenged to compete with the for-profit entities. All are taking measures to cut costs, and, in many instances, are adopting the methods of the for-profit HMOs. If this trend continues, it is possible that the distinction between for-profit and non-profit MCOs will blur. Moreover, for-profit organizations are rearranging themselves into new and unique forms at a rapid rate. Thus, as these new structures evolve, we must encourage the growth of those that foster the highest quality of patient care and physician satisfaction.

The HMO Physician's Duty to Cut Costs

William Edwards was 39 when a serious, potentially life-threatening ventricular heart arrhythmia (irregular contractions) was diagnosed during a routine physical examination. The cardiologist first prescribed quinidine, but it failed to bring the arrhythmia under control.

Diisopyramide was successful, but Mr. Edwards complained of severe blurred vision and dry mouth. When the medication was reduced, the side effects disappeared but the arrhythmia returned. At this point the cardiologist decided to combine the diisopyramide with propranolol, a common beta-blocker known to be effective in certain arrhythmias. This controlled the problem, without side effects.

Mr. Edwards continued with this medication regimen for five years until moving to a new town, where he joined a health maintenance organization (HMO). He immediately consulted Dr. Sam Forester, a cardiologist.

Dr. Forester agreed that medication was needed, but he was concerned about diisopyramide, since severe problems had been reported in some patients. Moreover,

Mr. Edwards and his original physician had never tried the obvious approach of using propranolol alone.

Both Dr. Forester and Mr. Edwards concluded that there were also risks in shifting to the single drug. Although it was generally safer than diisopyramide and probably should have been tried originally, there was a small chance of a fatal heart attack. On balance, both agreed that the status quo was slightly better for the patient.

Dr. Forester then noticed the financial ledger for Mr. Edwards's care, which included the cost of the medication paid for in full by the HMO. The yearly cost of the diisopyramide was $430; the propranolol cost $26 per year. He realized that even a significant increase in propranolol dosage, something that would involve little risk, would still reduce the HMO's medication bill by about $400.

Should Dr. Forester consider a change in medication, taking into account cost-saving for the HMO, or should he work solely on the basis of the welfare of the patient? If he should take into account the costs to the HMO, should he try to persuade the patient to agree to the change, or should he simply refuse to authorize any further prescriptions for the diisopyramide? Does Mr. Edwards have any moral obligation to take costs to the HMO into account in choosing a medication regimen?

From *Hastings Center Report* 15, no. 4 (August 1985): 13. Reproduced by permission. Copyright © 1985 The Hastings Center.

Fiscal Scarcity and the Inevitability of Bedside Budget Balancing

E. Haavi Morreim

While recognizing that cost containment will profoundly affect health care, many physicians and bioethicists insist that physicians can and should avoid directly compromising their patients' care to save third parties' money. "Physicians are required to do everything they believe may benefit each patient without regard to costs or other societal considerations";[1] "asking physicians to be cost-conscious . . . would be asking them to abandon their central commitment to their patients."[2-10] While the physician might assist in creating public

Archives of Internal Medicine 149 (1989): 1012–1015. Copyright © 1989 American Medical Association.

or hospital resource policies, and while he sometimes must ration—e.g., where there are too many patients for too few intensive care beds—on this traditional view he must never voluntarily say "no" to his own patient simply to cut costs.

A variant of this traditional view suggests that physicians can ethically participate in cost containment, but only if the health care system as a whole is morally just. A just system must at least assure all citizens a basic minimum of care, and must be "closed." Only if its total resources are fixed can the physician be sure that money saved in the care of one patient will actually help some needier patient, rather than reverting to taxpayers, stockholders, or munitions makers. Unless such criteria are satisfied, the physician may not ethically assist in economic rationing.[11,12]

I will argue that this prescription for aloofness is now untenable. The economic reorganization of health care has introduced a new kind of scarcity, requiring a different sort of rationing than that to which physicians are accustomed. Bedside trade-offs between one patient's welfare and other parties' competing needs, relatively rare in the past, are now inescapable.

THREE KINDS OF SCARCITY

Prior to the 1980s, limits on health care arose largely through two sources: (1) inadequate access to the health care system, either through the patient's inability to pay for care or through a regional shortage of personnel and facilities,[13] and (2) shortages of specific commodities, such as intensive care beds or hemodialysis units. Arising mainly around new or exotic technologies, serious "commodity scarcities" were otherwise uncommon. Government funding of capital improvements, combined with generous third-party reimbursement practices, generally meant that those who had access to the health care system at all could expect quite a full range of its benefits. Indeed, physicians and other providers had economic incentives not only to ignore costs (except where the patient himself was the payer), but to provide every possible benefit, as retrospective fee-for-service reimbursement rewarded maximal levels of intervention.[14–16]

In recent years, however, a third sort of scarcity has arisen: "fiscal scarcity," a general tightening of

health care dollars as government and business, who together pay three-fourths of the nation's health care bill, attempt to gain control over their skyrocketing expenditures. This tightening takes a variety of forms, such as prospective payment, utilization review, preferred provider arrangements, and managed care systems, but collectively signals a fundamental change in the nature of the allocation decisions physicians face.

In commodity scarcity, some discrete item is in limited supply, whether because of natural limits, as in the case of transplant organs, or through sheer cost, as with positron emission tomography. The list of patients needing that resource is usually fairly clear: only those with severe and irreversible hepatic disease are eligible for liver transplant. As a result, the consequences of allocation decisions are equally clear. We know not only the exact identity of those who receive the commodity, but also, reciprocally, the names, or at least the general description, of those who do not. If Mrs. Baker is admitted to the lone available intensive care bed, Mr. Abel, also in need, is not. But Mrs. Jones, recovering from pneumonia on another ward, is unaffected. Equally important, we can also be fairly sure that if one patient is denied the resource, some other needy person will nevertheless benefit. The difficult decision brings at least that consolation.

Because the consequences of commodity allocations are thus fairly clear, so are the trade-offs that must go into those decisions. To distribute transplant organs, we can assemble medical criteria to tell us which patients have the highest probability of living for what length of time, with what functional capacities and deficits.[17] And we can identify some nonmedical values that we can then choose either to include or to ignore. Should a criminal record disqualify one from eligibility for transplant? Should family responsibilities or occupational contributions count? During the early days of hemodialysis, some allocation committees decided that even after excluding, on "medical" grounds, applicants who were more than 40 years old or who suffered from mental illness, a surfeit of remaining candidates did require just such clearly nonmedical considerations.[18,19]

Fiscal scarcity is utterly different. Because every medical decision has its economic cost, literally every medical decision is now subject to scrutiny for its economic as well as its medical wisdom. Suddenly, not this or that item, but all of medicine, is an allocation issue—every laboratory test, every roentgenogram.

Unlike commodity scarcities, the consequences of fiscal allocation decisions are anything but clear. Obviously, the decision to order a $2,000 course of antibiotics rather than a $2 course means that this $2,000 will not be available for alternate use. But beyond that, consequences are amorphous. We cannot possibly name, or even describe generically, who will be denied what as a result of the expenditure. The diminution of funds may constrain future decisions to some degree, although it is rare for any single spending decision to be felt discernibly, even at the level of an individual hospital's finances, let alone at the statewide or national level. The collective impact of many spending decisions does not dictate which sorts of medical care will be constrained for which patients in the future. That is entirely a product of further decision making.

Because the consequences of fiscal allocation decisions cannot be specified, neither can the moral or medical trade-offs be precisely identified. To prescribe a cheaper but slightly less effective antibiotic may or may not affect the patient's outcome at all, and there is no assurance that the money saved will even be used to help other patients rather than be returned to stockholders or taxpayers.[11,12]

GUIDELINES

Commodity and fiscal scarcity can also be distinguished by the sort of criteria that can guide allocation decisions. Because the consequences and trade-offs of commodity decisions are fairly clear, and because decisions are episodic, required only when a particular patient(s) needs a specific item that is in short supply, it is possible to establish fairly explicit criteria, and to apply them fairly rigorously. One can consider whether an alcoholic ought to be denied a liver transplant,[20] and one can formulate a sorting system for allocating intensive care beds[21] or transplant organs.[17]

The decisions of fiscal allocation are not episodic, but chronic. Every decision has its price. As a result, criteria guiding fiscal allocation must ideally cover every detail of medical care,

whether to cull out useless interventions, or, under more stringent circumstances, to eliminate real benefits in some thoughtful, systematic way.

Actually, fiscal efficiency guidelines are now emerging throughout medicine. Many observers argue that physicians are morally obligated to eliminate from their clinical routines those interventions that are of little or no proven value, thereby conserving costs while preserving or even enhancing quality of care.[2,7,22–24] Thus, for example, the American College of Physicians, in collaboration with Blue Cross and Blue Shield, has issued "Diagnostic Testing Guidelines" for such common tests as arterial blood gas analysis, blood cultures, chest roentgenograms, and electrocardiograms. If used as bases on which to deny reimbursement, these guidelines could eventually save up to $10 million per year (James FE. Blue Cross Plans Coverage Limits on Many Tests. *Wall Street Journal.* April 10, 1987:29). Similarly, many health maintenance organizations have developed guidelines to suggest appropriate uses of hospitalization and sophisticated technologies, while many third-party payers use their own utilization review "cookbooks" to determine which medical interventions warrant reimbursement.

However, such efficiency protocols differ markedly from the kind of rationing criteria we develop for scarce commodities. They will not provide such clear guidance nor, more importantly, will they enable the physician to escape personal involvement in trade-offs between patients' welfare and economic considerations at the bedside. In both formulation and implementation, such guidelines will require some compromises in patient care.

FORMULATING GUIDELINES

Those who formulate efficiency protocols must eliminate not just utterly useless practices, but also some interventions of at least marginal value. Although physicians have occasionally been guilty of clear wastefulness as, for instance, admitting patients to the hospital on a Friday for an elective diagnostic workup that cannot begin until Monday, deleting such carelessness surely will not resolve the nation's entire health care challenge.[25] (If it could, then the medical profession would owe the nation a profound apology for triggering an economic crisis through sheer profligacy.)

But once we turn to interventions of marginal value, patient care will inevitably be compromised. Not all patients' care will be impaired, for many will actually be benefitted through reduced iatrogenesis and inconvenience. Nevertheless, to be of marginal benefit is, by definition, to be of some benefit.[14] The benefit may be small, as with palliative treatment of self-limited illness, or it may help only a few patients. Most commonly, marginal interventions reduce diagnostic or therapeutic uncertainty—the extra test to confirm clinical findings, the screening test to detect rare but serious and treatable maladies, the wide-spectrum antibiotic to cover for unidentified organisms.[26-28] In most cases, eliminating such interventions will do no harm. Yet some patients will be deprived of a real benefit, namely those few whose rare disease would have been detected by the now-eliminated diagnostic "zebra-hunt," or whose therapy would have been more effective with more potent agents. We may never know in advance which patients will be harmed and which patients will be helped as efficiency protocols eliminate marginal benefits. But the fact remains that some patients' welfare will have been exchanged for the health of other patients and for the wealth of third parties.

Such trade-offs require important value judgments. The move from "do anything that might help" to "do only what will help" represents a fundamental value shift from "interventionism" to "noninterventionism,"[29] a reversion from modern medicine's technological imperative to its older value, "do no harm." Further, to call a benefit "marginal" is to judge that its value is intrinsically small, or less important than alternative uses of the limited total resources.

This is not to say that physicians should therefore refuse to curb marginal practices. In times of resource scarcity it would be irresponsible to abdicate such essential, albeit difficult, "gray zone" decisions. Our point is only that one cannot "eliminate marginal benefits" without shifting a fundamental value of the profession and compromising at least some patients' care.

IMPLEMENTING GUIDELINES

Although they require important value judgments and will inevitably alter quality of care, efficiency protocols can at least be formulated away from the bedside. Unfortunately, physicians' cooperation with cost containment cannot be confined to just this "policy level."[30] Efficiency protocols will not save money until they are implemented at the bedside; and here the physician cannot escape directly saying "no" to his own patients in the name of resource conservation.

Each time an efficiency protocol would suggest suboptimal care for his patient, the physician has several choices. First, he can simply follow the protocol, refraining from any attempt to secure optimal care for his patient. In that case, he will have voluntarily done less than he could for his patient, a clear bedside trade-off.

Alternatively, he could avail himself of the flexibility that is necessarily built into such guidelines. No "cookbook" or computer program, however detailed, could possibly dictate exactly what should be done for each patient. Medical science is too uncertain, and patients too variable, to admit of such crisp determinacy. Any guideline must be tempered by the clinical judgment of a physician who personally knows the patient. Thus, though barium studies of the gastrointestinal tract can normally be safely completed on an outpatient basis, a frail elderly patient may well require inpatient observation. Further, third-party payers and others who apply such guidelines are unlikely to dictate medical decisions outright, lest they increase their own legal risks (*Wickline* v. *State of California*, 228 Cal Rptr 661 [Cal App 2 Dist, 1986]).

Such flexibility means that it is almost always possible for a physician to find some way to justify an exception for his patient any time the guideline might propose suboptimal care. Unfortunately, if the physician makes such an exception for literally every deprivation of even the smallest benefit, he will thwart the efficiency protocol completely. The very point of such guidelines is, after all, to eliminate (marginal) benefits and to distribute the resulting suboptimality of care in the most fair, medically benign way possible. If costs are to be contained, physicians must cooperate, by voluntarily doing less than they might for some of their own patients.

Because this compromise does threaten physicians' traditional fiduciary obligation to promote their own patients' interests above all others',[1] some observers have proposed a third alternative. Others, not the physician, should say "no."[4,8,9] However, although society can and should set basic health resource policies, legislators, bureaucrats, and judges have no business making individual patient care decisions. On another version, clinically knowledgeable hospital administrators or other local laymen would adjudicate requests for care not provided for within the guidelines, or which exceeded some designated threshold of expenditure.[2,3] As the physician pleads his patient's case while others allot or deny benefits, the physician can tell the patient that "they," not he, are rationing care. He maintains unsullied his loyalty to the patient. But at a terrible price.

He is no longer practicing medicine. Although outsiders can plausibly place firm controls, e.g., over the costliest technologies' proliferation and use, such supervision cannot invade the daily details of care. To the extent that others determine which patients will receive how many roentgenograms, which laboratory or radiologic studies, or how many days' hospitalization with what intensity of nursing care, those "others" are literally practicing medicine in the physician's stead, without a license, at that. The physician escapes saying "no" by becoming impotent to say "yes."

Firm guidelines and appeals procedures are initially attractive, perhaps because they are roughly feasible in the allocation of scarce commodities. As we have seen, commodity allocation decisions are episodic, the trade-offs fairly clear, the values often nonmedical, and the verdicts final. But, under fiscal scarcity, all of medicine is at stake. To dictate in advance the permissible economic impact of each health care decision is to dictate the medical decisions themselves, which is an unacceptable intrusion on clinical freedom.

Finally, the physician might try to ignore efficiency protocols and cost considerations altogether. By now this option is sorely tempting. When the physician cooperates with cost containment, he reneges on his fiduciary commitment to serve his patients' interests above all others'. If, on the other hand, he permits outsiders to impose all the economic trade-offs in his patients' care,

he has literally abdicated the practice of medicine. Perhaps he should simply ignore cost constraints as best he can, or at least wait until society has put in place a just allocation scheme in which his cooperation will not offend his patients' rights.[11,12]

THE INEVITABILITY OF BEDSIDE RATIONING

Unfortunately, ignoring economics is not an option either. Government and business are determined to control their health care expenditures. And not without justification. Government has other worthy projects to which it owes resources, and business will be less viable in the competitive international marketplace if it cannot control this important cost of production.[15,31,32] But controlling health care expenditures requires controlling spending decisions, and that, in turn, requires the control, or at least cooperation, of physicians, whose medical decisions largely determine health care expenditures.

In some cases, physicians' decisions and options are restricted through *direct controls*, as where a hospital pharmacy's formulary does not carry certain costly drugs, or where the primary care physician must obtain a subspecialist's approval to order an expensive test for his patient. While there is some room for such controls, however, we have already seen that excessive invasion into the daily details of medicine is untenable. Instead, physicians' economic cooperation is more commonly elicited through *incentives*. Whether through such "sticks" as administrators' letters of warning or threats to revoke hospital privileges,[33] or through "carrots" such as bonuses and profit-sharing, physicians are being systematically introduced to the economic consequences of their medical decisions. They are personally, professionally, and financially at risk for the level of care which they choose for their patients.[34]

COMMENT

My conclusion is unsavory, but its logic compelling. No matter how well we trim waste, regardless how efficiently we manage our resources, however generous our health care budget, our finite resources cannot possibly meet the limitless health care needs of the population. Limits necessitate decisions to deny benefits. If the physician has clinical authority to make medical (i.e., spending) decisions, then reciprocally he makes the decisions not to spend. Guidelines can help, but if flexible, they still leave final decisions in the physician's hands. Even where resource controls appear rigid, the physician must still make the decision whether to acquiesce or to challenge them on behalf of each particular patient. The physician remains free in any given case to render maximal care. Yet the requirement to limit the use of resources overall must ultimately translate into individual decisions to refrain from offering particular interventions to particular patients. The physician thus cannot escape reckoning with awkward decisions about when to offer everything and when to comply with the need to do less.

This is not to say that the quality of health care in the United States must decline substantially. Fiscal constraints are not yet dire, and there is still much "fat" to be trimmed from heavy administrative bureaucracy and from clinical routines of care. Further, competition and litigation constantly remind providers to maintain their standards. Neither does fiscal scarcity mean that physicians must now become principally agents of society, or that they must place their patients' interests simply on a par with the myriad of competing considerations. Nor does this constitute moral permission for hasty acquiescence to unpleasant financial or professional pressures, or an endorsement of ad hoc, idiosyncratic economic theorizing at the bedside. Collective research and reflection on optimal resource use is morally, medically, and economically preferable to solo cost-cutting.

Rather, fiscal scarcity means that physicians must now face rationing questions on an altogether different scale than before. Their moral question is no longer whether to participate in cost containment (that would be rather like asking "shall we abide by the law of gravity?"), but how to do so in morally credible ways. Although economic exigencies may force physicians to weigh more carefully the cost of each benefit and the value of the benefit to the patient, they do not require that the physician appraise the value of the patient himself or weigh his benefit to society. The physician can still be his patient's best advocate, even if he is not obligated to provide benefits without limit.

NOTES

1. Levinsky NG. The doctor's master. *N Engl J Med.* 1984;311:1573–1575.

2. Veatch RM. DRGs and the ethical reallocation of resources. *Hastings Cent Rep.* 1986;16:32–40.

3. Veatch RM. *A Theory of Medical Ethics.* New York, NY: Basic Books Inc; 1981.

4. Abrams FR. Patient advocate or secret agent? *JAMA.* 1986;256:1784–1785.

5. Swiryn S. The doctor as gatekeeper. *Arch Intern Med.* 1986;146:1789.

6. Pellegrino E, Thomasma D. *A Philosophical Basis of Medical Practice.* New York, NY: Oxford University Press Inc; 1981

7. Angell M. Cost containment and the physician. *JAMA.* 1985;254:1203–1207.

8. Hiatt H. Protecting the medical commons: who is responsible? *N Engl J Med.* 1975;293:235–241.

9. Fried C. Rights and health care: beyond equity and efficiency. *N Engl J Med.* 1975;293:241–245.

10. Beauchamp TL, Childress JF. *Principles of Biomedical Ethics.* 2nd ed. New York, NY: Oxford University Press Inc; 1983.

11. Cassel CK. Doctors and allocation decisions: a new role in the new medicare. *J Health Polit Policy Law.* 1985;10:549–564.

12. Daniels N. The ideal advocate and limited resources. *Theor Med.* 1987;8:69:80.

13. Komaroff AL. The doctor, the hospital, and the definition of proper medical practice. In: President's Commission, *Securing Access to Health Care.* Washington, D.C.: U.S. Government Printing Office; 1981;3:225–251.

14. Fuchs VR. The 'rationing' of medical care. *N Engl J Med.* 1984;311:1572–1573.

15. Thurow LC. Learning to say 'no'. *N Engl J Med.* 1984;311:1569–1572.

16. Thurow LC. Medicine versus economics. *N Engl J Med.* 1985;313:611–614.

17. Starzl TE, Hakala TR, Tzak A, et al. A multifactorial system for equitable selection of cadaver kidney recipients. *JAMA.* 1987;257:3073–3075.

18. Sanders D, Dukeminier J Jr. Medical advance and legal lag; hemodialysis and kidney transplantation. *UCLA Law Rev.* 1968;15:367–386.

19. Evans RW. Health care technology and the inevitability of resource allocation and rationing decisions. *JAMA.* 1983;249(pt 2):2208–2219.

20. Flavin DK, Niven RG, Kelsey JE. Alcoholism and orthotopic liver transplantation. *JAMA*. 1988; 259:1546–1547.
21. Engelhardt HT, Rie MA. Intensive care units, scarce resources, and conflicting principles of justice. *JAMA*. 1986;255:1159–1163.
22. Council on Ethical and Judicial Affairs. Recent opinions: economic incentives and levels of care. *JAMA*. 1986;256:224.
23. Wong ET, Lincoln TL. Ready! Fire! . . . Aim! *JAMA*. 1983;250:2510–2513.
24. Egdahl R. Ways for surgeons to increase efficiency of their use of hospitals. *N Engl J Med*. 1983;309:1184–1187.
25. Schwartz WB. The inevitable failure of current cost-containment strategies. *JAMA*. 1987;257:220–224.
26. Hardison JF. To be complete. *N Engl J Med*. 1979;300:193–194.
27. Reuben D. Learning diagnostic restraint. *N Engl J Med*. 1984;310:591–593.

28. Baily M. Rationing medical care: processes for defining adequacy. In: Agich GJ, Begley CE, eds. *The Price of Health*. Dordrecht, the Netherlands: D. Reidel Publishing Co; 1986;165–184.
29. Brett AS. Hidden ethical issues in clinical decision analysis. *N Engl J Med*. 1981;305:1150–1153.
30. Brett AS, McCullough LB. When patients request specific interventions. *N Engl J Med*. 1986; 315:1347–1351.
31. Aaron HJ, Schwartz WB. Hospital cost control: a bitter pill to swallow. *Harvard Bus Rev*. 1985; 64:160–167.
32. Board of Trustees. A proposal for financing health care of the elderly. *JAMA*. 1986;256:3379–3382.
33. Hershey N. Fourth-party audit organizations: practical and legal considerations. *Law Med Health Care*. 1986;14:54–65.
34. Egdahl RH, Taft CH. Financial incentives to physicians. *N Engl J Med*. 1986;315:59–61.

SECTION 4

Managed Care and Informed Consent

Informed Consent to Rationing Decisions*

Mark A. Hall

To ration health care spending among competing medical and societal uses raises profound legal and ethical dilemmas. Previous discussions analyze whether rationing is permissible in any form, whether patients, physicians, or insurers (government and private) should be the primary rationing decision maker, the proper criteria for rationing,

Milbank Quarterly, Vol. 71, No. 4, 1993. Copyright © 1993 Milbank Memorial Fund. Used with permission of Blackwell Publishers.
EDITORS' NOTE: All references and some footnotes have been deleted. Students who want to follow up on sources should consult the original article.

and the effect of cost containment on malpractice liability. Neglected in most of this legal–ethical discussion is the foundational doctrine of informed consent. There is little systematic analysis of how the physician's obligation to discuss the course of treatment and tailor it to individual patient desires is affected by public or private insurance that calls for the denial of marginally beneficial care because of costs. . . . The issue is a compelling one regardless of whether, and to what extent, physicians are forced to make rationing decisions by rules or are induced to do so by educational, professional, or financial incentives. In all events, the messenger who delivers the bad news is under a fiduciary obligation of candor, which the law of informed consent is designed to enforce.

Disclosure of rationing decisions can occur at two distinct points. General rationing rules and incentives can be disclosed to subscribers of health maintenance organizations (HMOs) and other limited insurance plans at the time of enrollment. Alternatively, particular, case-specific decisions not to contract for potentially beneficial care owing to excessive costs can be disclosed at the time of (non)treatment. This discussion addresses both stages, but the primary focus is on the second. A number of commentators have presented convincing arguments that enrollment disclosure should be required, even though no existing statute or case decision says so. Therefore, I will not elaborate on this position here, except to state my opinion that this glaring legal deficiency is inexcusable. HMO subscribers are clearly misled by the advertising slant that emphasizes their utopian features without mentioning the built-in incentives and constraints that can lead to the denial of beneficial care.

Although it is easy to agree on some global disclosure of rationing mechanisms at the time of enrollment (even if a consensus is lacking on exactly what to disclose and how to do it), we are still left with the thornier question of whether individual treatment options that are potentially beneficial but expensive must be disclosed precisely at the time the physician declines to order them, and, if so, whether the patient has a right to insist that the treatment be given. Beginning with James Blumstein's analysis, every commentator to consider the issue except two has concluded that the law indeed requires rationing decisions to be disclosed at the time of treatment, and several argue that it would constitute abandonment to deny beneficial care the patient desires.

This article explores whether the law in fact demands stringent adherence to individual patient autonomy or, instead, whether it is capable of absorbing economic constraints and how it would go about doing so. I begin by describing the technical requirements of existing law, and then proceed to analyze how these requirements could be adapted to the demands of limited forms of insurance. The essence of my analysis is to inquire whether adequate global disclosure at the time of enrollment (or re-enrollment) suffices to satisfy legal require-

ments of informed consent, either because it constitutes a prior consent to the bundle of nontreatment decisions implicit in a more conservative (i.e., cost-sensitive) treatment style or because it constitutes a valid waiver of the right to informed consent. I do not presume that, at present, such global enrollment disclosure in fact is adequately performed (indeed, I have just noted that it is not), nor do I attempt to articulate in any detail what such disclosure should contain. I mean only to lay the legal and analytic framework for constructive discussion of these important matters, in order to take us beyond the present extremes of requiring no disclosure on the one hand or, on the other, stipulating that only treatment-specific disclosures will suffice.

THE LAW OF INFORMED REFUSAL

To focus the discussion a bit more, suppose a 42-year-old, otherwise healthy male with high blood pressure asks his HMO primary-care physician for testing to determine the extent of his possible heart disease. The doctor orders a static electrocardiogram (EKG), which is an inexpensive test done on the spot. The test results are negative. Two months later, the patient suffers a nonfatal heart attack while jogging. His lawyer discovers that many respectable cardiac specialists would have performed a more accurate exercise stress test that costs far more and requires referral to a specialized facility; however, the prevailing standard of care allows only the simpler test for a younger, asymptomatic patient who is at low risk. Assuming that the patient has no legal basis to claim conventional malpractice, does he nevertheless have a valid informed consent claim for failure to disclose the existence of the more expensive alternative? Also, had the alternative been disclosed, could he have demanded that it be done and paid for by the HMO?

AN OVERVIEW OF THE LAW

On the surface, economically motivated decisions to decline marginally beneficial treatment do not readily appear to fit informed consent doctrine. That doctrine arose from battery law, a branch of tort law that compensates for harmful or offensive touchings. Therefore, it does not easily reach decisions not to treat. Moreover, the traditional focus of the negligence branch of informed consent law has been on medical risks, not economic costs. Thus, several courts have concluded that informed consent liability is "limited to those situations where the harm suffered arose from some affirmative violation of the patient's physical integrity such as surgical procedures, injections or invasive diagnostic tests."[1]

Nevertheless, a more fully developed version of informed consent doctrine and its rationale is easily capable of embracing a requirement that physicians disclose each decision to bypass, for economic or other reasons, a potentially beneficial treatment option. The central purpose of informed consent law is to enhance personal autonomy over decisions that affect physical and mental well-being. As Shultz has thoroughly and cogently argued, a medical decision can be equally vital regardless of whether it leads to treatment or nontreatment. As for the nature of the risk factors disclosed (medical versus economic), the California Supreme Court has held that the "concept of informed consent is broad enough to encompass . . . whether a physician has an economic interest that might affect the physician's professional judgment."[2] Other courts have held that physicians must disclose their alcoholism or their HIV-positive status.[3]

THE LAW'S POTENTIAL

Informed consent law has not yet reached its full, logical extension, however, because it remains tied to its traditional doctrinal moorings of battery and negligence. Battery law, as noted, requires some physical contact, whereas negligence law employs professional custom, not patient interests, as its standard for liability. In order for informed consent doctrine to shape itself into a fully actualized "dignitary tort," one that would thoroughly protect a patient's right to be involved in all forms of medical decision making, it would have to free itself from these constraining elements of traditional tort law.

Several commentators have argued for such an extension, observing that this is the logical end point of the path along which the informed consent doctrine has developed. They argue, first, that a full legal embodiment of patient autonomy

requires the standard of care to be elevated from simple disclosure of risk to one of true, epistemological understanding of the information conveyed (heightened duty). They also argue that plaintiffs should recover "dignitary" damages even though no physical harm resulted (no injury), even though it could not be shown they would have made any other decision if fully informed (no causation), and, most critical to our analysis, even though no treatment was rendered (no touching). . . .

MATERIALITY OF DISCLOSURE RECONSIDERED

. . . [W]e must return to the main line of analysis to inquire again whether the absence of insurance for an economically motivated treatment refusal makes disclosure immaterial to the patient's deliberations. As Menzel and Morreim have argued, it does not because the patient might pay out of pocket or seek to solicit donations. Even apart from the short-term possibility of acquiring the particular treatment, the information might be material to a longer-range decision of whether to switch doctors within the plan or to switch insurance plans at the next open-enrollment opportunity. Finally, nontreatment information might be considered material, even if it objectively has no effect on any medical decision, simply because the patient would want to know purely for the sake of knowledge. Few nontreatment decisions would clearly escape these standards of materiality. . . .

PRUDENTIAL CONSTRAINTS ON ECONOMIC INFORMED CONSENT

The law's ambivalence about extending informed consent requirements to rationing decisions may be caused by the deleterious effects that liability would cause for the practical workings of treatment relations under constrained insurance. Taken to its logical extreme, informed refusal law would require physicians to engage their patients in elaborate explanations for each discrete step in a complex tree of diagnostic and treatment options for even the most minor of ailments. In deciding to employ a single test, a physician might explicitly or elliptically pass over a dozen options. If informed consent theory applied with full vigor, doctors would have to engage their patients in an extensive, 14-point dialogue about each of these alternatives, periodically stopping along the way to test for full comprehension and videotaping these encounters to ensure proof of their sufficiently "prolonged conversation" and "shared decision making." This would have to be done for each branch in the decision tree, including every conceivable alternative encountered in a complex course of treatment.

Thoroughgoing disclosure of all economically motivated nontreatment decisions at the time they are made is also inconsistent with the nature of clinical judgment and the manner in which financial constraints are likely to be considered by physicians. Physicians are humans, not computers. Their judgmental processes are often more elliptical and heuristic than they are methodical and calculated. Like any other professional engaged with a complex body of knowledge and experience, physicians are subliminally affected by countless influences. Therefore, it has been observed that their practice styles develop more from habit and learned tradition than from rigorous, deductive logic. As resource constraints become more manifest, they are likely to induce physicians to alter their practice styles more or less subconsciously so that they engage in what is referred to as implicit rather than explicit rationing. Thus, physicians will not overtly consider that they are making marginal sacrifices in medical benefit. As demonstrated by the British experience, they will adjust their views of proper practice to fit within the constraints they face. Because implicit rationing will often occur without conscious deliberation, it is unrealistic to require physicians to disclose thought processes they in fact are not overtly engaged in.

Elsewhere, informed consent doctrine frequently compromises ideal theory to accommodate similar prudential concerns of administration in real world settings. This is witnessed even in the law's core standards of materiality and causation. Despite the purpose of informed consent law to actualize individual autonomy fully, the law employs an "objective test" of whether "reasonable" people would have viewed disclosure as important and whether the disclosure would have changed the "reasonable" patient's decision. The law compromises its purely subjective values in

order to prevent injured plaintiffs from playing unduly on the sympathies of a lay jury by asserting their after-the-fact regrets.

Even more telling is the fact that informed consent is routinely practiced in real-world settings only for invasive procedures and at major junctures in the treatment relationship, such as at the point of hospital admission. Despite the law's literal application to any treatment or nontreatment decision, and despite the defensive tendencies caused by physicians' hypersensitive liability concerns, rarely is written informed consent obtained to prescribe medication or perform a routine test. Never is it obtained for the multitude of injections, bodily inspections, and manipulations, midnight awakenings, and other personal invasions one encounters during the course of hospitalization. It is simply felt that, in practice, it is not worth carrying informed consent requirements to their logical extreme for minor, noninvasive steps, even on pain of the physician's liability or the patient's risk of harm.

Even more so would it be infeasible to apply informed consent literally to the vast multitude of nontreatment decisions. Great Britain has avoided this path, partly out of recognition that "the economics of the British National Health Service could not tolerate" total patient sovereignty. Even some of the commentators who advance the most stringent versions of informed consent *ethics* concede that the *law* is too blunt an instrument for behavioral control to strictly enforce ethical ideals through liability rules.

However, as convincing as this pragmatic reasoning may be, it still fails to supply a principled legal basis for suspending informed consent requirements. Filling in this analytic void will require developing a new theory of economic informed consent, which the remainder of this article undertakes in broad, conceptual outline. In the conclusion, I suggest some of the parameters that should shape the more detailed implementation of this legal theory in real-world settings, but I leave this further explication to future development.

PRIOR CONSENT TO RATIONING

A proper theory of economic informed consent requires us first to understand how patient autonomy, the fundamental value underlying informed consent, relates to economic constraints. Patient autonomy would be perfectly preserved despite resource constraints if there were no health insurance at all because patients would be free to purchase as much health care as they could afford, being fully informed along the way about the various options and their relative cost effectiveness. However, the exigencies of poor health and the anxiety of having to think about money when a patient or a family member is sick make the desire for some form of insurance compelling. The existence of insurance requires that, to some degree, spending decisions be delegated to treating physicians or to governing entities (whether corporate, government, professional, or consumer-oriented). This delegation of spending authority creates the dilemma that insured patients will lose control over rationing decision making.

Menzel [see Part Six, Section Three] and others have suggested the concept of prior consent to health care rationing as a way to reconcile the demands of patient autonomy with the need to preserve an affordable form of insurance. Prior consent reasons that enrolling with an HMO constitutes blanket advance consent to the subsequent denials of marginally beneficial care created by the rules, procedures, and incentives disclosed at the outset (and periodically reaffirmed through annual open enrollment decisions); thereafter, additional disclosure at the time of treatment is unnecessary.

PRESUMED CONSENT DISTINGUISHED

Prior consent should not be confused with presumed consent, a separate concept that Menzel develops. Presumed consent reasons that consent requirements are satisfied if it can be shown that, had the patient been asked, he or she would have consented. Menzel argues that presumed consent is an adequate substitute when actual consent is impossible or prohibitively costly as, for instance, where the patient is incompetent and in emergent need of care. He extends this absolute incapacity argument to the relative disabling effect that insurance has on economic rationality, or what economists call "moral hazard." In Menzel's view, the inability of insured patients to assess rationally which medical benefits are worth the costs paid by insurance is a form of incapacity that allows the

invocation of presumed consent. Because the ideal vantage point from which to gauge patients' cost-sensitive treatment preferences is when they choose how much to spend on an insurance premium, Menzel argues for allowing rationing decisions that reflect what the patient would have agreed to if asked before becoming ill, at the time of enrollment.

This controversial position need not be defended here. Instead, the position I wish to examine is whether a fully informed decision to enroll in a limited insurance plan constitutes *actual* consent to the subsequent treatment decisions. Under this position, there is nothing fictitious about the consent. Actual consent can be viewed as resulting from informed enrollment, even if all of the multitude of possible nontreatment decisions and their particular risks and benefits are not described to the patient, because he or she is informed of and consents to the broad parameters of a rationing *mechanism*. Advance agreement to a set of rationing rules and incentives binds the insured person by the treatment decisions that result from these mechanisms, much as a principal is bound by the contracts his agent forms.

THE LACK-OF-UNDERSTANDING OBJECTION

It might be objected that disclosure at the time of enrollment would rarely suffice to meet requirements of truly informed prior consent because the array of choices one must make at that stage are far too vast and complex for health policy experts, let alone ordinary subscribers, to comprehend adequately. Much the same objection can be made, however, about conventional applications of informed consent to invasive treatment decisions. Dozens of empirical studies have documented the frustrating reality that some people will never sufficiently comprehend the medical options they face regardless of how thorough the explanation because they simply lack the intellectual capacity or the experiential base. Despite this documented and persistent futility, we do not dispense with informed consent practices altogether, nor do we prohibit the performance of the procedure owing to the lack of true understanding. Instead, we reason that autonomy values are promoted simply by giving patients the opportunity to understand or to make their own mistakes.

However, this rationale provides no guidance on how much disclosure is required for consent to be truly informed because it concedes that being truly informed is largely a fiction and it argues that autonomy values are satisfied even in its absence. The sufficiency of patients' understanding and the rationality of their actual decision processes are not the talisman for the adequacy of disclosure. Instead, we decide when consent is sufficiently informed by a much more intuitive, pragmatic, and socially constructed judgment about how much effort at disclosure and education is appropriate in a given situation, for a specified range of decisions. In short, we do the best we can under the circumstances. In the present context, this means that the sufficiency of a global disclosure of rationing incentives, rules, and mechanisms at the time of enrollment can best be determined by examining how law and ethics regard similar instances of prior consent.

RECOGNIZED EXAMPLES OF BUNDLED, PRIOR CONSENT

Prior consent is the basis on which surrogates are allowed to refuse life-sustaining treatment. The patient's informed appointment of an agent satisfies consent requirements even for decisions as monumental as withdrawing life support. The argument here by analogy is that an informed enrollment decision in essence constitutes prior explicit consent to appointing the HMO medical director and the primary care physician as agents for a bundle of much less significant but nonspecific treatment refusal decisions. Although these agents may be affected by conflicting economic interests, so might family members, yet they are viewed as not only valid, but also as preferred agents for making explicitly life-and-death decisions.

Bundled consent is also how we conventionally view a single decision to be hospitalized or operated on as entailing consent to hundreds of discrete events of testing, medication, and bodily examination during the course of what may be a rather long and complex episode of treatment. Likewise, bundled consent applies to economically motivated refusals of marginally beneficial treatment because, when an insurance subscriber knowingly enrolls in a rationing system, he buys into an entire cost-constrained medical philosophy and set of practices.

An even more direct application of this reasoning that is widely accepted in bioethics and the law applies to "futile" treatment: care that falls outside the prevailing standard of care more because it lacks medical benefit than because it presents a medical risk. The conventional thinking is that informed consent law cannot be used to force physicians to provide or even discuss care that, in their view of medical benefit, has no utility whatsoever, such as laetrile for cancer patients, antibiotics for a viral respiratory infection, or megadoses of vitamin C for a common cold. No one even considers that doctors should inform patients as they silently bypass such generally disapproved alternatives, even though some other doctors indeed believe in the utility of these treatments. It is generally agreed that physicians are free to limit themselves to their chosen school of practice so long as that school is accurately reflected in their representations to the general patient community. Here, this same representation is made explicit by the global economic disclosures that should be made at the time of enrollment in a rationed insurance plan. . . .

WAIVER OF INFORMED CONSENT

It is perhaps easier to characterize an informed enrollment decision not as advance consent, but instead as a waiver of the right to be informed when a chosen rationing mechanism denies costly treatment of marginal benefit. Actual prior consent justifies silent rationing by arguing that global disclosure satisfies the primary informed consent duty; waiver invokes an affirmative defense to a prima facie violation of that duty. Under the waiver characterization, informed consent requirements are not satisfied—they are dispensed with at the patient's request. A number of legal authorities and commentators have observed in passing that informed consent can be waived, for to rule otherwise would undermine the very value of personal autonomy that the doctrine is intended to enforce. Allowing waiver is perfectly consistent with informed consent doctrine because the principal effect of consent is itself a waiver—of the right not to be touched. If the law is willing to allow the right of bodily integrity to be waived, it should be (and is) willing also to recognize the waiver of the secondary right to *information about* a bodily invasion, so long as the waiver itself is informed and freely given.

CONSTRAINTS ON FREE CHOICE

The success of this argument depends on whether, in fact, patients would prefer not to be told of long-shot, expensive treatment options that are not covered by their insurance. Whether patients in a real-world setting will agree to waive economic informed refusal disclosures naturally depends on what their options are. Quite a few more will demand full disclosure if that option comes at no cost or inconvenience to them in their choice of insurance plans, but they will have to think about it much harder if they learn that the least expensive or most comprehensive insurance (or both) demands this concession. However, can it be said that the right to informed consent is freely waived if the decision is made on pain of a substantial sacrifice in health benefits or increase in premiums? What if the *only* insurance available requires an informed refusal waiver, so that the only means to obtain full disclosure of nontreatment is to pay out of pocket?

Ideally, patients would be allowed to pick precisely the degree of disclosure they desire from any provider with no consequence to themselves. This could be accomplished, as Engelhardt suggests, by asking "subscribers to insurance programs . . . to check which standard of disclosure they wished used in their treatment . . . [and to] review their choices semiannually or annually." However desirable this may be, it may not be feasible, or, if it is, it is not required by the law. Doctors may find it difficult to employ multiple disclosure standards among their many patients and still satisfy the standard of proof required if their decisions are challenged in court. Doctors' bedside manner, like their basic medical practice style, tends to be fairly uniform across patients. Presumably, the law is lenient enough to allow a doctor to employ a single disclosure standard for all of his or her patients so long as it is sufficiently disclosed at the outset of the treatment relationship, leaving patients free to choose another provider if they wish.

Can the same be said for a group of doctors organized into an insurance plan? Choice might still be preserved, if not within the plan, then among plans, if a private employer offers a range of insurance options or a government program is administered through a managed competition system. We have already observed that a hospital can, without either violating fiduciary principles or being accused of coercion, insist that a patient cooperate with frequent, bothersome testing, medication, and other routine steps as a condition of treatment in that facility. Likewise, an HMO should be able to offer its services contingent on agreement to a reasonable disclosure standard, even one that is lower than the law ordinarily sets.

Some limitation of individual choice is particularly appropriate given the collective nature of insurance. An insurance subscriber joins a community of interest when pooling his or her risk with others. This necessarily requires a collective agreement on certain terms and conditions of coverage because demanding tailor-made insurance would destroy the risk-pooling function that makes insurance possible or affordable in the first place. Where the treatment function is integrated with the insurance function, as in HMOs, then subscribers necessarily must be bound by a collective agreement on certain aspects of the treatment relationship as well. To insist on a greater degree of disclosure than the rest of the pool is willing to tolerate is no more ethically justified than insisting on more treatment than the subscriber has paid for. In short, individual-rights-based informed consent principles derived from a solo practice, third-party-reimbursement setting do not automatically apply to the new forms of health care delivery. . . .

CONCLUSION

This analysis has mounted a relentless attack on full-bodied application of informed refusal liability to all rationing decisions. In doing so, I do not mean to argue that no legal duty exists or that consent (or waiver) should be blithely found in any enrollment decision. Instead, I mean only to sketch a theory of economic informed consent that articulates the conceptual parameters for constructive debate about the precise circumstances and extent of disclosure. Some global disclosure of rationing incentives, rules, and mechanisms is required at the outset of enrollment, although this presently is not done, and the details of what should be disclosed still have to be worked out. However, if such a disclosure can be accomplished, it serves to validate at least some subsequent rationing decisions, either under a prior, bundled consent conception, or under a waiver of consent conception. The extent of the required initial disclosure and the extent to which it encompasses subsequent treatment decisions are matters that are too complex and situation specific to prescribe in the present analysis, but the answers to these important inquiries should be shaped by the general principles I have advanced.

This freedom to engage in silent rationing is tempered, however, by a number of additional limitations that this article only touches on or has not mentioned at all:

1. Subscribers should be told that their doctors will not always point out when potentially beneficial treatment is not being offered because of its costs.
2. For this understanding to be enforceable, private employers must offer more than a single health insurance option and, more radically, public programs must be operated under principles of consumer choice that are common only in private markets.
3. Patients must always remain free to ask questions and, when they do, they must be answered thoroughly, including suggestions for where to obtain second opinions or optional, uninsured treatment.
4. Finally, some nontreatment decisions are so dramatic and high-stake, such as pulling the plug on life support or declining a life-saving operation for a terminally ill patient, that, if the plan imposes them, they should be specifically disclosed at the time of treatment. This could result either from the extension of informed consent doctrine or as the application of abandonment law, but legislative enactment or regulatory oversight might be preferable to the common law for drawing a justiciable line between dramatic and ordinary treatment refusals.

NOTES

1. *Karlsons v. Guerinot,* 57 A.D.2d 73, 394 N.Y.S.2d 933 (1977).
2. *Moore v. Regents of the University of California,* 793 P.2d 479, 483 (Cal. 1990).
3. *Hidding v. Williams,* 578 So.2d 1192 (La. App. 1991); *Behringer v. Princeton Medical Center,* 592 A.2d 1251 (N.J. Super. 1991).

Must We Forgo Informed Consent to Control Health Care Costs?
A Response to Mark A. Hall

Paul S. Appelbaum

Should physicians discuss openly with their patients the economic influences on their recommendations for care? Mark A. Hall argues that disclosure of alternative treatments precluded by patients' insurance coverage is not required by the law of informed consent. Morreim (1991), in contrast, looks to

Milbank Quarterly, Vol. 71, No. 4, 1993. Copyright © 1993 Milbank Memorial Fund. Used with permission of Blackwell Publishers.

patients' rights to self-determination, physicians' contractual obligations toward patients, and the fiduciary relationship that defines the doctor-patient interaction as bases for a contrary conclusion.

Before exploring some aspects of this debate, two preliminary points are worth clarifying. Although Hall frames his discussion in terms of whether informed consent law *would* require disclosure, his argument is more than a mere prediction of how the courts will apply existing law.

Legal doctrine is the embodiment of policy. When the courts created the law of informed consent, and as they subsequently modified it, they acted in pursuit of a set of policy goals that were partly directed toward altering the balance of power in physician–patient relationships (Appelbaum, Meisel, and Lidz 1987). If judges believe that disclosure of economic effects on treatment decisions is desirable, they will extend the law of informed consent to require such disclosure. Thus, I understand Hall's argument as prescriptive: that the courts should not apply consent law to require case-specific disclosure of economic constraints on medical recommendations.

Further, although the motivation for this position may be obvious, I do not find it stated overtly in Hall's article. When Hall and others argue against physicians' disclosure of options they have not recommended on economic grounds, they do so out of concern that such a requirement would undercut the effectiveness of reforms aimed at limiting health-care expenditures. Patients repeatedly confronted with real-life restrictions on treatment, in this view, would create irresistible demands for additional coverage that would undo any cost controls. Hall's suggestion that case-specific discussions be replaced by general disclosure of limitations on care at the time of enrollment in a health plan is designed to bolster the prospects of health reform, leaving patients unaware that they are being denied potentially beneficial care.

The worth of this decidedly utilitarian proposal depends on the correctness of several underlying presumptions, including the proposition that consumer ignorance is the only basis on which health care reform can rest. I focus, however, on two other issues that I find key to evaluating the reasonableness of this approach: the effectiveness of "global disclosure of rationing mechanisms at the time of enrollment"; and the likely effects of a failure to disclose economic components of decision making at the time a course of treatment is recommended.

Because there is substantial danger in allowing the discussion of health care reform to become too abstract, it may be useful to consider the following real-life case, around which the discussion can be structured:

Ms. Wickline, a woman hospitalized for vascular surgery, suffers several postoperative complications. As the period of hospitalization approved by her insurance plan draws to a close, her surgeon requests the insurer's approval for an additional eight days of inpatient care. Only four days are approved; the surgeon later maintains his belief that he had no choice but to discharge the patient after that period elapsed. Within a few days of leaving the hospital, the patient's leg begins to hurt and turn blue. She is not seen by a physician for nine days, by which time her leg requires amputation.[1]

Ms. Wickline's surgeon—as best I can tell from the reports of the case—appears not to have informed her that, in his judgment, four additional days of hospital care were desirable. Because the announcement of her insurer, California's public Medi-Cal program, that it would not pay for the extra days was the determining factor in the surgeon's decision, this would seem to be just the situation that Hall's proposal addresses. It is a "rationing decision," in his terms, because it involves a "decision to decline potentially beneficial care on account of excessive costs." Hall presumably would support the surgeon's failure to discuss the basis for his decision to discharge the patient as long as certain disclosures had been made at the time Ms. Wickline enrolled in the insurance plan.

EFFECTIVENESS OF DISCLOSURE AT TIME OF ENROLLMENT

What information, assuming it had been provided to Ms. Wickline prospectively, would have justified her surgeon's behavior? The answer, of course, depends on the goals of requiring that anything at all be disclosed to patients about the basis for physicians' recommendations. Informed consent law has been charged by different theorists with varying tasks, but the least controversial probably is to ensure that patients receive sufficient information to enable them to play a meaningful role in treatment decision making, if they so choose. What prospective disclosure would have allowed Ms. Wickline to function in this way?

Insurers currently offer limited information to subscribers about how decisions will be made on coverage of medical treatment. Some interventions (e.g., cosmetic plastic surgery) may be excluded outright; others (e.g., psychiatric hospitalization) often are subject to blanket caps on a calendar year or lifetime basis. In general, though, subscribers are told that all "medically necessary" care will be covered (Hall and Anderson 1992). Medical necessity, however, is a term that obscures as least as much as it reveals. Ms. Wickline's surgeon initially believed that eight additional days of hospitalization were medically necessary. Only when the insurer, with clear pecuniary interests of its own, disagreed, did the surgeon relent. Thus, at least in this case, medical necessity seems vulnerable to reinterpretation on the basis of economic pressures.

Clearly, some additional information must be provided to a subscriber like Ms. Wickline if she is to understand that the possibility of benefit to her medical condition—the plain meaning of medical necessity—is not a sufficient basis for decisions regarding her care. What might that information be? Havighurst (1992), who has struggled with this question, suggests two general approaches. The first would "assist consumers in economizing by surrendering legal rights that systematically induce or excuse excessive spending by physicians." Thus, subscribers might be told that their insurers and physicians would depart from customary treatment when to do so would not be unreasonable in benefit/cost terms, or that their rights to sue were limited to situations in which gross negligence could be demonstrated. Havighurst's second broad option would be to refer subscribers to sets of practice guidelines that would define the treatments for which insurers would be liable. Insureds might then know with some certainty what treatment they could expect to have covered.

Hall's approach to this question appears in greater detail elsewhere (Hall and Anderson 1992). He recommends that disclosure at the time of enrollment include enumeration of excluded treatments, general standards that would guide determinations of coverage, and the specification of entities that would apply these standards to medical treatments in general and to specific cases, like Ms. Wickline's, in particular.

To what extent would such disclosures help Ms. Wickline, lying in her hospital bed, to understand the basis for her surgeon's decision sufficiently for her to play a meaningful role in the outcome? Note that postulating an effect of disclosure at the time of enrollment depends on an interrelated set of highly questionable propositions: that disclosure is made in language sufficiently clear for a layperson

to understand; that subscribers are alerted to the importance of the information, such that they attend to its presentation, whether oral or written; that persons unsophisticated about medical concepts are able to appreciate the implications of the information for their future (unanticipated) medical conditions; and that, when faced with the need for medical treatment at some point in the indefinite future, subscribers are able to recall the provisions of their policies with clarity.

Even were all these desiderata to be achieved— an accomplishment students of informed consent in the real world would recognize as little short of miraculous—considerable doubt would remain as to whether patients still would grasp the impact of economic factors on their care. If Ms. Wickline, in a formidable act of will, had been able to recall that her insurer and physicians were authorized to depart from customary standards of care when warranted by benefit/cost considerations, would she have had any idea that her surgeon's initial recommendation for an extended stay had been modified in response to economic concerns? If practice guidelines covering vascular surgery, along with hundreds of other medical conditions, had been included by reference in her insurance contract, again assuming she read and recalled them, would they have been of sufficient detail to inform her of limits on length of stay in her peculiar circumstances, which involved several postoperative complications? If the policy had specified standards for determining when coverage was available and established independent bodies to apply them, would she have had any way of knowing that the discharge decision, among all others, had been affected by this process?

Only a cockeyed optimist is likely to respond to these queries in the affirmative. Moreover, most discussions of contractual mechanisms for limiting disclosure about and provision of potentially beneficial care assume, as does Hall, that patients' autonomy will be protected by allowing them to select among insurance plans, choosing the plan that provides the optimal combination of disclosure, coverage, and cost. Because options for health insurance are dwindling, however, as existing plans merge, this is increasingly unlikely to be the case. Indeed, many employers offer their workers only a single choice of plan, and Ms. Wickline, who relied on a public insurance program, also had no alternative but to accept the limitations imposed on her. Even with a choice of plans, the information costs of comparing plans according to provisions that are likely to affect discrete medical decisions will be, in almost all circumstances, prohibitive.

I conclude, therefore, that disclosure at the time of enrollment of an insurer's limitations on coverage based on economic considerations is unlikely to leave subscribers meaningfully informed about the ways in which their doctors' recommendations are being affected by concern over costs. Thus, whether one views their acceptance of enrollment as "prior consent" to rationing or as a "waiver" of consent, it is an action that for almost all persons will be taken in profound ignorance of its implications. Indeed, this should not be a surprising conclusion because keeping patients in the dark about the basis for particular rationing decisions is the motive force behind such proposals.

Even granting the ineffectiveness of prospective general disclosure, however, Hall and other advocates of this approach might well retort that the information in question will make little difference in any event—or, in legal terms, that it is not material to the patient's decision. If the insurer will not pay for the procedure, why require disclosure of particular rationing choices?

EFFECTS OF FAILURE TO DISCLOSE AT TIME OF TREATMENT

Hall himself offers a partial response to this question, noting that patients may elect to pay for treatment out of pocket if they are told that their physicians believe it is indicated. Moreover, patients might use such information to decide to switch doctors or insurance plans, or, Hall might have added, to advocate for alternative approaches to cost controls on medical care. As Hall notes, "Few nontreatment decisions would clearly escape these standards of materiality."

If I understand Hall's counterargument to these contentions, it is that physicians cannot be expected to inform patients of all the factors that influence the many decisions they make in the course of patient care. In addition, as physicians incorporate economic considerations into their decision making, they may not even be aware of the extent to which such influences are operative. These arguments have the feel of straw men. No one would contend that every factor entering into a treatment recommendation be disclosed to patients. But surely that is not the same as asking that physicians inform patients when, in their medical judgment, further treatment for which the patient's insurer will not pay is likely to be beneficial.

Nor have we exhausted the arguments that might be made in favor of such a practice. Although many patients, including Medi-Cal-insured Ms. Wickline, will not be able to pay out of pocket for noncovered care, they will always have the option of appealing the denial of benefits to the insurer. This was a step Ms. Wickline's surgeon, absent pressure from his patient, failed to pursue. The likelihood that appeals, particularly if supported by the physician, will be at least partially successful is demonstrated by advice given to insurers and managed-care companies to authorize care for an interim period while additional review (perhaps by a neutral third party) takes place (Hinden and Elden 1990).

Other beneficial effects may ensue from a discussion between physician and patient regarding the reasons why the additional, uncompensated care was thought desirable. Ms. Wickline, for example, neglected to seek medical attention after discharge, despite symptoms suggesting thrombosis in her leg. One can only speculate about the reasons for her inaction, but knowledge that her surgeon believed her condition warranted further hospitalization would have reinforced in her mind the importance of seeking follow-up care if complications developed.

Perhaps the most potent argument for disclosure at the time economic rationing decisions are made involves the probable effects of failure to disclose on the physician–patient relationship. The essence of that relationship always has been thought to be what Fried (1974) referred to as "personal care," the primary allegiance of the physician to the patient's well-being. It is undoubtedly true that this orientation is not absolute. Physicians long have been held to have obligations to protect the public health (e.g., by reporting communicable diseases), even when such action might be to the detriment of their patients. By and large, however, patients seem to understand and tolerate these uncommon exceptions to the general principle.

Were physicians, however, routinely to conceal their opinions that patients would benefit from additional medical care not covered by their insurers, the core of the physician-patient relationship would be in jeopardy. Patients legitimately would suspect all recommendations made by physicians, always concerned that they were being deceived regarding the care they needed. The medical treatment setting would be fully adversarialized, with wealthier patients seeking outside opinions of independently retained physicians on all matters of medical import. Indeed, even Hall is willing to compromise a bit here, allowing physicians to respond fully to questions patients ask—unwilling evidently to tolerate affirmative prevarication—although not forcing them to volunteer the information on their own. (Does this, by the way, not undo the entire effect of Hall's proposal? What is left of his plan once every patient learns to ask, "Are there any other treatments that you think would be beneficial for me, but are not recommending because of their cost?")

CONCLUSION

Although presented under the rubric of "prior consent," Hall's and similar proposals in fact sacrifice patient consent altogether. Subscribers are unlikely to understand or appreciate information provided at the time of enrollment, or to recall it when decisions are being made. Denying patients disclosure of the basis for medical recommendations therefore undermines any possibility of their playing a meaningful role in treatment decision making, with all the deleterious consequences outlined above. Is such institutionalized deception essential to cost-conscious health reform? I certainly hope not. At a minimum, however, there is no small irony in informed consent—a legal doctrine whose genesis and development were based on the desire to enhance patients' autonomous participation in medical decision making—being recruited for this purpose.

NOTES

1. *Wickline v. State,* 228 Cal. Rptr. 661 (Cal. App. 2 Dist. 1986).

REFERENCES

Appelbaum, P.S., A. Meisel, and C.W. Lidz. 1987. *Informed Consent: Legal Theory and Clinical Practice.* New York: Oxford University Press.

Fried, C. 1974. *Medical Experimentation: Personal Integrity and Social Policy.* New York: American Elsevier.

Hall, M.A., and G.E. Anderson. 1992. Health Insurers' Assessment of Medical Necessity. *University of Pennsylvania Law Review* 140: 1637–1712.

Havighurst, C.C. 1992. Prospective Self-denial: Can Consumers Contract Today to Accept Health Care Rationing Tomorrow? *University of Pennsylvania Law Review* 140:1755–1808.

Hinden, R.A., and D.L. Elden. 1990. Liability Issues for Managed Care Entities. *Seton Hall Legislative Journal* 14:1–63.

Morreim, E.H. 1991. Economic Disclosure and Economic Advocacy: New Duties in the Medical Standard of Care. *Journal of Legal Medicine* 12:275–329.

RECOMMENDED SUPPLEMENTARY READING

General Works

Ahronheim, Judith C., Moreno, Jonathan, and Zuckerman, Connie. *Ethics in Clinical Practice*. New York: Little, Brown and Co., 1994.

Annas, George J. *Standard of Care: The Law of American Bioethics*. Oxford: Oxford University Press, 1993.

Beauchamp, Tom L., and Childress, James F. *Principles of Biomedical Ethics*. 4th ed. New York: Oxford University Press, 1994.

Benjamin, Martin, and Curtis, Joy. *Ethics in Nursing*. New York: Oxford University Press, 1992.

Burt, Robert. *Taking Care of Strangers*. New York: Free Press, 1979.

Campbell, Alastair, Charlesworth, Max, Gillett, Grant, and Jones, Gareth. *Medical Ethics*. New York: Oxford University Press, 1997.

Caplan, Arthur. *If I Were a Rich Man Could I Buy a Pancreas?* Bloomington: Indiana University Press, 1992.

Cassell, Eric. *The Nature of Suffering and the Goals of Medicine*. New York: Oxford University Press, 1991.

Crigger, Bette-Jane, ed. *Cases in Bioethics*. 3rd ed. New York: St. Martin's Press, 1998.

Downie, R. S., and Calman, Kenneth C. *Healthy Respect: Ethics in Health Care*. New York: Oxford University Press, 1994.

Dubler, Nancy, and Nimmons, David. *Ethics on Call*. New York: Crown, 1992.

Dworkin, Roger B. *Limits: The Role of the Law in Bioethical Decision Making*. Bloomington: Indiana University Press, 1996.

Englehardt, H. Tristram, Jr. *The Foundations of Bioethics*. 2nd ed. New York: Oxford University Press, 1996.

Gert, Bernard, Culver, Charles M., and Clouser, K. Danner. *Bioethics: A Return To Fundamentals*. New York: Oxford University Press, 1997.

Gorovitz, Samuel. *Doctors' Dilemmas: Moral Conflict and Medical Care*. New York: Oxford University Press, 1982.

Herbert, Philip. *Doing Right: A Practical Guide for Physicians and Medical Trainees*. New York: Oxford University Press, 1996.

Holms, Helen, and Purdy, Laura, eds. *Feminist Perspectives in Medical Ethics*. Bloomington: Indiana University Press, 1992.

Jonsen, Albert. *The New Medicine and the Old Ethics*. Cambridge, MA: Harvard University Press, 1990.

Kass, Leon. *Toward a More Natural Science*. New York: Free Press, 1985.

Macklin, Ruth. *Mortal Choices: Bioethics in Today's World*. New York: Pantheon Books 1987.

May, William F. *The Patient's Ordeal*. Bloomington: Indiana University Press, 1991.

Moreno, Jonathan D. *Deciding Together*. New York: Oxford University Press, 1995.

Polansky, Ronald, and Kuczewski, Mark, eds. *Bioethics: Modern Problems, Classical Solutions*. Pittsburgh: Mathesis Publications, 1998.

Rothman, David J. *Strangers at the Bedside: A History of How Law and Bioethics Transformed Medical Decision Making*. New York: Basic Books, 1991.

Tong, Rosemarie. *Feminist Approaches to Bioethics*. Boulder, CA: Westview Press, 1997.

Veatch, Robert M. *A Theory of Medical Ethics*. New York: Basic Books, 1981.

Zaner, Richard. *Ethics and the Clinical Encounter*. Englewood Cliffs, NJ: Prentice-Hall, 1988.

Autonomy, Paternalism, and Medical Models

Agich, George J. *Autonomy and Long-Term Care*. Oxford: Oxford University Press, 1993.

Blustein, Jeffrey. "Doing What the Patient Orders: Maintaining Integrity in the Doctor-Patient Relationship." *Bioethics* 7, no. 4 (1993): 289–314.

Bok, Sissela. *Lying*. New York: Pantheon Books, 1978.

Brennan, Troy A. *Just Doctoring: Medical Ethics in the Liberal State*. Berkeley: University of California Press, 1991.

Brody, Howard. *The Healer's Power*. New Haven, CT: Yale University Press, 1992.

Childress, James F. *Who Should Decide? Paternalism and Health Care*. New York: Oxford University Press, 1982.

Churchill, Larry R. "Reviving a Distinctive Medical Ethic." *Hastings Center Report* (May–June 1989): 28–34.

Collopy, Bart J. "Autonomy in Long-Term Care: Some Crucial Distinctions" *Gerontologist* 28 (supplement, 1988): 10–17.

Collopy, Bart J., Dubler, Nancy, and Zuckerman, Connie. "The Ethics of Home Care: Autonomy and Accommodation." *Hastings Center Report* (special supplement, March–April 1990): 1–16.

Dworkin, Gerald. *The Theory and Practice of Autonomy*. Cambridge, UK: Cambridge University Press, 1988.

Halper, Thomas. "Privacy and Autonomy: From Warren and Brandeis to *Roe* and *Cruzan*." *Journal of Medicine and Philosophy* 21, no. 2 (April 1996): 121–135.

"Healthcare Relationships: Ties That Bind." *Cambridge Quarterly of Healthcare Ethics* 3, no. I (Winter 1994): 1–82.

Kane, Rosalie, and Caplan, Arthur, eds. *Ethical Conflicts in the Management of Home Care*. New York: Springer, 1993.

Kant, Immanuel. "On the Supposed Right to Lie from Altruistic Motives." In *Critique of Practical Reason*, trans. L. W. Beck. Chicago: University of Chicago Press, 1949.

Kleinig, John. *Paternalism*. Totowa, NJ: Rowman and Allanheld, 1984.

Kultgen, John. *Autonomy and Intervention: Paternalism in the Caring Life*. New York: Oxford University Press, 1995.

Lidz, Charles, Fischer, Lynn, and Arnold, Robert M. *The Erosion of Autonomy in Long-Term Care*. Oxford: Oxford University Press, 1992.

May, William F. "Code, Covenant, Contract, or Philanthropy." *Hastings Center Report* 5 (December 1975): 29–38.

Pellegrino, Edmund D., and Thomasma, David C. *For the Patient's Good: The Restoration of Beneficence in Health Care*. New York: Oxford University Press, 1988.

Shelp, Earl E., ed. *Virtue and Medicine*. Dordrecht, Holland: D. Reidel Publishing Co., 1985.

Strasser, Mark. "The New Paternalism." *Bioethics* 7, no. 2 (1988): 103–117.

VanDeVeer, Donald. *Paternalistic Intervention: The Moral Bounds of Benevolence*. Princeton, NJ: Princeton University Press, 1986.

Veatch, Robert M. "Models for Medicine in a Revolutionary Age." *Hastings Center Report* 2 (June 1972): 5–7.

Informed Consent

Appelbaum, Paul S., Lidz, Charles W., and Meisel, Alan. *Informed Consent: Legal Theory and Clinical Practice*. New York: Oxford University Press, 1987.

Brock, Dan. *Life and Death: Philosophical Essays in Biomedical Ethics*. New York: Cambridge University Press, 1993.

Cassell, Eric J. *Talking with Patients. Vol. 1. The Theory of Doctor-Patient Communication. Vol. 2, Clinical Technique*. Cambridge, MA: M.I.T. Press, 1985.

Faden, Ruth, and Beauchamp, Tom. A *History and Theory of Informed Consent*. New York: Oxford University Press, 1986.

Geller, Gail, et al. "'Decoding' Informed Consent." *Hastings Center Report* (March–April 1997): 28–33.

"In Case of Emergency: No Need for Consent." *Hastings Center Report* (Symposium, January–February, 1997): 7–12.

Katz, Jay. *The Silent World of Doctor and Patient*. New York: Free Press, 1984.

Kuczewski, Mark G. "Reconceiving the Family: The Process of Consent in Medical Decisionmaking." *Hastings Center Report* (March–April, 1996): 30–37.

Marta, Jan. "A Linguistic Model of Informed Consent." *Journal of Medicine and Philosophy* 21, no. 1 (February 1996): 41–60.

President's Commission for the Study of Ethical Problems in Medicine and Biomedical and Behavioral Research. *Making Health Care Decisions: The Ethical and Legal Implications of Informed Consent in the Patient-Practitioner Relationship*. Washington, DC: U.S. Government Printing Office, 1982.

Schuck, Peter H. "Rethinking Informed Consent." *Yale Law Journal* 103 (1994): 899 ff.

Veatch, Robert M. "Abandoning Informed Consent," *Hastings Center Report* (March–April 1995): 5–12.

Professional Responsibilities: Conflicts of Interest in Managed Care

Agich, George J., ed. *Responsibility in Health Care*. Dordrecht, Holland: D. Reidel Publishing Co., 1982.

Angell, Marcia. "The Doctor as Double Agent." *Kennedy Institute of Ethics Journal* 3, no. 3. (September 1993): 279.

"Conflicts of Interest in Health Care." *American Journal of Law and Medicine* 21, nos. 2 and 3 (1995).

Danis, Marion, and Churchill, Larry. "Autonomy and the Common Weal." *Hastings Center Report* (January–February 1991): 25–31.

Gray, Bradford H. *The Profit Motive and Patient Care: The Changing Accountability of Doctors and Hospitals*. Cambridge, MA: Harvard University Press, 1991.

———, ed. *For-Profit Enterprise in Health Care*. Washington, DC: National Academy Press, 1986.

"Health Care Capitated Payment Systems." *American Journal of Law and Medicine* 22, nos. 2 and 3 (1996).

Hoy, E. W. "Change and Growth in Managed Care." *Health Affairs*, 10 (Winter 1991): 19.

Latham, Stephen R. "Regulation of Managed Care Incentive Payments to Physicians." *American Journal of Law and Medicine* 22, no. 4 (1996): 399–432.

Macklin, Ruth. *The Enemies of Patients*. New York: Oxford University Press, 1993, chapter 7.

Martin, Julia A. and Bjerknes, Lisa K. "The Legal and Ethical Implications of Gag Clauses in Physician Contracts." *American Journal of Law and Medicine* 22, no. 4 (1996): 433–476.

Menzel, Paul T. "Double Agency and the Ethics of Rationing Health Care: A Response to Marcia Angell." *Kennedy Institute of Ethics Journal* 3, no. 3 (1993): 293–302.

Orentlicher, David. "Health Care Reform and the Patient-Physician Relationship." *Health Matrix: Journal of Law-Medicine* 5, no. 1 (1995): 141–180.

Rodwin, Marc A. *Medicine, Money and Morals: Physicians' Conflicts of Interest*. New York: Oxford University Press, 1993.

Spece, Roy G. Jr., Shimm, David S., and Buchanan, Allen E., eds. *Conflicts of Interest in Clinical Practice and Research*. New York: Oxford University Press, 1996.

Wolf, Susan M. "Health Care Reform and the Future of Physician Ethics." *Hastings Center Report* 24, no. 2 (March–April 1994): 28–41.

Managed Care and Informed Consent

Gunderson, Martin. "Eliminating Conflicts of Interest in Managed Care Organizations Through Disclosure and Consent." *Journal of Law, Medicine and Ethics* 25, no. 2/3 (Summer 1997): 192–198.

PART TWO

DEFINING DEATH, FORGOING LIFE-SUSTAINING TREATMENT, AND EUTHANASIA

Death remains as inevitable as always, yet somehow today it seems harder to achieve. In the past, diseases such as pneumonia, formerly called "the old man's friend," led to a speedy and fairly gentle death. Today such infections can be treated, and many of the more rapid causes of death can be staved off. Thus, the benefits of medical advances bring with them burdens, and here the burden is the possibility of a lingering death, surrounded not by loved ones in the home, but by medical hardware in an intensive care unit.

Indeed, it is now possible to sustain individuals for years in a "persistent vegetative state," a state in which they do not feel, think, or have any awareness of their surroundings. Some would argue that someone who lacks a capacity for *any* conscious activity is not, in any meaningful ethical sense, alive. This raises the first issue of this chapter: How do we define death?

THE DEFINITION OF DEATH AND THE PERSISTENT VEGETATIVE STATE

Before the development of high-technology forms of life support—in particular, the respirator—death was pretty straightforward. People were dead when they stopped breathing and their hearts stopped beating. Today, however, respiration can be artificially maintained, and when this is done, the heart can continue to beat even in the absence of any input from the brain. Hence, a patient with an intact heart can be maintained on a respirator even when his or her brain functions have ceased entirely.

This new state of affairs created the need for rethinking the meaning of death. In 1968, an ad hoc committee of the Harvard Medical School issued a report setting forth tests for identifying patients in whom brain function had completely and irreversibly ceased. The Committee recommended that such patients be declared dead, and then removed from the respirator. Despite opposition by some religious groups, this new standard—"whole brain death," or simply "brain death"—has been widely adopted in this country. The first reading in Section One is a selection from a report by the influential President's Commission for the Study of Ethical Problems in Medicine and Biomedical and Behavioral Research, endorsing the adoption of the brain-death standard. In endorsing brain death, the Commission at the same time rejects the more far-reaching suggestion that patients possessing brain stem activity, but without any of the higher brain functions necessary for consciousness, also be declared dead. In rejecting the "neocortical death" or "higher brain death" proposal, the Commission argues that whole brain death is not, as one might think, a wholly new concept of death. Rather, the Commission suggests, it is simply that artificial ventilation has made the traditional cardiopulmonary indicators of death invalid for a set of patients, and brain death substitutes new diagnostic measures for them.

According to the Commission, then, the *concept* of death remains the same, whatever the *criteria* for determining death are taken to be. However, others maintain that the decision about which set of criteria to use is not solely, or even primarily, a scientific matter; it is not a matter of choosing the most reliable criteria of death, for example. Rather, our understanding of what constitutes human death depends on our understanding of what it is to be a human being. If we think of the human being primarily as an organism, then the whole-brain theory provides the best account of death, for the organism dies when the entire brain permanently ceases functioning. But if we think of the human being primarily as a *person*, then the higher-brain criterion is the better view, for the person is gone when the capacities for awareness, thought, and social interaction are permanently lost. Whichever view is taken, the choice must be made on moral grounds; that is, a moral argument is needed to answer the question of why we ought to adopt a person-oriented conception, rather than an organism-oriented conception, of human death.

Robert Veatch tries to provide such a moral argument. He opts for a higher brain–oriented definition of death because he believes that the essence of a human being is integration of a mind and a body. Under such a definition, patients with irreversible loss of consciousness, such as patients in persistent vegetative state (PVS), as well as anencephalic babies, who are born without a cerebral cortex, would be considered dead. Veatch begins by arguing that the whole-brain definition of death has become obsolete. No one really believes anymore that literally all functions of the entire brain must be irreversibly lost for an individual to be dead, for individual, isolated brain cells can live even though integrated supercellular brain function is destroyed. Moreover, small amounts of electrical activity can be recorded on an EEG (electroencephalogram), even when the brain is permanently nonfunctioning. Adherents of whole-brain theory explain that these sorts of brain activity should be ignored in determining brain death because such activity does not contribute to the functioning of the organism as a whole. However, Veatch thinks that once whole-brain theorists make this response, they are well on the way to the higher brain–oriented approach he favors.

Perhaps the most difficult criticism for adherents of the higher brain–oriented definition of death is the danger of a "slippery slope." Defining categories of people as "dead" has serious implications; for example, such people could be used as organ donors. Should organs be taken from PVS patients and anencephalic babies? Moreover, are we likely to stop there? Or will we begin to treat senile elderly patients with only marginal consciousness as dead? Will we stop at using anencephalic babies as organ donors, or move on to using infants with other devastating impairments, such as hydranencephalic infants, whose cerebral hemispheres have been largely or entirely destroyed in utero by infection? Veatch thinks that the higher brain–oriented approach is not susceptible to slippery-slope arguments because, unlike the whole-brain approach, it has a principle for determining death: a living human being exists when, and only when, the capacities for organic (bodily) and mental function are present together in a single human entity. However, it is far from clear how to interpret "the capacities for organic and mental function." And even if that issue is settled, there remains considerable controversy about the application of the principle itself; whether, for example, anencephalics totally lack awareness, and whether human beings with other disorders also lack a capacity for mental function (Shinnar and Arras 1989; Capron 1987; Shewmon et al. 1989).

Veatch agrees with those who think that the debate about which criteria to use for determining death is a conceptual and moral debate. The debate about the definition of death is actually a debate about the moral status of human beings, a debate about when humans should be treated as full members of the moral community. However, recognizing that we are unlikely to get uniformity on this issue in a pluralistic society, Veatch supports (within limits) conscience clauses that would permit individuals to choose their own definition of death based on their religious and philosophical convictions.

The higher-brain approach favored by Veatch is not, at present, anywhere accepted as law or public policy. Current medical practice differentiates brain death and persistent vegetative state. Unfortunately, the public, the media, and even physicians continue to use terms describing various forms of neurological impairment in confusing and incorrect ways (Cranford 1988). For example, the distinction between coma and PVS is blurred in the unfortunate phrase "irreversible coma." This term is confusing because even today some physicians apply it to three different situations: whole-brain death, PVS, or general permanent unconsciousness. Even more confusing is the phrase "chronically and irreversibly comatose," since truly comatose patients usually have a life span of only weeks or months, and rarely years— hardly the duration appropriately characterized as chronic. It is, instead, PVS patients who are in a chronic condition of unconsciousness, as PVS patients can be sustained, with artificial nutrition, for decades.

Robert Truog agrees with Veatch that the concept of whole-brain death is incoherent in theory and confused in practice. However, where Veatch supports a higher-brain definition of death, Truog suggests we would be better off returning to the traditional criteria of death: the permanent cessation of respiration and circulation.

Truog stresses the importance of distinguishing among a definition of death, criteria to determine when the definition has been fulfilled, and tests for evaluating when the criteria have been satisfied. In whole-brain death, the definition of death is "permanent cessation of functioning of the organism as a whole." The criterion of death is "permanent cessation of functioning of the entire brain." The tests for determining a person is dead are either the traditional cardiorespiratory standard, or a battery of neurological tests.

The trouble with the whole-brain approach, Truog says, is inconsistency among the three levels. Many individuals who fulfill all of the tests for brain death do not have permanent cessation of functioning of the entire brain. Many retain clear evidence of integrated brain function at the level of the brainstem and midbrain; some may even have cortical function. Moreover, clinicians have observed that patients who fulfill the tests of brain death "frequently respond to surgical incision at the time of organ procurement with a significant rise in both heart rate and blood pressure. This suggests that integrated neurological function at a supraspinal level may be present in at least some patients diagnosed as brain-dead." In other words, using the criterion of "permanent cessation of functioning of the entire brain," these patients are not dead. Yet if we insist that only dead patients can be (vital) organ donors, this will reduce the supply of viable organs for transplantation.

Advocates of a higher-brain criterion of death argue that this approach solves the organ transplantation problem. But Truog rejects this approach, for two reasons. First, he questions whether it is possible to diagnose permanent unconsciousness with the level of certainty required for the determination of death. Second, he notes that PVS patients breathe (and, we might add, move their eyes and sometimes even make sounds). The thought of burying or cremating someone who is still breathing, moving, or moaning would be unacceptable to most people. One possibility is to acknowledge that the body of a patient in PVS continues to live (and must be either killed or allowed to die before disposal), although the patient is dead (Wikler 1988).

Truog does not consider Wikler's dual notion of death, whereby the body can live though the person has died. Instead, he suggests we separate the criterion of death from our policies regarding organ procurement. The standard of death would be the traditional one: the permanent absence of cardiac and respiratory function. However, death would no longer be a condition of organ donation. Instead, organ procurement would be permitted only with the consent of the donor or appropriate surrogate, and only when doing so would not harm the donor, because the donor is "permanently and irreversibly unconscious or imminently and irreversibly dying."

An advantage of the return to the traditional cardiopulmonary standard of death is that, as it is invariably accepted by different religious and cultural groups, it permits a common concept of death. With a lowest-common-denominator standard, there would be no need to let religious groups choose their own definition of death, as Veatch favors. It remains unclear whether Truog's approach solves the problem of organ donation. If his rejection of the higher-brain formulation is that it is not sufficiently certain for a determination of death, why is it sufficiently certain for the removal of vital organs, directly causing death? And if most people would prefer not to be buried or cremated while still breathing, would they not have a similar objection to having their vital organs removed?

One of the fundamental challenges for bioethics today is to decide when to terminate treatment for patients who are, by present definitions, alive. Competent patients have a well-established, common-law right to refuse even life-sustaining medical treatment. As articulated by Justice Cardozo in a rightly celebrated formulation, "Every adult human being of adult years and sound mind has a right to determine what shall be done with his own body. . . ." But what exactly do we mean by a "sound mind," and how are we to distinguish sound minds from unsound minds?

DECISIONAL CAPACITY AND THE RIGHT TO REFUSE TREATMENT

Although most patients either clearly possess or clearly lack the capacity for autonomous decision

*EDITORS' NOTE: Strictly speaking, "competence" is a legal term. Thus understood, only judges have the authority to declare a patient "incompetent." In the less formal context of this book, however, we define "competency" as the capacity for autonomous decision making.

making, a significant portion fall into a troublesome gray area between competence and incompetence.* In Section Two, the factual and conceptual difficulties involved in determining competency are well illustrated in the case of Mary Northern, a stubborn 72-year-old woman suffering from gangrene of both feet. Although Ms. Northern's physicians insisted that surgical amputation of her feet was required to save her life, she adamantly refused to grant them permission to operate. Contrary to the opinion of her physicians, she maintained that her feet were improving and that surgery was thus unnecessary. While her physicians characterized her refusal as irrational, a court-appointed guardian remarked on her good memory and overall coherence and intelligence. Her physicians found her to be "psychotic" with regard to discussions about her feet, but her guardian concluded that she was of "sound mind." Mary Northern's own testimony, delivered from her bed in an intensive care unit, supported both conclusions. Who was right? More importantly, what do we mean by "competency," and what standards of decision-making capacity should be imposed on patients like Mary Northern?

According to Allen Buchanan and Dan Brock in "Deciding for Others: Competency," competency ought to be understood not as a global attribute, but rather as a "decision-relative" concept. In other words, persons should be thought of as competent to do this or that, or to make this or that decision. Obviously, the same patient might thus be competent to refuse an easily explainable procedure but incompetent to manage her own complex finances.

In addition, Buchanan and Brock argue that our concept of competency encompasses not merely an assessment of the patient's actual psychological capacities, but also a complex societal weighting of the values of well-being and autonomy. Noting that our task is to avoid two diametrically opposed kinds of error—stripping capable patients of their autonomy or allowing impaired patients to make foolish and self-destructive decisions—Buchanan and Brock contend that our standard of competency must be *decided* rather than merely *discovered*. Contrary to those who argue for some minimal standard of competency in every case or judge a patient's choice according to some objective canon of normalcy, Buchanan and Brock focus our attention on the quality of the patient's process of reasoning and on the risks and benefits posed by the decision. In Mary Northern's case, for example, a situation involving a life or death decision by a woman of questionable competence, they would have insisted that the patient meet a high standard of decision-making capacity. We leave it to readers to decide whether this "sliding-scale" approach masks ethically problematic, paternalistic judgments as objective medical or psychiatric competency determinations; or whether it correctly avoids attributing autonomy to all conscious patients, regardless of cognitive impairment, whose decisions may be manifestly against their own best interests.

Some refusals of treatment cause consternation among physicians not because there is genuine doubt about the ability of the patient to understand his or her condition, treatment alternatives, possible outcomes, and the like, but rather because the patient's refusal seems patently irrational. Must all treatment refusals be honored, or only those that meet certain standards of rationality, legal competence, or professional medical ethics? Must doctors honor the refusal of any legally competent patient, no matter how irrational the choice might seem? What if sound medical practice offers a high probability of curing an otherwise fatal condition—should our medical ethic condone such self-destructive treatment refusals? Is the paternalistic imposition of therapy against the patient's will ever justified?

These questions converge in this section's case study. A freak accident left Don Cowart with severe burns on over 65 percent of his body. Despite the severity of his injuries, he was clearly competent, and he repeatedly asked to be allowed to die. Don's doctor at first dismissed his patient's pleas to stop treatment as the typical response of burn victims to the pain of their wounds and treatment. In time, however, he discussed Don's wish to die with Don, his mother, and his lawyer. Should Don have been allowed to discontinue his painful daily treatments in order to go home and die? Should his mother and lawyer have been able to block his treatment refusal? And is the ultimate outcome of Cowart's life—completing a law degree, passing the bar, and setting up a small practice—relevant to whether he should have been allowed to die?

ADVANCE DIRECTIVES

In Section One, we considered the proposal that permanently unconscious individuals should be considered dead. This would remove the problem of making medical decisions on their behalf, since dead people do not get medical attention. This is one advantage of the higher-brain conception of death, but higher-brain theory is, as we saw, still quite controversial. Moreover, there are many patients who are incapacitated because of temporary unconsciousness, and many others who are permanently incapacitated, although not completely unconscious. Someone must make medical decisions for such patients. Hence the problem of proxy decision making, which we explore in Section Three. If one individual is to be given life-or-death authority over another, on what basis should such a proxy make a decision?

The first, and still very important, legal decision in this area involved Karen Ann Quinlan, who slipped into a coma in April 1975. When it became clear that she was in a persistent vegetative state, her parents sought to have her respirator removed. Her doctors refused, and her parents took the case to court. The court found that Karen, were she competent, would have had a right to refuse treatment, and held that Karen's guardian could assert that right on Karen's behalf, provided that she would have wanted it exercised in such circumstances. The problem was that Karen had never specified what she would want done—she was, after all, a healthy 21-year-old prior to her sudden loss of consciousness. Despite this lack of evidence for implementing the standard that has come to be known as "the substituted judgment test," the court favored the right of Karen's family to make the decision to refuse her treatment. It stated that if *their* decision was that Karen would have wanted treatment stopped, they could exercise Karen's right of privacy. The court found such a choice permissible based on the medical prognosis—Karen had lost all chance of returning to a sapient, cognitive existence—and suggested that hospitals set up "ethics committees" to oversee such decisions and, in particular, confirm the prognoses.

The *Quinlan* case prompted the enactment of the nation's first living-will statute, California's Natural Death Act, in 1976. A living will is a document executed by a competent adult that directs medical treatment in the event of his or her future incapacitation. The California statute is very narrow. It allows the removal of life-sustaining treatment only after the patient has been diagnosed with a terminal illness that will cause death imminently. "Thus," as George Annas notes, "even though this statute was inspired by her story, it would have not helped Quinlan, because she was not terminally ill."

A living will is intended to provide clear evidence of what the person "would have wanted," thus providing a basis for proxy decision making. However, relatively few people (fewer than 10 percent of Americans) make living wills. Moreover, according to Annas, virtually all living-will statutes suffer from four major shortcomings: they are applicable only to those who are "terminally ill" (thus inapplicable to PVS patients who can survive for years); they limit the types of treatment that can be refused, usually allowing refusal only of "artificial" or "extraordinary" therapies; they make no provision for the designation of a decision maker to act on the person's behalf; and there is no penalty if health care providers do not honor these documents.

Another problem with living wills is that it is extremely difficult to foresee every medical problem and possible treatment that might arise. Living wills also require physicians to make treatment decisions based on their interpretation of the document, rather than on a discussion of the treatment options with a person acting on the patient's behalf.

The cases presented by Stuart Eisendrath and Albert Jonsen provide dramatic illustrations of these problems. For example, in Case 1, Mrs. T specified in a living will that if she should have a severe and disabling stroke, she wanted to be allowed to die if there was "no reasonable expectation of her recovery from physical or mental disability." The case highlights the vague nature of such phrases, and the difficulty of determining what a "reasonable expectation" is and what should count as "recovery."

A solution to the problems of foresight and interpretation is to replace living wills with durable-power-of-attorney forms, which would name a "health care proxy" or "surrogate" empowered to make medical decisions for the incapacitated person. Every state already has a durable-power-of-attorney law; however, the current trend is for states to enact additional proxy laws that deal specifically with health care. These laws authorize a proxy to make any decisions that the patient would have made if he or she were still competent. These decisions must prove consistent with the wishes of the patient, if known, or they must prove otherwise consistent with the patient's best interests.

Without some form of advance directive, either a living will or a health care proxy, individuals may find themselves receiving treatment that neither they nor their families want. Although nearly half the states follow *Quinlan* and permit family members to remove life-support systems for such patients, the rest do not give families this right. Consider the case of Joey Fiori, a 21-year-old Vietnam veteran who, due to medical negligence, suffered an epileptic seizure in 1976 that left him in a persistent vegetative state. In 1992, Joey's mother, Rosemarie Sherman, gave up hope that he would either recover or die on life support, and asked the nursing home to remove his feeding tube. The nursing home said it required a court order to do so. Prosecutors in the Pennsylvania Attorney General's office conceded that the law is unclear, but argued that Ms. Sherman could not have her son's life support removed unless she could prove, with "clear and convincing evidence," that he had expressed a preference, orally or in writing, for death if faced with this kind of condition ("Uncharted Law for a Man Between Life and Death," *New York Times*, Monday, 6 June 1994, B9). A living will or other advance directive by Joey, specifying that he did not want to be sustained in a persistent vegetative state, would have been considered "clear and convincing evidence" of his wishes.

Many people find the "clear and convincing" standard imposed in *Cruzan* and other cases far too stringent, especially in the case of individuals who are permanently and irreversibly unconscious. Such critics may ask whether life is of any benefit or value to someone who cannot hear, feel, think, or be aware of anything. A much more difficult decision arises in the case of minimally conscious patients, for they may get some benefit out of their lives, severely limited though they are. Some argue that a family, based on its intimate knowledge of the person over a lifetime, should have the right to terminate life support for a severely demented relative. However, in many cases it is extremely difficult even for family members to know what the patient "would have wanted."

Even if it is possible to ascertain what the patient would have wanted when he or she was competent, should this be the deciding factor? That is, should treatment decisions be made on the basis of the preferences and values of the once-competent individual, or on the basis of the interests of the patient as he or she is now? This issue is sharply highlighted in the scenarios by Norman Cantor and in Section Four, Choosing for Others.

CHOOSING FOR OTHERS

Admitting the limitations of the substituted judgment standard raises a serious problem: On what grounds does a proxy decide for an incompetent? *In the Matter of Claire C. Conroy*, a highly influential case decided by the same court that decided *Quinlan*, attempts to answer this. *Conroy* holds that when the subjective test is inapplicable, a patient's family can still terminate treatment if they meet an objective standard: if they can prove that the burdens of the patient's life clearly and markedly outweigh the benefits. The *Conroy* majority says these burdens should be measured in terms of physical pain and suffering, thus rendering the objective test very stringent. Justice Handler, in his partial dissent, would allow the benefits/burdens assessment to encompass more than physical pain, considering personal privacy, dignity, and bodily integrity as well. The point of disagreement between the majority and dissenting opinions is a crucial one: it can be seen as the difference between authorizing quality-of-life assessments limited to relatively objective factors such as pain, and authorizing quality-of-life assessments that include a variety of factors bearing upon the quality of someone's life.

John Arras reiterates the difficulties of determining what an incompetent person "would have wanted." Pulling out a feeding tube may indicate either a preference for death, or only irritation caused by the tube. Previous independence and avoidance of doctors may or may not mean that the patient would prefer death to being sustained by tube feedings. Given the problems with a subjective standard, it may seem that an objective best-interests standard is the appropriate test. However, the best-interests standard is not always applicable. For example, it is untenable for PVS patients who *have* no interests in the ordinary sense of the term. A best-interests standard would require that treatment always continue, given the very slight possibility of recovery or misdiagnosis, and the absence of pain or other burdens—a result Arras terms "paradoxical," since if anyone's life need not be maintained, surely PVS patients are at the top of the list. For PVS patients, a decision in favor of nontreatment should be based not on an objective weighing of benefits and burdens to the patient—since PVS patients cannot be benefited or burdened—but rather on a judgment that the patient has ceased to be a "person" in any meaningful sense.

Decision making is very different for marginally or moderately functional individuals who can think, feel, and relate to others. Even if such patients are incapable of rational decision making, they nevertheless are clearly persons with interests that can be either advanced or frustrated by their caregivers. These patients are, Arras says, entitled to a "patient-centered best-interests" medical analysis. However, applying a best-interests analysis to minimally functional patients, such as Arras's Mrs. Smith, is problematic. It is difficult to determine either the benefits or the burdens of continued existence in her condition. Nevertheless, Arras maintains that it is highly doubtful that the burdens of Mrs. Smith's life "clearly and markedly" outweigh the benefits; thus, a literal application of the *Conroy* formula would lead to the conclusion that the G-tube should be surgically implanted. The trouble with this conclusion is that it appears to leave out something important: namely, the patient's probable feelings about privacy, dependency, dignity, and bodily integrity. To focus solely on physical pain is to reduce Mrs. Smith "from the full-fledged person that she once was to a mere physical repository of pleasures and pains."

Considerations of this sort led Justice Handler to his eloquent dissent in *Conroy*. Arras notes, however, that Handler's dissent is also problematic. If we consider only Mrs. Smith's *present* interests, then these are indeed reduced to sensations of pleasure and pain. In her present state, she is not bothered by a lack of dignity or bodily integrity. If we consider the interests of the formerly competent Mrs. Smith, it is possible that she would have been appalled at being kept alive in her present condition. The trouble is that we cannot know this, since she left behind neither an advance directive nor a pattern of analogous choices that clearly demonstrate what she would have wanted under her present circumstances. Thus, the ambiguities of substituted judgment lead to the adoption of an objective best-interests standard, while the deficiencies of the objective standard—with its narrow focus on pain to the exclusion of other important values—send us back to the substituted judgment test. To get us out of this dilemma, Arras opts for a procedural solution, one that allows families or other trustworthy surrogates to make treatment decisions—including removing feeding tubes—for severely demented patients as they see fit, unless their decisions clearly violate the patient's best interests.

Opposed to Arras's "quality of life" approach is the statement from the U.S. Bishops' Pro-Life Committee, entitled "Nutrition and Hydration: Moral and Pastoral Reflections." It enumerates some basic principles of the Catholic moral tradition that apply to decisions about medically assisted nutrition and hydration. In a careful and nuanced discussion, the Bishops affirm their opposition to the deliberate taking of life, even permanently unconscious life, while at the same time they express support for the view that one is not obliged to prolong the life of a dying person by every possible means.

The section ends with an issue touched on by both Arras and Cantor: whether treatment decisions should be made on the basis of the interests of the once-competent patient, or only on the basis of the interests of the individual as he or she is now. Rebecca Dresser and John Robertson opt for basing treatment decisions on the actual interests of the incompetent patient. They criticize "the orthodox judicial approach," as enunciated in *Quinlan*, as both conceptually flawed and dangerous. In the orthodox approach, incompetent patients have the same right to refuse treatment as do competent ones, a right that may be exercised on their behalf by surrogates, or proxies. The proxy is to determine what the incompetent patient would have chosen, either by relying on advance directives or by using substituted judgment. The orthodox approach ostensibly promotes patient self-determination, protects individuals from overtreatment, recognizes a central role for family discretion, and avoids troublesome quality-of-life determinations. However, Dresser and Robertson fault the orthodox approach on all these

counts. The first issue, the autonomy of incompetent patients, cannot be respected because autonomy is literally a characteristic that belongs only to patients capable of making their own choices. Also, it is wrong to assume that the incompetent patient's prior preferences indicate the patient's current interests. Competent individuals have interests in work, family, friendships, and hobbies. They may feel that life without the possibility of pursuing these interests would be no longer worth living. However, severely demented individuals no longer have these interests. A life that may seem demeaning to a competent individual may still be of value to the incompetent patient. Why should the values and preferences of the person-while-competent prevail over the interests of the incompetent person? This is unlike the situation of a person making an ordinary will, since the testator no longer has interests after he or she is dead. By contrast, the maker of a living will may be authorizing decisions that are contrary to his or her own best interests.

The orthodox approach is dangerous, according to Dresser and Robertson, because it is likely to lead to undertreatment. They discuss several cases, including *Spring* and *Hier*, in which courts authorized nontreatment for elderly incompetent patients based on substituted judgment. Use of this standard "opens the door to non-treatment of nursing home residents and other severely debilitated persons" based on what others think they would have wanted. Instead, Dresser and Robertson recommend that such decisions be based on the patients' actual interests. Such an approach requires a forthright consideration of quality of life. If the patient is permanently unconscious, then treatment is not warranted, because some capacity to interact with the environment must be present for life to be of value to an individual. Moreover, when the patient has no interest in continued existence, then the family's burdens and financial costs may be taken into account. Treatment might also be withheld from barely conscious patients on the grounds that their lives are not of value to them. Like Arras, Dresser and Robertson would allow families to request nontreatment for minimally conscious individuals, not because the patient would prefer nontreatment, but rather on the grounds that such life does not clearly confer a genuine benefit. However, people differ on what kinds of life constitute a benefit. Some might argue that letting minimally conscious individuals die because others view their lives as having little worth violates the patients' right to life. They might view the current interests approach to be as likely to result in undertreatment for nursing home residents and other severely debilitated persons as a substituted judgment approach.

Nancy Rhoden attempts to answer the question posed by Dresser and Robertson: Why should the values and preferences of the once-competent person take precedence over the interests of the incompetent person? Her answer is that respect for persons requires us to adhere to the express and implicit wishes of individuals when they were competent. She says, "It is at least one, if not an overriding, component of treating persons with respect that we view them as they view themselves. If we are to do this, we must not ignore their prior choices and values." Applying this approach to the *Conroy* case, Rhoden suggests that the objective test strips the individual of his or her uniqueness and personality. She reminds us that Claire Conroy was not "just anyone"; she was a specific human being—Aunt Claire. While we can, and should, make quality-of-life assessments from a present-oriented perspective for individuals who were never competent (infants and severely retarded people), something is wrong, Rhoden argues, when we treat formerly competent patients as if they were never competent. She acknowledges that paying attention to advance directives and prior values does give primacy to the competent person, but this is not inexplicable or unjustifiable: "[I]t is, after all, competent persons who have the considered moral values, life plans, and treatment preferences that underlie our respect."

Rhoden also argues that the objective test endangers all of our choices, because any of us could become suddenly incapacitated. In the objective, current interests approach, a competent patient's "right" to refuse treatment will be upheld only for the time she remains competent. If she has a stroke that renders her incompetent, treatment decisions will be made on the basis of her present interests. Rhoden says, "Taken to an extreme, this could mean that a Jehovah's Witness could refuse a blood transfusion until he 'bled out,' after which he could be transfused."

EUTHANASIA AND PHYSICIAN-ASSISTED SUICIDE (PAS)

Whether life is always worthwhile, or whether there are times when death is preferable to life, is an issue that has become more pressing in recent years. One reason for the growing importance of this issue is the ability of modern medicine to keep people alive who would have died in earlier medical eras. The elongation of dying through modern medical technology has raised the issue of euthanasia even more persistently than in the past. Euthanasia (literally, a "beautiful death") means an easy or painless death, but has come to stand for deliberately bringing about such a death through action or inaction. On the one hand, euthanasia would appear to be antithetical to all that medical practice stands for (indeed, the Hippocratic Oath specifically enjoins inducing death, even if the patient requests it). On the other hand, if the purpose of medicine is not simply to prevent death but to alleviate suffering, then perhaps euthanasia is not entirely foreign to good, ethical, medical practice. Indeed, it has been practiced openly by physicians for several years in the Netherlands, with the acceptance of the country's highest court (Battin 1994).

Another reason for the recent attention to euthanasia, suicide, and physician-assisted suicide (PAS) is the AIDS epidemic. Many people with AIDS want the solace of knowing that they will be able to end their lives before either the pain becomes unbearable or they become demented. However, suicide is not always easily accomplished. According to a New York doctor with a large AIDS practice, "the reality is that most people with AIDS have very strong cardiovascular systems. Taking overdoses of most common prescription pills is not going to kill you" ("AIDS Patients Seek Solace in Suicide but Many Find Pain and Uncertainty," *New York Times*, Tuesday, 14 June 1994, C6). Also, people can develop a tolerance for morphine. A botched suicide attempt may leave a person alive, but without any brain function. When doctors are involved, things are less likely to go wrong. For this reason, many doctors say they favor changing laws that currently prohibit them from legally assisting in suicides of people with terminal illnesses; other doctors, however, still say they have qualms about assisted suicide, even in the case of AIDS.

There are two distinctions of fundamental importance to the moral assessment of euthanasia. The first is between active euthanasia (deliberately *bringing death about* through some action, such as administering a lethal injection) and passive euthanasia (deliberately *allowing death to occur* through some form of inaction, such as refraining from performing corrective surgery). Often this distinction has been characterized as the difference between "killing" and "letting die." A second distinction is made between voluntary euthanasia (actively requested by the patient) and nonvoluntary euthanasia, in which the patient (for example, a PVS patient) lacks the capacity to consent. Writers on the topic disagree as to whether all forms of euthanasia are permissible, or only some forms. Most people would agree that the voluntary/nonvoluntary distinction is at least relevant to, if not decisive in determining, the permissibility of euthanasia; some still maintain, however, that the distinction between active and passive euthanasia—if it can be coherently drawn at all—has no moral relevance (Steinbock and Norcross, 1994).

Legally, nevertheless, there is an important difference between actively causing someone's death and allowing him or her—even deliberately—to die. Liability for allowing to die depends on the relation between the "victim" and the one who allows him or her to die. A doctor who stops treatment at the request of a patient is unlikely to be liable for the patient's death, so long as the doctor acts within the bounds of accepted medical practice. Indeed, a doctor who continues treating a competent patient who has refused treatment is theoretically liable for battery (although few, if any, doctors have ever been successfully sued for treating without consent). Killing a patient, even at his or her request, is quite another matter. Assisting a suicide is a crime in most jurisdictions. In recent years, California and Washington have attempted initiatives to legalize doctor-assisted suicide; neither state succeeded. In 1994, Oregon became the only state to legalize PAS. Opponents sought to repeal the Death with Dignity Act, but this attempt was rejected by the voters in November 1997. As of this writing, three people have received suicide assistance under the Act (Pratt and Steinbock, 1998).

One of the few jurisdictions where there was no law, until recently, against assisting a suicide was

Michigan. For this reason, the controversial Dr. Jack Kevorkian chose Michigan as the place to perform several "medicides," as he calls them, using the "suicide machine" he invented for the purpose. Michigan quickly moved to pass a statute making assisted suicide a crime so that Dr. Kevorkian could be charged the next time he helped someone to die. However, on May 2, 1994, a Detroit jury acquitted Dr. Jack Kevorkian of charges that he had violated Michigan's law barring assisted suicide. Comments from jurors made it clear that the jury regarded Dr. Kevorkian as justified in helping terminally ill patients to die. As of this writing, Dr. Kevorkian has helped approximately 100 individuals to die.

Dr. Timothy Quill, the first author in Section Five, prescribed barbiturates for his longtime patient, Diane, who requested them to kill herself in order to avoid a lingering, painful (or drugged) death from leukemia. Many commentators have contrasted Dr. Quill with Dr. Kevorkian. Dr. Kevorkian is a retired pathologist; Dr. Quill a practicing internist. Dr. Kevorkian has helped about 100 people to die; Dr. Quill only one. Dr. Kevorkian does not know the individuals he helps to die, neither the details of their medical conditions nor their psychological states. Dr. Quill knew Diane very well, and met regularly with her over several months after she requested the barbiturates. Clearly, Dr. Quill is a conscientious, compassionate physician who had the deepest concern for his patient's well-being and the deepest respect for her choices. Having said that, did Dr. Quill do the right thing? And should such behavior be sanctioned by law?

During 1996, two federal appeals courts held that state laws criminalizing assisted suicide violated the Fourteenth Amendment to the United States Constitution. In June, 1997, the Supreme Court reversed the decisions in both *Washington* v. *Glucksberg* and *Vacco* v. *Quill,* holding that there is no constitutional right to physician-assisted suicide. This has settled (for the time being) the constitutional question. However, the moral and legal debate over whether one has a "right to die" is far from over. The Court's decision simply returns the question to the states.

One of the philosophically interesting claims made in the assisted-suicide cases was that laws prohibiting PAS wrongly distinguish between patients who are, and those who are not, on life-support systems. The law permits doctors to remove patients who request it from life support, thus hastening their deaths; whereas the law bars doctors from prescribing to patients who request it medication that would hasten their deaths. United States District Judge Barbara F. Rothstein viewed this discrepancy in Washington's law as untenable, saying, ". . . from a constitutional perspective, the court does not believe that a distinction can be drawn between refusing life-sustaining medical treatment and physician-assisted suicide by an uncoerced, mentally competent, terminally ill adult" (*Compassion in Dying* v. *Washington* 850 f. Supp. 1454 W. D. Wash. 1994).

The New York State Task Force on Life and the Law disagrees. In its supplement to its report, *When Death Is Sought*, the Task Force argues there are "compelling reasons to distinguish between the refusal of life-sustaining treatment and assisted suicide. . . ." One reason stems from the Hippocratic ethos, which has created in many physicians an unwillingness to forgo aggressive life-sustaining measures, despite patients' clear legal right to refuse such treatment. The result of equating withdrawal of life-sustaining measures with killing may be that physicians will "rethink their participation in the withholding and withdrawal of treatment. The result would be a disastrous setback for patient autonomy."

Another problem with equating the refusal of treatment with assisted suicide is that this makes limiting assisted suicide to competent, terminally ill patients impossible. The right to refuse treatment, even life-sustaining treatment, is not limited to terminally ill patients. Nor is the right to refuse treatment limited to competent individuals, as the decisions in *Quinlan* and *Cruzan* demonstrate. If the distinction between refusing treatment and other forms of hastening death is arbitrary, what justifies, in the case of PAS, cumbersome waiting periods, second opinions, and committee review? None of these procedural hurdles is imposed on individuals who seek to refuse life-sustaining treatment. Finally, the Task Force thinks it is important to retain the distinction between administering high doses of opioids, like morphine, to relieve pain, and PAS. The fact that morphine drips may accelerate patients' deaths in some cases does not make their use equivalent to assisted suicide or euthanasia: "Just as a surgeon might undertake risky heart surgery knowing that

the patient may die on the table, so the conscientious physician can risk suppressing the patient's respiratory drive and thus hastening death so long as she is pursuing a valid medical objective and there are no better (less risky) options at hand." Medical treatment sometimes requires trade-offs, and accepting negative consequences for legitimate medical purposes is not equivalent to causing those consequences for their own sake. Moreover, if physicians are told that adequate palliative treatment is equivalent to assisted suicide, the result may be an even greater lack of attention to pain relief than currently exists. The Task Force concludes that "advocates of legalizing assisted suicide should think carefully about the consequences of this argument for compassionate end-of-life care."

In "Physician-Assisted Suicide: A Tragic View," John D. Arras (who was a member of New York's Task Force on Life and the Law when its original report, *When Death Is Sought*, was written) lays out the pros and cons of legalizing PAS. Although Arras is "deeply sympathetic to the central values motivating the push for PAS and euthanasia," he ultimately concludes that the social risks of legalization outweigh the benefits. While there may be individual cases in which assisted suicide is the best choice, it does not follow that legalizing PAS is the wisest social policy. A better approach would be to improve radically the palliative care terminally ill patients receive. "At the end of this long and arduous process," Arras writes, "when we finally have an equitable, effective, and compassionate health care system in place . . . , then we might well want to reopen the discussion of PAS and active euthanasia."

The case in favor of assisted suicide is made by six well-known moral philosophers in the "The Philosophers' Brief," the third article in Section Five. The basis of their position is the general moral principle that every competent person has the right to make momentous personal decisions about life's value, including decisions about when life ceases to be worth living. At the same time, the authors acknowledge that people may make such momentous decisions impulsively or out of depression, and that the state has the right to adopt safeguards to ensure that a patient's decision for suicide is informed, competent, and free. The philosophers address the risk discussed by Arras that legalizing PAS might jeopardize vulnerable patients, and they conclude that such patients might be better, rather than less, well protected if assisted suicide were legalized with appropriate safeguards.

The "Brief" rejects the claim that there is always a morally and legally relevant difference between stopping life-sustaining treatment and prescribing lethal drugs to a patient; whether there is such a difference depends on the aim in both cases. If the rationale for stopping treatment is to bring about the patient's death, then stopping treatment is morally equivalent to prescribing lethal drugs. "If it is permissible for a doctor deliberately to withdraw medical treatment in order to allow death to result from a natural process, then it is equally permissible for him to help his patient hasten his own death more actively, if that is the patient's express wish."

Margaret Battin gives a cross-cultural comparison of end-of-life decisions in the Netherlands, Germany, and the United States. In the Netherlands, voluntary active euthanasia, while prohibited by statute, is nevertheless legally tolerated, provided the physician meets a rigorous set of guidelines. Euthanasia is infrequently chosen, but it is a "conspicuous option in terminal illness."

The painful history of Nazism in Germany, and the killing of mentally and physically handicapped patients (which led eventually to the Holocaust), has resulted in Germany's rejection of physician participation in causing death. "Euthanasia is viewed as always wrong, and the Germans view the Dutch as stepping out on a dangerously slippery slope." At the same time, assisted suicide is not a violation of the law, and the German Society for Humane Dying publishes a booklet listing drugs available by prescription, together with the specific dosages necessary for producing a certain, painless death. However, the removal of physicians from participating in assisted suicide means that decisions for suicide are not medically evaluated, either to confirm the patient's diagnosis or prognosis, or to rule out treatable depression as the motivating factor.

The United States differs from both the Netherlands and Germany in significant ways. We have no national health insurance, and cost increasingly plays a role in health care decisions. Battin, who generally supports voluntary euthanasia for the reasons given in the "Philosophers' Brief," concludes that PAS is a better alternative than euthanasia, given the cultural context in the United States, because PAS grants physicians a measure of control while it leaves the fundamental decision up to the patients themselves.

Forty years ago, in an influential article criticizing proposed "mercy-killing" legislation, Yale Kamisar warned against giving the choice of euthanasia to gravely ill patients, saying:

> Will we not sweep up, in the process, some who are not really tired of life, but think others are tired of them; some who do not really want to die, but who feel they should not live on, because to do so when there looms the legal alternative of euthanasia is to do a selfish or a cowardly act? Will not some feel an obligation to have themselves "eliminated" in order that funds allocated for their terminal care might be better used by their families or, financial worries aside, in order to relieve their families of the emotional strain involved? (Kamisar, 1958)

Most defenders of PAS try to argue that, with proper safeguards, Kamisar's fears will not materialize. By contrast, in what may be the most provocative article in this collection, John Hardwig suggests that there can be a moral obligation (not merely a right) to choose death. The basis of this obligation is the burden imposed on family members who care for sick and dying patients. It might seem that Hardwig is using a consequentialist analysis to derive a duty to die. In fact, his reasoning owes at least as much to Kantian ethics as to utilitarianism, for he says, "To think that my loved ones must bear whatever burdens my illness, debility, or dying process might impose upon them is to reduce them to means to my well-being. And that would be immoral." We leave it to the reader to decide whether Hardwig's claim of a duty to die is a moral advance—or the tragic fulfillment of Kamisar's prophetic warning.

SECTION 1

The Definition of Death and the Persistent Vegetative State

Defining Death*

President's Commission for the Study of Ethical Problems in Medicine and Biomedical and Behavioral Research

WHY UPDATE DEATH?

For most of the past several centuries, the medical determination of death was very close to the popular one. If a person fell unconscious or was found so, someone (often but not always a physician) would feel for the pulse, listen for breathing, hold a mirror before the nose to test for condensation, and look to see if the pupils were fixed. Although these criteria have been used to determine death since antiquity, they have not always been universally accepted.

DEVELOPING CONFIDENCE IN THE HEART-LUNG CRITERIA

In the eighteenth century, macabre tales of "corpses" reviving during funerals and exhumed skeletons found to have clawed at coffin lids led to widespread fear of premature burial. Coffins were developed with elaborate escape mechanisms and speaking tubes to the world above . . . , mortuaries employed guards to monitor the newly dead for signs of life, and legislatures passed laws requiring a delay before burial.

From the President's Commission for the Study of Ethical Problems in Medicine and Biomedical and Behavioral Research, *Defining Death: A Report on the Medical, Legal and Ethical Issues in the Determination of Death*, Washington, D.C.: U.S. Government Printing Office, 1981, 12–20, 31–43.
*Editors' Note: The notes have been omitted. Readers who wish to follow up on sources should consult the original article.

The medical press also paid a great deal of attention to the matter. In *The Uncertainty of the Signs of Death and the Danger of Precipitate Interments* in 1740, Jean-Jacques Winslow advanced the thesis that putrefaction was the only sure sign of death. In the years following, many physicians published articles agreeing with him. This position had, however, notable logistic and public health disadvantages. It also disparaged, sometimes with unfair vigor, the skills of physicians as diagnosticians of death. In reply, the French surgeon Louis published in 1752 his influential *Letters on the Certainty of the Signs of Death*. The debate dissipated in the nineteenth century because of the gradual improvement in the competence of physicians and a concomitant increase in the public's confidence in them.

Physicians actively sought to develop this competence. They even held contests encouraging the search for a cluster of signs—rather than a single infallible sign—for the diagnosis of death. One sign did, however, achieve prominence. The invention of the stethoscope in the mid–nineteenth century enabled physicians to detect heartbeat with heightened sensitivity. The use of this instrument by a well-trained physician, together with other clinical measures, laid to rest public fears of premature burial. The twentieth century brought even more sophisticated technological means to determine death, particularly the electrocardiograph (EKG), which is more sensitive than the stethoscope in detecting cardiac functioning.

THE INTERRELATIONSHIPS OF BRAIN, HEART, AND LUNG FUNCTIONS

The brain has three general anatomic divisions: the cerebrum, with its outer shell called the cortex; the cerebellum; and the brainstem, composed of the midbrain, the pons, and the medulla oblongata. . . . Traditionally, the cerebrum has been referred to as the "higher brain" because it has primary control of consciousness, thought, memory, and feeling. The brainstem has been called the "lower brain," since it controls spontaneous, vegetative functions such as swallowing, yawning, and sleep-wake cycles. It is important to note that these generalizations are not entirely accurate. Neuroscientists generally agree that such "higher brain" functions as cognition or consciousness probably are not mediated strictly by the cerebral cortex; rather, they probably result from complex interrelations between brainstem and cortex.

Respiration is controlled in the brainstem, particularly the medulla. . . . Neural impulses originating in the respiratory centers of the medulla stimulate the diaphragm and intercostal muscles, which cause the lungs to fill with air. Ordinarily, these respiratory centers adjust the rate of breathing to maintain the correct levels of carbon dioxide and oxygen. In certain circumstances, such as heavy exercise, sighing, coughing, or sneezing, other areas of the brain modulate the activities of the respiratory centers or even briefly take direct control of respiration.

Destruction of the brain's respiratory center stops respiration, which in turn deprives the heart of needed oxygen, causing it too to cease functioning. The traditional signs of life—respiration and heartbeat—disappear: the person is dead. The "vital signs" traditionally used in diagnosing death thus reflect the direct interdependence of respiration, circulation, and the brain.

The artificial respirator and concomitant life-support systems have changed this simple picture. Normally, respiration ceases when the functions of the diaphragm and intercostal muscles are impaired. This results from direct injury to the muscles or (more commonly) because the neural impulses between the brain and these muscles are interrupted. However, an artificial respirator (also called a ventilator) can be used to compensate for the inability of the thoracic muscles to fill the lungs with air. Some of these machines use negative pressure to expand the chest wall (in which case they are called "iron lungs"); others use positive pressure to push air into the lungs. The respirators are equipped with devices to regulate the rate and depth of "breathing," which are normally controlled by the respiratory centers in the medulla. The machines cannot compensate entirely for the defective neural connections since they cannot regulate blood gas levels precisely. But, provided that the lungs themselves have not been extensively damaged, gas exchange can continue and appropriate levels of oxygen and carbon dioxide can be maintained in the circulating blood.

Unlike the respiratory system, which depends on the neural impulses from the brain, the heart can pump blood without external control. Impulses from brain centers modulate the inherent rate and force of the heartbeat but are not required for the heart to contract at a level of function that is ordinarily adequate. Thus, when artificial respiration provides adequate oxygenation and associated medical treatments regulate essential plasma components and blood pressure, an intact heart will continue to beat, despite loss of brain functions. At present, however, no machine can take over the functions of the heart except for a very limited time and in limited circumstances (e.g., a heart-lung machine used during surgery). Therefore, when a severe injury to the heart or major blood vessels prevents the circulation of the crucial blood supply to the brain, the loss of brain functioning is inevitable because no oxygen reaches the brain.

LOSS OF VARIOUS BRAIN FUNCTIONS

The most frequent causes of irreversible loss of functions of the whole brain are (1) direct trauma to the head, such as from a motor vehicle accident or a gunshot wound, (2) massive spontaneous hemorrhage into the brain as a result of ruptured aneurysm or complications of high blood pressure, and (3) anoxic damage from cardiac or respiratory arrest or severely reduced blood pressure.

Many of these severe injuries to the brain cause an accumulation of fluid and swelling in the brain tissue, a condition called cerebral edema. In severe cases of edema, the pressure within the closed cavity increases until it exceeds the systolic blood pressure, resulting in a total loss of blood flow to both the upper and lower portions of the brain. If deprived of blood flow for at least 10 to 15 minutes, the brain, including the brainstem, will completely cease functioning. Other pathophysiologic mechanisms also result in a progressive and, ultimately, complete cessation of intracranial circulation.

Once deprived of adequate supplies of oxygen and glucose, brain neurons will irreversibly lose all activity and ability to function. In adults, oxygen and/or glucose deprivation for more than a few minutes causes some neuron loss. Thus, even in the absence of direct trauma and edema, brain functions can be lost if circulation to the brain is impaired. If blood flow is cut off, brain tissues completely self-digest (autolyze) over the ensuing days.

When the brain lacks all functions, consciousness is, of course, lost. While some spinal reflexes often persist in such bodies (since circulation to the spine is separate from that of the brain), all reflexes controlled by the brainstem as well as cognitive, affective, and integrating functions are absent. Respiration and circulation in these bodies may be generated by a ventilator together with intensive medical management. In adults who have experienced irreversible cessation of the functions of the entire brain, this mechanically generated functioning can continue only a limited time because the heart usually stops beating within two to ten days. (An infant or small child who has lost all brain functions will typically suffer cardiac arrest within several weeks, although respiration and heartbeat can sometimes be maintained even longer.)

Less severe injury to the brain can cause mild to profound damage to the cortex, lower cerebral structures, cerebellum, brainstem, or some combination thereof. The cerebrum, especially the cerebral cortex, is more easily injured by loss of blood flow or oxygen than is the brainstem. A 4 to 6 minute loss of blood flow—caused by, for example, cardiac arrest—typically damages the cerebral cortex permanently, while the relatively more resistant brainstem may continue to function.

When brainstem functions remain, but the major components of the cerebrum are irreversibly destroyed, the patient is in what is usually called a "persistent vegetative state" or "persistent noncognitive state." Such persons may exhibit spontaneous, involuntary movements such as yawns or facial grimaces, their eyes may be open, and they may be capable of breathing without assistance. Without higher brain functions, however, any apparent wakefulness does not represent awareness of self or environment (thus, the condition is often described as "awake but unaware"). The case of Karen Ann Quinlan has made this condition familiar to the general public. With necessary medical and nursing care—including feeding through intravenous or nasogastric tubes, and antibiotics for recurrent pulmonary infections—such patients can survive months or years, often without a respirator. (The longest survival exceeded 37 years.)

CONCLUSION: THE NEED FOR RELIABLE POLICY

Medical interventions can often provide great benefit in avoiding irreversible harm to a patient's injured heart, lungs, or brain by carrying a patient through a period of acute need. These techniques have, however, thrown new light on the interrelationship of these crucial organ systems. This has created complex issues for public policy as well.

For medical and legal purposes, partial brain impairment must be distinguished from complete and irreversible loss of brain functions or "whole brain death." The President's Commission regards the cessation of the vital functions of the entire brain—and not merely portions thereof, such as those responsible for cognitive functions—as the only proper neurologic basis for declaring death. This conclusion accords with the overwhelming consensus of medical and legal experts and the public.

Present attention to the "definition" of death is part of a process of development in social attitudes and legal rules stimulated by the unfolding of biomedical knowledge. In the nineteenth century increasing knowledge and practical skill made the public confident that death could be diagnosed reliably using cardiopulmonary criteria. The question now is whether, when medical intervention may be responsible for a patient's respiration and circulation, there are other equally reliable ways to diagnose death.

The Commission recognizes that it is often difficult to determine the severity of a patient's injuries, especially in the first few days of intensive care following a cardiac arrest, head trauma, or other similar event. Responsible public policy in this area requires that physicians be able to distinguish reliably those patients who have died from those whose injuries are less severe or are reversible. . . .

UNDERSTANDING THE "MEANING" OF DEATH

It now seems clear that a medical consensus about clinical practices and their scientific basis has emerged: certain states of brain activity and inactivity, together with their neurophysiological consequences, can be reliably detected and used to diagnose death. To the medical community, a sound basis exists for declaring death even in the presence of mechanically assisted "vital signs." Yet before recommending that public policy reflect this medical consensus, the Commission wished to know whether the scientific viewpoint was consistent with the concepts of "being dead" or "death" as they are commonly understood in our society. These questions have been addressed by philosophers and theologians, who have provided several formulations.

The Commission believes that its policy conclusions . . . including the [Uniform Determination of Death Act] must accurately reflect the social meaning of death and not constitute a mere legal fiction. The Commission has not found it necessary to resolve all of the differences among the leading concepts of death because these views all yield interpretations consistent with the recommended statute.

Three major formulations of the meaning of death were presented to the Commission: one focused upon the functions of the whole brain, one upon the functions of the cerebral hemispheres, and one upon non-brain functions. Each of these formulations (and its variants) is presented and evaluated.

THE "WHOLE BRAIN" FORMULATIONS

One characteristic of living things which is absent in the dead is the body's capacity to organize and regulate itself. In animals, the neural apparatus is the dominant locus of these functions. In higher animals and man, regulation of both maintenance of the internal environment (homeostasis) and interaction with the external environment occurs primarily within the cranium.

External threats, such as heat or infection, or internal ones, such as liver failure or endogenous lung disease, can stress the body enough to overwhelm its ability to maintain organization and regulation. If the stress passes a certain level, the organism as a whole is defeated and death occurs.

This process and its denouement are understood in two major ways. Although they are sometimes stated as alternative formulations of a "whole brain definition" of death, they are actually mirror images of each other. The Commission has found them to be complementary; together they enrich one's understanding of the "definition." The first focuses on the integrated functioning of the body's major organ systems, while recognizing the centrality of the whole brain, since it is neither revivable nor replaceable. The other identifies the functioning of the whole brain as the hallmark of life because the brain is the regulator of the body's integration. The two conceptions are subject to similar criticisms and have similar implications for policy.

The Concepts   The functioning of many organs—such as the liver, kidneys, and skin—and their integration is "vital" to individual health in the sense that if any one ceases and that function is not restored or artificially replaced, the organism as a whole cannot long survive. All elements in the system are mutually interdependent, so that the loss of any part leads to the breakdown of the whole, and eventually, to the cessation of functions in every part.

Three organs—the heart, lungs, and brain—assume special significance, however, because their interrelationship is very close and the irreversible cessation of any one very quickly stops the other two and consequently halts the integrated functioning of the organism as a whole. Because they were easily measured, circulation and respiration were traditionally the basic "vital signs." But breathing and heartbeat are not life itself. They are simply used as signs—as one window for viewing a deeper and more complex reality: a triangle of interrelated systems with the brain at its apex. As the biomedical scientists who appeared before the Commission made clear, the traditional means of diagnosing death actually detected an irreversible cessation of integrated functioning among the interdependent bodily systems. When artificial means of support mask this loss of integration as measured by the old methods, brain-oriented criteria and tests provide a new window on the same phenomenon.

On this view, death is that moment at which the body's physiological system ceases to constitute an integrated whole. Even if life continues in individual cells or organs, life of the organism as a whole requires complex integration, and without the latter, a person cannot properly be regarded as alive.

This distinction between systemic, integrated functioning and physiological activity in cells or individual organs is important for two reasons. First, a person is considered dead under this concept even if oxygenation and metabolism persist in some cells or organs. There would be no need to wait until all metabolism had ceased in every body part before recognizing that death has occurred.

More importantly, this concept would reduce the significance of continued respiration and heartbeat for the definition of death. This view holds that continued breathing and circulation are not in themselves tantamount to life. Since life is a matter of integrating the functioning of major organ systems, breathing and circulation are necessary but not sufficient to establish that an individual is alive. When an individual's breathing and circulation lack neurologic integration, he or she is dead.

The alternative "whole brain" explanation of death differs from the one just described primarily in the vigor of its insistence that the traditional "vital signs" of heartbeat and respiration were merely surrogate signs with no significance in themselves. On this view, the heart and lungs are not important as basic prerequisites to continued life but rather because the irreversible cessation of their functions shows that the brain had ceased functioning. Other signs customarily employed by physicians in diagnosing death, such as unresponsiveness and absence of pupillary light response, are also indicative of loss of the functions of the whole brain.

This view gives the brain primacy not merely as the sponsor of consciousness (since even unconscious persons may be alive), but also as the complex organizer and regulator of bodily functions. (Indeed, the "regulatory" role of the brain in the organism can be understood in terms of thermodynamics and information theory.) Only the brain can direct the entire organism. Artificial support for the heart and lungs, which is required only when the brain can no longer control them, cannot maintain the usual synchronized integration of the body. Now that other traditional indicators of cessation of brain functions (*i.e.*, absence of breathing), can be obscured by medical interventions, one needs, according to this view, some new standards for determining death—that is, more reliable tests for the complete cessation of brain functions.

Critique   Both of these "whole brain" formulations—the "integrated functions" and the "primary organ" views—are subject to several criticisms. Since both of these conceptions of death give an important place to the integrating or regulating capacity of the whole brain, it can be asked whether that characteristic is as distinctive as they would suggest. Other organ systems are also required for life to continue—for example, the skin to conserve fluid, the liver to detoxify the blood.

The view that the brain's functions are more central to "life" than those of the skin, the liver, and so on, is admittedly arbitrary in the sense of representing a choice. The view is not, however, arbitrary in the sense of lacking reasons. As discussed previously, the centrality accorded the brain reflects both its overarching role as "regulator" or "integrator" of other bodily systems and the immediate and devastating consequences of its loss for the organism as a whole. Furthermore, the Commission believes that this choice overwhelmingly reflects the views of experts and the lay public alike.

A more significant criticism shares the view that life consists of the coordinated functioning of the various bodily systems, in which process the whole brain plays a crucial role. At the same time, it notes that in some adult patients lacking all brain functions it is possible through intensive support to achieve constant temperature, metabolism, waste disposal, blood pressure, and other conditions typical of living organisms and not found in dead ones. Even with extraordinary medical care, these functions cannot be sustained indefinitely—typically, no longer than several days—but it is argued that this shows only that patients with nonfunctional brains are dying, not that they are dead. In this view, the respirator, drugs, and other resources of the modern intensive-care unit collectively substitute for the lower brain, just as a pump used in cardiac surgery takes over the heart's function.

The criticism rests, however, on a premise about the role of artificial support vis-à-vis the brainstem which the Commission believes is mistaken or at best incomplete. While the respirator and its associated medical techniques do substitute for the functions of the intercostal muscles and the diaphragm, which without neuronal stimulation from the brain cannot function spontaneously, they cannot replace the myriad functions of the brainstem or of the rest of the brain. The startling contrast between bodies lacking *all* brain functions and patients with intact brainstems (despite severe neocortical damage) manifests this. The former lie with fixed pupils, motionless except for the chest movements produced by their respirators. The latter can not only breathe, metabolize, maintain temperature and blood pressure, and so forth, *on their own* but also sigh, yawn, track light with their eyes, and react to pain or reflex stimulation.

It is not easy to discern precisely what it is about patients in this latter group that makes them alive while those in the other category are not. It is in part that in the case of the first category (*i.e.,* absence of all brain functions) when the mask created by the artificial medical support is stripped away what remains is not an integrated organism but "merely a group of artificially maintained subsystems." Sometimes, of course, an artificial substitute can forge the link that restores the organism as a whole to unified functioning. Heart or kidney transplants, kidney dialysis, or an iron lung used to replace physically impaired breathing ability in a polio victim, for example, restore the integrated functioning of the organism as they replace the failed function of a part. Contrast such situations, however, with the hypothetical of a decapitated body treated so as to prevent the outpouring of blood and to generate respiration: continuation of bodily functions in that case would not have restored the requisites of human life.

The living differ from the dead in many ways. The dead do not think, interact, autoregulate, or maintain organic identity through time, for example. Not all the living can always do *all* of these activities, however; nor is there one single characteristic (*e.g.,* breathing, yawning, etc.) the loss of which signifies death. Rather, what is missing in the dead is a cluster of attributes, all of which form part of an organism's responsiveness to its internal and external environment.

While it is valuable to test public policies against basic conceptions of death, philosophical refinement beyond a certain point may not be necessary. The task undertaken in this Report is to provide and defend a statutory standard for determining that a human being has died. In setting forth the standards recommended in this Report, the Commission has used "whole brain" terms to clarify the understanding of death that enjoys near-universal acceptance in our society. The Commission finds that the "whole brain" formulations give resonance and depth to the biomedical and epidemiological data presented in [a part of the study not reproduced here]. Further effort to search for a conceptual "definition" of death is not required for the purpose of public policy because, separately or together, the "whole brain" formulations provide a theory that is sufficiently precise, concise, and widely acceptable.

Policy Consequences   Those holding to the "whole brain" view—and this view seems at least implicit in most of the testimony and writing reviewed by the Commission—believe that when respirators are in use, respiration and circulation lose significance for the diagnosis of death. In a body without a functioning brain, these two functions, it is argued, become mere artifacts of the mechanical life supports. The lungs breathe and the heart circulates blood only because the respirator (and attendant medical interventions) cause them to do so, not because of any comprehensive integrated functioning. This is "breathing" and "circulation" only in an analogous sense: the function and its results are similar, but the source, cause, and purpose are different between those individuals with and those without functioning brains.

For patients who are not artificially maintained, breathing and heartbeat were, and are, reliable signs either of systemic integration and/or of continued brain functioning (depending on which approach one takes to the "whole brain" concept). To regard breathing and respiration as having diagnostic significance when the brain of a respirator-supported patient has ceased functioning, however, is to forget the basic reasoning behind their use in individuals who are not artificially maintained.

Although similar in most respects, the two approaches to "whole brain death" could have slightly different policy consequences. The "primary organ" view would be satisfied with a statute that contained only a single standard—the irreversible cessation of all functions of the entire brain. Nevertheless, as a practical matter, the view is also compatible with a statute establishing irreversible cessation of respiration and circulation as an alternative standard, since it is inherent in this view that the loss of spontaneous breathing and heartbeat are surrogates for the loss of brain functions.

The "integrated functions" view would lead one to a "definition" of death recognizing that collapse of the organism as a whole can be diagnosed through the loss of brain functions as well as through loss of cardiopulmonary functions. The latter functions would remain an explicit part of the policy statement because their irreversible loss will continue to provide an independent and wholly reliable basis for determining that death has occurred when respirators and related means of support are *not* employed.

The two "whole brain" formulations thus differ only modestly. And even conceptual disagreements have a context; the context of the present one is the need to clarify and update the "definition" of death in order to allow principled decisions to be made about the status of comatose respirator-supported patients. The explicit recognition of both standards—cardiopulmonary and whole brain—solves that problem fully. In addition, since it requires only a modest reformulation of the generally accepted view, it accounts for the importance traditionally accorded to heartbeat and respiration, the "vital signs" which will continue to be the grounds for determining death in the overwhelming majority of cases for the foreseeable future. Hence the Commission, drawing on the aspects that the two formulations share and on the ways in which they each add to an understanding of the "meaning" of death, concludes that public policy should recognize both cardiopulmonary and brain-based standards for declaring death.

THE "HIGHER BRAIN" FORMULATIONS

When all brain processes cease, the patient loses two important sets of functions. One set encompasses the integrating and coordinating functions, carried out principally but not exclusively by the cerebellum and brainstem. The other set includes the psychological functions which make consciousness, thought, and feeling possible. These latter functions are located primarily but not exclusively in the cerebrum, especially the neocortex. The two "higher brain" formulations of brain-oriented definitions of death discussed here are premised on the fact that loss of cerebral functions strips the patient of his psychological capacities and properties.

A patient whose brain has permanently stopped functioning will, by definition, have lost those brain functions which sponsor consciousness, feeling, and thought. Thus the higher brain rationales support classifying as dead bodies which meet "whole brain" standards, as discussed in the preceding section. The converse is not true, however. If there are parts of the brain which have no role in sponsoring consciousness, the higher brain formulation would regard their continued functioning as compatible with death.

The Concepts   Philosophers and theologians have attempted to describe the attributes a living being must have to be a person. "Personhood" consists of the complex of activities (or of capacities to engage in them) such as thinking, reasoning, feeling, and human intercourse which make the human different from, or superior to, animals or things. One higher brain formulation would define death as the loss of what is essential to a person. Those advocating the personhood definition often relate these characteristics to brain functioning. Without brain activity, people are incapable of these essential activities. A breathing body, the argument goes, is not in itself a person; and, without functioning brains, patients are merely breathing bodies. Hence personhood ends when the brain suffers irreversible loss of function.

For other philosophers, a certain concept of "personal identity" supports a brain-oriented definition of death. According to this argument, a patient literally ceases to exist as an individual when his or her brain ceases functioning, even if the patient's body is biologically alive. Actual decapitation creates a similar situation: the body might continue to function for a short time, but it would no longer be the "same" person. The persistent identity of a person as an individual from one moment to the next is taken to be dependent on the continuation of certain mental processes which arise from brain functioning. When the brain processes cease (whether due to decapitation or to "brain death") the person's identity also lapses. The mere continuation of biological activity in the body is irrelevant to the determination of death, it is argued, because after the brain has ceased functioning the body is no longer identical with the person.

Critique   Theoretical and practical objections to these arguments led the Commission to rely on them only as confirmatory of other views in formulating a definition of death. First, crucial to the personhood argument is acceptance of one particular concept of those things that are essential to being a person, while there is no general agreement on this very fundamental point among philosophers, much less physicians or the general public. Opinions about what is essential to personhood vary greatly from person to person in our society—to say nothing of intercultural variations.

The argument from personal identity does not rely on any particular conception of personhood, but it does require assent to a single solution to the philosophical problem of identity. Again, this problem has persisted for centuries despite the best attempts by philosophers to solve it. Regardless of the scholarly merits of the various philosophical solutions, their abstract technicality makes them less useful to public policy.

Further, applying either of these arguments in practice would give rise to additional important problems. Severely senile patients, for example, might not clearly be persons, let alone ones with continuing personal identities; the same might be true of the severely retarded. Any argument that classified these individuals as dead would not meet with public acceptance.

Equally problematic for the "higher brain" formulations, patients in whom only the neocortex or subcortical areas have been damaged may retain or regain spontaneous respiration and circulation. Karen Quinlan is a well-known example of a person who apparently suffered permanent damage to the higher centers of the brain but whose lower brain continues to function. Five years after being removed from the respirator that supported her breathing for nearly a year, she remains in a persistent vegetative state but with heart and lungs

that function without mechanical assistance.* Yet the implication of the personhood and personal identity arguments is that Karen Quinlan, who retains brainstem function and breathes spontaneously, is just as dead as a corpse in the traditional sense. The Commission rejects this conclusion and the further implication that such patients could be buried or otherwise treated as dead persons.

Policy Consequences   In order to be incorporated in public policy, a conceptual formulation of death has to be amenable to clear articulation. At present, neither basic neurophysiology nor medical technique suffices to translate the "higher brain" formulation into policy. First, as was discussed in [a part of the study not reproduced here], it is not known which portions of the brain are responsible for cognition and consciousness; what little is known points to substantial interconnections among the brainstem, subcortical structures, and the neocortex. Thus, the "higher brain" may well exist only as a metaphorical concept, not in reality. Second, even when the sites of certain aspects of consciousness can be found, their cessation often cannot be assessed with the certainty that would be required in applying a statutory definition.

Even were these difficulties to be overcome, the adoption of a higher brain "definition" would depart radically from the traditional standards. As already observed, the new standard would assign no significance to spontaneous breathing and heartbeat. Indeed, it would imply that the existing cardiopulmonary definition had been in error all along, even before the advent of respirators and other life-sustaining technology.

In contrast to this, the position taken by the Commission is deliberately conservative. The statutory proposal presented in [the Uniform Determination of Death Act] offers legal recognition for new diagnostic measures of death, but does not ask for acceptance of a wholly new concept of death. On a matter so fundamental to a society's sense of itself—touching deeply held personal and religious beliefs—and so final for the individuals involved, one would desire much

---

* EDITORS' NOTE: Karen Quinlan died on June 11, 1985.

greater consensus than now exists before taking the major step of radically revising the concept of death.

Finally, patients declared dead pursuant to the statute recommended by the Commission would be also considered dead by those who believe that a body without higher brain functions is dead. Thus, all the arguments reviewed thus far are in agreement that irreversible cessation of *all* brain functioning is sufficient to determine death of the organism.

THE NON-BRAIN FORMULATIONS

The Concepts The various physiological concepts of death so far discussed rely in some fashion on brain functioning. By contrast, a literal reading of the traditional cardiopulmonary criteria would require cessation of the flow of bodily "fluids," including air and blood, for death to be declared. This standard is meant to apply whether or not these flows coincide with any other bodily processes, neurological or otherwise. Its support derives from interpretations of religious literature and cultural practices of certain religious and ethnic groups, including some Orthodox Jews and Native Americans.

Another theological formulation of death is, by contrast, not necessarily related to any physiologic phenomenon. The view is traditional in many faiths that death occurs the moment the soul leaves the body. Whether this happens when the patient loses psychological capacities, loses all brain functions, or at some other point, varies according to the teachings of each faith and according to particular interpretations of the scriptures recognized as authoritative.

Critique The conclusions of the "bodily fluids" view lack a physiologic basis in modern biomedicine. While this view accords with the traditional criteria of death, as noted above, it does not necessarily carry over to the new conditions of the intensive care unit—which are what prompt the reexamination of the definition of death. The flow of bodily fluids could conceivably be maintained by machines in the absence of almost all other life processes; the result would be viewed by most as a perfused corpse, totally unresponsive to its environment.

Although the argument concerning the soul could be interpreted as providing a standard for secular action, those who adhere to the concept today apparently acknowledge the need for a more public and verifiable standard of death. Indeed, a statute incorporating a brain-based standard is accepted by theologians of all backgrounds.

Policy Consequences The Commission does not regard itself as a competent or appropriate forum for theological interpretation. Nevertheless, it has sought to propose policies consistent with as many as possible of the diverse religious tenets and practices in our society.

The statute set forth in the UDDA [Uniform Determination of Death Act] does not appear to conflict with the view that the soul leaves the body at death. It provides standards by which death can be determined to have occurred, but it does not prevent a person from believing on religious grounds that the soul leaves the body at a point other than that established as marking death for legal and medical purposes.

The concept of death based upon the flow of bodily fluids cannot be completely reconciled with the proposed statute. The statute is partially consistent with the "fluids" formulation in that both would regard as dead a body with no respiration and circulation. As noted previously, the overwhelming majority of patients, now and for the foreseeable future, will be diagnosed on such basis. Under the statute, however, physicians would declare dead those bodies in which respiration and circulation continued *solely* as a result of artificial maintenance, in the absence of all brain functions. Nonetheless, people who believe that the continued flow of fluids in such patients means they are alive would not be forced by the statute to abandon those beliefs nor to change their religious conduct. While the recommended statute may cause changes in medical and legal behavior, the Commission urges those acting under the statute to apply it with sensitivity to the emotional and religious needs of those for whom the new standards mark a departure from traditional practice. Determinations of death must be made in a consistent and evenhanded fashion, but the statute does not preclude flexibility in responding to individual circumstances after determination has been made.

The Impending Collapse of the Whole-Brain Definition of Death

Robert M. Veatch

For many years there has been lingering doubt, at least among theorists, that the currently fashionable "whole brain–oriented" definition of death has things exactly right. I myself have long resisted the term "brain death" and will use it only in quotation marks to indicate the still common, if ambiguous, usage. The term is ambiguous because it fails to distinguish between the biological claim that the brain is dead and the social/legal/moral claim that the individual as a whole is dead because the brain is dead. An even greater problem with the term arises from the lingering doubt that individuals with dead brains are really dead. Hence, even physicians are sometimes heard to say that the patient "suffered brain death" one day and "died" the following day. It is better to say that he "died" on the first day, the day the brain was determined to be dead, and that the cadaver's other bodily functions ceased the following day. For these reasons I insist on speaking of persons with dead brains as individuals who are dead, not merely persons who are "brain dead."

The presently accepted standard definition, the Uniform Determination of Death Act, specifies that an individual is dead who has sustained "irreversible cessation of all functions of the entire brain, including the brain stem."[1] It also provides an alternative definition specifying that an individual is also dead who has sustained "irreversible cessation of circulatory and respiratory functions." The President's Commission for the Study of Ethical Problems in Medicine and Biomedical and Behavioral Research made clear, however, that circulatory and respiratory function loss are important only as indirect indicators that the brain has been permanently destroyed (p. 74).

DOUBTS ABOUT THE WHOLE BRAIN–ORIENTED DEFINITION

It is increasingly apparent, however, that this consensus is coming apart. As long ago as the early 1970s some of us doubted that literally the entire brain had to be dead for the individual as a whole to be dead.[2]

From the early years it was known, at least among neurologists and theorists who read the literature, that individual, isolated brain cells could be perfused and continue to live even though integrated supercellular brain function had been destroyed. When the uniform definition of death said *all functions of the entire brain* must be dead, there was a gentleman's agreement that cellular-level functions did not count. The President's Commission recognized this, positing that "cellular activity alone is irrelevant" (p. 75). This willingness to write off cellular-level functions is more controversial than it may appear. After all, the law currently does not grant a dispensation to ignore cellular-level functions, no matter how plausible that may be. Keep in mind that critics of soon-to-be-developed higher brain definitions of death would need to emphasize that the model statute called for loss of *all* functions.

By 1977 an analogous problem arose regarding electrical activity. The report of a multicenter study that was funded by the National Institutes of Neurological Diseases and Stroke found that all of the functions it considered important could be lost irreversibly while very small (2 microvolt) electrical potentials could still be obtained on EEG. These were not artifact but real electrical activity from brain cells. Nevertheless, the committee concluded that there could be "electrocerebral silence" and therefore the brain could be considered "dead" even though these small electrical charges could be recorded.[3]

It is possible that the members of the committee believed that these were the result of nothing more than cellular-level functions, so that the same rea-

Hastings Center Report Vol. 23, No. 4, 1993, 18–24. Reprinted by permission. Copyright © 1993 The Hastings Center.

soning that permitted the President's Commission to write off little functions as unimportant would apply. However, no evidence was presented that these electrical potentials were arising exclusively from cellular-level functions. It could well be that the reasoning in this report expanded the existing view that cellular functions did not count to the view that some minor supercellular functions could be ignored as long as they were small.

More recently the neurologist James Bernat, a defender of the whole brain–oriented definition of death, has acknowledged that:

> the bedside clinical examination is not sufficiently sensitive to exclude the possibility that small nests of brain cells may have survived . . . and that their continued functioning, although not contributing significantly to the functioning of the organism as a whole, can be measured by laboratory techniques. Because these isolated nests of neurons no longer contribute to the functioning of the organism as a whole, their continued functioning is now irrelevant to the dead organism.[4]

The idea that functions of "isolated nests of neurons" can remain when an individual is declared dead based on whole brain–oriented criteria certainly stretches the plain words of the law that requires, without qualification, that *all functions of the entire brain* must be gone. That exceptions can be granted by individual private citizens based on their personal judgments about which functions are "contributing significantly" certainly challenges the integrity of the idea that the whole brain must be dead for the individual as a whole to be dead.

There is still another problem for those who favor what can now be called the "whole-brain definition of death." It is not altogether clear that the "death of the brain" is to be equated with the "irreversible loss of function." At least one paper appears to hold out not only for loss of function but also for destruction of anatomical structure.[5] Thus we are left with a severely nuanced and qualified whole brain–oriented definition of death. For it to hold as applied in the 1990s, one must assume that function rather than structure is irreversibly destroyed and that not only can certain cellular-level functions and microvolt-level electrical functions be ignored as "insignificant," but also certain

"nests of cells" and associated supercellular-level functions can as well.

By the time the whole brain–oriented definition of death is so qualified, it can hardly be referring to the death of the whole brain any longer. What is particularly troublesome is that private citizens—neurologists, philosophers, theologians, and public commentators—seem to be determining just which brain functions are insignificant.

THE HIGHER BRAIN–ORIENTED ALTERNATIVE

The problem is exacerbated when one reviews the early "brain death" literature. Writers trying to make the case for a brain-based definition of death over a heart-based one invariably pointed out that certain functions were irreversibly lost when the brain was gone. Then, implicitly or explicitly, they made the moral/philosophical/religious claim that individuals who have irreversibly lost these key functions should be treated as dead.

While this function-based defense of a brain-oriented definition of death served the day well, some of us realized that the critical functions cited were not randomly distributed throughout the brain. For instance, Henry Beecher, the chair of the Harvard Ad Hoc Committee, identified the following functions as critical: "the individual's personality, his conscious life, his uniqueness, his capacity for remembering, judging, reasoning, acting, enjoying, worrying, and so on."[6]

Of course, all these functions are known to require the cerebrum. If these are the important functions, the obvious question is why any lower brain functions would signal the presence of a living individual. This gave rise to what is now best called the *higher brain–oriented definition of death*: that one is dead when there is irreversible loss of all "higher" brain functions.[7] At first this was referred to as a cerebral or a cortical definition of death, but it seems clear that just as some brain stem functions may be deemed insignificant, likewise, some functions in the cerebrum may be as well. Moreover, it is not clear that the functions of the kind Beecher listed are always necessarily localized in the cerebrum or the cerebral cortex. At least in theory someday we may be able to build an artificial neurological organ that could replace some functions of the cerebrum. Someone who was thinking, feeling, reasoning, and carrying on a conversation through the use of an artificial brain would surely be recognized as alive even if the cerebrum that it had replaced was long since completely dead. I have preferred the purposely ambiguous term "higher brain function," as a way to make clear that the key philosophical issue is which of the many brain functions are really important.

Although that way of putting the question may offend the defenders of the more traditional whole-brain definition of death, once they have made the move of excluding the cellular, electrical, and supercellular functions they consider "insignificant," they are hardly in a position to complain about the project of sorting functions into important and unimportant ones.

CRITICISMS OF THE HIGHER BRAIN FORMULATIONS

Several defenders of the whole brain–oriented concept have claimed that defining death in terms of loss of certain significant brain functions involves a change in the concept of death. This, however, rests on the implausible claim of Alex Capron, the executive director of the President's Commission, that the move from a heart-oriented to a whole brain–oriented definition of death is not a change in concept at all, but merely the recognition of new diagnostic measures for the traditional concept of death (p. 41). It is very doubtful, however, that the move to a whole brain–oriented concept of death is any less of a fundamental change in concept than movement to a higher brain–oriented one. From the beginning of the debate many people with beating hearts and dead brains would have been alive under the traditional concept of death focusing on fluid flow, but are clearly dead based on a then-newer whole brain–oriented concept. Most understood this as a significant change in concept. In any case, even if there is a greater change in moving to a definition of death that identifies certain functions of the brain as significant, the mere fact that it is a conceptual change should not count against it. Surely, the critical question is which concept is right, not which concept squares with traditional views.

A second major charge against the higher brain–oriented formulations has been that we are unable to measure precisely the irreversible loss of these higher functions based on current neurophysiological techniques (p. 40). By contrast it has been assumed that the irreversible loss of all functions of the entire brain is measurable based on current techniques.

Although laypeople generally do not realize it, the measurement of death based on any concept can never be 100 percent accurate. The greatest error rates have certainly been with the heart-oriented concepts of death. Many patients have been falsely determined to have irreversibly lost heart functions. In earlier days we simply did not have the capacity to measure precisely. Even today there may be no reason to determine precisely whether the heart could be restarted in the case of a terminally ill, elderly patient who is ready to die.

There is even newly found ambiguity in the notion of irreversibility.[8] We are moving rapidly toward the day when organs for transplant will be obtained from non-heart-beating cadavers who have been determined to be dead based on heart function loss. It will be important for death to be pronounced as quickly as possible after the heart function has been found irreversibly lost. It is not clear, however, whether death should be pronounced when the heart has permanently stopped (say, following a decision based on an advance directive to withdraw a ventilator), but could be started again. In the minutes when it could be started, but will not be because the patient has refused resuscitation, can we say that the individual is dead?

Likewise, it is increasingly clear that we must acknowledge some, admittedly very small, risk of error in measuring the irreversible loss of all functions of the entire brain. Alan Shewmon has argued that the determination of the death of the entire brain cannot be made with as great a certainty as some neurologists would claim.[9] Some neurologists have persisted in claiming that brains are dead (or have irreversibly lost all function) even though electrical function still remains.[10] Clearly, brains with electrical function must have some living tissues; claims these brains are dead must rest on the assumption that remaining functions are insignificant.

None of this should imply that the death of the brain cannot be measured with great accuracy. But it is wrong to assume that similar or greater levels of accuracy cannot be obtained in measuring the irreversible loss of key higher functions, including consciousness. The literature on the persistent vegetative state repeatedly claims that we can know with great accuracy that consciousness is irreversibly lost.[11] The AMA's Councils on Scientific Affairs and Ethical and Judicial Affairs have concluded that the diagnosis can be made with an error rate of less than one in a thousand.[12] In fact the President's Commission itself said that "the Commission was assured that physicians with experience in this area can reliably determine that some patients' loss of consciousness is permanent."[13]

Even if we could not presently measure accurately the loss of key higher functions such as consciousness, that would have a bearing only on the clinical implementation of the higher brain–oriented definition, not the validity of the concept itself. Defenders of the higher brain formulation might continue to use the now old-fashioned measures of loss of all function, but only because of the assurance that if all functions are lost, the higher functions certainly are. Such a conservative policy would leave open the question of whether we could someday measure the loss of higher functions accurately enough to use the measures clinically.

Still another criticism is the claim that any higher brain formulation would rely on a concept of personhood or personal identity that is philosophically controversial (pp. 38–39). Personhood theories are notoriously controversial. It is simply wrong, however, to claim that any higher brain–oriented concept of death is based on either personhood or personal identity theories. I, for one, have acknowledged the possibility that there are living human beings who do not satisfy the various concepts of personhood. As long as the law is only discussing whether someone is a living individual, the personhood debate is irrelevant.

Perhaps the most serious charge against the higher brain–oriented formulations is that they are susceptible to the so-called slippery slope argument.[14] Once one yields on the insistence that all functions of the entire brain must be irreversibly gone before an individual is considered dead, there seems to be no stopping the slide of eliminating functions considered insignificant. The argument posits that once totally and permanently unconscious individuals who have some other brain functions (such as brain stem reflexes) remaining are considered dead, someone will propose that those with only marginal consciousness similarly lack significant function and soon all manner of functionally compromised humans will be defined as dead. Since being labelled dead is normally an indicator that certain moral and legal rights cease, such a slide toward considering increasing numbers of marginally functional humans as dead would be morally horrific.

But is the slippery slope argument plausible? In its most significant form, such an argument involves a claim that the same principle underlying one apparently tolerable judgment also entails other, clearly unacceptable judgments. For example, imagine we were trying to determine whether the elderly could be excluded from access to certain health care services based on the utilitarian principle of choosing the course that produced the maximum aggregate good for society. The slippery slope argument might be used to show that the same principle entails implications presumed clearly unacceptable, such as excluding health care from the socially unproductive. To the extent that one is certain that the empirical assumptions are correct (for example, that the utilitarian principle does entail excluding care from the unproductive) and one is confident that such an outcome would be morally unacceptable, then one might attempt to use slippery slope arguments to challenge the proposal to withhold health care from the elderly. The same principle used to support one policy also entails other policies that are clearly unacceptable.

The slippery slope argument is valid insofar as it shows that the principle used to support one policy under consideration entails clearly unacceptable implications when applied to different situations. In principle, there is no difference between the small, potentially tolerable move and the more dramatic, unacceptable move. However, as applied to the definition of death debate, the slippery slope argument can actually be used to show that the whole brain–oriented definition of death is less defensible than the higher brain–oriented one.

As we have seen, the whole brain–oriented definition of death rests on the claim that irreversible loss of all functions of the entire brain is necessary and sufficient for an individual to be dead. That, in effect, means drawing a sharp line between the top of the spinal cord and the base of the brain (i.e., the bottom of the brain stem). But is there any principled reason why one would draw a line at that point?

In the early years of the definition of death debate, the claim was made that an individual was dead when the central nervous system no longer retained the capacity for integration. It was soon discovered, however, that this could be taken to imply that one was "alive" as long as some spinal cord function remained. That was counterintuitive (and also made it more difficult to obtain organs for transplant). Hence, very early on it was agreed that simple reflexes of the spinal cord did not count as an indicator of life. Presumably the principle was that reflex arcs that do not integrate significant bodily functions are to be ignored.

But why then do brain stem reflexes mediated through the base of the brain stem count? By the same principle, if spinal reflexes can be ignored, it would seem that some brain stem reflexes might be as well. An effort to show that brain stem reflexes are more integrative of bodily function is doomed to fail. At most there are gradual, imperceptible gradations in complexity between the reflexes of the first cervical vertebra and those of the base of the brain stem. Some spinal reflexes that trigger extension of the foot while the contralateral arm is withdrawn certainly cover larger distances.

Whatever principle could be used to exclude the spinal reflexes surely can exclude some brain stem reflexes as well. We have seen that the defenders of the whole brain–oriented position admit as much when they start excluding cellular-level functions and electrical functions. Certainly, those who exclude "nests of cells" in the brain as insignificant have abandoned the whole-brain position and are already sliding along the slippery slope.

By contrast the defenders of the higher brain–oriented definition of death can articulate a principle that avoids such slipperiness. Suppose, for example, they rely on classical Judeo-Christian notions that the human is essentially the integration of the mind and body and that the existence of one without the other is not sufficient to constitute a living human being. Such a principle provides a

bright line that would clearly distinguish the total and irreversible loss of consciousness from serious but not total mental impairments.

Likewise, the integration of mind and body provides a firm basis for telling which functions of nests of brain cells count as significant. It avoids the hopeless task of trying to show why brain stem reflexes count more than spinal ones or trying to show exactly how many cells must be in a nest before it is significant. There is no subjective assessment of different bodily functions, no quibble about how much integration there must be for the organism to function as a whole. The principle is simple. It relies on qualitative considerations: when, and only when, there is the capacity for organic (bodily) and mental function present together in a single human entity is there a living human being. That, I would suggest, is the philosophical basis for the higher brain–oriented definition of death. It avoids the slippery slope on which the defenders of the whole brain–oriented position have found themselves; it, and only it, provides a principled reason for avoiding the slippery slope.

CONSCIENCE CLAUSES

There is one final development that signals the demise of the whole brain–oriented definition of death as the single basis for declaring death. It should be clear by now that the definition of death debate is actually a debate over the moral status of human beings. It is a debate over when humans should be treated as full members of the human community. When humans are living, full moral and legal human rights accrue. Saying people are alive is simply shorthand for saying that they are bearers of such rights. That is why the definition of death debate is so important. It is also why, in principle, there is no scientific way in which the debate can be resolved. The determination of who is alive—who has full moral standing as a member of the human community—is fundamentally a moral, philosophical, or religious determination, not a scientific one.

In a pluralistic society, we are not likely to reach agreement on such moral questions, which is why no one definition of death has carried the day thus far. When one realizes that there are many variants on each of the three major definitions of death, each of which has some group of adherents, it seems unlikely that any one position is likely to gain even a majority anytime soon. For example, defense of the higher brain–oriented position stands or falls on the claim that the essence of the human being is the integration of a mind and a body, a position reflecting religious and philosophical assumptions that are not beyond dispute. (Other defenders of the higher brain position, for example, are more Manichaean, holding that only the mind is important; they apparently are committed to a view that a human memory transferred to a computer with a capacity to continue mental function would still have all the essential ingredients of humanness and that the same living human being continues to live on the computer hard drive.) These are disputes not likely to be resolved soon.

As a society we have a method for dealing with fundamental disputes in religion and philosophy. We tolerate diversity and affirm the right of conscience to hold minority beliefs as long as actions based on those beliefs do not cause insurmountable problems for the rest of society. That is precisely what in 1976 I proposed doing in the dispute over the definition of death.[15] I proposed a definition of death with a conscience clause that would permit individuals to choose their own definition of death based on their religious and philosophical convictions. I did not say at the time, but should have, that the choices would have to be restricted to those that avoid violating the rights of others and avoid creating insurmountable social problems for the rest of society. For example, I assume that people would not be able to pick a definition that required society to treat them as dead even though they retained cardiac, respiratory, mental, and neurological integrating functions. Likewise, I assume that people would not be permitted to pick a definition that would insist that they be treated as alive when all these functions were absent. There are minimal public health considerations that would set limits on the choices available, but certainly the three major options would be tolerable: heart-, whole brain–, and higher brain–oriented definitions.

The state of New Jersey has gone part of the way recently by adopting a law with a conscience clause that would permit religious objectors to designate in advance that a heart-oriented defini-

tion should be used in pronouncing their deaths.[16] Since it is now widely accepted that anyone can write an advance directive mandating withdrawal of life support once one is permanently unconscious, any persons who favor a higher brain–oriented definition of death already have the legal right to make choices that end up with them dead in anyone's sense of the term very shortly after they had lost higher brain functions. Permitting them to designate that they be called dead when they are permanently unconscious changes very little.

There is a litany of worries over conscience clauses that defenders of the whole brain–oriented definitions cite. They worry about life insurance paying off at different times, depending on which definition is chosen, and about homicide charges being dependent on such choices, but these are already with us when people are permitted to use advance directives to control the timing of their deaths. They worry about health insurance costs, but for those who choose a higher brain–oriented formulation the only implication is lower costs. For those who choose a heart-oriented definition potentially higher health insurance costs could result, but that position is held only by a small minority, and it is technically so difficult to maintain a beating heart in someone whose brain is dead that the costs will probably not be significant. If they were, the problem could be addressed by clarifying that standard health insurance would not cover the medical costs for maintaining someone who is "alive with a dead brain." None of these problems has arisen in New Jersey, and none is likely to arise. In short, there is no reason to suspect that the use of a conscience clause will result in social chaos—only in greater respect for minority religious and philosophical views that would otherwise be suppressed by the tyranny of the majority. For convenience it would probably be prudent to adopt a single "default definition" favored by a majority; it would make little difference which definition is used as long as the minority who had strong preference for an alternative had the right to designate in advance its choice of another definition. As with surrogate decision making for terminal care and the procurement of cadaver organs, I think it would be reasonable for the next of kin to have the right of surrogate decision making in the case of minors or mentally incompetent individuals who had not expressed a preference while competent.

CRAFTING NEW PUBLIC LAW

Changing current law to conform to these suggestions will be complex and should be done with deliberate speed, but it should be done. Two changes would be needed in the current definition of death: (1) incorporating the higher brain function notion and (2) incorporating some form of the conscience clause.

Present law makes persons dead when they have lost all functions of the entire brain. It is uniformly agreed that the law should incorporate only this basic concept of death, not the precise criteria or tests needed to determine that the whole brain is dead. That is left up to the consensus of neurological experts.

All that would be needed to shift to a higher brain formulation is a change in the wording of the law to replace "all functions of the entire brain" with some relevant, more limited alternative. There are at least three options: references to higher brain functions, cerebral functions, or consciousness. While we could simply change the wording to read that an individual is dead when there is irreversible cessation of all higher brain functions, that poses a serious problem. We are now suffering from the problems created by the vagueness of the referring to "all functions of the entire brain." Even though referring to "all higher brain functions" would be conceptually correct, it would be even more ambiguous. It would lack needed specificity.

This specificity could be achieved by referring to irreversible loss of cerebral functions, but we have already suggested two problems with that wording. Just as we now know there are some isolated functions of the whole brain that should be discounted, so there are probably some isolated cerebral functions that most would not want to count either. For example, if, hypothetically, an isolated "nest" of cerebral motor neurons were perfused so that if stimulated the body could twitch, that would be a cerebral function, but not a significant one for determining life any more than a brain stem reflex is. Second, in theory some really significant functions such as consciousness might some-

day be maintainable even without a cerebrum—if, for example, a computer could function as an artificial center for consciousness. The term "cerebral function" adds specificity but is not satisfactory.

The language that seems best if integration of mind and body is what is critical is "irreversible cessation of the capacity for consciousness." That is, after all, what the defenders of the higher brain formulations really have in mind. (If someone were to claim that some other "higher" function is critical, that alternative could simply be plugged in.) As is the case now, the specifics of the criteria and tests for measuring irreversible loss of capacity for consciousness would be left up to the consensus of neurological expertise, even though measuring irreversible loss of capacity for a brain function such as consciousness involves fundamentally nonscientific value judgments. If the community of neurological expertise claims that irreversible loss of consciousness cannot be measured, so be it. We will at least have clarified the concept and set the stage for the day when it can be measured with sufficient accuracy. We have noted, however, that neurologists presently claim they can in fact measure irreversible loss of consciousness accurately.

A second significant change in the definition of death would be required to incorporate the conscience clause. It would permit individuals, while competent, to execute documents choosing alternative definitions of death that are, within reason, not threatening to significant interests of others. While the New Jersey law permits only the alternative of a heart-oriented definition, my proposal, assuming irreversible loss of consciousness were the default definition, would permit choosing either heart-oriented or whole brain–oriented definitions as alternatives.

The New Jersey law presently permits only competent adults to execute such conscience clauses. This, of course, excludes the possibility of parents choosing alternative definitions for their children. I had long ago proposed that, just as legal surrogates have the right to make medical treatment decisions for their wards provided that these decisions are within reason, so they should be permitted to choose alternative definitions of death provided the individual had never expressed a preference. This would, for example, permit Orthodox Jewish parents to require that the state continue to treat their child as alive even though he or she had suffered irreversible loss of consciousness or of total brain function. (Whether the state also requires insurers to continue paying for support of these individuals deemed living is a separate policy issue.) While the New Jersey law tolerates only variation with an explicitly religious basis, I would favor variation based on any conscientiously formulated position.

As a shortcut the law could state that patients who had clearly irreversibly lost consciousness because heart and lung function had stopped could continue to be pronounced dead based on criteria measuring heart and lung function. That this was simply an alternative means for measuring permanent loss of consciousness would have to be set out more clearly than in the present Uniform Determination of Death Act. I see no reason to continue including the alternative measurement in the legal definition. I would simply allow it to fall under the criteria to be articulated by the consensus of experts. This leads to a proposal for a new definition of death, which would read as follows:

> An individual who has sustained irreversible loss of consciousness is dead. A determination of death must be made in accordance with accepted medical standards.
> However, no individual shall be considered dead based on irreversible loss of consciousness if he or she, while competent, has explicitly asked to be pronounced dead based on irreversible cessation of all functions of the entire brain or based on irreversible cessation of circulatory and respiratory functions.
> Unless an individual has, while competent, selected one of these definitions of death, the legal guardian or next of kin (in that order) may do so. The definition selected by the individual, legal guardian, or next of kin shall serve as the definition of death for all legal purposes.

If one favored only the shift to consciousness as a definition of death without the conscience clause, only paragraph one would be necessary. One could also craft a similar definition using the whole brain–oriented definition of death as the default definition. Some have proposed an additional paragraph prohibiting a physician with a conflict of interest (such as an interest in the organs of the deceased) from pronouncing death. I am not convinced that paragraph is needed, however.

A PRINCIPLED REASON FOR DRAWING THE LINE

It has been puzzling why what at first seemed like a rather minor debate over when a human was dead should have persisted as long as it has. Many thought the definition of death debate was a technical argument that would be resolved in favor of the more fashionable, scientific, and progressive brain-oriented definition as soon as the old romantics attached to the heart died off. It is now clear that something much more complex and more fundamental is at stake. We have been fighting over the question of who has moral standing as a full member of the human moral community, a matter that forces on us some of the most basic questions of human existence: the relation of mind and body, the rights of religious and philosophical minorities, and the meaning of life itself.

I am not certain whether some version of the higher brain–oriented definition of death will be adopted in any legal jurisdiction anytime soon, but I am convinced that the now old-fashioned whole brain–oriented definition of death is becoming less and less plausible as we realize that no one really believes that literally all functions of the entire brain must be irreversibly lost for an individual to be dead. Unless there is some public consensus expressed in state or federal law conveying agreement upon exactly which brain functions are insignificant, we will all be vulnerable to a slippery slope in which private practitioners choose for themselves exactly where from the top of the cerebrum to caudal end of the spinal cord to draw the line. There is no principled reason to draw it exactly between the base of the brain and the top of the spine. Better that we have a principled reason for drawing it. To me, the principle is that for human life to be present—that is, for the human to be treated as a member in full standing of the human moral community—there must be integrated functioning of mind and body. That means some version of a higher brain–oriented formulation.

NOTES

1. President's Commission for the Study of Ethical Problems in Medicine and Biomedical and Behavioral Research, *Defining Death: Medical, Legal and Ethical Issues*

in the Definition of Death (Washington, D.C.: U.S. Government Printing Office, 1981), p. 2. Page numbers for subsequent citations are in the text.

2. Robert M. Veatch, "The Whole-Brain-Oriented Concept of Death: An Outmoded Philosophical Formulation," *Journal of Thanatology* 3 (1975): 13–30.

3. Earl A. Walker et al., "An Appraisal of the Criteria of Cerebral Death: A Summary Statement," *JAMA* 237 (1977): 982–86, at 983.

4. James L. Bernat, "How Much of the Brain Must Die on Brain Death?" *Journal of Clinical Ethics* 3, no. 1 (1992): 21–26, at 25.

5. Paul A. Byrne, Sean O'Reilly, and Paul M. Quay, "Brain Death: An Opposing Viewpoint," *JAMA* 242 (1979): 1985–90.

6. Cited in Robert M. Veatch, *Death, Dying, and the Biological Revolution* (New Haven: Yale University Press, 1976), p. 38.

7. Robert M. Veatch, "Whole-Brain, Neocortical, and Higher Brain Related Concepts," in *Death: Beyond Whole-Brain Criteria*, ed. Richard M. Zaner (Dordrecht, Holland: D. Reidel Publishing Company, 1988), pp. 171–86.

8. David J. Cole, "The Reversibility of Death," *Journal of Medical Ethics* 18 (1992): 26–30.

9. Alan D. Shewmon, "Caution in the Definition and Diagnosis of Infant Brain Death," in *Medical Ethics: A Guide for Health Professionals*, ed. John F. Monagle and David C. Thomasma (Rockville, Md.: Aspen Publishers, 1988), pp. 38–57.

10. Stephen Ashwal and Sanford Schneider, "Failure of Electroencephalography to Diagnose Brain Death in Comatose Patients," *Annals of Neurology* 6 (1979): 512–17.

11. Ronald B. Cranford and Harmon L. Smith, "Some Critical Distinctions between Brain Death and the Persistent Vegetative State," *Ethics in Science and Medicine* 6 (Winter 1979): 199–209; Phiroze L. Hansotia, "Persistent Vegetative State," *Archives of Neurology* 42 (1985): 1048–52.

12. Council on Scientific Affairs and Council on Ethical and Judicial Affairs, "Persistent Vegetative State and the Decision to Withdraw or Withhold Life Support," *JAMA* 263 (1990): 426–30, at 428.

13. President's Commission for the Study of Ethical Problems in Medicine and Biomedical and Behavioral Research, *Deciding to Forego Life-Sustaining Treatment: Ethical, Medical, and Legal Issues in Treatment Decisions* (Washington, D.C.: U.S. Government Printing Office, 1983), p. 177.

14. Bernat, "How Much of the Brain Must Die on Brain Death?" pp. 21–26.

15. Veatch, *Death, Dying, and the Biological Revolution*, pp. 72–76.

16. New Jersey Declaration of Death Act (1991), *New Jersey Statutes Annotated*, Title 26, 6A-1 to 6A-8.

Is It Time to Abandon Brain Death?*

Robert D. Truog

Over the past several decades, the concept of brain death has become well entrenched within the practice of medicine. At a practical level, this concept has been successful in delineating widely accepted ethical and legal boundaries for the procurement of vital organs for transplantation. Despite this success, however, there have been persistent concerns over whether the concept is theoretically coherent and internally consistent. Indeed, some have concluded that the concept is fundamentally flawed, and that it represents only a "superficial and fragile consensus."[1] In this analysis I will identify the sources of these inconsistencies, and suggest that the best resolution to these issues may be to abandon the concept of brain death altogether.

Hastings Center Report 27, No. 1, Jan./Feb. 1997, 29–37. Reprinted by permission. Copyright © 1997 The Hastings Center.

*EDITORS' NOTE: Some of the notes have been omitted and the remaining renumbered. Readers who wish to follow up on sources should consult the original article.

DEFINITIONS, CONCEPTS, AND TESTS

In its seminal work "Defining Death," the President's Commission for the Study of Ethical Problems in Medicine and Biomedical and Behavioral Research articulated a formulation of brain death that has come to be known as the "whole-brain standard." In the Uniform Determination of Death Act, the President's Commission specified two criteria for determining death: (1) irreversible cessation of circulatory and respiratory functions, or (2) irreversible cessation of all functions of the entire brain, including the brainstem."

Neurologist James Bernat has been influential in defending and refining this standard. Along with others, he has recognized that analysis of the concept of brain death must begin by differentiating between three distinct levels. At the most general level, the concept must involve a *definition*. Next, *criteria* must be specified to determine when the definition has been fulfilled. Finally, *tests* must be available for evaluating whether the criteria have been satisfied. As clarified by Bernat and colleagues, therefore, the concept of death under the whole brain formulation can be outlined as follows:

Definition of Death: The "permanent cessation of functioning of the organism as a whole."

Criterion for Death: The "permanent cessation of functioning of the entire brain."

Tests for Death: Two distinct sets of tests are available and acceptable for determining that the criterion is fulfilled:

(1) The cardiorespiratory standard is the traditional approach for determining death and relies upon documenting the prolonged absence of circulation or respiration. These tests fulfill the criterion, according to Bernat, since the prolonged absence of these vital signs is diagnostic for the permanent loss of all brain function.

(2) The neurological standard consists of a battery of tests and procedures, including establishment of an etiology sufficient to account for the loss of all brain functions, diagnosing the presence of coma, documenting apnea and the absence of brain-stem reflexes, excluding reversible conditions, and showing the persistence of these findings over a sufficient period of time.

CRITIQUE OF THE CURRENT FORMULATION OF BRAIN DEATH

Is this a coherent account of the concept of brain death? To answer this question, one must determine whether each level of analysis is consistent with the others. In other words, individuals who fulfill the tests must also fulfill the criterion, and those who satisfy the criterion must also satisfy the definition.[2]

First, regarding the tests-criterion relationship, there is evidence that many individuals who fulfill all of the tests for brain death do not have the "permanent cessation of functioning of the entire brain." In particular, many of these individuals retain clear evidence of integrated brain function at the level of the brainstem and midbrain, and may have evidence of cortical function.

For example, many patients who fulfill the tests for the diagnosis of brain death continue to exhibit intact neurohumoral function. Between 22 percent and 100 percent of brain-dead patients in different series have been found to retain free-water homeostasis through the neurologically mediated secretion of arginine vasopressin, as evidenced by serum hormonal levels and the absence of diabetes insipidus. Since the brain is the only source of the regulated secretion of arginine vasopressin, patients without diabetes insipidus do not have the loss of all brain function. Neurologically regulated secretion of other hormones is also quite common.

In addition, the tests for the diagnosis of brain death require the patient not to be hypothermic. This caveat is a particularly confusing catch 22, since the absence of hypothermia generally indicates the continuation of neurologically mediated temperature homeostasis. The circularity of this reasoning can be clinically problematic, since hypothermic patients cannot be diagnosed as brain-dead but the absence of hypothermia is itself evidence of brain function.

Furthermore, studies have shown that many patients (20 percent in one series) who fulfill the tests for brain death continue to show electrical activity on their electroencephalograms. While there is no way to determine how often this electrical activity represents true "function" (which would be incompatible with the criterion for brain death), in at least some cases the activity observed seems fully compatible with function.

Finally, clinicians have observed that patients who fulfill the tests for brain death frequently respond to surgical incision at the time of organ procurement with a significant rise in both heart rate and blood pressure. This suggests that integrated neurological function at a supraspinal level may be present in at least some patients diagnosed as brain-dead. This evidence points to the conclusion that there is a significant disparity between the standard tests used to make the diagnosis of brain death and the criterion these tests are purported to fulfill. Faced with these facts, even supporters of the current statutes acknowledge that the criterion of "whole-brain" death is only an "approximation."

If the tests for determining brain death are incompatible with the current criterion, then one way of solving the problem would be to require tests that always correlate with the "permanent cessation of functioning of the entire brain." Two options have been considered in this regard. The first would require tests that correlate with the actual destruction of the brain, since complete destruction would, of course, be incompatible with any degree of brain function. Only by satisfying these tests, some have argued, could we be assured that all functions of the entire brain have totally and permanently ceased. But is there a constellation of clinical and laboratory tests that correlate with this degree of destruction? Unfortunately, a study of over 500 patients with both coma and apnea (including 146 autopsies for neuropathologic correlation) showed that "it was not possible to verify that a diagnosis made prior to cardiac arrest by any set or subset of criteria would invariably correlate with a diffusely destroyed brain." On the basis of these data, a definition that required total brain destruction could only be confirmed at autopsy. Clearly, a condition that could only be determined after death could never be a requirement for declaring death.

Another way of modifying the tests to conform with the criterion would be to rely solely upon the cardiorespiratory standard for determining death. This standard would certainly identify the permanent cessation of all brain function (thereby fulfilling the criterion), since it is well established by common knowledge that prolonged absence of circulation and respiration results in the death of the entire brain (and every other organ). In addition, fulfillment of these tests would also convincingly demonstrate the cessation of function of the organism as a whole (thereby fulfilling the definition). Unfortunately, this approach for resolving the problem would also make it virtually impossible to obtain vital organs in a viable condition for transplantation, since under current laws it is generally necessary for these organs to be removed from a heart-beating donor.

These inconsistencies between the tests and the criterion are therefore not easily resolvable. In addition to these problems, there are also inconsistencies between the criterion and the definition. As outlined above, the whole-brain concept assumes that the "permanent cessation of functioning of the entire brain" (the criterion) necessarily implies the "permanent cessation of functioning of the organism as a whole" (the definition). Conceptually, this relationship assumes the principle that the brain is responsible for maintaining the body's homeostasis, and that without brain function the organism rapidly disintegrates. In the past, this relationship was demonstrated by showing that individuals who fulfilled the tests for the diagnosis of brain death inevitably had a cardiac arrest within a short period of time, even if they were provided with mechanical ventilation and intensive care. Indeed, this assumption had been considered one of the linchpins in the ethical justification for the concept of brain death. For example, in the largest empirical study of brain death ever performed, a collaborative group working under the auspices of the National Institutes of Health sought to specify the necessary tests for diagnosing brain death by attempting to identify a constellation of neurological findings that would inevitably predict the development of a cardiac arrest within three months, regardless of the level or intensity of support provided.

This approach to defining brain death in terms of neurological findings that predict the development of cardiac arrest is plagued by both logical and scientific problems, however. First, it confuses a prognosis with a diagnosis. Demonstrating that a certain class of patients will suffer a cardiac arrest within a defined period of time certainly proves that they are *dying*, but it says nothing about whether they are *dead*. This conceptual mistake can be clearly appreciated if one considers individuals who are dying of conditions not associated with severe neurological impairment. If a constellation of tests could identify a subgroup of patients with metastatic cancer who invariably suffered a cardiac arrest within a short period of time, for example, we would certainly be comfortable in concluding that they were dying, but we clearly could not claim that they were already dead.

Second, this view relies upon the intuitive notion that the brain is the principal organ of the body, the "integrating" organ whose functions cannot be replaced by any other organ or by artificial means. Up through the early 1980s, this view was supported by numerous studies showing that almost all patients who fulfilled the usual battery of tests for brain death suffered a cardiac arrest within several weeks.

The loss of homeostatic equilibrium that is empirically observed in brain-dead patients is almost certainly the result of their progressive loss of integrated neurohumoral and autonomic function. Over the past several decades, however, intensive care units (ICUs) have become increasingly sophisticated "surrogate brainstems," replacing both the respiratory functions as well as the hormonal and other regulatory activities of the damaged neuraxis. This technology is presently utilized in those tragic cases in which a pregnant woman is diagnosed as brain-dead and an attempt is made to maintain her somatic existence until the fetus reaches a viable gestation, as well as for prolonging the organ viability of brain-dead patients awaiting organ procurement. Although the functions of the brainstem are considerably more complex than those of the heart or the lungs, in theory (and increasingly in practice) they are entirely replaceable by modern technology. In terms of maintaining homeostatic functions, therefore, the brain is no more irreplaceable than any of the other vital organs. A definition of death predicated upon the "inevitable" development of a cardiac arrest within a short period of time is therefore inadequate, since this empirical "fact" is no longer true. In other words, cardiac arrest is inevitable only if it is allowed to occur, just as respiratory arrest in brain-dead patients is inevitable only if they are not provided with mechanical ventilation. This gradual development in technical expertise has unwittingly undermined one of the central ethical justifications for the whole-brain criterion of death.

In summary, then, the whole-brain concept is plagued by internal inconsistencies in both the tests-criterion and the criterion-definition relationships, and these problems cannot be easily solved. In addition, there is evidence that this lack of conceptual clarity has contributed to misunderstandings about the concept among both clinicians and laypersons. For example, Stuart Youngner and colleagues found that only 35 percent of physicians and nurses who were likely to be involved in organ procurement for transplantation correctly identified the legal and medical criteria for determining death. Indeed, most of the respondents used inconsistent concepts of death, and a substantial minority misunderstood the criterion to be the permanent loss of consciousness, which the President's Commission had specifically rejected, in part because it would have classified anencephalic newborns and patients in a vegetative state as dead. In other words, medical professionals who were otherwise knowledgeable and sophisticated were generally confused about the concept of brain death. In an editorial accompanying this study, Dan Wikler and Alan Weisbard claimed that this confusion was "appropriate," given the lack of philosophical coherence in the concept itself.[3] In another study, a survey of Swedes found that laypersons were more willing to consent to autopsies than to organ donation for themselves or a close relative. In seeking an explanation for these findings, the authors reported that "the fear of not being dead during the removal of organs, reported by 22 percent of those undecided toward organ donation, was related to the uncertainty surrounding brain death."[4]

On one hand, these difficulties with the concept might be deemed to be so esoteric and theoretical that they should play no role in driving the policy debate about how to define death and procure organs for transplantation. This has certainly been the predominant view up to now. In many other circumstances, theoretical issues have taken a back seat to practical matters when it comes to determining public policy. For example, the question of whether tomatoes should be considered a vegetable or a fruit for purposes of taxation was said to hinge little upon the biological facts of the matter, but to turn primarily upon the political and economic issues at stake. If this view is applied to the concept of brain death, then the best public policy would be that which best served the public's interest, regardless of theoretical concerns.

On the other hand, medicine has a long and respected history of continually seeking to refine the theoretical and conceptual underpinnings of its practice. While the impact of scientific and philosophical views upon social policy and public perception must be taken seriously, they cannot be the sole forces driving the debate. Given the evidence demonstrating a lack of coherence in the whole-brain death formulation and the confusion that is apparent among medical professionals, there is ample reason to prompt a look at alternatives to our current approach.

ALTERNATIVE APPROACHES TO THE WHOLE-BRAIN FORMULATION

Alternatives to the whole-brain death formulation fall into two general categories. One approach is to emphasize the overriding importance of those functions of the brain that support the phenomenon of consciousness and to claim that individuals who have permanently suffered the loss of all consciousness are dead. This is known as the "higher-brain" criterion. The other approach is to return to the traditional tests for determining death, that is, the permanent loss of circulation and respiration. As noted above, this latter strategy could fit well with Bernat's formulation of the definition of death, since adoption of the cardiorespiratory standard as the test for determining death is consistent with both the criterion and the definition. The problem with this potential solution is that it would virtually eliminate the possibility of procuring vital organs from heart-beating donors under our present system of law and ethics, since current requirements insist that organs be removed only from individuals who have been declared dead (the "dead-donor rule"). Consideration of this latter view would therefore be feasible only if it could be linked to fundamental changes in the permissible limits of organ procurement.

THE HIGHER-BRAIN FORMULATION

The higher-brain criterion for death holds that maintaining the potential for consciousness is the critical function of the brain relevant to questions of life and death. Under this definition, all individuals who are permanently unconscious would be considered to be dead. Included in this category would be (1) patients who fulfill the cardiorespiratory standard, (2) those who fulfill the current tests for whole-brain death, (3) those diagnosed as being in a permanent vegetative state, and (4) newborns with anencephaly. Various versions of this view

have been defended by many philosophers, and arguments have been advanced from moral as well as ontological perspectives.[5] In addition, this view correlates very well with many common-sense opinions about personal identity. To take a stock philosophical illustration, for example, consider the typical reaction of a person who has undergone a hypothetical "brain switch" procedure, where one's brain is transplanted into another's body, and vice versa. Virtually anyone presented with this scenario will say that "what matters" for their existence now resides in the new body, even though an outside observer would insist that it is the person's old body that "appears" to be the original person. Thought experiments like this one illustrate that we typically identify ourselves with our experience of consciousness, and this observation forms the basis of the claim that the permanent absence of consciousness should be seen as representing the death of the person.

Implementation of this standard would present certain problems, however. First, is it possible to diagnose the state of permanent unconsciousness with the high level of certainty required for the determination of death? More specifically, is it currently possible to definitively diagnose the permanent vegetative state and anencephaly? A Multi-Society Task Force recently outlined guidelines for diagnosis of permanent vegetative state and claimed that sufficient data are now available to make the diagnosis of permanent vegetative state in appropriate patients with a high degree of certainty. On the other hand, case reports of patients who met these criteria but who later recovered a higher degree of neurological functioning suggest that use of the term "permanent" may be overstating the degree of diagnostic certainty that is currently possible. This would be an especially important issue in the context of diagnosing death, where false positive diagnoses would be particularly problematic. Similarly, while the Medical Task Force on Anencephaly has concluded that most cases of anencephaly can be diagnosed by a competent clinician without significant uncertainty, others have emphasized the ambiguities inherent in evaluating this condition.

Another line of criticism is that the higher-brain approach assumes the definition of death should reflect the death of the *person*, rather than the death of the *organism*. By focusing on the person, this theory does not account for what is common to the death of all organisms, such as humans, frogs, or trees. Since we do not know what it would mean to talk about the permanent loss of consciousness of frogs or trees, then this approach to death may appear to be idiosyncratic. In response, higher-brain theorists believe that it is critical to define death within the context of the specific subject under consideration. For example, we may speak of the death of an ancient civilization, the death of a species, or the death of a particular system of belief. In each case, the definition of death will be different, and must be appropriate to the subject in order for the concept to make any sense. Following this line of reasoning, the higher-brain approach is correct precisely because it seeks to identify what is uniquely relevant to the death of a person.

Aside from these diagnostic and philosophical concerns, however, perhaps the greatest objections to the higher-brain formulation emerge from the implications of treating breathing patients as if they are dead. For example, if patients in a permanent vegetative state were considered to be dead, then they should logically be considered suitable for burial. Yet all of these patients breathe, and some of them "live" for many years. The thought of burying or cremating a breathing individual, even if unconscious, would be unthinkable for many people, creating a significant barrier to acceptance of this view into public policy.

One way of avoiding this implication would be to utilize a "lethal injection" before cremation or burial to terminate cardiac and respiratory function. This would not be euthanasia, since the individual would be declared dead before the injection. The purpose of the injection would be purely "aesthetic." This practice could even be viewed as simply an extension of our current protocols, where the vital functions of patients diagnosed as brain-dead are terminated prior to burial, either by discontinuing mechanical ventilation or by removing their heart and/or lungs during the process of organ procurement. While this line of argumentation has a certain logical persuasiveness, it nevertheless fails to address the central fact that most people find it counterintuitive to perceive a breathing patient as "dead." Wikler has suggested that this attitude is likely to change over time, and that eventually society will come to accept that the body of a patient in a permanent vegetative state is simply that person's "living remains." This opti-

mism about higher-brain death is reminiscent of the comments by the President's Commission regarding whole-brain death: "Although undeniably disconcerting for many people, the confusion created in personal perception by a determination of 'brain death' does not . . . provide a basis for an ethical objection to discontinuing medical measures on these dead bodies any more than on other dead bodies."[6] Nevertheless, at the present time any inclination toward a higher-brain death standard remains primarily in the realm of philosophers and not policymakers.

RETURN TO THE TRADITIONAL CARDIORESPIRATORY STANDARD

In contrast to the higher-brain concept of death, the other main alternative to our current approach would involve moving in the opposite direction and abandoning the diagnosis of brain death altogether. This would involve returning to the traditional approach to determining death, that is, the cardiorespiratory standard. In evaluating the wisdom of "turning back the clock," it is helpful to retrace the development of the concept of brain death back to 1968 and the conclusions of the Ad Hoc Committee that developed the Harvard Criteria for the diagnosis of brain death. They began by claiming:

> There are two reasons why there is need for a definition [of brain death]: (1) Improvements in resuscitative and supportive measures have led to increased efforts to save those who are desperately injured. Sometimes these efforts have only partial success so that the result is an individual whose heart continues to beat but whose brain is irreversibly damaged. The burden is great on patients who suffer permanent loss of intellect, on their families, and on those in need of hospital beds already occupied by these comatose patients. (2) Obsolete criteria for the definition of death can lead to controversy in obtaining organs for transplantation.[7]

These two issues can be subdivided into at least four distinct questions:

1. When is it permissible to withdraw life support from patients with irreversible neurological damage for the benefit of the patient?
2. When is it permissible to withdraw life support from patients with irreversible neurological damage for the benefit of society, where

the benefit is either in the form of economic savings or to make an ICU bed available for someone with a better prognosis?

3. When is it permissible to remove organs from a patient for transplantation?

4. When is a patient ready to be cremated or buried?

The Harvard Committee chose to address all of these questions with a single answer, that is, the determination of brain death. Each of these questions involves unique theoretical issues, however, and each raises a different set of concerns. By analyzing the concept of brain death in terms of the separate questions that led to its development, alternatives to brain death may be considered.

Withdrawal of life support. The Harvard Committee clearly viewed the diagnosis of brain death as a necessary condition for the withdrawal of life support: "It should be emphasized that we recommend the patient be declared dead before any effort is made to take him off a respirator . . . [since] otherwise, the physicians would be turning off the respirator on a person who is, in the present strict, technical application of law, still alive" (p. 339).

The ethical and legal mandates that surround the withdrawal of life support have changed dramatically since the recommendations of the Harvard Committee. Numerous court decisions and consensus statements have emphasized the rights of patients or their surrogates to demand the withdrawal of life-sustaining treatments, including mechanical ventilation. In the practice of critical care medicine today, patients are rarely diagnosed as brain-dead solely for the purpose of discontinuing mechanical ventilation. When patients are not candidates for organ transplantation, either because of medical contraindications or lack of consent, families are informed of the dismal prognosis, and artificial ventilation is withdrawn. While the diagnosis of brain death was once critical in allowing physicians to discontinue life-sustaining treatments, decisionmaking about these important questions is now appropriately centered around the patient's previously stated wishes and judgments about the patient's best interest. Questions about the definition of death have become virtually irrelevant to these deliberations.

Allocation of scarce resources. The Harvard Committee alluded to its concerns about having patients with a hopeless prognosis occupying ICU beds. In the years since that report, this issue has become even more pressing. The diagnosis of brain death, however, is of little significance in helping to resolve these issues. Even considering the unusual cases where families refuse to have the ventilator removed from a brain-dead patient, the overall impact of the diagnosis of brain death upon scarce ICU resources is minimal. Much more important to the current debate over the just allocation of ICU resources are patients with less severe degrees of neurological dysfunction, such as patients in a permanent vegetative state or individuals with advanced dementia. Again, the diagnosis of brain death is of little relevance to this central concern of the Harvard Committee.

Organ transplantation. Without question, the most important reason for the continued use of brain death criteria is the need for transplantable organs. Yet even here, the requirement for brain death may be doing more harm than good. The need for organs is expanding at an ever-increasing rate, while the number of available organs has essentially plateaued. In an effort to expand the limited pool of organs, several attempts have been made to circumvent the usual restrictions of brain death on organ procurement.

At the University of Pittsburgh, for example, a new protocol allows critically ill patients or their surrogates to offer their organs for donation after the withdrawal of life-support, even though the patients never meet brain death criteria. Suitable patients are taken to the operating room, where intravascular monitors are placed and the patient is "prepped and draped" for surgical incision. Life-support is then withdrawn, and the patient is monitored for the development of cardiac arrest. Assuming this occurs within a short period of time, the attending physician waits until there has been two minutes of pulselessness, and then pronounces the patient dead. The transplant team then enters the operating room and immediately removes the organs for transplantation.

This novel approach has a number of problems when viewed from within the traditional framework. For example, after the patient is pronounced dead, why should the team rush to remove the organs? If the Pittsburgh team truly believes that the patient is dead, why not begin chest compressions and mechanical ventilation, insert cannulae to place the patient on full cardiopulmonary bypass, and remove the organs in a more controlled fashion? Presumably, this is not done because two minutes of pulselessness is almost certainly not long enough to ensure the development of brain death. It is even conceivable that patients managed in this way could regain consciousness during the process of organ procurement while supported with cardiopulmonary bypass, despite having already been diagnosed as "dead." In other words, the reluctance of the Pittsburgh team to extend their protocol in ways that would be acceptable for dead patients could be an indication that the patients may really not be dead after all.

A similar attempt to circumvent the usual restrictions on organ procurement was recently attempted with anencephalic newborns at Loma Linda University. Again, the protocol involved manipulation of the dying process, with mechanical ventilation being instituted and maintained solely for the purpose of preserving the organs until criteria for brain death could be documented. The results were disappointing, and the investigators concluded that "it is usually not feasible, with the restrictions of current law, to procure solid organs for transplantation from anencephalic infants."

Why do these protocols strike many commentators as contrived and even somewhat bizarre? The motives of the individuals involved are certainly commendable: they want to offer the benefits of transplantable organs to individuals who desperately need them. In addition, they are seeking to obtain organs only from individuals who cannot be harmed by the procurement and only in those situations where the patient or a surrogate requests the donation. The problem with these protocols lies not with the motive, but with the method and justification. By manipulating both the process and the definition of death, these protocols give the appearance that the physicians involved are only too willing to draw the boundary between life and death wherever it happens to maximize the chances for organ procurement.

How can the legitimate desire to increase the supply of transplantable organs be reconciled with the need to maintain a clear and simple distinction between the living and the dead? One way would be to abandon the requirement for the death of the donor prior to organ procurement and, instead, focus upon alternative and perhaps more fundamental ethical criteria to constrain the procurement of organs, such as the principles of consent and nonmaleficence.

For example, policies could be changed such that organ procurement would be permitted only with the consent of the donor or appropriate surrogate and only when doing so would not harm the donor. Individuals who could not be harmed by the procedure would include those who are permanently and irreversibly unconscious (patients in a persistent vegetative state or newborns with anencephaly) and those who are imminently and irreversibly dying.

The American Medical Association's Council on Ethical and Judicial Affairs recently proposed (but has subsequently retracted) a position consistent with this approach.[8] The council stated that, "It is ethically permissible to consider the anencephalic as a potential organ donor, although still alive under the current definition of death," if, among other requirements, the diagnosis is certain and the parents give their permission. The council concluded, "It is normally required that the donor be legally dead before removal of their life-necessary organs . . . The use of the anencephalic neonate as a live donor is a limited exception to the general standard because of the fact that the infant has never experienced, and will never experience, consciousness" (pp.1617-18).

This alternative approach to organ procurement would require substantial changes in the law. The process of organ procurement would have to be legitimated as a form of justified killing, rather than just as the dissection of a corpse. There is certainly precedent in the law for recognizing instances of justified killing. The concept is also not an anathema to the public, as evidenced by the growing support for euthanasia, another practice that would have to be legally construed as a form of justified killing. Even now, surveys show that one-third of physicians and nurses do not believe brain-dead patients are actually dead, but feel comfortable with the process of organ procurement because the patients are permanently unconscious and/or imminently dying. In other words, many clinicians already seem to justify their actions on the basis of nonmaleficence and consent, rather than with the belief that the patients are actually dead.

This alternative approach would also eliminate the need for protocols like the one being used at the University of Pittsburgh, with its contrived and perhaps questionable approach to declaring death prior to organ procurement. Under the proposed system, qualified individuals who had given their consent could simply have their organs removed under general anesthesia, without first undergoing an orchestrated withdrawal of life support. Anencephalic newborns whose parents requested organ donation could likewise have the organs removed under general anesthesia, without the need to wait for the diagnosis of brain death.

The diagnosis of death.   Seen in this light, the concept of brain death may have become obsolete. Certainly the diagnosis of brain death has been extremely useful during the last several decades, as society has struggled with a myriad of issues that were never encountered before the era of mechanical ventilation and organ transplantation. As society emerges from this transitional period, and as many of these issues are more clearly understood as questions that are inherently unrelated to the distinction between life and death, then the concept of brain death may no longer be useful or relevant. If this is the case, then it may be preferable to return to the traditional standard and limit tests for the determination of death to those based solely upon the permanent cessation of respiration and circulation. Even today we uniformly regard the cessation of respiration and circulation as the standard for determining when patients are ready to be cremated or buried.

Another advantage of a return to the traditional approach is that it would represent a "common denominator" in the definition of death that virtually all cultural groups and religious traditions would find acceptable. Recently both New Jersey and New York have enacted statutes that recognize the objections of particular religious views to the concept of brain death. In New Jersey, physicians are prohibited from declaring brain death in persons who come from religious traditions that do not accept the concept. Return to a cardiorespiratory standard would eliminate problems with these objections.

Linda Emanuel recently proposed a "bounded zone" definition of death that shares some features with the approach outlined here.[9] Her proposal would adopt the cardiorespiratory standard as a "lower bound" for determining death that would apply to all cases, but would allow individuals to choose a definition of death that encompassed neurologic dysfunction up to the level of the permanent vegetative state (the "higher bound"). The practical implications of such a policy would be similar to some of those discussed here, in that it would (1) allow patients and surrogates to request organ donation when and if the patients were diagnosed with whole-brain death, permanent vegetative state, or anencephaly, and (2) it would permit rejection of the diagnosis of brain death by patients and surrogates opposed to the concept. Emanuel's proposal would not permit organ donation from terminal and imminently dying patients, however, prior to the diagnosis of death.

Despite these similarities, these two proposals differ markedly in the justifications used to support their conclusions. Emanuel follows the President's Commission in seeking to address several separate questions by reference to the diagnosis of death, whereas the approach suggested here would adopt a single and uniform definition of death, and then seek to resolve questions around organ donation on a different ethical and legal foundation.

Emanuel's proposal also provides another illustration of the problems encountered when a variety of diverse issues all hinge upon the definition of death. Under her scheme, some individuals would undoubtedly opt for a definition of death based on the "higher bound" of the permanent vegetative state in order to permit the donation of their vital organs if they should develop this condition. However, few of these individuals would probably agree to being cremated while still breathing, even if they were vegetative. Most likely, they would not want to be cremated until after they had sustained a cardiorespiratory arrest. Once again, this creates the awkward and confusing necessity of diagnosing death for one purpose (organ donation) but not for another (cremation). Only by abandoning the concept of brain death is it possible to adopt a definition of death that is valid for all purposes, while separating questions of organ donation from dependence upon the life/death dichotomy.

TURNING BACK

The tension between the need to maintain workable and practical standards for the procurement of transplantable organs and our desire to have a conceptually coherent account of death is an issue that must be given serious attention. Resolving these inconsistencies by moving toward a higher-brain definition of death would most likely create additional practical problems regarding accurate diagnosis as well as introduce concepts that are highly counterintuitive to the general public. Uncoupling the link between organ transplantation and brain death, on the other hand, offers a number of advantages. By shifting the ethical foundations for organ donation to the principles of nonmaleficence and consent, the pool of potential donors may be substantially increased. In addition, by reverting to a simpler and more traditional definition of death, the long-standing debate over fundamental inconsistencies in the concept of brain death may finally be resolved.

The most difficult challenge for this proposal would be to gain acceptance of the view that killing may sometimes be a justifiable necessity for procuring transplantable organs. Careful attention to the principles of consent and nonmaleficence should provide an adequate bulwark against slippery slope concerns that this practice would be extended in unforeseen and unacceptable ways. Just as the euthanasia debate often seems to turn less upon abstract theoretical concerns and more upon the empirical question of whether guidelines for assisted dying would be abused, so the success of this proposal could also rest upon factual questions of societal acceptance and whether this approach would erode respect for human life and the integrity of clinicians. While the answers to these questions are not known, the potential benefits of this proposal make it worthy of continued discussion and debate.

NOTES

1.   Stuart J. Youngner, "Defining Death: A Superficial and Fragile Consensus," *Archives of Neurology* 49 (1992): 570-72.

2.   Aspects of this analysis have been explored previously in Robert D. Truog and James C. Fackler, "Rethinking Brain Death," *Critical Care Medicine* 20 (1992):1705-13; Halevy and Brody, "Brain Death."

3.   Daniel Wikler and Alan J. Weisbard, "Appropriate Confusion over 'Brain Death,'" *JAMA* 261 (1989): 2246.

4.   Margareta Sanner, "A Comparison of Public Attitudes toward Autopsy, Organ Donation, and Anatomic Dissection: A Swedish Survey," *JAMA* 271 (1994): 284-88, at 287.

5.   Some of the many works defending this view include: Green and Wikler, "Brain Death and Personal Identity"; Gervais, *Redefining Death*; Truog and Fackler; "Rethinking Brain Death"; and Robert M. Veatch, *Death, Dying, and the Biological Revolution* (New Haven: Yale University Press, 1989).

6.   President's Commission for the Study of Ethical Problems in Medicine and Biomedical and Behavioral Research, *Defining Death* (Washington, D.C.: Government Printing Office, 1981), p. 84.

7.   Report of the Ad Hoc Committee of the Harvard Medical School to Examine the Definition of Brain Death, "A Definition of Irreversible Coma," *JAMA* 205 (1968): 337-40.

8.   AMA Council on Ethical and Judicial Affairs, "The Use of Anencephalic Neonates as Organ Donors," *JAMA* 273 (1995): 1614-18. After extensive debate among AMA members, the Council retracted this position statement. See Charles W. Plows, "Reconsideration of AMA Opinion on Anencephalic Neonates as Organ Donors," *JAMA* 275 (1996): 443-44.

9.   Linda L. Emanuel, "Reexamining Death: The Asymptotic Model and a Bounded Zone Definition," *Hastings Center Report* 25, no. 4 (1995): 27-35.

SECTION 2

Decisional Capacity and the Right to Refuse Treatment

State of Tennessee Department of Human Services v. Mary C. Northern

Court of Appeals of Tennessee, Middle Section, Feb. 7, 1978

On January 24, 1978, the Tennessee Department of Human Services filed this suit alleging that Mary C. Northern was 72 years old, with no available help from relatives; that Miss Northern resided alone under unsatisfactory conditions as a result of which she had been admitted to and was a patient in Nashville General Hospital; that the patient suffered from gangrene of both feet which required the removal of her feet to save her life; that the patient lacked the capacity to appreciate her condition or to consent to necessary surgery.

Attached to the complaint are identical letters from Drs. Amos D. Tackett and R. Benton Adkins, which read as follows:

> Mrs. Mary Northern is a patient under our care at Nashville General Hospital. She has gangrene of both feet probably secondary to frostbite and then thermal burning of the feet. She has developed infection along with the gangrene of her feet. This is placing her life in danger. Mrs. Northern does not understand the severity or consequences of her disease process and does not appear to understand that failure to amputate the feet at this time would probably result in her death. It is our recommendation as the physicians in charge of her case, that she undergo amputation of both feet as soon as possible.

On January 24, 1978, the Chancellor appointed a guardian ad litem to defend the cause and to receive service of process pursuant to Rule 4.04(2) T.R.C.P. On January 25, 1978, the guardian ad litem answered as follows:

> The Respondent, by and through her guardian ad litem, states as follows:
> 1. She is 72 years of age and a resident of Davidson County, Tennessee.
> 2. She is presently in the intensive care unit of General Hospital, Nashville, Tennessee, because of gangrenous condition in her two feet.
> 3. She feels very strongly that her present physical condition is improving, and that she will recover without the necessity of surgery.
> 4. She is in possession of a good memory and recall, responds accurately to questions asked her, is coherent and intelligent in her conversation, and is of sound mind.
> 5. She is aware that the Tennessee Department of Human Services has filed this complaint, knows the nature of the complaint, and does not wish for her feet to be amputated.

. . .

On January 26, 1978, there was filed in this cause a letter from Dr. John J. Griffin, reporting that he found the patient to be generally lucid and sane, but concluding:

> Nonetheless, I believe that she is functioning on a psychotic level with respect to ideas concerning her gangrenous feet. She tends to believe that her feet are black because of soot or dirt. She does not believe her physicians about the serious infection. There is an adamant belief that

EDITORS' NOTE: The suit was filed under the state "Protective Services for the Elderly" Act, which permits a court to appoint a guardian for the purposes of consent to medical treatment if an elderly person is in imminent danger of death without treatment and lacks capacity to consent to it.

her feet will heal without surgery, and she refused to even consider the possibility that amputation is necessary to save her life. There is no desire to die, yet her judgment concerning recovery is markedly impaired. If she appreciated the seriousness of her condition, heard her physicians' opinions, and concluded against an operation, then I would believe she understood and could decide for herself. But my impression is that she does not appreciate the dangers to her life. I conclude that she is incompetent to decide this issue. A corollary to this denial is seen in her unwillingness to consider any future plans. Here again I believe she was utilizing a psychotic mechanism of denial.

This is a schizoid woman who has been urged by everyone to have surgery. Having been self-sufficient previously (albeit a marginal adjustment), she is continuing to decide alone. The risks with surgery are great and her lifestyle has been permanently disrupted. If she has surgery there is a tremendous danger for physical and psychological complications. The chances for a post-operative psychosis are immense, yet the surgeons believe an operation is necessary to save her life. I would advise delaying surgery (if feasible) for a few days in order to attempt some work for strengthening her psychologically. Even if she does not consent to the operation after that time, however, I believe she is incompetent to make the decision.

. . .

On January 28, 1978, this Court entered an order reciting the following:

From all of the above the Court finds:

1. That the respondent is not now in 'imminent danger of death' in the extreme sense of the words, but that her present condition is such that 'imminent danger of death' may reasonably be expected during her continued hospitalization.
2. That both feet of respondent are severely necrotic and affected by wet gangrene, an infection which probably will result in death unless properly treated by amputation of the feet.
3. That the probability of respondent's survival without amputation is from 5 percent to 10 percent and the probability of survival after amputation is about 50 percent, with possible severe psychotic results.
4. That, with or without amputation, the prognosis of respondent's condition is poor.

5. That respondent is an intelligent, lucid, communicative, and articulate individual who does not accept the fact of the serious condition of her feet and is unwilling to discuss the seriousness of such condition or its fatal potentiality.
6. That, because of her inability or unwillingness to recognize the actual condition of her feet which is clearly observable by her, she is incompetent to make a rational decision as to the amputation of her feet.
7. That respondent has no wish to die, but is unable or unwilling to recognize an obvious condition which will probably result in her death if untreated.

This Court is therefore of the opinion that a responsible individual should be named with authority to consent to amputation of respondent's feet when urgently recommended in writing by respondent's physicians because of the development of (symptoms) indicating an emergency and severe imminence of death.

. . .

[Appellant's first assignment of error states:]

Such actions by the Court were injurious to the appellant because they deprived her of her right to make her own decisions—regardless as to whether death might be a probable consequence—as to whether she was willing to surrender control of her own person and life.

This controversy arises from the fact that Miss Northern's attending physicians have determined that all of the soft tissue of her feet has been killed by frostbite, that said dead tissue has become infected with gangrene, and that the feet must be removed to prevent loss of life from spreading of gangrene and its effects to the entire body. Miss Northern has refused to consent to the surgery.

The physicians have determined, and the Chancellor and this Court have found, that Miss Northern's life is critically endangered; that she is mentally incapable of comprehending the facts which constitute that danger; and that she is, to that extent, incompetent, thereby justifying State action to preserve her life.

As will be observed from the bill of exceptions, a member of this Court asked Miss Northern if she would prefer to die rather than lose her feet, and her answer was "possibly." This is the most definitive expression of her desires in this record.

The patient has *not* expressed a desire to die. She evidences a strong desire to live and an equally strong desire to keep her dead feet. She refuses to make a choice.

If the patient would assume and exercise her rightful control over her own destiny by stating that she prefers death to the loss of her feet, her wish would be respected. The doctors so testified; this Court so informed her; and this Court now reiterates its commitment to this principle.

The appellant has filed three supplemental assignments of error, of which the first is:

1. The statute, T.C.A. §§ 14-2301, *et seq.*, is impermissibly vague; and, therefore, void and unconstitutional. The two phrases used in the statute, 'imminent danger of death' and 'capacity to consent' have not been defined in the statute nor is the Court given any assistance to determine when either standard has been met in the legal context, rather than a medical context.

In the judgment of this Court, the words "imminent danger of death" are no more vague than is consistent with the nature of the subject matter.

. . .

The words, "imminent danger of death" mean conditions calculated to and capable of producing within a short period of time a reasonably strong probability of resultant cessation of life if such conditions are not removed or alleviated. Such is undoubtedly the legislative intent of the words.

"Imminent danger of death" should be reasonably interpreted to carry out the purposes of the statute. For an authorization to mildly encroach upon the freedom of the individual, a relatively mild imminence or danger of death may suffice. On the other hand, the authorization of a drastic encroachment upon personal freedom and bodily integrity would require a correspondingly severe imminence of death.

In the present case, the Chancellor was not called upon to act until the imminence of death was moderately severe. By the time of the hearing before this Court, the imminence of death had lessened somewhat but remained real and appreciable. Accordingly this Court, recognizing a present real and appreciable imminence of death, made provision for drastic emergency measures to be taken only in event of severe and urgent imminence of death.

Appellant also complains of vagueness of the meaning of "capacity to consent." Capacity means mental ability to make a rational decision, which includes the ability to perceive, to appreciate all relevant facts, and to reach a rational judgment upon such facts.

Capacity is not necessarily synonymous with sanity. A blind person may be perfectly capable of observing the shape of small articles by handling them, but not capable of observing the shape of a cloud in the sky.

A person may have "capacity" as to some matters and may lack "capacity" as to others.

In 44 C.J.S. Insane Persons § 2, pp. 17, 18, partial insanity is defined as follows:

Partial insanity. Although it is hard to define the invisible line that divides perfect and partial insanity, the law recognizes a state of mind called 'partial insanity,' that is, insanity on a particular subject only, sometimes denominating it 'insane delusion' or 'monomania.' The use of the term, however, has been criticized. Partial insanity has been said to be the derangement of one or more of the faculties of the mind, which prevents freedom of action. Ordinarily it is confined to a particular subject, the person being sane on every other. The degree of insanity, as partial or total, is to be measured by the extent and number of the delusions existing in the mind of the person in question. . . .

In the present case, this Court has found the patient to be lucid and apparently of sound mind generally. However, on the subjects of death and amputation of her feet, her comprehension is blocked, blinded, or dimmed to the extent that she is incapable of recognizing facts which would be obvious to a person of normal perception.

For example, in the presence of this Court, the patient looked at her feet and refused to recognize the obvious fact that the flesh was dead, black, shriveled, rotting, and stinking.

The record also discloses that the patient refuses to consider the eventuality of death which is, or ought to be, obvious in the face of such dire bodily deterioration.

As described by the doctors and observed by this Court, the patient wants to live and keep her dead feet, too, and refuses to consider the impossibility of such a desire. In order to avoid the unpleasant experience of facing death and/or loss of feet, her mind or emotions have resorted to the device of denying the unpleasant reality so that, to the patient, the unpleasant reality does not exist. This is the "delusion" which renders the patient incapable of making a rational decision as to whether to undergo surgery to save her life or to forgo surgery and forfeit her life.

The physicians speak of probabilities of death without amputation as 90 to 95 percent and the probability of death with surgery as 50–50 (1 in 2). Such probabilities are not facts, but the existence and expression of such opinions are facts which the patient is unwilling or unable to recognize or discuss.

If, as repeatedly stated, this patient could and would give evidence of a comprehension of the facts of her condition and could and would express her unequivocal desire in the face of such comprehended facts, then her decision, however unreasonable to others, would be accepted and honored by the Courts and by her doctors. The difficulty is that she cannot or will not comprehend the facts.

The first supplemental assignment of error is respectfully overruled.

The second supplemental assignment of error is as follows:

2. The Chancellor erred by denying the Appellant her rights to substantive and procedural due process. The entire legal proceedings involved in this case and on appeal are unprecedented; the order of the Chancellor granting the appeal but refusing the automatic stay of thirty days allowed by the Rules is one example of the procedural wrongs which was not in accordance with the established legal practice, and contrary to the expected procedure to be followed. The proposed amputation will not only permanently deprive the Appellant of her two limbs, but most likely will significantly and irreparably alter her personality for the worse, and make her mentally and physically dependent upon the State.

Whatever the propriety or impropriety of the action of the Chancellor in attempting to effectuate his action in spite of the appeal, the error, if any, has been rendered harmless by the action of this Court, after appeal, in reviewing and modifying his actions.

This Court does not recognize that it has been guilty of any improper deviation from correct procedure. The gravity of the condition of the patient and the resultant emergency in time required the unusual action of the Court under § 27-327 T.C.A. and the unusual acceleration of hearings and actions taken.

This Court is painfully and acutely aware of the possible tragic results of amputation. According to the doctors, the patient has only a 50 percent chance of surviving the surgery; and, if she survives, she will never be able to walk and may suffer severe mental and emotional problems.

On the other hand, the doctors testified, and this Court finds, that the patient's chances of survival without amputation are from 5 percent to 10 percent—a rather remote and fragile chance. Moreover, as testified by the doctors and found by this Court, even if the patient should survive without amputation, she will never walk because the dead flesh will fall off the bones of her feet leaving only bare bones.

IT IS, THEREFORE, ORDERED, ADJUDGED AND DECREED that

1. Mary C. Northern is in imminent danger of death if she does not receive surgical amputation of her lower extremities and she lacks the capacity to consent or refuse consent for such surgery.

2. That Honorable Horace Bass, Commissioner of Human Services of the State of Tennessee or his successor in office is hereby designated and authorized to act for and on behalf of said Mary C. Northern in consenting to surgical amputation of her lower extremities and of exercising such custodial supervision as is necessarily incident thereto at any time that Drs. Amos D. Tackett and R. Benton Adkins join in signing a written certificate that Mary C. Northern's condition has developed to such a critical stage as to demand immediate amputation to save her life. The previous order of this Court is likewise so modified.

As modified, the order of the Chancellor is affirmed. The cause is remanded for further appropriate proceedings.

·   ·   ·

Modified, Affirmed, and Remanded.*

*On May 1, 1978, Mary Northern died in a Nashville hospital as a result of a clot from the gangrenous tissue migrating through the bloodstream to a vital organ. Because of complications rendering surgery more dangerous, the proposed surgery was never performed.

Transcript of Proceedings: Testimony of Mary C. Northern

January 28, 1978

Testimony of Mary Northern: [The following interview took place at the bedside of Mary Northern in the Intensive Care Unit of the Nashville General Hospital. Present were Judge Todd, Judge Drowota, and the Reverend Palmer Sorrow, a friend and frequent visitor of the patient. Eds.]

JUDGE TODD: Now, Mrs. Mary, you know that there have been some proceedings in court about you, and that's the reason why the judges are here. And we wanted to see you and talk to you.

MISS NORTHERN: Yes.

JUDGE TODD: And give you a chance to talk to us.

MISS NORTHERN: Yeah.

JUDGE TODD: I understand that you had a little problem of getting too cold out there at your house.

MISS NORTHERN: Yes.

JUDGE TODD: That's right.

MISS NORTHERN: Yes. Well, now, it's a point of this, the swelling of my foot was—was very dangerous looking.

JUDGE TODD: Yes ma'am.

MISS NORTHERN: And so that's what caused most of the trouble, and the—it's starting to go down. Give it a chance, it is starting to go down, and it's almost . . . Well, these—these ankles and the—along on these legs have gone down wonderfully.

JUDGE TODD: Yes, now, Mrs. Mary, these doctors have been talking to us at great length about the condition of your feet.

MR. SORROW: I think it's okay.

MISS NORTHERN: Okay.

JUDGE TODD: —and they tell us this about your feet. Now, mind you . . . we don't know whether it's so or not, but I want you to know what they have told us. . . . They tell us that your feet have been frostbitten before, and that they got well.

MISS NORTHERN: Yes.

JUDGE TODD: What they tell us, that your feet were frostbitten a great deal worse this time than they were . . . before.

MISS NORTHERN: Yes.

JUDGE TODD: And they tell us this,—now I am going to say some things to you that might be a little uncomfortable, but I want—I don't believe these doctors have told it to you just like they told it to us.

MISS NORTHERN: Yeah.

JUDGE TODD: So I want to give it to you just like they have given it to us. They tell us that this time every bit of the flesh on your two feet is completely dead.

MISS NORTHERN: I know—No, it isn't, it will revive.

JUDGE TODD: I understand.

MISS NORTHERN: Four or five days ago it started to go down.

JUDGE TODD: All right. Now they tell us this, that when you came in . . . here that your feet were swollen. . . . And they tell us that the swelling has gone down.

MISS NORTHERN: Yes.

JUDGE TODD: But they tell us that your feet are shriveling up like a dead person's feet—

MISS NORTHERN: Unh-unh.

JUDGE TODD: —rather than a live person's feet.

MISS NORTHERN: No, no. . . . I can get and walk all the way down to the shopping places.

JUDGE TODD: Now they tell us—We questioned them very, very thoroughly about this thing, and they tell us that you can move your toes. And then I asked them how could a person move his toes if his foot was dead? You see? And here's what they tell us. They tell us that the ligaments that move the toes . . . are dead, but they are still just like strings,—

MISS NORTHERN: Yeah.

JUDGE TODD: —and that the muscles that move the toes are up here where they are still alive, and therefore a dead foot can move its toes.

MISS NORTHERN: Well, they are not going to—they are not going to take my legs away. They are not going to take my legs away from me, you understand this?

JUDGE TODD: Yes, ma'am.

MISS NORTHERN: And they are not going to—I think it's rather silly, because they all—all of em have gotten viable.

JUDGE TODD: Yes, ma'am. Yes, ma'am. Now here is the thing that disturbs us. The doctors tell us that you have a very heavy infection which they are keeping in control by antibiotics, but that your temperature has started to rise, that you have a hundred and one temperature . . . which indicates that the infection is increasing. And we questioned them very closely now, we have been a long time—

MISS NORTHERN: You understand they are going to do it. Now, does this have something to do with the Metropolitan Government, has it not? Well, the Metropolitan Government can't take anything—do me this way, you know?

JUDGE TODD: Yes, sir. Now, here is what I want to present to you. You are a very intelligent woman for your age. I want to compliment you on that, you really are. I said you were like my mother, but you do circles around my mother as far as talking and thinking.

Now, you are educated, and you know this business of "if," and I want to ask you an "if" question. If your feet, the flesh of your feet, really is dead, and if you have one chance in ten of living without surgery, that it is, if—if the feet are left on, that nine chances to one that you will not live, it will kill you,—

MISS NORTHERN: I am not going to have—

JUDGE TODD: —would you still say, "I want that one chance?"

MISS NORTHERN: Well, of course,—

JUDGE TODD: Ma'am?

MISS NORTHERN: —this is not going to do anything like this. All—All of these thing,—

JUDGE TODD: Yes, ma'am.

MISS NORTHERN: —and my feet have gone down.

JUDGE TODD: Yes, ma'am.

MISS NORTHERN: My ankles are—

JUDGE TODD: Yes, ma'am. Now, let me ask you one more question.

MISS NORTHERN: I am not going to—Let me tell you something. I am not going to argue any more with you, because I know you have a multiple of opinions.

JUDGE TODD: No, I haven't formed any opinions, that's the reason I came up to talk to you. I haven't decided.

MISS NORTHERN: It's an opinion you formed, and I am not going to let you tell me—

JUDGE TODD: I am just telling you what they told me. Now let me ask you one more little thing.

If the time comes that this infection gets so bad that you are practically unconscious and can't talk to anybody, would you then be willing for the doctors to go ahead and do what they think should be done? . . .

MR. SORROW: That's an "if"—That's an "if" question.

JUDGE TODD: "If."

MISS NORTHERN: I think that's an understandable idea.

JUDGE TODD: Yes, ma'am.

MISS NORTHERN: An amongst your—your own opinion former—opinion former.

JUDGE TODD: Yes. Now, if the time comes that you are so sick that you can't make the decision, are you willing for the doctors to make the decision for you then?

MISS NORTHERN: Well, I think that that's an unreasonable way to look at it because you want an opinion.

JUDGE TODD: Yes, ma'am.

MISS NORTHERN: And you see, that's—that—Groundhog Day and the—all the weather and everything else, now, it's an opinion.

JUDGE TODD: Judge, is there anything you would like to ask?

JUDGE DROWOTA: Well, I have the same questions, though, with the "if." And as Reverend Sorrow has said, if in fact at some day there is a feeling that—and you are unconscious and we can't ask you—

MR. SORROW: It's a question of whether to let you die.

JUDGE DROWOTA: —should we let you die, or would you rather live your life without your feet?

MISS NORTHERN: I am giving my feet a chance to get well.

MR. SORROW: Right, right. Okay. Let's say we have given it a chance to get well, and if the infection didn't get out of your system and you became unconscious, he is saying, would you rather—

MISS NORTHERN: I am not making any further . . . statement.

JUDGE TODD: In other words, you are not willing to admit that you might get unconscious?

MISS NORTHERN: No.

JUDGE TODD: I see. All right.

MISS NORTHERN: You are pretty handsome; it's rather nice to have all you handsome men come at you this morning.

MR. SORROW: Can they look at your feet?

MISS NORTHERN: No, no. Can you see me?

JUDGE TODD: I think maybe you better see your feet.

MISS NORTHERN: You know where they are? . . . They are there.

JUDGE TODD: I need to ask you this, Miss Mary. . . . When have you seen your feet?

MR. SORROW: Have you seen them recently? Have they let you see your feet real close?

MISS NORTHERN: They let me see my feet. I can see my feet.

JUDGE TODD: When did you see them, do you remember?

MISS NORTHERN: I seen them two or three times. Don't look at the feet. Let's don't look at the feet.

JUDGE TODD: I tell you what let's do.

MISS NORTHERN: Don't look at the feet.

JUDGE TODD: Let's don't look at the feet. I tell you what let's do. . . . Let's you and I look at them together at the same time and see what we can.

MISS NORTHERN: They are down there.

JUDGE TODD: I want you to look at them with me. Would you do it?

MISS NORTHERN: Isn't—I just don't understand, it's sadism about it. I can't understand it.

A NURSE: Let's all look at your feet.

MISS NORTHERN: Okay. All right, General.

A NURSE: All of us together. Let's get your gown down. There we go. Now—

MISS NORTHERN: That's all peeling off of that. It's all getting well. It's all going down.

JUDGE DROWOTA: Do you have feeling in your feet?

MISS NORTHERN: Oh, yes, they were knocking all around, and they're banging up against this thing and everything.

MR. SORROW: Can you feel it when you do that?

MISS NORTHERN: Yeah.

MR. SORROW: Is there feeling?

MISS NORTHERN: Yeah. . . .

JUDGE TODD: —Would you—would you just bear with us just for one more thing?

MISS NORTHERN: You want to establish your point.

JUDGE TODD: No, we don't. I am asking you—

MISS NORTHERN: You got your points all in writing and established it, according to your own—

JUDGE TODD: Yes, ma'am. If the time comes that you have to choose between losing your feet and dying, would you rather just go ahead and die than lose your feet? If that time comes?

MISS NORTHERN: It's possible—It's possible only if I—Just forget it. I—You are making me sick talking.

JUDGE TODD: I know. I know. And I am sorry. Would you be willing to say to me that you just don't want to live if you can't have your feet? Is that the way you feel?

MISS NORTHERN: I don't understand why it's so important to you people, why it's so important. . . .

JUDGE TODD: Mrs. Mary, you see a judge has to see both sides of the thing, and these people have come and told us something, and now we want you to tell us what you want to tell us so we can decide.

MISS NORTHERN: A billion of you have been here.

JUDGE TODD: I understand. And that's the reason we came out to see you, so we could let you—

MISS NORTHERN: I don't want to discuss it any more. I made my point.

JUDGE TODD: I believe, Mrs. Mary, that you have made your point that you would rather—that you don't want to live if you can't have your feet; isn't that about it?

MISS NORTHERN: That's possible. . . . It's possible to see it that way, to have that opinion. I don't want you all to change your opinion.

JUDGE TODD: No. I want you to tell me if you really feel that way. Tell me because I want to know it. I want to consider how you feel.

JUDGE DROWOTA: Or if you would rather live and have your feet. I mean, without your feet. See, you have got me confused, Miss Mary.

JUDGE TODD: She wants to live and have her feet.

MR. SORROW: That's exactly what she wants.

MISS NORTHERN: This is ridiculous. I am tired. And ridiculous, you know it is.

MR. SORROW: I think they are trying to look at your side of it and understand how you feel, and, of course, somebody else in your position, we don't know what we would do, and so I guess they are saying so many people have told these judges so much they want to see Miss Mary and say, "How do you feel, how do you feel?"

MISS NORTHERN: It's gotten a little roll.

MR. SORROW: Like a snowball.
MISS NORTHERN: This is—Let's leave it alone.
Let's leave it alone. And you keep your opinions. I
am through with it.
JUDGE TODD: I wish I could be through with it.
Let me leave you with a little thought, Miss Mary.
MISS NORTHERN: All right. . . .
JUDGE TODD: Did you ever read the Sermon on
the Mount?
MISS NORTHERN: Yes.

JUDGE TODD: You remember one thing the Good
Lord said?
MISS NORTHERN: What?
JUDGE TODD: If thy eye offend thee,—
MISS NORTHERN: Oh, yes, take the eye out.
JUDGE TODD: —cast it out. If thy hand offend
you, cut it off. Now, if and when your feet begin to
offend you, maybe, maybe, you will remember
that little verse.
MISS NORTHERN: I thank you.

Deciding for Others: Competency

Allen Buchanan and Dan W. Brock

COMPETENCE AND INCOMPETENCE

Discussions of competence have often been hampered by a failure to distinguish carefully among
the following questions:

- What is the appropriate *concept* of competence?
- Given an analysis of the appropriate concept
  of competence, what *standard* (or standards)
  of competence must be met if an individual is
  to be judged to be competent?
- What are the most reliable *operational measures* for ascertaining whether a given standard of competence is met?
- *Who* ought to make a determination of competence?
- What *sorts of institutional arrangements* are
  needed to assure that determinations of competence are made in an accurate and responsible way?

Each of these questions will be addressed separately. This section—which is concerned with the
theoretical underpinnings of determinations of com-

petence—will concentrate on the first three questions. The last two, which raise more practical and
concrete concerns, can only be addressed in detail
after the ethical framework has been laid out and the
realities of current practices have been described.

THE CONCEPT OF COMPETENCE

COMPETENCE AS DECISION-RELATIVE

The statement that a particular individual is (or is
not) competent is incomplete. Competence is
always competence *for some task*—competence *to
do something*. The concern here is with competence
to perform the task of making a decision. Hence,
competence is to be understood as *decision-making
capacity*. But the notion of decision-making capacity is itself incomplete until the nature of the
choice as well as the conditions under which it is
to be made are specified. Thus competence is decision-relative, not global. A person may be competent to make a particular decision at a particular
time, under certain circumstances, but incompetent to make another decision, or even the same
decision under different conditions. A competency
determination, then, is a determination of a particular person's capacity to perform a particular decision-making task at a particular time and under
specified conditions.

Any individual may be competent to perform
some tasks (e.g., drive a car), but not others (e.g.,

From *Milbank Quarterly,* 64:2, 1986, 67–80. Reprinted with
permission from Blackwell Publishers.

Editor's Note: References have been cut. Readers wishing to
follow up sources should consult the original article.

solve differential equations). The tasks relevant to this article vary substantially, and include making decisions about medical treatment, entering into contracts, deciding whether to continue to live on one's own in an unsupervised setting, and so forth. It is true, of course, that for some individuals, decision-making capacity is entirely lacking (for instance, when the individual is permanently unconscious), but these are the unproblematic cases.

Decision-making tasks vary substantially in the capacities they require for performance at an appropriate level of adequacy. For example, even restricted to medical treatment decisions, there is substantial variation in the complexity of information that is relevant to a particular treatment decision and that, consequently, must be understood by the decision maker. There is, therefore, variation in what might be called the *objective demands* of the task in question—here, the level of abilities to understand, reason, and decide about the options in question. But there is also variation of several sorts in a subject's ability to meet the demands of a particular decision. Many factors that diminish or eliminate competence altogether vary over time in their presence or severity in a particular person. For example, the effects of dementia on a person's cognitive capacities is at some stages commonly not constant, particularly in cases of borderline competence. Instead, mental confusion may come and go; periods of great confusion are sometimes followed by comparative lucidity.

In other cases, the environment and the behavior of others may affect the relative level of decision-making competence. For example, side effects of medications often impair competence, but a change of medication may reduce those effects. Behavior of others may create stresses for a person that diminish decision-making capacities, but that behavior can often be altered, or the situations in which it occurs can be avoided. Further, cognitive functioning can sometimes be enhanced by familiar surroundings and diminished by unfamiliar ones. A person may be competent to make a decision about whether to have an elective surgical procedure if the choice is presented in the familiar surroundings of home by someone known and trusted, but may be incompetent to make that same choice in what is found to be the intimidating, confusing, and unfamiliar environment of a hospital.

Factors such as these mean that even for a given decision, a person's competence may vary over time, and so be intermittent. The values that support the right of the competent person to participate in health care decisions also require that caretakers utilize periods of lucidity when they occur. Sometimes the emergency nature of the situation will not permit this, but it is no doubt possible to involve intermittently competent persons in decision making substantially more than is done at present. Sometimes, with opportune timing or other appropriate measures (such as medications), the intermittently competent person may be able to be involved in decision making at a time when he or she is clearly competent. Often, however, the person either consistently remains in, or can only be brought to, a state of borderline competence for the decision at hand. These borderline cases of questionable competence require more careful analysis of and clarity about the nature of the competency determination. They also illustrate the need for greater sophistication on the part of medical care providers and others about physical and mental problems that frequently affect the elderly.

CAPACITIES NEEDED FOR COMPETENCE

What capacities are necessary for a person competently to decide about such matters as health care, living arrangements, financial affairs, and so forth? As already noted, the demands of these different decisions will vary, but it is nevertheless possible to generalize about the necessary abilities. Two may be distinguished: the capacity for communication and understanding, and the capacity for reasoning and deliberation. Although these capacities are not entirely distinct, significant deficiencies in any of them can result in diminished decision-making competence. A third important element of competence is that the individual must have a set of values or conception of the good.

Under *communication and understanding* are included the various capacities that allow a person to take part in the process of becoming informed on and expressing a choice about a given decision. These include the ability to communicate and the possession of various linguistic, conceptual, and cognitive abilities necessary for an understanding of the particular information relevant to the decision at hand. The relevant cognitive abilities, in particular, are often impaired by disease processes to which the elderly are especially subject, including most obviously various forms of dementia, but also aphasia due to stroke and, in some cases, reduced intellectual performance associated with depression (pseudodementia). Even where cognitive function is only minimally impaired, ability to express desires and beliefs may be greatly diminished or absent (as in some patients with amyotrophic lateral sclerosis).

Understanding also requires the ability to appreciate the nature and meaning of potential alternative—what it would be and "feel" like to be in possible future states and to undergo various experiences. In young children this is often prevented by the lack of sufficient life experience. In the case of elderly persons facing diseases with progressive and extremely debilitating deterioration, it is hindered by people's generally limited ability to understand a kind of experience radically different from their own and by the inability of severely impaired individuals to communicate the character of their own experience to others. Major psychological blocks—such as fear, denial, and depression—can also significantly impair the appreciation of information about an unwanted or dreaded alternative. In general, communication and understanding require the capacities to receive, process, and make available for use the information relevant to particular decisions.

Competence also requires *capacities for reasoning and deliberation*. These include capacities to draw inferences about the consequences of making a certain choice and to compare alternative outcomes based on how they further one's good or promote one's ends. Some capacity to employ rudimentary probabilistic reasoning about uncertain outcomes will commonly be necessary, as well as the capacity to give due consideration to potential future outcomes in a present decision. Reasoning and deliberation obviously make use of both capacities mentioned earlier: understanding the information and applying the decision maker's values.

Finally, a competent decision maker also requires a *set of values or conception of what is good* that is reasonably consistent and stable. This is needed in order to be able to evaluate particular outcomes as benefits or harms, goods or evils, and to assign different relative weight or importance to them. Often what will be needed is the capacity to decide on the import and relative weight to be accorded different values, since that may not have

been fully determined before a particular choice must be made. Competence does not require a fully consistent set of goals, much less a detailed "life plan" to cover all contingencies. Sufficient internal consistency and stability over time in the values relative to a particular decision, however, are needed to yield a decision outcome. Although values change over time and although ambivalence is inevitable in the difficult choices faced by many persons of questionable competence concerning their medical care, living arrangements, and personal affairs, sufficient value stability is needed to permit, at the very least, a decision that can be stated and adhered to over the course of its discussion, initiation, and implementation.

COMPETENCE AS A THRESHOLD CONCEPT, NOT A COMPARATIVE ONE

Decision-making competence, and the skills and capacities necessary to it, is one of the three components in standard analyses of the requirements for informed consent in health care decision making. The informed-consent doctrine requires the free and informed consent of a competent patient to medical procedures that are to be performed. The idea underlying this doctrine is that of a patient deciding, in consultation with a physician, what health care, if any, will best serve the patient's aims and needs. If the decision is not voluntary, but instead coerced or manipulated, it will likely serve another's ends or another's view of the patient's good, not the patient's own view, and will, in a significant sense, originate with another and not the patient. If the appropriate information is not provided to the individual in a form the patient can understand, the patient will not be able to ascertain how available alternatives might serve his or her aims. Finally, if the patient is not competent, either the individual will be unable to decide at all or the decision-making process will be seriously flawed.

Sometimes incompetence will be uncontroversially complete, as with patients who are in a persistent vegetative state or who are in a very advanced state of dementia, unable to communicate coherently at all. Often, however, defects in the capacities and skills noted above as necessary to competence will be partial and a matter of degree, just as whether a patient's decision is voluntary or involuntary, informed or uninformed, is also often a matter of degree. Does this mean that competence itself should be thought of as sometimes partial and possessed in different degrees? It is certainly the case that persons are commonly thought of and said to be more or less competent to perform many tasks, not just decision making. Nevertheless, because of the role competency determinations play in health care generally, and in the legal process in particular, it is important to resist the notion that persons can be determined to be more or less competent, or competent to some degree. The difficulty with taking literally the notion that competence is a matter of degree can be seen clearly by looking at the function of the competency determination within the practice of informed consent for health care, or within other areas of the law in which it plays a role, such as conservatorship or guardianship for financial affairs.

That function is, first and foremost, to sort persons into two classes: (1) those whose voluntary decisions (about their health care, financial affairs, and so on) must be respected by others and accepted as binding, and (2) those whose decisions, even if uncoerced, will be set aside and for whom others will be designated as surrogate decision makers. The function of the competency determination, then, is to make an "all or nothing" classification of persons with regard to their competence to make particular decisions, not to make "matter of degree" findings about their decision-making capacities and skills. Persons are judged, both in the law and more informally in health care settings, to be either competent or incompetent to make a particular decision—even though the underlying capacities and skills forming the basis of that judgment are possessed in different degrees. Competence, then, is in this sense a threshold concept, not a comparative one.

The foregoing makes clear that the crucial question in the competency determination is *how* defective an individual's capacities and skills to make a particular decision must be for the individual to be found incompetent to make that decision, so that a surrogate decision maker becomes necessary. In keeping with the primary objective of this article, the analysis of that question focuses on medical decisions. Here, the familiar doctrine of informed consent provides considerable guidance.

The central purpose of assessing competence is to determine whether a patient may assert his or her

right to decide to accept or refuse a particular medical procedure, or whether that right shall be transferred to a surrogate. We must, therefore, ask what values are at stake in whether people are allowed to make such decisions for themselves. The informed-consent doctrine assigns the decision-making right to patients themselves; but what fundamental values are served by the practice of informed consent? In the literature dealing with informed consent, many different answers—and ways of formulating answers—to that question have been proposed, but we believe the most important values at stake are: (1) promoting and protecting the patient's well-being, and (2) respecting the patient's self-determination. It is in examining the effect of these two values that the answer to the proper standard of decision-making competence will be found.

STANDARDS OF COMPETENCE: UNDERLYING VALUES

PROMOTION OF INDIVIDUAL WELL-BEING

There is a long tradition in medicine that the physician's first and most important commitment should be to serve the well-being of the patient. The more recent doctrine of informed consent is consistent with that tradition, if it is assumed that, at least in general, competent individuals are better judges of their own good than others are. The doctrine recognizes that while the physician commonly brings to the physician-patient encounter medical training that the patient lacks, the patient brings knowledge that the physician lacks: knowledge of particular subjective aims and values that are likely to be affected by whatever decision is made.

As medicine's arsenal of possible interventions has dramatically expanded in recent decades, alternative treatments (and the alternative of no treatment) now routinely promise different mixes of benefits and risks to the patient. Moreover, since health is only one value among many, and is assigned different importance by different persons, there is commonly no one single intervention for a particular condition that is best for everyone. Which, if any, intervention best serves a particular patient's well-being will depend in part on that patient's aims and values. Health care decision making thus usually ought to be a joint undertaking between physician and patient, since each brings knowledge and experience that the other lacks, yet that is necessary for decisions that will best serve the patient's well-being.

In the exercise of their right to give informed consent, then, patients often decide in ways that they believe will best promote their own well-being as they conceive it. As is well known, and as physicians are frequently quick to point out, however, the complexity of many treatment decisions—together with the stresses of illness with its attendant fear, anxiety, dependency, and regression, not to mention the physical effects of illness itself—means that a patient's ordinary decision-making abilities are often significantly diminished. Thus, a patient's treatment choices may fail to serve his or her good or well-being, even as that person conceives it. Although one important value requiring patient participation in their own health care decision making is the promotion of patient well-being, that same value sometimes also requires persons to be protected from the harmful consequences to them of their own choices.

RESPECT FOR INDIVIDUAL SELF-DETERMINATION

The other principal value underlying the informed-consent doctrine is respect for a patient's self-determination, understood here as a person's interest in making important decisions about his or her own life. Although often conceived in the law under the right to privacy, the leading legal decisions in the informed-consent tradition appeal fundamentally to the right of individual self-determination. No attempt will be made here to analyze the complex of ideas giving context to the concept of individual self-determination, nor of the various values that support its importance. But it is essential to underline that many persons commonly want to make important decisions about their life for themselves, and that desire is in part independent of whether they believe that they are always in a position to make the best choice. Even when we believe that others may be able to decide for us better than we ourselves can, we sometimes prefer to decide for ourselves so as to be in charge of and responsible for our lives.

The interest in self-determination should not be overstated, however. People often wish to make such decisions for themselves simply because they believe that, at least in most cases, they are in a better position to decide what is best for themselves than others are. Thus, when in a particular case others are demonstrably in a better position to decide for us than we ourselves are, a part, but not all, of our interest in deciding for ourselves is absent.

CONFLICT BETWEEN THE VALUES OF SELF-DETERMINATION AND WELL-BEING

Because people's interest in making important decisions for themselves is not based solely on their concern for their own well-being, these two values of patient well-being and self-determination can sometimes conflict. Some people may appear to decide in ways that are contrary to their own best interests or well-being, even as determined by their own settled conception of their good, and others may be unable to convince them of their mistake. In other cases, others may know little of a person's own settled values, and the person may simply be deciding in a manner sharply in conflict with how most reasonable persons would decide. It may be difficult or even impossible to determine, however, whether this conflict is simply the result of a difference in values between this individual and most reasonable persons (for example, a difference in the weights assigned to various goods), or whether it results from some failure of the patient to assess correctly what will best serve his or her own interests or good.

In the conflict between the values of self-determination and patient well-being, a tradeoff between avoiding two kinds of errors should be sought. The first error is that of failing to protect a person from the harmful consequences of his or her decision when the decision is the result of serious defects in the capacity to decide. The second error is failing to permit someone to make a decision and turning the decision over to another, when the patient is able to make the decision him or herself. With a stricter or higher standard for competence, more people will be found incompetent, and the first error will be minimized at the cost of increasing the second sort of error. With a looser or more minimal standard for competence, fewer persons will be found incompetent, and the second sort of error is more likely to be minimized at the cost of increasing the first.

Evidence regarding a person's competence to make a particular decision is often uncertain, incomplete, and conflicting. Thus, no conceivable set of procedures and standards for judging competence could guarantee the elimination of all error. Instead, the challenge is to strike the appropriate balance and thereby minimize the incidence of either of the errors noted above. No set of procedures will guarantee that all and only the incompetent are judged to be incompetent.

But procedures and standards for competence are not merely inevitably imperfect. They are inevitably *controversial* as well. In the determination of competence, there is disagreement not only about which procedures will minimize errors, but also about the proper standard that the procedures should be designed to approximate. The core of the controversy derives from the different values that different persons assign to protecting individuals' well-being as against respecting their self-determination. We believe there is no uniquely "correct" answer to the relative weight that should be assigned to these two values, and in any event it is simply a fact that different persons do assign them different weight.

DECIDING ON STANDARDS OF COMPETENCE

Focusing only on the two values of patient well-being and self-determination is an oversimplification. Because other values are at stake, room for controversy about the proper standard of competence increases. For example, also important to the appropriate standard of competence is the value of maintaining public confidence in the integrity of the medical profession, so as to protect and foster the trust necessary to physician-patient relationships that function well.

The standard of competence, then, cannot be discovered. There is no reason to believe that there is one and only one optimal tradeoff to be struck between the competing values of well-being and self-determination, nor, hence, any one uniquely correct level of capacity at which to set the threshold of competence — even for a particular decision under specified circumstances. In this sense, setting a standard for competence is a value choice, not a scientific or factual matter. Nevertheless, the choice need not be and should not be arbitrary. Instead, it should be grounded in (1) a reflective appreciation of the values in question, (2) a clear

understanding of the goals that the determination of competence is to serve, and (3) an accurate prediction of the practical consequences of setting the threshold at this level rather than elsewhere.

People may disagree on exactly where the threshold should be set not only because they assign different weights to the values of self-determination and well-being, but also because they make different estimates of the probability that others will err in trying to promote a person's interests. Unanimous agreement on an optimal standard is not necessary, however, for workable social arrangements for determining competence, any more than it is for determining who may vote or who may drive an automobile.

DIFFERENT STANDARDS OF COMPETENCE

A number of different standards of competence have been identified and supported in the literature, though statutory and case law provide little help in articulating precise standards. It is not feasible to discuss here all the alternatives that have been proposed. Instead, the range of alternatives will be delineated and the difficulties of the main standards will be examined.

No single standard is adequate for all medical treatment decisions, much less so for decisions about living arrangements, financial affairs, participation in research, and so forth. It was argued above that a standard of competence must set a balance between the two principal values at stake in health care decision making: promoting and protecting the patient's well-being while respecting the patient's self-determination.

An example of a minimal standard of competence is that the patient merely be able to express a preference. This standard respects every expressed choice of a patient, and so is not, in fact, a criterion of *competent* choice at all. It entirely disregards whether defects or mistakes are present in the reasoning process leading to the choice, whether the choice is in accord with the patient's conception of his or her good, and whether the choice would be harmful to the patient. It thus fails to provide any protection for patient well-being, and it is insensitive to the way the value of self-determination itself varies with differences in people's capacities to choose in accordance with their conceptions of their own good.

At the other extreme are standards that look to the *content* or *outcome* of the decision, for example, the standard that the choice be a reasonable one, or be what other reasonable or rational persons would choose. On this view, failure of the patient's choice to match some such allegedly objective standard of choice entails that it is an incompetent choice. Such a standard maximally protects patient well-being—according to the standard's conception of well-being—but fails adequately to respect patient self-determination.

At bottom, a person's interest in self-determination is his or her interest in defining, revising over time, and pursuing his or her own particular conception of the good life. There are serious risks associated with any purportedly objective standard for the correct decision—the standard may ignore the patient's own distinctive conception of the good and may involve the substitution of another's conception of what is best for the patient. Moreover, even such a standard's claim to protect maximally a patient's well-being is only as strong as the objective account of a person's well-being on which the standard rests.

The issue is theoretically complex and controversial, but any standard of individual well-being that does not ultimately rest on an individual's own informed preferences is both problematic in theory and subject to intolerable abuse in practice. Thus, a standard that judges competence by comparing the content of a patient's decision to some objective standard for the correct decision may fail even to protect appropriately a patient's well-being. An adequate standard of competence will focus primarily not on the content of the patient's decision, but on the *process* of reasoning that leads up to that decision.

While an adequate competency evaluation and standard focuses on the patient's understanding and reasoning, rather than upon the particular decision that issues from them, the key issue remains. What level of reasoning is required for the patient to be competent? In other words, how well must the patient understand and reason to be competent? How much can understanding be limited or reasoning be defective and still be compatible with competence? It is important to emphasize another question faced by those evaluating competence. How certain must those persons evaluating competence be about how well the patient has understood and reasoned in coming to a decision? This last question is important because it is common in cases of marginal or questionable competence for there to be a significant degree of uncer-

tainty about the patient's decision-making process that can never be eliminated.

RELATION OF THE STANDARD OF COMPETENCE TO EXPECTED HARMS AND BENEFITS

Because the competency evaluation requires setting a balance between the two values of respecting patients' rights to decide for themselves and protecting them from the harmful consequences of their own choices, it should be clear that no single standard of competence—no single answer to the questions above—can be adequate. That is simply because the degree of expected harm from choices made at a given level of understanding and reasoning can vary from virtually none to the most serious, including major disability or death.

There is an important implication of this view that the standard of competence ought to vary with the expected harms or benefits to the patient of acting in accordance with a choice—namely, that just because a patient is competent to consent to a treatment, it does not follow that the patient is competent to refuse it, and vice versa. For example, consent to a low-risk life-saving procedure by an otherwise healthy individual should require a minimal level of competence, but refusal of that same procedure by such an individual should require the highest level of competence.

Because the appropriate level of competence properly required for a particular decision must be adjusted to the consequences of acting on that decision, no single standard of decision-making competence is adequate. Instead, the level of competence appropriately required for decision making varies along a full range from low/minimal to high/maximal. Table 1 illustrates this variation.

The presumed net balance of expected benefits and risks of patient choice in comparison with other alternatives refers to the physician's assessment of the expected effects in achieving the goals of prolonging life, preventing injury and disability, and relieving suffering from a particular treatment option as against its risks of harm. The table indicates that the relevant comparison is with other available alternatives, and the degree to which the net benefit/risk balance of the alternative chosen is better or worse than that for other treatment options. It should be noted that a choice might properly require only low/minimal competence,

Table 1. Decision-Making Competence and Patient Well-Being

Presumed net balance of expected benefits and risks of patient choice in comparison with other alternatives	Level of decision-making competence required	Grounds for believing patient's choice best promotes/protects own well-being
Net balance substantially better than for possible alternatives.	Low/minimal	Principally the benefit/risk assessment made by others.
Net balance roughly comparable to that of other alternatives.	Moderate/median	Roughly equally from the benefit/risk assessment made by others and from the patient's decision that the chosen alternative best fits patient's conception of own good.
Net balance substantially worse than for another alternative or alternatives.	High/maximal	Principally from patient's decision that the chosen alternative best fits own conception of own good.

although its expected risks exceeded its expected benefits, because all other available alternatives had substantially worse expected risk/benefit ratios.

Table 1 also indicates, for each level of competence, the grounds for believing that a patient's own choice best promotes his or her well-being. This brings out an important point. For all patient choices, other people responsible for deciding whether those choices should be respected should have grounds for believing that the choice, if it is to be honored, is reasonably in accord with the patient's good and does reasonably protect or promote the patient's well-being (though the choice need not, of course, *maximize* the patient's interests). When the patient's level of decision-making competence is only at the low/minimal level, the grounds derive only minimally from the fact that the patient has chosen the option in question; they principally stem from others' positive assessment of the choice's expected effects for life and health.

At the other extreme, when the expected effects of the patient's choice for life and health appear to be substantially worse than available alternatives, the requirement of a high/maximal level of competence provides grounds for relying on the patient's decision as itself establishing that the choice best fits the patient's good (his or her own particular aims and ends). That highest level of competence is required to rebut the presumption that if the choice seems not best to promote life

and health, then that choice is not, in fact, reasonably related to the patient's interests.

When the expected effects for life and health of the patient's choice are approximately comparable to those of alternatives, a moderate/median level of competence is sufficient to provide reasonable grounds that the choice promotes the patient's good and that his or her well-being is adequately protected. It is also reasonable to assume that as the level of competence increases (from minimal to maximal), the value or importance of respecting the patient's self-determination increases as well, since a part of the value of self-determination rests on the assumption that persons will secure their good when they choose for themselves. As competence increases, the likelihood of this happening increases.

Thus, according to the concept of competence endorsed here, a particular individual's decision-making capacity at a given time may be sufficient for making a decision to refuse a diagnostic procedure when forgoing the procedure does not carry a significant risk, although it would not necessarily be sufficient for refusing a surgical procedure that would correct a life-threatening condition. The greater the risk—where risk is a function of the severity of the expected harm and the probability of its occurrence—the greater the level of communication, understanding, and reasoning skills required for competence to make that decision. It is not always true, however, that if a person is competent to make one decision, then he or she is competent to make another decision so long as it involves equal risk. Even if this risk is the same, one decision may be more complex, and hence require a higher level of capacity for understanding options and reasoning about consequences.

RELATION OF REFUSAL OF TREATMENT TO DETERMINATION OF INCOMPETENCE

A common criticism of the way physicians actually practice is that patients' competence is rarely questioned until they refuse to consent to a physician's recommendation for treatment. It is no doubt true that patients' competence when they accept physicians' treatment recommendations should be questioned more often than it now is, because consent without understanding provides little basis for believing the choice is best for the patient, and because the physician's judgment about what is medically best is fallible. Nevertheless, treatment refusal does reasonably raise the question of a patient's competence in a way that acceptance of recommended treatment does not. It is a reasonable assumption that physicians' treatment recommendations are more often than not in the interests of their patients. Consequently, it is a reasonable presumption—though rebuttable in any particular instance—that a treatment refusal is contrary to the patient's interest. Exploration of the reasons for the patient's response, including determination of whether the decision was a competent one, are appropriate—though reassessment of the recommendation is often appropriate as well.

It is essential to distinguish here, however, between grounds for calling a patient's competence into question and grounds for a finding of incompetence. Treatment refusal does reasonably serve to trigger a competency evaluation. On the other hand, a disagreement with the physician's recommendation or refusal of a treatment recommendation is no basis whatsoever for a finding of incompetence. This conclusion follows from the premise noted earlier that the competency evaluation, as well as evidence in support of a finding of incompetence, should address the *process* of understanding and reasoning of the patient, *not* the *content* of a decision.

Another essential distinction is between two quite different types of treatment refusal: a refusal of all the treatment options offered, and refusing

the one treatment that the physician believes to be best while accepting an alternative treatment that lies within the range of medically sound options. If there is more than one medically sound treatment option—in the sense that competent medical judgment is divided as to which of two or more treatments would be optimal—then the patient's refusal to accept the option that the physician believes is optimal should not even raise the question of the patient's competence, much less entail a finding of incompetence, at least so long as the option the patient chooses lies within the range of medically sound options.

CONTRAST WITH FIXED MINIMUM THRESHOLD CONCEPTION OF COMPETENCE

Before elaborating the implications of this analysis for operational measurements of competence, it will be useful to contrast it with a widely held alternative conception that has been implicitly rejected here. According to this other conception—which may be called the "fixed minimal capacity" view—competence is *not* decision-relative. The simplest version of this view holds that a person is competent if he or she possesses the relevant decision-making capacities at some specified level, regardless of whether the decision to be made is risky or nonrisky, and regardless of whether the information to be understood or the consequences to be reasoned through are simple or complex. This concept of competence might also be called the "minimal threshold status concept," since the idea is that if a person's decision-making capacities meet or exceed the specified threshold, then the status of being a *competent individual* is to be ascribed to that person. According to this view, competence is an attribute of persons dependent solely on the level of decision-making capacities they possess (though these may vary, of course, from day to day or even from hour to hour, depending upon the effects of disease, medications, emotional states, and so on).

In contrast, according to the conception of competence espoused here, competence is a *relational* property. Whether a person is competent to make a given decision depends not only upon that person's own capacities but also upon certain features of the decision—including risk and information requirements. There are at least five points in favor of this approach.

First, a concept that allows a raising or lowering of the standard for decision-making capacities depending upon the risks of the decision in question is clearly more consonant with the way people actually make informal competency determinations in areas of judgment in which they have the greatest confidence and in which there is the most consensus. For example, you may decide that your 5-year-old child is competent to choose between a hamburger and a hotdog for lunch, but you would not think the child competent to make a decision about how to invest a large sum of money. This is because the risk in the latter case is greater, and the information required for reasoning about the relevant consequences of the options is much more complex. It is worth emphasizing that incompetence due to developmental immaturity, as in the case of a child, is in many respects quite different from the increasing incompetence due to a degenerative disease such as Alzheimer's. These and other cases of incompetence do have in common, however, the relevance of the degree of risk for determining the appropriate level of competence.

Second, the decision-relative concept of competence also receives indirect support from the doctrine of informed consent. The more risky the decision a patient must make, and the more complex the array of possible benefits and burdens, the greater the amount of information that must be provided and the higher the standard of understanding required on the part of the patient. For extremely low-risk procedures, with a clear and substantial benefit and an extremely small probability of significant harm, the information that must be provided to the patient is correspondingly less.

Third, perhaps the most important reason for preferring the decision-relative concept of competence is that it better coheres with our basic legal framework in two distinct respects. First, in its treatment of minors, the law has already tacitly adopted the decision-relative concept and rejected the minimum threshold concept. The courts as well as legislatures now recognize that a child can be competent to make some decisions but not others—that competence is not an all-or-nothing status—and that features of the decision itself (including risk) are relevant factors in determining whether the child is competent to make that decision. This approach is increasingly popular, and is utilized in, for example, "limited conservatorships," where some decision-making authority is expressly left with the conservatee.

In addition, the law in this country has, in general, steadfastly refused to recognize a right to interfere with a *competent* patient's voluntary choice on purely paternalistic grounds—that is, solely to prevent harms or to secure benefits for the competent patient him or herself. Instead, the law makes a finding of incompetence a necessary condition for justified paternalism. According to the decision-relative concept of competence, the greater the potential harm to the individual, the higher the standard of competence. From this it follows that a finding of incompetence is more likely in precisely those instances in which the case for paternalism is strongest—cases in which great harm can be easily avoided by taking the decision out of the individual's hands. Thus, the concept of competence favored here allows paternalism in situations in which the case for paternalism seems strongest, while at the same time preserving the law's fundamental tenet that, in general, people may be treated paternalistically only when they are incompetent to make their own decisions.

The fourth reason for preferring the decision-relative concept of competence is that it allows a finding of incompetence for a particular decision to be limited to that decision, and so it is not equivalent to a change in the person's overall status as a decision maker. Consequently, the decision-relative concept of competence contains a built-in safeguard to allay the fear that paternalism—even if justified in a particular case considered in isolation—is likely to spill over into other areas, eventually robbing the individual of all sovereignty over his or her own life. Further, any finding of incompetence is likely to evoke strong psychological reactions from some patients because to be labeled as "an incompetent" is to be returned to a childlike status. By making it clear that incompetence is decision-relative and hence may be limited to certain areas, the concept of competence used here can at least minimize the potentially devastating assault on self-esteem that a finding of incompetence represents to some individuals.

Finally, the decision-relative concept of competence has another clear advantage over the minimum threshold concept: It allows a better balance between the competing values of self-determination and well-being that are to be served by a determination of competence. The alternative concept, on its most plausible interpretation, also represents a balancing of these fundamental values, but in a cruder fashion (Brock 1983). Setting a minimal threshold of decision-making capacities represents a choice about the proper balance of tradeoff between respect for self-determination and concern for well-being, but it does so on the basis of an extremely sweeping, unqualified generalization—about the probability that unacceptable levels of harm will occur if individuals are left free to choose—over an indefinitely large number of highly diverse potential decisions.

But as indicated earlier, decisions can vary enormously in their information requirements, in the reasoning ability needed to draw inferences about relevant consequences, and in the magnitude of risk involved. Hence, any such sweeping general-

ization will be very precarious. If the generalization errs in one direction—by underestimating the overall harm that would befall individuals if the threshold for competence were set at one level—then the minimal threshold of decision-making capacities will be set so low that many people who are judged competent will make disastrous choices. If the generalization errs in the other direction—by overestimating the harm that would result if the threshold were set at a particular level—then many people will be interfered with for no good reason. Thus, regardless of where the minimal threshold is set, it seems likely that it will provide either too much protection or too little. The decision-relative concept of competence avoids relying upon such crude generalizations about harm and permits a finer balance to be struck between the goods of protecting well-being and respecting self-determination.

A Chronicle: Dax's Case As It Happened

Keith Burton

. . . *The story of Don Cowart is remarkable in some ways but commonplace in others. A man's wish to die is rather extraordinary in and of itself; but the pattern of events that shapes such a wish often is woven of the fabric of life's everyday occurrences. Such is the case with Cowart.*

Ray and Ada Cowart moved their family from the Rio Grande Valley to the small East Texas town of Henderson in the sixties. Ray prospered over the years as a rancher and real estate agent. Ada became a teacher in the Henderson school district. Their three children— Don, Jim, and Beth—were no different from other kids reared in a close-knit community. In fact, they were ordinary people living ordinary lives.

"Donny Boy," as he came to be called by his father, was popular in school and excelled in athletics. He was captain of his high school football team and performed in rodeos. He liked to take risks, a trait that often dismayed his mother. It was risk taking that would later lure him to skydiving, surfing, and other sports of chance.

Don Cowart left Henderson in 1966 to attend the University of Texas at Austin. He had planned to return home at his graduation three years later to join his father in business; however, when notified of his military draft selection, Cowart instead elected to join the U.S. Air Force. He became a pilot and served in Vietnam. He married a high school sweetheart in 1972, but they divorced eight months later. In May 1973 he was discharged from active duty and returned to Henderson, where he began working with his father in real estate.

July 23, 1973, seemed no different to Cowart from any other Wednesday. It was hot and sultry as the afternoon sun slipped low along the pine trees in the countryside near Henderson. Ray and Don had driven out to a ranch to look over some property being offered for sale by the owner. They parked their car on a bridge over a dry creek and took off by foot. They talked and laughed together as they surveyed points of interest on the land. Their business completed, the Cowarts then returned to their car to go home for dinner.

The accident happened with no warning. The Cowart men had returned to their car but had not been able to start the engine. Ray had lifted the hood and removed the air cleaner from the engine. He primed the

From *Dax's Case: Essays in Medical Ethics and Human Meaning,* edited by Lonnie D. Kliever, Southern Methodist University Press, 1989. Reprinted with permission.

carburetor by hand and instructed Don to try the ignition. Several tries failed. It seemed to Don that the battery was near exhaustion. A final attempt proved fateful, however, as a blue flame shot from the carburetor and ignited a terrible explosion and fire.

Ray Cowart was hurled into heavy underbrush by the force of the explosion. The blast rocked the car and showered window glass over Don's body. Around them, the fireball spread quickly, consuming pine trees and the scrub vegetation in the area. Don reacted quickly. He climbed from the burning car and began running toward the woods. But he was forced to stop by a fear that he would become entangled in the underbrush and slowly burn to death.

Don wheeled about and decided to chance the dirt road on which they had driven in. He ran through three walls of fire, emerged into a clearing, then fell to the ground and rolled his body to extinguish the flames. He got back to his feet and resumed running in search of help for his father.

It all seemed dreamlike. Don noticed his vision was blurred as though swimming under water. His eyes had been badly burned. Now the pain was coming in waves, and he knew it was real. He kept running.

Loud voices filtered through the woods. Don collapsed at the roadside as help arrived. He heard the footsteps of a man and then the exclamation, "Oh, my God!" when a farmer found him. Don sent the man after his father and lay wondering how badly he was burned. When the man returned, Don asked him to bring a gun—a gun he would use to kill himself. The farmer refused.

In shock, Don assumed he and his father had caused the explosion by igniting gasoline from the car's engine. Later he would learn that the explosion actually had been caused by a leaking propane gas transmission line in the area where they had parked. It was a freak event. A pocket of propane gas had formed in the dry creek bed. When the carburetor flamed up, it had ignited the gas.

Rescuers took the Cowart men to a hospital in nearby Kilgore. There, a decision was made to transport them by ambulance to a special burn unit at Dallas's Parkland Hospital. Ray Cowart died en route to Dallas. Don Cowart remembers incredible pain, his begging for pain medication, and the paramedic's refusal to administer drugs prior to their arrival in Dallas. By this time, Ada Cowart, too, was on her way to Dallas. She had returned home first to pack several changes of clothes. The radio had said the men were badly hurt. She didn't expect to return to Henderson any time soon.

Even as the ambulance sped the 140 miles from Kilgore to Dallas, Don Cowart's treatment regimen had begun. By telephone, Dr. Charles Baxter, head of Parkland's burn unit, had directed fluid therapies to help in preventing shock to vital organs. On examination in Dallas, Baxter found Cowart had severe burns over 65 percent of his body. His face suffered third-degree burns and both eyes were severely damaged. His ears and hands were also deeply burned. Fluid therapies continued and were aided by several other measures: the insertion of an intertracheal tube to control the airway, catheters placed in every body opening, treatment with antibiotics, cleansing the wounds with antibacterial drugs, and tetanus prophylaxis. Heavy doses of narcotics were given for the pain.

In the early days of Don's 232-day hospitalization at Parkland, doctors could not predict whether he would survive. It was touch and go for many weeks. Ada Cowart felt helpless; she could do little more than sit in the waiting area outside the intensive care unit with relatives of other burn victims, where she prayed and hoped for the best. Doctors permitted only short visits with her son. Don had given his mother power of attorney in the Parkland emergency room, and she in turn deferred to the medical professionals on treatment decisions.

For Cowart, there were countless whirlpool tankings in solutions to cleanse his wounds, procedures to remove dead tissue, grafts to protect living tissue, the amputation of badly charred fingers from both hands and the removal of his right eye. The damaged left eye was sewn shut. And there was terrible pain.

Through it all, Don had remained constant in his view that he did not want to live. His demands to die had started with the farmer at the accident site. They had continued at the Kilgore hospital, in the ambulance, and now at Parkland. He didn't want treatment that would extend his misery and he made this known to his mother and family, Dr. Charles Baxter, a nurse named Leslie Kerr, longtime friend Art Rousseau, attorney Rex Houston, and many others.

Baxter remained undaunted by Don's pleas to stop treatment, dismissing them at first as the typical response of burn victims to the pain of their wounds and treatment. In time, however, he openly discussed Cowart's wish to die with Don, his mother, and his lawyer, considering all the medical and legal ramifications. Failing to get Ada Cowart's and Rex Houston's consent to the withdrawal of treatment, Baxter continued to deliver it.

For her part, Ada Cowart understood her son's pain and anguish. She was haunted, nonetheless, by these thoughts: What if treatment were ceased and Don changed his mind in a near-death state? Would it be too late? Furthermore, her religious beliefs simply made mercy killing or suicide deplorable options. These religious constraints were reinforced by her fear that her son had not yet made his "peace with God."

Rex Houston also had mixed feelings about Don's wishes. On the one hand, he sympathized with Cowart's condition—being unable to so much as take medication to end his life without the assistance of others. On the other hand, it was Houston's duty to reach a favorable resolution of a lawsuit filed against the pipeline owners for Ray Cowart's death and for Don Cowart's disability. With regard to the latter, he needed a living plaintiff to achieve the best damage award for the Cowart family. Moreover, Houston believed that such an award would provide the financial means necessary for Don Cowart's ultimate rehabilitation. He therefore encouraged Cowart to see the legal proceedings through.

In February 1974, the lawsuit was settled out of court—one day prior to trial. Almost immediately, Don's demands to die quickened. There had been talk before with Art Rousseau of getting a gun. Don had asked Leslie Kerr if she would help him by injecting an overdose of medication. Now Cowart even talked with Houston about helping him get to a window of his sixth-floor hospital room, where presumably he would leap to his death. All listened but none agreed to help.

On March 12, 1974, Don was discharged from Parkland. He, his family, and his doctors agreed that his condition had improved sufficiently to warrant his transfer to the Texas Institute for Research and Rehabilitation in Houston. Nine months removed from his medical residency, Dr. Robert Meier of TIRR found Cowart to be a passive recipient of medical care, although the philosophy of treatment in this rehabilitation center encouraged patient involvement in treatment decisions. Previously Don had no say in his care; now he would be offered choices in his own treatment.

All seemed to go well during the first three weeks of his stay, until Cowart realized the pain he had endured might continue indefinitely, thanks to a careless comment by a resident plastic surgeon that his treatment would be years in completion. Faced with that prospect, Cowart refused treatment for his open burn areas and stopped taking food and water. In a matter of days, Cowart's medical condition deteriorated rapidly. Finding his patient in serious condition, Dr. Meier was deeply perplexed about what to do next. He believed it his duty to help Cowart achieve the highest measure of rehabilitation, but he was not inclined to force upon the patient care he did not wish to receive. Faced with this dilemma, he called for a meeting with Ada Cowart and Rex Houston to discuss with Don the future course of his treatment.

Ada Cowart was outraged by Don's condition. She had been discouraged from staying with her son at TIRR, and in her absence his burns had worsened. He was again near death, due to his refusal of whirlpool tankings and dressing changes. It was agreed in the meeting that Cowart would be transferred to the burn unit of John Sealy Hospital of the University of Texas Medical Branch in Galveston, where his injuries could again be treated by burn specialists.

On April 15, 1974, Don was admitted to the Galveston hospital, in chronic distress from infected wounds, poor nutrition, and severe depression. His right elbow and right wrist were locked tight. The stubs of his fingers on both hands were encased in grotesque skin "mittens." There was practically no skin on his legs. His right eye socket and closed left eye oozed infection. And excruciating pain remained his constant nemesis.

Active wound care was initiated immediately and further skin grafts were advised by Dr. Duane Larson to heal the open wounds on Cowart's chest, legs, and arms. But Cowart bitterly protested the daily tankings and refused to consent to surgery. One night he even crawled out of bed, hoping to throw himself through the window to his death, but he was discovered on the floor and returned to bed.

Frustrated by Cowart's behavior, Dr. Larson consulted Dr. Robert White of psychiatric services for an evaluation of Don's mental competency. White remembers being puzzled by Cowart: Was he a man who tolerated discomfort poorly or perhaps was profoundly depressed? Or was this an extraordinary man who had undergone such an incredible ordeal that he was frustrated beyond normal limits? White concluded, and a colleague confirmed, that Cowart was certainly not mentally incompetent. In fact, he was so impressed with the clarity of Cowart's expressed wish to die that he asked permission to do a videotape interview for classroom use in presenting the medical, ethical, and legal problems surrounding such cases. That filmed interview, which White entitled Please Let Me Die, eventually became a classic on patient rights in the field of medical ethics.

Having been declared mentally competent, Cowart still found it difficult to gain control over his treatment. He and his mother argued constantly over treatment procedures. Rex Houston helped get changes in his wound care but turned a deaf ear to Cowart's plea to go home to die from his wounds or to take his own life. In desperation, Cowart turned to other family members for assistance in securing legal representation, but without success. Finally, with White's help, Cowart reached an attorney who had represented Jehovah's Witnesses attempting to refuse medical treatment, but he was not optimistic that a lawsuit would free him from the hospital.

Rebuffed on every hand, Cowart reluctantly became more cooperative. White secured changes in Don's pain medication before and after the daily tankings, making treatments more bearable. Psychotherapy and medication helped improve his overall outlook by relieving his depression and improving his sleep. Encouraged that he might still regain sight in his left eye, Don more or less accepted his daily wound care and even agreed to surgical skin grafts early in June 1974. By July 15, his physical condition had improved enough to allow him to transfer out of the burn unit of the John Sealy Hospital to the psychiatric unit of the Jennie Sealy Hospital in the University of Texas Medical Branch under White's direct care while his wounds continued to heal.

Amid these changes there were still periodic conflicts between Cowart and those around him over his confinement in the hospital. There were reiterated demands to die and protests against treatment. A particularly explosive encounter between Cowart and Larson occurred on the day preceding his second and last major surgical procedure in the Galveston hospital. Cowart had agreed to undergo surgery to free up his hands, but the night before he changed his mind. The next morning, Larson angrily confronted Cowart with the challenge that, if he really wanted to die, he would agree to the surgery that would enable him to leave the hospital and go home where he could take his own life if he wished. Anxious to do exactly that, Cowart consented to the surgery, which was performed on July 31.

Don Cowart's stormy stay at Galveston finally ended on September 19, 1974. He had been hospitalized for a total of fourteen months, but at last he was going home. His prognosis upon dismissal was listed simply as "guarded."

Cowart was glad to be back in Henderson. The little things counted the most—sleeping in his own bed,

listening to music, visiting with friends. But it was different for him than before the accident. He was totally blind, his left eye having failed to recover. His hands and arms remained useless. He was badly scarred. A dropped foot now required that someone assist him in walking. Some of his burn sites still were not healed.

Everything he did required the help of others. Someone had to feed him, bathe him, and help with personal functions. The days seemed endless. He tried to find peace in sleep, but even this dark release was impossible without drugs. While he couldn't see himself, Don knew his appearance drew whispers and stares in restaurants.

He had his tapes, talking books, television, and CB radio. He could use his sense of hearing, though not as well as before due to the explosion and burns. And he could think. For a while, he could see in his mind's eye the memories of earlier times. Then the memories started to fade.

Ada Cowart had lost much, but she never lost her religious faith. There had been times when even she had admitted that maybe it would have been best if Don had died with her husband. She reconciled her doubt with the thought that no mother can give up the life of a son. Ada never gave up hope that Don could find new faith in God.

Homecoming brought peace for a time. As Don's early excitement for returning home gave way to deep depression and despair, however, conflict returned to their lives. They argued about how he could occupy himself, how he dressed, his personal habits, and his future. Frustration led to a veiled suicide attempt, Don stealing away from the house during the night to try throwing himself in the path of trucks hauling clay to a brick plant. The police found him and brought him home quietly.

For the next five years, Cowart lived in a shadow world of painful rehabilitation, chronic boredom, and failed relationships. His difficulties were not for want of trying. With Rex Houston's encouragement and assistance he tried pursuing a law degree. Fortunately, his legal settlement with the pipeline company provided the financial means for the nursing care and tutorial assistance which would be required because of his massive handicaps.

Cowart tested out his abilities as a blind student in two undergraduate courses at the University of Texas in Austin during the fall of 1975. He spent the spring at home in Henderson preparing for the tests that were required for admission to law school. In the summer of

1976, he enrolled for a part-time course load in Baylor University's School of Law.

Don handled his studies at Baylor in fine fashion despite his handicaps, but the strain was tremendous. He was forced to live with other people, his independence was limited, and his sleep problems persisted. When a special relationship with a woman ended abruptly in the spring of 1977, his life caved in. He tried to commit suicide by taking an overdose of pain and sleep medications, but he was discovered in time to have his stomach pumped at the hospital emergency room. He had trouble picking up his studies again, so he dropped out before the spring quarter was completed.

Cowart returned home defeated and discouraged, living with his mother for the next half year. He resumed his studies at Baylor in the spring of 1978, only to drop out again before he had completed the third quarter in the fall of 1979. He again retreated to his mother's home, filled with doubts that he would ever be able to pass the bar. By the spring of 1980, he was ready for another try at schooling, this time in a graduate program in building construction of Texas A&M University. Once again, the old patterns of sleepless nights and boring days got the best of him and he made a half hearted effort at slashing his wrists with a razor blade.

Looking back, Cowart saw his futile efforts to take his own life as a bitter human comedy. The doctors in Galveston had encouraged him to accept treatment that would free him of hospitalization and permit him to end his life, if that was his wish. But he found it difficult to find a way of killing himself without bringing further misery on himself—brain damage or further hospitalization. Ironically, he realized that he was no more successful in ending his life than in making his life work.

As a last resort, Cowart contacted White for help and was voluntarily readmitted under White's care to the Jennie Sealy Hospital on April 12, 1980. During his month-long stay, he met with White for psychotherapy treatments daily. Even more important, his sleep problems were finally resolved by weaning him away from the heavy sleep medications that he had taken for years. Cowart describes that experience as being like "coming out of a fog." For the first time since his harrowing burn treatment ordeal, his sleep became normal and his depression lifted.

It was during this stay that I met Don Cowart and we began early discussions of a film that would eventually come to be known as Dax's Case. I still call him Don because that is how I know him, but he legally changed his name to Dax in the summer of 1982. Some commentators on the film speculate that this change of name reflects some personal metamorphosis that Cowart went through during his lengthy rehabilitation period. But Cowart offers a simpler explanation. As a blind man with impaired hearing, he often found himself responding to comments addressed to others bearing the name of Don. I accepted his reasons for changing his name but asked him not to think the poorer of me for persisting in calling him Don.

It would be easy to believe that Dax's Case, more than five years in the making, served as a crucible for Don Cowart's rehabilitation. During this time, new hope and independence came into his life. He started a mail-order specialty foods business in Henderson using his creative powers. He moved into his own house. He became an articulate spokesperson for "the right to die" under auspices of Concern for Dying. And he married a former high school classmate in February 1983.

There is always another chapter, however. Even now, Don's life continues to shift. His first venture in business did not succeed financially. His second marriage ended unhappily. Amid failure has also come achievement. He returned to law school at Texas Tech University in Lubbock, where he completed his law degree in May and passed the bar in the summer of 1986. He set up a small law practice in Henderson and has recently taken in his first partner. He continues to represent his views on patient rights at educational symposiums and public forums. In time, he hopes to become a specialist in personal injury cases.

Commentary

Robert B. White

Donald's wish seemed in great measure logical and rational; as my psychiatric duties brought me to know him well, I could not escape the thought that if I were in his position I would feel as he did. I asked two other psychiatric colleagues to see the patient, and they came to the same conclusion. *Should his demand to die be respected?* I found myself in sympathy with his wish to put an end to his pathetic plight. On the other hand, the burden on his mother would be unthinkable if he left the hospital, and none of us who were responsible for his care could bring ourselves to say, "You're discharged; go home and die."

Another question occurred to me as I watched this blind, maimed, and totally helpless man defy and baffle everyone: could his adamant stand be the only way available for him to regain his independence after such a prolonged period of helplessness and total dependence?

Consequently, I decided to assist him in the one area where he did want help—obtaining legal assistance. He obviously had the right to legal recourse, and I told him I would help him obtain it. I also told him that I and the other doctors involved could not accede immediately to his demand to leave; we could not participate in his suicide. Furthermore, he was, I said, in no condition to leave unless his mother took him home, and that was an unfair burden to place on her. I urged him to have the surgery; then, when he was able to be up and about, he could take his own life if he wished without forcing others to arrange his death.

But Donald remained adamant, and the patient, his attorney, and I had several conferences. Finally, the attorney reluctantly agreed to represent the patient in court. The patient and I agreed that if the court ruled that he had the right to refuse further treatment, the life-sustaining daily trips to the Hubbard tank and all his other life-

sustaining treatment would be stopped. If he wished, he could remain in the hospital in order to be kept as free of pain as possible until he died.

Had Donald been burned a few years ago, before our increasingly exquisite medical and surgical technology became available, none of the moral, humanitarian, medical, or legal questions his case raised would have had time to occur; he would simply have died. But Donald lived, and never lost his courage or tenacity. He has imposed upon us the responsibility to explore the questions he has asked. On one occasion Donald put the matter very bluntly: "What gives a physician the right to keep alive a patient who wants to die?"

As we increase our ability to sustain life in a wrecked body we must find ways to assess the wishes of the person in that body as accurately as we assess the viability of his organs. We can no longer blindly hold to our instinctive tendency to regard death as an adversary to be defeated at any price. Nor must we accept immediately and at face value a patient's demand to be allowed to die. That demand may often be his only way to assert his will in the face of our unyielding determination to defeat death. The problem is relatively simple when brain death has occurred or when a patient refuses surgery for cancer. But what of the patient who has entered willingly on a prolonged and difficult course of treatment, and then, at the point at which he will obviously survive if the treatment is continued, decides that he does not want further treatment because he cannot tolerate the kind of future life that his injuries or illness will impose upon him?

The outcome of Donald's case does not resolve these questions but it should add to the depth of our reflections. Having won his point, having asserted his will, having thus found a way to counteract his months of total helplessness, Donald suddenly agreed to continue the treatment and to have the surgery on his hands. He remained in the hospital for five more months until medically ready to return home. In the six

Hastings Center Report, July 1975, 9–10. Copyright © 1975 The Hasting Center. Reprinted with permission.

months since he left, Donald has regained a considerable measure of self-sufficiency. Although still blind, he will soon have surgery on his eye, and it is hoped some degree of useful vision will be restored. He feeds himself, can walk as far as half a mile, and has become an enthusiastic operator of a citizen's band radio. When I told him of my wish to publish this case report, he agreed, and stated that he had been thinking of writing a paper about his remarkable experiences.

Commentary

H. Tristram Engelhardt, Jr.

This case raises a fundamental moral issue: how can one treat another person as free while still looking out for his best interests (even over his objections)? The issue is one of the bounds and legitimacy of paternalism. Paternalistic interventions are fairly commonplace in society: motorcyclists are required to wear helmets, no one may sell himself into slavery, etc. In such cases society chooses to intervene to maintain the moral agency of individuals so that their agency will not be terminated in death or in slavery. Society chooses in the purported best interest (i.e., to preserve the condition of self-determination itself—freedom) of the would-be reckless motorcyclist or slave. Or, in the paradigmatic case of paternalism, the choice by parents for their children is justifiable in that at a future time as adults, the children will say that their parents chose in their best interests (as opposed to the parents simply using their children for their own interests). That is, the paternalism involved in surrogate consent can be justified if the individual himself cannot choose, and one chooses in that individual's best interests so that if that person were (or is in the future) able to choose, he or she would (will) agree with the choice that has been made in his or her behalf.

Thus, one can justify treating a burned patient when first admitted even if that person protested: one might argue that the individual was not able to choose freely because of the pain and serious impact of the circumstances, and that by treating initially one gave the individual a reasonable chance to choose freely in the future. One would interpret the patient to be temporarily incompetent and have someone decide in his behalf. But once that initial time has passed, and once the patient is reasonably able to choose, should one respect a patient's request to refuse lifesaving therapy even if one has good reason to believe that later the patient might change his or her mind? This is the problem that this case presents.

Yet, what are the alternatives which are morally open: (1) to compel treatment, (2) at once to cease treatment, or (3) to convince the patient to persist, but if the patient does not agree, then to stop therapy. Simply to compel treatment is not to acknowledge the patient as a free agent (i.e., to vitiate the concept of *consent* itself), and simply to stop therapy at once may abandon the patient to the exigencies of unjustified despair. The third alternative recognizes the two values to be preserved in this situation: the freedom of the patient and the physician's commitment to preserve the life of persons.

But in the end, individuals, when able, must be allowed to decide their own destiny, even that of death. When the patient decides that the future quality of life open to him is not worth the investment of pain and suffering to attain that future quality of life, that is a decision proper to the patient. Such is the case *even if* one had good reasons to believe that once the patient attained that future state he would be content to live; one would have unjustifiably forced an investment of pain that was not agreed to. Of course, there are no easy answers. Physicians should not abandon patients when momentary pain overwhelms them; physicians

Hastings Center Report, June 1975, 9–10. Copyright © 1975 The Hastings Center. Reprinted with permission.

EDITORS' NOTE: This article explores the sparse secular morality that can bind moral strangers, not the thick morality that should guide all persons in their choices regarding dying and death. The first is not adequate for a good death.

should seek to gain consent for therapy. But when the patient who is able to give free consent does not, the moral issue is over. A society that will allow persons to climb dangerous mountains or do daredevil stunts with cars has no consistent grounds for paternalistic intervention here. Further, unlike the case of the motorcyclist or the would-be slave, in this case one would force unchosen pain and suffering on another in the name of their best interests, but in circumstances where their best interests are far from clear. That is, even if such paternalistic intervention may be justifiable in some cases (an issue which is different from the paternalism of surrogate decision-making, and which I will not contest at this point), it is dubious here, for the patient's choice is not a capricious risking on the basis of free action, but a deliberate choice to avoid considerable hardship. Further, it is a uniquely intimate choice

concerning the quality of life: the amount of pain which is worth suffering for a goal. Moreover, it is, unlike the would-be slave's choice, a choice which affirms freedom on a substantial point—the quality of one's life.

In short, one must be willing, as a price for recognizing the freedom of others, to live with the consequences of that freedom: some persons will make choices that they would regret were they to live longer. But humans are not only free beings, but temporal beings, and the freedom that is actual is that of the present. Competent adults should be allowed to make tragic decisions, if nowhere else, at least concerning what quality of life justifies the pain and suffering of continued living. It is not medicine's responsibility to prevent tragedies by denying freedom, for that would be the greater tragedy.

SECTION 3

Advance Directives

The Living Will: Help or Hindrance?

Stuart J. Eisendrath and Albert R. Jonsen

Physicians are accustomed to handing their patients' written instructions that prescribe a certain form of medical care, usually a medication. They are not accustomed to receiving from their patients written instructions that prescribe how they, the physicians, are to provide, or not provide, medical care. Yet the living will is just such a document, and it is appearing in the offices of physicians. It is one manifestation of the increasingly strong affirmation that patients should have substantial control over their medical care.

Journal of American Medical Association, Vol. 249:15, 1983, 2054–2058. Copyright © 1983 American Medical Association. Reprinted with permission.

As a legal doctrine and an ethical imperative, informed consent has become the central feature of that affirmation. Although often difficult to achieve and sometimes lightly treated, informed consent has become a standard of good practice and is, in principle, hardly controversial. Its obverse—"informed refusal"—is much more controversial. Although strong legal grounds and persuasive ethical justifications support the refusal of medical care by patients, the occasions of such refusal are frequently disruptive and disturbing. The living will has even more potential for such disruption and disturbance, since it is a refusal in writing rather than viva voce. Argument rages in the literature of medical ethics about the circumstances in which a refusal should itself be refused;

anxiety and uncertainty appear in the clinical setting. Psychiatric consultants, legal advisors, and ethicists are summoned.

The living will is a statement that directs the physicians to act in certain ways during the terminal phase of the patient's illness when he may no longer be mentally competent. The physician is instructed not to take measures that would prolong the life of the patient. This form of instruction was devised in 1969 by the Euthanasia Educational Council, now known as "Concern for Dying." This document was intended to be "a simple, reasonable statement of the belief in the right of the dying to die and not to be kept alive by artificial and heroic measures."[1] Within six years of its appearance, more than a half million copies had been distributed, frequently by churches and senior citizens groups. Different formulations of the living will have since appeared. Persons sometimes will write a living will in their own words.

The functions of the living will are multiple. The foremost idea has been to allow the patient maximal autonomy in deciding the extent of the medical interventions he would want for himself in the future should he become incompetent. Signing the living will before medical interventions, when the patient is healthy and of sound mind, presumably gives that individual control over the end of his life. Not only does such a device provide the patient autonomy, but it can also reduce futile pain and suffering. It may also assist the physician and the patient's family in the onerous and heartrending task of making decisions about the measure of care for the dying patient. Finally, as Bok suggests, it may lift the burden of choice from dying persons at a time when they have neither the strength nor will to worry about alternative forms of care. These many benefits contribute to the growing popularity of directions concerning care at the end of life.[2]

"Living will" is a phrase that sounds contradictory to persons trained in the law: a "will" is a document whose terms are to be executed after the death of the testator. The living will directs actions before the death of the testator that will usually hasten that death. When the living will first appeared, its standing was highly questionable. Not only was it a peculiar sort of "will," but its terms might direct acts that could be construed as illegal, and its language, which contains such words as *extraordinary* and *heroic,* was vague. Doubts might be cast on its

authenticity and on the persistence of the testator's intention at the time the will is to be executed.[3]

Acknowledging the legal questions about the living will, legislators in several states who were sympathetic with the purpose of such a document attempted to create a device with a more solid legal basis. Spearheaded by Walter Sackett, a physician legislator in Florida, legislative efforts were unsuccessful until the California Natural Death Act, sponsored by Senator Barry Keene of California, was signed by Governor Jerry Brown in 1976. At present, ten states have passed similar legislation (Arkansas, California, Idaho, Kansas, New Mexico, North Carolina, Oregon, Texas, and Washington). Inevitably, passage of such legislation is accompanied by controversy. At the extremes, proponents of mercy killing are pitted against right-to-life advocates. In the center, physicians object that laws are unnecessary and intrusive; patients argue their rights are ignored without legislation.[4] Some thoughtful commentators worry that when such laws are passed, patients who have signed and witnessed living wills will be maintained alive for unreasonable periods of time because of physicians' fear of malpractice.[5]

The California law is strictly drawn. It requires the patient to sign a document in which the words are prescribed exactly in the law. This document directs the physician to refrain from life-sustaining procedures when "in the judgment of the attending physician, death is imminent whether or not such procedures are utilized." The letter of the law seems to make the Act irrelevant for many clinical situations where it might be expected to be helpful.[6] However, the letter of the law does not seem to deter physicians. A survey of 275 physicians showed that few of them were familiar with the precise provisions of the Act. At the same time, two thirds of the respondents said they had patients who had signed the Act and two thirds said the Act had made a difference in their clinical decisions about those patients.[7] Another survey reported that California physicians who were familiar with the Act considered its principal value to lie less in having a legal directive than in the opportunity it provided to discuss appropriate care during terminal illness while the patient was still alert and competent.[8]

Whether a patient presents a legally sanctioned document or an unofficial living will to the physician, questions of interpretation are certain to arise. If the physician and patient can discuss together the document's wishes and intentions, agreement can be reached about the extent and nature of care during terminal illness. It is, of course, highly desirable that such common agreement be reached. However, the living will or its legal counterpart may appear in the clinical situation after the patient has ceased to be an active participant. Either it may be given to the physician at an earlier time, without its intent ever being clarified, or relatives may produce it during the course of a serious illness. Difficulties of interpretation can then become extreme. Even those physicians who sincerely desire to follow their patients' wishes may be uncertain how to do so. Case 1 illustrates this problem. In contrast, case 2 demonstrates that the presence of a living will can facilitate clinical decision (as it is intended to do).

REPORT OF CASES

CASE 1.—Mrs T. was a 65-year-old woman who was admitted to the vascular surgery service for evaluation of an asymptomatic carotid bruit. The bruit had been discovered on a routine physical examination when the patient had seen her personal physician with a fracture of her right humerus, which had occurred while playing golf. Arteriography disclosed a high-grade stenosis of her left carotid, and a thromboendarterectomy was suggested as a prophylactic procedure to prevent a disabling stroke. The patient consented to the operation but stated to a house officer before the procedure that she had signed a living will four years earlier, shortly after her husband had died of a lingering illness. The patient reaffirmed on the day before surgery that she wished the living will to be carried out should she experience a severe and disabling stroke as a sequela of the surgery. She knew that a stroke was a possibility from the surgery, since several months earlier a friend of hers had had a severe stroke after an endarterectomy. She stated that she felt life was worth living only if she could be healthy and independent.

She presented the following living will (The Concern for Dying format) to the house officer:

To my family, my physician, my lawyer, and to any medical facility in whose care I happen to be,

or to any individual who may become responsible for my health and welfare or affairs. Death is as much a reality as birth, maturity, and old age. It is the one certainty of life. If the time comes when I, Mrs T., can no longer take part in decisions for my own future, let this statement stand as an expression of my wishes while I am of sound mind. If a situation should arise in which there is no reasonable expectation of my recovery from physical or mental disability, I request that I be allowed to die and not be kept alive by artificial means or heroic measures. I do not fear death itself as much as the indignities of deterioration, dependence, and hopeless pain. I therefore ask that medications be mercifully administered to me to alleviate suffering, even though this may hasten the moment of death. This request is made after careful consideration. I hope that you who care for me will feel morally bound to follow its mandate. I recognize that this appears to place a heavy responsibility upon you, but it is with the intention of relieving you of such responsibility and of placing it upon myself, in accordance with my strong convictions, that this statement is made. Signed (by the patient).

The patient underwent surgery, which was uneventful. She awoke and had full neurological functioning. Approximately 30 minutes later, however, she began to experience progressive right-sided weakness and a neurological picture compatible with a dense stroke in the distribution of the left middle cerebral artery. She was taken back to the operating room and reexplored, and an extensive clot formation was removed from her carotid artery.

After this reoperation, the patient continued to have a profound neurological deficit manifested by right-sided paresis and responsiveness to deep pain only. She was transferred from the recovery room to the Intensive Care Unit and received assisted ventilation. The patient's lack of responsiveness persisted for several days, and it appeared that she might be left with a permanent, profound neurological impairment. Added to this, aspiration pneumonia developed. It was decided that a tracheostomy should be done to control her ventilation over a long term. This procedure was performed electively. Certain staff members raised the question, "Why are we doing this to this lady? Wasn't her living will specific in spelling out what she didn't want to have happen?" In answer to this question, her attending physicians stated that one week after her stroke, it was impossible to tell how much function the patient would regain: "We must continue acute care, hoping for the best at this point." Others questioned this approach, stating that if they persisted, the patient would end up trapped in a poorly functioning body, unable even to take her own life should she desire to do so. As a previously vigorous woman, this is precisely what she did not want, they asserted. The patient's respiratory status improved considerably with antibiotic treatment, and she was transferred to the vascular surgery floor.

At this point, the patient's brother questioned the patient's attending physician about the appropriateness of continuing medical treatment. He suggested, with the most sincere intention, that the patient be sedated and, in essence, be allowed to die. In a letter to the patient's attending surgeon, the brother referred to her living will and implied that he might begin litigation if the patient was allowed to continue living in this neurologically impaired state. Nonetheless, the nurses persisted in encouraging the patient to make rehabilitative efforts. An ethics consultation was requested.

A medical ethics committee exists at this institution. It is used for consultation in difficult cases, and, while neither binding nor having legal force, its advice is usually found helpful.[9,10] The medical ethics committee gathered information. The patient's neurological status was meticulously reviewed. Neurology consultants could not be definitive in stating the patient's prognosis for recovery, stating that it would take several months for the ultimate prognosis to become certain. As part of the ethics consultation, a psychiatric consultation was obtained to clarify the patient's current level of competence to make decisions as well as to estimate the validity of her previously signed living will. The psychiatrist found the patient to be globally aphasic and unable to communicate by any means. From history gathered from the patient's family, however, it became clear that she had never had any psychiatric disorder, nor was there any family history of such. It was also apparent that the patient's decision to sign a living will had not been the result of any discernible psychiatric illness, e.g., a depressive suicidal wish.

On the basis of information provided by neurology and psychiatric consultants, the medical ethics committee suggested to the attending physician that the living will not be acted on at this point in time. The committee suggested that respiratory support not be withdrawn and there be no authorization of an order not to resuscitate the patient if she developed cardiopulmonary arrest. The reason for this conclusion was the uncertainty of the prognosis. It was simply impossible, on the basis of the medical evidence, to predict to what extent the conditions stated in the living will ("deterioration, dependence, and hopeless pain") would become manifest. In view of the psychiatric evidence and the history, the will could be taken as a valid expression of the patient's wishes, but, at the same time, the conditions envisioned by those wishes could not be reliably predicted. Thus, the will should not determine the clinical decisions, at least until the picture about future levels of function became more certain. This conclusion ran the risk, of course, of leaving this woman alive in the condition which she wanted to avoid. Faced with this dilemma, the ethics consultants followed the venerable rule of thumb, "in cases of doubt, favor life."[11] It should be noted that if the patient had presented a California Natural Death Act Directive, the condition required by this law, "imminent death whether or not treatment is provided," would certainly not be fulfilled, making the directive inoperative according to its strict letter.

Ten days after her transfer to the vascular surgery floor, the patient became capable of written and verbal communication. The tracheostomy was capped, and she began speaking short phrases and was able to understand verbal and written questions and instructions. In a few days, her ability to speak increased remarkably. This improvement occurred approximately three weeks after the onset of her stroke. Improvement continued at a dramatic rate, and within a week, plans were made to discharge the patient to a rehabilitation center. Before leaving the medical center, the patient was asked about having signed the living will and her views of her recent medical care. She responded by saying that the living will was "a good thing in certain conditions." She did not feel, however, that she herself had been in a condition in which such a document should have been invoked. She stated, "I didn't want to be a vegetable."

This statement highlighted the quandary that the staff had found themselves in several weeks earlier. What had the patient meant in her living will when she used the term "no reasonable expectation of my recovery from physical or mental disability?" Who would define what the term "reasonable" would mean? Who would define what the term "recovery" would mean? Had the patient meant by her recovery that she should be in a condition in which she'd be able to play her usual game of golf or move around in a wheelchair? What level of disability was the patient describing in her living will? At the patient's discharge, the staff felt satisfied that they had not misinterpreted the patient's desires from her living will document. Almost universally, they believed that they had carried out the most appropriate medical treatment for this patient.

As a postscript to this case, several months after the patient's discharge, the patient's brother wrote a note to the medical and nursing staff who had treated the patient. In his note, he stated that both he and the patient were glad that the staff had stood firm in providing the patient with maximal therapeutic efforts in the face of his demands for reduced care. He described her progress in her rehabilitation efforts. He thanked the staff for being "so helpful" during the critical decision-making period.

CASE 2—Mrs Z. was a 55-year-old woman who was a foreign language teacher. She was admitted to the Intensive Care Unit with an aspiration pneumonia, which was believed caused by a diminished gag reflex secondary to her 20-year history of multiple sclerosis. For several days, the patient received appropriate antibiotic therapy, and her pneumonia cleared. The patient seemed to be at continuous risk for a recurrence of aspiration, since her diminished gag reflex was presumably caused by irreversible nerve damage.

The question of what preventive measures could be used was explored by staff members. One member suggested oversewing the patient's epiglottis to prevent recurrent aspirations. This procedure would require a permanent tracheostomy, and the patient would lose laryngeal speech capability. This intervention would have profound implications for this patient, because she had been grossly debilitated by the years of multiple sclerosis and was confined to a bed at home. Her only interaction with friends involved speech. She was an articulate and highly educated person. Her major pastime was as a foreign language tutor for university students. Thus, the loss of verbal communication would have a major and unique impact on this patient. In presenting the option of permanent tracheostomy v the possibility of recurrent aspiration pneumonia, it was pointed out to the patient that she had essentially no pulmonary reserve and that future episodes of aspiration would almost certainly be fatal. She stated that she would rather die than be unable to speak.

In discussing the options with the patient, the attending physicians were unclear how well she comprehended the decision before her. They obtained a psychiatric consultation to evaluate the patient's mental status and competence to make this major decision. In reviewing the history, the psychiatric consultant found that the patient had been hospitalized for urinary tract infections six weeks before the current hospitalization. At that time, a psychiatric consultation had been obtained, since the patient had been noted to be "hallucinating and paranoid." Antipsychotic medication had been recommended but never administered. In evaluating the patient's current mental status, the psychiatrist found her to be guarded in her responses and uncooperative with formal cognitive testing. It appeared that the patient might have a mild organic brain syndrome. Although there was no clear-cut evidence of any psychosis, it was difficult to determine whether the patient fully understood the implications of the choices she was to make regarding her medical care. At this point, the patient's sole surviving sister came from a distant city. The sister brought forth the following living will, which the patient had signed four years earlier:

TO WHOM THIS MAY CONCERN: The undersigned hereby directs all doctors and hospitals that she does not wish to be kept alive artificially, in the event that the outcome and prognosis is such that undersigned will not be able to lead a useful life, and with the prognosis as such, in the opinion of competent medical practitioners, that the medical treatment being rendered is just prolonging life without the possibility of reasonable recovery. Signed (by the patient).

According to the sister, the patient had clarified to her that a "useful life" meant the ability to relate to others meaningfully by verbal communication. From the sister's description, it was clear that the patient was mentally lucid at the time she had signed this document. With this information, it was much easier for the attending physician to rest with the patient's decision not to have a tracheostomy. Although she seemed to have a general understanding of what the tracheostomy would mean, the living will supported the idea that the patient would not want to be kept alive in the condition in which she would exist indefinitely but be unable to speak—her criteria for a useful life.

In this case, the living will substantially helped the staff to make a reasonable decision that they felt comfortable with. The patient did not receive a tracheostomy and was transferred to a rehabilitation facility for further treatment. Should she aspirate again, her probable death would be the result of a decision she herself had participated in both by word and by living will. Several months after the transfer, she remained in the same medical condition.

COMMENT

It is clear legally and ethically that a competent patient's refusal of treatment should be honored. The living will is an attempt to carry the patient's wishes into the time when the patient is no longer able to be a spokesman on his or her behalf. Yet the first case raises many of the difficulties inherent in implementing a living will. Although one of the living will's main purposes is to promote patient autonomy, this case illustrates how difficult it can be to achieve this in the clinical setting. The medical staff had a difficult time deciding on the proper treatment of this patient, not because they wished to impose their will on her, but rather because they could not interpret exactly what her desires would be given her medical condition. Her living will was not specific enough to assist the medical staff in attempting to fulfill her desires. Although her document used terms like "a reasonable expectation of recovery," these terms are open to a variety of interpretations. The ambiguity allows the staff to project their own attitudes and feelings onto a given statement, setting the stage for conflict and controversy.[12]

In Mrs T.'s case, for example, some of the staff members believed a great injustice was being done when the patient was given a tracheostomy tube,

stating that Mrs T.'s living will spoke against such procedures. Medical indications for the tracheostomy, and, indeed, for rehabilitative care after her neurological insult, were clear. Nonetheless, the split in the staff's response to the patient's document made the pursuit of clinically appropriate treatment controversial. Projection of staff's attitudes is not uncommon in critically ill patients. This phenomenon has been well described in the psychiatric consultation literature.[13,14] Conflicting attitudes were aired in the discussion of the patient's treatment, because the staff had to guess at what the specific conditions were that the patient alluded to in her document.

Hindrance of staff management highlights one of the drawbacks of a living will, ie, in cases where it is most needed—for example, when the patient's communication is grossly if not totally impaired, then the living will can become a source of confusion because of variably interpretable phrases included in the document.

In contrast to the first case, the second case illustrates how a living will can be extremely helpful. In this case, the document signed by the patient alleviated the burden of decision making for the family and attending physicians. This case differed considerably from the first in that the prognosis was much more certain (although less favorable). In addition, the patient appeared to have a reasonable idea of what decision she was making by signing this document, since she had lived with the disabling effects of multiple sclerosis for approximately 15 years.

There is little question in this case of the patient having full control of her faculties at the time she signed the will, which was several years before hospitalization. Even though during her current hospitalization there was uncertainty as to her ability to comprehend fully the medical decisions facing her, it did seem that she had a general understanding of what her options were. That impression was greatly enhanced when her sister brought in the supporting document. It should be noted that if the physicians had determined that the surgery was the most appropriate treatment and they regarded the patient as incompetent, a judicial authorization would have been a prerequisite.

The second case was also clearer than the first in that the possible long-term outcomes were more sharply defined, ie, the value of the surgical procedure to oversew the patient's epiglottis had the definite outcome of ensuring the prolongation of her life, whereas, the failure to do so carried the serious risk of reaspiration and almost certain death. For this patient, the ability to speak was critical for her desire to continue living.

These two cases point out the advantages and disadvantages of the living will in a clinical situation. The advantages are that patients' autonomy can be honored with greater certainty, unacceptable pain and suffering avoided, and physicians absolved from doing what might be medically possible but personally, to patient and physician, undesirable. The disadvantages arise from the lack of specificity in written documents and the uncertainty of prognosis. These disadvantages can be alleviated in part if physicians undertake to clarify the patient's intention by detailed conversation in advance of the situation when the terms of the will must be interpreted. In the first case, the patient presented the living will to the anesthesiology resident the night before the surgery. The resident accepted it, put it in the record, but did not discuss it. In the second case, the physicians, with the help of the patient's sister, were able to interpret the patient's intentions, but it would have been desirable for the patient herself to discuss the matter with her physician (which she had not) during the long course of her illness.

The presence of a relative or friend who can be relied on to interpret faithfully and honestly the patient's wishes is invaluable. While such people have no legal standing as a surrogate, their advice can be helpful and should be readily accepted unless there is some suspicion of bias. One attempt has been made to provide, by legislative means, standing for a person appointed by the patient, but it failed to pass.[15] Even without such standing, a patient who writes a living will might be advised to indicate in the document those persons who might serve as its interpreter. Naturally, physicians should be aware of the law regarding proxy decisions for incompetent patients that prevail in the jurisdiction in which they practice.[16]

Whenever possible, a frank discussion of the terms of the living will is always advisable. It may happen that such a discussion leads the physician to judge that the restrictions placed on clinical discretion are unacceptable. If this were to happen, the physician would be obliged to inform the patient that he or she cannot fulfill the conditions of the living will in good conscience. Should the patient insist, it would be necessary to withdraw from the case after timely notice and referral.

Some physicians might find the living will contrary to their personal ethic;[11] others might have religious objections to its terms. Catholic physicians should not be troubled, since their moral theology permits withdrawing from "extraordinary treatments" at the patient's request; however, some Catholic physicians might find objections to what they consider an antilife tone.[17] Orthodox Jewish physicians are more likely to find the living will objectionable on this ground.[18] However, most religious doctrines, as well as the current common opinion in medical ethics, justify the living will in principle. The difficulties lie largely in its application, as we have tried to show in this article.

In the absence of opportunities for clarification by discussion, the living will can be, at best, one piece of evidence among others about the patient's wishes. It needs to be weighed, along with medical indications, estimates of future quality of life, and other expressions of the patient's preferences contributed by friends and family, in reaching a suitable clinical decision.[19] The living will, despite its difficulties, should always be taken seriously as an expression of the patient's autonomy. Although it might not be decisive in certain circumstances, it is always deserving of consideration.

NOTES

1. Bass AN: Euthanasia to date. *Vassar Qrtly* 1975, p 72.
2. Bok S: Personal directions for care at the end of life. *N Engl J Med* 1976;295:367–369.
3. Keene B: Can we make the Natural Death Act a better law? Read before the California Medical Association annual scientific assembly, San Francisco, March 19, 1978.
4. Garland M: The right to die in California. *Hastings Cent Rep* 1976;6:5–7.
5. Lebacqz K: Against the California Natural Death Act. *Hastings Cent Rep* 1977;7:14–15.
6. Jonsen AR: Dying right in California: The Natural Death Act. *Clin Res* 1978;26:55–60.
7. Redleaf D, Schmitt S: Natural Death Act study: Some surprising results. *Santa Clara Med Soc Bull* Jan 1979.

8. Klutch M: Survey results after one year's experience with the Natural Death Act. *West J Med* 1978; 128:329–330.

9. Veatch RM: Hospital ethics committees: Is there a role? *Hastings Cent Rep* 1977;6:22–25.

10. Levine C: Hospital ethics committees: A guarded prognosis. *Hastings Cent Rep* 1977;7:25–27.

11. Epstein F: The role of the physician in the prolongation of life, in Ingelfinger FJ, Relman AS, Finland M (eds): *Controversy in Internal Medicine II.* Philadelphia, WB Saunders Co, 1974, pp 103–109.

12. Jackson DL, Youngner S: Patient autonomy and 'death with dignity.' *N Engl J Med* 1979;301:404–408.

13. Eisendrath SJ, Dunkel J: Psychological issues in inten-

sive care unit staff. *Heart Lung* 1979;8:751–758.

14. McCartny JR: Refusal of treatment: Suicide or competent choice? *Gen Hosp Psychiatry* 1979;1:338–344.

15. Relman AS: Michigan's sensible 'living will.' *N Engl J Med* 1979;300:1270–1271.

16. Meyers DW: *Medico-Legal Implications of Death and Dying.* San Francisco, Bancroft-Whitney Co, 1981.

17. Hellegers AE, Wakin E: Is the right to die wrong? *US Catholic* 1978;43:13–17.

18. Horowitz E: The California Natural Death Act and us. *Sh'ma* 1977;7:93–103.

19. Jonsen AR, Siegler M, Winslade WJ: *Clinical Ethics.* New York, Macmillan Publishing Co, 1982.

The Health Care Proxy and the Living Will

George J. Annas

American medicine is awash in forms: insurance forms, disability forms, informed-consent forms, and forms for various examinations, to name just a few. Forms can help make the practice of medicine more efficient, but they can also make it more routinized, impersonal, and bureaucratic. Congress and the President have decreed that beginning December 1, 1991, all hospitals, nursing facilities, hospice programs, and health maintenance organizations that serve Medicare or Medicaid patients must provide all their new adult patients with written information describing the patients' rights under state law to make decisions about medical care, including their right to execute a living will or durable power of attorney. New forms will be routinely added to the practice of medicine. Their purpose is to help implement a right that has been universally recognized: the right to refuse any and all medical interventions, even life-sustaining inter-

ventions. The challenge is to use these forms to foster communication between doctor and patient, as well as respect for the patient's autonomy.

HISTORICAL CONTEXT

The term "living will" was coined by Luis Kutner in 1969 to describe a document in which a competent adult sets forth directions regarding medical treatment in the event of his or her future incapacitation. The document is a will in the sense that it spells out the person's directions. It is "living" because it takes effect before death. Public interest in this document has always been high, and a national organization, Concern for Dying, has devoted most of its resources for the past 20 years to educating the public and professionals about the living will. A sister organization, Society for the Right to Die (which has merged with Concern for Dying to form the National Council for Death and Dying), simultaneously devoted its primary efforts to encouraging states to pass legislation giving formal legal recognition to the living will.

In 1976 the country's attention focused on the case of Karen Ann Quinlan, a young woman in a persistent vegetative state, and her parents'

New England Journal of Medicine 324, No. 17, April 25, 1991: 1210–1213. Copyright © 1991, Massachusetts Medical Society. All rights resererrd. Reprinted with permission.

EDITORS' NOTE: The notes have been omitted. Readers wishing to follow up on sources should consult the original article.

attempts to have her ventilator removed so she could die a natural death. The New Jersey Supreme Court granted the parents' petition and held that an "ethics committee" could grant all parties concerned legal immunity for their actions. The court did this because it believed that it was the fear of legal liability that prevented Quinlan's physicians from honoring her parents' request. Her story prompted the enactment of the nation's first living-will statute, California's Natural Death Act, in 1976. The California statute is very narrow. A legally enforceable declaration can be executed only 14 days or more after a person is diagnosed as having a terminal illness, defined as one that will cause the patient's death "imminently," whether or not life-sustaining procedures are continued. Thus, even though this statute was inspired by her story, it would not have helped Quinlan, because she was not terminally ill.

By 1991, more than 40 states had enacted living-will statutes. All these laws provide immunity to physicians and other health care professionals who follow the patient's wishes as expressed in a living will. Virtually all of them also suffer from four major shortcomings, however: they are applicable only to those who are "terminally ill"; they limit the types of treatment that can be refused, usually to "artificial" or "extraordinary" therapies; they make no provision for the person to designate another person to make decisions on his or her behalf, or set forth the criteria for such decisions; and there is no penalty if health care providers do not honor these documents.

ADDRESSING THE LIMITATIONS OF THE LIVING WILL

These problems led to calls for second-generation legislation on the living will. Other shortcomings were also noted. Living wills require a person to predict accurately his or her final illness or injury and what medical interventions might be available to postpone death, and living wills require physicians to make decisions on the basis of their interpretation of a document, rather than a discussion of the treatment options with a person acting on behalf of the patient. The proposed solution to these problems was not to modify the living will

but to replace it with another form, one assigning a durable power of attorney to a designated person (known, in this context, as appointing a health care proxy). The person named in the document (also called the health care proxy) is variously known as the attorney, the agent, the surrogate, or the proxy—four terms that are synonyms in this context.

Every state has a durable-power-of-attorney law that permits persons to designate someone to make decisions for them if they become incapacitated. Although these statutes were enacted primarily to permit the agent to make financial decisions, no court has ever invalidated a durable power of attorney specifically designed to enable the designated person to make health care decisions. In the recent *Cruzan* case—in which Nancy Cruzan's parents, basing their attempt on their daughter's previous statements, sought to have her tube feeding discontinued after she had been left in a persistent vegetative state by an automobile accident—Justice Sandra Day O'Connor advised citizens to employ this device. In her concurring opinion, O'Connor observed that the decision in *Cruzan* "does not preclude a future determination that the Constitution requires the States to implement the decisions of a duly appointed surrogate." The *Cruzan* case itself, which involved facts essentially identical to those in *Quinlan*, gave impetus to the concept of a health care proxy, just as the *Quinlan* case had previously increased interest in the living will. Physicians are legally and ethically bound to respect the directions of a patient set forth in a living will, but living wills are limited because no one can accurately foretell the future, and interpretation may be difficult. Attempts to make the living will less ambiguous by developing comprehensive checklists with alternative scenarios may be too confusing and abstract to be useful to either patients or heath care providers, although opinions on this differ.

THE MOVE TO DESIGNATE HEALTH CARE PROXIES

Although new laws are not necessary in any state (because of existing laws regarding the assignment of a durable power of attorney), the current trend in the United States is for states to enact additional proxy laws that specifically deal with health care. Such laws generally specify the information that must be included in the proxy form and the standards on which treatment decisions must be based and grant good-faith immunity for all involved in carrying out the treatment decision. Two of the best-written proxy laws have recently become effective in New York (in January 1991) and Massachusetts (in December 1990). The New York law is based on a recommendation of the New York State Task Force on Life and the Law, and that group's statement of its rationale is still the best introduction to the concept of the health care proxy. The Massachusetts proxy law is largely modeled on the New York law.

The heart of both laws (and all proxy laws) is the same: to enable a competent adult (the "principal") to choose another person (the "proxy" or "agent") to make treatment decisions for him or her if he or she becomes incompetent to make them. The agent has the same authority to make decisions that the patient would have if he or she were still competent. Instead of having to decipher a document, the physician is able to discuss treatment options with a person who has the legal authority to grant or withhold consent on behalf of the patient. The manner in which the agent must exercise this authority is also crucial. The agent must make decisions that are consistent with the wishes of the patient, if these are known, and otherwise that are consistent with the patient's best interests.

Proxy laws also permit the principal to limit the authority of the agent in the document (for example, by not granting authority to refuse cardiopulmonary resuscitation or tube feeding), but the more limitations the principal puts on the agent, the more the document appointing a health care proxy resembles a living will. In addition, because every limitation is subject to interpretation, the likelihood that a dispute will arise about the meaning of the document is increased. One compromise is to give the agent blanket authority to make decisions and to detail one's values and wishes with as much precision as possible in a private letter to the agent. The agent could use this letter when it was relevant to the actual decision and keep it private when it was not relevant.

IMPLEMENTING LAWS REGARDING HEALTH CARE PROXIES

The goal of appointing a proxy is to simplify the process of making decisions and to make it more likely that the patient's wishes will be followed—not to complicate existing problems. If hospitals and hospital lawyers cooperate, this goal will be attained, because the vast majority of physicians will welcome the ability to discuss treatment options with a person, chosen by the patient, who has the legal authority to give or withhold consent. Hospitals can help their patients by making a simple proxy form available, by educating their medical, nursing, and social-service staffs about the laws governing health care proxies, and by supporting decisions made by the agents. Hospitals can impede the process of making good decisions, however, if they concentrate on the paperwork rather than on the way in which decisions are made. Some Massachusetts attorneys, for example, have already drafted a 13-page, singlespaced proxy form that is all but unintelligible to nonlawyers. Others have begun to explore and to catalogue all the reasons why physicians and hospitals might want to seek judicial review before honoring the decision of a health care agent. Neither of these strategies is constructive. The use of complex forms and obstructive strategies makes it likely that treatment decisions will actually be made by the hospital's lawyers and the agent's lawyers, not by the agent and the physician. If this happens, the trend to designating a health care agent will be frustratingly counterproductive, since, instead of encouraging a focus on the patient and the patient's wishes, where it belongs, the new proxy forms will add another layer of bureaucracy and another outsider to the decision process.

The most useful form for both patients and providers is a simple one-page document that sets forth all necessary information in easily comprehensible language. The one-page form in the Appendix, which is easily understood and meets all the requirements of the new Massachusetts proxy law (as well as those of the New York law) was developed by a broad-based task force made up of representatives of all the major health care organizations in the state, including the Massachusetts Medical Society, the Massachusetts Hospital Association, the Massachusetts Nurses

Association, the Massachusetts Federation of Nursing Homes, and also the Massachusetts Department of Public Health, as well as the Massachusetts Executive Office of Elder Affairs and the Massachusetts Bar Association. This model form (available in bulk from Massachusetts Health Decisions, 101 Tremont St., No. 600, Boston, MA 02108), which also includes instructions and spaces for the optional signatures of the agent and an alternate (naming an alternate is not required), will be distributed across the state. The degree of cooperation in its development was virtually unprecedented and may provide a model for future efforts.

ADDING TO THE DOCUMENT DESIGNATING A PROXY

Perhaps out of concern for efficiency, some commentators have advocated combining an organ-donor form with the form designating a health care proxy. This is a serious error for at least two reasons. First, much effort has been expended over the past 20 years to separate the issues of organ donation and treatment decisions in the public's mind, since the main reason people do not sign organ-donor cards is that they believe doctors might "do something to me before I'm really dead." Tying organ donation to treatment refusals that might lead to death only heightens this concern and is likely to lead people to use neither form. Second, the proxy form takes effect when the patient becomes incompetent; in contrast, the organ-donor form takes effect only on the patient's death. The health care agent can have nothing to say about organ donation, because the agent can make only treatment decisions, an authority that dies with the patient. Organ donation is laudable, but it is not related to the designation of a health care agent, and the principal should authorize donation on a separate form designed for that purpose. Organ-donor forms may teach another lesson as well. No physician in the United States will honor an organ-donor form over the objections of the patient's family. Similarly, physicians have difficulty honoring a patient's living will over the family's objections. Because it identifies a person with legal authority to talk with the physician, the health care proxy is likely to be a more effective mechanism to implement the patient's wishes.

It should be stressed that forms naming a health care proxy do not substantively change existing law; they merely make it procedurally easier for a person to designate an agent who is authorized to make whatever health care decisions the person could legally make if competent, and they give health care providers legal immunity for honoring such decisions. The patient can, for example, give the agent the authority to refuse any and all medical care, but the agent has no more legal authority than the principal to insist on assisted suicide or to demand a lethal injection. The naming of an agent also solves the problem of a dispute among family members concerning treatment, since the agent has the legal and ethical right and responsibility to make the decision. When a long-lost relative arrives and demands that "everything be done or I'll sue," the physician can refer that person to the agent, rather than try to achieve a consensus.

LIMITS OF THE CONCEPT OF THE HEALTH CARE PROXY

Only competent adults who actually execute a document can name a health care agent. Since fewer than 10 percent of Americans have either living wills or organ-donor cards, few may use this mechanism. It has no application to children, the mentally retarded, or others unable to appreciate the nature and consequences of their decisions. Treatment decisions for these groups will continue to be governed by the vague "best interests" standard, which is the functional equivalent of "reasonable medical care," "appropriate medical care," or "indicated medical care." The document will also be of limited use in the emergency department, although in rare cases the health care agent may arrive with the principal and there may be time for consultation and informed consent before a specific intervention is tried. Nor will the document solve problems of futility. Physicians will retain the right not to offer treatment that is contraindicated, useless, or futile.

THE RESPONSIBILITY OF PHYSICIANS

I have encouraged members of both the Boston Bar Association and the Massachusetts Bar Association to make health care–proxy forms available to the public and their clients free of charge as a public service. Many have agreed. It will also be useful to the public if physicians make such forms available to their patients and encourage them to fill them out. Physicians may also be more comfortable about relying on the decisions of the designated agent if patients are willing to discuss their choice of agent with the physician, although this is not a requirement. Any form that is used must be written in language that both patients and health care providers can easily understand; the form need not be written by a lawyer and should not require a lawyer to interpret.

Like soldiers in past wars, Americans serving in the Persian Gulf wrote their wills. This time, however, many also wrote living wills or executed durable powers of attorney. As one reporter observed, "In the process, the soldiers had to clarify ambiguous personal relationships, chart out their children's lives, and, in some cases, confront their own mortality for the first time." Designating a health care agent gives us all the opportunity to confront our mortality and to determine who among our friends and relatives we want to make treatment decisions on our behalf when we are unable to make them ourselves. A clear focus on these substantive issues, rather than on forms or formalities, could help patients feel more secure that their wishes regarding medical treatment will be respected, and could help health care professionals be more secure that the treatment decisions made for incompetent patients actually reflect the patients' wishes. These are certainly worthy goals.

Testing the Limits of Prospective Autonomy: Five Scenarios

Norman L. Cantor

Several examples will help crystallize the potential tension between an advance directive and the contemporaneous interests of an incompetent patient. In the following scenarios, assume that all patients were fifty years old at the time of making an advance directive and that the critical medical decisions are confronted five years later. Assume also that no evidence exists that the patient changed his or her mind or wavered in resolve between preparation of the advance directive and losing competence.

Scenario 1: Person A, a Jehovah's Witness, prescribes in an advance directive that blood transfusions should not be administered regardless of the life-saving potential of such medical intervention. She is aware of the life and death implications of this religiously motivated instruction. Later, A becomes prematurely senile and incompetent. Still later, the senile patient develops bleeding ulcers

which demand blood transfusions. With a blood transfusion, she will survive and continue to live as a "pleasantly senile" person for a number of years. The senile A no longer has recollection of, or interest in, religion; however, she remained an avid Jehovah's Witness up until the time of incompetency. Should the attending physician administer a life-saving blood transfusion?

Scenario 2: Person B believes both that life should be preserved to the maximum extent possible and that suffering is preordained and carries redemptive value in an afterlife. B prepares an advance directive in which all possible life-extending medical intervention is requested and all pain relief is rejected. At the time of the preparation of the directive, B has a conversation with a physician in which the physician explicitly warns B that many terminal illnesses entail excruciating pain. Despite that admonition, B directs that all means to preserve life be utilized and that analgesics be omitted. Subsequently, B suffers from cancer, which both affects his brain, rendering him incompetent, and causes him to suffer excruciating pain.

From Advanced Directives and the Pursuit of Death with Dignity by Norman L. Cantor, Indiana University Press, 1993. Reprinted with permisssion from the publisher.

Further medical treatment such as radiation or chemotherapy will extend B's life but will not itself relieve the pain or cause any remission in which competence would return. Should the attending physician sedate the patient, or cease the life-prolonging medical intervention, or both?

Scenario 3: Person C is an individual with chronic heart problems. Physicians have informed C that at some stage he will need a heart transplant in order to survive. C prepares an advance directive stating that if he becomes incompetent and survival becomes dependent on a heart transplant, then such a transplant should be rejected because of its expense. C prefers to leave a substantial monetary legacy to his children. Later, C becomes prematurely senile and incompetent. Still later, C's heart deteriorates and a heart transplant becomes necessary to preserve C's life. With the transplant, C will very likely continue to live for three to five years. Without it, C will die within a few months. The transplant will cost $100,000 and is not covered by any insurance or government benefit program. C's estate totals $100,000. Should a life-extending heart transplant be performed?

Scenario 4: Person D is a health-care professional sensitive to society's needs for organ and tissue donations. In her advance directive, D provides that if she should become incompetent but remain physically healthy, then she wishes to donate a kidney and bone marrow to needy recipients. Later, D is afflicted with Alzheimer's disease and reaches a point of profound dementia. Needy recipients for kidney and bone-marrow transplants have been located. The prospective transplant operations will pose only a slight risk to D and entail only mild pain. At the same time, the now incompetent D has no recollection of her prior instruction and no appreciation of the altruism involved in donating an organ or tissue. She will derive no contemporaneous gain from the contemplated operations. Should the transplants be performed in accord with D's advance directive?

Scenario 5: Person E is a sociology professor known for her intellectual sharpness. E takes enormous pride in that intellectual acuity. E drafts an advance directive prescribing that if she should become mentally impaired and incompetent to the point where she can no longer read and comprehend a sociology text, then all life-preserving medical intervention should be withheld. When reminded by her spouse about the potential for happiness in an incompetent state, E replies that she deems significant mental dysfunction to be degrading and personally distasteful. For her, such a debilitated existence is a fate worse than death. Later, E suffers a serious stroke which renders her permanently incompetent and incapable of reading or performing intellectual tasks. E is also unable to swallow and is therefore dependent on artificial nutrition. At the same time, E does not appear to be in any pain and seems to derive some pleasure from listening to music. Should the life-preserving nasogastric tube be continued?

In each of the above situations, people have issued advance directives which effectuate their personal values and concepts of dignity. Yet implementation of those prior instructions conflict in some measure with the contemporaneous interests or well-being of the incompetent persona. Can the advance directive prevail? Does prospective autonomy encompass the prerogative to impact negatively on the incompetent persona?

SECTION 4

Choosing for Others

In the Matter of Claire C. Conroy

Supreme Court of New Jersey. 98 N.J. 321, 486 A. 2d 1209, decided Jan. 17, 1985

SCHREIBER, J.

At issue here are the circumstances under which life-sustaining treatment may be withheld or withdrawn from incompetent, institutionalized, elderly patients suffering from severe and permanent mental and physical impairments and a limited life expectancy.

Plaintiff, Thomas C. Whittemore, nephew and guardian of Claire Conroy, an incompetent, sought permission to remove a nasogastric feeding tube, the primary conduit for nutrients, from his ward, an eighty-four-year-old bedridden woman with serious and irreversible physical and mental impairments, who resided in a nursing home. John J. Delaney, Jr., Conroy's guardian *ad litem*, opposed the guardian's petition. The trial court granted the guardian permission to remove the tube, and the Appellate Division reversed. . . .

At the time of trial, Ms. Conroy was no longer ambulatory and was confined to bed, unable to move from a semi-fetal position. She suffered from arteriosclerotic heart disease, hypertension, and diabetes mellitus; her left leg was gangrenous to her knee; she had several necrotic decubitus ulcers (bed sores) on her left foot, leg, and hip; an eye problem required irrigation; she had a urinary catheter in place and could not control her bowels; she could not speak; and her ability to swallow was very limited. On the other hand, she interacted with her environment in some limited ways: she could move her head, neck, hands, and arms to a minor extent; she was able to scratch herself,

and had pulled at her bandages, tube, and catheter; she moaned occasionally when moved or fed through the tube, or when her bandages were changed; her eyes sometimes followed individuals in the room; her facial expressions were different when she was awake from when she was asleep; and she smiled on occasion when her hair was combed, or when she received a comforting rub.

Dr. Kazemi and Dr. Davidoff, a specialist in internal medicine who observed Ms. Conroy before testifying as an expert on behalf of the guardian, testified that Ms. Conroy was not brain dead, comatose, or in a chronic vegetative state. They stated, however, that her intellectual capacity was very limited, and that her mental condition probably would never improve. Dr. Davidoff characterized her as awake, but said that she was severely demented, was unable to respond to verbal stimuli, and, as far as he could tell, had no higher functioning or consciousness. Dr. Kazemi, in contrast, said that although she was confused and unaware, "she responds somehow."

The medical testimony was inconclusive as to whether, or to what extent, Ms. Conroy was capable of experiencing pain. Dr. Kazemi thought that Ms. Conroy might have experienced some degree of pain from her severely contracted limbs, or that the contractures were a reaction to pain, but that she did not necessarily suffer pain from the sores on her legs. According to Dr. Davidoff, it was unclear whether Ms. Conroy's feeding tube caused her pain, and it was "an open question whether she [felt] pain" at all; however, it was possible that she was experiencing a great deal of pain. Dr. Davidoff further testified that she responded to noxious or painful stimuli by moaning. The trial

---

EDITORS' NOTE: Case has been shortened and most legal references have been omitted.

court determined that the testimony of a neurologist who had examined Ms. Conroy would not be necessary, since it believed that it had sufficient evidence about her medical condition on which to base a decision.

Both doctors testified that if the nasogastric tube were removed, Ms. Conroy would die of dehydration in about a week. Dr. Davidoff believed that the resulting thirst could be painful but that Ms. Conroy would become unconscious long before she died. Dr. Kazemi concurred that such a death would be painful. . . .

Ms. Conroy's only surviving blood relative was her nephew, the guardian, Thomas Whittemore. He had known her for over fifty years, had visited her approximately once a week for four or five years prior to her commitment to the nursing home, and had continued to visit her regularly at the nursing home for some time. The record contained additional evidence about the nephew's and aunt's financial situations and the history of their relationship. Based on the details of that record, there was no question that the nephew had good intentions and had no real conflict of interest due to possible inheritance when he sought permission to remove the tube.

Mr. Whittemore testified that Ms. Conroy feared and avoided doctors and that, to the best of his knowledge, she had never visited a doctor until she became incompetent in 1979. He said that on the couple of occasions that Ms. Conroy had pneumonia, "[y]ou couldn't bring a doctor in," and his wife, a registered nurse, would "try to get her through whatever she had." He added that once, when his wife took Ms. Conroy to the hospital emergency room, "as foggy as she was she snapped out of it, she would not sign herself in, and she would have signed herself out immediately." According to the nephew, "[a]ll [Ms. Conroy and her sisters] wanted was to . . . have their bills paid and die in their own house." He also stated that he had refused to consent to the amputation of her gangrenous leg in 1982 and that he now sought removal of the nasogastric tube because, in his opinion, she would have refused the amputation and "would not have allowed [the nasogastric tube] to be inserted in the first place."

.   .   .

The trial court decided to permit removal of the tube. It reasoned that the focus of inquiry should be whether life has become impossibly and permanently burdensome to the patient. If so, the court held, prolonging life becomes pointless and perhaps cruel. It determined that removal of the tube would lead to death by starvation and dehydration within a few days, and that the death might be painful. Nevertheless, it found that Ms. Conroy's intellectual functioning had been permanently reduced to a very primitive level, that her life had become impossibly and permanently burdensome, and that removal of the feeding tube should therefore be permitted.

The guardian *ad litem* appealed. While the appeal was pending, Ms. Conroy died with the nasogastric tube intact. Nevertheless, the Appellate Division decided to resolve the meritorious issues, finding that they were of significant public importance and that this type of case was capable of repetition but would evade review because the patients involved frequently die during litigation.

.   .   .

The Appellate Division . . . held that the right to terminate life-sustaining treatment based on a guardian's judgment was limited to incurable and terminally ill patients who are brain dead, irreversibly comatose, or vegetative, and who would gain no medical benefit from continued treatment. As an alternative ground for its decision, it held that a guardian's decision may never be used to withhold nourishment, as opposed to the treatment or attempted curing of a disease, from an incompetent patient who is not comatose, brain dead, or vegetative, and whose death is not irreversibly imminent. Depriving a patient of a basic necessity of life, such as food, under those circumstances, the court stated, would hasten death rather than simply allow the illness to take its natural course. The court concluded that withdrawal of Ms. Conroy's nasogastric tube would be tantamount to killing her—not simply letting her die—and that such active euthanasia was ethically impermissible. The Appellate Division therefore reversed the trial court's judgment.

We granted the guardian's petition for certification, despite Ms. Conroy's death, since we agree with the Appellate Division that the matter is of substantial importance and is capable of repetition but evades review. . . .

I

This case requires us to determine the circumstances under which life-sustaining treatment may be withheld or withdrawn from an elderly nursing-home resident who is suffering from serious and permanent mental and physical impairments, who will probably die within approximately one year even with the treatment, and who, though formerly competent, is now incompetent to make decisions about her life-sustaining treatment and is unlikely to regain such competence. . . .

The *Quinlan* decision dealt with a special category of patients: those in a chronic, persistent vegetative or comatose state. In a footnote, the opinion left open the question whether the principles it enunciated might be applicable to incompetent patients in "other types of terminal medical situations . . . , not necessarily involving the hopeless loss of cognitive or sapient life." We now are faced with one such situation: that of elderly, formerly competent nursing-home residents who, unlike Karen Quinlan, are awake and conscious and can interact with their environment to a limited extent, but whose mental and physical functioning is severely and permanently impaired and whose life expectancy, even with the treatment, is relatively short. The capacities of such people, while significantly diminished, are not as limited as those of irreversibly comatose persons, and their deaths, while no longer distant, may not be imminent. Large numbers of aged, chronically ill, institutionalized persons fall within this general category.

Such people (like newborns, mentally retarded persons, permanently comatose individuals, and members of other groups with which this case does not deal) are unable to speak for themselves on life-and-death issues concerning their medical care. This does not mean, however, that they lack a right to self-determination. The right of an adult who, like Claire Conroy, was once competent, to determine the course of her medical treatment remains intact even when she is no longer able to assert that right or to appreciate its effectuation. As one commentator has noted:

> Even if the patient becomes too insensate to appreciate the honoring of his or her choice, self-determination is important. After all, law respects testamentary dispositions even if the testator never views his gift being bestowed. [Cantor, 30 *Rutgers L.Rev.* at 259.] . . .

Any other view would permit obliteration of an incompetent's panoply of rights merely because the patient could no longer sense the violation of those rights. [*Id.* at 252.]

Since the condition of an incompetent patient makes it impossible to ascertain definitively his present desires, a third party acting on the patient's behalf often cannot say with confidence that his treatment decision for the patient will further rather than frustrate the patient's right to control his body. Nevertheless, the goal of decision-making for incompetent patients should be to determine and effectuate, insofar as possible, the decision that the patient would have made if competent. Ideally, both aspects of the patient's right to bodily integrity—the right to consent to medical intervention and the right to refuse it—should be respected.

In light of these rights and concerns, we hold that life-sustaining treatment may be withheld or withdrawn from an incompetent patient when it is clear that the particular patient would have refused the treatment under the circumstances involved. The standard we are enunciating is a subjective one, consistent with the notion that the right that we are seeking to effectuate is a very personal right to control one's own life. The question is not what a reasonable or average person would have chosen to do under the circumstances but what the particular patient would have done if able to choose for himself.

The patient may have expressed, in one or more ways, an intent not to have life-sustaining medical intervention. Such an intent might be embodied in a written document, or "living will," stating the person's desire not to have certain types of life-sustaining treatment administered under certain circumstances. It might also be evidenced in an oral directive that the patient gave to a family member, friend, or health care provider. It might consist of a durable power of attorney or appointment of a proxy authorizing a particular person to make the decisions on the patient's behalf if he is no longer capable of making them for himself. It might take the form of reactions that the patient voiced regarding medical treatment administered to others. *See, e.g., Storar*, 52 N.Y.2d 363, 420 N.E.2d 64, 438 N.Y.S.2d 266 (withdrawal of respirator was justified as an effectuation of patient's stated wishes when patient, as member of Catholic religious order, had stated more than once in formal discussions concerning the moral implications of the *Quinlan* case, most recently two months before he suffered cardiac arrest that left him in an irreversible coma, that he would not want extraordinary means used to keep him alive under similar circumstances). It might also be deduced from a person's religious beliefs and the tenets of that religion, or from the patient's consistent pattern of conduct with respect to prior decisions about his own medical care. Of course, dealing with the matter in advance in some sort of thoughtful and explicit way is best for all concerned.

Any of the above types of evidence, and any other information bearing on the person's intent, may be appropriate aids in determining what course of treatment the patient would have wished to pursue. In this respect, we now believe that we were in error in *Quinlan*, to disregard evidence of statements that Ms. Quinlan made to friends concerning artificial prolongation of the lives of others who were terminally ill. Such evidence is certainly relevant to shed light on whether the patient would have consented to the treatment if competent to make the decision.

Although all evidence tending to demonstrate a person's intent with respect to medical treatment should properly be considered by either surrogate decision-makers, or by a court in the event of any judicial proceedings, the probative value of such evidence may vary depending on the remoteness, consistency, and thoughtfulness of the prior statements or actions and the maturity of the person at the time of the statements or acts. Thus, for example, an offhand remark about not wanting to live under certain circumstances made by a person when young and in the peak of health would not in itself constitute clear proof twenty years later that he would want life-sustaining treatment withheld under those circumstances. In contrast, a carefully considered position, especially if written, that a person had maintained over a number of years or that he had acted upon in comparable circumstances might be clear evidence of his intent.

Another factor that would affect the probative value of a person's prior statements of intent would be their specificity. Of course, no one can predict with accuracy the precise circumstances with which he ultimately might be faced. Nevertheless, any details about the level of impaired functioning and the forms of medical treatment that one would find tolerable should be incorporated into advance directives to enhance their later usefulness as evidence.

Medical evidence bearing on the patient's condition, treatment, and prognosis, like evidence of the patient's wishes, is an essential prerequisite to decision-making under the subjective test. The medical evidence must establish that the patient fits within the Claire Conroy pattern: an elderly, incompetent nursing-home resident with severe and permanent mental and physical impairments and a life expectancy of approximately one year or less. In addition, since the goal is to effectuate the patient's right of informed consent, the surrogate decision-maker must have at least as much medical information upon which to base his decision about what the patient would have chosen as one would expect a competent patient to have before consenting to or rejecting treatment. Such information might include evidence about the patient's present level of physical, sensory, emotional, and cognitive functioning; the degree of physical pain resulting from the medical condition, treatment, and termination of treatment, respectively; the degree of humiliation, dependence, and loss of dignity probably resulting from the condition and treatment; the life expectancy and prognosis for recovery with and without treatment; the various treatment options; and the risks, side effects, and benefits of each of those options. Particular care should be taken not to base a decision on a premature diagnosis or prognosis.

We recognize that for some incompetent patients it might be impossible to be clearly satisfied as to the patient's intent either to accept or reject the life-sustaining treatment. Many people may have spoken of their desires in general or casual terms, or, indeed, never considered or resolved the issue at all. In such cases, a surrogate decision-maker cannot presume that treatment decisions made by a third party on the patient's behalf will further the patient's right to self-determination, since effectuating another person's right to self-determination presupposes that the substitute decision-maker knows what the person would have wanted. Thus, in the absence of adequate proof of the patient's wishes, it is naive to pretend that the right to self-determination serves as the basis for substituted decision-making.

We hesitate, however, to foreclose the possibility of humane actions, which may involve termination of life-sustaining treatment, for persons who never clearly expressed their desires about life-sustaining treatment but who are now suffering a prolonged and painful death. An incompetent, like a minor child, is a ward of the state, and the state's *parens patriae* power supports the authority of its courts to allow decisions to be made for an incompetent that serve the incompetent's best interests, even if the person's wishes cannot be clearly established. This authority permits the state to authorize guardians to withhold or withdraw life-sustaining treatment from an incompetent patient if it is manifest that such action would further the patient's best interests in a narrow sense of the phrase, even though the subjective test that we articulated above may not be satisfied. We therefore hold that life-sustaining treatment may also be withheld or withdrawn from a patient in Claire Conroy's situation if either of two "best interests" tests—a limited-objective or a pure-objective test— is satisfied.

Under the limited-objective test, life-sustaining treatment may be withheld or withdrawn from a patient in Claire Conroy's situation when there is some trustworthy evidence that the patient would have refused the treatment, and the decision-maker is satisfied that it is clear that the burdens of the patient's continued life with the treatment outweigh the benefits of that life for him. By this we mean that the patient is suffering, and will continue to suffer throughout the expected duration of his life, unavoidable pain, and that the net burdens of his prolonged life (the pain and suffering of his life with the treatment less the amount and duration of pain that the patient would likely experience if the treatment were withdrawn) markedly outweigh any physical pleasure, emotional enjoyment, or intellectual satisfaction that the patient may still be able to derive from life. This limited-objective standard permits the termination of treatment for a patient who had not unequivocally expressed his desires before becoming incompetent, when it is clear that the treatment in question would merely prolong the patient's suffering.

Medical evidence will be essential to establish that the burdens of the treatment to the patient in terms of pain and suffering outweigh the benefits that the patient is experiencing. The medical evidence should make it clear that the treatment would merely prolong the patient's suffering and not provide him with any net benefit. Information

is particularly important with respect to the degree, expected duration, and constancy of pain with and without treatment, and the possibility that the pain could be reduced by drugs or other means short of terminating the life-sustaining treatment. The same types of medical evidence that are relevant to the subjective analysis, such as the patient's life expectancy, prognosis, level of functioning, degree of humiliation and dependency, and treatment options, should also be considered.

This limited-objective test also requires some trustworthy evidence that the patient would have wanted the treatment terminated. This evidence could take any one or more of the various forms appropriate to prove the patient's intent under the subjective test. Evidence that, taken as a whole, would be too vague, casual, or remote to constitute the clear proof of the patient's subjective intent that is necessary to satisfy the subjective test—for example, informally expressed reactions to other people's medical conditions and treatment—might be sufficient to satisfy this prong of the limited-objective test.

In the absence of trustworthy evidence, or indeed any evidence at all, that the patient would have declined the treatment, life-sustaining treatment may still be withheld or withdrawn from a formerly competent person like Claire Conroy if a third, pure-objective test is satisfied. Under that test, as under the limited-objective test, the net burdens of the patient's life with the treatment should clearly and markedly outweigh the benefits that the patient derives from life. Further, the recurring, unavoidable, and severe pain of the patient's life with the treatment should be such that the effect of administering life-sustaining treatment would be inhumane. Subjective evidence that the patient would not have wanted the treatment is not necessary under this pure-objective standard. Nevertheless, even in the context of severe pain, life-sustaining treatment should not be withdrawn from an incompetent patient who had previously expressed a wish to be kept alive in spite of any pain that he might experience.

Although we are condoning a restricted evaluation of the nature of a patient's life in terms of pain, suffering, and possible enjoyment under the limited-objective and pure-objective tests, we expressly decline to authorize decision-making based on assessments of the personal worth or social utility of another's life, or the value of that life to others. We do not believe that it would be appropriate for a court to designate a person with the authority to determine that someone else's life is not worth living simply because, to that person, the patient's "quality of life" or value to society seems negligible. The mere fact that a patient's functioning is limited or his prognosis dim does not mean that he is not enjoying what remains of his life or that it is in his best interests to die. But see *President's Commission Report*, at 135 (endorsing termination of treatment whenever the surrogate decision-maker in his discretion believes it is in the patient's best interests, defined broadly to "take into account such factors as the relief of suffering, the preservation or restoration of functioning, and the quality as well as the extent of life sustained"). More wide-ranging powers to make decisions about other people's lives, in our view, would create an intolerable risk for socially isolated and defenseless people suffering from physical or mental handicaps.

We are aware that it will frequently be difficult to conclude that the evidence is sufficient to justify termination of treatment under either of the "best interests" tests that we have described. Often, it is unclear whether and to what extent a patient such as Claire Conroy is capable of, or is in fact, experiencing pain. Similarly, medical experts are often unable to determine with any degree of certainty the extent of a nonverbal person's intellectual functioning or the depth of his emotional life. When the evidence is insufficient to satisfy either the limited-objective or pure-objective standard, however, we cannot justify the termination of life-sustaining treatment as clearly furthering the best interests of a patient like Ms. Conroy.

The surrogate decision-maker should exercise extreme caution in determining the patient's intent and in evaluating medical evidence of the patient's pain and possible enjoyment, and should not approve withholding or withdrawing life-sustaining treatment unless he is manifestly satisfied that one of the three tests that we have outlined has been met. When evidence of a person's wishes or physical or mental condition is equivocal, it is best to err, if at all, in favor of preserving life. . . .

II

We emphasize that in making decisions whether to administer life-sustaining treatment to patients such as Claire Conroy, the primary focus should be the patient's desires and experience of pain and enjoyment—not the type of treatment involved. Thus, we reject the distinction that some have made between actively hastening death by terminating treatment and passively allowing a person to die of a disease as one of limited use in a legal analysis of such a decision-making situation.

Characterizing conduct as active or passive is often an elusive notion, even outside the context of medical decision-making.

> Saint Anselm of Canterbury was fond of citing the trickiness of the distinction between "to do" (*facere*) and "not to do" (*non facere*). In answer to the question "What's he doing?" we say "He's just sitting there" (positive), really meaning something negative: "He's not doing anything at all." [*D. Walton*, at 234 (footnote omitted).]

The distinction is particularly nebulous, however, in the context of decisions whether to withhold or withdraw life-sustaining treatment. In a case like that of Claire Conroy, for example, would a physician who discontinued nasogastric feeding be actively causing her death by removing her primary source of nutrients, or would he merely be omitting to continue the artificial form of treatment, thus passively allowing her medical condition, which includes her inability to swallow, to take its natural course? The ambiguity inherent in this distinction is further heightened when one performs an act within an overall plan of nonintervention, such as when a doctor writes an order not to resuscitate a patient.

> Consequently, merely determining whether what was done involved a fatal act or omission does not establish whether it was morally acceptable. . . . [In fact, a]ctive steps to terminate life-sustaining interventions may be permitted, indeed required, by the patient's authority to forego therapy even when such steps lead to death. [*President's Commission Report*, at 67, 72.]

For a similar reason, we also reject any distinction between withholding and withdrawing life-sustaining treatment. Some commentators have suggested that discontinuing life-sustaining treatment once it has been commenced is morally more problematic than merely failing to begin the treatment. Discontinuing life-sustaining treatment, to some, is an "active" taking of life, as opposed to the more "passive" act of omitting the treatment in the first instance. In the words of one writer, "[T]he difference between taking away that which one has come to count on as normal support for life and not instituting therapy when a new crisis begins . . . fits nicely a basic moral distinction throughout life—we are not morally obligated to help another person, but we are morally obligated not to interfere with his life-sustaining routines."

This distinction is more psychologically compelling than logically sound. As mentioned above, the line between active and passive conduct in the context of medical decisions is far too nebulous to constitute a principled basis for decision-making. Whether necessary treatment is withheld at the outset or withdrawn later on, the consequence—the patient's death—is the same. Moreover, from a policy standpoint, it might well be unwise to forbid persons from discontinuing a treatment under circumstances in which the treatment could permissibly be withheld. Such a rule could discourage families and doctors from even attempting certain types of care and could thereby force them into hasty and premature decisions to allow a patient to die.

Some commentators, as indeed did the Appellate Division here, have made yet a fourth distinction, between the termination of artificial feedings and the termination of other forms of life-sustaining medical treatment. According to the Appellate Division:

> If, as here, the patient is not comatose and does not face imminent and inevitable death, nourishment accomplishes the substantial benefit of sustaining life until the illness takes its natural course. Under such circumstances nourishment always will be an essential element of ordinary care which physicians are ethically obligated to provide. [190 *N.J.Super.* at 473, 464, A.2d 303.]

Certainly, feeding has an emotional significance. As infants we could breathe without assistance, but we were dependent on others for our lifeline of nourishment. Even more, feeding is an expression of nurturing and caring, certainly for infants and children, and in many cases for adults as well.

Once one enters the realm of complex, high-technology medical care, it is hard to shed the "emotional symbolism" of food. However, artificial feedings such as nasogastric tubes, gastrostomies, and intravenous infusions are significantly different from bottle-feeding or spoon-feeding—they are medical procedures with inherent risks and possible side effects, instituted by skilled health-care providers to compensate for impaired physical functioning. Analytically, artificial feeding by means of a nasogastric tube or intravenous infusion can be seen as equivalent to artificial breathing by means of a respirator. Both prolong life through mechanical means when the body is no longer able to perform a vital bodily function on its own.

Furthermore, while nasogastric feeding and other medical procedures to ensure nutrition and hydration are usually well tolerated, they are not free from risks or burdens; they have complications that are sometimes serious and distressing to the patient.

Nasogastric tubes may lead to pneumonia, cause irritation and discomfort, and require arm restraints for an incompetent patient. The volume of fluid needed to carry nutrients itself is sometimes harmful.

Finally, dehydration may well not be distressing or painful to a dying patient. For patients who are unable to sense hunger and thirst, withholding of feeding devices such as nasogastric tubes may not result in more pain than the termination of any other medical treatment. Indeed, it has been observed that patients near death who are not receiving nourishment may be more comfortable than patients in comparable conditions who are being fed and hydrated artificially. Thus, it cannot be assumed that it will always be beneficial for an incompetent patient to receive artificial feeding or harmful for him not to receive it.

Under the analysis articulated above, withdrawal or withholding of artificial feeding, like any other medical treatment, would be permissible if there is sufficient proof to satisfy the subjective, limited-objective, or pure-objective test. A competent patient has the right to decline any medical treatment, including artificial feeding, and should retain that right when and if he becomes incompetent. In addition, in the case of an incompetent patient who has given little or no trustworthy indication of an intent to decline treatment and for whom it becomes necessary to engage in balancing under the limited-objective or pure-objective test, the pain and invasiveness of an artificial feeding device, and the pain of withdrawing that device, should be treated just like the results of administering or withholding any other medical treatment.

III

The decision-making procedure for comatose, vegetative patients suggested in *Quinlan*, namely, the concurrence of the guardian, family, attending physician, and hospital prognosis committee, is not entirely appropriate for patients such as Claire Conroy, who are confined to nursing homes. . . .

Because of the special vulnerability of mentally and physically impaired, elderly persons in nursing homes and the potential for abuse with unsupervised institutional decision-making in such homes, life-sustaining treatment should not be withdrawn or withheld from a nursing-home resident like Claire Conroy in the absence of a guardian's decision, made in accordance with the procedure outlined below, that the elements of the subjective, limited-objective, or pure-objective test have been satisfied. A necessary prerequisite to surrogate decision-making is a judicial determination that the patient is incompetent to make the decision for himself and designation of a guardian for the incompetent patient if he does not already have one.

As noted above, the guardian will resolve the issues in these matters and make the ultimate decision with such concurrences as we have required. Ordinarily, court involvement will be limited to the determination of incompetency, and the appointment of a guardian unless a personal guardian has been previously appointed, who will determine whether the standards we have prescribed have been satisfied. The record in this case did not satisfy those standards. The evidence that Claire Conroy would have refused the treatment, although sufficient to meet the lower showing of intent required under the limited-objective test, was certainly not the "clear" showing of intent contemplated under the subjective test. More information should, if possible, have been obtained by the guardian with respect to Ms. Conroy's intent. What were her ethical, moral, and religious beliefs? She did try to refuse initial hospi-

talization, and indeed had "scorned medicine." However, she allowed her nephew's wife, a registered nurse, to care for her during several illnesses. It was not clear whether Ms. Conroy permitted the niece to administer any drugs or other forms of medical treatment to her during these illnesses. Although it may often prove difficult, and at times impossible, to ascertain a person's wishes, the Conroy case illustrates the sources to which the guardian might turn. For example, in more than eight decades of life in the same house, it is possible that she revealed to persons other than her nephew her feelings regarding medical treatment, other values, and her goals in life. Some promising avenues for such an inquiry about her personal values included her response to the illnesses and deaths of her sisters and others, and her statements with respect to not wanting to be in a nursing home.

Moreover, there was insufficient information concerning the benefits and burdens of Ms. Conroy's life to satisfy either the limited-objective or pure-objective test. Although the treating doctor and the guardian's expert testified as to Claire Conroy's condition, neither testified conclusively as to whether she was in pain or was capable of experiencing pain or thirst. There was medical agreement that removal of the tube would have caused pain during the period of approximately one week that would have elapsed before her death, or at least until she were to lapse into a coma. On the other hand, there was little, if any, evidence of the discomfort, suffering, and pain she would endure if she continued to be fed and medicated through the tube during her remaining life—contemplated to be up to one year. Apparently her feedings sometimes occasioned moaning, but it remains unclear whether these were reflex responses or expressions of discomfort. Moreover, although she tried to remove the tube, it is not clear that this was intentional, and there was little evidence that she was in distress. Her treating physician also offered contradictory views as to whether the contractures of her legs caused pain or whether, indeed, they might be the result of pain, without offering any evidence on that issue. The trial court rejected as superfluous the offer to present as an expert witness a neurologist, who might have been able to explain what Ms. Conroy's reactions to the environment indicated about her perception of pain.

The evidence was also unclear with respect to Ms. Conroy's capacity to feel pleasure, another issue as to which the information supplied by a neurologist might have been helpful. What was known of her awareness of the world? Although Ms. Conroy had some ability to smile and scratch, the relationship of these activities to external stimuli apparently was quite variable.

The trial transcript reveals no exploration of the discomfort and risks that attend nasogastric feedings. A casual mention by the nurse/administrator of the need to restrain the patient to prevent the removal of the tube was not followed by an assessment of the detrimental impact, if any, of those restraints. Alternative modalities, including gastrostomies, intravenous feeding, subcutaneous or intramuscular hydration, or some combination, were not investigated. Neither of the expert witnesses presented empirical evidence regarding the treatment options for such a patient.

It can be seen that the evidence at trial was inadequate to satisfy the subjective, the limited-objective, or the pure-objective standard that we have set forth. Were Claire Conroy still alive, the guardian would have been required to explore these issues prior to reaching any decision. Guardians—and courts, if they are involved—should act cautiously and deliberately in deciding these cases. The consequences are most serious—life or death. . . .

The judgment of the Appellate Division is reversed. In light of Ms. Conroy's death, we do not remand the matter for further proceedings.

HANDLER, J., concurring in part and dissenting in part. . . .

In my opinion, the Court's objective tests too narrowly define the interests of people like Miss Conroy. While the basic standard purports to account for several concerns, it ultimately focuses on pain as the critical factor. The presence of significant pain in effect becomes the sole measure of such a person's best interests. "Pain" thus eclipses a whole cluster of other human values that have a proper place in the subtle weighing that will ultimately determine how life should end.

The Court's concentration on pain as the exclusive criterion in reaching the life-or-death decision in reality transmutes the best-interests determination into an exercise of avoidance and nullification rather than confrontation and fulfillment. In most

cases the pain criterion will dictate that the decision be one not to withdraw life-prolonging treatment and not to allow death to occur naturally. First, pain will not be an operative factor in a great many cases. "[P]resently available drugs and techniques allow pain to be reduced to a level acceptable to virtually every patient, usually without unacceptable sedation." *President's Commission Report*, at 50–51. *See id.* at 19 n. 19 *citing* Saunders, "Current Views on Pain Relief and Terminal Care," in *The Therapy of Pain* 215 (Swerdlow, ed. 1981) (a hospice reports complete control of pain in over 99% of its dying patients). Further, as was true in Miss Conroy's case, health care providers frequently encounter difficulty in evaluating the degree of pain experienced by a patient. Finally, "[o]nly a minority of patients—fewer than half of those with malignancies, for example—have substantial problems with pain. . . ." *President's Commission Report*, at 278. Thus, in a great many cases, the pain test will become an absolute bar to the withdrawal of life-support therapy.

The pain requirement, as applied by the Court in its objective tests, effectively negates other highly relevant considerations that should appropriately bear on the decision to maintain or to withdraw life-prolonging treatment. The pain standard may dictate the decision to prolong life despite the presence of other factors that reasonably militate in favor of the termination of such procedures to allow a natural death. The exclusive pain criterion denies relief to that class of people who, at the very end of life, might strongly disapprove of an artificially extended existence in spite of the absence of pain. Thus, some people abhor dependence on others as much, or more, than they fear pain. Other individuals value personal privacy and dignity, and prize independence from others when their personal needs and bodily functions are involved. Finally, the ideal of bodily integrity may become more important than simply prolonging life at its most rudimentary level. Persons, like Miss Conroy, "may well have wished to avoid . . . '[t]he ultimate horror [not of] death but the possibility of being maintained in limbo, in a sterile room, by machines controlled by strangers.'" *In re Torres*, 357 N.W.2d at 340, quoting Steel, "The Right to Die: New Options in California," 93 *Christian Century* [July–Dec. 1976].

Clearly, a decision to focus exclusively on pain as the single criterion ignores and devalues other important ideals regarding life and death. Consequently, a pain standard cannot serve as an indirect proxy for additional and significant concerns that may bear on the decision to forgo life-prolonging treatments. . . .

I would therefore have the Court adopt a test that does not rely exclusively on pain as the ultimately determinative criterion. Rather, the standard should consist of an array of factors to be medically established and then evaluated by the decision-maker both singly and collectively to reach a balance that will justify the determination to withdraw or to continue life-prolonging treatment. The withdrawal of life-prolonging treatment from an unconscious or comatose, terminally ill individual near death, whose personal views concerning life-ending treatment cannot be ascertained, should be governed by such a standard.

Several important criteria bear on this critical determination. The person should be terminally ill and facing imminent death. There should also be present the permanent loss of conscious thought processes in the form of a comatose state or profound unconsciousness. Further, there should be the irreparable failure of at least one major and essential bodily organ or system. Obviously the presence or absence of significant pain is highly relevant.

In addition, the person's general physical condition must be of great concern. Progressive, irreversible, extensive, and extreme physical deterioration, such as ulcers, lesions, gangrene, infection, incontinence, and the like, which frequently afflict the bedridden, terminally ill, should be considered

in the formulation of an appropriate standard. The medical and nursing treatment of individuals in *extremis* and suffering from these conditions entails the constant and extensive handling and manipulation of the body. At some point, such a course of treatment upon the insensate patient is bound to touch the sensibilities of even the most detached observer. Eventually, pervasive bodily intrusions, even for the best motives, will arouse feelings akin to humiliation and mortification for the helpless patient. When cherished values of human dignity and personal privacy, which belong to every person living or dying, are sufficiently transgressed by what is being done to the individual, we should be ready to say: enough.

In my view, our understanding as to how life should end must be infused with the fundamental human moral values that serve us while we live. As we have faced life, so should we be able to face death. When an individual's personal philosophy or moral values cannot otherwise be brought to bear to resolve the dilemma of whether to live or die, then factors that generally and normally shape basic human moral values should be taken into account. These factors should be assessed reasonably and fairly from the patient's perspective. They should be weighed and balanced by an appropriate, responsible surrogate decision-maker in reaching the final awesome decision whether to withdraw life-prolonging treatment from the unfortunate and hapless patient. I believe that a decision informed by these considerations would be conducive to the humane, dignified, and decent ending of life.

The Severely Demented, Minimally Functional Patient: An Ethical Analysis

John D. Arras

Mrs. Smith, an 85-year-old resident of a nursing home, was transferred to the hospital for treatment of pneumonia. Although she has respond-

From *Journal of the American Geriatrics Society* 36 (1988): 938–944. Reprinted with permission.

ed well to antibiotic therapy, her overall condition and prognosis remain grim. For the past 3 years her mental state has been steadily deteriorating due to a series of strokes which have finally rendered her severely demented. She is now nonambulatory, incapable of sitting up in bed, and uncommunicative most of the time. When she does talk, her speech is completely incoherent and repetitive. Mrs. Smith shows no signs of recognizing or remembering her family and primary caregivers. The nurses in charge of her care assert that she appears to experience pleasure only when her hair is combed or her back rubbed.

During her recovery from the pneumonia, Mrs. Smith began to have problems with swallowing food. Following a precipitous decline in her caloric intake, her son and daughter (the only involved family members) consented to the placement of a nasogastric tube. Mrs. Smith continually pulled out the tube, however, and continues to resist efforts to reinsert it.

The health care team faces difficult choices regarding Mrs. Smith's care. Foremost among them is whether her physicians should surgically insert a gastrostomy tube in spite of her aversive behavior. Mrs. Smith has neither left behind a living will nor has she indicated to family or friends at the nursing home what her preferences would be regarding life-sustaining care in this sort of circumstance. Both her son and daughter have stated that she would nevertheless not have wanted a gastrostomy tube inserted and would, if she could presently decide, prefer an earlier death to being sustained indefinitely in the twilight of her minimally functional condition. In defense of this claim, they note that she has always been a very active, independent person who avoided doctors whenever possible.

PROBING THE PATIENT'S SUBJECTIVITY

The first order of business in deciding for incompetent patients is to inquire, whenever possible, what the patient would want were she presently able to communicate. In the absence of a designated proxy or living will that speaks with rare precision about which modes of treatment are to be forgone under which circumstances, this task is more difficult than many commentators and jurists would have us think. The case before us yields two distinct sources of revelation bearing on the patient's putative subjective wishes regarding the present decision. As we shall see, neither provides evidence sufficiently compelling for us to conclude

with moral certitude that she would not allow the insertion of a G-tube.

EXTRAPOLATING FROM THE PATIENT'S PRIOR VALUES

First, we have the testimony of family members who claim that the patient's character traits of independence and aloofness from physicians point to the conclusion that she would not want to be sustained by a G-tube. Although this claim may well be *plausible* and at least *consistent* with Mrs. Smith's previously held attitudes and behaviors, it would require a great leap of both faith and logic to conclude that evidence of this sort *entails* a negative decision on life-sustaining treatment. As several commentators have pointed out, there is a great difference between the degree of respect owed to a patient's *actual choices*, even choices made prior to the advent of incompetency, and to his or her preferences or tastes.[1-4] It is one thing to have negative attitudes toward aggressive life support, but it is quite another to actually refuse it in your own case. By doing so, a person *commits* himself or herself to a particular course of action and it is this commitment, rather than mere attitudes or generalized preferences abstracted from the particular details of choosing situations, that commands especially stringent respect.

Even if someone's generalized views about life, dependency, and doctors deserve the status of right claims, which they do not, they usually do not yield unequivocal answers to treatment dilemmas. Supposing that Mrs. Smith was indeed fiercely independent and skeptical of the medical profession, does this necessarily mean that she would prefer death to her present "twilight state" sustained by tube feedings? Conversely, if Mrs. Smith were an exceptionally dependent sort of person who actively sought and followed the advice of physicians, would that mean that she would presently prefer an indefinite extension of her barely conscious existence to an early death? Although such character traits indisputably have *some* evidentiary value, they appear to be compatible with a range of possible responses.[4] In Mrs. Smith's case, it is certainly *plausible* that she would decline the insertion of a G-tube, but that is not the only plausible interpretation. For all we know, she might have been content, were she miraculously lucid and communicative for an instant, to accede to the operation rather than go peacefully into that dark night. The question for Mrs. Smith's caregivers, then—and we shall explore this point more fully later on—is not whether her loved ones have provided a uniquely correct extrapolation of her previous values to her present situation, for in most cases that will simply be an unattainable goal; rather, the question is whether their plausible invocations of her values and character traits should be given the benefit of the doubt.

THE EVIDENTIARY VALUE OF AVERSIVE BEHAVIOR

Mrs. Smith has been constantly pulling out her nasogastric tube and waving off the attentions of her caregivers. What are we to make of this behavior? In contrast to the patient's previous preferences and attitudes, which are ill-matched in their generality to the concreteness of the present situation, Mrs. Smith's aversive behavior at least has the advantage of being contemporaneous. She is extubating herself right here and now. According to Daniel Callahan,[5] a philosopher who generally sees no justification for terminating food and fluids in severely demented patients, such behavior constitutes a "clear signal" mandating withdrawal of the tube.

But a clear signal of what? It is crucial to remember at this juncture that Mrs. Smith is severely demented and completely incompetent. Even though her aversive behavior occurs in the present, it is the behavior of a woman who has completely lost her rational capacity. She cannot even recognize her family, let alone engage in sophisticated deliberations bearing on the respective benefits and burdens of continued tube feeding in her minimally functional state versus an earlier death. Aphasic but otherwise competent patients might be able to send clear signals under such circumstances, but not Mrs. Smith, whose behavior appears to be freighted with a variety of possible meanings.

It is possible that her tube-pulling represents a firm and fixed present desire to forgo aggressive life-sustaining treatments in favor of an early death. It is also possible that it signals some kind of deeply sedimented personal desire manifested in spite of her present incompetence. But it is equally possible that her aversive behavior is nothing more than an elemental reflex signalling only her transient irritation from the tube. Nasogastric tubes *are* bothersome and sometimes painful intrusions, and one need not entertain sophisticated benefit-burden calculations to wish merely to be rid of such noxious stimuli. Thus, the interpretive options range from deeply intentional options for death in the face of minimally functional existence to reflexes of an almost exclusively physiological nature.

Mrs. Smith's "signal" is thus anything but clear, and this is a significant fact for her caregivers to ponder. While aversive behavior expressive of deeply sedimented personal values should be accorded the same degree of respect allotted to general character traits and attitudes, aversive reflexes to unpleasant stimuli should command little, if any, deference from surrogate decision-makers. Small children extubate themselves all the time, but no one would view such actions as a "clear signal" of a wish to die. The real problem facing Mrs. Smith's physicians is that they have no reliable way of discerning the "real meaning" behind her ongoing resistance to feeding tubes. It would certainly help if Mrs. Smith had been known to shun tube feeding even while she was competent, for that would at least provide some plausible evidence connecting her presently aversive behavior to sedimented preferences. But in the absence of such a record, the meaning of her "rejection" remains profoundly unclear.

Given the inconclusiveness of this inquiry into the patient's previous attitudes and present behavior, her caregivers might reasonably shift their focus of attention away from the patient's elusive subjectivity and toward a more objective assessment of her "best interests."

THE BEST-INTERESTS STANDARD

In the absence of reliable indicators of the patient's actual or hypothetical preferences, courts and commentators recommend an inquiry into the best interests of the patient.[6,7] What course of action (or inaction) will bring about the best overall result for the patient? Rather than finding this "objective" path an easier route to the correct decision, caregivers attempting to apply such a test to the case of a severely demented, minimally functional patient such as Mrs. Smith will immediately confront a series of equally perplexing questions. What will be the actual impact of placing a G-tube on Mrs. Smith's well-being? What definition of the good will ground their assessments of her best interests? And, given her low level of functioning, is it quite accurate even to describe Mrs. Smith as a full-fledged "person" with actual, discernable interests? Since these exceedingly difficult questions lack intuitively obvious answers, perhaps the best way to proceed is to examine categories of patients on either side of Mrs. Smith on the continuum of incompetency, categories that do yield fairly firm moral intuitions, and then attempt to locate a proper response to her case by means of "moral triangulation." Needless to say, the clarity and distinctness of these idealized categories often become somewhat blurred in real clinical situations, but there is still considerable theoretical value in discussing our responses to clear-cut cases.

PATIENTS IN PERSISTENT VEGETATIVE STATES

What if, instead of being minimally functional, Mrs. Smith were completely nonfunctional? (We shall call this hypothetical patient Mrs. Jones.) What if, instead of slowly declining into a twilight of consciousness, she were to have experienced a protracted period of anoxia that consigned her to a persistently vegetative condition? Although still alive, Mrs. Jones would subsist on brain-stem activity alone, her neocortex—the physical substratum of her capacity for consciousness—having been completely destroyed. She would thus persist in countless sleep-wake cycles, unable to connect with the world and with her past through conscious awareness, unable to plan or hope for better circumstances, unable even to perceive pleasure or pain. What rights, if any, would Mrs. Jones have, and what duties would be owed her by caregivers?

If we were to apply straightforwardly the best-interests test to the case of Mrs. Jones, we would be hard-pressed to discover actual interests that could be meaningfully imputed to her. Lacking consciousness, she lacks a conception of herself as a moral agent with real interests in continued life and in the pursuit of her own vision of the good. Lacking the ability to experience pleasure and pain, she cannot be physically benefitted or harmed.[8] Indeed, as several commentators have pointed out, her only remaining interest in staying alive is based on the miniscule possibility that she has been misdiagnosed and could possibly regain some degree of consciousness in the future.[9] Apart from that slimmest of chances, she has no interests that might be assessed through a best-interests test.

If we seek a solution to the problem of Mrs. Jones in an examination of her best interests, we discover the paradoxical result that her best interests will probably be served by further treatment. True, except for the possibility of misdiagnosis, she cannot be benefitted in any way by continued existence, but her lack of capacity for conscious experience renders her equally incapable of being harmed by further treatments and the extension of her life. Thus, we cannot say, as the best-interests test would appear to require, that Mrs. Jones is being excessively burdened by her treatments or that she would be "better-off dead." This result is indeed paradoxical, because if anyone's life need not be maintained, one would think that patients in persistently vegetative conditions must be at the top of the list.

Given the vanishingly small likelihood of misdiagnosis, especially after the passage of several weeks, I would argue that it is ethically appropriate to treat all PVS patients as though they had no interests either for or against treatment. Since continued medical interventions cannot realistically be thought to benefit them in any way, since caregivers cannot realistically be thought to have duties toward patients who cannot be helped or harmed, and since such treatments entail considerable costs—including the expenditure of huge sums of money, the time and energy of caregivers, and emotional strains on survivors—they may be ethically forgone.

The important lesson here is that although a rigorously patient-centered best-interests test might be ethically appropriate in most cases involving incompetent patients, it cannot be meaningfully applied when the patient under consideration lacks all fundamentally human capacities. In cases such as this, a judgment in favor of nontreatment must be based not on an objective weighing of benefits and burdens to the patient—for such patients are capable of neither benefit nor burden—but rather upon a judgment that the patient has ceased to be a "person" in any meaningful moral sense. Once this determination has been made, it is then ethically permissible to consider the financial and emotional impact of continued treatment upon other interested parties.[10] Certainly some families will, for religious or other personal reasons, continue to request life-sustaining treatments for their persistently vegetative relations; but others would be acting ethically to request the termination of all medical care, including artificially administered food and fluids.

MARGINALLY FUNCTIONAL PATIENTS

On the other side of Mrs. Smith are those patients who might usefully be described as "marginally functional." Mr. Black, for example, is a 90-year-old man presenting with rectal bleeding and suspected colon cancer who refuses a laparotomy to confirm the diagnosis. "I have lived a good life," he says, "and I don't want any surgery." His daughter, to whom he appears very close, concurs with his decision. Although Mr. Black appears on the surface to be sufficiently competent to make this decision, subsequent examinations by liaison psychiatrists reveal a glaring absence of short-term memory and significant confusion about his medical diagnosis and surroundings. He is described as "pleasantly demented."

Although patients like Mr. Black are strictly speaking incapable of rational decision-making most or all of the time, they differ from Mrs. Jones in their ability to reason, albeit rather poorly, in their ability to relate to other persons, and in their capacities to experience emotions, pain, and pleasure. Notwithstanding their inability to make most health care decisions, these patients are clearly "persons" with a multitude of interests that can be advanced or frustrated by their caregivers. In spite of their deficits and relatively low quality of life, such moderately functional patients have every right to a patient-centered best-interests analysis. While invasive, painful, and risky surgery may or may not eventually be deemed to be in Mr. Black's best interests, his capacities for experiencing the world are sufficiently intact to rule out any thought of forgoing other sorts of life-sustaining therapies, such as artificial nutrition and hydration.

THE MINIMALLY FUNCTIONAL PATIENT

Returning now to the example of Mrs. Smith, we find her to fall squarely between the permanently vegetative and moderately functional patient. Like the totally nonfunctional, vegetative patient, she is so demented that she lacks most of the criteria of "moral personhood."[11] Unfortunately, she appears to have been reduced to a mere shell of her former self. She can no longer reason, communicate (except in the most rudimentary, reflexive manner), relate to her family, or experience manifestations of love. Indeed, it is doubtful that she can be accurately described as a self-conscious, moral agent whose identity through time is cemented by the bonds of memory. There is, in cases such as this where the psychological glue of memory has given out, simply no enduring "self" there.[12] Formerly a self-conscious moral agent with a well-defined idea of the good, hopes and plans for the future, Mrs. Smith has been reduced to a mere locus of transient sensations. As philosopher James Rachels[13] puts it, she continues to have biological life, but her *biographical* life has come to an end.

On the other hand, Mrs. Smith resembles Mr. Black at least in her possession of some conscious life, albeit on a very low level, and in her ability to experience pleasure, pain, and perhaps some rudimentary emotions. Although she is not a "person" in the strict sense, she does have some interests. Insofar as she is open to pleasure and pain, she has a definite interest in experiencing the former and avoiding the latter. How might a "best-interests" test be applied to someone like Mrs. Smith?

Better-Off Dead?   In order to justify the termination of food and fluids under a best-interests test, decision-makers would have to show that the burdens of a patient's life with the proposed treatment would clearly and markedly outweigh whatever benefits she might derive from continued life.[7] In other words, they would have to show that the patient would be "better-off dead."

The most influential formulation of this best-interests test, the majority opinion in the Conroy case, requires not merely that the burdens of life clearly outweigh the benefits, but also that further treatment would be inhumane due to the presence of severe and uncontrollable pain.[7] The court's motivation in establishing such a strict standard is not hard to grasp. While people might disagree about the desirability of persisting in a minimally functional condition, severe and intractable pain is presumably something that just about everyone would prefer to avoid. It is this nearly universal sentiment that death would be preferable to a life of unmitigated pain and suffering that gives this test an air of "objectivity," as opposed to the subjectivity of tests based upon the patient's past preferences.

How then would this strict formula apply to Mrs. Smith? As we have seen, there isn't much to place in the "benefits" column. No longer able to take food by mouth or to interact meaningfully with her family and caregivers, it appears that Mrs. Smith experiences few pleasures apart from an occasional rub or combing. The only possible benefit to be derived from further treatment would appear to be the indefinite continuation of this twilight existence. And although the patient might conceivably derive some pleasure merely from lying in bed and dwelling in her alien world, it is highly doubtful that such a patient—bereft of memory, a sense of continuing selfhood, hopes, and plans—could possibly have an interest in, or be benefitted by, *continued* existence.

Given Mrs. Smith's low level of existence, it is equally difficult to discern the burdens of continued treatment. To be sure, she will experience some degree of pain and discomfort from the surgical insertion of a G-tube, but this pain will not approximate the kind of prolonged, severe, and intractable pain required by the Conroy best-interests formula.

Another possible source of pain and suffering would be the forcible imposition of medical treatment against the wishes of the incompetent patient. Even incompetent patients can have strong preferences for or against treatment or diagnostic procedures, and even if these preferences are not well grounded in medical reality or in the patient's previously authentic value system, forcible treatment will often be experienced as a painful and humiliating violation. Although this kind of coercion need not be thought of as a violation of the patient's autonomy, which may have already been destroyed by dementia, the pain, humiliation, distrust, and hostility it engenders must nevertheless be counted in any best-interests calculation. In some cases, Mr. Black's for example, the negative consequences of forcing treatment may not be worth the gains.

In Mrs. Smith's case, however, the side effects of coercive treatment are likely to be nonexistent. As we have already seen, her aversive reaction to NG tube feeding could just as easily be ascribed to immediate physical discomfort as to some deep-seated desire to die through the refusal of life-sustaining treatment. Mrs. Smith is probably too demented at this point to have preferences about tube feedings or to acknowledge the forcible imposition of surgery over against her aversive behavior. It is highly unlikely, then, that she would experience the insertion of a G-tube as a violation of her wishes (no matter how distorted) or as a painful humiliation.

In the absence of any persistent and severe pain underlying her condition, it would appear highly doubtful that the burdens of Mrs. Smith's continued existence clearly and markedly outweigh the benefits, even when the benefits approach zero. A literal reading and application of the Conroy formula would thus lead to the conclusion that the G-tube should be surgically implanted and that she should be maintained indefinitely with artificial nutrition and hydration.

Limitations of the Best-Interests Standard   Not everyone will be satisfied with this result. Those who believe that quality of life should never affect treatment decisions will no doubt applaud this conclusion, but others might well think that something important has been left out of our deliberations. Judge Handler,[7] the lone dissenter in *Conroy*, identifies this missing factor as a legitimate concern for the patient's probable feelings about broader issues, such as privacy, dependency, dignity, and bodily integrity. By focusing the entire best-interests discussion upon the narrow issue of pain, we tend to reduce the patient from the full-fledged person that she once was to the status of a mere physical repository of pleasures and pains. Is this crudely hedonistic notion of the good an adequate or desirable measure of humane treatment decisions for minimally functional patients? Should we simply ignore the patient's probable responses to such abject dependency and daily violations of dignity?

Although Judge Handler's dissent eloquently pinpoints a major shortcoming of the *Conroy* best-interests formula, it is problematical in its own right. Specifically, it is unclear how Judge Handler's concerns for these larger issues of privacy and dignity might be grafted onto the *Conroy* best-interests formula. That test, let us recall, attempts to ascertain the *present* best interests of patients; it asks about the present and future benefits and burdens likely to be experienced by the patient. The obvious problem for Judge Handler's proposed enlargement of this formula is that severely demented, minimally functional patients like Mrs. Smith are presently incapable of experiencing what more functional patients would describe as insults to their privacy, dignity, and physical integrity. Although it is quite possible that the formerly competent Mrs. Smith would have been appalled at the loss of dignity entailed by her present situation, the present Mrs. Smith knows nothing of dignitary insults or violations of privacy. She is so demented that she cannot be affected, one way or the other, by solicitude for her present responses to these larger, humanistic issues.

In order to vindicate Judge Handler's concerns, we will have to reintroduce them at the stage of our inquiry into the patient's prior preferences (i.e., the substituted judgment test). Under that test, we would have to show that Mrs. Smith would have clearly viewed continued treatment under these circumstances as an indignity, and that she would have preferred an early death to the insertion of a G-tube. The problem with this move is that, as we have already seen, Mrs. Smith left behind neither a precise advance directive nor a pattern of analogous choices that clearly demonstrate what she would have wanted under present circumstances. Indeed, our earlier failure to provide this sort of clear evidence mandated our present effort to find a solution in terms of Mrs. Smith's best interests.

So we have come full circle. Our inability to satisfy a rigorous substituted judgment test required us to search for a solution in terms of Mrs. Smith's best interests. But the best-interests test, at least as articulated in *Conroy*, led to an unacceptably narrow focus on pain that excluded important values. Mrs. Smith's present lack of capacity to appreciate such values finally led us back again to the substituted judgment test. Clearly, something has gone wrong here.

A PROCEDURAL SOLUTION

According to lawyer-bioethicist Nancy Rhoden,[4] the problem lies not in our inability to come up with better evidence of a patient's wishes or level of pain and suffering, but rather in the questions we are asking. She argues convincingly that both the substituted judgment and best-interests tests set the standard of evidence far too high. By requiring *clear and convincing* evidence either that a patient's prior values would dictate the withdrawal of life-sustaining treatment or that the burdens of a patient's life outweigh the benefits, these tests establish a standard that cannot realistically be met by the kinds of evidence we are likely to have at our disposal. As we have seen, in the absence of a carefully drafted living will, a durable power of attorney, or severe and intractable pain, it will rarely be *clear* either that a patient would have refused treatment or that death is in her best interests. Given the usual evidentiary materials at hand, in most cases the best we can do is conclude that forgoing treatment is *probably* what the patient would have wanted, or that death is *likely* to be in the patient's best interests, although we will never know for sure in either case.

To be sure, there are some easy cases where a patient's best interests are clearly and perceptibly being violated. For example, greedy relatives might request the termination of treatment that could realistically return the patient to a good quality of life; or guilt-ridden relatives might press for full resuscitative measures on a moribund patient riddled with metastatic cancer. But apart from such clear-cut cases of unmistakable undertreatment and overtreatment, most of the truly problematical cases (like Mrs. Smith's) fall into a vast gray area between these extremes where the patient's best interests will remain unclear and largely inscrutable. Our problem, then, is that we have been asking questions for which there exist, in most of the hard cases at least, no clearly correct answers.

Rhoden's solution, in which I concur, is to bypass this substantive impasse with a procedural solution. Taking her cue from the President's Commission report[6] addressed to the problem of severely impaired newborns, she argues that when a proposed course of action falls into the gray area of uncertainty, involved and well-intentioned family members should have discretion to decide as they see fit. Presumably, they will invoke precisely the same kinds of evidence bearing on the patient's value system, religious affiliation, quality of life, and the potential benefits and burdens of treatment, but they would not be held to a standard of evidence requiring that their choice be uniquely correct.

To be sure, many caring and well-meaning family members will also want to weigh the impact of continued treatment upon themselves and the family unit. Sometimes the ongoing provision of care and treatment to severely demented patients like Mrs. Smith can impose great burdens, both financial and emotional, upon families. I believe that such concerns are for the most part inevitable and that they often subtly color treatment decisions even when officially banished under the auspices of the usual ethical-legal standards. This is to be expected and should not give us grounds for concern so long as the case originally falls within the gray area of ethical ambiguity, and so long as the interests of family do not *clearly* violate the best interests of the patient.

The correct question for us, then, is not whether forgoing treatment is clearly the right answer, but rather whether Mrs. Smith's case falls into the problematical gray area. If it does, then the decision of a trustworthy surrogate should prevail over objections from caregivers, unless the latter can show a clear violation of best interests. Since a case must exhibit considerable ethical ambiguity to fall into this gray zone in the first place, we should expect that well-meaning and ethically sensitive people will reach different conclusions about the care of such patients. The opinions of trustworthy surrogates should be given priority simply because they are usually in the best position to assess the prior wishes and best interests of incompetent patients, and because their familial and emotional bonding to patients usually gives them a greater claim than members of the health care team.[6]

What, then, are the boundaries of the gray area? When is a case sufficiently ambiguous to warrant our trust in surrogate decision-making? We can begin with a reassertion of the *Conroy* case's best-interests formula. If a patient's capacity for benefitting from continued life appears to be eclipsed by the constant presence of severe and intractable pain, then the case falls either in the gray area or the clear-cut zone of nontreatment. I would add that this imbalance of burdens over benefits need not be conclusively proven by clear and convincing evidence. It should be sufficient merely for the surrogate to make a strong case that the burdens are disproportionate to the benefits. In Mrs. Smith's case, however, no such claim can be made.

In the absence of severe pain, we must ask whether the patient is genuinely capable of benefitting from continued existence. Does she recognize and interact with other persons, including her family and caregivers? Does she have a sufficiently intact self to conceive of the future and to care about what happens in it? If the answers to these questions are negative, even if the patient is capable of some rudimentary physical pleasures, I would argue that the patient has no real interest in either continued life or the administration of life-sustaining treatments and thus falls squarely into the gray area.

Mrs. Smith fits this profile. She is so demented that she cannot recognize family or caregivers. Her memory is so depleted, and her sense of self so fractured, that she cannot be said to have genuinely human interests.

Since the boundaries of this morally ambiguous zone will inevitably correspond to the limits of societal toleration, it will often be helpful to ask what most reasonable people would want for themselves in this circumstance. Although this question is generally not allowed in more patient-centered inquiries into the patient's prior preferences or best interests, it should be allowable here, where we are merely trying to determine whether a case is sufficiently morally problematic to fit into the gray zone. If we ask the question with regard to Mrs. Smith, I think that the overwhelming majority of persons would say that they would rather die than continue to live in such a physically, emotionally, and socially impoverished state.

Another useful clue is to ask how we would have responded to Mrs. Smith's death from lack of adequate nutrition had it occurred prior to the advent of artificial feeding. No doubt there would have been the inevitable sadness associated with the death of any human being, but there would have been no shock, no outrage, no sense of tragedy, nor even any feeling that death had deprived her of any real benefits. The predominant response to such a death would most likely have been relief, both for the sake of the patient and for her loved ones.

In such cases, the only apparent rationale for the imposition of life-sustaining technologies is that since they exist, they must be used. And the more they are used, the more pervasive their presence in hospital and long-term care facilities, the more their expanded use assumes the necessity of a moral imperative. But it is precisely here, in cases such as Mrs. Smith's, that we must pause to ask about the proper uses of such technologies. If they do nothing to further the real interests of patients, if all they do is to prolong the biological existence of patients whose biographical lives have long since come to an end, then biomedical technologies assume the status of idols—i.e., inanimate objects worshipped by the human beings who created them, objects that return to dominate us rather than serving our purposes.

NOTES

1. Dworkin R: Autonomy and the Demented Self. *Milbank Quarterly* 64: supp. 2, 4–16, 1986.
2. Buchanan A, Brock DW: Deciding for Others. *Milbank Quarterly* 64:supp. 2, 71, 1986.

3. Dresser R: Life, Death, and Incompetent Patients: Conceptual Infirmities and Hidden Values in the Law. *Arizona Law Review* 28: 376–379, 1986.
4. Rhoden NK: Litigating Life and Death. *Harvard Law Review* 102: 2, 375–446, Dec. 1988.
5. Callahan D: *Setting Limits: Medical Goals in an Aging Society.* New York, Simon & Schuster, 1987, p. 192.
6. President's Commission for the Study of Ethical Problems in Medicine and Biomedical and Behavioral Research: Deciding to Forego Life Sustaining Treatment. Washington, D.C., U.S. Government Printing Office, 1983, p. 134 ff.
7. In re Conroy, 98 N.J. 321, 486 A.2d 1209 (1985).
8. Cranford RE: The Persistent Vegetative State: The Medical Reality (Getting the Facts Straight). *Hastings Cent Rep* 18:27–32, Feb./Mar. 1988.
9. Feinberg J: The Rights of Animals and Unborn Generations, in *Rights, Justice, and the Bounds of Liberty.* Princeton, Princeton University Press, 1980, pp. 176–177.
10. Arras JD: Quality of Life in Neonatal Ethics: Beyond Denial and Evasion, in Weil WB, Benjamin M, (eds): *Ethical Issues at the Outset of Life.* Boston, Blackwell, 1987, pp. 151–186.
11. Engelhardt HT: *The Foundations of Bioethics.* New York, Oxford University Press, 1986.
12. Brock DW: Justice and the Severely Demented Elderly. *J Med Philos* 13:1, 73–99, Feb. 1988.
13. Rachels J: *The End of Life.* New York, Oxford University Press, 1986.

Nutrition and Hydration: Moral and Pastoral Reflections

U.S. Bishops' Pro-Life Committee

INTRODUCTION

Modern medical technology seems to confront us with many questions not faced even a decade ago.

EDITORS' NOTE: The article has been edited and all footnotes omitted. Readers wishing to follow up on sources should consult the original article.

Corresponding changes in medical practice have benefited many, but have also prompted fears by some that they will be aggressively treated against their will or denied the kind of care that is their due as human persons with inherent dignity. Current debates about life-sustaining treatment suggest that our society's moral reflection is having difficulty keeping pace with its technological progress.

A religious view of life has an important contribution to make to these modern debates. Our Catholic tradition has developed a rich body of thought on these questions, which affirms a duty to preserve human life but recognizes limits to that duty.

Our first goal in making this statement is to reaffirm some basic principles of our moral tradition, to assist Catholics and others in making treatment decisions in accord with respect for God's gift of life.

These principles do not provide clear and final answers to all moral questions that arise as individuals make difficult decisions. Catholic theologians may differ on how best to apply moral principles to some questions not explicitly resolved by the church's teaching authority. Likewise, we understand that those who must make serious healthcare decisions for themselves or for others face a complexity of issues, circumstances, thoughts and emotions in each unique case.

This is the case with some questions involving the medically assisted provision of nutrition and hydration to helpless patients—those who are seriously ill, disabled or persistently unconscious. These questions have been made more urgent by widely publicized court cases and the public debate to which they have given rise.

Our second purpose in issuing this statement, then, is to provide some clarification of the moral issues involved in decisions about medically assisted nutrition and hydration. We are fully aware that such guidance is not necessarily final, because there are many unresolved medical and ethical questions related to these issues and the continuing development of medical technology will necessitate ongoing reflection. But these decisions already confront patients, families and health-care personnel every day. They arise whenever competent patients make decisions about medically assisted nutrition and hydration for their own present situation, when they consider signing an advance directive such as a "living will" or health-care proxy document, and when families or other proxy decision-makers make decisions about those entrusted to their care. We offer guidance to those who, facing these issues, might be confused by opinions that at times threaten to deny the inherent dignity of human life. We therefore address our reflections first to those who share our Judeo-Christian traditions, and secondly to others concerned about the dignity and value of human life who seek guidance in making their own moral decisions.

MORAL PRINCIPLES

The Judeo-Christian moral tradition celebrates life as the gift of a loving God and respects the life of each human being because each is made in the image and likeness of God. As Christians we also believe we are redeemed by Christ and called to share eternal life with him. From these roots the Catholic tradition has developed a distinctive approach to fostering and sustaining human life. Our church views life as a sacred trust, a gift over which we are given stewardship and not absolute dominion. The church thus opposes all direct attacks on innocent life. As conscientious stewards we have a duty to preserve life, while recognizing certain limits to that duty:

(1) Because human life is the foundation for all other human goods, it has a special value and significance. Life is "the first right of the human person" and "the condition of all the others."

(2) All crimes against life, including "euthanasia or willful suicide," must be opposed. Euthanasia is "an action or an omission which of itself or by intention causes death, in order that all suffering may in this way be eliminated." Its terms of reference are to be found "in the intention of the will and in the methods used." Thus defined, euthanasia is an attack on life which no one has a right to make or request, and which no government or other human authority can legitimately recommend or permit. Although individual guilt may be reduced or absent because of suffering or emotional factors that cloud the conscience, this does not change the objective wrongfulness of the act. It should also be recognized that an apparent plea for death may really be a plea for help and love.

(3) Suffering is a fact of human life, and has special significance for the Christian as an opportunity to share in Christ's redemptive suffering. Nevertheless there is nothing wrong in trying to relieve someone's suffering; in fact it is a positive good to do so, as long as one does not intentionally cause death or interfere with other moral and religious duties.

(4) Everyone has the duty to care for his or her own life and health and to seek necessary medical care from others, but this does not mean that all possible remedies must be used in all circumstances. One is not obliged to use either "extraordinary" means or "disproportionate" means of preserving

life—that is, means which are understood as offering no reasonable hope of benefit or as involving excessive burdens. Decisions regarding such means are complex, and should ordinarily be made by the patient in consultation with his or her family chaplain or pastor and physician when that is possible.

(5) In the final stage of dying one is not obliged to prolong the life of a patient by every possible means: "When inevitable death is imminent in spite of the means used, it is permitted in conscience to take the decision to refuse forms of treatment that would only secure a precarious and burdensome prolongation of life, so long as the normal care due to the sick person in similar cases is not interrupted."

(6) While affirming life as a gift of God, the church recognizes that death is unavoidable and that it can open the door to eternal life. Thus, "without in any way hastening the hour of death," the dying person should accept its reality and prepare for it emotionally and spiritually.

(7) Decisions regarding human life must respect the demands of justice, viewing each human being as our neighbor and avoiding all discrimination based on age or dependency. A human being has "a unique dignity and an independent value, from the moment of conception and in every stage of development, whatever his or her physical condition." In particular, "the disabled person (whether the disability be the result of a congenital handicap, chronic illness or accident, or from mental or physical deficiency, and whatever the severity of the disability) is a fully human subject, with the corresponding innate, sacred and inviolable rights." First among these is "the fundamental and inalienable right to life."

(8) The dignity and value of the human person, which lie at the foundation of the church's teaching on the right to life, also provide a basis for any just social order. Not only to become more Christian, but to become more truly human, society should protect the right to life through its laws and other policies.

While these principles grow out of a specific religious tradition, they appeal to a common respect for the dignity of the human person. We commend them to all people of good will.

QUESTIONS ABOUT MEDICALLY ASSISTED NUTRITION AND HYDRATION

In what follows we apply these well-established moral principles to the difficult issue of providing medically assisted nutrition and hydration to persons who are seriously ill, disabled or persistently unconscious. We recognize the complexity involved in applying these principles to individual cases and acknowledge that, at this time and on this particular issue, our applications do not have the same authority as the principles themselves.

1. IS THE WITHHOLDING OR WITHDRAWING OF MEDICALLY ASSISTED NUTRITION AND HYDRATION ALWAYS A DIRECT KILLING?

In answering this question one should avoid two extremes.

First, it is wrong to say that this could not be a matter of killing simply because it involves an omission rather than a positive action. In fact a deliberate omission may be an effective and certain way to kill, especially to kill someone weakened by illness. Catholic teaching condemns as euthanasia "an action or an omission which of itself or by intention causes death, in order that all suffering may in this way be eliminated." Thus "euthanasia includes not only active mercy killing but also the omission of treatment when the purpose of the omission is to kill the patient."

Second, we should not assume that all or most decisions to withhold or withdraw medically assisted nutrition and hydration are attempts to cause death. To be sure, any patient will die if all nutrition and hydration are withheld. But sometimes other causes are at work—for example, the patient may be imminently dying, whether feeding takes place or not, from an already existing terminal condition. At other times, although the shortening of the patient's life is one foreseeable result of an omission, the real purpose of the omission was to relieve the patient of a particular procedure that was of limited usefulness to the patient or unreasonably burdensome for the patient and the patient's family or caregivers. This kind of decision should not be equated with a decision to kill or with suicide.

The harsh reality is that some who propose withdrawal of nutrition and hydration from certain patients do directly intend to bring about a patient's death and would even prefer a change in the law to allow for what they see as more "quick and painless" means to cause death. In other words, nutrition and hydration (whether orally administered or medically assisted) are sometimes withdrawn not because a patient is dying, but precisely because a patient is not dying (or not dying quickly) and someone believes it would be better if he or she did, generally because the patient is perceived as having an unacceptably low "quality of life" or as imposing burdens on others.

When deciding whether to withhold or withdraw medically assisted nutrition and hydration, or other forms of life support, we are called by our moral tradition to ask ourselves: What will my decision do for this patient? And what am I trying to achieve by doing it? We must be sure that it is not our intent to cause the patient's death—either for its own sake or as a means to achieving some other goal such as the relief of suffering.

2. IS MEDICALLY ASSISTED NUTRITION AND HYDRATION A FORM OF "TREATMENT" OR "CARE"?

Catholic teaching provides that a person in the final stages of dying need not accept "forms of treatment that would only secure a precarious and burdensome prolongation of life," but should still receive "the normal care due to the sick person in similar cases." . . . But the teaching of the church has not resolved the question whether medically assisted nutrition and hydration should always be seen as a form of normal care.

Almost everyone agrees that oral feeding, when it can be accepted and assimilated by a patient, is a form of care owed to all helpless people. . . . But our obligations become less clear when adequate nutrition and hydration require the skills of trained medical personnel and the use of technologies that may be perceived as very burdensome— that is, as intrusive, painful or repugnant. Such factors vary from one type of feeding procedure to another, and from one patient to another, making it difficult to classify all feeding procedures as either "care" or "treatment."

Perhaps this dilemma should be viewed in a broader context. Even medical "treatments" are morally obligatory when they are "ordinary" means—that is, if they provide a reasonable hope of benefit and do not involve excessive burdens. Therefore we believe people should make decisions in light of a simple and fundamental insight: Out of respect for the dignity of the human person we are obliged to preserve our own lives and help others preserve theirs, by the use of means that have a reasonable hope of sustaining life without imposing unreasonable burdens on those we seek to help, that is, on the patient and his or her family and community.

We must therefore address the question of benefits and burdens next, recognizing that a full moral analysis is only possible when one knows the effects of a given procedure on a particular patient.

3. WHAT ARE THE BENEFITS OF MEDICALLY ASSISTED NUTRITION AND HYDRATION?

. . .

Nutrition and hydration, whether provided in the usual way or with medical assistance . . . benefit patients in several ways. First, for all patients who can assimilate them, suitable food and fluids sustain life, and providing them normally expresses loving concern and solidarity with the helpless. Second, for patients being treated with the hope of a cure, appropriate food and fluids are an important element of sound health care. Third, even for patients who are imminently dying and incurable, food and fluids can prevent the suffering that may arise from dehydration, hunger and thirst.

. . . But sometimes even food and fluids are no longer effective in providing this benefit because a patient has entered the final stage of a terminal condition. At such times we should make the dying person as comfortable as possible and provide nursing care and proper hygiene as well as companionship and appropriate spiritual aid. Such a person may lose all desire for food and drink and even be unable to ingest them. Initiating medically assisted feeding or intravenous fluids in this case may increase the patient's discomfort while providing no real benefit; ice chips or sips of water may instead be appropriate to provide comfort and counteract the adverse effects of dehydration. Even in the case of the imminently dying patient, of course, any action or omission that of itself or by intention causes death is to be absolutely rejected. . . .

4. WHAT ARE THE BURDENS OF MEDICALLY ASSISTED NUTRITION AND HYDRATION?

. . .

The risks and objective complications of medically assisted nutrition and hydration will depend on the procedure used and the condition of the patient. In a given case a feeding procedure may become harmful or even life-threatening. . . .

If the risks and burdens of a particular feeding procedure are deemed serious enough to warrant withdrawing it, we should not automatically deprive the patient of all nutrition and hydration but should ask whether another procedure is feasible that would be less burdensome. We say this because some helpless patients, including some in a "persistent vegetative state," receive tube feedings not because they cannot swallow food at all but because tube feeding is less costly and difficult for health-care personnel. . . .

Many people see feeding tubes as frightening or even as bodily violations. Assessments of such burdens are necessarily subjective; they should not be dismissed on that account, but we offer some practical cautions to help prevent abuse.

First, in keeping with our moral teaching against the intentional causing of death by omission, one should distinguish between repugnance to a particular procedure and repugnance to life itself. The latter may occur when a patient views a life of helplessness and dependency on others as itself a heavy burden, leading him or her to wish or even to pray for death. Especially in our achievement-oriented society, the burden of living in such a condition may seem to outweigh any possible benefit of medical treatment and even lead a person to despair. But we should not assume that the burdens in such a case always outweigh the benefits; for the sufferer, given good counseling and spiritual support, may be brought again to appreciate the precious gift of life.

Second, our tradition recognizes that when treatment decisions are made, "account will have to be taken of the reasonable wishes of the patient and the patient's family, as also of the advice of the doctors who are specially competent in the matter." . . .

Third, we should not assume that a feeding procedure is inherently repugnant to all patients without specific evidence. In contrast to Americans' general distaste for the idea of being supported by "tubes and machines," some studies indicate surprisingly favorable views of medically assisted nutrition and hydration among patients and families with actual experience of such procedures. . . .

While some balk at the idea, in principle cost can be a valid factor in decisions about life support. For example, money spent on expensive treatment for one family member may be money otherwise needed for food, housing and other necessities for the rest of the family. Here, also, we offer some cautions. . . . Even for altruistic reasons a patient should not directly intend his or her own death by malnutrition or dehydration, but may accept an earlier death as a consequence of his or her refusal of an unreasonably expensive treatment.

. . . Individual decisions about medically assisted nutrition and hydration should [not] be determined by macroeconomic concerns such as national budget priorities and the high cost of health care. These social problems are serious, but it is by no means established that they require depriving chronically ill and helpless patients of effective and easily tolerated measures that they need to survive.

Third, tube feeding alone is generally not very expensive and may cost no more than oral feeding. What is seen by many as a grave financial and emotional burden on caregivers is the total long-term care of severely debilitated patients, who may survive for many years with no life support except medically assisted nutrition and hydration and nursing care. . . .

In the context of official church teaching, it is not yet clear to what extent we may assess the burden of a patient's total care rather than the burden of a particular treatment when we seek to refuse "burdensome" life support. On a practical level, those seeking to make good decisions might assure themselves of their own intentions by asking: Does my decision aim at relieving the patient of a particularly grave burden imposed by medically assisted nutrition and hydration? Or does it aim to avoid the total burden of caring for the patient? If so, does it achieve this aim by deliberately bringing about his or her death?

Rather than leaving families to confront such dilemmas alone, society and government should improve their assistance to families whose financial and emotional resources are strained by long-term care of loved ones.

5. WHAT ROLE SHOULD "QUALITY OF LIFE" PLAY IN OUR DECISIONS?

Financial and emotional burdens are willingly endured by most families to raise their children or to care for mentally aware but weak and elderly family members. It is sometimes argued that we need not endure comparable burdens to feed and care for persons with severe mental and physical disabilities, because their low "quality of life" makes it unnecessary or pointless to preserve their lives.

But this argument—even when it seems motivated by a humanitarian concern to reduce suffering and hardship—ignores the equal dignity and sanctity of all human life. Its key assumption—that people with disabilities necessarily enjoy life less than others or lack the potential to lead meaningful lives—is also mistaken. Where suffering does exist, society's response should not be to neglect or eliminate the lives of people with disabilities, but to help correct their inadequate living conditions. Very often the worst threat to a good "quality of life" for these people is not the disability itself, but the prejudicial attitudes of others—attitudes based on the idea that a life with serious disabilities is not worth living.

This being said, our moral tradition allows for three ways in which the "quality of life" of a seriously ill patient is relevant to treatment decisions:

(1) Consistent with respect for the inherent sanctity of life, we should relieve needless suffering and support morally acceptable ways of improving each patient's quality of life.

(2) One may legitimately refuse a treatment because it would itself create an impairment imposing new serious burdens or risks on the patient. This decision to avoid the new burdens or risks created by a treatment is not the same as directly intending to end life in order to avoid the burden of living in a disabled state.

(3) Sometimes a disabling condition may directly influence the benefits and burdens of a specific treatment for a particular patient. For example, a confused or demented patient may find medically assisted nutrition and hydration more frightening and burdensome than other patients do because he or she cannot understand what it is. The patient may even repeatedly pull out feeding tubes, requiring burdensome physical restraints if this form of feeding is to be continued. In such cases, ways of alleviating such special burdens should be explored before concluding that they justify withholding all food and fluids needed to sustain life.

These humane considerations are quite different from a "quality of life" ethic that would judge individuals with disabilities or limited potential as not worthy of care or respect. It is one thing to withhold a procedure because it would impose new disabilities on a patient, and quite another thing to say that patients who already have such disabilities should not have their lives preserved. A means considered ordinary or proportionate for other patients should not be considered extraordinary or disproportionate for severely impaired patients solely because of a judgment that their lives are not worth living.

In short, while considerations regarding a person's quality of life have some validity in weighing the burdens and benefits of medical treatment, at the present time in our society judgments about the quality of life are sometimes used to promote euthanasia. The church must emphasize the sanctity of life of each person as a fundamental principle in all moral decision-making.

6. DO PERSISTENTLY UNCONSCIOUS PATIENTS REPRESENT A SPECIAL CASE?

Even Catholics who accept the same basic moral principles may strongly disagree on how to apply them to patients who appear to be persistently unconscious—that is, those who are in a permanent coma or a "persistent vegetative state" (PVS). Some moral questions in this area have not been explicitly resolved by the church's teaching authority.

On some points there is wide agreement among Catholic theologians:

(1). An unconscious patient must be treated as a living human person with inherent dignity and value. Direct killing of such a patient is as morally reprehensible as the direct killing of anyone else. Even the medical terminology used to describe these patients as "vegetative" unfortunately tends to obscure this vitally important point, inviting speculation that a patient in this state is a "vegetable" or a subhuman animal.

(2) The area of legitimate controversy does not concern patients with conditions like mental retardation, senility, dementia or even temporary unconsciousness. Where serious disagreement begins is with the patient who has been diagnosed as completely and permanently unconscious after careful testing over a period of weeks or months.

Some moral theologians argue that a particular form of care or treatment is morally obligatory only when its benefits outweigh its burdens to a patient or the care providers. In weighing burdens, they say, the total burden of a procedure and the consequent requirements of care must be taken into account. If no benefit can be demonstrated, the procedure, whatever its burdens, cannot be obligatory. These moralists also hold that the chief criterion to determine the benefit of a procedure cannot be merely that it prolongs physical life, since physical life is not an absolute good but is relative to the spiritual good of the person. They assert that the spiritual good of the person is union with God, which can be advanced only by human acts, i.e., conscious, free acts. Since the best current medical opinion holds that persons in the persistent vegetative state (PVS) are incapable now or in the future of conscious, free human acts, these moralists conclude that, when careful diagnosis verifies this condition, it is not obligatory to prolong life by such interventions as a respirator, antibiotics or medically assisted hydration and nutrition. To decide to omit non-obligatory care, therefore, is not to intend the patient's death, but only to avoid the burden of the procedure. Hence, though foreseen, the patient's death is to be attributed to the patient's pathological condition and not to the omission of care. Therefore, these theologians conclude, while it is always wrong directly to intend or cause the death of such patients, the natural dying process which would have occurred without these interventions may be permitted to proceed.

While this rationale is convincing to some, it is not theologically conclusive and we are not persuaded by it. In fact, other theologians argue cogently that theological inquiry could lead one to a more carefully limited conclusion.

These moral theologians argue that while particular treatments can be judged useless or burdensome, it is morally questionable and would create a dangerous precedent to imply that any human life is not a positive good or "benefit." They emphasize that while life is not the highest good, it is always and everywhere a basic good of the human person and not merely a means to other goods. They further assert that if the "burden" one is trying to relieve by discontinuing medically assisted nutrition and hydration is the burden of remaining alive in the allegedly undignified condition of PVS, such a decision is unacceptable because one's intent is only achieved by deliberately ensuring the patient's death from malnutrition or dehydration. Finally, these moralists suggest that PVS is best seen as an extreme form of mental and physical disability—one whose causes, nature and prognosis are as yet imperfectly understood—and not as a terminal illness or fatal pathology from which patients should generally be allowed to die. Because the patient's life can often be sustained indefinitely by medically assisted nutrition and hydration that is not unreasonably risky or burdensome for that patient, they say, we are not dealing here with a case where "inevitable death is imminent in spite of the means used." Rather, because the patient will die in a few days if medically assisted nutrition and hydration are discontinued, but can often live a long time if they are provided, the inherent dignity and worth of the human person obligates us to provide this patient with care and support.

Further complicating this debate is a disagreement over what responsible Catholics should do in the absence of a final resolution of this question. Some point to our moral tradition of probabilism, which would allow individuals to follow the appropriate moral analysis that they find persuasive. Others point to the principle that in cases where one might risk unjustly depriving someone of life, we should take the safer course.

In the face of the uncertainties and unresolved medical and theological issues, it is important to defend and preserve important values. On the one hand, there is a concern that patients and families should not be subjected to unnecessary burdens, ineffective treatments and indignities when death is approaching. On the other hand, it is important to ensure that the inherent dignity of human persons, even those who are persistently unconscious, is respected and that no one is deprived of nutrition and hydration with the intent of bringing on his or her death.

It is not easy to arrive at a single answer to some of the real and personal dilemmas involved in this issue. In study, prayer and compassion we continue to reflect on this issue and hope to discover additional information that will lead to its ultimate resolution.

In the meantime, at a practical level we are concerned that withdrawal of all life support, including nutrition and hydration, not be viewed as appropriate or automatically indicated for the entire class of PVS patients simply because of a judgment that they are beyond the reach of medical treatment that would restore consciousness. We note the current absence of conclusive scientific data on the causes and implications of different degrees of brain damage, on the PVS patient's ability to experience pain and on the reliability of prognoses for many such patients. We do know that many of these patients have a good prognosis for long-term survival when given medically assisted nutrition and hydration, and a certain prognosis for death otherwise—and we know that many in our society view such an early death as a positive good for a patient in this condition. Therefore we are gravely concerned about current attitudes and policy trends in our society that would too easily dismiss patients without apparent mental faculties as non-persons or as undeserving of human care and concern. In this climate, even legitimate moral arguments intended to have a careful and limited application can easily be misinterpreted, broadened and abused by others to erode respect for the lives of some of our society's most helpless members. . . .

Quality of Life and Non-Treatment Decisions for Incompetent Patients: A Critique of the Orthodox Approach

Rebecca S. Dresser and John A. Robertson

Since the Quinlan decision in 1976, courts and legislatures have made substantial progress in defining rules to govern non-treatment of dying and debilitated patients. For example, the right of the competent patient to refuse necessary care is now widely established, and the legality of withdrawing respirators and even nutrition and hydration from permanently unconscious patients is increasingly recognized.

More difficult questions arise, however, when the patient is neither competent nor permanently unconscious, but instead is in a conscious, severely demented and debilitated state, with experiences that appear quite limited. Thousands of patients in this condition are cared for in private homes, hospitals, and nursing homes, the victims of stroke, senility, Alzheimer's disease, and other illnesses. Even though they usually require only low-tech, minimally supportive care, such patients can

Rebecca S. Dresser and John A. Robertson, "Quality of Life and Non-Treatment Decisions for Incompetent Patients," *Law, Medicine & Health Care* 17, no. 3 (Fall 1989):234–244. Reprinted by permission of Professors Dresser and Robertson and the American Society of Law, Medicine & Ethics.

EDITORS' NOTE: Notes have been omitted. Readers wishing to follow up on sources should consult the original article.

impose great stress on their families and high financial costs on the health care system.

As the population of frail elderly and demented patients grows, determining the limits of family and societal obligations to sustain them has become a major ethical, legal, and policy issue. Its resolution requires balancing the importance of life in such compromised conditions against the social and familial burdens that prolonging such lives entails. A conflict between a patient-centered and other-directed approach inevitably arises, testing the scope of society's respect for vulnerable and debilitated persons.

Unfortunately, the orthodox judicial approach to non-treatment decisions is not an adequate guide to resolution of these issues. Judicial analysis is too focused on the model of a competent person refusing treatment, even when the case involves a person who is incompetent and unable to choose. Although many of the decided cases have produced defensible results, the courts' efforts to fit incompetent patients to the model of a competent decision-maker are seriously flawed and ultimately threaten harm to many incompetent patients.

Courts, legislators, and physicians would do better to focus directly on the interests of the incompetent patient before them. Competing interests, such as family distress and financial costs, may then be directly evaluated and their role in such decisions properly assigned. Such an approach has the best chance of respecting incompetent persons, while giving due regard to the interests of families and society.

THE ORTHODOX APPROACH: ADVANCE DIRECTIVES AND SUBSTITUTED JUDGMENT

Starting with *In re Quinlan*, and continuing with such cases as *Superintendent of Belchertown* v. *Saikewicz, Eichner* v. *Dillon, Barber* v. *Superior Court, In re Conroy, Brophy* v. *New England Sinai Hospital, Inc.*, and *In re Jobes*, the courts have found that life-sustaining treatment may be withheld or withdrawn from incompetent patients in certain circumstances.

The cases adopt the same general pattern of reasoning. Adopting a patient-centered approach, they require that patient choices concerning their medical care be respected. The basic legal premise, derived from common law and constitutional rights to self-determination and privacy, is that competent patients have a right to refuse necessary medical care when they face intrusive treatment or life in a compromised state. Countervailing state interests in preserving life, preventing suicide, and upholding the integrity of the medical profession are then found insufficient to override the patient's objection to treatment.

What, however, if the patient is incompetent and cannot make a choice about treatment? Here the courts in most jurisdictions make a conceptual move that determines the structure of subsequent analysis. They assume that respect for incompetent patients requires according such patients the same right to refuse treatment accorded competent patients. This assumption requires that the incompetent patient be viewed as a choosing individual and leads the courts to find or construct a competent person as decision-maker to determine the incompetent patient's choice.

Determining what the fictional competent person in the incompetent patient's situation would choose entails further moves. An incompetent patient's prior oral or written directive concerning treatment when incompetent is given great weight in determining that hypothetical choice. If no directive exists, courts typically adopt the substituted judgment doctrine and allow the family or other proxy to choose as they think the patients would have chosen when or if competent.

This approach to decision-making for incompetent patients was first enunciated in the landmark New Jersey Supreme Court case, *In re Quinlan*, when the court stated that the patient's guardian and family should determine whether she would herself choose non-treatment in her present circumstances: ". . . the only practical way to prevent destruction of the right [of privacy] is to permit the guardian and family of Karen to render their best judgment . . . as to whether she would exercise it in these circumstances."

This approach has shaped the reasoning and analysis in every subsequent non-treatment case involving incompetent patients. Indeed, eleven years later the New Jersey Supreme Court forcefully reiterated the accepted view in *Jobes*:

. . . the patient's right to self-determination is the guiding principle in determining whether to continue or withdraw life-sustaining treatment;

... therefore the goal of a surrogate decision-maker for an incompetent patient must be to determine and effectuate what that patient, if competent, would want.

The strategy of relying on prior expressed wishes or proxy inferred competent treatment preferences to determine treatment choices for incompetent patients has wide currency in ethical and policy analysis involving incompetent patients. Authoritative bodies such as the President's Commission for the Study of Ethical Problems in Medicine and the Hastings Center have also endorsed it. Living-will and durable-power-of-attorney legislation embodies a further acceptance of the theme. Health professionals and ethicists hail it as the best solution to the difficult problem of deciding when treatment should be withheld from incompetent patients. It has also been extended to govern medical treatment for patients who never were competent, psychiatric treatment for civilly committed persons, sterilization of retarded persons, and organ donation by incompetent persons.

THE ALLURE OF THE ORTHODOX APPROACH

The orthodox judicial approach of relying on the patient's prior directive or choice inferred by a proxy's substituted judgment has a strong allure for several reasons. One is the appearance on consistency with widely shared values of personal autonomy. When we look to what incompetent patients formerly wanted, or what we infer they would desire, if known, the patient as competent appears to be deciding. This position purportedly extends the freedom and autonomy of competent persons to situations of incompetency.

A second attraction is that the orthodox approach has generally operated to protect incompetent patients from overzealous medical interventions. Until recently, applications of the test in most jurisdictions have found that patients would have refused treatment if they were competent, and have thus permitted intrusive, expensive treatments to be forgone. Also, by ostensibly treating incompetent patients as choice-makers who control whether treatment occurs, the orthodox approach denies others the power, at least explicitly, to override the incompetent patient's interests for the sake of others.

The orthodox approach also attracts because it recognizes a central role for family discretion in treatment decisions for incompetent patients. Since families are so directly involved in the illness of loved ones, an approach that reposes authority in the family seems to respect present social mores. Although this discretion is couched in terms of ascertaining what the patient would choose if competent, or what the patient in fact once said, the family is usually the source of this information and hence is in a position to control it. Close scrutiny of the family's assessment of these questions is frequently omitted, thus giving them ultimate discretion to decide the matter.

Finally, the orthodox approach is attractive because it is comfortable. It enables decision-makers to finesse the dilemmas or tragic choices that make decisions for incompetent patients so difficult. By shifting the inquiry to what the patient when competent had or would have decided, it absolves decision-makers of the need to confront directly the value of debilitated life versus the burdens such life places on families, physicians, and society. It enables the courts to say, as they do in *Saikewicz* and *Brophy*, that they are not making quality of life choices or privileging other-directed interests but simply honoring what the patient has or would have chosen.

With these advantages, it is no surprise that the orthodox approach of treating the incompetent patient as a competent decision-maker so dominates legal and ethical thinking in this area. But its conceptual flaws and contradictions emerge when it is applied to the conscious, demented, and debilitated patients who now claim judicial and policy attention. When extended to this diverse group of individuals, the orthodox approach risks giving excessive and unexamined power to family and cost considerations in the guise of respecting patient autonomy.

THE ERRORS OF THE ORTHODOX APPROACH

Despite its allure and wide acceptance, the orthodox approach to non-treatment decisions for incompetent patients is conceptually confused and threatens to harm conscious incompetent patients. The problems arise from its concept of the incompetent patient, which excludes the patient's current needs, and from its implementation method, which allows family and other interests to take control. To demonstrate these points, we examine three erroneous assumptions of the orthodox approach.

1. Incompetent Persons Must Be Treated as Autonomous Choice-Makers.

A major error in the orthodox approach is the assumption that equal respect for incompetent patients requires that they be treated as competent patients—that is, as choice-making actors. Equal respect for incompetent patients requires that their interests be protected and that they not be abused simply because they are incompetent. However, it does not follow that they must be treated as if they were exercising autonomy.

Choice is irrelevant if one lacks the capacity to choose, and incompetent persons are by definition incapable of exercising choice or self-determination. Rather than engage in the fiction of asking what they would choose, we should determine what interests, if any, they currently have in receiving life-sustaining treatment. As we will show, the interests of incompetent patients are not respected by an approach that analyzes their situations as if they were competent individuals exercising choice about treatment and continued life.

2. Expressed or Inferred Prior Choices Are an Accurate Indicator of Incompetent Persons' Current Interests.

A second conceptual error implicit in the orthodox approach is the assumption that the incompetent patient's own treatment choice, if known, would incorporate the preferences the patient had as a competent person. It is wrong to assume that the incompetent patient's prior competent preferences are the best indicator of the patient's current interests. If we could determine the choice that these patients would make if suddenly able to speak—if they could tell us what their interests in their compromised states are—such choices would reflect their current and future interests as incompetent individuals, not their past preferences.

Linking incompetent patients' past competent treatment preferences to their existing welfare is highly problematic. The desires competent persons have concerning their future medical care reflect the activities and goals that make life worthwhile for them as competent, choosing individuals. To

most competent persons, work, family, friendships, exercise, hobbies, and related pursuits seem integral to a life worth living. Self-determination, bodily integrity, and personal privacy are also matters of deep concern. Many competent persons would refuse life-sustaining treatment that severely compromised those interests.

When people become incompetent and seriously ill, however, their interests may radically change. With their reduced mental and physical capacities, what was once of extreme importance to them no longer matters, while things that were previously of little moment assume much greater significance. An existence that seems demeaning and unacceptable to the competent person may still be of value to the incompetent patient, whose abilities, desires, and interests have so greatly narrowed.

It is difficult, if not impossible, for competent individuals to predict their interests in future treatment situations when they are incompetent because their needs and interests will have so radically changed. As a result, the directives they issue for future situations of incompetency, though they reflect their current needs and interests, may have little relevance to their needs and interests once they become incompetent. Indeed, their advance directives may even be detrimental to their interests once in that state.

Philosophical concepts of personal identity are relevant to this analysis. One contemporary theory, which is articulated most clearly by the British philosopher Derek Parfit, holds that a person's life can be a series of successive selves, with a new self emerging as the individual undergoes significant changes in beliefs, desires, memories, and intentions. According to this theory, advance directives for non-treatment could be issued by a different person than the subsequently incompetent individual. In such a situation, the former self's preferences would have no particular authority to govern the incompetent patient's treatment.

Yet our analysis does not depend on acceptance of Parfit's theory of personal identity, which could have radical implications for contract, criminal, and other rules of law. According to an alternate widely held view of personal identity, an essential core of the individual persists over time. Persons retain a unitary identity during their entire lives, even though a person's interests may change dramatically as new personal situations arise. The position that a person's interests may change drastically once incompetency develops is consistent with this theory of a more unitary personal identity, and argues against taking the prior directive as an indication of the patient's current interests.

3. Personal Autonomy Includes the Right to Control the Future by Advance Directives.

Some persons might argue that the orthodox approach, especially in its reliance on advance directives, follows from the generally recognized right of autonomous persons to order their future in various ways. The advance directive against medical treatment is simply another way to exert control over one's fate, by minimizing the risk that one will be kept alive unnecessarily. If persons control their future by contract, will, and other self-binding arrangements, should they not also have the right to control their medical future by advance directives against life-prolonging treatment?

At the outset it should be noted that the argument from autonomy only partially supports the orthodox approach to non-treatment decisions regarding incompetent patients. Even if accepted, it would apply only to situations in which the person had issued an explicit directive concerning future conditions that have come to exist. This argument gives no support to the substituted judgment approach to decision-making for incompetent patients, for the proxy decision-maker is not then relying on an explicit directive issued by a person trying to exercise autonomy over her future. Instead, the proxy infers from general statements and behavior what the incompetent patient would have chosen if she had made a decision when competent or could now express a competent preference.

Even with this proviso, it is not clear why a person's directions concerning situations that arise when incompetent should be followed. Such directives are very different from ordering the future by contract or will. For example, unlike contracts, advance treatment directives are not promises on which other parties rely, in return for their own promise of performance or other consideration. Other persons may have their own interests in enforcement of an advance directive, but they have no contractual right to enforcement, since they have not promised performance in return. Thus, an obligation to honor advance directives does not follow from the obligation to enforce contracts.

The advance directive is also dissimilar to a devise by will. At the time that a will takes effect the testator is dead and no longer has interests that can be harmed by a decision to honor the prior instructions. By contrast, honoring the advance directive occurs at a time when the maker is still alive and can very much be harmed by adherence to its provisions. Failing to honor a "living will" is, therefore, not inconsistent with honoring a "property will."

The argument from autonomy in effect represents a normative judgment that it is more important to give persons the advance certainty that they will not be overtreated than to prevent mistakes of undertreatment which their directives may cause. The security gained in empowering persons to control their medical future in this way is not cost-free. The cost—too often overlooked—is that adherence to the directive will lead to the death of incompetent patients who retain significant interests in continued life. Because interests change over time and the person executing the directive may not be assessing the situation from the perspective of the future incompetent patient, the interests of the competent person contemplating a hypothetical future and the interests of the incompetent person once that future occurs, may diverge. A policy favoring advance directives is not justified unless it recognizes and chooses to run this risk.

A recent New York case, *Evans* v. *Bellevue Hospital*, shows that this concern is more than theoretical. In *Evans*, an incompetent patient diagnosed with AIDS-related complex had when competent executed a document stating that life-sustaining treatment should be forgone if he suffered from "illness, disease or injury or experienced extreme mental deterioration, such that there is no reasonable expectation of recovering or regaining a meaningful quality of life." He also had executed a power of attorney authorizing another individual to make all medical decisions on his behalf.

The court case arose after physicians observed that the patient had multiple brain lesions, which they attributed to toxoplasmosis, a type of infection. The patient's proxy decision-maker asked physicians to withhold antibiotic treatment for the infection. They refused, arguing that the treatment was expected to produce recovery from toxoplasmosis and restore the patient's ability to communicate. The court authorized the treatment, on grounds that the document's reference to "meaningful quality of life" was too ambiguous to sanction non-treatment in this case. The judge noted, however, that if the document had specified conditions that clearly applied to the patient's situation, the proxy would have been permitted to decline the treatment.

Evans sheds light on several major problems with the advance treatment directive. First is the document's imprecision. Living wills and other non-treatment directives tend to consist of broad statements that may supply little guidance on specific treatment questions. In fact they may have no binding effect at all simply because they are too vague or general to be construed to authorize non-treatment in a variety of circumstances never explicitly contemplated by the maker.

A second problem is the strong possibility that individuals who execute directives are unaware that they may be authorizing actions or omissions that conflict with their subsequent well-being. The argument for enforcing a prior directive even when it conflicts with the incompetent patient's interests is hardly compelling if the person, when competent, had not been made aware that his future interests may radically change, and thus be in conflict with what he judged—through the eyes of his previously competent self—to be in his interest.

The *Evans* decision also raises the more serious policy issue of whether to honor advance directives that appear clearly to conflict with the incompetent patient's existing interests. (Of course, many competent patients' advance directives will represent the patients' current interests as well, but in those cases there is no real need for an advance directive to justify forgoing treatment.) Although there is insufficient information to determine if a conflict between past wishes and present interests existed in the *Evans* case, the scenario illustrates the need for courts and legislatures to address this issue.

Avoiding unnecessary, nonbeneficial treatment is clearly a valid individual, family, and policy concern. Patients should not be treated unnecessarily whether or not they have issued a prior directive against such treatment. Withholding treatment in those cases is thus not dependent on issuing an advance directive. As we discuss below, the need to treat should be assessed independently in each case regardless of a directive. Since the

directive is unnecessary to this end and may in other situations threaten the welfare of incompetent patients, the policy judgment in its favor is open to serious question. Respect for autonomy thus does not automatically include an obligation to adopt the orthodox approach on prior directives.

THE DANGERS OF THE ORTHODOX APPROACH: UNDERTREATMENT AND INAPPROPRIATE ATTENTION TO COSTS AND FAMILY DISTRESS

The orthodox approach threatens incompetent patients with undertreatment, because it overlooks the interests they may have in continued life in their diminished state. Prior directives made when patients were competent, as well as choices proxy decision-makers infer patients would make under substituted judgment, may conflict with patients' current interests, thus leading to non-treatment decisions that harm incompetent patients.

The potential for conflict with patient interests is heightened under the substituted judgment doctrine. This standard will affect many more people than the advance directive approach, given that few people issue explicit treatment directives. In most applications of substituted judgment, there is no express evidence speaking to the situation at hand. Instead, the family is asked what the formerly competent person would have wanted, if confronted with a choice about this situation. The patient's relatives are seen as having an "intimate understanding of the patient's medical attitudes and general world view." But in answering the treatment question, strong pressures may also move the family to focus on considerations other than the needs of the patient before them.

First, the question itself shifts attention to the patient at another time—to the preferences and needs the patient had as a competent person. As we noted previously, these can differ from the incompetent patient's existing interests. Second, families often have their own interests in being relieved of the distress of seeing their loved ones in a chronic debilitated state. Although not conscious or directly influential, such distress may push the family to determine that the patient "would certainly have wanted treatment forgone." After all, they themselves would not want to be treated in those circumstances. Is it not reasonable to assume that the patient as a competent person would have wanted the same?

When the treatment decision is made, however, the patient is no longer competent, and thus, in most cases, lacks interests in privacy, dignity, and other values that presuppose some conscious appreciation of those concerns. Assigning these factors weight when they are no longer relevant to the patient actually gives priority to family interests and to generally held values of competent persons. Indeed, the real offense in maintaining debilitated patients is to competent observers, whose own concepts of what constitutes dignified and respectful medical treatment for seriously compromised human beings have been violated. Perhaps, as Justice Handler argued in his *Conroy* and *Jobes* opinions, these interests should be influential in the treatment setting. The orthodox approach, however, formally proclaims that they have no role while simultaneously permitting them *sub silentio* to shape non-treatment decisions that may conflict with the patient's current welfare.

The possibility of conflict between patients' interests and the outcomes permitted under the substituted judgment standard is not merely theoretical. Although the proxy's assumptions about the incompetent patient's choices "if competent" may coincide with the incompetent patient's current interests, they may also diverge in crucial ways. A key difference between the approaches emerges when the patient's current interests would seem to require treatment, contrary to the patient's inferred competent wishes.

This difficulty is evident in *Spring* and *Hier*, two Massachusetts cases that permitted life-sustaining care to be withheld from conscious incompetent patients. These cases illustrate how courts applying the substituted judgment approach have failed to examine and protect the actual interests of the individual incompetent patients before them. Both these opinions gave the patients' interests as incompetent individuals short shrift, focusing instead on their alleged interests in privacy and dignity, interests they appeared incapable of possessing at the time due to their incapacity. Moreover, the decisions are vulnerable to charges that family distress and cost considerations influenced the substituted judgment inquiry.

In re Spring concerned a 78-year-old senile but fully conscious nursing-home resident whose end-stage renal disease was being treated with dialysis. He sometimes resisted the procedure and required sedation during its administration. His family asked the court to authorize cessation of the dialysis. The court applied the substituted judgment test and, relying on the family's claim that if Spring were competent he would have refused treatment, held that the dialysis could be discontinued.

The judgment that Spring's competent decision would be to refuse dialysis ignored the possibility that in his incompetent state he obtained sufficient countervailing pleasure and satisfaction to make the benefits of continued life outweigh the discomforts of the dialysis necessary to preserve that life. Nor was there any examination of whether the burdens of dialysis could be reduced by less drastic means, such as behavior modification techniques. The court accepted with little scrutiny the family's view that the patient would have wanted treatment withheld because he had previously been an active outdoorsman.

While Spring's family might have been sincere in their assessment, they were really focusing on what some (certainly not all) competent persons in Spring's situation might choose, and not on what would serve the interests of a person who no longer was competent. The court also failed to consider the possibility that the family's own distress and expense in such a situation influenced their assessment of what the patient would have wanted. The opinion dispenses with any need to assess these possibilities by simply assuming that they would not influence the wishes of a family faced with chronic nursing-home care of a senile husband and father.

Similar conceptual weaknesses characterize the opinion in *In re Hier*, a case involving a 92-year-old nonterminally ill incompetent patient who required feeding by gastrostomy tube. When she pulled out the tube and resisted its reinsertion, the hospital sought judicial guidance. The Court refused to order the minor surgery necessary to replace the tube, stressing the procedure's risk and interpreting Hier's behavior as a "plea for privacy and personal dignity for a 92-year-old person who is seriously ill and for whom life has little left to offer."

The determination that Hier's resistance to feeding manifested a desire for privacy and personal dignity attributed the concerns of a competent individual to an incompetent patient who was probably expressing a simple response, such as irritation with the feeding apparatus or a demand for attention. As in *Spring*, the major deficiencies in this opinion are its omission of a systematic analysis of the patient's current capacities and experiences, and its failure to weigh and balance these elements in determining whether the patient had significant contemporaneous interests in continued life.

Particularly troubling is the *Hier* court's neglect of the pain and distress a conscious patient could experience if she were denied nourishment, as well as its omission of any inquiry into the possibility that she obtained pleasure and enjoyment from her restricted life. There also was evidence that one physician who testified against performing the surgery did so because Hier had already consumed "enough" health care resources. (After the appellate court decision, Hier's legal representative returned to the trial court, presented additional medical testimony, and convinced the lower court to order the surgery.)

These cases illustrate how the court's application of the substituted judgment standard opens the door to non-treatment of nursing-home residents and other severely debilitated persons based on what competent persons believe they would want in those situations, or on what meets the needs of their families and others, rather than on what serves the needs of the incompetent patients themselves. The more recent *Brophy* case reinforces this possibility. Although *Brophy* involved a patient who was irreversibly comatose, the court formulated the substituted judgment doctrine in broad terms that could affect all incompetent patients. The result is that respirators, antibiotics, nutrition, or any other treatment could be withheld from conscious incompetent patients whenever the family asserts that the incompetent patients would have found their current lives "degrading and without human dignity" when they were competent. Since many competent persons might so view such a diminished existence, *Brophy* opens the door legally to withdrawing treatment from any conscious, incompetent nursing-home resident.

THE ORTHODOX APPROACH AND THE RISKS OF OVERTREATMENT

Although the orthodox approach has been generally favorable to family requests for non-treatment, sometimes granting such requests even when unjustified, it could as easily be interpreted to deny proxy requests for non-treatment that should be granted. In *re O'Connor*, decided last year by New York's highest court, exemplifies this problem. Ms. O'Connor was an elderly woman who had suffered a series of strokes that left her paralyzed and bedridden. The court described her as "severely demented" and "profoundly incapacitated," able to respond to some simple commands, but with severe, irreparable neurological damage. Yet the court ruled against removal of a nasogastric tube because the evidence of her past preferences was insufficient to establish that she would have opted against such treatment if she were competent. Similarly, in *Cruzan v. Harmon*, the Missouri Supreme Court recently prohibited cessation of tube feeding for a permanently unconscious patient, emphasizing the lack of evidence that she had expressed desires to avoid such treatment.

As in *Spring* and *Hier*, these courts failed to inquire systematically into the patients' current interests in continued life. Instead, they sought to apply the orthodox approach, but took a stricter approach to what counted as sufficient evidence of the patients' competent wishes. Since it is difficult to know what an incompetent patient "if competent" would have wanted, the standard of proof applied to answering that question will control the outcome. Unlike the *Spring* and *Hier* judges, the courts in *O'Connor* and *Cruzan* applied a higher standard of proof to answering that question, finding insufficient evidence that they would have chosen non-treatment.

These cases illustrate the ultimate indeterminacy of the fiction of treating the incompetent patient as a self-determining individual. While the predominant danger of the orthodox approach is undertreatment, it also poses a risk that unjustified overtreatment will occur whenever the courts impose a strict standard for inferring the patient's choice if competent. In that case, medical zeal and rigid concern with right to life values may override patient and other interests. In either case, by focusing on the wrong question—the wishes of a past or hypothetical competent person—the interests of the incompetent patient as they now exist are ignored.

TOWARD A NEW LEGAL STANDARD: THE INCOMPETENT PATIENT'S CURRENT INTERESTS

The orthodox approach to non-treatment decisions for incompetent patients is seriously flawed and should be scrapped. It mistakenly assumes that incompetent patients should be regarded as choice-makers when they are incapable of decision, and then constructs a hypothetical competent decision-maker that confuses past or inferred preferences of patients with their current interests. By overlooking the conflict between past directives and current interests, it allows concerns with family stress and costs to override the real needs of incompetent patients, without an adequate evaluation of each. Alternatively, the test can be manipulated to require such a high standard of proof for inferring competent choice, that treatment can seldom be withheld, no matter how justified in terms of the patient's current interests.

An alternative approach that is more likely to protect conscious incompetent patients and to give factors external to patient welfare their proper role is to ask whether treatment actually serves the incompetent patient's existing interests. If treatment cannot succeed in supplying patients with an acceptable quality of life, then external considerations should be permitted to affect the decision. If treatment would serve patient interests but would impose heavy burdens on family or society, the conflict can be faced openly. Society's commitment to a patient-centered position can be reaffirmed or modified on the merits, not in the guise of determining what the incompetent patient would have chosen if competent.

To develop defensible standards governing the care of incompetent patients, legal decision-makers must directly assess the value to patients of their diminished or marginalized lives. The most appropriate method is to adopt a variation of the "best interests" standard and to ask whether treatment will advance the current and future welfare of the patient. This approach requires a systematic evaluation of the incompetent patient's personal contemporaneous interests, rather than the interests competent persons might have in those situations. Assessing these interests requires observers to evaluate, from the incompetent patient's perspective, indications of the patient's subjective state, and ultimately, to judge whether this state of existence is a sufficient good to justify further treatment of the patient. The question is not how a competent person would feel in such states, but whether these experiences are of value to a person in the incompetent person's situation. The important question is whether patients who cannot experience the richness of normal life still have experiences that make continued existence from their own perspective better than no life at all.

Such an approach has several advantages that recommend its adoption for all decision-making regarding incompetent patients. First, it is respectful of the individual whose treatment is at issue. The ethical commitment to a patient-centered approach requires a focus on the patient as she now is, and not on the desires that she previously had when her interests were quite different. This approach will better protect a debilitated patient's existing interests in continued life.

Second, it will permit non-treatment to occur when justified, e.g., when the patient cannot reasonably be said to have any continued interest in living because her level of awareness is so minimal that the patient is unable to appreciate being alive. For life to be of value to an individual, some capacity to interact with the environment must be present. Thus, incompetent patients with minimal "relational capacity," such as Nancy Cruzan, Claire Conroy, or Mary O'Connor, lack significant interests in having their lives maintained, and might have further treatment withheld under this test.

Third, the current-interests approach acknowledges the role of costs, family stress, and similar concerns, thus preventing them from influencing non-treatment decisions in an uncontrolled or unprincipled way. By focusing on the incompetent patient's current interests, room is given for these competing concerns when no significant patient interests are affected. Thus, for example, in cases involving permanently unconscious and barely conscious individuals, the family's burdens and financial costs may be taken into account because no interests of the patient are directly affected.

Fourth, a focus on current interests of the incompetent patient sharpens the conflict between a patient-centered and other-directed approach, thus requiring explicit consideration of the normative judgments supporting either approach. The desire to relieve family stress and reduce costs may operate at some level in treatment decisions affecting many severely debilitated patients. Unless these factors are candidly confronted, they risk influencing treatment decisions in an unprincipled fashion, potentially overriding the significant interests some incompetent patients have in obtaining life-sustaining treatment. While such directness may be discomforting, facing the question openly will keep other-directed concerns from operating subterraneously and hold them in check.

Finally, a current-interests approach still permits the family to be the initial or primary decision-maker—an important ingredient of any public policy. The family or other proxy will, in effect, be asked to determine whether the patient's life is so diminished that the patient has no further interests in living, not whether continued living is what the patient would have chosen. Doctors, courts, and others reviewing family decisions, however, will then explicitly apply a current-interests test to the proxy's choice. Ultimately a societal judgment about what states of diminished life are worth protecting will be brought to bear on those decisions.

Such an approach is not as radical a departure as it might initially sound, and is inevitable once the inability of the orthodox approach to handle more difficult cases becomes clear. Indeed, variations on this approach have already appeared. In *Saikewicz*, for example, the court purportedly applied the substituted judgment standard, couching its decision in terms of the patient's privacy and self-determination rights. In reality it performed a best interests analysis and concluded that in light of the patient's capacity to understand the pain that would be imposed to gain a few extra months of living, a decision against treatment would best serve his interests. Similarly, although its decision to require treatment might be questioned, the New York Court of Appeals in *Storar* based its decision on an individualized assessment of the burdens and benefits of continued treatment for the patient. Unfortunately it chose not to follow that lead in *O'Connor*, where a judgment that

further treatment was not in the patient's interests could reasonably have been reached.

The New Jersey Supreme Court in *Conroy* partially accepted this approach when no explicit treatment directive or other clear evidence of a patient's past preferences was available. According to the court, if "the net burdens of the patient's life with the treatment . . . clearly and markedly outweigh the benefits that the patient derives from life" and "the recurring, unavoidable, and severe pain of the patient's life [are] such that the effect of administering life-sustaining treatment would be inhumane," life-sustaining treatment may be forgone.

In our view, however, *Conroy* articulates the benefit-burden analysis too narrowly to protect incompetent patients adequately, for it fails to include such factors as lack of awareness and relational capacity. Thus, it does not authorize nontreatment of permanently unconscious or barely conscious patients who obtain negligible benefits from life, but experience no pain and suffering. Moreover, *Conroy, Saikewicz,* and *Storar* limit the benefit-burden analysis to cases in which reliable evidence of the patients' competent treatment preferences is lacking, thus overlooking the possibility of conflict between such evidence and current interests. Nevertheless, the courts' partial recognition of the need to examine the incompetent patient's contemporaneous interests is encouraging, and may facilitate expanded acceptance of the current-interests standard.

DIFFICULTIES OF A CURRENT-INTERESTS APPROACH

The major difficulty in applying a current-interests approach lies in obtaining reliable information about a patient's subjective experiences and in evaluating their significance. The danger is that arbitrary assessments of patient interests will occur, to the detriment of patients and society's respect for life.

However, the difficulty in obtaining and evaluating data about the patient and thus determining her interests is surmountable in many cases. Even though these patients typically can furnish us with little or no verbal data on how they experience their lives, the observer can gain this information from assessing their behavior and physical condition. Evidence bearing on patients' perception of pain and other physical sensations, ability to interact with other persons and the environment, and ability to engage in cognitive activity are all relevant to the examination of what these patients' lives are like for them.

More daunting is the next step: to determine whether these experiences provide "a life worth living" to the patient and a corresponding obligation by family or society to preserve it, despite the burdens that doing so entails. Yet here too it is possible to make considerable progress before facing the toughest questions about quality of life and trade-offs with other interests.

For example, a wide consensus already exists that certain states of being are not in a patient's interest, and therefore need not be provided if the family requests non-treatment. One such situation exists when the patient can experience only unremitting pain, without any countervailing pleasure and enjoyment. With modern techniques of pain relief, however, few patients may be in this category.

Permanently unconscious patients comprise a larger agreed-upon category of individuals lacking significant interests in prolonged life. All available medical evidence indicates that these individuals have no mental awareness. Although they suffer no pain or distress, they cannot experience any benefit from continued life. For them, there is only the remote possibility of restoration in the event of a mistaken diagnosis or an as yet undiscovered cure that supplies a reason for maintenance. With the exception of the *Cruzan* case in Missouri, every state court that has faced the question has permitted non-treatment of these individuals under the orthodox approach. It is likely that these decisions were influenced by the view that continued life fails to confer a significant benefit on such patients, although the opinions fail explicitly to incorporate this analysis.

Assessment of current interests of other groups of patients may also reasonably occur. "Barely conscious" individuals who cannot initiate purposeful activity, whose experiences are limited to physical sensations, and whose medical prognosis holds no reasonable chance of improvement, have clear interests in avoiding pain and discomfort. Their interests in continued life seem small, however, because they lack the cognitive capacity to interact with others and to appreciate being alive. Although some will argue that any minimally conscious human being has a significant stake in being maintained, it is difficult to see how life without greater awareness of self and others can confer a genuine benefit on these patients. Families who take this position and request non-treatment would not therefore be violating the right to life of such patients.

In contrast, conscious incompetent patients who can experience enjoyment and pleasure, and whose conditions and necessary treatment interventions impose on them small or moderate burdens, have more significant interests in obtaining life-sustaining care. The "pleasantly senile" and other debilitated individuals who appear to receive benefits from their restricted lives fall into this category. Even though their activities may seem unduly limited to some observers, these individuals appear to retain sufficient mental capacity for continued life to hold material value for them. If society is committed to a patient-centered approach, it should be willing to provide the resources necessary to protect these patients' lives. It should also find that these patients' former competent preferences against treatment and family distress are inadequate to override the patients' interests in receiving continued care.

The hardest cases will fall between those who are barely conscious and the pleasantly senile. For those patients it may be difficult to ascertain or meaningfully discuss their interests in living from their own limited perspective. "Objective" quality of life assessments are inevitably crude and subject to dispute. Disagreement and controversy may be unavoidable. In some cases, it will be impossible to reach a clear decision on what outcome would best serve the patient's existing interests. Moreover, extensive debate may be required to determine what level of awareness and benefit is sufficient to give incompetent patients a significant interest in continued life, notwithstanding the patients' former competent preferences against treatment and the burdens imposed on family and society.

But these problems are no greater than the problems under the orthodox approach of determining what the patient would choose if competent when that approach is scrupulously applied. The comparative advantage of the current-interests standard is that quality of life assessments and the conflicts they pose with other interests are faced openly, rather than in the guise of family or proxy decision of what the patient would choose if competent. In our view this openness constitutes a great advantage.

THE INEVITABILITY OF QUALITY OF LIFE ASSESSMENTS

Applying the current-interests test necessarily involves assessing the value of a particular existence to the incompetent patient in question, and its value relative to the burdens that providing it poses for family and society. Ultimately, the current-interests test brings us to the controversial task of making quality of life judgments—of deciding whether the duty to sustain life in marginalized states is obligatory, notwithstanding the burdens on others of doing so.

Although balancing patient quality of life against other interests has long been a taboo subject, we believe that an honest, direct approach to these issues is both warranted and manageable. Since quality of life judgments must inevitably be made, it is preferable to make them openly so that arbitrary or unjustified assessments can be identified. The alternative is a conceptually flawed approach that allows those judgments to be made covertly, thus risking even greater likelihood of damage to incompetent patients, their families, and society.

How do these considerations apply to actual decision-making for incompetent patients? Families will still retain primary decision-making authority, deciding whether the patient has further interests in living. In the great majority of instances their choices will reflect general societal judgments about the value to patients of greatly diminished states of existence. In cases that are less clear, the family or proxy's choice should be reviewed in light of the current-interests standard. If an objective viewer finds that the patient has significant interests in continued existence, then treatment providing that existence should continue unless the community at large reevaluates its overriding commitment to a patient-centered approach to these questions.

CONCLUSION

As the non-treatment debate moves to hard questions concerning conscious incompetent patients, it is essential that the issues be clearly posed and carefully analyzed. The orthodox judicial approach, which substitutes the fiction of a competent decision-maker for the reality of an incompetent person, is inadequate to this task and should be abandoned. That fiction confuses the issue, misleads families, doctors, and others struggling with treatment decisions, and harms the patients and families most directly affected.

An approach that focuses on the current interests of the incompetent patient—on her quality of life—is far preferable. Open assessment of quality of life will give incompetent patients their due, while at the same time acknowledging a proper role for family and cost concerns. While difficult questions will remain, the central normative questions will be directly faced. What quality of diminished life should be protected? At what cost? These are the questions that must be faced in decision-making at the margins of life.

The Limits of Legal Objectivity

Nancy K. Rhoden

PRIOR DIRECTIVES AND THE OBJECTIVE ENTERPRISE

The objective standard as articulated in *Conroy* was, of course, intended only for those situations in which the patient's prior beliefs were not determinative. If taken to its logical extension, however, the quest for a person-neutral standard may come to clash with the widespread acceptance of clear-cut prior directives as controlling. This conflict arises because if we focus solely on the incompetent's present interests, we so radically distinguish her from the author of the prior directive that it's hard to see why the prior choice should govern.

To illustrate how a completely present-oriented test can undermine the justification for honoring living wills, imagine for a moment that after the court evaluated Ms. Conroy objectively, her nephew discovered a valid and clearly applicable living will rejecting all medical treatment if "barely conscious." Given its preference for a subjective test, the *Conroy* court almost certainly would want to reconsider and let the document control. But this hypothetical discovery creates a "past-present" conflict, in which Ms. Conroy's present interests support treatment, while her prior choice is to forgo it. Although the court could simply hold that an applicable living will trumps current interests,

North Carolina Review 68, no. 5, June 1990: 845–865. Copyright © 1990 North Carolina Law Review Association. Reprinted with permission.

EDITORS' NOTE: Professor Rhoden's article has been substantially edited and most of the footnotes have been omitted. Readers wishing to follow up on sources should consult the original article. Deleted sections noted the problems with the "subjective" tests articulated in the Conroy case (reprinted in this section) and challenged the adequacy of the "objective" tests on the grounds that they (1) set a standard that can almost never be met, and (2) focus narrowly on pain to the exclusion of other important subjective values. In the sections reprinted here, Rhoden argues that the objective approach advocated in the preceding article by Professors Dresser and Robertson also threatens the validity of prior directives.

this decision procedure seems rather arbitrary in light of the just-completed assessment of current interests. Why, one might ask, should a prior directive control if it thwarts a patient's present interests?

One answer to this is that it should not. Dresser, as the most logical and consistent advocate of a present best interests test, essentially rejects living wills, except to the extent they provide useful reassurance in cases in which the objective choice would be to terminate treatment, so that the wills are largely redundant.[1] Hence my first task is to analyze her arguments and rebut them by setting forth a rights-based justification for honoring prior directives. . . .

THE IMPAIRMENT OF THE INCOMPETENT'S INTERESTS

. . . [Dresser argues] that honoring a living will can compromise unacceptably the interests of an incompetent person. One cannot be sure that what the person chose then is what he would choose now, because views about what constitutes an acceptable level of functioning may change radically as function declines. Active, healthy persons often say they would never want to live if wheelchair-bound, on dialysis, or whatever, and then later embrace life despite their disabilities. Likewise, once capacity for complex intellectual pleasures is gone, simpler things take on greater importance. As Dresser and Robertson put it:

> If we truly could determine the choice that these patients would make if suddenly able to speak—if they could tell us what their interests in their compromised states are—such choices would be most likely to reflect their current and future interests as incompetent individuals, not their past preferences.[2]

Thus prior directives reflect competent persons' former interests, but the better, more caring way to make choices for incompetents is to focus on their current interests. The law should not allow someone to make a binding future choice for death, because to do so gives an unacceptable degree of primacy to the interests of competent persons over incompetent ones.

The strength of this argument is reinforced by a very troubling sort of example. Suppose a highly intellectual person makes a prior directive stating that if he becomes even somewhat mentally impaired, he wants no medical treatment. He then suffers a mild stroke and is in a nursing home. While he cannot comprehend his prior directive, and hence can neither affirm nor rescind it, he appears to enjoy his simple existence, watching television and sharing meals with other patients. Then he gets pneumonia. His directive clearly rejects antibiotics. If it is controlling, the staff must simply watch him die. But, Dresser quite reasonably argues, he has substantial present interests in life, and they must prevail. This sort of case may well incline us toward a Parfit-type view*—that this happy incompetent person *is* someone different from the intellectual who made the document—or, at least, should make us question the wisdom of necessarily subordinating present interests to prior choices, no matter how explicit and strongly held.

All this makes a strong case against prior directives. It suggests that the reason living wills have been so widely accepted is not that we have an abiding faith in future-oriented choices, but that the substantive choice in most living wills is an objectively reasonable one (to avoid prolongation of the dying process, or treatment when persistently vegetative). Hence a prior directive may well help bolster a decision to stop treatment for a patient who lacks present interests in living, but it should not justify termination when the patient has such interests. I will later deal with the case in which the incompetent patient has clear-cut and substantial interests in living and will suggest that the right to make binding future choices should be less absolute than the right to make present ones. But first I must resurrect prior directives in general as reflecting a moral preference for individual choice rather than merely reinforcing objective decisions. To do so, I will show that rejecting future-oriented choices threatens present ones.

THE CONTINUUM WITH CONTEMPORANEOUS CHOICES

Assume that George is a Christian Scientist who rejects all surgical interventions. He makes a prior directive refusing surgery at any time for any condition. He subsequently develops a brain tumor which impairs his cognitive processes so that he is incapable of either affirming or rejecting his prior directive. He is happily watching television, and the brain tumor could be removed, extending his life (though not restoring his competency). Dresser undoubtedly would say that decision makers should authorize surgery, on the grounds that the prior religious faith is no longer relevant and that his present interests in his happy, albeit limited, life should control.

George's case seems very similar to the intellectual's, except of course that his prior beliefs are religious rather than "merely" secular. A truly "hard-core" believer in prior directives may feel that in even these cases, the directive should prevail. Some proponents of precedent autonomy may feel otherwise, because the incompetent patients: (1) have such clear-cut interests in life; and (2) are so unlikely to retain beliefs in the primacy of the intellect or the tenets of the Christian Science faith. Hence some supporters of prior directives may wish to disavow them in one or both of these cases. To show, however, that this should not lead to a wholesale rejection of precedent autonomy, we merely need alter one of two variables. The first is the time frame; the second is the patient's mental status at the time of initial diagnosis and decision making.

First, the time frame. Assume our intellectual is also psychic—or at least aware that his blood pressure is 210 over 190. He anticipates his stroke and one day before it makes his prior directive. Although the stroke affects only his brain, one week later he contracts pneumonia. Despite his recent choice, made in anticipation of disability, a proponent of current interests undoubtedly still would protect the incompetent's present interests. After all, interests can change gradually over twenty years, or in one fell swoop when one's neocortex is damaged.

If this feels somewhat less comfortable to the proponent of patient autonomy, it is because the rapidity of the developments has blurred the distinction between present-and future-oriented choice. We can blur this distinction even further if, returning to George, the brain tumor is diagnosed while he is still competent. As a Christian Scientist, he refuses surgery. Because he knows incompetency may soon ensue, he makes a prior directive. One week later, he is incompetent. Rethinking his choice now seems to me like a wrong to George—the George who competently chose, based on considered religious beliefs, to reject treatment. Yet from the present-oriented perspective, I cannot see why this is any different from the other cases. *Now* George is an incompetent whose life could be prolonged by medical intervention. And *now* he lacks the mental structure to hold his former beliefs. Under a present-oriented view, we would respect choice as long as the person was competent, but then, once his powers dimmed, we would rethink it if treatment was still potentially efficacious. In other words, a competent choice will lose its force once the person is incapable of realizing it has been made, because now—whether this occurs gradually or suddenly—the incompetent is the only player in town.

If we accept this present focus, then the competent patient's "right" to refuse treatment will be upheld only for the few months, weeks, days, or hours she remains competent. After that, the treatment decision will be made on the basis of the objectively assessed present interests of the incompetent. Taken to an extreme, this could mean that a Jehovah's Witness could refuse a blood transfusion until he "bled out" and became incompetent, after which he could be transfused.

However an objective test would decide cases of intermittent incompetency, such as the typical Jehovah's Witness scenario, it seems to commit us to a wholesale reassessment of contemporaneous treatment refusals upon subsequent incompetency. Not all refusals will impair the interests of the now-incompetent: if he is terminally ill, he may be better-off dying more quickly. But many treatment refusals will, especially those based upon minority views about religion or modern medicine. Minority beliefs are usually considered to be precisely those for which protection of autonomy is most crucial. Once we recognize that present autonomy and precedent autonomy are simply two ends of a continuum, along which are choices initially made when competent, reaffirmed repeat-

edly, but subject to reexamination after the person becomes incompetent, we see that rejecting precedent autonomy threatens a fairly broad spectrum of present, prior, and mixed present/prior choices.

VIEWING THE INCOMPETENT

This returns us to the dilemma of how to view incompetent patients. They can, of course, be viewed just in the present, with only their current, highly truncated interests taken into account. As so viewed, the prior directive clearly impairs the incompetent's interests. Back when the directive was made, however, the person was acting as a moral agent, and it is harder to take a completely present-oriented view toward moral agents and their interests. As Christine Korsgaard, who criticizes Parfit for viewing persons in a peculiarly passive sense as essentially the experiencers of various sensations, puts it:

> Perhaps it is natural to think of the present self as necessarily concerned with present satisfaction. But it is mistaken. In order to make deliberative choices, your present self must identify with something from which you will derive your reasons, but not necessarily with something present. The sort of thing you identify yourself with may carry you automatically into the future; and I have been suggesting that this will very likely be the case. Indeed, the choice of any action, no matter how trivial, takes you some way into the future. And to the extent that you regulate your choices by identifying yourself as the one who is implementing something like a particular plan of life, you need to identify with your future in order to be *what you are even now*. When the person is viewed as an agent, no clear content can be given to the idea of a merely present self.[3]

Dresser criticizes prior directives as giving moral and legal primacy to competent persons over incompetent ones. While incompetent persons of course warrant respect, I think it is nonetheless perfectly appropriate to give primacy to competent persons—at least if the incompetent person inhabits the formerly competent person's body. The competent person's primacy derives from his status as moral agent. Moral agency is inherently future-directed, and the future may, unfortunately, encompass one's incompetency.

Prior directives are the tools for projecting one's moral and spiritual values into the future. These values seem to me worthy of respect even when they conflict with the subsequent, purely physical, interests of an incompetent. (I must admit here, though, that there may be an irreconcilable clash of instincts about whether the incompetent should be viewed as the moral agent he was or the more passive experiencer of physical sensations he is now.)

Another problem with the purely present perspective is that prior directives reflect concern for others. Many people make living wills because they do not want their family's resources to be consumed in sustaining a barely sentient existence. Consider another example of other-directed values. Suppose a pregnant woman is stricken with cancer. Her prognosis is better if she aborts, but she refuses, because having this baby is the most important thing to her. She makes out a document specifying this, and then lapses into incompetency. An abortion still could be performed. Someone who rejects prior directives would, it seems, have to reopen the issue of the abortion and endorse it if it promoted the now-incompetent woman's physical interests. Yet just as it is difficult to view moral agents only in the present, it is difficult to view them in total isolation. Surely it is misleading to view *this* woman in complete isolation. Her most cherished goal—to leave the legacy of a child—is attainable only via a prior directive that harms the incompetent. It reflects the values of the competent person she was, and these values warrant a degree of moral primacy.

All this suggests that while it may be true that the incompetent person, if suddenly able to speak, would choose based on her current interests, this should not be determinative, because her former values, though no longer consciously held, have not lost their moral force. Among other reasons, such values are still important because the formerly competent person made a choice—an exercise of her autonomy. Her living will should not be seen simply as evidence of what she (as an incompetent) might now want. Seen as mere evidence, a prior directive inevitably will fail, because even the most devastatingly impaired patient could now, at least hypothetically, want something else. Viewed as an actual choice, a living will can function fairly well. It of course has limitations, as do other prior choices such as testamentary wills. Much as one cannot know one's precise medical plight in advance, one cannot anticipate the changes in conduct, lifestyle, or fortune of one's heirs. A regular will clearly is not evidence of most recent desires, but is an actual choice, and a change in circumstances is simply the risk one runs in making future choices. The alternative is not to make such choices (or to designate a proxy rather than make a substantive choice). But if we believe in the right to make future choices, we should not complain about their inherent and inescapable limitations.

The analogy with testamentary wills, however, returns us to the troubling example of the intellectual's idiosyncratic directive, because a living will, unlike a testamentary will, can severely compromise a person's present interests. Are there no limits to the harmful future choices a person can make? It does not seem inconsistent with accepting precedent autonomy to place some limits on it. In a few cases, competent contemporaneous choices are overruled, because, for example, they place medical professionals in such an untenable position. This was the impetus for denying Elizabeth Bouvia the relief sought in her first lawsuit—the right to refuse food and water by mouth while receiving hygienic care in the psychiatric ward of a hospital. The court held, essentially, that individual autonomy could not transform medical professionals into attendants at a suicide parlor. Prior directives are made with far less knowledge of the medical situation and the patient's future interests than are current choices. Hence some restrictions could be placed on them (as the law currently does), so that the former intellectual could not demand that nursing home staff let a happy, otherwise healthy, but "pleasantly senile" person die. We can thus concede that such an unusual prior directive need not control—because other concerns can override our prima facie duty to honor it—without rejecting the basic principle of prior control. After all, challenging as this philosophical puzzle is, no one (at least at present) makes such directives. People make prior directives to avoid being tethered to medical technology when unconscious or in a state such as Claire Conroy's. When they start saying, "If I can't do higher mathematics, kill me," we will have to worry in earnest about the limits of precedent autonomy.

Finally, I do not deny that we can, when pressed, make quality-of-life assessments from a present-oriented perspective. Decision makers must do this for infants and for the never-competent. Something is wrong, however, when we treat formerly competent patients as if they were never competent. Someone who makes a prior directive sees herself as the unified subject of a human life. She sees her concern for her body, her goals, or her family as transcending her incapacity. It is at least one, if not an overriding, component of treating persons with respect, that we view them as they view themselves. If we are to do this, we must not ignore their prior choices and values.

Actual prior choices are an exercise of autonomy and hence deserve far more weight than informally expressed preferences. This is not only because of evidentiary concerns, but because a person who makes a living will has exercised her right to decide—a right that imposes upon others a prima facie duty to honor her choice. We have, however, no similar right that informally expressed preferences be honored. Yet many of the same reasons that make prior directives morally relevant also make prior preferences relevant. Primary among them is the sense that most persons, when competent, see their preferences, goals, and values as relevant to future choices about them, because they see themselves as unified subjects of their lives. Were we all Parfitians, this conclusion would change. But, I hazard to say, we are not. Hence, when making moral choices for formerly competent persons who left no explicit directives we should still consider their probable desires, although we should avoid succumbing to the illusion that such desires will necessarily be unambiguous or determinative.

THE ANALOGY TO WILLS AND THE PROBLEM OF THE SUBJECT

Someone might object that all this boils down to the claim that because many people feel that if they become incompetent they would want others to think of them as they were in their prime, the law should accept and reinforce this delusion. In other words, if there is no competent person there who will notice the dishonoring of his prior wishes, then thinking we must honor them is just as silly as thinking of the dead as they were when alive and imagining we have duties to them. The "problem of the subject"—the question of just who is harmed by posthumous betrayals—has received substantial philosophical consideration. I cannot treat it adequately here, but can offer some suggestions that relate back to the unconscious or barely conscious. One solution that is easy—perhaps too easy—is just to emphasize that competent people care about their future, and if word gets out that choices will be reassessed upon incompetency, everyone will be anxious and uneasy. This rule-utilitarian approach does yield a duty to honor prior directives, albeit one that does not run to anyone in particular. It clearly would be acceptable to someone whose general moral theory is a rule-utilitarian one. It is less satisfactory to a rights-based theorist, because it means that while failure to honor a present choice wrongs the chooser, failure to honor a prior choice is, in Joel Feinberg's words, merely a "diffuse public harm."

Because Feinberg believes that the dead can be wronged (and, indeed, harmed), he tackles this problem of who is harmed by a posthumous betrayal. Feinberg distinguishes two ways of conceptualizing the dead: as dead bodies ("postmortem persons") and as the persons they were when alive ("antemortem persons"). Postmortem persons cannot be harmed; they are mere corpses. But, Feinberg argues, antemortem persons can be harmed, because they can have "surviving interests" that can be invaded. Hence posthumous betrayals can count as harms to antemortem persons. Holding that the subject of the harm is the antemortem person is an attempt, and probably a successful one, to solve the problem of the subject.

Joan Callahan argues that although in postulating antemortem persons, Feinberg has devised a proper subject of harm, he faces another problem—that of "backward causation," or the implication that an event after a person's death can harm him prior to his death.[4] Feinberg seeks to avoid this implication by holding that the antemortem subject of posthumous harm was harmed all along, or at least at the point when he acquired the interest that would subsequently be defeated. It is just that until the harmful event actually occurs, no one could know of his harmed condition. As Feinberg puts it:

[T]he financial collapse of the life-insurance company through which I have protected my loved dependents, occurring, let us imagine, five minutes after my death, several years in the future, makes it true that my present interest in my children's security is harmed, and therefore, that *I* am harmed too, though I know it not. When that time comes, my friends might feel sorry not only for my children but for me too, though I am dead.[5]

According to Feinberg, believing that the ante-mortem person is harmed before the event is no different from believing that a father whose son has just been killed is immediately harmed, even though he has not yet received the bad news.

Several closely related and, it seems, telling criticisms have been made of this notion that a person whose interests will be defeated after his death is in a harmed state from the time he acquires such interests. W. J. Waluchow notes that we do not think this way about future harms to existing persons; we do not consider ourselves already harmed by events that will happen in the future.[6] It seems he is correct that future harms should have the same logical structure whether the victim will be dead or alive when the harmful event occurs. As Callahan points out, Feinberg's theory implies that a person who will later perform a harmful action is, long before doing so, responsible for placing the victim in a harmed (though as-of-yet unrecognizably so) position. Sympathetic as I find Feinberg's overall approach, this particular aspect does seem to smack of predestination. If before a decedent's demise his future betrayer had not even formed his evil intent, it seems very strange to maintain that the decedent while alive was in a harmed state. Despite Feinberg's attempt to equate this with a father's lack of awareness of his son's recent death, there does seem to be a crucial asymmetry between being unaware of an event that has occurred, and being unaware of a future event that, unless we are fatalists, may not happen after all.

Even if Feinberg's attempted solution to the problem of backward causation fails, I believe that the basic moral intuition that we wrong the promisee when we breach a promise, even posthumously, remains firm, as Callahan's discussion itself illustrates. Callahan first tries to defend this duty by claiming that testamentary bequests gen-

erally merit respect in their own right; that we feel obligated to honor them because they usually coincide with other values we hold important, such as the good of individual heirs. To support this, she notes that we would feel less obligation to carry out an iniquitous or wasteful request (that all the paintings of a great artist be burned). But surely we don't feel that giving an estate to the decedent's spoiled, self-indulgent son (to whom it was bequeathed) is objectively preferable to giving it to his hard-working, saintly (but disinherited) daughter. If honoring his will is morally obligatory, this is because we believe the deceased had a right to distribute his estate as he saw fit, even if we abhor the end result. If truly heinous requests are not binding upon us, it is simply because other moral principles can sometimes override prima facie rights.

Callahan does admit that the independent moral value of bequests cannot fully account for what she recognizes as the genuine moral conviction that persons have a right to dispose of their property as they see fit. However, she claims that right yields a duty not to the decedent, but only to his heirs. That sounds initially plausible, but how would it apply to other promises made to a decedent? Suppose I leave my friend ten thousand dollars in my will in return for his promise to care for my cat. If, as soon as I die, he has my cat euthanized, it is hard not to think that he has breached a duty to me, rather than to my cat. It becomes even harder if the promise was to nurture my stamp collection. Moreover, when we turn to living wills, holding that the duty runs to the relatives is clearly unworkable, because surely the absence of family would not negate the duty to respect the prior directive. (And suggesting that duties run to persistently vegetative patients, viewed just in the present, is no more plausible than saying they run to corpses.) Thus Callahan is left recognizing the moral force of the duty to honor wills, but failing either to ground or direct such a duty.

The perplexities about harm predating the harmful event, and the opposite problem of being unable to justify the belief that there are duties to the dead, can each be avoided if we simply extrapolate from the observation that a right-holder need not have either the capacity or potential to discover a breach of duty. Clearly, if a person who has contracted for a statue to be erected in her honor moves to Australia, failure of the promisor to erect the statue is a breach of duty to the person in Australia, even if she never finds out. Why should the analysis change if the promisor procrastinates and breaches the contract after the emigrant has died? It is still a breach of duty, and of a duty that ran to the person who, while alive, held the right to performance. In other words, rights and duties, although correlative, need not be temporally coextensive.

This analysis relates back to the various ways persons can view themselves. Someone seeking a future-oriented promise sees herself as caring how her body, or property, or heirs, are treated. The promisor in turn incurs a duty of performance that entails an obligation to see the promisee as she envisioned herself. Thus the promisor cannot legitimately focus only upon the consequences of a breach (reasoning "she's a corpse now, she cannot care"), but instead must think of the promisee as she was in the past, and as she projected her goals and interests into the future. This duty in some sense runs backward: the object of its fulfillment or breach is most appropriately viewed as the person as she was when alive (Feinberg's "ante-mortem person"). But recognizing duties to ante-mortem persons does not mean we have to agree that dead persons can be harmed or that future victims of harms are harmed from the moment they acquire interests that will be defeated. All we need affirm is that living persons can have rights of future performance, and that breaches of duties to perform after death count as wrongs to the right-holder, thought of as she was when alive.

Although duties to persons who previously held the correlative right but who no longer exist are admittedly an unusual case, we might think of this as similar to other future-oriented promises made in anticipation of incapacity. Suppose Joe, a manic-depressive given to extravagant and disastrous business deals in his manic phase, makes a contract (during a lucid period) with a friend whereby the friend promises not to let him make any business deals while manic. Then Joe becomes manic. In adhering to the contract, the friend is upholding his duty to view Joe (and Joe's interests) as Joe saw things when lucid. This case differs from wills or living wills, because Joe himself will benefit in the future from having his present desires thwarted. But the cases are not so completely different,

because each involves a duty to act upon wishes of a person that are no longer held and indeed to view the person, for moral purposes, as he viewed himself at a previous time, and as he projected the values held then into the future. The solution of saying a duty exists *now*, and breach of it is a breach of duty, and thus a wrong, to the person as he was *then*, is not unproblematic. If one accepts a rights-based justification for present and precedent autonomy, however, the backward-looking solution seems preferable to holding that upon death or incapacity, a formerly grounded duty suddenly runs in no direction at all.

CONCLUSION

Thus we must reject the premise of the present-oriented objective test—that if a subjective analysis does not yield a definitive answer, a fully objective approach must be used. Viewing the patient only in the present divides her from her history, her values, and her relationships—from all those things that made her a moral agent. It likewise undermines living wills. Living wills are not as unproblematic as often assumed: they are subject to the criticism that they subjugate the interests of incompetent persons to the values of competent ones. But as we have seen, many or most autonomous choices take the chooser some way into the future. Denying the right of future choice thus threatens the right of present choice. Hence the mirror image of the asserted problem with living wills is giving so much primacy to incompetents that one acts as if they never were competent. If a person has stated, "Treat me, when incompetent, as if my competent values still hold," respect for persons demands that we do so. This does give primacy to the competent person, but it is, after all, competent persons who have the considered moral values, life plans, and treatment preferences that underlie our respect. Finally, this analysis can apply, albeit less strongly, to formerly competent patients who did not make prior directives, because they, too, most likely held relevant views. If we believe that a competent person is, more likely than not, to see her values as still being relevant during incapacity, then respect for persons suggests that we consider those values in making treatment decisions, even while recognizing that they may be more difficult to assess, and hence far less determinative, than actual prior choices.

NOTES

1. R. Dresser, "Life, Death, and Incompetent Patients: Conceptual Infirmities and Hidden Values in the Law," 373 *Ariz. L. Rev.* at 379–82, 394–95; Dresser, "Relitigating Life and Death," 51 *Ohio St. L. J.* 425 (1990), at 433.
2. "Quality of Life and Non-Treatment Decisions for Incompetent Patients: A Critique of the Orthodox Approach," 17 *Law, Med. & Health Care* 234, 236–37 (1989) [*supra* this section].
3. Korsgaard, "Personal Identity and the Unity of Agency: A Kantian Response to Parfit," 18 *Phil. & Pub. Aff.* 101, 113–14 (1989) (footnotes omitted).
4. *See* Callahan, "On Harming the Dead," 97 *Ethics* 341, 345 (1987).
5. J. Feinberg, *Harm to Others.* 91 (1984).
6. Waluchow, "Feinberg's Theory of 'Preposthumous' Harm," 25 *Dialogue* 727, 732–33 (1986).

SECTION 5

Euthanasia and Physician-Assisted Suicide

Death and Dignity: A Case of Individualized Decision Making

Timothy E. Quill

Diane was feeling tired and had a rash. A common scenario, though there was something subliminally worrisome that prompted me to check her blood count. Her hematocrit was 22, and the white-cell count was 4.3 with some metamyelocytes and unusual white cells. I wanted it to be viral, trying to deny what was staring me in the face. Perhaps in a repeated count it would disappear. I called Diane and told her it might be more serious than I had initially thought—that the test needed to be repeated and that if she felt worse, we might have to move quickly. When she pressed for the possibilities, I reluctantly opened the door to leukemia. Hearing the word seemed to make it exist. "Oh, shit!" she said. "Don't tell me that." Oh, shit! I thought, I wish I didn't have to.

Diane was no ordinary person (although no one I have ever come to know has been really ordinary). She was raised in an alcoholic family and had felt alone for much of her life. She had vaginal cancer as a young woman. Through much of her adult life, she had struggled with depression and her own alcoholism. I had come to know, respect, and admire her over the previous eight years as she confronted these problems and gradually overcame them. She was an incredibly clear, at

New England Journal of Medicine 324, No. 10, March 7, 1991: 691–694. Copyright © 1991, Massachusetts Medical Society. Reprinted by permission of the publisher.

times brutally honest, thinker and communicator. As she took control of her life, she developed a strong sense of independence and confidence. In the previous three-and-one-half years, her hard work had paid off. She was completely abstinent from alcohol, she had established much deeper connections with her husband, college-age son, and several friends, and her business and her artistic work were blossoming. She felt she was really living fully for the first time.

Not surprisingly, the repeated blood count was abnormal, and detailed examination of the peripheral blood smear showed myelocytes. I advised her to come into the hospital, explaining that we needed to do a bone marrow biopsy and make some decisions relatively rapidly. She came to the hospital knowing what we would find. She was terrified, angry, and sad. Although we knew the odds, we both clung to the thread of possibility that it might be something else.

The bone marrow confirmed the worst: acute myelomonocytic leukemia. In the face of this tragedy, we looked for signs of hope. This is an area of medicine in which technological intervention has been successful, with cures 25 percent of the time—long-term cures. As I probed the costs of these cures, I heard about induction chemotherapy (three weeks in the hospital, prolonged neutropenia, probable infectious complications, and hair loss; 75 percent of patients respond, 25 percent do not). For the survivors, this is followed by consolidation chemotherapy (with similar side effects; another 25 percent die, for a net survival of 50 percent). Those still alive, to have a reasonable chance of long-term survival, then need bone marrow transplantation (hospitalization for two months and whole-body irradiation, with complete killing of the bone marrow, infectious complications, and the possibility for graft-versus-host disease—with a survival of approximately 50 percent, or 25 percent of the original group). Though hematologists may argue over the exact percentages, they don't argue about the outcome of no treatment—certain death in days, weeks, or at most a few months.

Believing that delay was dangerous, our oncologist broke the news to Diane and began making plans to insert a Hickman catheter and begin induction chemotherapy that afternoon. When I saw her shortly thereafter, she was enraged at his presumption that she would want treatment, and

devastated by the finality of the diagnosis. All she wanted to do was go home and be with her family. She had no further questions about treatment and in fact had decided that she wanted none. Together we lamented her tragedy and the unfairness of life. Before she left, I felt the need to be sure that she and her husband understood that there was some risk in delay, that the problem was not going to go away, and that we needed to keep considering the options over the next several days. We agreed to meet in two days.

She returned in two days with her husband and son. They had talked extensively about the problem and the options. She remained very clear about her wish not to undergo chemotherapy and to live whatever time she had left outside the hospital. As we explored her thinking further, it became clear that she was convinced she would die during the period of treatment and would suffer unspeakably in the process (from hospitalization, from lack of control over her body, from the side effects of chemotherapy, and from pain and anguish). Although I could offer support and my best effort to minimize her suffering if she chose treatment, there was no way I could say any of this would not occur. In fact, the last four patients with acute leukemia at our hospital had died very painful deaths in the hospital during various stages of treatment (a fact I did not share with her). Her family wished she would choose treatment but sadly accepted her decision. She articulated very clearly that it was she who would be experiencing all the side effects of treatment and that odds of 25 percent were not good enough for her to undergo so toxic a course of therapy, given her expectations of chemotherapy and hospitalization and the absence of a closely matched bone marrow donor. I had her repeat her understanding of the treatment, the odds, and what to expect if there were no treatment. I clarified a few misunderstandings, but she had a remarkable grasp of the options and implications.

I have been a longtime advocate of active, informed patient choice of treatment or nontreatment, and of a patient's right to die with as much control and dignity as possible. Yet there was something about her giving up a 25 percent chance of long-term survival in favor of almost certain death that disturbed me. I had seen Diane fight and use her considerable inner resources to overcome alcoholism and depression, and I half expected her to change her mind over the next week. Since the window of time in which effective treatment can be initiated is rather narrow, we met several times that week. We obtained a second hematology consultation and talked at length about the meaning and implications of treatment and nontreatment. She talked to a psychologist she had seen in the past. I gradually understood the decision from her perspective and became convinced that it was the right decision for her. We arranged for home hospice care (although at that time Diane felt reasonably well, was active, and looked healthy), left the door open for her to change her mind, and tried to anticipate how to keep her comfortable in the time she had left.

Just as I was adjusting to her decision, she opened up another area that would stretch me profoundly. It was extraordinarily important to Diane to maintain control of herself and her own dignity during the time remaining to her. When this was no longer possible, she clearly wanted to die. As a former director of a hospice program, I know how to use pain medicines to keep patients comfortable and lessen suffering. I explained the philosophy of comfort care, which I strongly believe in. Although Diane understood and appreciated this, she had known of people lingering in what was called relative comfort, and she wanted no part of it. When the time came, she wanted to take her life in the least painful way possible. Knowing of her desire for independence and her decision to stay in control, I thought this request made perfect sense. I acknowledged and explored this wish but also thought that it was out of the realm of currently accepted medical practice and that it was more than I could offer or promise. In our discussion, it became clear that preoccupation with her fear of a lingering death would interfere with Diane's getting the most out of the time she had left until she found a safe way to ensure her death. I feared the effects of a violent death on her family, the consequences of an ineffective suicide that would leave her lingering in precisely the state she dreaded so much, and the possibility that a family member would be forced to assist her, with all the legal and personal repercussions that would follow. She discussed this at length with her family. They believed that they should respect her choice. With this in mind, I told Diane that

information was available from the Hemlock Society that might be helpful to her.

A week later she phoned me with a request for barbiturates for sleep. Since I knew that this was an essential ingredient in a Hemlock Society suicide, I asked her to come to the office to talk things over. She was more than willing to protect me by participating in a superficial conversation about her insomnia, but it was important to me to know how she planned to use the drugs and to be sure that she was not in despair or overwhelmed in a way that might color her judgment. In our discussion, it was apparent that she was having trouble sleeping, but it was also evident that the security of having enough barbiturates available to commit suicide when and if the time came would leave her secure enough to live fully and concentrate on the present. It was clear that she was not despondent and that in fact she was making deep, personal connections with her family and close friends. I made sure that she knew how to use the barbiturates for sleep, and also that she knew the amount needed to commit suicide. We agreed to meet regularly, and she promised to meet with me before taking her life, to ensure that all other avenues had been exhausted. I wrote the prescription with an uneasy feeling about the boundaries I was exploring—spiritual, legal, professional, and personal. Yet I also felt strongly that I was setting her free to get the most out of the time she had left, and to maintain dignity and control on her own terms until her death.

The next several months were very intense and important for Diane. Her son stayed home from college, and they were able to be with one another and say much that had not been said earlier. Her husband did his work at home so that he and Diane could spend more time together. She spent time with her closest friends. I had her come into the hospital for a conference with our residents, at which she illustrated in a most profound and personal way the importance of informed decision making, the right to refuse treatment, and the extraordinarily personal effects of illness and interaction with the medical system. There were emotional and physical hardships as well. She had periods of intense sadness and anger. Several times she became very weak, but she received transfusions as an outpatient and responded with marked improvement of symptoms. She had two serious infections that responded surprisingly well to empirical courses of oral antibiotics. After three tumultuous months, there were two weeks of relative calm and well-being, and fantasies of a miracle began to surface.

Unfortunately, we had no miracle. Bone pain, weakness, fatigue, and fevers began to dominate her life. Although the hospice workers, family members, and I tried our best to minimize the suffering and promote comfort, it was clear that the end was approaching. Diane's immediate future held what she feared the most—increasing discomfort, dependence, and hard choices between pain and sedation. She called up her closest friends and asked them to come over to say goodbye, telling them that she would be leaving soon. As we had agreed, she let me know as well. When we met, it was clear that she knew what she was doing, that she was sad and frightened to be leaving, but that she would be even more terrified to stay and suffer. In our tearful goodbye, she promised a reunion in the future at her favorite spot on the edge of Lake Geneva, with dragons swimming in the sunset.

Two days later her husband called to say that Diane had died. She had said her final goodbyes to her husband and son that morning, and asked them to leave her alone for an hour. After an hour, which must have seemed an eternity, they found her on the couch, lying very still and covered by her favorite shawl. There was no sign of struggle. She seemed to be at peace. They called me for advice about how to proceed. When I arrived at their house, Diane indeed seemed peaceful. Her husband and son were quiet. We talked about what a remarkable person she had been. They seemed to have no doubts about the course she had chosen or about their cooperation, although the unfairness of her illness and the finality of her death were overwhelming to us all.

I called the medical examiner to inform him that a hospice patient had died. When asked about the cause of death, I said, "acute leukemia." He said that was fine and that we should call a funeral director. Although acute leukemia was the truth, it was not the whole story. Yet any mention of suicide would have given rise to a police investigation and probably brought the arrival of an ambulance crew for resuscitation. Diane would have become a "coroner's case," and the decision to perform an autopsy would have been made at the discretion of the medical examiner. The family or I could have been subject to criminal prosecution, and I to professional review, for our roles in support of Diane's choices. Although I truly believe that the family and I gave her the best care possible, allowing her to define her limits and directions as much as possible, I am not sure the law, society, or the medical profession would agree. So I said "acute leukemia" to protect all of us, to protect Diane from an invasion into her past and her body, and to continue to shield society from the knowledge of the degree of suffering that people often undergo in the process of dying. Suffering can be lessened to some extent, but in no way eliminated or made benign, by the careful intervention of a competent, caring physician, given current social constraints.

Diane taught me about the range of help I can provide if I know people well and if I allow them to say what they really want. She taught me about life, death, and honesty and about taking charge and facing tragedy squarely when it strikes. She taught me that I can take small risks for people that I really know and care about. Although I did not assist in her suicide directly, I helped indirectly to make it possible, successful, and relatively painless. Although I know we have measures to help control pain and lessen suffering, to think that people do not suffer in the process of dying is an illusion. Prolonged dying can occasionally be peaceful, but more often the role of the physician and family is limited to lessening but not eliminating severe suffering.

I wonder how many families and physicians secretly help patients over the edge into death in the face of such severe suffering. I wonder how many severely ill or dying patients secretly take their lives, dying alone in despair. I wonder whether the image of Diane's final aloneness will persist in the minds of her family, or if they will remember more the intense, meaningful months they had together before she died. I wonder whether Diane struggled in that last hour, and whether the Hemlock Society's way of death by suicide is the most benign. I wonder why Diane, who gave so much to so many of us, had to be alone for the last hour of her life. I wonder whether I will see Diane again, on the shore of Lake Geneva at sunset, with dragons swimming on the horizon.

Assisted Suicide: The Philosophers' Brief

Ronald Dworkin

INTRODUCTION

The laws of all but one American state now forbid doctors to prescribe lethal pills for patients who want to kill themselves.· These cases[1] began when groups of dying patients and their doctors in Washington State and New York each sued asking that these prohibitions be declared unconstitutional so that the patients could be given, when and if they asked for it, medicine to hasten their death. The pleadings described the agony in which the patient plaintiffs were dying, and two federal Circuit Courts of Appeal—the Ninth Circuit in the Washington case and the Second Circuit in the New York case—agreed with the plaintiffs that the Constitution forbids the government from flatly prohibiting doctors to help end such desperate and pointless suffering.[2]

Washington State and New York appealed these decisions to the Supreme Court, and a total of sixty amicus briefs were filed, including briefs on behalf of the American Medical Association and the United States Catholic Conference urging the Court to reverse the circuit court decisions, and on behalf of the American Medical Students Association and the Gay Men's Health Crisis urging it to affirm them. The justices' comments during oral argument persuaded many observers that the Court would reverse the decisions, probably by a lopsided majority. The justices repeatedly cited

two versions—one theoretical, the other practical—of the "slippery slope" argument: that it would be impossible to limit a right to assisted suicide in an acceptable way, once that right was recognized.

The theoretical version of the argument denies that any principled line can be drawn between cases in which proponents say a right of assisted suicide is appropriate and those in which they concede that it is not. The circuit courts recognized only a right for competent patients already dying in great physical pain to have pills prescribed that they could take themselves. Several justices asked on what grounds the right once granted could be so severely limited. Why should it be denied to dying patients who are so feeble or paralyzed that they cannot take pills themselves and who beg a doctor to inject a lethal drug into them? Or to patients who are not dying but face years of intolerable physical or emotional pain, or crippling paralysis or dependence? But if the right were extended that far, on what ground could it be denied to anyone who had formed a desire to die—to a sixteen-year-old suffering from a severe case of unrequited love, for example?

The philosophers' brief answers these questions in two steps. First, it defines a very general moral and constitutional principle—that every competent person has the right to make momentous personal decisions which invoke fundamental religious or philosophical convictions about life's value for himself. Second, it recognizes that people may make such momentous decisions impulsively or out of emotional depression, when their act does not reflect their enduring convictions; and it therefore allows that in some circumstances a state has the constitutional power to override that right in order to protect citizens from mistaken but irrevocable acts of self-destruction. States may be allowed to prevent assisted suicide by people who—it is plausible to think—would later be grateful if they were prevented from dying.

That two-step argument would justify a state's protecting a disappointed adolescent from himself. It would equally plainly not justify forcing a com-

Introduction to "Assisted Suicide: The Philosophers' Brief" by Ronald Dworkin, *The New York Review of Books*, Vol. XLIV, No. 5, March 27, 1997, 41–47. Reprinted with permission from The New York Review of Books. Copyright © 1997 NYREV, Inc.

Editors' Note: In June 1997 the Supreme Court decided two cases (State of Washington v. Glucksberg and Vacco v. Quill) posing the question whether dying patients have a right to physician-assisted suicide. We present here the amicus curiae brief of six moral philosophers, with an introduction by Ronald Dworkin.

* In November 1997, Oregon voters rejected Measure 51, which would have reversed Measure 16 (approved by the voters in 1994), thereby legalizing physician-assisted suicide in that state.

petent dying patient to live in agony a few weeks longer. People will of course disagree about the cases in between these extremes, and if the Court adopted this argument, the federal courts would no doubt be faced with a succession of cases in years to come testing whether, for example, it is plausible to assume that a desperately crippled patient in constant pain but with years to live, who has formed a settled and repeatedly stated wish to die, would one day be glad he was forced to stay alive. But though two justices dwelled, during the oral argument, on the unappealing prospect of a series of such cases coming before the courts, it seems better that the courts do assume that burden, which they could perhaps mitigate through careful rulings, than that they be relieved of it at the cost of such terrible suffering. The practical version of the slippery slope argument is more complex. If assisted suicide were permitted in principle, every state would presumably adopt regulations to insure that a patient's decision for suicide is informed, competent, and free. But many people fear that such regulations could not be adequately enforced, and that particularly vulnerable patients—poor patients dying in overcrowded hospitals that had scarce resources, for example—might be pressured or hustled into a decision for death they would not otherwise make. The evidence suggests, however, that such patients might be better rather than less well protected if assisted suicide were legalized with appropriate safeguards.

More of them could then benefit from relief that is already available—illegally—to more fortunate people who have established relationships with doctors willing to run the risks of helping them to die. The current two-tier system—a chosen death and an end of pain outside the law for those with connections and stony refusals for most other people—is one of the greatest scandals of contemporary medical practice. The sense many middle-class people have that if necessary their own doctor "will know what to do" helps to explain why the political pressure is not stronger for a fairer and more open system in which the law acknowledges for everyone what influential people now expect for themselves.

For example, in a recent study in the State of Washington, which guaranteed respondents anonymity, 26 percent of doctors surveyed said they had received explicit requests for help in dying, and had provided, overall, lethal prescriptions to 24 percent of patients requesting them.[3] In other studies, 40 percent of Michigan oncologists surveyed reported that patients had initiated requests for death, 18 percent said they had participated in assisted suicide, and 4 percent in "active euthanasia"—injecting lethal drugs themselves. In San Francisco, 53 percent of the 1,995 responding physicians said they had granted an AIDS patient's request for suicide assistance at least once.[4] These statistics approach the rates at which doctors help patients die in Holland, where assisted suicide is in effect legal.

The most important benefit of legalized assisted suicide for poor patients however, might be better care while they live. For though the medical experts cited in various briefs disagreed sharply about the percentage of terminal cases in which pain can be made tolerable through advanced and expensive palliative techniques, they did not disagree that a great many patients do not receive the relief they could have. The Solicitor General who urged the Court to reverse the lower court judgments conceded in the oral argument that 25 percent of terminally ill patients actually do die in pain. That appalling figure is the result of several factors, including medical ignorance and fear of liability, inadequate hospital funding, and (as the Solicitor General suggested) the failure of insurers and health care programs to cover the cost of special hospice care. Better training in palliative medicine, and legislation requiring such coverage, would obviously improve the situation, but it seems perverse to argue that the patients who would be helped were better pain management available must die horribly because it is not; and, as Justice Breyer pointed out, the number of patients in that situation might well increase as medical costs continue to escalate.

According to several briefs, moreover, patients whose pain is either uncontrollable or uncontrolled are often "terminally sedated"—intravenous drugs (usually barbiturates or benzodiazepenes) are injected to induce a pharmacologic coma during which the patient is given neither water nor nutrition and dies sooner than he otherwise would.[5] Terminal sedation is widely accepted as legal, though it advances death.[6] But it is not subject to regulations nearly as stringent as those that a state forced to allow assisted suicide would enact, because such regulations would presumably include a requirement that hospitals, before accepting any request for assistance in suicide, must demonstrate that effective medical care including state-of-the art pain management had been offered. The guidelines recently published by a network of ethics committees in the Bay Area of California, for example, among other stringent safeguards, provide that a primary care physician who receives a request for suicide must make an initial referral to a hospice program or to a physician experienced in palliative care, and certify in a formal report filed in a state registry, signed by an independent second physician with expertise in such care, that the best available pain relief has been offered to the patient.[7]

Doctors and hospitals anxious to avoid expense would have very little incentive to begin a process that would focus attention on their palliative care practices. They would be more likely to continue the widespread practice of relatively inexpensive terminal care which is supplemented, perhaps, with terminal sedation. It is at least possible, however, that patients' knowledge of the possibility of assisted suicide would make it more difficult for such doctors to continue as before. That is the view of the Coalition of Hospice Professionals, who said, in their own amicus brief, "Indeed, removing legal bans on suicide assistance will enhance the opportunity for advanced hospice care for all patients because regulation of physician-assisted suicide would mandate that all palliative measures be exhausted as a condition precedent to assisted suicide."

So neither version of the slippery slope argument seems very strong. It is nevertheless understandable that Supreme Court justices are reluctant, particularly given how little experience we have so far with legalized assisted suicide, to declare that all but one of the states must change their laws to allow a practice many citizens think abominable and sacrilegious But as the philosophers' brief that follows emphasizes, the Court is in an unusually difficult position. If it closes the door to a constitutional right to assisted suicide it will do substantial damage to constitutional practice and precedent, as well as to thousands of people in great suffering. It would face a dilemma in justifying any such decision, because it would be forced to choose between the two unappealing strategies that the brief describes.

The first strategy—declaring that terminally ill patients in great pain do not have a constitutional right to control their own deaths, even in principle—seems alien to our constitutional system, as the Solicitor General himself insisted in the oral argument. It would also undermine a variety of the Court's own past decisions, including the carefully constructed position on abortion set out in its 1993 decision in Casey. Indeed some amicus briefs took the occasion of the assisted suicide cases to criticize the abortion decisions—a brief filed on behalf of Senator Orrin Hatch of Utah and Representatives Henry Hyde of Illinois and Charles Canady of Florida, for example, declared that the abortion decisions were "of questionable legitimacy and even more questionable prudence." Protecting the abortion rulings was presumably one of the aims of the Clinton administration in arguing, through the Solicitor General, for the second strategy instead.

The first strategy would create an even more evident inconsistency within the practice of terminal medicine itself. Since the Cruzan decision discussed in the brief, lawyers have generally assumed that the Court would protect the right of any competent patient to have life sustaining equipment removed from his body even though he would then die. In the oral argument, several justices suggested a "common-sense" distinction between the moral significance of acts, on the one hand, and omissions, on the other. This distinction, they suggested, would justify a constitutional distinction between prescribing lethal pills and removing life support; for, in their view, removing support is only a matter of "letting nature take its course," while prescribing pills is an active intervention that brings death sooner than natural processes would.

The discussion of this issue in the philosophers' brief is therefore particularly significant. The brief insists that such suggestions wholly misunderstand the "common-sense" distinction, which is not between acts and omissions, but between acts or omissions that are designed to cause death and those that are not. One justice suggested that a patient who insists that life support be disconnected is not committing suicide. That is wrong: he is committing suicide if he aims at death, as most such patients do, just as someone whose wrist is cut in an accident is committing suicide if he refuses to try to stop the bleeding. The distinction between acts that aim at death and those that do not cannot justify a constitutional distinction between assisting in suicide and terminating life support. Some doctors, who stop life support only because the patient so demands, do not aim at death. But neither do doctors who prescribe lethal pills only for the same reason, and hope that the patient does not take them. And many doctors who terminate life support obviously do aim at death, including those who deny nutrition during terminal sedation, because denying nutrition is designed to hasten death, not to relieve pain.

There are equally serious objections, however, to the second strategy the philosophers' brief discusses. This strategy concedes a general right to assisted suicide but holds that states have the power to judge that the risks of allowing any exercise of that right are too great. It is obviously dangerous for the Court to allow a state to deny a constitutional right on the ground that the state lacks the will or resource to enforce safeguards if it is exercised, particularly when the case for the practical version of the "slippery slope" objection seems so weak and has been little examined.

NOTES

1. *State of Washington et al.* v. *Glucksberg et al.* and *Vacco et al.* v. *Quill et al.*, argued January 8, 1997.

2. I described the circuit court decisions in an earlier article, "Sex and Death in the Courts," *The New York Review*, August 8, 1996.

3. Anthony L. Back et al., "Physician-Assisted Suicide and Euthanasia in Washington State," *Journal of the American Medical Association*, Volume 275, No. 2, pp. 919, 920, 922 (1996).

4. See David I. Doukas et al., "Attitudes and Behaviors on Physician Assisted Death: A Study of Michigan Oncologists," *Clinical Oncology*, Volume 13, p. 1055 (1995); and L. Slome et al., "Attitudes Toward Assisted Suicide in AIDS: A Five Year Comparison Study," conference abstract now available on the World Wide Web (1996). The amicus brief of the Association of Law School Professors offers other statistics to the same effect taken from other states and from nurses.

5. According to one respondent's brief, "Despite some imprecision in the empirical evidence, it has been estimated that between 5 percent and 52 percent of dying patients entering home palliative care units have been terminally sedated." The brief cites Paul Rousseau, "Terminal Sedation In The Care of Dying Patients," *Archives of Internal Medicine*, Volume 156, p.1785 (1996).

6. The amicus brief of the Coalition of Hospice Professionals raised a frightening question about terminal sedation. "Unfortunately, while a terminally sedated patient exhibits an outwardly peaceful appearance, medical science cannot verify that the individual ceases to experience pain and suffering. To the contrary, studies of individuals who have been anaesthetized (with the same kinds of drugs used in terminal sedation) for surgery (and who are in a deeper comatose state than terminally sedated patients since their breathing must be sustained by a respirator) have demonstrated that painful stimuli applied to the patient will cause a significant increase in brain activity, even though there is no external physical response." See, e.g., Orlando R. Hung et al., "Thiopental Pharmacodynamics: Quantitation of Clinical and Electroencephalographic Depth of Anesthesia," *Anesthesiology*, Volume 77, p. 237 (1992).

7. *BANEC-Generated Guidelines for Comprehensive Care of the Terminally Ill*. Bay Area Network of Ethics Committees, September, 1996.

The Philosophers' Brief

Ronald Dworkin, Thomas Nagel, Robert Nozick, John Rawls, Thomas Scanlon, and Judith Jarvis Thomson

Amici are six moral and political philosophers who differ on many issues of public morality and policy. They are united, however, in their conviction that respect for fundamental principles of liberty and justice, as well as for the American constitutional tradition, requires that the decisions of the Courts of Appeals be affirmed.

INTRODUCTION AND SUMMARY OF ARGUMENT

These cases do not invite or require the Court to make moral, ethical, or religious judgments about how people should approach or confront their death or about when it is ethically appropriate to hasten one's own death or to ask others for help in doing so. On the contrary, they ask the Court to recognize that individuals have a constitutionally protected interest in making those grave judgments for themselves, free from the imposition of any religious or philosophical orthodoxy by court or legislature. States have a constitutionally legitimate interest in protecting individuals from irrational, ill-informed, pressured, or unstable decisions to hasten their own death. To that end, states may regulate and limit the assistance that doctors may give individuals who express a wish to die. But states may not deny people in the position of the patient-plaintiffs in these cases the opportunity to demonstrate, through whatever reasonable procedures the state might institute—even procedures that err on the side of caution—that their decision to die is indeed informed, stable, and fully free. Denying that opportunity to terminally ill patients who are in agonizing pain or otherwise doomed to an existence they regard as intolerable could only be justified on the basis of a religious or ethical conviction about the value or meaning of life itself. Our Constitution forbids government to impose such convictions on its citizens.

Petitioners [i.e., the state authorities of Washington and New York] and the amici who support them offer two contradictory arguments. Some deny that the patient-plaintiffs have any constitutionally protected liberty interest in hastening their own deaths. But that liberty interest flows directly from this Court's previous decisions. It flows from the right of people to make their own decisions about matters "involving the most intimate and personal choices a person may make in a lifetime, choices central to personal dignity and autonomy." *Planned Parenthood* v. *Casey*, 505 U.S. 833, 851(1992).

The Solicitor General, urging reversal in support of Petitioners, recognizes that the patient-plaintiffs do have a constitutional liberty interest at stake in these cases. *See* Brief for the United States as Amicus Curiae Supporting Petitioners at 12, *Washington* v. *Vacco* (hereinafter Brief for the United States) ("The term 'liberty' in the Due Process Clause . . . is broad enough to encompass an interest on the part of terminally ill, mentally competent adults in obtaining relief from the kind of suffering experienced by the plaintiffs in this case, which includes not only severe physical pain, but also the despair and distress that comes from physical deterioration and the inability to control basic bodily functions."); *see also id.* at 13 ("*Cruzan* . . . supports the conclusion that a liberty interest is at stake in this case.").

The Solicitor General nevertheless argues that Washington and New York properly ignored this profound interest when they required the patient-plaintiffs to live on in circumstances they found intolerable. He argues that a state may simply declare that it is unable to devise a regulatory scheme that would adequately protect patients whose desire to die might be ill informed or unstable or foolish or not fully free, and that a state may therefore fall back on a blanket prohibition. This Court has never accepted that patently dangerous rationale for denying protection altogether to a conceded fundamental constitutional interest. It would be a serious mistake to do so now. If that rationale were accepted, an interest acknowledged to be constitutionally protected would be rendered empty.

ARGUMENT

I. THE LIBERTY INTEREST ASSERTED HERE IS PROTECTED BY THE DUE PROCESS CLAUSE

The Due Process Clause of the Fourteenth Amendment protects the liberty interest asserted by the patient-plaintiffs here.

Certain decisions are momentous in their impact on the character of a person's life decisions about religious faith, political and moral allegiance, marriage, procreation, and death, for example. Such deeply personal decisions pose controversial questions about how and why human life has value. In a free society, individuals must be allowed to make those decisions for themselves, out of their own faith, conscience, and convictions. This Court has insisted, in a variety of contexts and circumstances, that this great freedom is among those protected by the Due Process Clause as essential to a community of "ordered liberty." *Palko* v. *Connecticut*, 302 U.S. 319, 325 (1937). In its recent decision in *Planned Parenthood* v. *Casey*, 505 U.S. 833, 851 (1992), the Court offered a paradigmatic statement of that principle:

> matters [] involving the most intimate and personal choices a person may make in a lifetime, choices central to a person's dignity and autonomy, are central to the liberty protected by the Fourteenth Amendment.

That declaration reflects an idea underlying many of our basic constitutional protections. As the Court explained in *West Virginia State Board of Education* v. *Barnette*, 319 U.S. 624, 642 (1943):

> If there is any fixed star in our constitutional constellation, it is that no official . . . can prescribe what shall be orthodox in politics, nationalism, religion, or other matters of opinion or force citizens to confess by word or act their faith therein.

A person's interest in following his own convictions at the end of life is so central a part of the more general right to make "intimate and personal choices" for himself that a failure to protect that particular interest would undermine the general right altogether. Death is, for each of us, among the most significant events of life. As the Chief Justice said in *Cruzan* v. *Missouri*, 497 U.S. 261, 281(1990), "[t]he choice between life and death is a deeply personal decision of obvious and overwhelming finality." Most of us see death—whatever we think will follow it—as the final act of life's drama, and we want that last act to reflect our own convictions, those we have tried to live by, not the convictions of others forced on us in our most vulnerable moment.

Different people, of different religious and ethical beliefs, embrace very different convictions about which way of dying confirms and which contradicts the value of their lives. Some fight against death with every weapon their doctors can devise. Others will do nothing to hasten death even if they pray it will come soon. Still others, including the patient-plaintiffs in these cases, want to end their lives when they think that living on, in the only way they can, would disfigure rather than enhance the lives they had created. Some people make the latter choice not just to escape pain. Even if it were possible to eliminate all pain for a dying patient—and frequently that is not possible—that would not end or even much alleviate the anguish some would feel at remaining alive, but intubated, helpless, and often sedated near oblivion.

None of these dramatically different attitudes about the meaning of death can be dismissed as irrational. None should be imposed, either by the pressure of doctors or relatives or by the fiat of government, on people who reject it. Just as it would be intolerable for government to dictate that doctors never be permitted to try to keep someone alive as long as possible, when that is what the patient wishes, so it is intolerable for government to dictate that doctors may never, under any circumstances, help someone to die who believes that further life means only degradation. The Constitution insists that people must be free to make these deeply personal decisions for themselves and must not be forced to end their lives in a way that appalls them, just because that is what some majority thinks proper.

II. THIS COURT'S DECISIONS IN *CASEY* AND *CRUZAN* COMPEL RECOGNITION OF A LIBERTY INTEREST HERE

A. Casey *Supports the Liberty Interest Asserted Here.* In *Casey*, this Court, in holding that a state cannot constitutionally proscribe abortion in all cases, reiterated that the Constitution protects a sphere of autonomy in which individuals must be permitted to make certain decisions for themselves. The Court began its analysis by pointing out that "[a]t the heart of liberty is the right to define one's own concept of existence, of meaning, of the universe, and of the mystery of human life." 505 U.S. at 851. Choices flowing out of these conceptions, on matters "involving the most intimate and personal choices a person may make in a lifetime, choices central to personal dignity and autonomy, are central to the liberty protected by the Fourteenth Amendment." *Id.* "Beliefs about these matters," the Court continued, "could not define the attributes of personhood were they formed under compulsion of the State." *Id.*

In language pertinent to the liberty interest asserted here, the Court explained why decisions about abortion fall within this category of "personal and intimate" decisions. A decision whether or not to have an abortion, "originat[ing] within the zone of conscience and belief," involves conduct in which "the liberty of the woman is at stake in a sense unique to the human condition and so unique to the law." *Id.* at 852. As such, the decision necessarily involves the very "destiny of the woman" and is inevitably "shaped to a large extent on her own conception of her spiritual imperatives and her place in society." *Id.* Precisely because of these characteristics of the decision, "the State is [not] entitled to proscribe [abortion] in all instances." *Id.* Rather, to allow a total prohibition on abortion would be to permit a state to impose one conception of the meaning and value of human existence on all individuals. This the Constitution forbids.

The Solicitor General nevertheless argues that the right to abortion could be supported on grounds other than this autonomy principle, grounds that would not apply here. He argues, for example, that the abortion right might flow from the great burden an unwanted child imposes on its mother's life. Brief for the United States at 14-15. But whether or not abortion rights could be defended on such grounds, they were not the grounds on which this Court in fact relied. To the contrary, the Court explained at length that the right flows from the constitutional protection accorded all individuals to "define one's own concept of existence, of meaning, of the universe, and of the mystery of human life." *Casey*, 505 U.S. at 851.

The analysis in *Casey* compels the conclusion that the patient-plaintiffs have a liberty interest in this case that a state cannot burden with a blanket prohibition. Like a woman's decision whether to have an abortion, a decision to die involves one's very "destiny" and inevitably will be "shaped to a large extent on (one's] own conception of [one's] spiritual imperatives and [one's] place in society." *Id.* at 852. Just as a blanket prohibition on abortion would involve the improper imposition of one conception of the meaning and value of human existence on all individuals, so too would a blanket prohibition on assisted suicide. The liberty interest asserted here cannot be rejected without undermining the rationale of *Casey*. Indeed, the lower court opinions in the Washington case expressly recognized the parallel between the liberty interest in *Casey* and the interest asserted here. *See Compassion in Dying* v. *Washington*, 79 F.3d 790, 801(9th Cir. 1996) (en banc) ("In deciding right-to-die cases, we are guided by the Court's approach to the abortion cases. *Casey* in particular provides a powerful precedent, for in that case the Court had the opportunity to evaluate its past decisions and to determine whether to adhere to its original judgment."), *aff'g*, 850 F. Supp. 1454,1459 (W. D. Wash. 1994) ("[T]he reasoning in *Casey* [is] highly instructive and almost prescriptive . . ."). This Court should do the same.

B. Cruzan *Supports the Liberty Interest Asserted Here*
We agree with the Solicitor General that this Court's decision in "*Cruzan* . . . supports the conclusion that a liberty interest is at stake in this case." Brief for the United States at 8. Petitioners, however, insist that the present cases can be distinguished because the right at issue in *Cruzan* was limited to a right to reject an unwanted invasion of one's body.[1] But this Court repeatedly has held that in appropriate circumstances a state may require individuals to accept unwanted invasions of the body. *See, e.g., Schmerber* v. *California*, 384 U.S. 757 (1966) (extraction of blood sample from individual suspected of driving while intoxicated, notwithstanding defendant's objection, does not violate privilege against self-incrimination or other constitutional rights); *Jacobson* v. *Massachusetts*, 197 U.S. 11 (1905) (upholding compulsory vaccination for smallpox as reasonable regulation for protection of public health).

The liberty interest at stake in *Cruzan* was a more profound one. If a competent patient has a constitutional right to refuse life-sustaining treatment, then, the Court implied, the state could not override that right. The regulations upheld in *Cruzan* were designed only to ensure that the individual's wishes were ascertained correctly. Thus, if *Cruzan* implies a right of competent patients to refuse life-sustaining treatment, that implication must be understood as resting not simply on a right to refuse bodily invasions but on the more profound right to refuse medical intervention when what is at stake is a momentous personal decision, such as the timing and manner of one's death. In her concurrence, Justice O'Connor expressly recognized that the right at issue involved a "deeply personal decision" that is "inextricably intertwined" with our notion of "self-determination." 497 U.S. at 287–89.

Cruzan also supports the proposition that a state may not burden a terminally ill patient's liberty interest in determining the time and manner of his death by prohibiting doctors from terminating life support. Seeking to distinguish *Cruzan*, Petitioners insist that a state may nevertheless burden that right in a different way by forbidding doctors to assist in the suicide of patients who are not on life-support machinery. They argue that doctors who remove life support are only allowing a natural process to end in death whereas doctors who prescribe lethal drugs are intervening to cause death. So, according to this argument, a state has an independent justification for forbidding doctors to assist in suicide that it does not have for forbidding them to remove life support. In the former case though not the latter, it is said, the state forbids an act of killing that is morally much more problematic than merely letting a patient die.

This argument is based on a misunderstanding of the pertinent moral principles. It is certainly true that when a patient does not wish to die, different acts, each of which foreseeably results in his death, nevertheless have very different moral status. When several patients need organ transplants and organs are scarce, for example, it is morally permissible for a doctor to deny an organ to one patient, even though he will die without it, in order to give it to another. But it is certainly not permissible for a doctor to kill one patient in order to use his organs to save another. The morally sig-

nificant difference between those two acts is not, however, that killing is a positive act and not providing an organ is a mere omission, or that killing someone is worse than merely allowing a "natural" process to result in death. It would be equally impermissible for a doctor to let an injured patient bleed to death, or to refuse antibiotics to a patient with pneumonia—in each case the doctor would have allowed death to result from a "natural" process—in order to make his organs available for transplant to others. A doctor violates his patient's rights whether the doctor acts or refrains from acting, against the patient's wishes, in a way that is designed to cause death.

When a competent patient does want to die, the moral situation is obviously different, because then it makes no sense to appeal to the patient's right not to be killed as a reason why an act designed to cause his death is impermissible. From the patient's point of view, there is no morally pertinent difference between a doctor's terminating treatment that keeps him alive, if that is what he wishes, and a doctor's helping him to end his own life by providing lethal pills he may take himself, when ready, if that is what he wishes—except that the latter may be quicker and more humane. Nor is that a pertinent difference from the doctor's point of view. If and when it is permissible for him to act with death in view, it does not matter which of those two means he and his patient choose. If it is permissible for a doctor deliberately to withdraw medical treatment in order to allow death to result from a natural process, then it is equally permissible for him to help his patient hasten his own death more actively, if that is the patient's express wish.

It is true that some doctors asked to terminate life support are reluctant and do so only in deference to a patient's right to compel them to remove unwanted invasions of his body. But other doctors, who believe that their most fundamental professional duty is to act in the patient's interests and that, in certain circumstances, it is in their patient's best interests to die, participate willingly in such decisions: they terminate life support to cause death because they know that is what their patient wants. *Cruzan* implied that a state may not absolutely prohibit a doctor from deliberately causing death, at the patient's request, in that way and for that reason. If so, then a state may not prohibit doctors from deliberately using more direct and often more humane means to the same end when that is what a patient prefers. The fact that failing to provide life-sustaining treatment may be regarded as "only letting nature take its course" is no more morally significant in this context, when the patient wishes to die, than in the other, when he wishes to live. Whether a doctor turns off a respirator in accordance with the patient's request or prescribes pills that a patient may take when he is ready to kill himself, the doctor acts with the same intention: to help the patient die.

The two situations do differ in one important respect. Since patients have a right not to have life-support machinery attached to their bodies, they have, in principle, a right to compel its removal. But that is not true in the case of assisted suicide: patients in certain circumstances have a right that the state not forbid doctors to assist in their deaths, but they have no right to compel a doctor to assist them. The right in question, that is, is only a right to the help of a willing doctor.

III. STATE INTERESTS DO NOT JUSTIFY A CATEGORICAL PROHIBITION ON ALL ASSISTED SUICIDE

The Solicitor General concedes that "a competent, terminally ill adult has a constitutionally cognizable liberty interest in avoiding the kind of suffering experienced by the plaintiffs in this case." Brief for the United States at 8. He agrees that this interest extends not only to avoiding pain, but to avoiding an existence the patient believes to be one of intolerable indignity or incapacity as well. *Id.* at 12. The Solicitor General argues, however, that states nevertheless have the right to "override" this liberty interest altogether, because a state could reasonably conclude that allowing doctors to assist in suicide, even under the most stringent regulations and procedures that could be devised, would unreasonably endanger the lives of a number of patients who might ask for death in circumstances when it is plainly not in their interests to die or when their consent has been improperly obtained.

This argument is unpersuasive, however, for at least three reasons. *First,* in *Cruzan,* this Court noted that its various decisions supported the

recognition of a general liberty interest in refusing medical treatment, even when such refusal could result in death. 497 U.S. at 278–79. The various risks described by the Solicitor General apply equally to those situations. For instance, a patient kept alive only by an elaborate and disabling life-support system might well become depressed, and doctors might be equally uncertain whether the depression is curable: such a patient might decide for death only because he has been advised that he will die soon anyway or that he will never live free of the burdensome apparatus, and either diagnosis might conceivably be mistaken. Relatives or doctors might subtly or crudely influence that decision, and state provision for the decision may (to the same degree in this case as if it allowed assisted suicide) be thought to encourage it.

Yet there has been no suggestion that states are incapable of addressing such dangers through regulation. In fact, quite the opposite is true. In *McKay v. Bergstedt,* 106 Nev. 808, 801 P.2d 617 (1990), for example, the Nevada Supreme Court held that "competent adult patients desiring to refuse or discontinue medical treatment" must be examined by two nonattending physicians to determine whether the patient is mentally competent, understands his prognosis and treatment options, and appears free of coercion or pressure in making his decision. *Id.* at 827–28, 801 P.2d at 630. See also: *id.* (in the case of terminally ill patients with natural life expectancy of less than six months, [a] patient's right of self-determination shall be deemed to prevail over state interests, whereas [a] non-terminal patient's decision to terminate life-support systems must first be weighed against relevant state interests by trial judge); [and] *In re Farrell,* 108 N.J. 335, 354, 529 A.2d 404, 413 (1987) ([which held that a] terminally-ill patient requesting termination of life-support must be determined to be competent and properly informed about [his] prognosis, available treatment options and risks, and to have made decision voluntarily and without coercion). Those protocols served to guard against precisely the dangers that the Solicitor General raises. The case law contains no suggestion that such protocols are inevitably insufficient to prevent deaths that should have been prevented.

Indeed, the risks of mistake are overall greater in the case of terminating life support. *Cruzan* implied that a state must allow individuals to make such decisions through an advance directive stipulating either that life support be terminated (or not initiated) in described circumstances when the individual was no longer competent to make such a decision himself, or that a designated proxy be allowed to make that decision. All the risks just described are present when the decision is made through or pursuant to such an advance directive, and a grave further risk is added: that the directive, though still in force, no longer represents the wishes of the patient. The patient might have changed his mind before he became incompetent, though he did not change the directive, or his proxy may make a decision that the patient would not have made himself if still competent. In *Cruzan,* this Court held that a state may limit these risks through reasonable regulation. It did not hold—or even suggest—that a state may avoid them through a blanket prohibition that, in effect, denies the liberty interest altogether.

Second, nothing in the record supports the [Solicitor General's] conclusion that no system of rules and regulations could adequately reduce the risk of mistake. As discussed above, the experience of states in adjudicating requests to have life-sustaining treatment removed indicates the opposite. The Solicitor General has provided no persuasive reason why the same sort of procedures could not be applied effectively in the case of a competent individual's request for physician-assisted suicide.

Indeed, several very detailed schemes for regulating physician-assisted suicide have been submitted to the voters of some states and one has been enacted. In addition, concerned groups, including a group of distinguished professors of law and other professionals, have drafted and defended such schemes. *See, e.g.,* Charles H. Baron, *et. al, A Model State Act to Authorize and Regulate Physician-Assisted Suicide,* 33 Harv. J. Legis. 1 (1996). Such draft statutes propose a variety of protections and review procedures designed to insure against mistakes, and neither Washington nor New York attempted to show that such schemes would be porous or ineffective. Nor does the Solicitor General's brief: it relies instead mainly on flat and conclusory statements. It cites a New York Task Force report, written before the proposals just described were drafted, whose findings have been widely disputed and were implicitly

rejected in the opinion of the Second Circuit below. *See generally Quill* v. *Vacco,* 80 F.3d 716 (2d Cir. 1996). The weakness of the Solicitor General's argument is signaled by his strong reliance on the experience in the Netherlands which, in effect, allows assisted suicide pursuant to published guidelines. Brief for the United States at 23–24. The Dutch guidelines are more permissive than the proposed and model American statutes, however. The Solicitor General deems the Dutch practice of ending the lives of people like neonates who cannot consent particularly noteworthy, for example, but that practice could easily and effectively be made illegal by any state regulatory scheme without violating the Constitution.

The Solicitor General's argument would perhaps have more force if the question before the Court were simply whether a state has any rational basis for an absolute prohibition; if that were the question, then it might be enough to call attention to risks a state might well deem not worth running. But as the Solicitor General concedes, the question here is a very different one: whether a state has interests sufficiently compelling to allow it to take the extraordinary step of altogether refusing the exercise of a liberty interest of constitutional dimension. In those circumstances, the burden is plainly on the state to demonstrate that the risk of mistakes is very high, and that no alternative to complete prohibition would adequately and effectively reduce those risks. Neither of the Petitioners has made such a showing.

Nor could they. The burden of proof on any state attempting to show this would be very high. Consider, for example, the burden a state would have to meet to show that it was entitled altogether to ban public speeches in favor of unpopular causes because it could not guarantee, either by regulations short of an outright ban or by increased police protection, that such speeches would not provoke a riot that would result in serious injury or death to an innocent party. Or that it was entitled to deny those accused of crime the procedural rights that the Constitution guarantees, such as the right to a jury trial, because the security risk those rights would impose on the community would be too great. One can posit extreme circumstances in which some such argument would succeed. *See, e.g., Korematsu* v. *United States,* 323 U.S, 214 (1944) (permitting United States to detain individuals of Japanese ancestry during wartime). But these circumstances would be extreme indeed, and the *Korematsu* ruling has been widely and severely criticized.

Third, it is doubtful whether the risks the Solicitor General cites are even of the right character to serve as justification for an absolute prohibition on the exercise of an important liberty interest. The risks fall into two groups. The first is the risk of medical mistake, including a misdiagnosis of competence or terminal illness. To be sure, no scheme of regulation, no matter how rigorous, can altogether guarantee that medical mistakes will not be made. But the Constitution does not allow a state to deny patients a great variety of important choices, for which informed consent is properly deemed necessary, just because the information on which the consent is given may, in spite of the most strenuous efforts to avoid mistake, be wrong. Again, these identical risks are present in decisions to terminate life support, yet they do not justify an absolute prohibition on the exercise of the right.

The second group consists of risks that a patient will be unduly influenced by considerations that the state might deem it not in his best interests to be swayed by, for example, the feelings and views of close family members. Brief for the United States at 20. But what a patient regards as proper grounds for such a decision normally reflects exactly the judgments of personal ethics—of why his life is important and what affects its value—that patients have a crucial liberty interest in deciding for themselves. Even people who are dying have a right to hear and, if they wish, act on what others might wish to tell or suggest or even hint to them, and it would be dangerous to suppose that a state may prevent this on the ground that it knows better than its citizens when they should be moved by or yield to particular advice or suggestion in the exercise of their right to make fateful personal decisions for themselves. It is not a good reply that some people may not decide as they really wish—as they would decide, for example, if free from the "pressure" of others. That possibility could hardly justify the most serious pressure of all—the criminal law which tells them that they may not decide for death if they need the help of a doctor in dying, no matter how firmly they wish it.

There is a fundamental infirmity in the Solicitor General's argument. He asserts that a state may reasonably judge that the risk of "mistake" to some persons justifies a prohibition that not only risks but insures and even aims at what would undoubtedly be a vastly greater number of "mistakes" of the opposite kind—preventing many thousands of competent people who think that it disfigures their lives to continue living, in the only way left to them, from escaping that—to them—terrible injury. A state grievously and irreversibly harms such people when it prohibits that escape. The Solicitor General's argument may seem plausible to those who do not agree that individuals are harmed by being forced to live on in pain and what they regard as indignity. But many other people plainly do think that such individuals are harmed, and a state may not take one side in that essentially ethical or religious controversy as its justification for denying a crucial liberty.

Of course, a state has important interests that justify regulating physician-assisted suicide. It may be legitimate for a state to deny an opportunity for assisted suicide when it acts in what it reasonably judges to be the best interests of the potential suicide, and when its judgment on that issue does not rest on contested judgments about "matters involving the most intimate and personal choices a person may make in a lifetime, choices central to personal dignity and autonomy." *Casey,* 505 U.S. at 851. A state might assert, for example, hat people who are not terminally ill, but who have formed a desire to die, are, as a group, very likely later to be grateful if they are prevented from taking their own lives. It might then claim that it is legitimate, out of concern for such people, to deny any of them a doctor's assistance [in taking their own lives].

This Court need not decide now the extent to which such paternalistic interests might override an individual's liberty interest. No one can plausibly claim, however—and it is noteworthy that neither Petitioners nor the Solicitor General does claim—that any such prohibition could serve the interests of any significant number of terminally ill patients. On the contrary, any paternalistic justification for an absolute prohibition of assistance to such patients would of necessity appeal to a widely contested religious or ethical conviction many of them, including the patient-plaintiffs, reject. Allowing *that* justification to prevail would vitiate the liberty interest.

Even in the case of terminally ill patients, a state has a right to take all reasonable measures to insure that a patient requesting such assistance has made an informed, competent, stable and uncoerced decision. It is plainly legitimate for a state to establish procedures through which professional and administrative judgments can be made about these matters, and to forbid doctors to assist in suicide when its reasonable procedures have not been satisfied. States may be permitted considerable leeway in designing such procedures. They may be permitted, within reason, to err on what they take to be the side of caution. But they may not use the bare possibility of error as justification for refusing to establish any procedures at all and relying instead on a flat prohibition.

CONCLUSION

Each individual has a right to make the "most intimate and personal choices central to personal dignity and autonomy." That right encompasses the right to exercise some control over the time and manner of one's death.

The patient-plaintiffs in these cases were all mentally competent individuals in the final phase of terminal illness and died within months of filing their claims.

Jane Doe described how her advanced cancer made even the most basic bodily functions such as swallowing, coughing, and yawning extremely painful and that it was "not possible for [her] to reduce [her] pain to an acceptable level of comfort and to retain an alert state." Faced with such circumstances, she sought to be able to "discuss freely with [her] treating physician [her] intention of hastening [her] death through the consumption of drugs prescribed for that purpose." *Quill* v. *Vacco*, 80 F.2d 716, 720 (2d Cir. 1996) (quoting declaration of Jane Doe).

George A. Kingsley, in advanced stages of AIDS which included, among other hardships, the attachment of a tube to an artery in his chest which made even routine functions burdensome and the development of lesions on his brain, sought advice from his doctors regarding prescriptions which could hasten his impending death. *Id.*

Jane Roe, suffering from cancer since 1988, had been almost completely bedridden since 1993 and experienced constant pain which could not be alleviated by medication. After undergoing counseling for herself and her family, she desired to hasten her death by taking prescription drugs. *Compassion in Dying* v. *Washington,* 850 F. Supp. 1454, 1456 (1994).

John Doe, who had experienced numerous AIDS-related ailments since 1991, was "especially cognizant of the suffering imposed by a lingering terminal illness because he was the primary caregiver for his long-term companion who died of AIDS" and sought prescription drugs from his physician to hasten his own death after entering the terminal phase of AIDS. *Id.* at 1456–57.

James Poe suffered from emphysema which caused him "a constant sensation of suffocating" as well as a cardiac condition which caused severe leg pain. Connected to an oxygen tank at all times but unable to calm the panic reaction associated with his feeling of suffocation even with regular doses of morphine, Mr. Poe sought physician-assisted suicide. *Id.* at 1457.

A state may not deny the liberty claimed by the patient-plaintiffs in these cases without providing them an opportunity to demonstrate, in whatever way the state might reasonably think wise and necessary, that the conviction they expressed for an early death is competent, rational, informed, stable, and uncoerced.

Affirming the decisions by the Courts of Appeals would establish nothing more than that there is such a constitutionally protected right in principle. It would establish only that some individuals, whose decisions for suicide plainly cannot be dismissed as irrational or foolish or premature, must be accorded a reasonable opportunity to show that their decision for death is informed and free. It is not necessary to decide precisely which patients are entitled to that opportunity. If, on the other hand, this Court reverses the decisions below, its decision could only be justified by the momentous proposition—a proposition flatly in conflict with the spirit and letter of the Court's past decisions—that an American citizen does not, after all, have the right, even in principle, to live and die in the light of his own religious and ethical beliefs, his own convictions about why his life is valuable and where its value lies.

NOTE

1. In that case, the parents of Nancy Cruzan, a woman who was in a persistent vegetative state following an automobile accident, asked the Missouri courts to authorize doctors to end life support and therefore her life. The Supreme Court held that Missouri was entitled to demand explicit evidence that Ms. Cruzan had made a decision that she would not wish to be kept alive in those circumstances, and to reject the evidence the family had offered as inadequate. But a majority of justices assumed, for the sake of the argument, that a competent patient has a right to reject life-preserving treatment, and it is now widely assumed that the Court would so rule in an appropriate case.

The Distinction Between Refusing Medical Treatment and Suicide

New York State Task Force on Life and the Law

The distinction between the refusal of life-sustaining medical treatment and suicide has been a critical component of all of our recommendations on end-of-life care. In our report on do-not-resuscitate orders, we grounded our legal analysis on the premise that suicide relates only to self-inflicted deaths and "not to a decision to refuse life-sustaining treatment." We reaffirmed this position in our report on the health care proxy, which found that "as a matter of public policy the taking of human life must not be granted legal sanction." Based on that conclusion, the health care proxy law, as enacted by the New York State Legislature, provides that "[t]his article is not intended to permit or promote suicide, assisted suicide, or euthanasia." Our proposed legislation on surrogate decision-making for incapacitated patients without advance directives contains a similar statement; the report accompanying the proposed legislation expressly states that surrogate decision-making is "not intended either as a step on the road to assisted suicide or as a vehicle to extend the authority of family members beyond the traditional boundaries established by consent to provide treatment or not to treat." Most recently, our report on assisted suicide and euthanasia proposed "a clear line for public policies and medical practice between forgoing medical interventions and assistance to commit suicide or euthana-

sia," and outlined the legal, ethical, and policy considerations distinguishing the two practices.

We recognize that "the moral distinction between assisting to die and withdrawing treatment is hard to discern in certain cases." The alleged distinction between "acts" and "omissions," for example, is "particularly nebulous," given that physicians who comply with requests to refuse treatment are often required to undertake affirmative acts, such as disconnecting respirators or feeding tubes. Resting the distinction on a difference in intent is also not always persuasive, because "[i]n the act of disconnecting a life-sustaining ventilator . . . some physicians actually intend, not just to rid the patient of unwelcome technology, but to help the patient end her suffering by dying sooner.[1] Finally, as an empirical matter, it is undeniable that withdrawing or withholding life-sustaining treatment, at least in some cases, can play a causal role in any death that ensues. "When a doctor detaches a feeding tube from a patient who could have lived for an additional decade, albeit in a profoundly diminished state, she is certainly 'the cause' of death insofar as she determines when and how the patient dies.[2]

Nonetheless, the fact that the refusal of life-sustaining treatment and assisted suicide are similar in certain aspects does not mean that the practices implicate identical legal, clinical, ethical, and public policy concerns. The following factors, taken together, present compelling reasons to distinguish between the refusal of life-sustaining treatment and assisted suicide for law and public policy, despite the similarities that might exist in individual cases.

From The New York State Task Force on Life and the Law, *When Death Is Sought: Assisted Suicide. and Euthanasia in the Medical Context* (Supplement to Report, April 1997).

Although these distinctions may not, in themselves, compel the conclusion that assisted suicide should remain illegal, they undermine the claim that the legal recognition of a broad right to refuse treatment requires recognition of a right to assisted suicide as a matter of constitutional law.

THE RIGHT TO REFUSE MEDICAL TREATMENT IS BASED ON THE LONG-STANDING RIGHT TO RESIST UNWANTED PHYSICAL INVASIONS, NOT ON A RIGHT TO "HASTEN DEATH."

Critics of the distinction between the refusal of life-sustaining treatment and assisted suicide contend that both practices are based on the position that dying patients have a right to "hasten death." For example, in *Glucksberg*, Judge Reinhardt characterized the judicial recognition of the right to refuse life-sustaining treatment as a "drastic change regarding acceptable medical practices," reflecting the courts' belief "that terminally ill persons are entitled . . . to hasten their deaths, and that . . . physicians may assist in the process.[3] This description of the development of the right to refuse treatment simply cannot be reconciled with the cases originally recognizing that right.

Courts that affirmed the right to refuse treatment, including life-sustaining measures, consistently grounded that right in the long-standing doctrine of informed consent, which forbids physicians from performing invasive medical procedures without the patient's knowing and voluntary agreement. That doctrine is based on the common-law concept of battery, under which any nonconsensual "touching" is a "tort"—a legal wrong—providing grounds for the victim to sue. While patients who refuse treatment may become sicker, and sometimes will die, that result has always been regarded as an unavoidable consequence of applying the doctrine of informed consent consistently and without exception, not as a reason to recognize individuals' right to refuse treatment capable of prolonging life. Contrary to Judge Reinhardt's assertion, the fact that courts did not explicitly recognize the right to refuse life-sustaining treatment until relatively recently does not mean that the right represented a "drastic change." Rather, the courts' recognition of the right to refuse life-sustaining treatment was simply an application of the long-standing prohibition of battery to "the advance of medical technology capable of sustaining life well past the point where natural forces would have brought certain death in earlier times." Until the widespread use of devices such as respirators, dialysis machines, and feeding tubes, there was simply no occasion for courts to consider the right to refuse life-sustaining treatment, outside the narrow context of "patients who refused medical treatment forbidden by their religious beliefs."

The fact that courts grounded the right to refuse treatment in the long-standing right to resist unwanted physical invasions, rather than in a broader "right" to "hasten death," strongly undermines the claim that the refusal of treatment and assisted suicide are legally and ethically the same. Prohibiting individuals from refusing medical treatment would represent "a violation of personal autonomy and physical integrity totally incompatible with the deepest meaning of our traditional respect for liberty. In some cases, such prohibitions would violate sincerely-held religious beliefs opposing certain medical interventions, such as the belief among Jehovah's Witnesses against receiving transfusions of blood. Decisions about assisted suicide do not implicate these interests. For this reason alone, assisted suicide is fundamentally different from the right to refuse treatment; moreover, the difference is not simply in degree but in kind.

CHARACTERIZING THE REFUSAL OF MEDICAL TREATMENT AS "THE CAUSE" OF ANY DEATHS THAT RESULT WOULD UNDERMINE SOCIETY'S COMMITMENT TO RESPECTING PATIENTS' DECISIONS ABOUT MEDICAL CARE.

In case after case, courts have concluded that deaths following the refusal of treatment are caused primarily by the patient's underlying disease, not the patient's decision or act. As the New Jersey Supreme Court has held, "a patient does not die because of the withdrawal of a kidney dialysis machine, but because his underlying disease has destroyed the proper functioning of his kidney." Likewise, a patient does not die "from the withdrawal of a nasogastric tube, but because of her underlying medical problem, i.e., an inability to swallow."[4] If these statements were meant to suggest that the refusal of treatment plays absolutely no causal role in the patient's death, they would obviously be untrue. For example, when a physician withdraws a respirator or disconnects a feeding tube from a seriously ill patient, it is undeniable that these actions causally contribute to the patient's death: but for the withdrawal of treatment, the patient would probably have continued to live. This empirical question of "but-for" causation, however, is clearly not what the courts had in mind. Instead, the law's traditional analysis of the cause of deaths following the refusal of life-sustaining treatment reflects important judgments about the nature and goals of medicine, which society should be extremely hesitant to revise, particularly in the guise of constitutional interpretation.

The law has long distinguished between the determination of causation as a factual matter and the determination of causation for the purpose of assessing legal and ethical accountability. When a variety of factual causes are necessary, but not individually sufficient, to bring about a particular result, the determination of which among them are properly cited as causative for legal purposes becomes a policy judgment, reflecting underlying assumptions about rights, duties, and moral blame. This is precisely the case when patients die following the refusal of life-sustaining treatment. In contrast to patients who take lethal drugs, patients who refuse life-sustaining treatment will not die unless they are suffering from a condition that makes it impossible to live without invasive medical support (such as an inability to breath, or an inability to swallow or assimilate food taken orally). As Daniel Callahan has put it, "there must be an underlying fatal pathology if allowing to die is even possible."[5] In light of the multiple causes of death following the refusal of life-sustaining treatment, the determination of legal causation cannot be based on simple empirical observation, but requires a deliberate judgment about legal and ethical accountability. The traditional view that the disease, not the refusal of treatment, is the primary cause of death affirms widely-shared beliefs about the nature of medical care—in particular, that consent to medical treatment is not obligatory, but a matter of individual choice. Because the technology is optional, patients who refuse it are not considered to be accountable for causing their own deaths.

By claiming that patients who refuse life-sustaining treatment are the primary cause of any deaths that result, the Second and Ninth Circuits unfairly stigmatize patients who choose not to submit to every available technology capable of prolonging life. The implication of assigning causal accountability to the patient, rather than the underlying injury or disease, is that consent to life-sustaining treatment is expected, and that those who refuse treatment are therefore responsible for bringing about their own deaths. In *Quill*, Judge Miner actually states that deaths following the refusal of life-sustaining treatment are unnatural: "[b]y ordering the discontinuance of . . . artificial life-sustaining processes or refusing to accept them in the first place, a patient hastens his death by means that are not natural in any sense."[6] This statement reflects a curious—and, we believe, dangerous—view of the relationship between nature and technology. Until the development of respirators and feeding tubes, patients who lost the ability to breathe or swallow would inevitably die, and no one would think to argue that such deaths were self-inflicted or anything but natural consequences of injury or disease. If, as Judge Miner claims, it is now "unnatural" to die from an inability to breathe or swallow, it is only because technologies have been developed that can forestall many of these deaths. The invention of new technology, however, does not make the choice to allow events to proceed without the technology "unnatural." To claim otherwise is to establish a "technological imperative," in which the very existence of technology becomes a mandate for its use. Such reasoning is actually more consistent with the claim that the use of life-sustaining treatment should be obligatory, and should be disturbing to those who support patients' right to control their own medical care.

Indeed, if patients who refuse life-sustaining treatment are responsible for "causing" the deaths that result, few deaths could be attributed to natural causes. Death often follows a decision to forgo an available medical treatment that could potentially prolong the patient's life. For example, death is typically preceded by the cessation of breathing and heartbeat, and only sometimes are efforts made to resuscitate dying patients by performing CPR. If deaths resulting from the failure to provide medical treatment are "nothing more nor less than assisted suicide," the consensual failure to perform CPR is a form of assisted suicide, and the doctor who does nothing when a patient's heart has stopped has "caused" the patient's death.[7] Likewise, patients who refuse chemotherapy, because they are unwilling to endure the painful and debilitating side effects, would no longer be victims of cancer, but of their own "unnatural" acts. While some might distinguish these examples of withholding life-sustaining treatment from more active instances of turning off respirators or disconnecting feeding tubes, it is widely accepted that "withdrawing" and "withholding" medical treatment implicate identical legal and ethical concerns. Thus, if turning off a respirator is suicide, so too is refusing to be connected to the respirator in the first place. And if refusing a respirator is suicide, the same must be true for refusing an organ transplant, or refusing any other grueling procedure with an uncertain outcome. Such characterizations defy common sense. There is an obvious difference between refusing invasive technologies that have the potential to prolong life long after the body is able to survive on its own, and deciding to commit suicide by causing the body to stop functioning before death would otherwise occur.

Finally, as a practical matter, telling physicians that they are the primary cause of death when patients refuse medical treatment is likely to backfire, by leading physicians, especially those opposed to assisted suicide, to question their participation in the withdrawal and withholding of medical care. Despite patients' clear legal right to refuse life-sustaining treatment, many doctors—particularly those who are opposed to any participation in efforts to "hasten death"—must still be persuaded to comply with patients' requests to forgo aggressive measures. By assuring doctors that they are not the legal cause of death when patients refuse treatment—in other words, by affirming that withholding and withdrawing treatment are not assisted suicide—existing legal and ethical standards allow physicians to honor patients' wishes about treatment without having to feel responsible for causing the patient's death. If physicians are told that deaths following the refusal of treatment are "unnatural," and that the refusal of treatment is the primary legal and ethical "cause of death," many physicians are likely to rethink their participation in the withholding and

withdrawal of treatment. The result would be a disastrous setback for patient autonomy.

EQUATING THE REFUSAL OF TREATMENT WITH SUICIDE WOULD MAKE IT IMPOSSIBLE TO LIMIT PHYSICIAN-ASSISTED SUICIDE TO COMPETENT, TERMINALLY ILL PATIENTS, OR TO LEGALIZE PHYSICIAN-ASSISTED SUICIDE WITHOUT ALSO LEGALIZING EUTHANASIA.

Equating the refusal of treatment with assisted suicide is also inconsistent with the claim that assisted suicide could be limited to competent, terminally ill patients, or that assisted suicide could be legalized while physician-administered lethal injections remain illegal. These practical consequences of abandoning the distinction between the refusal of treatment and suicide should not be ignored. In contrast to the broad right to refuse medical treatment, few proponents of legalizing assisted suicide argue that the practice should be available to anyone on demand. Instead, advocates of legalization have argued that assisted suicide should be treated as a "nonstandard medical practice reserved for extraordinary circumstances,"[8] or as a "response to medical failure," for those "few patients" who "will face a bad death despite all medical efforts.[9] In fact, most advocates of legalization acknowledge that laws prohibiting assisted suicide serve valuable societal interests, especially when applied to healthy individuals suffering from reversible physical or psychological problems. As Judge Reinhardt observed in *Glucksberg,* "the state has a clear interest in preventing anyone, no matter what age, from taking his own life in a fit of desperation, depression, or loneliness or as a result of any other problem, physical or psychological, which can be significantly ameliorated." In such cases, he wrote, "the heartache of suicide is the senseless loss of a life ended prematurely," and the state can legitimately take steps to prevent these suicides from taking place.[10]

Recognizing the need for limits, the plaintiffs in *Glucksberg* and *Quill* propose a right to physician-assisted suicide only for competent patients who are terminally ill. In addition, they argue that recognizing a right to a prescription for lethal drugs does not mean that patients should be permitted to direct their physicians to administer a lethal injection, even if they are unable to commit suicide by any other means. Legislative proposals to legalize assisted suicide now pending in many states contain similar limitations. In fact, these distinctions were critical to the success of the referendum to legalize physician-assisted suicide in Oregon.

Characterizing the refusal of life-sustaining treatment as a form of assisted suicide, however, would make it impossible (and probably unconstitutional) to limit assisted suicide to these narrow categories of cases. First, the claim that assisted suicide could be limited to terminally ill patients ignores the fact that the right to refuse treatment has not been limited to patients who are terminally ill. For example, in *Bouvia* v. *Superior Court*,[11] the California Court of Appeals authorized the removal of a feeding tube from a young woman afflicted with severe cerebral palsy, who had years of life ahead of her, rejecting efforts to limit the right to refuse treatment to patients who are terminally ill. As the Bouvia court observed, "if [the] right to choose may not be exercised because there remains to [the patient], in the opinion of a court, a physician or some committee, a certain arbitrary number of years, months, or days, [the] right will have lost its value and meaning." Other state courts have also rejected terminal illness as a constitutional benchmark, and the opinions of the Supreme Court justices in *Cruzan*—a case involving a patient who was not terminally ill—suggest that the United States Supreme Court would do the same thing if it were directly confronted with the question. If terminal illness is not an appropriate prerequisite for the refusal of life-sustaining treatment, and the refusal of treatment "is nothing more nor less than assisted suicide,"[12] how can other forms of assisted suicide be limited to patients who are terminally ill?

The same is true for the claim that assisted suicide could be limited to competent patients who make a contemporaneous request for physician-assisted death. As the New Jersey Supreme Court observed in the case of Karen Ann Quinlan, if a patient's decision to forgo life-sustaining treatment is deserving of legal recognition, "it should not be discarded solely on the basis that her condition prevents her conscious exercise of the choice."[13] To

protect individuals' right to refuse unwanted life-sustaining treatment after a loss of capacity, the law has created mechanisms like living wills, health care proxies, and surrogate decision-making, all of which rely on a good-faith assessment of the incapacitated patient's wishes and/or best interests by health care professionals, family members, and close friends. If the refusal of treatment is a form of suicide, and it is permitted for patients without decision-making capacity, other forms of suicide would have to be permitted for incapacitated patients as well. At a minimum, it would be impossible to deny the right to incapacitated patients who have specifically requested assisted suicide as part of an advance directive, or who have given a relative or friend explicit decision-making authority over treatment decisions by signing a health care proxy. In fact, a footnote in Judge Reinhardt's opinion in *Glucksberg* directly opens the door to such practices, by stating that "a decision of a duly appointed surrogate decision maker is for all legal purposes the decision of the patient himself."[14] What this means is that, even if the law is never changed to legalize euthanasia for the incapacitated, surrogate decision-makers could authorize the provision of lethal drugs to incapacitated patients by consenting to assisted suicide on the patient's behalf.

Moreover, characterizing the refusal of life-sustaining treatment as a form of suicide is inconsistent with the claim that physicians could be allowed to help patients commit suicide by prescribing lethal drugs, but not by providing lethal injections at a patient's request. If it is unfair to distinguish between "hastening death" by refusing life-sustaining treatment and "hastening death" by self-administering lethal drugs, how can it be acceptable to distinguish between *self-administering* lethal drugs and instructing a *physician* to administer those same drugs directly? Allowing physicians to prescribe lethal drugs but not to provide lethal injections would discriminate against patients who want to commit suicide but are physically unable to pick up or swallow a pill. These patients may in fact be suffering more than their able-bodied counterparts, and their claims for assistance may therefore appear more deserving of societal respect.

Finally, even what are characterized as "procedural" limitations on the right to physician-assisted suicide, approved by the Second and Ninth Circuits and endorsed by virtually all supporters of legalization, would be difficult to defend if the refusal of life-sustaining treatment is seen as a form of assisted suicide as a matter of law. If, as Judge Miner claims, any distinctions between the refusal of treatment and other forms of "hastening death" are arbitrary and unconstitutional, there would be no basis for requiring candidates for assisted suicide to submit to waiting periods, second opinions, and committee review. Such requirements are not imposed on individuals who seek to refuse life-sustaining treatment, and any effort to introduce them would undoubtedly be seen as burdensome and intrusive. "[I]f there is really no moral or legal difference between 'allowing to die' and 'assisting suicide'—if, as Judge Miner opines, adding [physician-assisted suicide] to our repertoire of choices would not add one iota of additional risk to individuals or society over and above those we already countenance—then it would seem that encumbering the choice for [physician-assisted suicide] with all sorts of extra protective devices would lack constitutional validity."[15]

THE BALANCE BETWEEN THE BENEFITS AND RISKS LIKELY TO RESULT FROM THE LEGALIZATION OF PHYSICIAN-ASSISTED SUICIDE IS EXTREMELY DIFFERENT FROM A SIMILAR BALANCING IN THE CONTEXT OF DECISIONS TO REFUSE MEDICAL TREATMENT.

In *When Death is Sought,* we concluded that the legalization of assisted suicide would create insurmountable risks of mistake and abuse. To the extent the Second and Ninth Circuit recognized these risks, they dismissed them as irrelevant, on the theory that similar risks apply when patients refuse life-sustaining medical treatment. The fact that similar risks exist in both situations, however, does not mean that the risks have the same implications for law and clinical practice. The critical question is whether the risks can be mitigated through careful regulation, and, if not, whether they outweigh the reasons advanced for changing the law. On both of these grounds, the risks associated with legalizing assisted suicide are fundamentally different from those involved in respecting patients' refusals of life-sustaining medical treatment.

First, the risks associated with legalizing assisted suicide would be far more difficult to regulate than the risks involved in refusing life-sustaining treatment. Many decisions to refuse life-sustaining treatment—particularly decisions to withdraw respirators and feeding tubes—take place in hospitals and nursing homes. By contrast, decisions about assisted suicide are likely to take place at home or in a physician's office. It is comparatively easy to require second opinions, committee oversights, and retrospective monitoring in institutional settings. Outside of hospitals and nursing homes, "effective oversight to minimize error or abuse would be more difficult, if not unrealizable."[16]

Second, with the refusal of treatment, the balance between the risks and the underlying individual right at stake yields different results from a similar balancing in the context of assisted suicide. On the risk side of the ledger, any harms that might result from the inappropriate refusal of treatment extend only to individuals who are suffering from an underlying condition that makes it impossible to live without invasive medical support. The size of this group, although not negligible, is inherently limited, and just about everyone in this category must be very bad off indeed. With assisted suicide, by contrast, the risk of mistake and abuse is considerably larger, because anyone who takes lethal drugs will die, regardless of any underlying pathology. As Seth Kreimer has argued, "[t]he quantitative distinction between some and all can be a legitimate predicate for the qualitative distinction between permission and prohibition."[17]

At the same time, the individual and societal need for a broad right to refuse treatment is far greater than the need for changing the law to allow physicians to help patients commit suicide with lethal drugs. If the law did not permit patients to refuse life-sustaining treatment, dying patients would be forced to submit to any procedure that might potentially extend their lives, no matter how burdensome. The result—strapping patients down, pumping them with drugs, sticking tubes into them, and cutting them open to perform surgery—would be a brutal assault on individual rights and, in many cases, sincerely-held religious beliefs. By contrast, the legal prohibition of assisted suicide prevents patients from obtaining a physician's assistance in escaping a situation imposed by nature, but does not impose any additional harm not caused by the patient's own injury or disease. Moreover, "to the extent that laws prohibiting assisted suicide and euthanasia impose a burden, they do so only for individuals who make an informed, competent choice to have their lives artificially shortened, and who cannot do so without another person's aid. As studies have confirmed, very few individuals fall into this group, particularly if appropriate pain relief and supportive care are provided." The refusal of treatment, by contrast, is an integral part of everyday medical practice. Prohibiting such decisions would therefore constitute a burden to individual autonomy in a significantly larger number of cases.

THE DISTINCTION BETWEEN ADMINISTERING HIGH DOSES OF OPIOIDS TO RELIEVE PAIN AND "PHYSICIAN-ASSISTED DEATH"

Some proponents of legalizing assisted suicide argue that the practice is indistinguishable from another, widely-accepted, aspect of medical care: the use of morphine and other opioids to relieve pain. In a 1994 article in *The New York Times*, Thomas Preston, a cardiologist, stated that the use of morphine drips "is undeniably euthanasia, hidden by the cosmetics of professional tradition and language." According to Dr. Preston, the continuous injection of morphine into a patient's vein will inevitably lead to the patient's death by "curtailing her breathing." Acceptance of the practice, he wrote, is "society's wink to euthanasia," and demonstrates that, despite existing legal prohibitions, "euthanasia is widespread now."[18]

Judge Reinhardt relied heavily on this argument in his opinion in *Glucksberg*. "As part of the tradition of administering comfort care," he wrote, "doctors have been supplying the causal agent of patients' deaths for decades." When physicians administer morphine drips for the relief of pain, "the actual cause of the patient's death is the drug administered by the physician or by a person acting under his supervision or direction. Because physicians are already causing patients' deaths by administering morphine drips, Judge Reinhardt concluded, the

State cannot assert an interest in preventing physicians from causing death by prescribing lethal drugs for patients to self-administer.[19] The court dismissed the State's reliance on differences in intention, because "one of the known effects in each case is to hasten the end of the patient's life."[20]

The effort to characterize morphine drips as a form of covert euthanasia is extremely misguided. First, as a factual matter, the causal relationship between morphine drips and patients' deaths is far less clear than Dr. Preston or Judge Reinhardt contend. While high doses of morphine can depress respiration when administered to patients who have not developed tolerance to the drug, physicians who treat patients with morphine for the relief of pain increase the doses gradually, so that tolerance can develop. Dr. Kathleen Foley, chief of the pain service at Memorial Sloan-Kettering Cancer Center, has concluded that "[t]he rapid development of tolerance to the respiratory depressant effects allows for escalation of the opioid dose in some patients to very high doses.," and that "[t]here appears to be no limit to tolerance" when the drug is administered properly.[21] The claim that the use of morphine at properly titrated levels "hastens" patients' deaths, based on the effects of high doses of morphine on patients who have not developed tolerance, is entirely unfounded. It represents one of many myths about the consequences of using narcotics in the clinical setting, which have themselves contributed to the undermedication of patients experiencing treatable pain.

Second, and more importantly, the fact that morphine drips may accelerate patients' deaths in some cases does not make their use equivalent to assisted suicide or euthanasia. "Just as a surgeon might undertake risky heart surgery knowing that the patient may die on the table, so the conscientious physicians can risk suppressing the patient's respiratory drive and thus hastening death so long as she is pursuing a valid medical objective and there are no better (less risky) options at hand."[22] As the President's Commission observed, "the moral issue is whether or not the decisionmakers have considered the full range of foreseeable effects, have knowingly accepted whatever risk of death is entailed, and have found the risk to be justified in light of the paucity and undesirability of other options."[23] These observations are consistent with the legal concept of recklessness, which is defined as the conscious disregard of a substantial and "unjustifiable" risk. "This definition necessarily excludes situations where the benefit of taking action outweighs the likelihood that the action will cause harm." Thus, physicians are not permitted to prescribe morphine for minor headaches, when ordinary aspirin would work as well, but they can (and indeed, should) for the pain associated with terminal illness, assuming that no other less risky options exist. This does not mean that the physician can administer opioids indiscriminately: the doctrine of recklessness requires the physician to undertake a good-faith balancing of the benefits and risks. Instead, it recognizes that medical treatment sometimes requires significant trade-offs, and that acceptance of negative consequences for legitimate medical purposes is not equivalent to causing those consequences for their own sake.

Just as conflating the refusal of treatment with assisted suicide is likely to undermine patients' ability to control their medical treatment, telling physicians that an unintended death resulting from the provision of necessary palliative treatment is a form of covert euthanasia is likely to result in many more patients experiencing unrelieved pain. As John Arras has pointed out, "many physicians would sooner give up their allegiance to adequate pain control than their opposition to assisted suicide and euthanasia."[24] Characterizing the provision of pain relief as a form of euthanasia may well lead to an increase in needless suffering at the end of life. Advocates of legalizing assisted suicide should think carefully about the consequences of this argument for compassionate end-of-life care.

NOTES

1. J. Arras, "Physician-Assisted Suicide: A Tragic View," *J. Contemp. Health Law & Pol.* 13: 361-389 (1997). In this volume, pp. 274–280.
2. *Id.*
3. 79 F.3d at 821–22.
4. *In re Peter,* 108 N.J. 365, 529 A.2d 419 (1987).
5. D. Callahan, *The Troubled Dream of Life: In Search of a Peaceful Death* (New York: Simon & Schuster, 1993): 77.
6. 80 F.3d at 729.
7. G.J. Annas, "The Promised End—Constitutional Aspects of Physician-Assisted Suicide," *N. Eng. J. Med.* 335 (1996): 683-87 ("Since the failure to perform cardiopulmonary resuscitation always 'hastens death', . . . patients who refuse cardiopulmonary resuscitation would always be committing suicide (and doctors who write do-not-resuscitate orders would always be assisting suicide).").
8. F.G. Miller, T.E. Quill, H. Brody, J.C. Fletcher, L.O. Gostin, and D.E. Meier, "Regulating Physician-Assisted Death," *N. Eng. J. Med.* 331(1994): 119-23, at 119.
9. H. Brody, "Assisted Death—A Compassionate Response to a Medical Failure," *N. Eng. J Med* 327 (1992): 1384-88, at 1385.
10. 79 F.3d at 820.
11. 225 Cal. Rptr. 297 (Cal. Ct. App. 1986).
12. *Quill,* 80 F.3d at 729.
13. 70 N.J. at 4l, 335 A.2d at 664.
14. 79 F.3d at 832, n.120.
15. Arras, "Physician-Assisted Suicide: A Tragic View."
16. C.H. Coleman & T.E. Miller, "Stemming the Tide: Assisted Suicide and the Constitution," *J. Law, Med. & Ethics* 23 (1995): 389-97. at 394
17. S. Kreimer, "Does Pro-Choice Mean Pro-Kevorkian? An Essay on *Roe, Casey,* and the Right to Die," *Am. U. L. Rev.* 44 (1995): 803, 841.
18. T.A. Preston. "Killing Pain, Ending Life," *The New York Times,* Nov. 1, 1994, at A27.
19. 79 F.3d at 823.
20. *Id.* at 824 (emphasis added).
21. K.M. Foley, "Controversies in Cancer Pain: Medical Perspectives," *Cancer* 63 (1989): 2257-65, at 2261-62; see also W.C. Wilson. N.G. Smedira, & C. Fink, "Ordering and Administering of Sedatives and Analgesics During the Withholding and Withdrawal of Life Support From Critically Ill Patients," *JAMA* 267 (1992):949–53 (finding "no evidence that death actually was hastened by the administration of drugs," and that, "if anything," the data "suggest that death occurred earlier in the patient who did not receive drugs").
22. Arras, "Physician-Assisted Suicide: A Tragic View."
23. President's Commission for the Study of Ethical Problems in Medicine and Biomedical and Behavioral Research, *Deciding to Forgo Life-Sustaining Treatment* (Washington: U.S. Government Printing Office, 1983)
24. Arras, "Physician-Assisted Suicide: A Tragic View."

Physician-Assisted Suicide: A Tragic View

John D. Arras

INTRODUCTION

For many decades now, the call for physician-assisted suicide (PAS) and euthanasia have been perennial lost causes in American society. Each generation has thrown up an assortment of earnest reformers and cranks who, after attracting their fifteen minutes of fame, inevitably have been defeated by the combined weight of traditional law and morality. Incredibly, two recent federal appellate court decisions suddenly changed the legal landscape in this area, making the various states within their respective jurisdictions the first governments in world history, excepting perhaps the Nazi regime in Germany, to officially sanction PAS. Within the space of a month, both an eight to three majority of the United States Court of Appeals 'or the Ninth Circuit[1] on the West Coast, and a three-dge panel in the United States Court of Appeals for ' Second Circuit,[2] in the Northeast, struck down r-standing state laws forbidding physicians to aid et their patients in acts of suicide. Within a virtu-k of an eye, the unthinkable had come to pass: nd euthanasia had emerged from their exile the pale of law to occupy center stage in a public debate that eventually culminated in States Supreme Court's unanimous rever-lower court decisions in June 1997....[3]

n believer in patient autonomy, I find deeply sympathetic to the central values e case for PAS and euthanasia; I have wever, that these practices pose too the rights and welfare of too many alized in this country at the present ny argument in this paper will be recently overturned decisions of mploy a form of case-based rea-ed to the development of sound

social policy in this area. I shall argue that in order to do justice to the very real threats posed by the widespread social practices of PAS and euthanasia, we need to adopt precisely the kind of policy perspective that the circuit courts rejected on principle. Thus, this essay thus presents the case for a forward-looking, legislative approach to PAS and euthanasia, as opposed to an essentially backward-looking, judicial or constitutional approach.[4] Although I suggest below that the soundest legislative policy at the present time would be to extend the legal prohibition of PAS into the near future, I remain open to the possibility that a given legislature, presented with sufficient evidence of the reliability of various safeguards, might come to a different conclusion.

ARGUMENTS AND MOTIVATIONS IN FAVOR OF PAS/EUTHANASIA

Let us begin, then, with the philosophical case for PAS and euthanasia, which consists of two distinct prongs, both of which speak simply, directly, and powerfully to our commonsensical intuitions. First, there is the claim of autonomy, that all of us possess a right to self-determination in matters profoundly touching on such religious themes as life, death, and the meaning of suffering. . . . Second, PAS and/or euthanasia are merciful acts that deliver terminally ill patients from painful and protracted death. . . . For patients suffering from the final ravages of end-stage AIDS or cancer, a doctor's lethal prescription or injection can be, and often is, welcomed as a blessed relief. Accordingly, we should treat human beings at least as well as we treat grievously ill or injured animals by putting them, at their own request, out of their misery.

These philosophical reflections can be supplemented with a more clinical perspective addressed to the motivational factors lying behind many requests to die. Many people advocate legalization because they fear a loss of control at the end of life. They fear falling victim to the technological imperative; they fear dying in chronic and uncontrolled

al
ral
ent
82.
v."

rary Health Law and Policy 13: permission.

as been heavily edited. Many nd the remainder have been g to follow up on sources e.

pain; they fear the psychological suffering attendant upon the relentless disintegration of the self; they fear, in short, a bad death. All of these fears, it so happens, are eminently justified. Physicians routinely ignore the documented wishes of patients and all-too-often allow patients to die with uncontrolled pain.[5] Studies of cancer patients have shown that over fifty percent suffer from unrelieved pain,[6] and many researchers have found that uncontrolled pain, particularly when accompanied by feelings of hopelessness and untreated depression, is a significant contributing factor for suicide and suicidal ideation.

Clinical depression is another major factor influencing patients' choice of suicide. Depression, accompanied by feelings of hopelessness, is the strongest predictor of suicide for both individuals who are terminally ill and those who are not. Yet most doctors are not trained to notice depression, especially in complex cases such as the elderly suffering from terminal illnesses. Even when doctors succeed in diagnosing depression, they often do not successfully treat it with readily available medications in sufficient amounts.

Significantly, the New York Task Force found that the vast majority of patients who request PAS or euthanasia can be treated successfully both for their depression and their pain, and that when they receive adequate psychiatric and palliative care, their requests to die usually are withdrawn.[7] In other words, patients given the requisite control over their lives and relief from depression and pain usually lose interest in PAS and euthanasia.

With all due respect for the power of modern methods of pain control, it must be acknowledged that a small percentage of patients suffer from conditions, both physical and psychological, that currently lie beyond the reach of the best medical and humane care. Some pain cannot be alleviated short of inducing a permanent state of unconsciousness in the patient, and some depression is unconquerable. For such unfortunate patients, the present law on PAS/euthanasia can represent an insuperable barrier to a dignified and decent death.[8]

OBJECTIONS TO PAS/EUTHANASIA

Opponents of PAS and euthanasia can be grouped into three main factions. One strongly condemns both practices as inherently immoral, as violations of the moral rule against killing the innocent. Most members of this group tend to harbor distinctly religious objections to suicide and euthanasia, viewing them as violations of God's dominion over human life. They argue that killing is simply wrong in itself, whether or not it is done out of respect for the patient's autonomy or out of concern for her suffering. Whether or not this position ultimately is justifiable from a theological point of view, its imposition on believers and non-believers alike is incompatible with the basic premises of a secular, pluralistic political order.

A second faction primarily objects to the fact that physicians are being called upon to do the killing. While conceding that killing the terminally ill or assisting in their suicides might not always be morally wrong for others to do, this group maintains that the participation of physicians in such practices undermines their role as healers and fatally compromises the physician-patient relationship.

Finally, a third faction readily grants that neither PAS nor active euthanasia, practiced by ordinary citizens or by physicians, are always morally wrong. On the contrary, this faction believes that in certain rare instances early release from a painful or intolerably degrading existence might constitute both a positive good and an important exercise of personal autonomy for the individual. Indeed, many members of this faction concede that should such a terrible fate befall them, they would hope to find a thoughtful, compassionate, and courageous physician to release them from their misery. But in spite of these important concessions, the members of this faction shrink from endorsing or regulating PAS and active euthanasia due to fears bearing on the social consequences of liberalization. This view is based on two distinct kinds of so-called "slippery slope" arguments: one bears on the inability to cabin PAS/euthanasia within the confines envisioned by its proponents; the other focuses on the likelihood of abuse, neglect, and mistake.

AN OPTION WITHOUT LIMITS

The first version of the slippery slope argument contends that a socially sanctioned practice of PAS would in all likelihood prove difficult, if not impossible, to cabin within its originally anticipated boundaries. Proponents of legalization usually begin with a wholesomely modest policy agenda, limiting their suggested reforms to a narrow and highly specified range of potential candidates and practices. "Give us PAS," they ask, "not the more controversial practice of active euthanasia, for presently competent patients who are terminally ill and suffering unbearable pain." But the logic of the case for PAS, based as it is upon the twin pillars of patient autonomy and mercy, makes it highly unlikely that society could stop with this modest proposal once it had ventured out on the slope. As numerous other critics have pointed out, if autonomy is the prime consideration, then additional constraints based upon terminal illness or unbearable pain, or both, would appear hard to justify. Indeed, if autonomy is crucial, the requirement of unbearable suffering would appear to be entirely subjective. Who is to say, other than the patient herself, how much suffering is too much? Likewise, the requirement of terminal illness seems an arbitrary standard against which to judge patients' own subjective evaluation of their quality of life. If my life is no longer worth living, why should a terminally ill cancer patient be granted PAS but not me, merely because my suffering is due to my "non-terminal" amyotrophic lateral sclerosis (ALS) or intractable psychiatric disorder?

Alternatively, if pain and suffering are deemed crucial to the justification of legalization, it is hard to see how the proposed barrier of contemporaneous consent of competent patients could withstand serious erosion. If the logic of PAS is at all similar to that of forgoing life-sustaining treatments, and we have every reason to think it so, then it would seem almost inevitable that a case soon would be made to permit PAS for incompetent patients who had left advance directives. That would then be followed by a "substituted judgment" test for patients who "would have wanted" PAS, and finally an "objective" test would be developed for patients (including newborns) whose best interests would be served by PAS or active euthanasia even in the absence of any subjective intent (see Part Two, Section Four above).

In the same way, the joint justifications of autonomy and mercy combine to undermine the plausibility of a line drawn between PAS and active euthanasia. As the authors of one highly publicized proposal have come to see, the logic of justification for active euthanasia is identical to that of PAS.[9] Legalizing PAS, while continuing to ban active euthanasia, would serve only to discriminate unfairly against patients who are suffering and wish to end their lives, but cannot do so because of some physical impairment. Surely these patients, it will be said, are "the worst-off group," and therefore they are the most in need of the assistance of others who will do for them what they can no longer accomplish on their own.

None of these initial slippery slope considerations amount to knock-down objections to further liberalization of our laws and practices. After all, it is not obvious that each of the highly predictable shifts (e.g., from terminal to "merely" incurable, from contemporaneous consent to best interests, and from PAS to active euthanasia), are patently immoral and unjustifiable. Still, in pointing out this likely slippage, the consequentialist opponents of PAS/euthanasia are calling on society to think about the likely consequences of taking the first tentative step onto the slope. If all of the extended practices predicted above pose substantially greater risks for vulnerable patients than the more highly circumscribed initial liberalization proposals, then we need to factor in these additional risks even as we ponder the more modest proposals.[10]

THE LIKELIHOOD OF ABUSE

The second prong of the slippery slope argument argues that whatever criteria for justifiable PAS and active euthanasia ultimately are chosen, abuse of the system is highly likely to follow. In other words, patients who fall outside the ambit of our justifiable criteria will soon be candidates for death. This prong resembles what I have elsewhere called an "empirical slope" argument, as it is based not on the close logical resemblance of concepts or justifications, but rather on an empirical prediction of what is likely to happen when we insert a particular social practice into our existing social system.

In order to reassure skeptics, the proponents of PAS/euthanasia concur that any potentially justifiable social policy in this area must meet at least the following three requirements. The policy would have to insist first, that all requests for death be truly voluntary; second, that all reasonable alternatives to PAS and active euthanasia must be explored before acceding to a patient's wishes; and, third, that a reliable system of reporting all cases must be established in order to effectively monitor these practices and respond to abuses. As a social pessimist on these matters, I believe, given social reality as we know it, that all three assumptions are problematic.

With regard to the voluntariness requirement, we pessimists contend that many requests would not be sufficiently voluntary. In addition to the subtly coercive influences of physicians and family members, perhaps the most slippery aspect of this slope is the highly predictable failure of most physicians to diagnose reliably and treat reversible clinical depression, particularly in the elderly population. As one geriatric psychiatrist testified before the New York Task Force, we now live in the "golden age" of treating depression, but the "lead age" of diagnosing it. We have the tools, but physicians are not adequately trained and motivated to use them. Unless dramatic changes are effected in the practice of medicine, we can predict with confidence that many instances of PAS and active euthanasia will fail the test of voluntariness.

Second, there is the lingering fear that any legislative proposal or judicial mandate would have to be implemented within the present social system marked by deep and pervasive discrimination against the poor and members of minority groups. We have every reason to expect that a policy that worked tolerably well in an affluent community like Scarsdale or Beverly Hills, might not work so well in a community like Bedford-Stuyvesant or Watts, where your average citizen has little or no access to basic primary care, let alone sophisticated care for chronic pain at home or in the hospital. There is also reason to worry about any policy of PAS initiated within our growing system of managed care, capitation, and physician incentives for delivering less care. Expert palliative care no doubt is an expensive and time-consuming proposition, requiring more, rather than less, time spent just talking with patients and providing them with humane comfort. It is highly doubtful that the context of physician-patient conversation within this new dispensation of "turnstile medicine" will be at all conducive to humane decisions untainted by subtle economic coercion.

In addition, given the abysmal and shameful track record of physicians in responding adequately to pain and suffering,[11] we also can confidently predict that in many cases all reasonable alternatives will not have been exhausted. Instead of vigorously addressing the pharmacological and psychosocial needs of such patients, physicians no doubt will continue to ignore, undertreat or treat many of their patients in an impersonal manner. The result is likely to be more depression, desperation, and requests for physician-assisted death from patients who could have been successfully treated. The root causes of this predictable failure are manifold, but high on the list is the inaccessibility of decent primary care to over thirty-seven million Americans. Other notable causes include an appalling lack of training in palliative care among primary care physicians and cancer specialists alike; discrimination in the delivery of pain control and other medical treatments on the basis of race and economic status; various myths shared by both physicians and patients about the supposed ill effects of pain medications; and restrictive state laws on access to opioids.

Finally, with regard to the third requirement, pessimists doubt that any reporting system would adequately monitor these practices. A great deal depends here on the extent to which patients and practitioners will regard these practices as essentially private matters to be discussed and acted upon within the privacy of the doctor-patient relationship. As the Dutch experience has conclusively demonstrated, physicians will be extremely loath to report instances of PAS and active euthanasia to public authorities, largely for fear of bringing the harsh glare of publicity upon the patients' families at a time when privacy is most needed. The likely result of this predictable lack of oversight will be society's inability to respond appropriately to disturbing incidents and long-term trends. In other words, the practice most likely will not be as amenable to regulation as the proponents contend.

The moral of this story is that deeply seated inadequacies in physicians' training, combined with structural flaws in our health care system, can be reliably predicted to secure the premature deaths of many people who would in theory be excluded by the criteria of most leading proposals to legalize PAS. If this characterization of the status quo is at all accurate, then the problem will not be solved by well meaning assurances that abuses will not be tolerated, or that patients will, of course, be offered the full range of palliative care options before any decision for PAS is ratified.[12] While such regulatory solutions are possible in theory, and may well justly prevail in the future, we should be wary of legally sanctioning any negative right to be let alone by the state when the just and humane exercise of that right will depend upon the provision of currently nonexistent services. The operative analogy here, I fear, is our failed and shameful policy of "deinstutionaliza-tion," which left thousands of vulnerable and defenseless former residents of state psychiatric hospitals to fend for themselves on the streets, lit-erally "rotting with their rights on." It is now gen-erally agreed that the crucial flaw in this well-intended but catastrophic policy was our society's willingness to honor such patients' negative right to be free of institutional fetters without having first made available reliable local alternatives to institutionalization. The operative lesson for us here is that judges and courts are much better at enunciating negative rights than they are at pro-viding the services required for their successful implementation. . . .

TOWARD A POLICY OF PRUDENT (LEGAL) RESTRAINT AND AGGRESSIVE (MEDICAL) INTERVENTION

In contrast to the judicial approach, which totally vindicates the value of patient autonomy at the expense of protecting the vulnerable, my own pre-ferred approach to a social policy of PAS and euthanasia conceives of this debate as posing an essentially "tragic choice."[13] It frankly acknowl-edges that whatever choice we make, whether we opt for a reaffirmation of the current legal restraints or for a policy of legitimization and reg-ulation, there are bound to be "victims." The vic-tims of the current policy are easy to identify: They are on the news, the talk shows, the documen-taries, and often on Dr. Kevorkian's roster of so-called "patients." The victims of legalization, by contrast, will be largely hidden from view; they will include the clinically depressed eighty-year-old man who could have lived for another year of good quality if only he had been adequately treat-ed, and the fifty-year-old woman who asks for death because doctors in her financially stretched HMO cannot, or will not, effectively treat her unrelenting, but mysterious, pelvic pain. Perhaps eventually, if we slide far enough down the slope, the uncommunicative stroke victim, whose distant children deem an earlier death to be a better death, will fall victim. There will be others besides these, many coming from the ranks of the uninsured and the poor. To the extent that minorities and the poor already suffer from the effects of discrimina-tion in our health care system, it is reasonable to expect that any system of PAS and euthanasia will exhibit similar effects, such as failure to access ade-quate primary care, pain management, and psy-chiatric diagnosis and treatment. Unlike Dr. Kevorkian's "patients," these victims will not get their pictures in the papers, but they all will have faces and they will all be cheated of good months or perhaps even years.

This "tragic choice" approach to social policy on PAS/euthanasia takes the form of the following argument formulated at the legislative level. First, the number of "genuine cases" justifying PAS, active euthanasia, or both, will be relatively small. Patients who receive good personal care, good pain relief, treatment for depression, and adequate psycho-social supports tend not to persist in their desire to die.

Second, the social risks of legalization are seri-ous and highly predictable. They include the expansion of these practices to nonvoluntary cases, the advent of active euthanasia, and the wide-spread failure to pursue readily available alterna-tives to suicide motivated by pain, depression, hopelessness, and lack of access to good primary medical care.

Third, rather than propose a momentous and dangerous policy shift for a relatively small num-ber of "genuine cases"—a shift that would surely involve a great deal of persistent social division and strife analogous to that involved in the abor-tion controversy—we should instead attempt to redirect the public debate toward a goal on which we can and should all agree, namely the manifest and urgent need to reform the way we die in America. Instead of pursuing a highly divisive and dangerous campaign for PAS, we should attack the problem at its root with an ambitious program of reform in the areas of access to primary care and the education of physicians in palliative care. At least as far as the "slippery slope" opponents of PAS are concerned, we should thus first see to it that the vast majority of people in this country have access to adequate, affordable, and nondiscriminatory primary and palliative care. At the end of this long and arduous process, when we finally have an equitable, effective, and compassionate health care system in place, one that might be compared favorably with that in the Netherlands, then we might well want to reopen the discussion of PAS and active euthanasia.

Finally, there are those few unfortunate patients who truly are beyond the pale of good palliative, hospice, and psychiatric care. The opponents of legalization must face up to this suffering remnant and attempt to offer creative and humane solutions. One possibility is for such patients to be rendered permanently unconscious by drugs until such time, presumably not a long time, as death finally claims them. Although some will find such an option to be aesthetically unappealing, many would find it a welcome relief. Other patients beyond the reach of the best palliative and hospice care could take their own lives, either by well-known traditional means, or with the help of a physician who could sedate them while they refused further food and (life extending) fluids. Finally, those who find this latter option to be unacceptable might still be able to find a compassionate physician who, like Dr. Timothy Quill, will ultimately be willing, albeit in fear and trembling, to "take small risks for people they really know and care about." Such actions will continue to take place within the privacy of the patient-physician relationship, however, and thus will not threaten vulnerable patients and the social fabric to the same extent as would result from full legalization and regulation.

As the partisans of legalized PAS correctly point out, the covert practice of PAS will not be subject to regulatory oversight, and is thus capable of generating its own abuses and slippery slope. Still, I believe that the ever-present threat of possible criminal sanctions and revocation of licensure will continue to serve, for the vast majority of physicians, as powerful disincentives to abuse the system. Moreover, as suggested earlier, it is highly unlikely that the proposals for legalization would result in truly effective oversight.

CONCLUSION

Instead of conceiving this momentous debate as a choice between, on the one hand, legalization and regulation with all of their attendant risks, and on the other hand, the callous abandonment of patients to their pain and suffering, enlightened opponents must recommend a positive program of clinical and social reforms. On the clinical level, physicians must learn how to really listen to their patients, to unflinchingly engage them in sensitive discussions of their needs and the meaning of their requests for assisted death, to deliver appropriate palliative care, to distinguish fact from fiction in the ethics and law of pain relief, to diagnose and treat clinical depression, and finally, to ascertain and respect their patients' wishes for control regarding the forgoing of life-sustaining treatments. On the social level, opponents of PAS must aggressively promote major initiatives in medical and public education regarding pain control, in the sensitization of insurance companies and licensing agencies to issues of the quality of dying, and in the reform of state laws that currently hinder access to pain-relieving medications.

In the absence of an ambitious effort in the direction of aggressive medical and social reform, I fear that the medical and nursing professions will have lost whatever moral warrant and credibility they might still have in continuing to oppose physician-assisted suicide and active euthanasia. As soon as these reforms are in place, however, we might then wish to proceed slowly and cautiously with experiments in various states to test the overall benefits of a policy of legalization. Until that time, however, we are not well served as a society by court decisions allowing for legalization of PAS. The Supreme Court has thus reached a sound decision in ruling out a constitutional right to PAS. As the Justices acknowledged, however, this momentous decision will not end the moral debate over PAS and euthanasia. Indeed, it should and hopefully will intensify it.

NOTES

1. *Compassion in Dying* v. *Washington*, 79 F.3d 790, 838 (9th Cir. 1996).
2. *Quill* v. *Vacco*, 80 F.3d 716, 731(2nd Cir. 1996).

3. *Vacco, Attorney General of New York. et al. v. Quill et al.* certiorari to the United States Court of Appeals for the Second Circuit, No. 95-1858. Argued January 8, 1997— Decided June 26, 1997. *Washington et al. v. Glucksberg et al.,* certiorari to the United States Court of Appeals for the Ninth Circuit, No. 96-110. Argued January 8, 1997— Decided June 26, 1997.

4. My stance on these issues has been profoundly influenced by my recent work with the New York State Task Force on Life and the Law (hereinafter "Task Force") to come to grips with this issue.

5. "A Controlled Trial to Improve Care for Seriously Ill Hospitalized Patients: The Study to Understand Prognoses and Preferences for Outcomes and Risks of Treatments" (SUPPORT), *Journal of the American Medical Association* 274 Nov. 22, 1995): 1591-92.

6. Task Force, *When Death is Sought*, x-xi.

7. Task Force, *When Death Is Sought*, xiv.

8. The preceding section thus signals two important points of agreement with the so-called "Philosophers' Brief" submitted to the Supreme Court in *Compassion in Dying* and *Vacco* by Ronald Dworkin, Thomas Nagel, Robert Nozick, John Rawls, Thomas Scanlon, and Judith Jarvis Thomson [in this volume, pp. 254–66]. I agree that individuals in the throes of a painful or degrading terminal illness may well have a very strong moral and even legal interest in securing PAS. I also agree that the pain and suffering of a small percentage of dying patients cannot be adequately controlled by currently available medical interventions. As we shall see, however, I disagree with the philosophers' conclusion that this interest is sufficiently strong in the face of current medical and social inadequacies as to justify a legal right that would void the reasonably cautious prohibitions of PAS and euthanasia in effect in every state.

9. Cassel et al., "Care of the Hopelessly Ill," 1380-84. See also Franklin G. Miller et al., "Regulating Physician-Assisted Death," *New England Journal of Medicine* 331(1994): 199-23 (conceding by the untenability of the previous distinction).

10. Professors Dworkin, et al. consistently fail to mention the possibility, let alone the high likelihood, of this first sort of slippage; I take this to be a serious omission both in their joint brief and in Dworkin's individually authored articles on this subject. These authors simply assume (with the plaintiffs and circuit court majority opinions) that this right will be restricted by means of procedural safeguards to presently competent, incurably ill individuals manifesting great pain and suffering due to physical illness. (For evidence of Dworkin's continuing failure to acknowledge this problem, see his assessment of the Supreme Court opinions in "Assisted Suicide: What the Court Really Said," *New York Review of Books* 44, no. 14 (Sept.25, 1997): 40-44. Failure to notice this sort of dynamic might be due either to the philosophers' lack of familiarity with the recent history of bioethics or to their belief that the social risks of PAS are equivalent to the risks inherent in the widely accepted practice of forgoing life-sustaining treatments, and thus that such slippage would not present any additional risk. The latter assumption is, of course, vigorously contested by the opponents of PAS and euthanasia.

11. Task Force, *When Death Is Sought*, 43-47. "Despite dramatic advances in pain management, the delivery of pain relief is grossly inadequate in clinical practice. . . Studies have shown that only 2 to 60 percent of cancer pain is treated adequately." *Ibid.*, 43.

12. See, e.g., Ronald Dworkin, "Introduction to the Philosophers' Brief," *New York Review of Books*, 41-42 [in this volume, 255–56]; and Dworkin. "Assisted Suicide: What the Court Really Said," 44.

13. For an explication of the notion of a "tragic choice" in the sense that I employ here, see Guido Calabresi and Philip Bobbit, *Tragic Choices* (New York: W.W. Norton, 1978).

Euthanasia: The Way We Do It, the Way They Do It

Margaret P. Battin

INTRODUCTION

Because we tend to be rather myopic in our discussions of death and dying, especially about the

Reprinted by permission of Elsevier Science from "Euthanasia" by Margaret Battin, *Journal of Pain and Symptom Management*, Vol. 6, No. 5, 1991, 298–305.

issues of active euthanasia and assisted suicide, it is valuable to place the question of how we go about dying in an international context. We do not always see that our own cultural norms may be quite different from those of other nations and that our background assumptions and actual practices differ dramatically. Thus, I would like to examine the perspectives on end-of-life dilemmas in three countries: the Netherlands, Germany, and the United States.

The Netherlands, Germany, and the United States are all advanced industrial democracies. They all have sophisticated medical establishments and life expectancies over 70 years of age; their populations are all characterized by an increasing proportion of older persons. They are all in what has been called the fourth stage of the epidemiologic transition[1]—that stage of societal development in which it is no longer the case that most people die of acute parasitic or infectious diseases. In this stage, it is no longer the case that most people die of diseases with rapid, unpredictable onsets and sharp fatality curves; rather, the majority of the population—as much as perhaps 70–80%—die of degenerative diseases, especially delayed-degenerative diseases that are characterized by late, slow onset and extended decline. Most people in highly industrialized countries die from cancer; atherosclerosis; heart disease (by no means always suddenly fatal); chronic obstructive pulmonary disease; liver, kidney, or other organ disease; or degenerative neurological disorders; with the principal exception of AIDS, they die not so much from attack by outside diseases but from gradual disintegration. Thus, all three of these countries are alike in facing a common problem: how to deal with the characteristic new ways in which we die.

DEALING WITH DYING IN THE UNITED STATES

In the United States, we have come to recognize that the maximal extension of life-prolonging treatment in these late-life degenerative conditions is often inappropriate. Although we could keep the machines and tubes—the respirators, intravenous lines, feeding tubes—hooked up for extended periods, we recognize that this is inhumane, pointless, and financially impossible. Instead, as a society we have developed a number of mechanisms for dealing with these hopeless situations, all of which involve withholding or withdrawing various forms of treatment.

Some mechanisms for withholding or withdrawing treatments are exercised by the patient who is confronted by such a situation or who anticipates it. These include refusal of treatment, the patient-executed Do Not Resuscitate (DNR) order, the Living Will, and the Durable Power of Attorney. Others are mechanisms for decision by second parties about a patient who is no longer competent or never was competent. The latter are reflected in a long series of court cases, including *Quinlan; Saikewicz; Spring; Eichner; Barber; Bartling; Conroy; Brophy;* the trio *Farrell, Peter,* and *Jobes;* and *Cruzan.* These are cases that attempt to delineate the precise circumstances under which it is appropriate to withhold or withdraw various forms of therapy, including respiratory support, chemotherapy, antibiotics in intercurrent infections, and artificial nutrition and hydration. Thus, during the past 20 years or so, roughly since *Quinlan* (1976), we have developed an impressive body of case law and state statutes that protects, permits, and facilitates our characteristic American strategy of dealing with end-of-life situations. These cases provide a framework for withholding or withdrawing treatment when we believe there is no medical or moral point in going on. This is sometimes termed *passive euthanasia;* more often, it is simply called *allowing to die,* and it is ubiquitous in the United States.

For example, a study by Miles and Gomez indicates that some 85% of deaths in the United States occur in health care institutions, including hospitals, nursing homes, and other facilities, and of these, about 70% involve electively withholding some form of life-sustaining treatment.[2] A 1989 study cited in the *Journal of the American Medical Association* claims that 85–90% of critical care professionals state that they are withholding and withdrawing life-sustaining treatments from patients who are "deemed to have irreversible disease and are terminally ill."[3] Still another study identified some 115 patients from whom care was withheld or withdrawn in two intensive-care units; 110 were already incompetent by the time the decision to limit care was made. The 89 who died while still in the intensive-care unit accounted for 45% of all deaths there."[4] It is estimated that 1.3 million American deaths a year follow decisions to withhold life support;[5] this is a majority of the just over 2 million American deaths per year.

In recent years, the legitimate practice of withholding and withdrawing treatment has increasingly been understood to include highly specific forms certain to result in death, such as withholding or withdrawing artificial nutrition and hydration. The administration of escalating doses of morphine, which, though it will depress respiration and so hasten death, is acceptable under the (Catholic) principle of double effect, "foreseen but not intended" to result in death; it is thus said to be distinguished from killing. At least in theory, withholding and withdrawing treatment is the way we in the United States go about dealing with dying. A number of recent studies have shown that many physicians do receive requests for assistance in suicide or active euthanasia and that a substantial number of these physicians have complied with one or more such requests; however, this more direct assistance in dying takes place entirely out of sight of the law. *Allowing to die,* but not *causing to die,* has been the only legally protected alternative to maximal treatment legally recognized in the United States.

In very recent years, the United States has seen considerable ferment over the legalization of physician-assisted suicide. In November 1994, voters in Oregon passed a ballot initiative known as Measure 16, permitting a physician to prescribe a lethal medication for a terminally ill patient who requests it, subject to a number of safeguards; this measure was tied up in court challenges for several years. In 1996, the 9th and 2nd circuit federal courts of appeal independently held that state laws prohibiting physician-assisted suicide were unconstitutional; in 1997 the U.S. Supreme Court unanimously overturned these ruling in *Washington v. Glucksberg* and *Vacco v. Quill,* holding that there is no constitutional right to physician-assisted suicide. These rulings had the effect of allowing the individual states to prohibit or permit physician-assisted suicide; active euthanasia was not at issue in these cases. As of early 1998, the majority of states retained statutory, case law, or common law prohibitions of assisted suicide, and only Oregon—whose Measure 16 survived a repeal challenge in 1997—had made it legal. Reliance on "allowing to die" remains American medicine's official posture in the face of death.

DEALING WITH DYING IN THE NETHERLANDS

In the Netherlands, although the practice of withholding and withdrawing treatment is similar to that in the United States, voluntary active euthanasia and physician assistance in suicide are also available responses to end-of-life situations.[6] Although active euthanasia and assistance in suicide remain technically prohibited by statutory law, they are protected by a series of lower and supreme court decisions and are widely regarded as legal, or, more precisely, *gedogen,* legally "tolerated." Euthanasia is the more frequent form of assistance in dying and most discussion has concerned euthanasia rather than assistance in suicide, though the conceptual difference is not always regarded as great: many cases of what the Dutch term *voluntary active euthanasia* involve initial self-administration of the lethal dose by the patient and so would count for Americans as physician-assisted suicide, though in either case, the physician is prepared to be present to assist in preventing any unwanted side effects and, if necessary, to ensure that the lethal process is complete. The Dutch court decisions have the effect of protecting the physician who performs euthanasia or provides assistance in suicide from prosecution, provided a rigorous set of guidelines are met.

These guidelines, variously stated, contain five central provisions:

1. that the patient's request be voluntary and enduring
2. that the patient be undergoing intolerable suffering
3. that the alternatives acceptable to the patient for relieving the suffering have been tried
4. that the patient have full information
5. that the physician consult with a second physician whose judgment can be expected to be independent

Of these criteria, it is the first that is central: euthanasia may be performed only at the voluntary request of the patient. This criterion is also understood to require that the patient's request be a stable, enduring, reflective one—not the product of a transitory impulse. Every attempt is to be made to rule out depression, psychopathology, pressures from family members, unrealistic fears, and other factors compromising voluntariness.

In 1990, a comprehensive, nationwide study requested by the Dutch government, popularly known as the Remmelink Commission report, provided the first objective data about the incidence of euthanasia.[7] This study also provided information about other medical decisions at the end of life: withholding or withdrawal of treatment; the use of life-shortening doses of opioids for the control of pain; and direct termination, including not only voluntary active euthanasia and physician-assisted suicide but life-ending procedures not termed euthanasia. The Remmelink study was supplemented by a second empirical examination, focusing particularly carefully on the characteristics of patients and the nature of their euthanasia requests.[8] Five years later, the researchers from these two studies jointly conducted a major new nationwide study replicating much of the previous Remmelink inquiry, providing empirical data both about current practice in the Netherlands and change over a five-year period.[9]

About 130,000 people die in the Netherlands every year, and of these deaths, about 30% are acute and unexpected, while about 70% are predictable and foreseen, usually the result of degenerative illnesses comparatively late in life. Of the total deaths in the Netherlands, about 20% involve decisions to withhold or withdraw treatment in situations where continuing treatment would probably have prolonged life; another 20% involved the "double effect" use of opioids to relieve pain but in dosages probably sufficient to shorten life.[10]

The 1990 study revealed that about 2,300 people, 1.8% of the total deaths in the Netherlands, died by euthanasia—understood as the termination of the life of the patient at the patient's explicit and persistent request; another 400 people, 0.3% of the total, chose physician-assisted suicide. However, the study also revealed that another 0.8% of patients who died did so as the result of life-terminating procedures not technically called euthanasia, without explicit, current requests. These cases, known as "the 1000 cases," unleashed highly exaggerated claims that patients were being killed against their wills. In fact, in about half of these cases, euthanasia had been previously discussed with the patient or the patient had expressed in a previous phase of the disease a wish for euthanasia if his or her suffering became unbearable ("Doctor, please don't let me suffer too long"); and in the other half, the patient was no longer competent and was near death, clearly suffering grievously although verbal contact had become impossible.[11] In 91% of these cases without explicit, current request, life was shortened by less than a week, and in 33% by less than a day.

By 1995, although the proportion of cases of assisted suicide had remained about the same, the proportion of cases of euthanasia had risen to about 2.4% (associated, the authors conjectured, with the aging population and in increase in the proportion of deaths due to cancer, that condition in which euthanasia is most frequent). However, the proportion of cases of life termination without current explicit request had declined slightly to 0.7%. In 1990, a total of 2.9% of all deaths had involved euthanasia and related practices; by 1995 this total was 3.3%. Only about 41% of cases are reported to the coroner as required, though there has been a dramatic gain since the physician has no longer been required to report them directly to the police or the Ministry of Justice. However, there are no major differences between reported and unreported cases in terms of the patient's characteristics, clinical conditions, or reasons for the action.[12] Euthanasia is performed in about 1:25 of the deaths that occur in the home, about 1:75 of hospital deaths, and about 1:800 of nursing home deaths.

Although euthanasia is thus not frequent, a small fraction of the total annual mortality, it is nevertheless a conspicuous option in terminal illness, well-known to both physicians and the general public. There has been very widespread public discussion of the issues that arise with respect to euthanasia during the last two decades, and surveys of public opinion show that public support for a liberal euthanasia policy has been growing: from 40% in 1966 to 81% in 1988.[13] Doctors, too, support the practice, and although there has been a vocal opposition group, it has remained in the clear minority. Some 53% of Dutch physicians say that they have performed euthanasia or provided assistance in suicide, including 63% of general practitioners. An additional 35% of all physicians said that although they had not actually done so, they could conceive of situations in which they would be prepared to do so. Nine percent say they would never perform it, and just 3% say they not only would not do so themselves but would not refer a patient who requested it to a physician who would. Thus, although many physicians who had practiced euthanasia mentioned that they would be most reluctant to do so again and that "only in the face of unbearable suffering and with no alternatives would they be prepared to take such action,"[14] both the 1990 and 1995 studies showed that the majority of Dutch physicians accept the practice in some cases. Surveying the changes over the 5-year period between 1990–1995, the study authors also commented that the data do not support claims of a slippery slope.

In general, pain alone is not the basis for deciding upon euthanasia, since pain can, in most cases, be effectively treated. Rather, the "intolerable suffering" mentioned in the second criterion is understood to mean suffering that is intolerable in the patient's (rather than the physician's) view and can include a fear of or unwillingness to endure *entluistering,* that gradual effacement and loss of personal identity that characterizes the end stages of many terminal illnesses. In very exceptional circumstances, the Supreme Court ruled in the Chabot case of 1994, physician-assisted suicide, about 80% have cancer, while just 3% have cardiovascular disease and 4% neurological disease.

In a year, almost 35,000 patients seek reassurance from their physicians that they will be granted euthanasia if their suffering becomes severe; there are about 9,700 explicit requests, and about two-thirds of these are turned down, usually on the grounds that there is some other way of treating the patient's suffering. In 14% of cases in 1990, the denial was based on the presence of depression or psychiatric illness.

In the Netherlands, many hospitals now have protocols for the performance of euthanasia; these serve to ensure that the court-established guidelines have been met. However, euthanasia is often practiced in the patient's home, typically by the general practitioner who is the patient's long-term family physician. Euthanasia is usually performed after aggressive hospital treatment has failed to arrest the patient's terminal illness; the patient has come home to die, and the family physician is prepared to ease this passing. Whether practiced at home or in the hospital, it is believed that euthanasia usually takes place in the presence of the family members, perhaps the visiting nurse, and often the patient's pastor or priest. Many doctors say that performing euthanasia is never easy but that it is something they believe a doctor ought to do for his or her patient when nothing else can help.

Thus, in the Netherlands a patient who is facing the end of life has an option not openly practiced in the United States: to ask the physician to bring his or her life to an end. Although not everyone does so—indeed, almost 97% of people who die in a given year do not do so—it is a choice widely understood as available.

FACING DEATH IN GERMANY

In part because of its very painful history of Nazism, Germany appears to believe that doctors should have no role in causing death. Although societal generalizations are always risky, it is fair, I think, to say that there is vigorous and nearly universal opposition in Germany to the notion of active euthanasia. Euthanasia is viewed as always wrong, and the Germans view the Dutch as stepping out on a dangerously slippery slope.

However, it is an artifact of German law that, whereas killing on request (including voluntary euthanasia) is prohibited, assisting suicide is not a violation of the law, provided the person is *tatherrschaftsfähig,* capable of exercising control over his or her actions, and also acting out of *freiverantwortliche Wille,* freely responsible choice. In response to this situation, a private organization, the *Deutsche Gesellschaft für Humanes Sterben* (DGHS), or German Society for Humane Dying, has been providing support to its very extensive membership (over 50,000 persons) in choosing suicide as an alternative to terminal illness.

Although for legal reasons the DGHS no longer publishes its own book of drug dosages for ending life, a person who has been a member of the DGHS for at least a year, provided he or she has not received medical or psychotherapeutic treatment for depression or other psychiatric illness during the last two years, can order a copy of *Departing Drugs* (German title, *Selbsterlösung durch Medikamente*). This booklet, published in Scotland by an international working group, provides a list of prescription drugs, together with the specific dosages necessary for producing a certain, painless death. DGHS recommended that the member approach a physician for a prescription for the drug desired, asking, for example, for a barbiturate to help with sleep. If necessary, the DGHS would also arrange for someone to obtain drugs from neighboring countries, including France, Italy, Spain, Portugal, and Greece, where they may be available without prescription. In unusual cases, the DGHS would also provide what it calls *Sterbebegleitung* (accompaniment in dying), which involved arranging for a companion to remain with the person during the often extended period that is required for the lethal drug to take full effect. However, the *Sterbebegleiter* was typically a layperson, not someone medically trained, and physicians played no role in assisting in these cases of suicide.

To preclude suspicion by providing evidence of the person's intentions, the DGHS also provided a form—printed on a single sheet of distinctive purple paper—to be signed once when joining the organization, documenting that the person has reflected thoroughly on the possibility of "free death" (*Freitod*) or suicide in terminal illness as a way of releasing oneself from severe suffering, and expressing the intention to determine the time and character of one's own death. The person then signs this form again at the time of the suicide, leaving it beside the body as evidence that the act is not an impetuous one. The form also requests that, if the person discovered before the suicide is complete, no rescue measures be undertaken. Because assisting suicide is not illegal in Germany, provided the person is competent and in control of his or her own will, there is no legal risk for family members, the *Sterbebegleiter*, or others in reporting information about the methods and effectiveness of suicide attempts, and the DGHS encouraged its network of regional bureaus, located in major cities throughout the country, to facilitate feedback. On this basis, it has regularly updated and revised the drug information it provides to the international consortium that publishes *Departing Drugs*.

Open, legal assistance in suicide is supported by a feature of the German language that makes it possible to conceptualize it in a comparatively benign way. While English, French, Spanish, and many other languages have just a single primary word for suicide, German has four: *Selbstmord, Selbsttötung, Suizid*, and *Freitod*, of which the latter has comparatively positive, even somewhat heroic connotations.[15] Thus German-speakers can think about the deliberate termination of their lives in a linguistic way not easily available to speakers of other languages. The DGHS has consistently used *Freitod* rather than German's other, more negative terms to describe the practice with which it provides assistance. No reliable figures are available

about the number of available suicides with which the organization has assisted, but it is fair to say, both because of the legal differences and the different conceptual horizons of German-speakers, that the option of self-produced death outside the medical system is more clearly open in Germany than it has been in the Netherlands or the United States.

In the wake of the 1992 scandal that engulfed the original founder and president of the DGHS, Hans Hennig Atrott, who was convicted for violations of drug laws and tax evasion for selling some members cyanide for exorbitant sums, the DGHS has gone through a period of considerable introspection and reassessment. It has turned much of its attention to the development of other measures for protecting the rights of the terminally ill. It now also distributes newly legalized advance directives, including the Living Will and the Durable Power of Attorney as well as detailed organ-donation documents. Yet it remains steadfast in defense of the right to suicide as a part of the right to self-determination, and continues to be supportive of patients who make this choice.

To be sure, assisted suicide is not the only option open to the terminally ill patient in Germany, nor is there clear evidence concerning its frequency. Reported suicide rates in Germany are not dramatically higher than in the Netherlands or the United States, though there is reason to think that many terminal-illness suicides in all countries are reported as deaths from the underlying disease. Germany is also seeing increasing emphasis on help in dying that does not involve direct termination, and organizations like Omega, which offers hospice-style care and an extensive program of companionship, are attracting increasing attention. Nevertheless, the DGHS is a conspicuous, widely known organization, and many Germans appear to be aware that assisted suicide is available and not illegal even if they do not use its services.

OBJECTIONS TO THE THREE MODELS OF DYING

In response to the dilemmas raised by the new circumstances of death, in which the majority of the population in each of the advanced industrial nations dies of degenerative diseases after an extended period of terminal deterioration, different countries develop different practices. Except in

Oregon, at this moment, the United States legally permits only withholding and withdrawal of treatment, though of course physician-assisted suicide and active euthanasia do occur. The Netherlands also permits voluntary active euthanasia, and although Germany rejects euthanasia, it permits non-physician-assisted suicide. To be sure, all of these practices are currently undergoing evolution, and in some ways they are becoming more alike: Germany is paying new attention to the right of patients to execute advance directives and thus to have treatment withheld and withdrawn. A 1995 policy statement of the Royal Dutch Medical Association expressed a careful preference for physician-assisted suicide in preference to euthanasia, urging that physicians encourage patients who request euthanasia to administer the lethal dose themselves as a further protective of voluntary choice. And, in the United States, the Supreme Court's ruling there is no constitutional right to physician-assisted suicide has been understood to countenance the emergence of a "state-by-state laboratory" as individual states, following Oregon, move to legalize physician-assisted suicide. Nevertheless, there remain substantial differences among these three countries in their approaches to dying, and while each recognizes advantages to its approach, there are also serious moral objections to be made to each of them, objections to be considered before resolving the issue of which practices our own culture ought to permit.

OBJECTIONS TO THE GERMAN PRACTICE

German law does not prohibit assisting suicide, but postwar German culture discourages physicians from taking an active role in death. This gives rise to distinctive moral problems. For one thing, it appears that there is little professional help or review provided for patients' choices about suicide; because the patient makes this choice essentially outside the medical establishment, medical professionals are not in a position to detect or treat impaired judgment on the part of the patient, especially judgment impaired by depression. Similarly, if the patient must commit suicide assisted only by persons outside the medical profession, there are risks that the patient's diagnosis and prognosis will be inadequately confirmed, that the means chosen for suicide will be

unreliable or inappropriately used, that the means used for suicide will fall into the hands of other persona, and that the patient will fail to recognize or be able to resist intrafamilial pressures and manipulation. After the 1992 scandal, even the DGHS itself was accused of promoting rather than simply supporting choices of suicide. Finally, as the DGHS now emphasizes, assistance in suicide can be a freely chosen option only in a legal context that also protects the many other choices a patient may make about how his or her life shall end, including those involving the withholding or withdrawal of treatment.

OBJECTIONS TO THE DUTCH PRACTICE

The Dutch practice of physician-performed active voluntary euthanasia also raises a number of ethical issues, many of which have been discussed vigorously both in the Dutch press and in commentary on the Dutch practices front abroad. For one thing, it is sometimes said that the availability of physician-performed euthanasia creates a disincentive for providing good terminal care. There is no evidence that this is the case; on the contrary, Peter Admiraal, the anesthesiologist who has been perhaps the Netherlands' most vocal defender of voluntary active euthanasia, insists that pain should rarely or never be the occasion for euthanasia, as pain (in contrast to suffering) is comparatively easily treated.[16] In fact, pain is the primary reason for the request in only about 5% of cases. Instead, it is a refusal to endure the final stages of deterioration, both mental and physical, that primarily motivates the majority of requests.

It is also sometimes said that active euthanasia violates the Hippocratic oath. The original Greek version of the Oath does prohibit the physician from giving a deadly drug, even when asked for it; but the original version also prohibits the physician from performing surgery and from taking fees for teaching medicine, neither of which prohibition has survived into contemporary medical practice. Dutch physicians often say that they see performing euthanasia—where it is genuinely requested by the patient and nothing else can be done to relieve the patient's condition—as part of their duty to the patient, not as a violation of it. As the 1995 Remmelink report commented, "a large majority of Dutch physicians consider euthanasia an exceptional but accepted part of medical practice."[17]

The Dutch are also often said to be at risk of starting down the slippery slope, that is, that the practice of voluntary active euthanasia for patients who meet the criteria will erode into practicing less-than-voluntary euthanasia on patients whose problems are not irremediable and perhaps by gradual degrees will develop into terminating the lives of people who are elderly, chronically ill, handicapped, mentally retarded, or otherwise regarded as undesirable. This risk is often expressed in vivid claims of widespread fear and wholesale slaughter—claims based on misinterpretation of the 1,000 cases of life-ending treatment without explicit, current request, claims that are often repeated in the right-to-life press in both Holland and the United States though they are simply not true. However, it is true that the Dutch are now beginning to agonize over the problems of the incompetent patient, the mentally ill patient, the newborn with serious deficits, and other patients who cannot make voluntary choices, though these are largely understood as issues about withholding or withdrawing treatment, not about direct termination.[18]

What is not often understood is that this new and acutely painful area of reflection for the Dutch—withholding and withdrawing treatment from incompetent patients—has already led in the United States to the development of a vast, highly developed body of law: namely, that series of cases cited earlier in the chapter, beginning with *Quinlan* and culminating in *Cruzan*. Americans have been discussing these issues for a long time and have developed a broad set of practices that are regarded as routine in withholding and withdrawing treatment from persons who are no longer or never were competent. The Dutch see Americans as much further out on the slippery slope than they are, because Americans have already become accustomed to second-party choices that result in death for other people. Issues involving second-party choices are painful to the Dutch in a way they are not to us precisely because *voluntariness* is so central in the Dutch understanding of choices about dying. Concomitantly, the Dutch see the Americans' squeamishness about first-party choices—voluntary euthanasia, assisted suicide—as evidence that

we are not genuinely committed to recognizing voluntary choice after all. For this reason, many Dutch commentators believe that the Americans are at a much greater risk of sliding down the slippery slope into involuntary killing than they are. (I fear, I must add, that they are right about this.)

OBJECTIONS TO THE AMERICAN PRACTICE

The German, Dutch, and American practices all occur within similar conditions—in industrialized nations with highly developed medical systems where a majority of the population die of illnesses exhibiting characteristically extended downhill courses—but the issues raised by our own response to this situation, relying on withholding and withdrawal of treatment, may be even more disturbing than those of the Dutch or the Germans. We Americans often assume that our approach is "safer" because it involves only letting someone die, not killing him or her; but it, too, raises very troubling questions.

The first of these issues is a function of the fact that withdrawing and especially withholding treatment are typically less conspicuous, less pronounced, less evident kinds of actions than direct killing, even though they can equally well lead to death. Decisions about nontreatment have an invisibility that decisions about directly causing death do not have, even though they may have the same result, and hence there is a much wider range of occasions in which such decisions can be made. One can decline to treat a patient in many different ways, at many different times—by not providing oxygen, by not instituting dialysis, by not correcting electrolyte imbalances, and so on—all of which will cause the patient's death; open medical killing also brings about death but is much more overt and conspicuous. Consequently, letting die also invites many fewer protections. In contrast to the standard slippery-slope argument, which sees killing as riskier than letting die, the more realistic slippery-slope argument warns that because our culture relies primarily on decisions about nontreatment, grave decisions about living or dying are not as open to scrutiny as they are under more direct life-terminating practices and hence are more open to abuse.

Second, reliance on withholding and withdrawal of treatment invites rationing in an extremely strong way, in part because of the comparative invisibility of these decisions. When a health care provider does not offer a specific sort of care, it is not always possible to discern the motivation; the line between believing that it would not provide benefit to the patient and that it would not provide benefit worth the investment of resources in the patient can be very thin. This is a particular problem where health care financing is decentralized and profit-oriented, as in the United States, and where rationing decisions without benefit of principle are not always available for easy review.

Third, relying on withholding and withdrawal of treatment can often be cruel. It requires that the patient who is dying from one of the diseases that exhibits a characteristic extended, downhill course (as the majority of patients in the Netherlands, Germany, and the United States all do) must, in effect, wait to die until the absence of a certain treatment will cause death. For instance, the cancer patient who forgoes chemotherapy or surgery does not simply die from this choice; he or she continues to endure the downhill course of the cancer until the tumor finally destroys some crucial bodily function or organ. The patient with amyotrophic lateral sclerosis who decides in advance to decline respiratory support does not die at the time this choice is made but continues to endure increasing paralysis until breathing is impaired and suffocation occurs. We often try to ameliorate these situations by administering pain medication or symptom control at the same time we are withholding treatment, but these are all ways of disguising the fact that we are letting the disease kill the patient rather than directly bringing about death. But the ways diseases kill people are far more cruel than the ways physicians kill patients when performing euthanasia or assisting in suicide.

THE PROBLEM: A CHOICE OF CULTURES

Thus we see three similar cultures and countries and three similar sets of circumstances, but while much of medical practice in them is similar, they do offer three quite different basic options in approaching death. All three of these options generate moral problems; none of them, nor any others we might devise, is free of moral difficulty. But the question that faces us is this: which of these options is best?

It is not possible to answer this question in a less-than-ideal world without more attention to the specific characteristics and deficiencies of the society in question. In asking which of these practices is best, we must ask which is best *for us*. That we currently employ one set of these options rather than others does not prove that it is best for us; the question is, would practices developed in other cultures or those not yet widespread in any culture be better for our own culture than that which has developed here? Thus, it is necessary to consider the differences between our own society and these European cultures that have real bearing on which model of approach to dying we ought to adopt.

First, notice that different cultures exhibit different degrees of closeness between physicians and patients—different patterns of contact and involvement. The German physician is sometimes said to be more distant and more authoritarian than the American physician; on the other hand, the Dutch physician is often said to be closer to his or her patients than either the American or the German is. In the Netherlands, basic primary care is provided by the *huisarts*, the general practitioner or family physician, who typically lives in the neighborhood, makes house calls frequently, and maintains an office in his or her own home. This physician usually provides care for the other members of the patient's family and will remain the family's physician throughout his or her practice. Thus, the patient for whom euthanasia becomes an issue—say, the terminal cancer patient who has been hospitalized in the past but who has returned home to die—will be cared for by the trusted family physician on a regular basis. Indeed, for a patient in severe distress, the physician, supported by the visiting nurse, may make house calls as often as once a day, twice a day, or even more frequently (after all, the physician's office is right in the neighborhood) and is continuous contact with the family. In contrast, the traditional American institution of the family doctor who makes house calls is rapidly becoming a thing of the past, and although some patients who die at home have access to hospice services and receive house calls from their long-term physician, many have no such long-term care and receive most of it from staff at a clinic or from house staff rotating through the services of a hospital. Some 78% of Americans die in institutions, 61% in hospitals and 17% in nursing homes; in the Netherlands, over 40% of deaths occur at home. The degree of continuing contact that the patient can have with a familiar, trusted physician and the degree of institutionalization clearly influence the nature of his or her dying and also play a role in whether physician-performed active euthanasia, assisted suicide, and/or withholding and withdrawing treatment is appropriate.

Second, the United States has a much more volatile legal climate than either the Netherlands or Germany; our medical system is increasingly litigious, much more so than that of any other country in the world. Fears of malpractice actions or criminal prosecution color much of what physicians do in managing the dying of their patients. We also tend to develop public policy through court decisions and to assume that the existence of a policy puts an end to any moral issue. A delicate legal and moral balance over the issue of euthanasia, as is the case in the Netherlands, would hardly be possible here.

Third, we in the United States have a very different financial climate in which to do our dying. Both the Netherlands and Germany, as well as virtually every other industrialized nation, have systems of national health insurance or national health care. Thus the patient is not directly responsible for the costs of treatment, and consequently the patient's choices about terminal care and/or euthanasia need not take personal financial considerations into account. Even for the patient who does have health insurance in the United States, many kinds of services are not covered, whereas the national health care or health insurance programs of many other countries provide multiple relevant services, including at-home physician care, home-nursing care, home respite care, care in a nursing home or other long-term facility, dietitian care, rehabilitation care, physical therapy, psychological counseling, and so on. The patient in the United States needs to attend to the financial aspects of dying in a way that patients in many other countries do not, and in this country both the patient's choices and the recommendations of the physician are very often shaped by financial considerations.

There are many other differences between the United States, on the one hand, and the Netherlands and Germany, with their different options for dying, on the other hand, including differences in degrees of paternalism in the medical establishment, in racism, sexism, and ageism in the general culture, and in awareness of a problematic historical past, especially Nazism. All of these cultural, institutional, social, and legal differences influence the appropriateness or inappropriateness of practices such as active euthanasia and assisted suicide. For instance, the Netherlands' tradition of close physician-patient contact, its absence of malpractice-motivated medicine, and its provision of comprehensive health insurance, together with its comparative lack of racism and ageism and its experience in resistance to Nazism, suggest that this culture is able to permit the practice of voluntary active euthanasia, performed by physicians, without risking abuse. On the other hand, it is sometimes said that Germany still does not trust its physicians, remembering the example of Nazi experimentation, and given a comparatively authoritarian medical climate in which the contact between physician and patient is quite distanced, the population could not be comfortable with the practice of active euthanasia or physician-assisted suicide. There, only a wholly patient-controlled response to terminal situations, as in non-physician-assisted suicide, is a reasonable and prudent practice.

But what about the United States? This is a country where (1) sustained contact with a personal physician has been decreasing, (2) the risk of malpractice action is perceived as substantial, (3) much medical care is not insured, (4) many medical decisions are financial decisions as well, (5) racism has been on the rise, and (6) the public has not experienced direct contact with Nazism or similar totalitarian movements. Thus, the United States is in many respects an untrustworthy candidate for practicing active euthanasia. Given the pressures on individuals in an often atomized society, encouraging solo suicide, assisted if at all only by non-professionals, might well be open to considerable abuse too.

However, there are several additional differences between the United States and both the Netherlands and Germany that may seem peculiarly relevant here. First, American culture is more confrontational than many others, including Dutch culture. While the Netherlands prides itself rightly on a long tradition of rational discussion of public issues and on toleration of others' views and practices, the United States (and to some degree also Germany) tends to develop highly partisan, moralizing oppositional groups, especially over social issues like abortion. In general, this is a disadvantage, but in the case of euthanasia it may serve to alert the public to issues and possibilities it might not otherwise consider, especially to the risks of abuse. Here the role of religious groups may be particularly strong, since in discouraging or prohibiting suicide and euthanasia (as many, though by no means all, religious groups do), they may invite their members to reinspect the reasons for such choices and encourage families, physicians, and health care institutions to provide adequate, humane alternatives.

Second, though this may at first seem to be not only a peculiar but trivial difference, it is Americans who are particularly given to self-analysis. This tendency not only is evident in America's high rate of utilization of counseling services, including religious counseling, psychological counseling, and psychiatry, but also is more clearly evident in its popular culture: its diet of soap operas, situation comedies, and pop psychology books. It is here that the ordinary American absorbs models for analyzing his or her personal relationships and individual psychological characteristics. While, of course, things are changing and our cultural tastes are widely exported, the fact remains that the ordinary American's cultural diet contains more in the way of professional and do-it-yourself amateur psychology and self-analysis than anyone else's. This long tradition of self-analysis may put us in a better position for certain kinds of end-of-life practices than many other cultures. Despite whatever other deficiencies we have, we live in a culture that encourages us to inspect our own motives, anticipate the impact of our actions on others, and scrutinize our own relationships with others, including our physicians. This disposition is of importance in euthanasia and assisted-suicide contexts because these are the kinds of fundamental choices about which one may have somewhat mixed motives, be subject to various interpersonal and situational pressures, and so on. If the voluntary character of choices about one's own dying is to be protected, it may be a good thing to inhabit a culture in which self-inspection of one's own mental habits and motives, not to mention those of one's family, physician, and others who

might affect one's choices, is culturally encouraged. Counseling specifically addressed to end-of-life choices is not yet easily or openly available, especially if physician-assisted suicide is at issue, but I believe it will become more frequent in the future as people facing terminal illnesses characterized by long downhill, deteriorative courses consider how they want to die.

Finally, the United States population, varied as it is, is characterized by a kind of do-it-yourself ethic, an ethic that devalues reliance on others and encourages individual initiative and responsibility. (To be sure, this ethic is little in evidence in the series of court cases cited earlier, but these were all cases about patients who had become or always were incapable of decision making.) This ethic seems to be coupled with a sort of resistance to authority that perhaps also is basic to the American temperament. If this is really the case, Americans might be especially well-served by end-of-life practices that emphasize self-reliance and resistance to authority.

These, of course, are mere conjectures about features of American culture that would support appropriate use of euthanasia or assisted suicide. These are the features that one would want to reinforce should these practices become general, in part to minimize the effects of the negative influences. But, of course, these positive features will differ from one country and culture to another, just as negative features do. In each country, a different architecture of antecedent assumptions and cultural features develops around end-of-life issues, and in each country the practices of euthanasia and assisted or physician-assisted suicide, if they are to be free from abuse, must be adapted to the culture in which they take place.

What, then, is appropriate for our own cultural situation? Physician-performed euthanasia, even if not in itself morally wrong, is morally jeopardized where legal, time-related, and especially financial pressures on both patients and physicians are severe; thus, it is morally problematic in our culture in a way that it is not in the Netherlands. Solo suicide outside the institution of medicine (as in Germany) may be problematic in a country (like the United States) that has an increasingly alienated population, offers deteriorating and uneven social services, is increasingly racist and classist, and in other ways imposes unusual pressures on individuals, despite opportunities for self-analysis. Reliance only on withholding and withdrawing treatment (as in the United States) can be cruel, and its comparative invisibility invites erosion under cost-containment and other pressures. These are the three principal alternatives we have considered, but none of them seems wholly suited to our actual situation for dealing with the new fact that most of us die of extended-decline, deteriorative diseases.

Perhaps, however, there is one that would best suit the United States, certainly better than its current reliance on only withholding and withdrawing, and better than the Netherlands' more direct physical involvement or Germany's practices entirely outside medicine. The "arm's-length" model of physician-assisted suicide—permitting physicians to supply their terminally ill patients who request it with the means for ending their own lives (as has become legal under Oregon's Measure 16) still grants physicians some control over the circumstances in which this can happen— only, for example, when the prognosis is genuinely grim and the alternatives for symptom control are poor—but leaves the fundamental decision about whether to use these means to the patient alone. It is up to the patient then—the independent, confrontational, self-analyzing, do-it-yourself, authority-resisting patient—and his or her advisors, including family members, clergy, the physician, and other health care providers, to be clear about whether he or she really wants to use these means or not. Thus, the physician is involved but not directly, and it is the patient's decision, although the patient is not making it alone. Thus also it is the patient who performs the action of bringing his or her own life to a close, though where the patient is physically incapable of doing so or where the process goes awry the physician must be allowed to intercede. We live in an imperfect world, but of the alternatives for facing death—which we all eventually must—I think that the practice of permitting this somewhat distanced though still medically supported form of physician-assisted suicide is the one most nearly suited to the current state of our own flawed society. This is a model not yet central in any of the three countries examined here—the Netherlands, Germany, or (except in Oregon) the United States—but it is the one, I think, that suits us best.

NOTES

1. S. J. Olshansky and A. B. Ault, "The Fourth Stage of the Epidemiological Transition: The Age of Delayed Degenerative Diseases," *Milbank Memorial Fund Quarterly Health and Society* 64 (1986): 355–91.

2. S. Miles and C. Gomez, *Protocols for Elective Use of Life-Sustaining Treatment* (New York: Springer-Verlag, 1988).

3. C. L. Sprung, "Changing Attitudes and Practices in Forgoing Life-Sustaining Treatments," *JAMA* 262 (1990): 2213.

4. N. G. Smedira et al., "Withholding and Withdrawal of Life Support from the Critically Ill," *New England Journal of Medicine* 322 (1990): 309–15.

5. *New York Times,* 23 July 1990. A13.

6. For a fuller account, see my remarks "A Dozen Caveats Concerning the Discussion of Euthanasia in the Netherlands," in Margaret P. Battin, *The Least Worst Death: Essays in Bioethics on the End of Life* (New York and London: Oxford University Press, 1994): 130–44.

7. P. J. van der Maas, J. J. M. van Delden, L. Pijnenborg, "Euthanasia and Other Medical Decisions Concerning the End of Life," published in full in English as a special issue of *Health Policy,* 22, nos. 1–2 (1992) and, with C. W. N. Looman, in summary in *The Lancet* 338 (1991): 669–674.

8. G. van der Wall et al., "Euthanasie en hulp bij zelfdoding door artsen in de thuissituatie," parts 1 and 2, *Nederlands Tijdschrift voor Geneesekunde* 135 (1991): 1593–98, 1600–03.

9. P. J. van der Maas, G. van der Wal, et al., "Euthanasia, Physician-Assisted Suicide, and Other Medical Practices Involving the End of Life in the Netherlands, 1990–1995," *New England Journal of Medicine* 335:22 (1996): 1699–1705.

10. The precise figures are 17.9% (1990) and 20.2% (1995) deaths involving decisions to forgo treatment; 18.8% (1990) and 19.1% (1995) deaths involving opioids in large doses; 1.7% (1990) and 2.4% (1995) euthanasia; 0.2% (1990) and 0.2 (1995) physician-assisted suicide; and 0.8% (1990) and 0.7% (1995), life-ending without patient's explicit request. Source: van der Maas et al., Table 1, p. 1701.

11. L. Pijnenborg, P. J. van der Maas, J. J. M. van Delden, C. W. N. Looman, "Life Terminating Acts without Explicit Request of Patient," *The Lancet* 341 (1993): 1196–99.

12. G. van der Wal et al., "Evaluation of the Notification Procedure for Physician-Assisted Death in the Netherlands," *New England Journal of Medicine* 335:22 (1996): 1706–1711.

13. E. Borst-Eilers, "Euthanasia in the Netherlands: Brief Historical Review and Present Situation," in Robert I. Misbin, ed., *Euthanasia: The Good of the Patient, the Good of Society* (Frederick, Md.: University Publishing Group, 1992): 59.

14. van der Maas et al., "Euthanasia and Other Medical Decisions Concerning the End of Life," 673.

15. See my "Assisted Suicide: Can We Learn from Germany?" in Margaret P. Battin, *The Least Worst Death: Essays in Bioethics on the End of Life* (New York and London: Oxford University Press, 1994): 254–70.

16. P. Admiraal, "Euthanasia in a General Hospital," paper read at the Eighth World Congress of the

International Federation of Right-to-Die Societies, Maastricht, the Netherlands, June 8, 1990.

17. van der Maas et al., "Euthanasia, Physician-Assisted Suicide, and Other Medical Practices," 1705.

18. H. ten Have, "Coma: Controversy and Consensus," *Newsletter of the European Society for Philosophy of Medicine and Health Care* (May 1990): 19–20.

Is There a Duty to Die?

John Hardwig

Many people were outraged when Richard Lamm claimed that old people had a duty to die. Modern medicine and an individualistic culture have seduced many to feel that they have a right to health care and a right to live, despite the burdens and costs to our families and society. But in fact there are circumstances when we have a duty to die. As modern medicine continues to save more of us from acute illness, it also delivers more of us over to chronic illnesses, allowing us to survive far longer than we can take care of ourselves. It may be that our technological sophistication coupled with a commitment to our loved ones generates a fairly widespread duty to die.

When Richard Lamm made the statement that old people have a duty to die, it was generally shouted down or ridiculed. The whole idea is just too preposterous to entertain. Or too threatening. In fact, a fairly common argument against legalizing physician-assisted suicide is that if it were legal, some people might somehow get the idea that they have a duty to die. These people could only be the victims of twisted moral reasoning or vicious social pressure. It goes without saying that there is no duty to die.

But for me the question is real and very important. I feel strongly that I may very well some day have a duty to die. I do not believe that I am idiosyncratic, mentally ill, or morally perverse in think-

ing this. I think many of us will eventually face precisely this duty. But I am first of all concerned with my own duty. I write partly to clarify my own convictions and to prepare myself. Ending my life might be a very difficult thing for me to do.

This notion of a duty to die raises all sorts of interesting theoretical and metaethical questions. I intend to try to avoid most of them because I hope my argument will be persuasive to those holding a wide variety of ethical views. Also, although the claim that there is a duty to die would ultimately require theoretical underpinning, the discussion needs to begin on the normative level. As is appropriate to my attempt to steer clear of theoretical commitments, I will use "duty" "obligation," and "responsibility" interchangeably, in a pretheoretical or preanalytic sense.[1]

CIRCUMSTANCES AND A DUTY TO DIE

Do many of us really believe that no one ever has a duty to die? I suspect not. I think most of us probably believe that there is such a duty, but it is very uncommon. Consider Captain Oates, a member of Admiral Scott's expedition to the South Pole. Oates became too ill to continue. If the rest of the team stayed with him, they would all perish. After this had become clear, Oates left his tent one night, walked out into a raging blizzard, and was never seen again.[2] That may have been a heroic thing to do, but we might be able to agree that it was also

Hastings Center Report, Vol. 27, No. 2, 1997, 34-42. Copyright © 1997 The Hastings Center.

no more than his duty. It would have been wrong for him to urge—or even to allow—the rest to stay and care for him.

This is a very unusual circumstance—a "lifeboat case"—and lifeboat cases make for bad ethics. But I expect that most of us would also agree that there have been cultures in which what we would call a duty to die has been fairly common. These are relatively poor, technologically simple, and especially nomadic cultures. In such societies, everyone knows that if you manage to live long enough, you will eventually become old and debilitated. Then you will need to take steps to end your life. The old people in these societies regularly did precisely that. Their cultures prepared and supported them in doing so.

Those cultures could be dismissed as irrelevant to contemporary bioethics; their circumstances are so different from ours. But if that is our response, it is instructive. It suggests that we assume a duty to die is irrelevant to us because our wealth and technological sophistication have purchased exemption for us . . . except under very unusual circumstances like Captain Oates's.

But have wealth and technology really exempted us? Or are they, on the contrary, about to make a duty to die common again? We like to think of modern medicine as all triumph with no dark side. Our medicine saves many lives and enables most of us to live longer. That is wonderful, indeed. We are all glad to have access to this medicine. But our medicine also delivers most of us over to chronic illnesses and it enables many of us to survive longer than we can take care of ourselves, longer than we know what to do with ourselves, longer than we even are ourselves.

The costs—and these are not merely monetary—of prolonging our lives when we are no longer able to care for ourselves are often staggering. If further medical advances wipe out many of today's "killer diseases"—cancers, heart attacks, strokes,—ALS, AIDS, and the rest—then one day most of us will survive long enough to become demented or debilitated. These developments could generate a fairly widespread duty to die. A fairly common duty to die might turn out to be only the dark side of our life-prolonging medicine and the uses we choose to make of it.

Let me be clear. I certainly believe that there is a duty to refuse life-prolonging medical treatment and also a duty to complete advance directives refusing life-prolonging treatment. But a duty to die can go well beyond that. There can be a duty to die before one's illnesses would cause death, even if treated only with palliative measures. In fact, there may be a fairly common responsibility to end one's life in the absence of any terminal illness at all. Finally, there can be a duty to die when one would prefer to live. Granted, many of the conditions that can generate a duty to die also seriously undermine the quality of life. Some prefer not to live under such conditions. But even those who want to live can face a duty to die. These will clearly be the most controversial and troubling cases; I will, accordingly, focus my reflections on them.

THE INDIVIDUALISTIC FANTASY

Because a duty to die seems such a real possibility to me, I wonder why contemporary bioethics has dismissed it without serious consideration. I believe that most bioethics still shares in one of our deeply embedded American dreams: the individualistic fantasy. This fantasy leads us to imagine that lives are separate and unconnected, or that they could be so if we chose. If lives were unconnected, things that happened in my life would not or need not affect others. And if others were not (much) affected by my life, I would have no duty to consider the impact of my decisions on others. I would then be free morally to live my life however I please, choosing whatever life and death I prefer for myself. The way I live would be nobody's business but my own. I certainly would have no duty to die if I preferred to live.

Within a health care context, the individualistic fantasy leads us to assume that the patient is the only one affected by decisions about her medical treatment. If only the patient were affected, the relevant questions when making treatment decisions would be precisely those we ask: What will benefit the patient? Who can best decide that? The pivotal issue would always be simply whether the patient wants to live like this and whether she would consider herself better off dead.[3] "Whose life is it, anyway?" we ask rhetorically.

But this is morally obtuse. We are not a race of hermits. Illness and death do not come only to those who are all alone. Nor is it much better to think in terms of the bald dichotomy between "the interests of the patient" and "the interests of society" (or a third-party payer), as if we were isolated individuals connected only to "society" in the abstract or to the other, faceless members of our health maintenance organization.

Most of us are affiliated with particular others and most deeply, with family and loved ones. Families and loved ones are bound together by ties of care and affection, by legal relations and obligations, by inhabiting shared spaces and living units, by interlocking finances and economic prospects, by common projects and also commitments to support the different life projects of other family members, by shared histories, by ties of loyalty. This life together of family and loved ones is what defines and sustains us; it is what gives meaning to most of our lives. We would not have it any other way. We would not want to be all alone, especially when we are seriously ill, as we age, and when we are dying.

But the fact of deeply interwoven lives debars us from making exclusively self-regarding decisions, as the decisions of one member of a family may dramatically affect the lives of all the rest. The impact of my decisions upon my family and loved ones is the source of many of my strongest obligations and also the most plausible and likeliest basis of a duty to die. "Society," after all, is only very marginally affected by how I live, or by whether I live or die.

A BURDEN TO MY LOVED ONES

Many older people report that their one remaining goal in life is not to be a burden to their loved ones. Young people feel this, too: when I ask my undergraduate students to think about whether their death could come too late, one of their very first responses always is, "Yes, when I become a burden to my family or loved ones." Tragically, there are situations in which my loved ones would be much better off—all things considered, the loss of a loved one notwithstanding—if I were dead.

The lives of our loved ones can be seriously compromised by caring for us. The burdens of providing care or even just supervision twenty-four hours a day, seven days a week are often overwhelming.[4]

When this kind of caregiving goes on for years, it leaves the caregiver exhausted, with no time for herself or life of her own. Ultimately, even her health is often destroyed. But it can also be emotionally devastating simply to live with a spouse who is increasingly distant, uncommunicative, unresponsive, foreign, and unreachable. Other family members' needs often go unmet as the caring capacity of the family is exceeded. Social life and friendships evaporate, as there is no opportunity to go out to see friends and the home is no longer a place suitable for having friends in.

We must also acknowledge that the lives of our loved ones can be devastated just by having to pay for health care for us. One part of the recent SUPPORT study documented the financial aspects of caring for a dying member of a family. Only those who had illnesses severe enough to give them less than a 50 percent chance to live six more months were included in this study. When these patients survived their initial hospitalization and were discharged about one-third required considerable caregiving from their families; in 20 percent of cases a family member had to quit work or make some other major lifestyle change; almost one-third of these families lost all of their savings; and just under 30 percent lost a major source of income.[5]

If talking about money sounds venal or trivial, remember that much more than money is normally at stake here. When someone has to quit work, she may well lose her career. Savings decimated late in life cannot be recouped in the few remaining years of employability, so the loss compromises the quality of the rest of the caregiver's life. For a young person, the chance to go to college may be lost to the attempt to pay debts due to an illness in the family, and this decisively shapes an entire life.

A serious illness in a family is a misfortune. It is usually nobody's fault; no one is responsible for it. But we face choices about how we will respond to this misfortune. That's where the responsibility comes in and fault can arise. Those of us with families and loved ones always have a duty not to make selfish or self-centered decisions about our lives. We have a responsibility to try to protect the lives of loved ones from serious threats or greatly impoverished quality, certainly an obligation not to make choices that will jeopardize or seriously compromise their futures. Often, it would be wrong to do just what we want or just what is best for ourselves; we should choose in light of what is best for all concerned. That is our duty in sickness as well as in health. It is out of these responsibilities that a duty to die can develop.

I am not advocating a crass, quasi-economic conception of burdens and benefits, nor a shallow, hedonistic view of life. Given a suitably rich understanding of benefits, family members sometimes do benefit from suffering through the long illness of a loved one. Caring for the sick or aged can foster growth, even as it makes daily life immeasurably harder and the prospects for the future much bleaker. Chronic illness or a drawn-out death can also pull a family together, making the care for each other stronger and more evident. If my loved ones are truly benefiting from coping with my illness or debility, I have no duty to die based on burdens to them.

But it would be irresponsible to blithely assume that this always happens, that it will happen in my family, or that it will be the fault of my family if they cannot manage to turn my illness into a positive experience. Perhaps the opposite is more common: a hospital chaplain once told me that he could not think of a single case in which a family was strengthened or brought together by what happened at the hospital.

Our families and loved ones also have obligations, of course—they have the responsibility to stand by us and to support us through debilitating illness and death. They must be prepared to make significant sacrifices to respond to an illness in the family. I am far from denying that. Most of us are aware of this responsibility and most families meet it rather well. In fact, families deliver more than 80 percent of the long-term care in this country, almost always at great personal cost. Most of us who are a part of a family can expect to be sustained in our time of need by family members and those who love us.

But most discussions of an illness in the family sound as if responsibility were a one-way street. It is not, of course. When we become seriously ill or debilitated, we too may have to make sacrifices. To think that my loved ones must bear whatever burdens my illness, debility, or dying process might impose upon them is to reduce them to means to my well-being. And that would be immoral.

Family solidarity, altruism, bearing the burden of a loved one's misfortune, and loyalty are all important virtues of families, as well. But they are all also two-way streets.

OBJECTIONS TO A DUTY TO DIE

To my mind, the most serious objections to the idea of a duty to die lie in the effects on my loved ones of ending my life. But to most others, the important objections have little or nothing to do with family and loved ones. Perhaps the most common objections are: (1) there is a higher duty that always takes precedence over a duty to die; (2) a duty to end one's own life would be incompatible with a recognition of human dignity or the intrinsic value of a person; and (3) seriously ill, debilitated, or dying people are already bearing the harshest burdens and so it would be wrong to ask them to bear the additional burden of ending their own lives.

These are all important objections; all deserve a thorough discussion. Here I will only be able to suggest some moral counterweights—ideas that might provide the basis for an argument that these objections do not always preclude a duty to die.

An example of the first line of argument would be the claim that a duty to God, the giver of life, forbids that anyone take her own life. It could be argued that this duty always supersedes whatever obligations we might have to our families. But what convinces us that we always have such a religious duty in the first place? And what guarantees that it always supersedes our obligations to try to protect our loved ones?

Certainly, the view that death is the ultimate evil cannot be squared with Christian theology. It does not reflect the actions of Jesus or those of his early followers. Nor is it clear that the belief that life is sacred requires that we never take it. There are other theological possibilities.[6] In any case, most of us—bioethicists, physicians, and patients alike—do not subscribe to the view that we have an obligation to preserve human life as long as possible. But if not, surely we ought to agree that I may legitimately end my life for other-regarding reasons, not just for self-regarding reasons.

Secondly, religious considerations aside, the claim could be made that an obligation to end one's own life would be incompatible with human dignity or would embody a failure to recognize the intrinsic value of a person. But I do not see that in thinking I had a duty to die I would necessarily be failing to respect myself or to appreciate my dignity or worth. Nor would I necessarily be failing to respect you in thinking that you had a similar duty. There is surely also a sense in which we fail to respect ourselves if in the face of illness or death, we stoop to choosing just what is best for ourselves. Indeed, Kant held that the very core of human dignity is the ability to act on a self-imposed moral law, regardless of whether it is in our interest to do so.[7] We shall return to the notion of human dignity.

A third objection appeals to the relative weight of burdens and thus, ultimately, to considerations of fairness or justice. The burdens that an illness creates for the family could not possibly be great enough to justify an obligation to end one's life—the sacrifice of life itself would be a far greater burden than any involved in caring for a chronically ill family member.

But is this true? Consider the following case:

An 87-year-old woman was dying of congestive heart failure. Her APACHE score predicted that she had less than a 50 percent chance to live for another six months. She was lucid, assertive, and terrified of death. She very much wanted to live and kept opting for rehospitalization and the most aggressive life-prolonging treatment possible. That treatment successfully prolonged her life (though with increasing debility) for nearly two years. Her 55-year-old daughter was her only remaining family, her caregiver, and the main source of her financial support. The daughter duly cared for her mother. But before her mother died, her illness had cost the daughter all of her savings, her home, her job, and her career.

This is by no means an uncommon sort of case. Thousands of similar cases occur each year. Now, ask yourself which is the greater burden:

(a) To lose a 50 percent chance of six more months of life at age 87?

(b) To lose all your savings, your home, and your career at age 55?

Which burden would you prefer to bear? Do we really believe the former is the greater burden? Would even the dying mother say that (a) is the greater burden? Or has she been encouraged to believe that the burdens of (b) are somehow morally irrelevant to her choices?

I think most of us would quickly agree that (b) is a greater burden. That is the evil we would more hope to avoid in our lives. If we are tempted to say that the mother's disease and impending death are the greater evil, I believe it is because we are taking a "slice of time" perspective rather than a "lifetime perspective."[8] But surely the lifetime perspective is the appropriate perspective when weighing burdens. If (b) is the greater burden, then we must admit that we have been promulgating an ethics that advocates imposing greater burdens on some people in order to provide smaller benefits for others just because they are ill and thus gain our professional attention and advocacy.

A whole range of cases like this one could easily be generated. In some, the answer about which burden is greater will not be clear. But in many it is. Death—or ending your own life—is simply not the greatest evil or the greatest burden.

This point does not depend on a utilitarian calculus. Even if death were the greatest burden (thus disposing of any simple utilitarian argument), serious questions would remain about the moral justifiability of choosing to impose crushing burdens on loved ones in order to avoid having to bear this burden oneself. The fact that I suffer greater burdens than others in my family does not license me simply to choose what I want for myself, nor does it necessarily release me from a responsibility to try to protect the quality of their lives.

I can readily imagine that, through cowardice, rationalization, or failure of resolve, I will fail in this obligation to protect my loved ones. If so, I think I would need to be excused or forgiven for what I did. But I cannot imagine it would be morally permissible for me to ruin the rest of my partner's life to sustain mine or to cut off my sons' careers, impoverish them, or compromise the quality of their children's lives simply because I wish to live a little longer. This is what leads me to believe in a duty to die.

WHO HAS A DUTY TO DIE?

Suppose, then, that there can be a duty to die. Who has a duty to die? And when? To my mind, these are the right questions, the questions we should be asking. Many of us may one day badly need answers to just these questions.

But I cannot supply answers here, for two reasons. In the first place, answers will have to be very particular and contextual. Our concrete duties are often situated, defined in part by the myriad details of our circumstances, histories, and relationships. Though there may be principles that apply to a wide range of cases and some cases that yield pretty straightforward answers, there will also be many situations in which it is very difficult to discern whether one has a duty to die. If nothing else, it will often be very difficult to predict how one's family will bear up under the weight of the burdens that a protracted illness would impose on them. Momentous decisions will often have to be made under conditions of great uncertainty.

Second and perhaps even more importantly, I believe that those of us with family and loved ones should not define our duties unilaterally, especially not a decision about a duty to die. It would be isolating and distancing for me to decide without consulting them what is too much of a burden for my loved ones to bear. That way of deciding about my moral duties is not only atomistic, it also treats my family and loved ones paternalistically. They must be allowed to speak for themselves about the burdens my life imposes on them and how they feel about bearing those burdens.

Some may object that it would be wrong to put a loved one in a position of having to say, in effect, "You should end your life because caring for you is too hard on me and the rest of the family." Not only will it be almost impossible to say something like that to someone you love, it will carry with it a heavy load of guilt. On this view, you should decide by yourself whether you have a duty to die and approach your loved ones only after you have made up your mind to say good-bye to them. Your family could then try to change your mind, but the tremendous weight of moral decision would be lifted from their shoulders.

Perhaps so. But I believe in family decisions. Important decisions for those whose lives are interwoven should be made together, in a family discussion. Granted, a conversation about whether I have a duty to die would be a tremendously difficult conversation. The temptations to be dishonest could be enormous. Nevertheless, if I am con-templating a duty to die, my family and I should, if possible, have just such an agonizing discussion. It will act as a check on the information, perceptions, and reasoning of all of us. But even more importantly, it affirms our connectedness at a critical juncture in our lives and our life together. Honest talk about difficult matters almost always strengthens relationships.

However, many families seem unable to talk about death at all, much less a duty to die. Certainly most families could not have this discussion all at once, in one sitting. It might well take a number of discussions to be able to approach this topic. But even if talking about death is impossible, there are always behavioral clues—about your caregiver's tiredness, physical condition, health, prevailing mood, anxiety, financial concerns, outlook, overall well-being, and so on. And families unable to talk about death can often talk about how the caregiver is feeling, about finances, about tensions within the family resulting from the illness, about concerns for the future. Deciding whether you have a duty to die based on these behavioral clues and conversation about them honors your relationships better than deciding on your own about how burdensome you and your care must be.

I cannot say when someone has a duty to die. Still, I can suggest a few features of one's illness, history, and circumstances that make it more likely that one has a duty to die. I present them here without much elaboration or explanation.

(1) A duty to die is more likely when continuing to live will impose significant burdens—emotional burdens, extensive caregiving, destruction of life plans, and, yes, financial hardship—on your family and loved ones. This is the fundamental insight underlying a duty to die.

(2) A duty to die becomes greater as you grow older. As we age, we will be giving up less by giving up our lives, if only because we will sacrifice fewer remaining years of life and a smaller portion of our life plans. After all, it's not as if we would be immortal and live forever if we could just manage to avoid a duty to die. To have reached the age of, say, seventy-five or eighty years without being ready to die is itself a moral failing, the sign of a life out of touch with life's basic realities.[9]

(3) A duty to die is more likely when you have already lived a full and rich life. You have already had a full share of the good things life offers.

(4) There is greater duty to die if your loved ones' lives have already been difficult or impoverished, if they have had only a small share of the good things that life has to offer (especially if through no fault of their own).

(5) A duty to die is more likely when your loved ones have already made great contributions—perhaps even sacrifices—to make your life a good one. Especially if you have not made similar sacrifices for their well-being or for the well-being of other members of your family.

(6) To the extent that you can make a good adjustment to your illness or handicapping condition, there is less likely to be a duty to die. A good adjustment means that smaller sacrifices will be required of loved ones and there is more compensating interaction for them. Still, we must also recognize that some diseases—Alzheimer or Huntington chorea—will eventually take their toll on your loved ones no matter how courageously, resolutely, even cheerfully you manage to face that illness.

(7) There is less likely to be a duty to die if you can still make significant contributions to the lives of others, especially your family. The burdens to family members are not only or even primarily financial, neither are the contributions to them. However, the old and those who have terminal illnesses must also bear in mind that the loss their family members will feel when they die cannot be avoided, only postponed.

(8) A duty to die is more likely when the part of you that is loved will soon be gone or seriously compromised. Or when you soon will no longer be capable of giving love. Part of the horror of dementing disease is that it destroys the capacity to nurture and sustain relationships, taking away a person's agency and the emotions that bind her to others.

(9) There is a greater duty to die to the extent that you have lived a relatively lavish lifestyle instead of saving for illness or old age. Like most upper middle-class Americans, I could easily have saved more. It is a greater wrong to come to your family for assistance if your need is the result of having chosen leisure or a spendthrift lifestyle. I may eventually have to face the moral consequences of decisions I am now making.

These, then, are some of the considerations that give shape and definition to the duty to die. If we can agree that these considerations are all relevant, we can see that the correct course of action will often be difficult to discern. A decision about when I should end my life will sometimes prove to be every bit as difficult as the decision about whether I want treatment for myself.

CAN THE INCOMPETENT HAVE A DUTY TO DIE?

Severe mental deterioration springs readily to mind as one of the situations in which I believe I could have a duty to die. But can incompetent people have duties at all? We can have moral duties we do not recognize or acknowledge, including duties that we never recognized. But can we have duties we are unable to recognize? Duties when we are unable to understand the concept of morality at all? If so, do others have a moral obligation to help us carry out this duty? These are extremely difficult theoretical questions. The reach of moral agency is severely strained by mental incompetence.

I am tempted to simply bypass the entire question by saying that I am talking only about competent persons. But the idea of a duty to die clearly raises the specter of one person claiming that another—who cannot speak for herself—has such a duty. So I need to say that I can make no sense of the claim that someone has a duty to die if the person has never been able to understand moral obligation at all. To my mind, only those who were formerly capable of making moral decisions could have such a duty.

But the case of formerly competent persons is almost as troubling. Perhaps we should simply stipulate that no incompetent person can have a duty to die, not even if she affirmed belief in such a duty in an advance directive. If we take the view that formerly competent people may have such a duty, we should surely exercise extreme caution when claiming a formerly competent person would have acknowledged a duty to die or that any formerly competent person has an unacknowledged duty to die. Moral dangers loom regardless of which way we decide to resolve such issues.

But for me personally, very urgent practical matters turn on their resolution. If a formerly competent person can no longer have a duty to die (or if other people are not likely to help her carry out this duty), I believe that my obligation may be to die while I am still competent, before I become unable to make and carry out that decision for myself. Surely it would be irresponsible to evade my moral duties by temporizing until I escape into incompetence. And so I must die sooner than I otherwise would have to. On the other hand, if I could count on others to end my life after I become incompetent, I might be able to fulfill my responsibilities while also living out all my competent or semicompetent days. Given our society's reluctance to permit physicians, let alone family members, to perform aid-in-dying, I believe I may well have a duty to end my life when I can see mental incapacity on the horizon.

There is also the very real problem of sudden incompetence—due to a serious stroke or automobile accident, for example. For me, that is the real nightmare. If I suddenly become incompetent, I will fall into the hands of a medical-legal system that will conscientiously disregard my moral beliefs and do what is best for me, regardless of the consequences for my loved ones. And that is not at all what I would have wanted!

SOCIAL POLICIES AND A DUTY TO DIE

The claim that there is a duty to die will seem to some a misplaced response to social negligence. If our society were providing for the debilitated, the chronically ill, and the elderly as it should be, there would be only very rare cases of a duty to die. On this view, I am asking the sick and debilitated to step in and accept responsibility because society is derelict in its responsibility to provide for the incapacitated

This much is surely true: there are a number of social policies we could pursue that would dramatically reduce the incidence of such a duty.

Most obviously, we could decide to pay for facilities that provided excellent long-term care (not just health care!) for all chronically ill, debilitated, mentally ill, or demented people in this country. We probably could still afford to do this. If we did, sick, debilitated, and dying people might still be morally required to make sacrifices for their families. I might, for example, have a duty to forgo personal care by a family member who knows me and really does care for me. But these sacrifices would only rarely include the sacrifice of life itself The duty to die would then be virtually eliminated.

I cannot claim to know whether in some abstract sense a society like ours should provide care for all who are chronically ill or debilitated. But the fact is that we Americans seem to be unwilling to pay for this kind of long-term care, except for ourselves and our own. In fact, we are moving in precisely the opposite direction—we are trying to shift the burdens of caring for the seriously and chronically ill onto families in order to save costs for our health care system. As we shift the burdens of care onto families, we also dramatically increase the number of Americans who will have a duty to die.

I must not, then, live my life and make my plans on the assumption that social institutions will protect my family from my infirmity and debility. To do so would be irresponsible. More likely, it will be up to me to protect my loved ones.

A DUTY TO DIE AND THE MEANING OF LIFE

A duty to die seems very harsh, and often it would be. It is one of the tragedies of our lives that someone who wants very much to live can nevertheless have a duty to die. It is both tragic and ironic that it is precisely the very real good of family and loved ones that gives rise to this duty. Indeed, the genuine love, closeness, and supportiveness of family members is a major source of this duty: we could not be such a burden if they did not care for us. Finally, there is deep irony in the fact that the very successes of our life-prolonging medicine help to create a widespread duty to die. We do not live in such a happy world that we can avoid such tragedies and ironies. We ought not to close our eyes to this reality or pretend that it just doesn't exist. We ought not to minimize the tragedy in any way.

And yet, a duty to die will not always be as harsh as we might assume. If I love my family, I will want to protect them and their lives. I will want not to make choices that compromise their futures. Indeed, I can easily imagine that I might want to avoid compromising their lives more than I would want anything else. I must also admit that I am not necessarily giving up so much in giving up my life: the conditions that give rise to a duty to die would usually already have compromised the quality of the life I am required to end. In any case, I personally must confess that at age fifty-six, I have already lived a very good life, albeit not yet nearly as long a life as I would like to have.

We fear death too much. Our fear of death has led to a massive assault on it. We still crave after virtually any life-prolonging technology that we might conceivably be able to produce. We still too often feel morally impelled to prolong life—virtually any form of life—as long as possible. As if the best death is the one that can be put off longest.

We do not even ask about meaning in death, so busy are we with trying to postpone it. But we will not conquer death by one day developing a technology so magnificent that no one will have to die. Nor can we conquer death by postponing it ever longer. We can conquer death only by finding meaning in it.

Although the existence of a duty to die does not hinge on this, recognizing such a duty would go some way toward recovering meaning in death. Paradoxically, it would restore dignity to those who are seriously ill or dying. It would also reaffirm the connections required to give life (and death) meaning. I close now with a few words about both of these points.

First, recognizing a duty to die affirms my agency and also my moral agency. I can still do things that make an important difference in the lives of my loved ones. Moreover, the fact that I still have responsibilities keeps me within the community of moral agents. My illness or debility has not reduced me to a mere moral patient (to use the language of the philosophers). Though it may not be the whole story, surely Kant was onto something important when he claimed that human dignity rests on the capacity for moral agency within a community of those who respect the demands of morality.

By contrast, surely there is something deeply insulting in a medicine and an ethic that would ask only what I want (or would have wanted) when I become ill. To treat me as if I had no moral responsibilities when I am ill or debilitated implies that my condition has rendered me morally incompetent. Only small children, the demented or insane, and those totally lacking in the capacity to act are free from moral duties. There is dignity, then, and a kind of meaning in moral agency, even as it forces extremely difficult decisions upon us.

Second, recovering meaning in death requires an affirmation of connections. If I end my life to spare the futures of my loved ones, I testify in my death that I am connected to them. It is because I love and care for precisely these people (and I know they care for me) that I wish not to be such a burden to them. By contrast, a life in which I am free to choose whatever I want for myself is a life unconnected to others. A bioethics that would treat me as if I had no serious moral responsibilities does what it can to marginalize, weaken, or even destroy my connections with others.

But life without connection is meaningless. The individualistic fantasy, though occasionally liberating, is deeply destructive. When life is good and vitality seems unending, life itself and life lived for yourself may seem quite sufficient. But if not life, certainly death without connection is meaningless. If you are only for yourself, all you have to care about as your life draws to a close is yourself and your life. Everything you care about will then perish in your death. And that—the end of everything you care about—is precisely the total collapse of meaning. We can, then, find meaning in death only through a sense of connection with something that will survive our death.

This need not be connections with other people. Some people are deeply tied to land (for example, the family farm), to nature, or to a transcendent reality. But for most of us, the connections that sustain us are to other people. In the full bloom of life, we are connected to others in many ways—through work, profession, neighborhood, country, shared faith and worship, common leisure pursuits, friendship. Even the guru meditating in isolation on his mountain top is connected to a long tradition of people united by the same religious quest.

But as we age or when we become chronically ill, connections with other people usually become much more restricted. Often, only ties with family and close friends remain and remain important to us. Moreover, for many of us, other connections just don't go deep enough. As Paul Tsongas has reminded us, "When it comes time to die, no one says, 'I wish I had spent more time at the office.'"

If I am correct, death is so difficult for us partly because our sense of community is so weak. Death seems to wipe out everything when we can't fit it into the lives of those who live on. A death motivated by the desire to spare the futures of my loved ones might well be a better death for me than the one I would get as a result of opting to continue my life as long as there is any pleasure in it for me. Pleasure is nice, but it is meaning that matters.

. . .

I don't know about others, but these reflections have helped me. I am now more at peace about facing a duty to die. Ending my life if my duty required might still be difficult. But for me, a far greater horror would be dying all alone or stealing the futures of my loved ones in order to buy a little more time for myself. I hope that if the time comes when I have a duty to die, I will recognize it, encourage my loved ones to recognize it too, and carry it out bravely.

ACKNOWLEDGMENTS

I wish to thank Mary English, Hilde Nelson, Jim Bennett, Tom Townsend, the members of the Philosophy Department at East Tennessee State University, and anonymous reviewers of the *Report* for many helpful comments on earlier versions of this paper. In this paper, I draw on material in John Hardwig, "Dying at the Right Time; Reflections on (Un)Assisted Suicide" in *Practical Ethics*, ed. H. LaFollette (London: Blackwell, 1996), with permission.

NOTES

1. Given the importance of relationships in my thinking, "responsibility"—rooted as it is in "respond"—would perhaps be the most appropriate word. Nevertheless, I often use "duty" despite its legalistic overtones, because

Lamm's famous statement has given the expression "duty to die" a certain familiarity. But I intend no implication that there is a law that grounds this duty, nor that someone has a right corresponding to it.

2. For a discussion of the Oates case, see Tom L. Beauchamp, "What Is Suicide?" in *Ethical Issues in Death and Dying*, ed. Tom L. Beauchamp and Seymour Perlin (Englewood Cliffs, N.J.: Prentice-Hall, 1978).

3. Most bioethicists advocate a "patient-centered ethics"—an ethics which claims only the patient's interests should be considered in making medical treatment decisions. Most health care professionals have been trained to accept this ethic and to see themselves as patient advocates. For arguments that a patient-centered ethics should be replaced by a family-centered ethics see John Hardwig, "What About the Family?" *Hastings Center Report* 20, no. 2 (1990): 5-10; Hilde L. Nelson and James L. Nelson, *The Patient in the Family* (New York: Routledge. 1995).

4. A good account of the burdens of caregiving can be found in Elaine Brody, *Women in the Middle: Their Parent-Care Years* (New York: Springer Publishing Co., 1990). Perhaps the best article-length account of these burdens is Daniel Callahan, "Families as Caregivers; the Limits of Morality" in *Aging and Ethics: Philosophical Problems in Gerontology*, ed. Nancy Jecker (Totowa N.J.: Humana Press, 1991).

5. Kenneth E. Covinsky et al., "The Impact of Serious Illness on Patients' Families," *JAMA* 272 (1994): 1839-44.

6. Larry Churchill, for example, believes that Christian ethics takes us far beyond my present position: "Christian doctrines of stewardship prohibit the extension of one's own life at a great cost to the neighbor . . . And such a gesture should not appear to us a sacrifice, but as the ordinary virtue entailed by a just, social conscience." Larry Churchill, *Rationing Health Care in America* (South Bend, Ind.: Notre Dame University Press, 1988), p. 112.

7. Kant, as is well known, was opposed to suicide. But he was arguing against taking your life out of self-interested motives. It is not clear that Kant would or we should consider taking your life out of a sense of duty to be wrong. See Hilde L. Nelson, "Death with Kantian Dignity," *Journal of Clinical Ethics* 7 (1996): 215-21.

8. Obviously, I owe this distinction to Norman Daniels. Norman Daniels, *Am I My Parents' Keeper? An Essay on Justice Between the Young and the Old* (New York: Oxford University Press, 1988). Just as obviously, Daniels is not committed to my use of it here.

9. Daniel Callahan, *The Troubled Dream of Life* (New York: Simon & Schuster, 1993).

RECOMMENDED SUPPLEMENTARY READING

General Works

Annas, George J. *Standard of Care: The Law of American Bioethics*. Oxford: Oxford University Press, 1993.

Battin, Margaret Pabst. *The Last Worst Death: Essays in Bioethics on the End of Life*. New York: Oxford University Press, 1994.

Beauchamp, Tom L., and Veatch, Robert M. *Ethical Issues in Death and Dying*. 2nd ed. Upper Saddle River, NJ: Prentice-Hall, 1996.

Brock, Dan. *Life and Death: Philosophical Essays in Biomedical Ethics*. New York: Cambridge University Press, 1993.

Brody, Baruch. *Life and Death Decision Making*. New York: Oxford University Press, 1988.

Buchanan, Allen, and Brock, Dan. *Deciding for Others: The Ethics of Surrogate Decision Making*. Cambridge: Cambridge University Press, 1989.

Byock, Ira. *Dying Well: The Prospect for Growth at the End of Life*. New York: Riverhead Books, 1997.

Cantor, Norman. *Legal Frontiers of Death and Dying*. Bloomington: Indiana University Press, 1987.

Dworkin, Ronald. *Life's Dominion: An Argument about Abortion, Euthanasia, and Individual Freedom*. New York: Alfred A. Knopf, 1993.

Gorovitz, Samuel. *Drawing the Line: Life, Death, and Ethical Choice in an American Hospital*. Oxford: Oxford University Press, 1991.

Kamm, F.M. *Morality, Mortality*. 2 vols. New York: Oxford University Press, 1993–1996.

Meisel, Alan. *The Right to Die*. New York: John Wiley and Sons, 1989.

Moller, David Wendell. *Confronting Death*. New York: Oxford University Press, 1996.

President's Commission for the Study of Ethical Problems in Medicine and Biomedical and Behavioral Research. *Deciding to Forego Life-Sustaining Treatment*. Washington, DC: U.S. Government Printing Office, 1983.

Ramsey, Paul. *Ethics at the Edges of Life, Part Two*. New Haven, CT: Yale University Press, 1978.

Veatch, Robert. *Death, Dying, and the Biological Revolution*. 2nd ed. New Haven, CT: Yale University Press, 1989.

Weir, Robert F. *Abating Treatment with Critically Ill Patients*. New York: Oxford University Press, 1989.

———. ed. *Ethical Issues in Death and Dying*. 2nd ed. New York: Columbia University Press, 1986.

The Definition of Death and the Persistent Vegetative State

Agich, George, and Jones, Royce P. "Personal Identity and Brain Death: A Critical Response." *Philosophy and Public Affairs* 15 (Summer 1986): 267–274.

Brody, Baruch. "Special Ethical Issues in the Management of PVS Patients." *Law, Medicine & Health Care* 20 (1992): 104–115.

Capron, Alexander. "Anencephalic Donors: Separate the Dead from the Dying." *Hastings Center Report* 17, no. 1 (1987): 5–9.

Cole, David. "Statutory Definitions of Death and the Management of Terminally Ill Patients Who May Become Organ Donors after Death." *Kennedy Institute of Ethics Journal* 3, no. 2 (1993): 145–155.

Cranford, Ronald E. "The Persistent Vegetative State: The Medical Reality (Getting the Facts Straight)," *Hastings Center Report* 18, no. 1 (1988): 27–32.

Emanuel, Linda L. "Reexamining Death: The Asymptomatic Model and a Bounded Zone Definition." *Hastings Center Report* (July–August 1995): 27-35.

Englehardt, H. Tristram, Jr. *The Foundations of Bioethics*. New York: Oxford University Press, 1986.

Gervais, Karen Grandstrand. "Advancing the Definition of Death: A Philosophical Essay," *Medical Humanities Review* 3, no. 2 (1989): 7–19.

Gervais, Karen Grandstrand. *Redefining Death*. New Haven, CT: Yale University Press, 1986.

Green, Michael, and Wikler, Daniel. "Brain Death and Personal Identity." *Philosophy and Public Affairs* 9, no. 2 (Winter 1980): 105–133.

Harvard Medical School Ad Hoc Committee to Examine the Definition of Brain Death. "A Definition of Irreversible Coma." *Journal of the American Medical Association* 205, no. 6 (August 5, 1968): 337–340.

McMahan, Jeff. "The Metaphysics of Brain Death." *Bioethics* 9, no. 2 (April 1995): 91–126.

Shewmon, D. Alan; Capron, A. M.; Peacock, W.J.; and Shulman, B.L. "The Use of Anencephalic Infants as Organ Sources: A Critique." *Journal of the American Medical Association* 261, no. 12 (March 24–31, 1989): 1773–1781.

Shinnar, Shlomo, and Arras, John. "Ethical Issues in the Use of Anencephalic Infants as Organ Donors." *Neurologic Clinics* 7, no. 4 (November 1989): 729–743.

Steinbock, Bonnie. "Recovery from Persistent Vegetative State? The Case of Carrie Coons." *Hastings Center Report* 19, no. 4 (1989): 14–15.

Tomlinson, Tom. "The Irreversibility of Death: Reply to Cole." *Kennedy Institute of Ethics Journal* 3, no. 2 (1993): 157–165.

Wikler, Daniel. "Brain Death: A Durable Consensus?" *Bioethics* 7, nos. 2–3 (1993): 239–246.

Wikler, Daniel. "Not Dead, Not Dying? Ethical Categories and Persistent Vegetative State," *Hastings Center Report* 18, no. 1 (1988): 41–47.

Youngner, Stuart; Arnold, Robert; Shapiro, Renie, eds. *Defining Death.* Baltimore: Johns Hopkins University Press, 1999.

Youngner, Stuart, et al. "'Brain Death' and Organ Retrieval: A Cross-Sectional Survey of Knowledge and Concepts among Health Professionals." *Journal of the American Medical Association* 261 (1989): 2205–2210.

Zaner, Richard M., ed. *Death: Beyond Whole-Brain Criteria.* Dordrecht, Holland: Kluwer Academic Press, 1988.

Decisional Capacity and the Right to Refuse Treatment

Abernethy, Virginia. "Compassion, Control, and Decisions about Competency." *American Journal of Psychiatry* 141, no. 1 (January 1984): 53–60.

Brink, Susan. "Taking Charge," *U.S. News & World Report* (July 28, 1997): 17–21 (An update on the Dax Cowart Story.)

Brock, Dan W. "Decision-Making Competence and Risk." *Bioethics* 5, no. 2 (1991): 105–112.

Burt, Robert. *Taking Care of Strangers: The Rule of Law in Doctor-Patient Relations.* New York: Free Press, 1979, chapter 1.

Callahan, Daniel. "Terminating Life-Sustaining Treatment of the Demented." *Hastings Center Report* (November–December 1995): 25–31.

Connors, Russell B., Jr., and Smith, Martin L. "Religious Insistence on Medical Treatment: Christian Theology and Imagination." *Hastings Center Report* (July–August 1996): 23–30.

Drane, James. "The Many Faces of Competency." *Hastings Center Report* 17, no. 15 (April 1985): 17–21.

Freedman, Benjamin. "Competence, Marginal and Otherwise: Concepts and Ethics." *International Journal of Law and Psychiatry* 4 (1981): 53–72.

Jehovah's Witnesses and the Question of Blood. New York: Watchtower Bible and Tract Society of New York, 1977.

Jonsen, Albert R. "Blood Transfusions and Jehovah's Witnesses." *Critical Care Clinics* 2, no. 1 (January 1986): 91–100.

Kliever, Lonnie D., ed. *Dax's Case: Essays in Medical Ethics and Human Meaning.* Dallas, TX: Southern Methodist University Press, 1989.

Kopelman, Loretta M. "On the Evaluative Nature of Competency and Capacity Judgments." *International Journal of Law and Psychiatry* (1990): 309–329.

Macklin, Ruth. "Consent, Coercion and Conflicts of Rights." *Perspectives in Biology and Medicine* 20, no. 3 (1977): 360–371.

May, Larry. "Challenging Medical Authority: The Refusal of Treatment by Christian Scientists." *Hastings Center Report* (January–February 1995): 15–21.

Meisel, Alan. "Legal Myths about Terminating Life Support." *Archives of Internal Medicine* 109 (1991): 1497–1502.

Powell, Tia, and Lowenstein, Bruce. "Refusing Life-Sustaining Treatment after Catastrophic Injury: Ethical Implications." *Journal of Law, Medicine and Ethics* 24, no. 1 (Spring 1996): 54–61.

Roth, Loren H.; Meisel, Alan; and Lidz, Charles, "Tests of Competency to Consent to Treatment." *American Journal of Psychiatry* 134, no. 3 (March 1977): 279–284.

Sheldon, Mark. "Ethical Issues in the Forced Transfusion of Jehovah's Witness Children," *The Journal of Emergency Medicine* 14, no. 2 (1996): 251–257.

Skene, Loane. "Risk-Related Standard Inevitable in Assessing Competence." *Bioethics* 5, no. 2 (1991): 113–122.

Wicclair, Mark R. "Patient Decision-Making Capacity and Risk." *Bioethics* 5, no. 2 (1991): 91–104.

Advance Directives

"Advance Directives: Expectations, Experience, and Future Practice." *Journal of Clinical Ethics* 4, no. 1 (1993): 1–104.

Brett, Allan S. "Limitations of Listing Specific Medical Interventions in Advance Directives." *Journal of the American Medical Association* 266, no. 6 (August 14, 1991): 825–828.

———. "Advance Directives and the Personal Identity Problem." *Philosophy and Public Affairs* 17 (Fall 1988): 277–302.

Cantor, Norman. *Advance Directives and the Pursuit of Death with Dignity.* Bloomington: Indiana University Press, 1993.

Hackler, C. R.; Moseley, R.; and Vawter, D. E., eds. *Advance Directives in Medicine.* New York: Praeger Publishers, 1989.

"Patient Self-Determination Act." *Cambridge Quarterly of Healthcare Ethics* 2, no. 2 (special section, 1992): 97–126.

Robertson, John. "Second Thoughts on Living Wills." *Hastings Center Report* 21, no. 6 (1991): 6–9.

Teno, Joan, et al. "Do Formal Advance Directives Affect Resuscitation Decisions and the Use of Resources for Seriously Ill Patients?" *Journal of Clinical Ethics* 5, no. 1 (Spring 1994): 23–30.

Choosing for Others

Arras, John. "Beyond *Cruzan:* Individual Rights, Family Autonomy and the Persistent Vegetative State." *Journal of the American Geriatrics Society* 39 (1991): 1018–1024.

Blustein, Jeffrey. "The Family in Medical Decisionmaking." *Hastings Center Report* 23, no. 3 (May–June 1993): 6–13.

Capron, Alexander M., ed. "Medical Decision-Making and the 'Right to Die' after *Cruzan.*" *Law, Medicine & Health Care* 19, nos. 1–2 (Spring/Summer 1991): 5–104.

"Children and Bioethics: Uses and Abuses of the Best Interests Standard." *Journal of Medicine and Philosophy* 22, no. 3 (symposium, June 1997).

Dresser, Rebecca. "Missing Persons: Legal Perceptions of Incompetent Patients." *Rutgers Law Review* 46, no. 2 (Winter 1994): 609–719.

———. "Dworkin on Dementia: Elegant Theory, Questionable Policy." *Hastings Center Report* (November–December 1995): 32–38.

Emanuel, Ezekiel J. *The Ends of Human Life: Medical Ethics in a Liberal Polity.* Cambridge, MA: Harvard University Press, 1991.

Emanuel, Ezekiel J., and Linda L. "Decisions at the End of Life: Guided by Communities of Patients." *Hastings Center Report* 23, no. 5 (1993): 6–14.

Freedman, Benjamin "Respectful Service and Reverent Obedience: A Jewish View on Making Decisions for Incompetent Parents." *Hastings Center Report* (July–August 1996): 31–37.

Kadish, Sanford H. "Letting Patients Die: Legal and Moral Reflections." *California Law Review* 80, no. 4 (1992): 857–888.

Lynn, Joanne, ed. *By No Extraordinary Means: The Choice to Forego Life-Sustaining Food and Water.* Bloomington: Indiana University Press, 1986.

May, William E., et al. "Feeding and Hydrating the Permanently Unconscious and Other Vulnerable Persons." *Issues in Law and Medicine* 3, no. 3 (1987): 203–211.

Meisel, Alan. "The Legal Consensus about Forgoing Life-Sustaining Treatment: Its Status and Prospects." *Kennedy Institute of Ethics Journal* 2, no. 4 (December 1992): 309–342.

Nelson, James Lindermann. "Taking Families Seriously." *Hastings Center Report* 22, no. 4 (1992): 6–12.

———. "Critical Interests and Sources of Familial Decision-Making Authority for Incapacitated Patients." *Journal of Law, Medicine and Ethics* 23, no 2 (Summer 1995): 143–148.

New York State Task Force on Life and the Law. *Life-Sustaining Treatment: Making Decisions and Appointing a Health Care Agent.* 1987.

———. *When Others Must Choose: Deciding for Patients without Capacity.* 1992.

"Pediatric Decision Making." *Journal of Law, Medicine and Ethics* 23, no. 1 (symposium, Spring 1995).

Rhoden, Nancy K. "Litigating Life and Death." *Harvard Law Review* 102, no. 2 (December 1988): 375–446.

Solomon, Mildred Z., et al. "Decisions Near the End of Life: Professional Views on Life-Sustaining Treatments." *American Journal of Public Health* 83, no. 1 (January 1993): 14–23.

Veatch, Robert M. "Forgoing Life-Sustaining Treatment: Limits to the Consensus." *Kennedy Institute of Ethics Journal* 3, no. 1 (March 1993): 1–19.

White, Patricia D., ed. "Essays in the Aftermath of *Cruzan.*" *Journal of Medicine and Philosophy* 17, no. 6 (December 1992): 563ff.

Euthanasia and Physician-Assisted Suicide

"Aid in Dying: The Supreme Court and the Public Response." *Hastings Center Report* (September–October, 1997).

Arras, John D. "The Right to Die on the Slippery Slope." *Social Theory and Practice* 8, no. 3 (Fall 1982): 285–328.

Battin, Margaret P. *The Death Debate: Ethical Issues in Suicide.* Englewood Cliffs, NJ: Prentice Hall, 1996.

———. *The Least-Worst Death: Essays in Bioethics on the End of Life.* New York: Oxford University Press, 1994.

Battin, Margaret P., ed. *Ethical Issues in Suicide.* Englewood Cliffs, NJ: Prentice Hall, 1995.

Battin, Margaret P.; Rhodes, Rosamond; and Silvers, Anita. "A Dozen Caveats Concerning the Discussion of Euthanasia in the Netherlands." In *Managing Morality: Ethics, Euthanasia, and the Termination of Medical Treatment,* edited by Ronald Cranford and Arthur Caplan. Forthcoming.

———. eds. *Physician-Assisted Suicide: Expanding the Debate.* London: Routledge, 1998.

Beauchamp, Tom L., ed. *Intending Death: The Ethics of Assisted Suicide and Euthanasia.* Upper Saddle River, NJ: Prentice Hall, 1996.

Brock, Dan W. "Voluntary Active Euthanasia." *Hastings Center Report* (March–April 1992).

Brody, Baruch. *Suicide and Euthanasia.* Dordrecht, Holland: Kluwer Academic Press, 1989.

Brody, Howard. "Assisted Death: A Compassionate Response to Medical Failure." *New England Journal of Medicine* 327, no. 19 (November 5, 1992): 1384–1388.

Callahan, Daniel. *The Troubled Dream of Life: Living with Mortality.* New York: Simon & Schuster, 1993.

Cohen, Cynthia B. "Christian Perspectives on Assisted Suicide and Euthanasia: The Anglican Tradition." *Journal of Law, Medicine and Ethics* 24, no. 4 (Winter 1996): 369–379.

"Dying Well? A Colloquy on Euthanasia and Assisted Suicide." *Hastings Center Report* 22, no. 2 (special issue, 1992): 6–55.

"Euthanasia and Physician-Assisted Suicide: Murder or Mercy." *Cambridge Quarterly of Healthcare Ethics* 2, no. 1 (special section, 1993): 9–88.

Feinberg, Joel. "Voluntary Euthanasia and the Inalienable Right to Life." *Philosophy and Public Affairs* 7, no. 2 (Winter 1978): 93–123.

Foot, Philippa. "Euthanasia." *Philosophy and Public Affairs* 6, no. 2 (Winter 1977): 85–112.

Gaylin, Willard, et al. "Doctors Must Not Kill." *Journal of the American Medical Association* 259, no. 14 (April 8, 1988): 2139–2140.

Glover, Jonathan. *Causing Death and Saving Lives.* New York: Penguin Books, 1977.

Jennings, Bruce. "Active Euthanasia and Forgoing Life-Sustaining Treatment: Can We Hold the Line?" *Journal of Pain and Symptom Management* 6, no. 5 (July 1991): 312–316.

Kamisar, Yale. "Are Laws against Assisted Suicide Unconstitutional?" *Hastings Center Report* 23, no. 3 (1993): 32–41.

———. "Some Non-Religious Views against Proposed 'Mercy-Killing' Legislation." *Minnesota Law Review* 42 (1958): 969–1042.

Kass, Leon. "Is There a Right to Die?" *Hastings Center Report* 23, no. 1 (1993): 34–43.

Kevorkian, Jack. *Prescription Medicine: The Goodness of Planned Death.* Buffalo, NY: Prometheus Books, 1991.

Momeyer, Richard. "Does Physician-Assisted Suicide Violate the Integrity of Medicine?" *Journal of Medicine and Philosophy* 20, no. 1 (February 1995): 13–24.

New York State Task Force on Life and the Law. *When Death Is Sought: Assisted Suicide and Euthanasia in the Medical Context.* May 1994.

————. *When Death Is Sought: Assisted Suicide and Euthanasia in the Medical Context, Supplement to Report.* April 1997.

Orentlicher, David. "The Legalization of Physician-Assisted Suicide: A Very Modest Revolution." *Boston College Law Review* 38, no. 3 (1997): 443–475.

"Physician-Assisted Suicide in Context: Constitutional, Regulatory, and Professional Challenges." *Journal of Law, Medicine & Ethics* 24, no. 3 (symposium, Fall 1996): 181–242.

Pratt, David A. and Steinbock, Bonnie. "Too Many Physicians: Physician-Assisted Suicide After *Washington/Quill*," *Albany Law Journal of Science and Technology* 8, no. 2 (1998).

Quill, Timothy E. "The Ambiguity of Clinical Intentions." *New England Journal of Medicine* 329 (1992): 1039–1040.

————. *Death and Dignity: Making Choices and Taking Charge.* New York: Oxford University Press, 1986.

————. *A Midwife Through the Dying Process: Stories of Healing and Hard Choices at the End of Life.* Baltimore: Johns Hopkins University Press, 1996.

Quill, Timothy E.; Cassel, Christine K.; and Meier, Diane E. "Care of the Hopelessly Ill: Proposed Clinical Criteria for Physician-Assisted Suicide." *New England Journal of Medicine* 327, no. 19 (November 5, 1992): 1380–1384.

Rachels, James. *The End of Life: Euthanasia and Morality.* New York: Oxford University Press, 1986.

Steinbock, Bonnie, and Norcross, Alastair, eds. *Killing and Letting Die.* 2nd ed. New York: Fordham University Press, 1994.

Symposium on Assisted Suicide. *Hastings Center Report* (May–June 1995).

Velleman, J. David. "Against the Right to Die." *Journal of Medicine and Philosophy* 17, no. 6 (December 1992): 664–681.

Weir, R. F. "The Morality of Physician-Assisted Suicide." *Law, Medicine & Health Care* 20 (1992): 116–126.

PART THREE

CONTRACEPTION, ABORTION, AND PRENATAL DIAGNOSIS

CONTROVERSIES OVER CONTRACEPTION

It may seem incredible to today's youth, but contraception was once as controversial as abortion is today (Garrow 1994). Contraception was opposed both by traditionalists, who feared (rightly, as it turned out) that liberating women from unwanted pregnancies would irrevocably change sexual roles, and by some feminists, who feared that men, freed from concern about pregnancy, would make insatiable sexual demands on their wives. The feminists' fear seems less plausible than that of the traditionalists, since it stems from a Victorian misconception that women are less interested in sex than men.

Today, contraception is not controversial except in the case of young people. Conservatives generally oppose sex education in schools, including disseminating information about contraception. They believe such sex education contributes to earlier sexual activity, although studies have found no conclusive evidence for this claim, and "in-depth studies of a few specific sex education programs have shown that some approaches contribute to greater delay in teenagers becoming sexually active, at least in the short term" (Alan Guttmacher Institute 1992). Contraceptive use by adults is widely regarded as morally permissible and noncontroversial, despite continued opposition by the Roman Catholic Church. Many opponents of abortion point to the existence of contraception as an argument against the need for abortion. Sexually active adults who wish to avoid pregnancy are *supposed* to use contraception, and failure to use it, or to use it regularly and correctly, is interpreted by many as irresponsible behavior.

The pendulum has swung from a condemnation of contraception to suggestions from some that contraception should be required—or at least heavily encouraged—for those who, for whatever reason, would be unable to care properly for their offspring. The idea of mandating contraception received greater impetus in 1990 when the Food and Drug Administration (FDA) approved the contraceptive Norplant. A highly effective birth control method, Norplant consists of six small hormone-releasing rods that are inserted in a woman's upper arm and last up to five years.

A few months after the FDA approved Norplant, a California judge presiding over a case of a woman convicted of child abuse imposed implantation of Norplant in lieu of a prison sentence. Shortly thereafter, a bill was introduced in the Kansas legislature that offered women on welfare a cash bonus if they agreed to use the contraceptive (Moskowitz and Jennings 1996). In response, there was an outcry from an informal coalition of civil libertarians, feminists, and members of minority groups that such legislation is unconstitutional, racist, sexist, unduly coercive, and generally poor public policy. In the first selection of Section One, Stuart Taylor, Jr., argues that the critics are wrong. He maintains that offering welfare bonuses to women who agree to use Norplant is a good way to break the bleak cycle of teen pregnancy and welfare dependency. It is more humane than current welfare reform proposals which, he claims, will simply take millions of mothers and children off the welfare rolls, leaving them to beg, starve, and sleep on the streets.

Taylor assumes that teenage pregnancy is a large social problem that contributes to poverty and welfare dependency. This idea has been challenged recently by the sociologist Kristin Luker (Luker 1996). Luker argues that the focus on teen pregnancy is more a reflection of the public mood than a demographic reality. The data show that the rate of teenage pregnancy has not changed very much during this century. What has changed is the number of *unmarried* teenage mothers. In 1970, the proportion of teenage mothers who were unmarried at the time of birth was 30 percent; in 1995 it was 70 percent. While the number of single teenage mothers is increasing at a rapid rate, so is the number of single mothers at every age; fewer than a third of single mothers are teenagers. Single

parenthood is a social problem, but scapegoating teenagers does not address that issue.

Moreover, Luker says, it is simply not true that delaying childbirth for a few years would benefit those at the bottom of the income scale, whose life prospects would not significantly change even if they did postpone parenthood. Nor would the life chances of a teenage mother improve much if the father of her child married her, since he is likely to be young, poor, and without prospects himself. Early childbearing may make a bad situation worse, Luker acknowledges, but early childbearing is not the problem. It is not a cause of poverty, but a symptom—"an indicator of the extent to which so many young people have been excluded from the American dream. . . ." Luker would regard Taylor's proposal as a misguided and short-term fix to the entrenched problems of racism, poverty, and the existence of an underclass. A better, although more difficult, solution would be to provide young women with "a rich array of choices, so that having a baby is not the only or most attractive one on the horizon." (Luker 1996, pp. 182–183).

In the second selection, Bonnie Steinbock looks at the concept of coercion in order to evaluate the criticism that certain uses of Norplant are unethical because they are coercive. She argues that "coercive" has become a generalized term of abuse that is not always appropriately applied. In part, this has occurred because the concept of coercion is complex and difficult to apply. In addition, critics have not always distinguished between a policy that coerces, exploits, violates equality, or infringes on autonomy. Such intellectual sloppiness both undercuts the charge of coercion where the criticism is apt and blinds us to other, equally important, grounds for objecting to policies.

THE MORALITY OF ABORTION

Abortion is an issue that will not go away. Twenty-five years have passed since the Supreme Court struck down restrictive abortion statutes in 1973, yet the battle rages on with no end in sight. At the extremes are two hostile camps, each demanding total moral and political victory. Antiabortionists insist that fetuses are helpless unborn children, as deserving of the law's protection as are newborn infants. Animating their crusade is a single moral principle: the unborn child's right to life. To accomplish the abolition of abortion, these "pro-life" groups have mounted an impressive grassroots political movement that has effectively blocked the public funding of abortion in many states. Their attempt to pass a constitutional amendment that would recognize fetuses as persons failed, but there have been several important cases aimed at overturning *Roe v. Wade* (including *Webster* and *Casey*). With each new case, commentators predicted the end of the right to abortion. Yet despite the increasingly conservative turn of the Supreme Court during the Reagan-Bush years, *Roe v. Wade* was not overturned, although some restrictions, such as waiting periods and parental notification, were instituted. Despite these restrictions, the basic principle of *Roe v. Wade*—that a woman has the right to terminate pregnancy up until viability, and thereafter when necessary to protect her life or health—has been upheld (Robertson 1992, p. 24).

Pro-life groups have battled on many other fronts as well. They have mounted a public-relations war, carrying posters with pictures of dismembered and bloody fetuses. They have distributed films, like *The Silent Scream,* that claim that fetuses experience pain during abortion. They have staged sit-ins, rallies, and demonstrations, some aimed at preventing patients from entering abortion clinics. Doctors who perform abortions have been subjected to harassment, and several doctors and clinic workers have been killed by antiabortion fanatics. In the wake of violence directed at abortion clinics, Congress passed a law that imposes severe penalties on anyone attempting to prevent people from obtaining medical services. Pro-lifers objected that they were being singled out for punishment not given to other protest groups, and that their First Amendment rights were violated by the law.

Most recently, anti-abortion forces have focused on a particular late-term abortion technique they call "partial-birth abortion" (known medically as intact dilation and extraction), in which a fetus is partly delivered and its brain suctioned out in order to collapse the skull so that it can pass through the cervix. Opponents of the procedure describe it as horrific, brutal, grisly, and a form of infanticide. Polls indicate that 78 percent of Americans want the procedure banned. Congress

twice attempted to ban partial-birth abortions, and twice the legislation was vetoed by President Clinton. At this writing, seventeen states have passed laws banning the procedure; these laws have been successfully challenged on constitutional grounds in ten states. In New Jersey, Governor Christie Whitman vetoed a ban on partial-birth abortions only to have the state legislature override her veto on December 15, 1997. The next day, U.S. District Judge Anne E. Thompson issued a temporary restraining order that she extended on Christmas Eve, pending a trial June 3, 1998.

Physicians are divided on whether the procedure is ever medically indicated. Some physicians call it "a rogue procedure" that is not in any textbook or taught in medical school. The American Medical Association (AMA) voted in June 1997 to support a ban on partial-birth abortions. The vote was only the second in the organization's 150-year history in which it supported making a medical procedure a crime. The first vote was in 1996, when the AMA urged Congress to outlaw the genital mutilation of women.

Other physicians maintain that the technique may sometimes be medically necessary—that using a different method of termination could sometimes endanger a woman's health or future reproductive capacity. They argue that the method of abortion should be determined by the woman's doctor, not by elected officials. Abortion rights advocates also maintain that the statutes are worded so vaguely that they could apply to virtually all second-trimester, and even some late first-trimester, abortions. They suspect this is precisely the intention of the sponsors of bans on partial-birth abortion: to galvanize public support against one method of termination, and then use this support to overturn abortion rights generally.

On the other side, "pro-choice" advocates have continued to press for women's rights to control their own bodies. They have consistently opposed every restriction on abortion, such as waiting periods, information about the fetus, or parental notification. Some pro-choice advocates have opposed any attempts to control or influence a woman's behavior during pregnancy, on the grounds that such attempts threaten the right to abortion. For example, in 1991, the New York State chapter of the National Organization for Women (NOW) joined liquor sellers in lobbying against a bill that would require bars, restaurants, and liquor stores to post signs warning pregnant women of the dangers of alcohol consumption to fetal development. The New York NOW called the proposed legislation an attack on women's right to choose, arguing that it places the rights of a fetus ahead of the rights of the woman carrying it (Steinbock 1992, 238, n. 18). For many in the pro-choice camp, there is but one operative moral principle: a woman should have the right to control her reproductive activity.

For a long time, the two sides weren't even willing to talk to each other, let alone compromise. But an increasingly centrist position is emerging, which wants to keep abortion safe and legal, but acknowledges that it is a morally regrettable taking of human life (see, for example, Dworkin 1993).

The selections in Section Two are designed both to present a representative sampling of conservative, moderate, and liberal views on abortion, and to suggest the necessity of moving beyond the impasse of absolute and contradictory rights. At the *least,* an honest and sympathetic reading of these selections should foster rational discussion of this thorny issue, by making each of us more aware of the strengths of the other side's argument; at the *most,* these readings could help us transcend this sterile contest of rights, and move toward a reasonable moral and political compromise.

MORAL PERSPECTIVES

The six selections in Section Two offer philosophical discussions that illuminate the basic moral structure behind the issue of abortion. The abortion controversy poses two fundamental and extraordinarily difficult ethical questions. The first question—is the fetus a "human being" or "person," thus having a right to life?—relates to the moral status of the fetus. The second question—does the fetus's purported right to life outweigh the rights of the mother to both life and liberty?—concerns the resolution of conflicting moral rights and claims.

While all of the parties to the dispute over abortion seem to agree that it is usually morally wrong to kill an innocent human being, there is considerable disagreement over the ontological and moral

status of the fetus. This much seems clear: *If* the fetus is a full-fledged person, then it surely possesses a right to life that cannot be easily overridden. Moreover, the usual reasons for supporting abortion—that the world is already overpopulated, that children are better-off if they are wanted, that bearing and raising unwanted children imposes serious burdens on women—all presuppose that the fetus does not have the moral status of a born human being. It would scarcely be thought morally right to combat overpopulation by killing some segment of the population, say, the elderly or the sick. Nor would it be morally acceptable to ensure that every child is a wanted child by killing unwanted newborns. As for the burdens imposed on women by unwanted pregnancies, other situations also impose burdens on women. Women are the primary caretakers of elderly parents, but no one suggests that we ought to kill old and senile people to relieve the burden on their daughters.

The traditional conservative position against abortion is represented by a selection from the *Evangelium Vitae* by Pope John Paul II: Abortion is an "unspeakable crime." It is "the deliberate and direct killing of a human being." The Pope acknowledges that the decision to have an abortion is often made not for selfish reasons or out of convenience, but to protect important values such as the woman's own health, or to procure a decent standard of living for her family. Nevertheless, he maintains that such reasons "can never justify the deliberate killing of an innocent human being." The Pope then considers the objection that a fertilized egg is not yet "a human life," and he concludes that it must be: "It would never be made human if it were not human already." Nor does this claim rest on religious views such as the occurrence of ensoulment. Rather, "modern genetic science" demonstrates that at fertilization there is a new, individual human being. This human being is to be respected and treated as a person, with a right to life, from the moment of conception.

Judith Jarvis Thomson attempts to defend a prochoice position by claiming that the conservative argument is *invalid;* that is, that the conclusion that abortion is always wrong does not follow from the argument's premises. Thomson's argument is novel because she does not attempt to rebut the conservative premise that the fetus is a human being with a subsequent right to life. Instead, she argues that abortion would be morally permissible in most cases *even if we allow that the fetus has a right to life*. The core of her argument is that a right to life does not carry with it the right to whatever one may need to stay alive. Arguing by analogy, Thomson maintains that a person's right to life does not give him or her a right to use another person's body to uphold that right. If a fetus does not have a right to use a woman's body, then even if it has a right to life, abortion does not *violate* its right to life; thus, abortion is not unjust killing. Much of Thomson's article discusses whether the woman's (partial) responsibility for the fetus's existence in her body *does* give the fetus-person a right to use her body. Somewhat ironically, although Thomson's article is intended as a defense of abortion, her argument has great appeal for people who think that abortion is generally wrong, but make an exception for abortion in the case of rape. In the traditional conservative view, it does not matter how the fetus came into existence, whether due to voluntary intercourse or rape; the fact that its father was a rapist does not change the fetus's status as an innocent human being. According to Thomson's argument, however, the woman's responsibility for getting pregnant makes a big difference. If the woman was clearly not responsible for her pregnancy, as in the case of rape, then she cannot be said to have tacitly given the fetus a right to use her body. Thus, abortion in the case of rape would not be unjust killing.

Thomson tries to show that non-responsibility extends beyond the rape scenario; that, for example, a woman who has a contraceptive failure also has not given the fetus a right to use her body. She then goes on to consider whether a woman *ought*—out of common decency—to allow the fetus-person to use her body, even if it has no right to do so. Thomson rejects this suggestion, however, saying that the sacrifice on the part of the pregnant woman is too great. No one is morally required to make large sacrifices in order to keep another person alive. This part of Thomson's article inspired an "equal protection" argument against restrictive abortion laws, on the grounds that requiring women, but not men, to be "Good Samaritans" violates equal protection (Regan 1979). Thomson's arguments are of particular interest, since they attempt to provide a rigorous philosophical defense for one of the central claims of the feminist movement—that a woman has a right to use her own body as she chooses. Despite its title, Thomson's article is *not* a full-blown defense of abortion, but a focused critique of the argument against abortion based entirely on the fetus's personhood and consequent right to life. Even if Thomson is correct about the limitations of rights in general, and the right to life in particular, it would still be possible to argue that abortion is morally wrong on some other grounds, such as the moral obligation of a mother to nurture and protect her child.

It is precisely the limits of Thomson's anti-abortion argument that Mary Anne Warren finds objectionable. Warren looks for a defense of abortion that does not depend on how the woman became pregnant or whether her getting pregnant was, in some way, "her fault." To do this, Warren claims that one must mount a convincing argument to show that, contrary to the Pope's *Evangelium Vitae*, the fetus is not a person, not a member of the moral community. Conservatives, Warren argues, fail to recognize that the term "human" is ambiguous; it can refer either to a being's membership in the species *homo sapiens* (which Warren calls "genetic humanity"), or it can refer to a being's moral standing (which she calls "moral humanity"). The conservative's mistake, Warren argues, is to confuse these two concepts and to think therefore that all—and only—genetic humans are also moral humans. However, she claims, it is not true that only genetic humans can be full-fledged members of the moral community. Consider the character "E.T." from the movie of the same name. E.T. is highly intelligent, emotionally sensitive, and morally responsible. To deny him full membership in the moral community, and a right to life, would be completely arbitrary. If this is so, then being genetically human is not a condition of moral humanity or, to use the term Warren prefers, "personhood." By the same token, not all genetic humans are persons: those who are permanently unconscious, for example, are no longer persons. To be a person, in Warren's view, has nothing to do with species membership, but rather with criteria such as consciousness, self-consciousness, reasoning, and the capacity to communicate. Since fetuses, even late-gestation fetuses, have relatively few of these person-making characteristics, fetuses are not persons. Fetuses "cannot be said to have any more right to life than, let us say, a newborn guppy, . . . and . . . a right of that magnitude could never override a woman's right to obtain an abortion, at any stage of her pregnancy."

A difficulty with Warren's "person view" of moral status is that it appears to have extremely counterintuitive results. If even a fully viable nine-month-old fetus fails to be a member of the moral community, and entitled to its protection, does not the same exclusion apply to newborns and most infants? Does not Warren's logic lead us to conclude that infanticide is perfectly acceptable? In order to head off such a conclusion, Warren has appended a "Postscript" to her article, in which she contends that even if killing infants does not amount to murder (that is, the wrongful killing of a *person*), infanticide is immoral on the straightforward utilitarian ground that it forecloses the possibility of happiness for prospective adoptive parents.

Whatever else might be said for this argument, it certainly does not seem to square with or explain our moral repugnance to infanticide. For this reason, a number of theorists (Sumner 1981, Steinbock 1992) have suggested a weaker criterion of moral status, namely, sentience—the ability to experience pain and pleasure. Sentience theorists maintain that sentience is necessary for having moral status, because nonsentient beings, such as trees, rocks, and cars, do not have interests. That is, it cannot matter to a nonsentient being what happens to it. Since they have no interests, their interests cannot be considered, which is another way of saying that they lack moral status. (It does not follow that it is morally permissible to do whatever you like to a nonsentient being; it could be morally wrong to slash a beautiful painting or chop down an old oak tree. The wrongness, however, does not stem from the interests of the *painting* in not being slashed or the interests of the *tree* in not being chopped down.) Sentience is also considered sufficient for moral status. That is, if a being has experiences, such as the experience of pain, those experiences provide reasons for us to treat it in certain ways, for example, not to inflict pain on it.

Applied to fetuses, the sentience view denies that fetuses, throughout most of gestation, are sen-

tient. Therefore, they lack moral status. Killing them is not seriously wrong and can be justified by appealing to the rights and interests of the pregnant woman. After the fetus becomes sentient (probably during the last half of the second trimester), it acquires moral status, and its interests (for example, avoiding pain and having pleasurable experiences, for which continued existence is a prerequisite) should be balanced against those of the pregnant woman. This accords with a moderate view on abortion in which the reasons for having an abortion must be proportionately more compelling as the fetus develops and acquires more of the characteristics of born human beings.

The biggest difficulty for sentience theorists is the status of nonhuman animals. Just as the challenge for person theorists is to explain why it would be wrong to kill human infants, the challenge for sentience theorists is to explain why it is not seriously wrong to kill (most) animals. Some theorists in both camps are willing to "bite the bullet" and accept the counterintuitive implications of their views. Michael Tooley, a person theorist, thinks infanticide is not generally wrong (Tooley 1983), and Peter Singer, a sentience theorist, thinks the killing of animals is usually wrong (Singer 1975). Those who are not willing to accept these conclusions need to explain how their rejection is consistent with their general view of moral status.

Don Marquis is a conservative with a difference. Like traditional conservatives, Marquis thinks that abortion is immoral, as wrong as killing an innocent adult human being. However, his view significantly differs from the standard conservative position. Marquis analyzes the difficulties facing the traditional arguments on both sides of the abortion issue. Anti-abortionists who base their position on the fetus's being *human* find it hard to explain why it is reasonable to base moral status on something as arbitrary as species membership. Pro-choicers who adopt the person view avoid this problem, since such characteristics as consciousness, rationality, and moral agency do seem morally relevant. However, adherents of the person view are in the embarrassing position of having to explain why their principle does not also justify the killing of infants, young children, and the severely mentally impaired. Sentience theorists do not face this problem, but they have the equally difficult task of explaining why it is rational to accord greater moral status, and a right to life, only to some sentient beings, namely, human beings.

The way out of this dialectical quandary, Marquis suggests, is to develop a general account of the wrongness of killing. What makes killing wrong is the loss of the victim's future—in particular, a future like ours. This principle differs from the usual "pro-life" position in two ways. First, it is not based on the special value of human life; it is not "speciesist." If there are nonhuman aliens or animals with "a future like ours," they too have a right to life. Second, Marquis's principle does not entail that euthanasia is always wrong, since incurably ill people who are in great pain and wish to die do not suffer a loss if they are killed.

Marquis emphasizes that his argument does not rely on the "invalid inference" that, since it is wrong to kill persons, it is also wrong to kill potential persons. Marquis avoids this logical error because the central category in his argument is not *personhood* at all, but rather the category of having a valuable future like ours. Nevertheless, critics may argue that Marquis is offering another version of the argument from potential (based on the potential to have a future like ours, rather than the potential to become a person), and that his argument is therefore vulnerable to the standard criticism against all potentiality theorists; namely, that their argument makes contraception and abortion equally wrong. Since this conclusion is unacceptable to virtually all potentiality theorists, they must differentiate between contraception and abortion by arguing that fertilized eggs have futures of which they can be deprived, while gametes do not. The success of Marquis's antiabortion position depends heavily on the plausibility of this ontological and highly criticized distinction (Norcross 1990).

The arguments of Marquis and others focus mainly on the status of the fetus. Feminists have found this emphasis on the fetus pathetically one-sided, reducing women to mere fetal containers. As we saw, Thomson focuses the issue on the woman's right to her own body. However, some feminists find Thomson's approach deeply unsatisfying. They reject "masculinist" conceptions of privacy, choice, and property rights that do not meet the needs and interests of many women. Susan Sherwin contrasts Thomson's approach with a feminist approach that takes into account the woman's situation, her relation to other people, and her feelings about the fetus. Feminists are also concerned with women's position in society, and the impact abortions (or restrictive abortion laws) have on the status of women. Sherwin criticizes traditional pro-choice arguments for focusing on the moral status of the fetus, and giving only secondary consideration to the pregnant woman. She argues that it is a mistake to treat fetuses as physically, ontologically, or socially separate from the women whose bodies they inhabit. "Because of this inexorable biological reality, the responsibility and privilege of determining a fetus's specific social status and value must rest with the woman carrying it."

Not all feminists agree with Sherwin's analysis. Sidney Callahan offers a "pro-life feminism" which she considers to be more faithful to the basic tenets of feminism than a pro-choice approach. While Callahan acknowledge women's rights to control their own bodies, she denies that this includes a right to kill defenseless human beings. Just as feminists have fought for justice for themselves and other oppressed individuals, so too they should empathize with the fetus who cannot defend itself. Feminism, Callahan argues, is inconsistent with the characteristically male tendencies toward aggression and killing. A society in which abortion is a "necessity," she asserts, is a male-dominated society that feminists should reject. Only pro-life feminism can accord adequate respect and support to women and their reproductive capacities.

PROCREATIVE AUTONOMY AND RESPONSIBILITY

In Section Three, we addressed the question of whether, and under what conditions, abortion is morally *permissible*. In this section, we turn to the issue of whether it can be morally irresponsible to procreate. Are there times when having children is immoral?

In a case study of the McCaughey septuplets, Bonnie Steinbock discusses both parental and professional responsibility in multiple pregnancies resulting from the use of fertility drugs. Multiple pregnancies pose serious health risks, both to the mother and the babies. Is it fair to the offspring to impose such risks on them? Is this consistent with being responsible parents? And should fertility doctors provide treatment that can result in "litters"? How should the desire of couples for children be balanced against the possibility of premature death, cerebral palsy, blindness, and mental retardation for the children who are born?

The same question arises for couples who may pass on genetic disorders to their offspring. Prior to the late 1960s, couples had no way of knowing whether their children would be born with genetic disorders. Today, prenatal diagnosis primarily in the form of amniocentesis and, more recently, chorionic villus sampling, allows the couple to find out if the fetus is affected with a genetic abnormality. Armed with this knowledge, the prospective parents can choose whether to continue the pregnancy, or to terminate it and "try again." Many couples use prenatal diagnosis for reassurance that their fetus is not affected with a particular disorder. Some couples who are carriers of a genetic disease, such as Tay-Sachs, would not attempt pregnancy without prenatal testing, and many women would choose abortion upon becoming pregnant. For these couples, prenatal testing allows them to risk pregnancy, and thus enhances their procreative options. However, Barbara Katz Rothman challenges the view that prenatal testing for genetic disease broadens procreative liberty. She thinks that both the choice to have or forgo prenatal testing, and the choice to continue or terminate a pregnancy if the fetus is affected, are illusory because a lack of social resources would make it impossible for most women to care for a child with special needs. In addition, the deep stigma attached to disability in our society makes some women feel guilty about bringing a handicapped child into the world. By presenting prenatal diagnosis and subsequent abortion as a "personal choice," society ignores the social pressures imposed on women to make these difficult choices, and avoids collective responsibility for disabled children.

Adrienne Asch takes Rothman's argument a step further. While supporting the legal right to abort for any reason, including fetal defects, she questions the moral justification for acting on this right. Abortion for fetal defects is, Asch suggests, much like abortion for sex selection, at least when the defect is not severe enough to cause either a speedy death or a life of intractable pain for the child. Persons with Down's syndrome, spina bifida, cystic fibrosis, and many other disorders can live happy, productive, and in many cases lengthy, lives. Many of their problems stem not from their physical disabilities, but from social barriers to equal treatment and access for the handicapped. Prenatal detection and termination of such potential lives may suggest to people living with these disabilities that they should not exist. Moreover, Asch suggests, the woman who aborts for fetal defects wants a child, but has decided that she does not want *this* child. Being a parent, however, is not an activity subject to complete control; one cannot select the characteristics one desires in a child. Asch argues that people should not seek made-to-order children, but should be willing to love and accept the children they bear, perfect or not.

Asch's position is certainly compatible with a "pro-life" stance that regards fetuses as morally equivalent to already born children, for parents do have obligations to love and accept their children, perfect or not. It is less clear that Asch's argument coheres with a generally pro-choice position on abortion. Pro-choicers may argue that women do not have the same obligations of love and care to their fetuses as they do to their born children. They may deny that the mere *intention* to have a child imposes the moral obligation to assume the burdens and sacrifices that typically accompany raising a severely disabled child. If this stance is right, then abortion for fetal defects is as justifiable as abortion to avoid other foreseen burdens of childbearing and childrearing.

Bonnie Steinbock and Ron McClamrock ask whether it might not be positively wrong to bear children who will have serious diseases or disabilities. Following the reasoning of Joel Feinberg (1984), Steinbock and McClamrock explain how someone could have a right not to be born. However, they note that Feinberg's analysis is limited to those rare cases in which *all* of the interests of the disabled child are *completely* "doomed to defeat." Steinbock and McClamrock argue that the "doomed-to-defeat" test is too stringent. They also consider it wrong to bring children into the world when they are destined to have lives that will fall below a decent quality-of-life minimum. Moreover, they insist that the test for whether it would be unfair to bring a child into the world is *not* whether the child itself will be glad to have been born. The test is rather whether the child's life is likely to be one that caring parents would want for their child. Steinbock and McClamrock propose a principle of parental responsibility that requires people who cannot give their children even a decent chance at a life well worth living to refrain (when possible) from procreating. They then discuss under what conditions it might be wrong deliberately to procreate, giving as an example a woman who knows that she is HIV-positive. However, they caution that the principle of parental responsibility does not imply that only people who can assure their children ideal lives should procreate. Nor does it suggest that disabled children cannot lead happy lives. The principle of parental responsibility asks only that before embarking on an enterprise as serious as parenting, prospective parents take into consideration the kinds of lives their children are likely to have.

In the last selection, Dan Brock delves more deeply into the question of whether it is wrong to bring children into the world under harmful conditions, such as genetically transmitted diseases. As Derek Parfit has pointed out, there seems to be a systematic difficulty in maintaining that such cases could ever be examples of immoral or irresponsible reproduction, namely, that the child has no other way of being born. Avoiding conception or terminating a pregnancy cannot provide a child with a healthy life, but rather provides no life at all. Assuming that the child will have a worthwhile life, even with a genetic disease, how can it be wrong to bring the child into existence? How can procreation under these conditions be "unfair to the child"? Brock concludes that although it *is* wrong to bring children with serious handicaps into the world when it can be prevented by avoiding conception or terminating a pregnancy, it is *not* a wrong to the child who is born and has a worthwhile life. Any attempt to characterize the wrongness as a wrong done to the child misconceives the situation. However, this is not a problem, according to Brock, because we can appeal to "non–person-affecting principles" to explain why it would be wrong to pass on serious genetic diseases when this can be prevented by avoiding procreation.

SECTION 1

Controversies over Contraception

The Norplant Option

Stuart Taylor, Jr.

Now that Congress and President Clinton have opted to use the threat of utter destitution to dissuade poor teen-agers and women from having children on the public dole, it's time to revive a more humane, and perhaps more effective, proposal with the same objective.

This idea surfaced briefly and spectacularly in 1990, when the *Philadelphia Inquirer* suggested in an editorial that perhaps some welfare mothers should be "offered an increased benefit" if they would agree to practice effective birth control—specifically, to use the then-new Norplant contraceptive, which prevents pregnancy for five years after being implanted under the skin of the upper arm.

An uproar followed. The editorial writers—who had insensitively suggested a desire to reduce births of poor black babies in particular—were savaged by many *Inquirer* staffers and others as racist advocates of eugenics, even of "genocide." They also caught it from some abortion-rights zealots, who are suspicious of any government efforts to influence reproductive choices, and from conservatives, who think the only proper way to discourage teen pregnancy is to preach abstinence. The newspaper abjectly apologized for a "misguided and wrongheaded editorial opinion." And ever since, the whole subject has been taboo.

But it's still a good idea, for poor girls and women themselves, and for the rest of us. Millions of babies are being born to poor teen-agers so lacking in elementary skills, work habits, and self-disci-

pline that they are unlikely to be either responsible parents or self-supporting providers. Many of these babies grow up in squalor and themselves become dependent denizens of the welfare culture.

The only realistic hope for breaking the bleak cycle of teen pregnancy and welfare dependency is to find ways to persuade poor teen-agers not to have babies—at least not until they are old enough, and capable enough, and self-supporting enough to provide a decent home life. But nobody—nobody—has any great ideas for realizing this hope, short of reverting to the cruelest, let-'em-starve brand of social Darwinism.

Thoughtful progressives like Sen. Daniel Patrick Moynihan, D-N.Y., have properly stressed the need to push welfare mothers into jobs and job-training programs. This makes sense because some of these women will rise to the occasion, learn the work ethic, and become self-supporting. And others may be dissuaded from having children by the prospect of being required to work. But (as Moynihan acknowledges) many welfare mothers are so crippled by their own early childhood environments as to be essentially unemployable, no matter how well-financed and well-run the jobs programs and related counseling, training, and child-care programs.

And under the harsh new welfare reform, the jobs programs will not be well financed. It appears that millions of welfare mothers and children will simply be cut off—unable to get or hold jobs, and left to beg from relatives and strangers, to steal what they can, even to sleep on the streets, depending on how much Calcutta-style misery the taxpayers are willing to tolerate.

Given the stark ugliness of trying to end the welfare culture by spreading homelessness and

---

The Legal Times, August 19, 1996, pp. 23–26. Reprinted with permission of Legal Times, 1730 M Street, N.W., Suite 802, Washington, D.C. 20036. Phone: 202-457-0686. Copyright © 1996 Legal Times.

hunger, it's especially striking that one pretty good, pretty humane idea has been virtually ignored in the welfare debate of the past year.

In a small effort to reopen discussion of this option, here's a specific proposal: States should experiment with programs in which all qualifying teen-agers and women would be offered lump-sum $1,000 cash payments—on top of any other benefits they receive—to have Norplant (or another long-term contraceptive) implanted at government expense. They would be free to have it removed whenever they chose, but would be rewarded with additional payments (of say, $30) for each month in which they kept it.

The category of qualifying teen-agers and women could include all recipients of welfare or other public assistance (including daughters of recipients) who are competent to give informed consent to the implant procedure. Or the program could be restricted in various ways in order to blunt possible objections. For example, you could require parental consent. Or eligibility could be restricted to those who have already been pregnant, or at least sexually active; to those over age 13, or under age 21; or some combination thereof.

Why Norplant? Because it requires no ongoing effort or supervision to be effective, and it can be discontinued only after some (rather small) effort. As such, Norplant is the only contraceptive the government could pay people to use with any hope of affecting those who aren't strongly motivated to either become pregnant or avoid pregnancy.

How much good the Norplant option would do is debatable. But the arguments that it would do harm seem unpersuasive. Here's a quick review of possible objections, left and right:

Bribing poor women and girls to implant Norplant would coerce them into not having children, thus violating their rights to reproductive choice, like the one-child-per-family policy and coerced abortions in China.

To the contrary, a government offer of money is not coercion—and not even remotely comparable to what goes on in China. Existing benefits would not be reduced for anyone declining Norplant. This means that nobody who really wanted a child would be prevented from having one. To be sure, the government would be trying to influence reproductive choices. But the same is true of existing policies promoting free contraception, and of laws like the Hyde Amendment, which denies Medicaid funding for abortions—not to mention the still extant statutes making it a crime to commit statutory rape (sex with a consenting minor), fornication (premarital sex), and adultery.

In its groveling 1990 editorial apology, the *Inquirer* said: "Our critics countered that to dangle cash or some other benefit in front of a desperately poor woman is tantamount to coercion. They're right." No, they were wrong, and the *Inquirer* was right in its initial Norplant editorial, when it noted that women would be free to "change their minds at any point and become fertile again."

"Many people," David Boldt, then-editor of the Inquirer's *editorial page, noted in a subsequent commentary, "saw the editorial as part of an ongoing white conspiracy to carry out genocide of blacks in America."*

This is pernicious nonsense, no matter how many people say it. The original *Inquirer* editorial unwittingly invited such smears by linking its Norplant proposal to race—specifically, to a report that nearly half the nation's black children are living in poverty. But nobody is proposing that race be a factor in any program promoting Norplant to welfare recipients, most of whom are white. Nobody is proposing to sterilize women or forbid them from having children. And while a disproportionate percentage of welfare mothers and children are black, black America, like white America, can only benefit from any program that rewards people for avoiding pregnancy unless and until they are old enough and self-supporting enough to provide decently for children.

Girls and women on Norplant may be at greater risk of contracting and spreading AIDS, because they will be less likely to demand that their sex partners use condoms.

A 1994 study reported in *The New England Journal of Medicine* found that Norplant had no effect on recipients' decisions whether to use condoms or visit doctors—and was 19 times as effective as the pill in preventing pregnancy. Any Norplant incentive program should include vigorous counseling about the need to use condoms against disease. But even now, how many women and girls are so much more afraid of pregnancy than of death that they use condoms solely to avoid the former, and would stop once on Norplant? Not many, I suspect.

Norplant itself may be unhealthy.

The possibility of serious long-term health damage from any relatively new contraceptive like Norplant must be taken seriously, and the risks should, of course, be fully disclosed to women considering using it. But no contraceptive is risk-free. And the available evidence indicates that the risks inherent in pregnancy and childbirth—and in abortion—are at least as great as the risks inherent in Norplant.

Plaintiffs' tort lawyers have nearly killed off Norplant, scaring away many women and doctors, by a torrent of personal-injury suits against its manufacturer. The lawyers include many of the same folks who created a tidal wave of litigation based on the apparently bogus claim about the dangers of silicone breast implants. But the Food and Drug Administration has repeatedly found Norplant to be safe and effective. More than a million women have used it with only minor side effects, such as changing menstrual bleeding patterns, reported.

There have been complaints by a small percentage of Norplant users of severe pain or scarring from having it removed. But the apparent reason was inadequate training of physicians in the (usually quick and painless) removal procedure—an easily remedied problem—and not any inherent defect in the product.

It is sexist to seek to thrust contraception only upon women.

Sexism has nothing to do with it. First, almost all welfare checks are written to women—not to men, who don't get pregnant. Second, the only forms of contraception now available for men are condoms and vasectomies. It would hardly make sense to hand out $1,000 payments to men for taking home a bunch of condoms, or to try to police their use. And a vasectomy—unlike a Norplant implant— cannot always be reversed.

Giving teen-agers contraceptives encourages promiscuity, and bribing them to use Norplant will encourage it even more.

The weight of the evidence suggests that teen-agers' decisions whether or not to engage in sexual activity don't have much to do with whether the government gives them contraceptives. Many have unprotected sex, and almost all can get con-

traceptives if they want them. As I have suggested, one possible restriction (although not one I would favor) on any Norplant incentive program would be to limit eligibility to teen-agers who have already been pregnant or, at least, sexually active. Norplant counselors could also stress the benefits of abstinence, while presenting the contraceptive as a backup safeguard.

Teen-agers should learn about sex and contraception from their parents, not the government.

A parental-consent requirement would answer this objection. I would not advocate such a requirement, however, because of the overwhelming evidence that many parents have little or no constructive communication with their children about such matters. I hope that my own two daughters (now 12 and nine years old) would consult with me and my wife before getting Norplant or becoming sexually active. But if they end up deciding to go their own ways, I'd rather that they have unrestricted access to Norplant than that they risk pregnancy.

Would a Norplant program be thwarted by the fact that many poor teen-agers actually want to get pregnant and have a child? I don't think so. First, there are about 3 million unwanted pregnancies in the United States every year, half of which end in abortion. Many of these involve teen-agers and women who are (or will be) on welfare. Norplant could stop almost all these. Second, the allure of pregnancy for many other poor teen-agers may be so slight, or so fleeting, or so fraught with ambivalence, that a $1,000 Norplant incentive would have plenty of takers.

And even if such a program only delayed pregnancies a few years, that would be a very good thing. Most 15-year-olds would be better mothers, and have a better chance of making something of their own lives, if they waited five or seven years before having babies.

Norplant is no panacea for poverty; nothing is. The question is whether a Norplant incentive program might do some good. There's only one way to find out: Give it a try. If it fails, the cost—in terms of numbers of teen-agers and women taking the $1,000 offer—will be tiny. And it just might help.

Coercion and Contraception

Bonnie Steinbock

The ability to control one's fertility has long been recognized to be essential to women's equality and self-determination. In some parts of the world, where death from childbirth or unsafe abortions is relatively common, it is a vital matter of health as well. Yet the choices available in contraception have been limited, and most methods have disadvantages. The newest long-acting contraceptive on the scene, and the one that has received the greatest attention, is Norplant. After it was approved for use in the United States in December 1990, Norplant was widely hailed as a breakthrough, a nearly ideal contraceptive: safe, effective, easy to use. Yet Norplant has created bitter controversy. Precisely those features that help make it a nearly ideal contraceptive (its effectiveness and the fact that it works without having to think about it) make it ideal for mandated contraception. Since Norplant is implanted on the inside of the upper arm, where it can be felt, and since it cannot be safely removed except by a trained practitioner, its continued usage can be monitored. This being the case, it is hardly surprising that within a few weeks of its approval by the FDA, an editorial in the *Philadelphia Inquirer* suggested that Norplant could be a useful tool for "reducing the underclass," by offering welfare mothers incentives to use Norplant. (The paper later apologized for the editorial and its racist overtones after protests from people inside and outside the paper.) Norplant's originator, Sheldon Segal, expressed outrage that a device intended to enhance reproductive freedom might be used coercively to restrict it.

Similar concerns about coercion were soon raised when bills were introduced in Kansas, Louisiana, Mississippi, Tennessee, and Ohio offering incentives to women on public assistance for using Norplant. Bills were also introduced in Kansas,

Ohio, South Carolina, and Washington, all generally providing for the involuntary implantation of Norplant in substance-abusing women who had given, or might give, birth to drug-addicted children. Most of these bills died in committee. The most famous court case involving Norplant occurred in Tulare County, California, in January 1991, when Superior Court Judge Howard Broadman ordered Darlene Johnson, who was convicted of child abuse, to use Norplant for three years as a condition of her probation. In April 1991, a trial judge in Indiana ordered a defendant to use Norplant after she allowed her boyfriend to kill her six-month-old son. Since 1966, there have been at least twenty cases in which judges have ordered criminal defendants to be sterilized, to practice contraception, or to refrain from becoming pregnant.

A number of commentators view such legislation and court orders as examples of an assault on reproductive rights. They see parallels between past occurrences of sterilization abuse and the potential for coercive uses of Norplant. As an article in *The New York Times* expressed it:

> The same qualities that make Norplant a boon to women may be a two-edged sword: some public health groups and women's advocates worry that the contraceptive could easily become an instrument of social control, forced on poor women and others whose fertility is seen as more of a threat to society than a blessing.[1]

Incentives aimed at women on public assistance, such as those proposed in Louisiana and Kansas, have been characterized as "clearly coercive, discriminatory, and a violation of those women's reproductive rights."[2]

However, it is often far from clear whether a given policy or program is coercive because the concept is complex, controversial, and often difficult to apply. For example, should we understand coercion narrowly, as involving only physical threats of force? Or can the offering of benefits and incentives to get people to do things they would otherwise not do be coercive? Intuitions differ as

From Coerced Contraception, Ellen Moskovitz and Bruce Jennings, eds., Georgetown University Press, 1996, pp. 53–78. Used with permission from publisher.

EDITORS' NOTE: Some footnotes have been omitted; those wishing to follow up on sources should consult the original.

to whether a proposal *expands* or *constricts* a person's options, and so enhances or limits freedom. Moreover, the essentially normative nature of coercion claims entails that judgments about whether a policy is coercive embody substantive moral arguments, about which reasonable people can disagree.

Despite the problematic nature of many coercion claims, the concept of coercion can be useful in evaluating social policies, if the concept is carefully and appropriately used. To label a policy "coercive" is to make a *prima facie* objection to it. However, it should be remembered that coercion is not always unjustified or improper: for example, the coercive sanctions attached to the law to force individuals to obey. Moreover, some socially desirable ends can only be achieved through mutually agreed-on coercive policies, such as taxation and immunization. Another problem is that too often coercion is used as a generalized term of abuse, without sufficient attention paid to the identifiable dimensions of the concept. Such intellectual sloppiness has two unfortunate results. First, it undercuts the charge of coercion where this is an apt and important moral criticism. Second, the overuse of coercion as a criticism creates the impression that there are no other reasons for objecting to social policies. Even if a policy is not correctly characterized as coercive, there may be other, equally important, objections to it. Incentives for birth control, for example, might be criticized as violating autonomy, equal protection, or informed consent, even if offering such incentives is not coercive.

After analyzing the concept of coercion in the first part of this article, I apply the analysis in the second part to two cases: (1) mandated birth control for probationers, and (2) financial incentives for women on public assistance. In both cases, the claim that such policies are coercive, while plausible, is not obviously correct. In any event, coerciveness may not be their most objectionable feature.

THE CONCEPT OF COERCION

COERCION, VOLUNTARINESS, AND RESPONSIBILITY

Coercion plays an important role in morality and the law because coercion typically acts as a *dis-claimer of responsibility*. It has this role because coercion deprives people of free choice and thus makes what they do, to some extent, nonvoluntary.

The most clearcut examples of coercion involve physical force or constraint. In the paradigm coercion situation, A says to B, brandishing a pistol, "Your money or your life." In what sense is B not acting according to his own free will? It is not that A deprives B of volition, as when A gets B to sign a contract by physically moving his hand, or by hypnotizing B. When B gives A his money, he does so deliberately and intentionally. He does what he most wants to do, given the situation. The coercion in this example is not the absence of volition, but rather *constrained volition*. Although intentional and deliberate, B's action is not done freely or autonomously.

The mere existence of external pressure or influence does not establish coercion. The influence or pressure exerted must be of a kind and amount that diminishes free choice. The central question for understanding the concept of coercion, then, is *how much, and what kind of, influence or pressure deprives actions and decisions of their autonomous character.* As we will see, the question does not have a simple or straightforward answer. Moreover, pressure or influence that does not qualify as coercive may also be morally objectionable, for example if it exploits a person's desperate situation.

While the highwayman example is a clear case of coercion, we need a general theory of coercion to help us decide more controversial cases. Such a theory is given by Alan Wertheimer in his book, *Coercion.*[3]

WERTHEIMER'S TWO-PRONGED THEORY

This theory consists of two independent tests for coercion or duress, each of which is necessary and which are together jointly sufficient. The two prongs are:

1. The choice prong. A's proposal is coercive only if B has *no reasonable alternative but to succumb* to A's proposal.

2. The proposal prong. A's proposal is coercive only if it is *wrongful* (and not simply because it deprives B of free will and judgment). In general, if A has a right to do what he proposes, then his proposal is not

wrongful (although it may be morally objectionable on other grounds).

COERCION AS NORMATIVE

Note that the two-pronged theory is a moralized theory. That is, its conditions of application contain an ineliminable reference to moral rightness and wrongness. We cannot decide whether a proposal is coercive without talking about what A and B have a right to do, or should do. Although a few philosophers have attempted to give morally neutral analyses of coercion, there appears to be general agreement that the concept of coercion is inescapably normative.[4] To take a recent example from the law, a woman was convicted of homicide after she participated in the kidnapping of an executive who died. She claimed to be a battered wife, and said that she was forced by her husband to participate. The judge rejected her argument, saying that being slapped and yelled at doesn't justify torture and murder. His judgment that she was not coerced derives from his conviction that her actions were unjustifiable; therefore she was morally responsible. In many situations, the judgment that someone was coerced, or had "no choice," depends on whether we think the person was justified in acting as he or she did.

OFFERS AND THREATS

Both offers and threats are proposals that provide an external influence or impetus to action. Yet threats coerce, whereas offers generally do not. How can threats be distinguished from offers? The intuitive answer is that threats limit freedom, whereas offers enhance it; that one acts involuntarily in response to a threat, whereas one voluntarily accepts an offer; that the recipient of an offer is free to decline, whereas the recipient of a threat is not. Wertheimer characterizes the distinction between threats and offers this way: A threatens B by proposing to make B worse off relative to some baseline. A makes an offer when, if B does not accept A's proposal, B will be no worse off than in the relevant baseline position.

However, sometimes it seems that A's proposal can make B better off than he would have been, relative to his baseline situation, and still be coercive. Consider this example from Robert Nozick:

The Slave Case. A beats B, his slave, each morning, for reasons having nothing to do with B's behavior. A proposes not to beat B the next morning, if B will do X, which is distasteful to him.

Assume that B would rather do X than get beaten. If we think of B's baseline as being set by what *normally happens* (call this the "statistical test"), A is making an offer (noncoercive). B expects to be beaten each morning, and relative to that expectation, A is proposing to make B better off. However, we can also think of the baseline as being set by what is *morally required* (call this the "moral test"). Under the moral test, A is making a threat (coercive). For A is morally required not to beat B, indeed, not to own slaves at all, and relative to that baseline, A is proposing to make B worse off. In addition to the statistical and moral tests, Wertheimer says there is also a "phenomenological test": how it seems to B. A's proposal may *feel like* a threat to B. Consider the following example:

Each week, A calls B and asks her for a date. They have grown fond of each other, but they have not had sexual intercourse. After three months, A tells B that unless she has sexual intercourse with him, he will stop dating her.

Wertheimer comments that under the statistical and phenomenological tests, B may or may not regard A's proposal as a threat. "That would depend upon the history of their relationship and B's expectations."[5] Applying the moral test is complicated, but Wertheimer thinks that it is clear that B has no right that A continue to date her, and on B's preferred terms. Relative to that moral baseline, A's proposal is an offer.

It is by no means clear that Wertheimer has applied the moral test correctly. One might equally argue that A is not entitled to expect sexual intercourse from B, and is wrong to insist on sex as a condition of the relationship continuing. Relative to that moral baseline, A's proposal is a threat. The correct application of the moral test would depend on factual details not given, such as the age of the parties, their views on the morality of extramarital sexual intercourse, and so forth.

Wertheimer maintains that it is because there are these different tests, all of which can be used to characterize A's proposal as an offer or a threat, that intuitions about the coerciveness of proposals often conflict. What looks like an offer may really be a threat. It depends on what test is used—and, I would add, how the test is applied—to set the baseline. Moreover, Wertheimer doesn't think there's any way to decide which is *the* correct test to determine the baseline. This often makes it difficult to say, with any certitude, that a proposal is coercive (and so objectionable). Consider the following intriguing example.

> *The Lecherous Millionaire:* B's child will die without expensive surgery which her insurance doesn't cover, and for which the state will not pay. A, a millionaire, offers to pay for the surgery if B will agree to become his mistress.

Wertheimer says that this is an offer under either the statistical or the moral test: B does not expect A to pay for her child's surgery, nor is A morally required to do so.

Some philosophers argue that offers, as well as threats, can be "coercive." Joel Feinberg argues that the Lecherous Millionaire's proposal is a "coercive offer" because it manipulates B's options in such a way that B has no choice but to comply, or else suffer an unacceptable alternative. Wertheimer responds that A also "manipulates" B's options when he offers him a job at three times his present salary. This may well be "an offer he cannot refuse," yet surely such an offer is not coercive. Moreover, what if it was the child's mother who proposed to the millionaire, knowing of his lecherous propensities, that she become his mistress if he will pay for the surgery? Surely that wouldn't be a coercive offer, Wertheimer says, so why is it coercive when A makes the offer to B? A's proposal may be "unseemly," according to Wertheimer, but it is not coercive, because it expands rather than reduces B's options.

It appears that, for Wertheimer, the phenomenological test is not really a test of coerciveness at all. The fact that someone feels threatened is not conclusive evidence, if it is evidence at all, that the proposal is coercive. The true test, for Wertheimer, is whether the recipient's options have been expanded or reduced. This bears further examination. Can an offer which expands one's options nevertheless be coercive? Consider the proposal made in the fairy tale, *Rumpelstiltskin.* According to the story, the miller's daughter will be put to death if she doesn't spin a roomful of straw into gold. Twice Rumpelstiltskin saves the miller's daughter by spinning the straw into gold in return for trinkets she gives him. The third time, however, the miller's daughter has nothing left to give him. Rumpelstiltskin then offers to spin the straw into gold in return for her firstborn child. The girl reluctantly accepts.

Has the miller's daughter been coerced? Feinberg would say yes. The decision to give up her child is not one she makes freely or willingly or voluntarily. She makes it because otherwise she will be killed. Admittedly, the miller's daughter prefers relinquishing her child to being put to death, but the fact that she prefers one alternative to the other doesn't prevent the offer from being coercive. The robbery victim also prefers giving up his money to being killed. What makes both of these examples cases of coercion is that the choosers reasonably see themselves as having no choice.

Wertheimer would say that the miller's daughter was not coerced, because if she declines Rumpelstiltskin's offer, she will be no worse off than she was before the offer was made. Admittedly, she will be put to death, but she would have been put to death anyway, regardless of whether Rumpelstiltskin made his proposal. On Wertheimer's analysis, then, Rumpelstiltskin's offer (distasteful as it may be) expands the maiden's options, and therefore is noncoercive.

Is there a way to reconcile the persuasive intuition that there can be "coercive offers" (and that the offers made by the Lecherous Millionaire and Rumpelstiltskin are such offers) with Wertheimer's analysis of coercion? One possibility is to reconsider the moral baseline. Under the moral test, whether Rumpelstiltskin is making an offer or a threat will depend on whether Rumpelstiltskin has an obligation to spin the straw into gold for the miller's daughter. It might seem that he has no such obligation. Individuals are not generally obligated to do work for others, especially without compensation. However, morality requires that we help others when they will die otherwise, and when giving the help is not terribly onerous. We might not want such moral obligations to be made into law, but it is certainly plausible that there are such obligations. On this basis, it could be argued that Rumpelstiltskin ought to help the miller's daughter, even though she has nothing left to give him, because she needs his help so desperately, and helping her isn't terribly burdensome to him.

Relative to that moral baseline, he is proposing to make her worse off. His proposal is therefore a threat, and by definition coercive.

However, this move will not help us with the Lecherous Millionaire. His offer can be seen as a threat only if we maintain that the millionaire has a moral obligation to pay for the child's expensive surgery. It does not seem plausible to maintain that a person—even a very wealthy person—is morally required to lay out large sums of money to meet the medical expenses of strangers. What's objectionable about the millionaire's behavior is not that he fails to help someone he could have helped; rather, it is that he exploits the woman's desperate situation in a particularly nasty way. That his offer is exploitive is unquestionable. The question is whether such exploitation should be regarded as coercive (because, under the circumstances, the child's mother has "no choice") or whether it should be regarded as noncoercive (because the millionaire does not create, but merely takes advantage of, the woman's plight). In my opinion, this is an example of a difference that does not make a moral difference, since—as the examples show—an exploitive (but not coercive) offer can be as morally reprehensible as a coercive one.

INCENTIVES

Incentives, like threats, are ways of trying to get people to do things. Unlike threats, incentives are typically welcome offers that seem morally unobjectionable. Yet sometimes inducements and incentives are alleged to be coercive. For example, A offers B, who is desperately poor, a large sum of money for his kidney. Why is this thought to be coercive? It isn't just that B is being offered a lot of money; generous offers are not coercive. Perhaps the objection is that B's impoverished situation may make him unable fully to weigh the costs and benefits of the proposal. He may be inclined to weigh too heavily the short-term benefits of having the money, versus the long-term risks of not having an extra kidney. Offering a poor person money for a body part exploits or takes advantage of his poverty, but it is not clear that it forces or coerces him.

Incentives to do things that people ordinarily would not consider doing appear to be in the same category as exploitive offers. Whether they are

coercive is unclear. However, even if they are not coercive, they may be morally impermissible. Only a detailed substantive analysis can determine this. To determine the morality of offering incentives, we have to ask other questions, such as, Can persons in such conditions make intelligent judgments about their interests? Does society have an obligation to provide them with better alternatives? If society has not provided them with better alternatives, should such persons be allowed to improve their situations anyway?

The next section applies the above discussion of the concept of coercion to several issues: court-ordered birth control as a condition of probation, financial incentives for welfare mothers to use long-term contraception, the "Dollar-a-Day" program in Colorado, and the decision to offer Norplant in a Baltimore high school.

APPLYING THE CONCEPT OF COERCION

PEOPLE V. JOHNSON

Darlene Johnson was a 27-year-old African-American woman with a criminal record for check fraud, petty theft, disturbing the peace, battery, and burglary. At the time of her conviction for child abuse, she had four children and was pregnant with the fifth. Her 11-year-old son was living with her mother and stepfather, and she had custody of her three daughters, aged 3, 5, and 6.

On Sept. 13, 1990, Johnson's stepfather contacted the police to report that she was physically abusing her children. The five- and six-year-old girls told the police that their mother and her boyfriend had beaten them with a belt, sometimes using the buckle end, and an electrical cord. They had significant bruises on their backs, arms, necks, and legs. The state removed all of the children and placed them in foster care.

On December 13, Johnson pleaded guilty to three counts of inflicting corporal injury on children, and appeared before Judge Howard Broadman, a judge known for his creative sentencing.[6] Because of her prior convictions, Johnson could have been sentenced to six years in prison but, because her past crimes were unrelated to child abuse, the judge felt enhancement was inappropriate. Her application for probation was granted, and her prison sentence was suspended for three years. Included in the conditions of probation were that she attend counseling and parenting programs; that she refrain from striking her children; and that she abstain from alcohol, tobacco, or drugs during her pregnancy. Finally, her probation was conditioned on her agreement to use Norplant for three years, after she delivered. She was instructed to see her own doctor for insertion.

On January 10, 1991, Johnson's attorney moved for reconsideration of the Norplant condition, claiming that it violated her right to privacy, and that by imposing such a condition the court was practicing medicine without a license. Johnson said that she had agreed out of fear of being sent back to prison and that she didn't know enough about Norplant to make an informed decision. Furthermore, she declared that she suffered from high blood pressure, heart murmurs, and diabetes, conditions that made her an unsuitable candidate for Norplant.

Judge Broadman denied the motion, holding that Johnson had given her informed consent to Norplant, and maintaining that the terms of her probation were reasonably related to the compelling state interest in reformation, rehabilitation, and public safety. Acknowledging that the Norplant condition did impinge her right to procreate, the judge noted that the right is not absolute and may be balanced against the need to prevent child abuse. Johnson appealed, but on the eve of oral argument, her probation was revoked after she tested positive for cocaine on three occasions. She was sent to state prison for five years.

PROBATION AND COERCION

Was the imposition of Norplant as a condition of probation coercive? To decide this, we must ask whether Johnson's consent was given freely and autonomously. Two factors are pertinent to answering this question: first, whether Johnson was given information about Norplant necessary for her informed consent, and second, whether the threat of prison is an external influence or pressure that deprives decisions of their autonomous character.

Despite Judge Broadman's ruling, it is clear that Johnson did not give anything remotely resem-

bling informed consent. Judge Broadman gave Johnson virtually no information about Norplant, beyond telling her that it was like the pill. She was not informed that the drug is not advised for women with diabetes, nor that some doctors will not prescribe Norplant for women with heart disease, blood clots, or high blood pressure. She was not told of any side effects of Norplant. In sum, she received none of the counseling recommended by Wyeth-Ayerst Laboratories (Norplant's American manufacturer), nor was she given the recommended thorough physical examination to screen for conditions that would contraindicate the use of Norplant. Nor was she given a chance to reflect on her decision, nor to consult with her lawyer. A decision made in such utter ignorance cannot be considered free or autonomous.

Suppose Judge Broadman had provided Ms. Johnson with more information about Norplant. What if he had made the order contingent upon her consent given after she had consulted with her doctor? Some would argue that she would still not have given genuine informed consent, because her consent was based on the fear of going to jail. However, this is true of all probation conditions. Defendants agree to them because they want to avoid being sent to jail. Probation conditions thus meet Wertheimer's "choice prong": defendants have "no reasonable alternative" but to agree. If this makes probation conditions coercive, then probation itself is problematic, not just birth control as a condition of probation. Critics of Judge Broadman's sentence, however, have not objected to probation in general, but only the imposition of Norplant.

Opposition to Judge Broadman's sentence in particular, and not probation in general, can be explained if we remember that, on Wertheimer's analysis, coercion involves *two* tests, each of which is necessary. All probation conditions fulfill the choice prong, but what about the proposal prong? The proposal prong stipulates that the proposal is *wrongful*, independently of its deprivation of free choice. To call a proposal "wrongful" is not merely to claim that there are objections to it. For example, there could be decisive utilitarian objections to a social policy. Such a policy would be a bad idea, but not necessarily wrongful. To call a proposal wrongful implies that the proposer has no right to make it, that the very making of the proposal violates the rights of the person to whom it is made. Wrongful proposals include ones that violate fundamental rights or due process, or discriminate against individuals on specious grounds.

It seems clear that the institution of probation does not qualify as a wrongful proposal, and so probation conditions in general are not coercive. However, it could be argued that imposing Norplant *is* wrongful, that this differs from typical probation conditions, such as restricting travel or freedom of association—even though these are both constitutionally protected rights. The difference is that Norplant is medical treatment. It is especially wrong, it may be said, to impose invasive medical treatment as a condition of probation. The wrongness derives in part from a conception of the doctor-patient relationship, which is supposed to be based on good faith and mutual trust. In addition, the imposition of Norplant requires bodily invasion and has the potential for harmful side effects and contraindications. These features distinguish the imposition of forced medical treatment from other probation conditions. It is doubtful that someone could be sentenced to donate bone marrow, or even a pint of blood, even if such donation were plausibly related to a legitimate aim of probation, such as rehabilitation. Note that these arguments are not based on the wrongness of restricting the probationer's fertility (an argument which is vulnerable to the counterargument that a prison term also restricts fertility), but rather based on the special wrongness of administering punishment that violates the doctor-patient relationship, involves bodily invasion, and has potentially harmful side effects.

There are other serious problems with such sentences which merit consideration. For example, issues of race and class cannot be ignored. The women who are targeted for forced use of contraception, in particular, Norplant, are most often poor women and women of color. Ms. Johnson's prosecution and sentence were very likely influenced by her race.

A recent Florida study found that black women are ten times more likely than white women to be referred for prosecution for substance abuse while pregnant, even though a comparable percentage of women of both races have been documented as using harmful drugs. Child abuse prosecutions are similarly influenced by race. It follows, therefore, that when women of color are convicted of child abuse or drug use while pregnant, and are subsequently forced to use Norplant, the decision is very likely to be racially motivated.[7]

In addition to race and class, gender is also an issue. Men procreate, men abuse children, yet it is only women whose procreative liberty is restricted. Darlene Johnson's boyfriend also allegedly beat her children, yet he was not even indicted, much less sentenced to use birth control. It might be argued that it is not so easy to mandate birth control for men, since there is no male equivalent of Norplant. However, judges have been willing to require that women—but not men—consent to sterilization, even though vasectomy is an available option. In January 1993, a Tennessee woman and her husband were convicted of molesting the woman's two sons. They were each sentenced to 10 years in prison, but the judge said he would give them probation if the *woman* would consent to a tubal ligation. The judge's offer did not require her husband to be sterilized. *The New York Times* called the order "sexism at its most flagrant":

> If he [Judge Brown] *really* believed that sterilization was sound punishment for molestation, shouldn't he have given the husband the same choice he gave the wife? Since when is it only women who are responsible for pregnancy?[8]

An issue relating to discrimination concerns contraception and religious beliefs. Some religions (e.g., Roman Catholicism) prohibit the use of contraceptives. Women who are offered a choice between prison and contraception are thus forced to choose between their freedom and their religion. Mandatory use of Norplant may therefore violate the First Amendment.

In addition to informed consent and discrimination, mandated birth control is likely to create problems with procedural due process. Due process is violated when a court imposes a sentence that is vague or indefinite. The probationer must be able to tell whether she is conforming with the probation condition, and the court must be able to determine whether she has violated its command. In addition, probation conditions must be one with which the probationer is able to comply.

Sometimes judges have ordered convicted child abusers "not to conceive." Such orders are so vague as to violate due process. Is the order intended to require the probationer to abstain from having sex? In *Johnson* and other cases, the judges expressly noted that the sentences were not intended to interfere with the defendants' rights to sexual expression. However, if courts do not intend to mandate abstinence, an order not to conceive demands the impossible, because no contraceptive method is 100 percent effective. Perhaps the order is intended as requiring a good faith effort to avoid conception. However, this is also indefinite and vague. There may be medical reasons why a woman cannot use a very reliable form of contraception, such as the pill or Norplant. Her doctor may recommend against an IUD, out of concern for future fertility. If she faithfully uses a diaphragm, and becomes pregnant anyway (the failure rate is 10 percent), has she violated her probation? And how does a court intend to monitor her use of such methods to determine compliance?

Mandating a specific form of birth control, such as Norplant, avoids the problem of violating procedural due process. To comply with the probation condition, the probationer need only have Norplant implanted and leave it in for the requisite period of time. Because Norplant is inserted in the upper arm, compliance can be determined without invading her privacy. If she should become pregnant, it would clearly be due to product failure, not to any lapse on her part.

However, Norplant is not for every woman. It has a range of side effects which make it unacceptable to some women. Moreover, women who smoke heavily, who experience abnormal vaginal bleeding, blood clots, or any circulation or heart problems or liver disease, or who have had breast cancer or any condition for which they were treated with hormones are strongly advised against using Norplant. Women who have diabetes, high blood pressure, migraines or frequent headaches, depression, epilepsy, or gall bladder or kidney disease should consider Norplant use with extreme caution. To mandate Norplant for a woman who has one of these conditions, especially if her doctor advises against it, would violate every principle of informed consent and the right to refuse medical treatment.

Thus, judges who wish to prevent convicted child abusers from having babies are caught between a rock and a hard place. As Stacey Arthur puts it:

> If a court complies with standards of due process by prescribing the contraceptive method to be used with clarity and precision, it may violate a probationer's right to give informed consent before receiving medical treatment. However, if a court chooses the less intrusive path and orders a defendant to consult with her physician and freely select the method of birth control that she prefers, it runs the risk that (1) she will choose none, or (2) that her choice will create insurmountable procedural due process problems.[9]

The likelihood that informed consent to medical treatment will not be obtained; the bodily invasiveness; the damage to the doctor-patient relationship; the potential for discrimination based on race, gender, or religion; and the violation of procedural due process make a powerful case for regarding as wrongful the imposition of Norplant as a condition of probation. Thus, such sentences fulfill both prongs and are properly denounced as coercive. Even if one takes the position that mandated birth control is no more coercive than other probation conditions, these additional objections are decisive reasons for rejecting mandated birth control as a condition of probation. I conclude that, despite the legitimate concern with a rising tide of child abuse, judges should not impose birth control as a condition of probation. At the same time, drug and psychological counselors, as well as teachers of parenting classes, will undoubtedly and properly urge women who are not yet capable of caring for themselves to get their lives in order before having more children. To do this, they will need access to substance abuse programs and contraception, as well as protection from abusive husbands and boyfriends who force or intimidate them into sexual relations without contraceptives.

FINANCIAL INCENTIVES FOR USING BIRTH CONTROL

After Norplant was approved in December 1990, states moved rapidly to add Norplant to their Medicaid programs. All states except Massachusetts now reimburse poor women for all or part of the cost of Norplant. In 1991, a new kind of assistance program appeared: offering a cash bonus to women on public assistance if they use birth control (usually Norplant). In Kansas, a bill was introduced in 1991 that would have provided any woman on public assistance with a one-time grant of $500 for getting Norplant implanted, as well as $50 a year for each year she kept it in. Representative David Duke introduced a bill in 1991 that would have given Louisiana women on public assistance $100 a year if they used Norplant. It was amended in committee to provide $100 a year to any woman on public assistance who used any method of birth control, including abstinence. Then it was amended to remove cash incentives for the use of contraception. The final version of the bill simply provided that Norplant would be given free of charge to women on public assistance.

In Mississippi, a bill was introduced in 1992 that would have required women with four or more biological children to have Norplant implanted in order to be eligible to receive state assistance. In Tennessee, a bill was introduced in 1992 that would have provided a payment of $500 to women on public assistance if they agreed to be implanted with Norplant and additional payments of $50 annually at checkup time to ensure that the drug was still working. A similar bill was introduced in the state of Washington. All of these bills were either defeated or (more commonly) died in committee.

A bill introduced in Ohio would have provided a new welfare mother with a one-time payment of $1,000 and an increase of her monthly cash assistance to 150 percent of her base subsidy if she would agree to be sterilized by tubal ligation. If she agreed to have a long-acting contraceptive, such as Depo-Provera or Norplant, she would get a $500 payment and a 10 percent increase of her base subsidy every six months until it reached the 150-percent level. Under the bill's provisions, the welfare mother would be required to identify the father of the child. He could elect to pay child support, perform community service work, be sterilized and receive $1,000, or be sent to prison for two years. Also, a new welfare mother would have to pass a test prepared by the state Department of Human Services to show she has appropriate parenting skills. The newborn of a person who refuses to take the test or who fails could be placed with relatives or in a foster home.

Under the bill, the child could be put up for adoption if the parent doesn't pass within a year.[10]

It is difficult to imagine anyone dreaming up such a cruel law. Even if we had reason to think that tests could be devised that would reliably indicate which individuals will be neglectful or abusive parents—which is very dubious—it would be outrageous to remove a newborn simply because its mother failed the test. She might have difficulty reading or comprehending the questions. She might not speak English well. She might simply have been nervous. Children are harmed when they are taken from their mothers, harmed when they are put in foster care, especially an overburdened foster care system. Taking a newborn away from a mother who wants to keep it should be a last resort. Moreover, if society wants to ensure that children are cared for by people with adequate parenting skills, why focus on poor people? Child abuse exists in all classes and income levels. It is discriminatory to single out women on public assistance and force them to take tests to demonstrate their parenting skills, on pain of losing their babies.

Leaving aside the Ohio bill, with its nightmarish conditions, are Norplant bonus programs in general coercive? Or are they a logical extension of other kinds of incentive programs, such as those that offer incentives for welfare recipients to stay in school? In Ohio, for example, an experimental program paid teenage mothers on welfare a bonus of $62 a month if they attended school. It deducted $62 a month from their monthly checks if they skipped classes or dropped out. Researchers found that 61 percent of the teenage mothers already in school remained enrolled when they were offered incentives, as opposed to 51 percent who were not offered incentives. Among those who had already dropped out of school, 47 percent returned to classes under the incentive program, compared with 33 percent who were not given an incentive. Senator Daniel Patrick Moynihan was so impressed with the results that he is urging the Clinton Administration to offer the same education incentives nationwide.[11]

Most commentators have no objection to educational incentives. It is pointed out that financial gain motivates the poor like everyone else, and that there is nothing wrong with such incentives. If it is acceptable to offer tax breaks to the rich to get them to act in socially responsible ways (e.g., donating their art to museums rather than selling them), it is equally acceptable to offer cash incentives to young mothers to get them to stay in school.

By contrast, many regard incentives to persuade women on public assistance not to get pregnant as coercive. They argue that women are not free to reject the extra money and that it is intrinsically wrongful to ask them to curb their fertility. Let us look more closely at the arguments against this kind of incentive.

THE UNCONSTITUTIONAL CONDITIONS DOCTRINE

As Kathleen Sullivan explains it, "The doctrine of unconstitutional conditions holds that government may not grant a benefit on the condition that the beneficiary surrender a constitutional right, even if the government may withhold that benefit altogether."[12] A law that forced women to use birth control would clearly be unconstitutional. The right of privacy gives individuals the right to use, or not use, contraceptives without government intervention. If the government cannot compel women to use birth control, then it would seem that the unconstitutional conditions doctrine does not allow the government to condition a benefit, such as a cash bonus, on the use of birth control.

However, substantial uncertainty remains about the rationale for and application of the doctrine. The Supreme Court has repeatedly suggested that the problem with unconstitutional conditions is their coercive effect. However, earlier we distinguished offers, which are supposedly not coercive, from threats, which are. The question, then, is whether monetary incentives to use birth control are offers or threats. The answer to that question depends on whether the proposal makes the intended recipient worse off. It might be argued that Norplant bonus programs do not make anyone worse off, since while those who choose to participate are given extra benefits, the benefits of those who opt not to take the offer are not reduced. They remain in the same economic position they had prior to the offer. On Wertheimer's analysis, such an offer appears not to be coercive.

Sullivan argues that coercion cannot serve as the ordering principle of unconstitutional conditions doctrine. Because coercion is an inescapably normative concept, we would have to agree on the appropriate baselines in order to be able to distinguish offers from threats. Since the government does not have to offer any welfare benefits at all, it is impossible to construct or identify a normative baseline that would distinguish threats from offers.

In any event, Sullivan thinks that focusing on coercion alone misses the point:

> There is good reason to turn elsewhere in a search for the rationale of unconstitutional conditions doctrine, both because the necessary baselines are elusive, once government benefits in this context are conceded to be gratuitous, and because government, which differs significantly from any given individual, can burden rights to autonomy through means other than coercion. Coercion thus begins rather than ends the inquiry.[13]

According to Sullivan, unconstitutional conditions cases raise issues of equality as well as liberty. These cases inherently classify potential beneficiaries into two groups: those who comply with the condition, and thereby get better treatment, and those who do not. "Background inequalities of wealth and resources necessarily determine one's bargaining position in relation to government. . . . The poor may have nothing to trade but their liberties."[14]

The Supreme Court acknowledged this problem in its decision in *Skinner* v. *Oklahoma*, when it invalidated, on equal protection grounds, a state requirement of sterilization for recidivist thieves but not embezzlers. Sullivan argues that this decision implies that some rights (such as the right to procreate) are too important to be reserved for selected privileged groups. She suggests a "strict scrutiny" test for "any government benefit condition whose primary purpose or effect is to pressure recipients to alter a choice about exercise of a preferred constitutional liberty in a direction favored by government."[15] This does not mean that government could never burden a preferred liberty, since some burdens may ultimately survive strict scrutiny. The question would be whether the state's interests to be achieved by imposing the condition are sufficiently compelling to justify the burden on the preferred liberty.

What are the state's interests in offering Norplant bonuses? Obviously, saving the state money by reducing the number of children on welfare is a prime motivation, but this interest is not sufficiently compelling to justify restricting a fundamental right. Another reason is offered by David Coale:

> The most visible reason is growing discontent with the current welfare system. Decades of "antipoverty" programs have been widely criticized for failing to elevate living standards and instead creating an intergenerational cycle of welfare dependency. Those critics advocate reforms that would encourage welfare recipients to break that cycle. Examples of reforms include incentives for welfare recipients to attend school and restructuring AFDC benefits to discourage large families. Proposals to encourage Norplant use seem a natural outgrowth of this movement.[16]

The attempt to help people out of poverty is certainly a legitimate, perhaps even a compelling, state interest. It is not clear, however, that the state can try to achieve this goal through incentives for using birth control. It can be argued that linking Norplant to welfare benefits goes beyond legitimate attempts toward helping the poor improve their lives. Providing people with information about birth control, making contraceptives accessible and affordable (or even free), paying for abortion as well as childbirth—all of these activities are acceptable because they enhance individual choice. Offering fairly large sums of money to use Norplant is a different matter. A bonus of $500 to a woman on public assistance may mean the difference between the rent getting paid or not; $50 may mean the children have shoes or Christmas presents. Norplant bonuses specifically target poor women by offering them relatively large sums of money in order to influence and pressure their procreative decisions. Even if such programs are not clearly coercive, they pose a threat to the values of autonomy and equality, and should be rejected for these reasons.

CONCLUSION

Long-acting contraceptives, like Norplant, which are easy to monitor and do not require user-compliance, clearly have a potential for coercive use. However,

the charge of coercion is not always warranted. It remains controversial whether incentives paid to women on public assistance who get Norplant are coercive. Those who think they are not coercive point to the fact that the women who opt not to have Norplant are no worse off for refusing than they would be if there were no incentive program. The program thus expands, rather than contracts, their options. Those who think they are coercive maintain that poor women have no choice but to accept Norplant, or else suffer an unacceptable alternative, that is, go without desperately needed money. This dispute may be unresolvable if, as Wertheimer and Sullivan maintain, there isn't any way to decide which is the correct baseline, and therefore no way to decide whether the proposal is coercive. However, coercion is not the only possible objection. Focusing entirely on whether such programs are coercive may mask other important objections to such programs, such as their targeting of vulnerable groups, creating and reinforcing inequality.

The clearest example of the coercive use of Norplant is mandatory birth control as a condition of probation. Such sentences are not coercive solely because defendants agree to them in order to avoid going to jail; all probation conditions share this feature. However, because such sentences are potentially discriminatory and violative of religious freedom, due process, and norms of informed consent, they are morally and legally objectionable. Calling them coercive alludes to the features that make such probation conditions wrongful.

NOTES

1. Tamar Lewin, "5-Year Contraceptive Implant Seems Headed for Wide Use," *New York Times*, November 29, 1991, A1.
2. Barbara Feringa, Sarah Iden, and Allan Rosenfield, "Norplant: Potential for Coercion," in *Dimensions of New Contraceptives: Norplant and Poor Women*, ed. Sarah E. Samuels and Mark D. Smith (Henry J. Kaiser Family Foundation, 1992), p. 58.
3. Alan Wertheimer, *Coercion* (Princeton, N.J.: Princeton University Press, 1987).
4. See Kathleen M. Sullivan, "Unconstitutional Conditions," *Harvard Law Review* 102:7 (1989), pp. 1413-1506.
5. Wertheimer, *Coercion*, p. 211.

6. Stacey L. Arthur, "The Norplant Prescription: Birth Control, Woman Control, or Crime Control?" *University of California Los Angeles Law Review* 40 (1992), p. 34.

7. Julia R. Scott, "Norplant and Women of Color," in *Norplant and Poor Women*, p. 46.

8. *New York Times*, February 10, 1993.

9. Ibid., p. 99.

10. Ohio House Bill 343 (1993).

11. Jason DeParle, "Ohio Welfare Bonuses Keep Teenage Mothers in School," *New York Times*, April 12, 1993, A14.

12. Sullivan, "Unconstitutional Conditions," p. 1415.

13. Ibid., p. 1456.

14. Ibid., pp. 1497–98.

15. Ibid., pp. 1499–1500.

16. Coale, "Norplant Bonuses," pp. 196–97.

SECTION 2

The Morality of Abortion

The Unspeakable Crime of Abortion

Pope John Paul II

Among all the crimes which can be committed against life, procured abortion has characteristics making it particularly serious and deplorable. The Second Vatican Council defines abortion, together with infanticide, as an "unspeakable crime."[1]

But today, in many people's consciences, the perception of its gravity has become progressively obscured. The acceptance of abortion in the popular mind, in behaviour and even in law itself, is a telling sign of an extremely dangerous crisis of the moral sense, which is becoming more and more incapable of distinguishing between good and evil, even when the fundamental right to life is at stake. Given such a grave situation, we need now more than ever to have the courage to look the truth in the eye and *to call things by their proper name*, without yielding to convenient compromises or to the temptation of self-deception. In this regard the reproach of the Prophet is extremely straightforward: "Woe to those who call evil good and good evil, who put darkness for light and light for darkness" (*Is* 5:20). Especially in the case of abortion there is a widespread use of ambiguous terminology, such as "interruption of pregnancy," which tends to hide abortion's true nature and to attenuate its seriousness in public opinion. Perhaps this linguistic phenomenon is itself a symptom of an uneasiness of conscience. But no word has the power to change the reality of things: procured abortion is *the deliberate and direct killing, by whatever means it is carried out, of a human being in the initial phase of his or her existence, extending from conception to birth.*

The moral gravity of procured abortion is apparent in all its truth if we recognize that we are dealing with murder and, in particular, when we consider the specific elements involved. The one eliminated is a human being at the very beginning of life. No one more absolutely *innocent* could be imagined. In no way could this human being ever be considered an aggressor, much less an unjust aggressor! He or she is *weak*, defenseless, even to the point of lacking that minimal form of defence consisting in the poignant power of a newborn baby's cries and tears. The unborn child is *totally entrusted* to the protection and care of the woman carrying him or her in the womb.

From John Paul II. *Evangelium Vitae*, Encyclical Letter, August 16, 1993. Copyright © 1993 Libreria Editrice Vaticana.

And yet sometimes it is precisely the mother herself who makes the decision and asks for the child to be eliminated, and who then goes about having it done.

It is true that the decision to have an abortion is often tragic and painful for the mother, insofar as the decision to rid herself of the fruit of conception is not made for purely selfish reasons or out of convenience, but out of a desire to protect certain important values such as her own health or a decent standard of living for the other members of the family. Sometimes it is feared that the child to be born would live in such conditions that it would be better if the birth did not take place. Nevertheless, these reasons and others like them, however serious and tragic, *can never justify the deliberate killing of an innocent human being.*

As well as the mother, there are often other people too who decide upon the death of the child in the womb. In the first place, the father of the child may be to blame, not only when he directly pressures the woman to have an abortion, but also when he indirectly encourages such a decision on her part by leaving her alone to face the problems of pregnancy:[2] in this way the family is thus mortally wounded and profaned in its nature as a community of love and in its vocation to be the "sanctuary of life." Nor can one overlook the pressures which sometimes come from the wider family circle and from friends. Sometimes the woman is subjected to such strong pressure that she feels psychologically forced to have an abortion: certainly in this case moral responsibility lies particularly with those who have directly or indirectly obliged her to have an abortion. Doctors and nurses are also responsible, when they place at the service of death skills which were acquired for promoting life.

But responsibility likewise falls on the legislators who have promoted and approved abortion laws, and, to the extent that they have a say in the matter, on the administrators of the health-care centres where abortions are performed. A general and no less serious responsibility lies with those who have encouraged the spread of an attitude of sexual permissiveness and a lack of esteem for motherhood, and with those who should have ensured—but did not—effective family and social policies in support of families, especially larger families and those with particular financial and educational needs. Finally, one cannot overlook the network of complicity which reaches out to include international institutions, foundations and associations which systematically campaign for the legalization and spread of abortion in the world. In this sense abortion goes beyond the responsibility of individuals and beyond the harm done to them, and takes on a distinctly social dimension. It is a most serious *wound* inflicted on society and its culture by the very people who ought to be society's promoters and defenders. As I wrote in my *Letter to Families*, "we are facing an immense threat to life: not only to the life of individuals but also to that of civilization itself."[3] We are facing what can be called a *"structure of sin"* which opposes human life not yet born.

Some people try to justify abortion by claiming that the result of conception, at least up to a certain number of days, cannot yet be considered a personal human life. But in fact, "from the time that the ovum is fertilized, a life is begun which is neither that of the father nor the mother; it is rather the life of a new human being with his own growth. It would never be made human if it were not human already. This has always been clear, and . . . modern genetic science offers clear confirmation. It has demonstrated that from the first instant there is established the programme of what this living being will be: a person, this individual person with his characteristic aspects already well determined. Right from fertilization the adventure of a human life begins, and each of its capacities requires time—a rather lengthy time—to find its place and to be in a position to act."[4] Even if the presence of a spiritual soul cannot be ascertained by empirical data, the results themselves of scientific research on the human embryo provide "a valuable indication for discerning by the use of reason a personal presence at the moment of the first appearance of a human life: how could a human individual not be a human person?"[5]

Furthermore, what is at stake is so important that, from the standpoint of moral obligation, the mere probability that a human person is involved would suffice to justify an absolutely clear prohibition of any intervention aimed at killing a human embryo. Precisely for this reason, over and above all scientific debates and those philosophical affirmations to which the Magisterium has not expressly committed itself, the Church has always taught and continues to teach that the result of human procreation, from the first moment of its existence, must be guaranteed that unconditional respect which is morally due to the human being in his or her totality and unity as body and spirit: *"The human being is to be respected and treated as a person fom the moment of conception*; and therefore from that same moment his rights as a person must be recognized, among which in the first place is the inviolable right of every innocent human being to life."[6] . . .

NOTES

1. Pastoral Constitution on the Church in the Modern World *Gaudium et Spes*, 51: "Abortius necnon infanticidium nefanda sunt crimina."
2. Cf. John Paul II. Apostolic Letter *Muliens Dignitatem* 15 August 1988), 14:*AAS* 8O (1988), 1686.
3. No. 21:*AAS* 86 (1994), 920.
4. Congregation for the Doctrine of the Faith, *Declaration on Procured Abortion* (18 November 1974), Nos. 12–13: *AAS* 66 (1974), 738.
5. Congregation for the Doctrine of the Faith, Instruction on Respect for Human Life in Its Origin and on the Dignity of Procreation *Donum vitae* (22 February 1987), I, No. 1:*AAS*80 (1988), 78–79.
6. *Ibid., loc.* cit:., 79.

A Defense of Abortion[1]

Judith Jarvis Thomson

Most opposition to abortion relies on the premise that the fetus is a human being, a person, from the moment of conception. The premise is argued for, but, as I think, not well. Take, for example, the most common argument. We are asked to notice that the development of a human being from conception through birth into childhood is continuous; then it is said that to draw a line, to choose a point in this development and say "before this point the thing is not a person, after this point it is a person" is to make an arbitrary choice, a choice for which in the nature of things no good reason can be given. It is concluded that the fetus is, or anyway that we had better say it is, a person from the moment of conception. But this conclusion does not follow. Similar things might be said about the development of an acorn into an oak tree, and it does not follow that acorns are oak trees, or that we had better say they are. Arguments of this form are sometimes called "slippery slope arguments"—the phrase is perhaps self-explanatory—and it is dismaying that opponents of abortion rely on them so heavily and uncritically.

I am inclined to agree, however, that the prospects for "drawing a line" in the development of the fetus look dim. I am inclined to think also that we shall probably have to agree that the fetus has already become a human person well before birth. Indeed, it comes as a surprise when one first learns how early in its life it begins to acquire human characteristics. By the tenth week, for example, it already has a face, arms and legs, fingers and toes; it has internal organs, and brain activity is detectable.[2] On the other hand, I think that the premise is false, that the fetus is not a person from the moment of conception. A newly fertilized ovum, a newly implanted clump of cells, is no more a person than an acorn is an oak tree. But I shall not discuss any of this. For it seems to me to be of great interest to ask what happens if, for the sake of argument, we allow the premise. How, precisely, are we supposed to get from there to the conclusion that abortion is morally impermissible? Opponents of abortion commonly spend most of their time establishing that the fetus is a person, and hardly any time

From *Philosophy and Public Affairs* Vol. 1, No. 1, 47–66. Copyright © 1971 by Princeton University Press. Reprinted by permission of Princeton University Press.

explaining the step from there to the impermissibility of abortion. Perhaps they think the step too simple and obvious to require much comment. Or perhaps instead they are simply being economical in argument. Many of those who defend abortion rely on the premise that the fetus is not a person, but only a bit of tissue that will become a person at birth; and why pay out more arguments than you have to? Whatever the explanation, I suggest that the step they take is neither easy nor obvious, that it calls for closer examination than it is commonly given, and that when we do give it this closer examination we shall feel inclined to reject it.

I propose, then, that we grant that the fetus is a person from the moment of conception. How does the argument go from here? Something like this, I take it. Every person has a right to life. So the fetus has a right to life. No doubt the mother has a right to decide what shall happen in and to her body; everyone would grant that. But surely a person's right to life is stronger and more stringent than the mother's right to decide what happens in and to her body, and so outweighs it. So the fetus may not be killed; an abortion may not be performed.

It sounds plausible. But now let me ask you to imagine this. You wake up in the morning and find yourself back to back in bed with an unconscious violinist. A famous unconscious violinist. He has been found to have a fatal kidney ailment, and the Society of Music Lovers has canvassed all the available medical records and found that you alone have the right blood type to help. They have therefore kidnapped you, and last night the violinist's circulatory system was plugged into yours, so that your kidneys can be used to extract poisons from his blood as well as your own. The director of the hospital now tells you, "Look, we're sorry the Society of Music Lovers did this to you—we would never have permitted it if we had known. But still, they did it, and the violinist now is plugged into you. To unplug you would be to kill him. But never mind, it's only for nine months. By then he will have recovered from his ailment, and can safely be unplugged from you." Is it morally incumbent on you to accede to this situation? No doubt it would be very nice of you if you did, a great kindness. But do you *have* to accede to it? What if it were not nine months, but nine years? Or longer still? What if the director of the hospital

says, "Tough luck, I agree, but you've now got to stay in bed, with the violinist plugged into you, for the rest of your life. Because remember this. All persons have a right to life, and violinists are persons. Granted you have a right to decide what happens in and to your body, but a person's right to life outweighs your right to decide what happens in and to your body. So you cannot ever be unplugged from him." I imagine you would regard this as outrageous, which suggests that something really is wrong with that plausible-sounding argument I mentioned a moment ago.

In this case, of course, you were kidnapped; you didn't volunteer for the operation that plugged the violinist into your kidneys. Can those who oppose abortion on the ground I mentioned make any exception for a pregnancy due to rape? Certainly. They can say that persons have a right to life only if they didn't come into existence because of rape; or they can say that all persons have a right to life, but that some have less of a right to life than others, in particular, that those who came into existence because of rape have less. But these statements have a rather unpleasant sound. Surely the question of whether you have a right to life at all, or how much of it you have, shouldn't turn on the question of whether or not you are the product of a rape. And in fact the people who oppose abortion on the ground I mentioned do not make this distinction, and hence do not make an exception in case of rape.

Nor do they make an exception for a case in which the mother has to spend the nine months of her pregnancy in bed. They would agree that would be a great pity, and hard on the mother; but all the same, all persons have a right to life, the fetus is a person, and so on. I suspect, in fact, that they would not make an exception for a case in which, miraculously enough, the pregnancy went on for nine years, or even the rest of the mother's life.

Some won't even make an exception for a case in which continuation of the pregnancy is likely to shorten the mother's life; they regard abortion as impermissible even to save the mother's life. Such cases are nowadays very rare, and many opponents of abortion do not accept this extreme view. All the same, it is a good place to begin: a number of points of interest come out in respect to it.

1. Let us call the view that abortion is impermissible even to save the mother's life "the extreme view." I want to suggest first that it does not issue from the argument I mentioned earlier without the addition of some fairly powerful premises. Suppose a woman has become pregnant, and now learns that she has a cardiac condition such that she will die if she carries the baby to term. What may be done for her? The fetus, being a person, has a right to life, but as the mother is a person too, so has she a right to life. Presumably they have an equal right to life. How is it supposed to come out that an abortion may not be performed? If mother and child have an equal right to life, shouldn't we perhaps flip a coin? Or should we add to the mother's right to life her right to decide what happens in and to her body, which everybody seems to be ready to grant—the sum of her rights now outweighing the fetus's right to life?

The most familiar argument here is the following. We are told that performing the abortion would be directly killing[3] the child, whereas doing nothing would not be killing the mother, but only letting her die. Moreover, in killing the child, one would be killing an innocent person, for the child has committed no crime, and is not aiming at his mother's death. And then there are a variety of ways in which this might be continued. (1) But as directly killing an innocent person is always and absolutely impermissible, an abortion may not be performed. Or, (2) as directly killing an innocent person is murder, and murder is always and absolutely impermissible, an abortion may not be performed.[4] Or, (3) as one's duty to refrain from directly killing an innocent person is more stringent than one's duty to keep a person from dying, an abortion may not be performed. Or, (4) if one's only options are directly killing an innocent person or letting a person die, one must prefer letting the person die, and thus an abortion may not be performed.[5]

Some people seem to have thought that these are not further premises which must be added if the conclusion is to be reached, but that they follow from the very fact that an innocent person has a right to life.[6] But this seems to me to be a mistake, and perhaps the simplest way to show this is to bring out that while we must certainly grant that innocent persons have a right to life, the theses in (1) through (4) are all false. Take (2), for example. If directly killing an innocent person is

murder, and thus is impermissible, then the mother's directly killing the innocent person inside her is murder, and thus is impermissible. But it cannot seriously be thought to be murder if the mother performs an abortion on herself to save her life. It cannot seriously be said that she *must* refrain, that she *must* sit passively by and wait for her death. Let us look again at the case of you and the violinist. There you are, in bed with the violinist, and the director of the hospital says to you "It's all most distressing, and I deeply sympathize, but you see this is putting an additional strain on your kidneys, and you'll be dead within the month. But you *have* to stay where you are all the same. Because unplugging you would be directly killing an innocent violinist, and that's murder, and that's impermissible." If anything in the world is true, it is that you do not commit murder, you do not do what is impermissible, if you reach around to your back and unplug yourself from that violinist to save your life. . . .

2. The extreme view could of course be weakened to say that while abortion is permissible to save the mother's life, it may not be performed by a third party, but only by the mother herself. But this cannot be right either. For what we have to keep in mind is that the mother and the unborn child are not like two tenants in a small house which has, by an unfortunate mistake, been rented to both: the mother *owns* the house. The fact that she does adds to the offensiveness of deducing that the mother can do nothing from the supposition that third parties can do nothing. But it does more than this: it casts a bright light on the supposition that third parties can do nothing. Certainly it lets us see that a third party who says "I cannot choose between you" is fooling himself if he thinks this is impartiality. If Jones has found and fastened on a certain coat, which he needs to keep him from freezing, but which Smith also needs to keep him from freezing, then it is not impartiality that says "I cannot choose between you" when Smith owns the coat. Women have said again and again "This body is *my* body!" and they have reason to feel angry, reason to feel that it has been like shouting into the wind. Smith, after all, is hardly likely to bless us if we say to him, "Of course it's your coat, anybody would grant that it is. But no one may choose between you and Jones who is to have it."

We should really ask what it is that says "no one may choose" in the face of the fact that the body that houses the child is the mother's body. It may be simply a failure to appreciate this fact. But it may be something more interesting, namely the sense that one has a right to refuse to lay hands on Jones, a right to refuse to do physical violence to people, even where it would be just and fair to do so, even where justice seems to require that somebody do so. Thus justice might call for somebody to get Smith's coat back from Jones, and yet you have a right to refuse to be the one to lay hands on Jones, a right to refuse to do physical violence to him. This, I think, must be granted. But then what should be said is not "no one may choose" but only "I cannot choose," and indeed not even this, but "I will not *act*," leaving it open that somebody else can or should, and in particular that anyone in a position of authority, with the job of securing people's rights, both can and should. So this is no difficulty. I have not been arguing that any given third party must accede to the mother's request that he perform an abortion to save her life, but only that he may.

I suppose that in some views of human life the mother's body is only on loan to her, the loan not being one which gives her any prior claim to it. One who held this view might well think it impartiality to say "I cannot choose." But I shall simply ignore this possibility. My own view is that if a human being has any just, prior claim to anything at all, he has a just, prior claim to his own body. And perhaps this needn't be argued for here anyway, since, as I mentioned, the arguments against abortion we are looking at do grant that the woman has a right to decide what happens in and to her body.

But although they do grant it, I have tried to show that they do not take seriously what is done in granting it. I suggest the same thing will reappear even more clearly when we turn away from cases in which the mother's life is at stake, and attend, as I propose we now do, to the vastly more common cases in which a woman wants an abortion for some less weighty reason than preserving her own life.

3. Where the mother's life is not at stake, the argument I mentioned at the outset seems to have a much stronger pull. "Everyone has a right to life, so the unborn person has a right to life." And isn't the child's right to life weightier than anything other than the mother's own right to life, which she might put forward as ground for an abortion?

This argument treats the right to life as if it were unproblematic. It is not, and this seems to me to be precisely the source of the mistake.

For we should now, at long last, ask what it comes to, to have a right to life. In some views having a right to life includes having a right to be given at least the bare minimum one needs for continued life. But suppose that what in fact *is* the bare minimum a man needs for continued life is something he has no right at all to be given? If I am sick unto death, and the only thing that will save my life is the touch of Henry Fonda's cool hand on my fevered brow, then all the same, I have no right to be given the touch of Henry Fonda's cool hand on my fevered brow. It would be frightfully nice of him to fly in from the West Coast to provide it. It would be less nice, though no doubt well meant, if my friends flew out to the West Coast and carried Henry Fonda back with them. But I have no right at all against anybody that he should do this for me. Or again, to return to the story I told earlier, the fact that for continued life that violinist needs the continued use of your kidneys does not establish that he has a right to be given the continued use of your kidneys. He certainly has no right against you that *you* should give him continued use of your kidneys. For nobody has any right to use your kidneys unless you give him such a right; and nobody has the right against you that you shall give him this right—if you do allow him to go on using your kidneys, this is a kindness on your part, and not something he can claim from you as his due. Nor has he any right against anybody else that *they* should give him continued use of your kidneys. Certainly he had no right against the Society of Music Lovers that they should plug him into you in the first place. And if you now start to unplug yourself, having learned that you will otherwise have to spend nine years in bed with him, there is nobody in the world who must try to prevent you, in order to see to it that he is given something he has a right to be given.

Some people are rather stricter about the right to life. In their view, it does not include the right to be given anything, but amounts to, and only to, the right not to be killed by anybody. But here a related difficulty arises. If everybody is to refrain from killing that violinist, then everybody must refrain from doing a great many different sorts of things. Everybody must refrain from slitting his throat, everybody must refrain from shooting him—and everybody must refrain from unplugging you from him. But does he have a right against everybody that they shall refrain from unplugging you from him? To refrain from doing this is to allow him to continue to use your kidneys. It could be argued that he has a right against us that *we* should allow him to continue to use your kidneys. That is, while he has no right against us that we should give him the use of your kidneys, it might be argued that he anyway has a right against us that we shall not now intervene and deprive him of the use of your kidneys. I shall come back to third-party interventions later. But certainly the violinist has no right against you that *you* shall allow him to continue to use your kidneys. As I said, if you do allow him to use them, it is a kindness on your part, and not something you owe him.

The difficulty I point to here is not peculiar to the right to life. It reappears in connection with all the other natural rights; and it is something which an adequate account of rights must deal with. For present purposes it is enough just to draw attention to it. But I would stress that I am not arguing that people do not have a right to life—quite to the contrary, it seems to me that the primary control we must place on the acceptability of an account of rights is that it should turn out in that account to be a truth that all persons have a right to life. I am arguing only that having a right to life does not guarantee having either a right to be given the use of or a right to be allowed continued use of another person's body—even if one needs it for life itself. So the right to life will not serve the opponents of abortion in the very simple and clear way in which they seem to have thought it would.

4. There is another way to bring out the difficulty. In the most ordinary sort of case, to deprive someone of what he has a right to is to treat him unjustly. Suppose a boy and his small brother are jointly given a box of chocolates for Christmas. If the older boy takes the box and refuses to give his brother any of the chocolates, he is unjust to him, for the brother has been given a right to half of them. But suppose that, having learned that otherwise it means nine years in bed with that violinist, you unplug yourself from him. You surely are not being unjust to him, for you gave him no right to use your kidneys, and no one else can have given him any such right. But we have to notice that in unplugging yourself, you are killing him; and violinists, like everybody else, have a right to life, and thus in the view we were considering just now, the right not to be killed. So here you do what he supposedly has a right you shall not do, but you do not act unjustly to him in doing it.

The emendation which may be made at this point is this: the right to life consists not in the right not to be killed, but rather in the right not to be killed unjustly. This runs a risk of circularity, but never mind: it would enable us to square the fact that the violinist has a right to life with the fact that you do not act unjustly toward him in unplugging yourself, thereby killing him. For if you do not kill him unjustly, you do not violate his right to life, and so it is no wonder you do him no injustice.

But if this emendation is accepted, the gap in the argument against abortion stares us plainly in the face: it is by no means enough to show that the fetus is a person, and to remind us that all persons have a right to life—we need to be shown also that killing the fetus violates its right to life, i.e., that abortion is unjust killing. And is it?

I suppose we may take it as a datum that in a case of pregnancy due to rape the mother has not given the unborn person a right to the use of her body for food and shelter. Indeed, in what pregnancy could it be supposed that the mother has given the unborn person such a right? It is not as if there were unborn persons drifting about the world, to whom a woman who wants a child says "I invite you in."

But it might be argued that there are other ways one can have acquired a right to the use of another person's body than by having been invited to use it by that person. Suppose a woman voluntarily indulges in intercourse, knowing of the chance it will issue in pregnancy, and then she does become pregnant; is she not in part responsible for the presence, in fact the very existence, of the unborn person inside her? No doubt she did not invite it in. But doesn't her partial responsibility for its being there itself give it a right to the use of her body?[7] If so, then her aborting it would be more like the boy's taking away the chocolates, and less like your unplugging yourself from the violinist—doing so would be depriving it of what it does have a right to, and thus would be doing it an injustice.

And then, too, it might be asked whether or not she can kill it even to save her own life: If she voluntarily called it into existence, how can she now kill it, even in self-defense?

The first thing to be said about this is that it is something new. Opponents of abortion have been so concerned to make out the independence of the fetus, in order to establish that it has a right to life, just as its mother does, that they have tended to overlook the possible support they might gain from making out that the fetus is *dependent* on the mother, in order to establish that she has a special kind of responsibility for it, a responsibility that gives it rights against her which are not possessed by any independent person—such as an ailing violinist who is a stranger to her.

On the other hand, this argument would give the unborn person a right to its mother's body only if her pregnancy resulted from a voluntary act, undertaken in full knowledge of the chance a pregnancy might result from it. It would leave out entirely the unborn person whose existence is due to rape. Pending the availability of some further argument, then, we would be left with the conclusion that unborn persons whose existence is due to rape have no right to the use of their mothers' bodies, and thus that aborting them is not depriving them of anything they have a right to and hence is not unjust killing.

And we should also notice that it is not at all plain that this argument really does go even as far as it purports to. For there are cases and cases, and the details make a difference. If the room is stuffy, and I therefore open a window to air it, and a burglar climbs in, it would be absurd to say, "Ah, now he can stay, she's given him a right to the use of her house—for she is partially responsible for his presence there, having voluntarily done what enabled him to get in, in full knowledge that there are such things as burglars, and that burglars burgle." It would be still more absurd to say this if I had had bars installed outside my windows, precisely to prevent burglars from getting in, and a burglar got in only because of a defect in the bars. It remains equally absurd if we imagine it is not a burglar who climbs in, but an innocent person who blunders or falls in. Again, suppose it were like this: people-seeds drift about in the air like pollen, and if you open your windows, one may drift in and take root in your carpets or upholstery. You don't want children, so you fix up your windows with fine mesh screens, the very best you can buy. As can happen, however, and on very, very rare occa-sions does happen, one of the screens is defective; and a seed drifts in and takes root. Does the person-plant who now develops have a right to the use of your house? Surely not—despite the fact that you voluntarily opened your windows, you knowingly kept carpets and upholstered furniture, and you knew that screens were sometimes defective. Someone may argue that you are responsible for its rooting, that it does have a right to your house, because after all you *could* have lived out your life with bare floors and furniture, or with sealed windows and doors. But this won't do—for by the same token anyone can avoid a pregnancy due to rape by having a hysterectomy, or anyway by never leaving home without a (reliable!) army.

It seems to me that the argument we are looking at can establish at most that there are *some* cases in which the unborn person has a right to the use of its mother's body, and therefore *some* cases in which abortion is unjust killing. There is room for much discussion and argument as to precisely which, if any. But I think we should sidestep this issue and leave it open, for at any rate the argument certainly does not establish that all abortion is unjust killing.

5. There is room for yet another argument here, however. We surely must all grant that there may be cases in which it would be morally indecent to detach a person from your body at the cost of his life. Suppose you learn that what the violinist needs is not nine years of your life, but only one hour: all you need do to save his life is to spend one hour in that bed with him. Suppose also that letting him use your kidneys for that one hour would not affect your health in the slightest. Admittedly you were kidnapped. Admittedly you did not give anyone permission to plug him into you. Nevertheless it seems to me plain you *ought* to allow him to use your kidneys for that hour—it would be indecent to refuse.

Again, suppose pregnancy lasted only an hour, and constituted no threat to life or health. And suppose that a woman becomes pregnant as a result of rape. Admittedly she did not voluntarily do anything to bring about the existence of a child. Admittedly she did nothing at all which would give the unborn person a right to the use of her body. All the same it might well be said, as in the newly emended violinist story, that she *ought* to allow it to remain for that hour—that it would be indecent of her to refuse.

Now some people are inclined to use the term "right" in such a way that it follows from the fact that you ought to allow a person to use your body for the hour he needs, that he has a right to use your body for the hour he needs, even though he has not been given that right by any person or act. They may say that it follows also that if you refuse, you act unjustly toward him. This use of the term is perhaps so common that it cannot be called wrong; nevertheless it seems to me to be an unfortunate loosening of what we would do better to keep a tight rein on. Suppose that box of chocolates I mentioned earlier had not been given to both boys jointly, but was given only to the older boy. There he sits, stolidly eating his way through the box, his small brother watching enviously. Here we are likely to say "You ought not to be so mean. You ought to give your brother some of those chocolates." My own view is that it just does not follow from the truth of this that the brother has any right to any of the chocolates. If the boy refuses to give his brother any, he is greedy, stingy, callous—but not unjust. I suppose that the people I have in mind will say it does follow that the brother has a right to some of the chocolates, and thus that the boy does act unjustly if he refuses to give his brother any. But the effect of saying this is to obscure what we should keep distinct, namely the difference between the boy's refusal in this case and the boy's refusal in the earlier case, in which the box was given to both boys jointly, and in which the small brother thus had what was from any point of view clear title to half.

A further objection to so using the term "right" that from the fact that A ought to do a thing for B, it follows that B has a right against A that A do it for him, is that it is going to make the question of whether or not a man has a right to a thing turn on how easy it is to provide him with it; and this seems not merely unfortunate, but morally unacceptable. Take the case of Henry Fonda again. I said earlier that I had no right to the touch of his cool hand on my fevered brow even though I needed it to save my life. I said it would be frightfully nice of him to fly in from the West Coast to provide me with it, but that I had no right against him that he should do so. But suppose he isn't on the West Coast. Suppose he has only to walk across the room, place a hand briefly on my brow—and lo, my life is saved. Then surely he

ought to do it; it would be indecent to refuse. Is it to be said, "Ah, well, it follows that in this case she has a right to the touch of his hand on her brow, and so it would be an injustice for him to refuse"? So that I have a right to it when it is easy for him to provide it, though no right when it's hard? It's rather a shocking idea that anyone's rights should fade away and disappear as it gets harder and harder to accord them to him.

So my own view is that even though you ought to let the violinist use your kidneys for the one hour he needs, we should not conclude that he has a right to do so—we should say that if you refuse, you are, like the boy who owns all the chocolates and will give none away, self-centered and callous, indecent in fact, but not unjust. And similarly, that even supposing a case in which a woman pregnant due to rape ought to allow the unborn person to use her body for the hour he needs, we should not conclude that he has a right to do so; we should conclude that she is self-centered, callous, indecent, but not unjust, if she refuses. The complaints are no less grave; they are just different. However, there is no need to insist on this point. If anyone does wish to deduce "he has a right" from "you ought," then all the same he must surely grant that there are cases in which it is not morally required of you that you allow that violinist to use your kidneys, and in which he does not have a right to use them, and in which you do not do him an injustice if you refuse. And so also for mother and unborn child. Except in such cases as the unborn person has a right to demand it—and we were leaving open the possibility that there may be such cases—nobody is morally *required* to make large sacrifices, of health, of all other interests and concerns, of all other duties and commitments, for nine years, or even for nine months, in order to keep another person alive.

6. We have in fact to distinguish between two kinds of Samaritan: the Good Samaritan and what we might call the Minimally Decent Samaritan. The story of the Good Samaritan, you will remember, goes like this:

> A certain man went down from Jerusalem to Jericho, and fell among thieves, which stripped him of his raiment, and wounded him, and departed, leaving him half dead.
> And by chance there came down a certain priest that way; and when he saw him, he passed by on the other side.

And likewise a Levite, when he was at the place, came and looked on him, and passed by on the other side.

But a certain Samaritan, as he journeyed, came where he was; and when he saw him he had compassion on him.

And went to him, and bound up his wounds, pouring in oil and wine, and set him on his own beast, and brought him to an inn, and took care of him.

And on the morrow, when he departed, he took out two pence, and gave them to the host, and said unto him, "Take care of him; and whatsoever thou spendest more, when I come again, I will repay thee."

(Luke 10:30–35)

The Good Samaritan went out of his way, at some cost to himself, to help one in need of it. We are not told what the options were, that is, whether or not the priest and the Levite could have helped by doing less than the Good Samaritan did, but assuming they could have, then the fact they did nothing at all shows they were not even Minimally Decent Samaritans, not because they were not Samaritans, but because they were not even minimally decent.

These things are a matter of degree, of course, but there is a difference, and it comes out perhaps most clearly in the story of Kitty Genovese, who, as you will remember, was murdered while thirty-eight people watched or listened, and did nothing at all to help her. A Good Samaritan would have rushed out to give direct assistance against the murderer. Or perhaps we had better allow that it would have been a Splendid Samaritan who did this, on the ground that it would have involved a risk of death for himself. But the thirty-eight not only did not do this, they did not even trouble to pick up a phone to call the police. Minimally Decent Samaritanism would call for doing at least that, and their not having done it was monstrous.

After telling the story of the Good Samaritan, Jesus said, "Go, and do thou likewise." Perhaps he meant that we are morally required to act as the Good Samaritan did. Perhaps he was urging people to do more than is morally required of them. At all events it seems plain that it was not morally required of any of the thirty-eight that he rush out to give direct assistance at the risk of his own life, and that it is not morally required of anyone that he give long stretches of his life—nine years or nine months—to sustaining the life of a person who has no special right (we were leaving open the possibility of this) to demand it.

Indeed, with one rather striking class of exceptions, no one in any country in the world is *legally* required to do anywhere near as much as this for anyone else. The class of exceptions is obvious. My main concern here is not the state of the law in respect to abortion, but it is worth drawing attention to the fact that in no state in this country is any man compelled by law to be even a Minimally Decent Samaritan to any person; there is no law under which charges could be brought against the thirty-eight who stood by while Kitty Genovese died. By contrast, in most states in this country women are compelled by law to be not merely Minimally Decent Samaritans, but Good Samaritans to unborn persons inside them. This doesn't by itself settle anything one way or the other, because it may well be argued that there should be laws in this country—as there are in many European countries—compelling at least Minimally Decent Samaritanism.[8] But it does show that there is a gross injustice in the existing state of the law. And it shows also that the groups currently working against liberalization of abortion laws, in fact working toward having it declared unconstitutional for a state to permit abortion, had better start working for the adoption of Good Samaritan laws generally, or earn the charge that they are acting in bad faith.

I should think, myself, that Minimally Decent Samaritan laws would be one thing, Good Samaritan laws quite another, and in fact highly improper. But we are not here concerned with the law. What we should ask is not whether anybody should be compelled by law to be a Good Samaritan, but whether we must accede to a situation in which somebody is being compelled—by nature, perhaps—to be a Good Samaritan. We have, in other words, to look now at third-party interventions. I have been arguing that no person is morally required to make large sacrifices to sustain the life of another who has no right to demand them, and this even where the sacrifices do not include life itself; we are not morally required to be Good Samaritans or anyway Very Good Samaritans to one another. But what if a man cannot extricate himself from such a situation? What if he appeals to us to extricate him? It seems to me plain that there are cases in which we can, cases in which a Good Samaritan would extricate him. There you are, you were kidnapped, and nine years in bed with that violinist lie ahead of you. You have your own life to lead. You are sorry, but you simply cannot see giving up so much of your life to the sustaining of his. You cannot extricate yourself, and ask us to do so. I should have thought that—in light of his having no right to the use of your body—it was obvious that we do not have to accede to your being forced to give up so much. We can do what you ask. There is no injustice to the violinist in our doing so.

7. Following the lead of the opponents of abortion, I have throughout been speaking of the fetus merely as a person, and what I have been asking is whether or not the argument we began with, which proceeds only from the fetus's being a person, really does establish its conclusion. I have argued that it does not.

But of course there are arguments and arguments, and it may be said that I have simply fastened on the wrong one. It may be said that what is important is not merely the fact that the fetus is a person, but that it is a person for whom the woman has a special kind of responsibility issuing from the fact that she is its mother. And it might be argued that all my analogies are therefore irrelevant—for you do not have that special kind of responsibility for that violinist, Henry Fonda does not have that special kind of responsibility for me. And our attention might be drawn to the fact that men and women both *are* compelled by law to provide support for their children.

I have in effect dealt (briefly) with this argument in section 4 above; but a (still briefer) recapitulation now may be in order. Surely we do not have any such "special responsibility" for a person unless we have assumed it, explicitly or implicitly. If a set of parents do not try to prevent pregnancy, do not obtain an abortion, and then at the time of birth of the child do not put it out for adoption, but rather take it home with them, then they have assumed responsibility for it, they have given it rights, and they cannot *now* withdraw support from it at the cost of its life because they now find it difficult to go on providing for it. But if they have taken all reasonable precautions against having a child, they do not simply by virtue of their biological relationship to the child who comes into existence have a special

responsibility for it. They may wish to assume responsibility for it, or they may not wish to. And I am suggesting that if assuming responsibility for it would require large sacrifices, then these parents may refuse. A Good Samaritan would not refuse— or anyway, a Splendid Samaritan, if the sacrifices that had to be made were enormous. But then so would a Good Samaritan assume responsibility for that violinist; so would Henry Fonda, if he is a Good Samaritan, fly in from the West Coast and assume responsibility for me.

8. My argument will be found unsatisfactory on two counts by many of those who want to regard abortion as morally permissible. First, while I do argue that abortion is not impermissible, I do not argue that it is always permissible. There may well be cases in which carrying the child to term requires only Minimally Decent Samaritanism of the mother, and this is a standard we must not fall below. I am inclined to think it a merit of my account precisely that it does *not* give a general yes or a general no. It allows for and supports our sense that, for example, a sick and desperately frightened fourteen-year-old schoolgirl, pregnant due to rape, may *of course* choose abortion, and that any law which rules this out is an insane law. And it also allows for and supports our sense that in other cases resort to abortion is even positively indecent. It would be indecent in the woman to request an abortion, and indecent in a doctor to perform it, if she is in her seventh month, and wants the abortion just to avoid the nuisance of postponing a trip abroad. The very fact that the arguments I have been drawing attention to treat all cases of abortion, or even all cases of abortion in which the mother's life is not at stake, as morally on a par ought to have made them suspect at the outset.

Secondly, while I am arguing for the permissibility of abortion in some cases, I am not arguing for the right to secure the death of the unborn child. It is easy to confuse these two things in that up to a certain point in the life of the fetus it is not able to survive outside the mother's body; hence removing it from her body guarantees its death. But they are importantly different. I have argued that you are not morally required to spend nine months in bed, sustaining the life of that violinist; but to say this is by no means to say that if, when you unplug yourself, there is a miracle and he survives, you then have a right to turn round and slit his throat. You may detach yourself even if this costs him his life; you have no right to be guaranteed his death, by some other means, if unplugging yourself does not kill him. There are some people who will feel dissatisfied by this feature of my argument. A woman may be utterly devastated by the thought of a child, a bit of herself, put out for adoption and never seen or heard of again. She may therefore want not merely that the child be detached from her, but more, that it die. Some opponents of abortion are inclined to regard this as beneath contempt—thereby showing insensitivity to what is surely a powerful source of despair. All the same, I agree that the desire for the child's death is not one which anybody may gratify, should it turn out to be possible to detach the child alive.

At this place, however, it should be remembered that we have only been pretending throughout that the fetus is a human being from the moment of conception. A very early abortion is surely not the killing of a person, and so is not dealt with by anything I have said here.

NOTES

1. I am very much indebted to James Thomson for discussion, criticism, and many helpful suggestions.
2. Daniel Callahan, *Abortion: Law, Choice and Morality* (New York, 1970), p. 373. This book gives a fascinating survey of the available information on abortion. The Jewish tradition is surveyed in David M. Feldman, *Birth Control in Jewish Law* (New York, 1968), Part 5, the Catholic tradition in John T. Noonan, Jr., "An Almost Absolute Value in History," in *The Morality of Abortion*, ed. John T. Noonan, Jr. (Cambridge, Mass., 1970).

3. The term "direct" in the arguments I refer to is a technical one. Roughly, what is meant by "direct killing" is either killing as an end in itself, or killing as a means to some end; for example, the end of saving someone else's life. See note 5 below, for an example of its use.
4. Cf. *Encyclical Letter of Pope Pius XI on Christian Marriage*, St. Paul Editions (Boston, n.d.), p. 32: "however much we may pity the mother whose health and even life is gravely imperiled in the performance of the duty allotted to her by nature, nevertheless what could ever be a sufficient reason for excusing in any way the direct murder of the innocent? This is precisely what we are dealing with here." Noonan (*The Morality of Abortion*, p. 43) reads this as follows: "What cause can ever avail to excuse in any way the direct killing of the innocent? For it is a question of that."
5. The thesis in (4) is in an interesting way weaker than those in (1), (2), and (3): they rule out abortion even in cases in which both mother *and* child will die if the abortion is not performed. By contrast, one who held the view expressed in (4) could consistently say that one needn't prefer letting two persons die to killing one.
6. Cf. the following passage from Pius XII, *Address to the Italian Catholic Society of Midwives*: "The baby in the maternal breast has the right to life immediately from God.—Hence there is no man, no human authority, no science, no medical, eugenic, social, economic or moral 'indication' which can establish or grant a valid juridical ground for a direct deliberate disposition of an innocent human life, that is a disposition which looks to its destruction either as an end or as a means to another end perhaps in itself not illicit.—The baby, still not born, is a man in the same degree and for the same reason as the mother" (quoted in Noonan, *The Morality of Abortion*, p. 45).
7. The need for a discussion of this argument was brought home to me by members of the Society for Ethical and Legal Philosophy, to whom this paper was originally presented.
8. For a discussion of the difficulties involved, and a survey of the European experience with such laws, see *The Good Samaritan and the Law*, ed. James M. Ratcliffe (New York, 1966).

On the Moral and Legal Status of Abortion

Mary Anne Warren

We will be concerned with both the moral status of abortion, which for our purposes we may define as the act which a woman performs in voluntarily terminating, or allowing another person to terminate, her pregnancy, and the legal status which is appropriate for this act. I will argue that, while it is not possible to produce a satisfactory defense of a woman's right to obtain an abortion without showing that a fetus is not a human being, in the morally relevant sense of that term, we ought not to conclude that the difficulties involved in determining whether or not a fetus is human make it impossible to produce any satisfactory solution to the problem of the moral status of abortion. For it is possible to show that, on the basis of intuitions which we may expect even the opponents of abortion to share, a fetus is not a person, and hence not the sort of entity to which it is proper to ascribe full moral rights.

Of course, while some philosophers would deny the possibility of any such proof,[1] others will deny that there is any need for it, since the moral permissibility of abortion appears to them to be too obvious to require proof. But the inadequacy of this attitude should be evident from the fact that both the friends and the foes of abortion consider their position to be morally self-evident. Because proabortionists have never adequately come to grips with the conceptual issues surrounding abortion, most if not all, of the arguments which they advance in opposition to laws restricting access to abortion fail to refute or even weaken the traditional antiabortion argument, i.e., that a fetus is a human being, and therefore abortion is murder.

These arguments are typically of one of two sorts. Either they point to the terrible side effects of the restrictive laws, e.g., the deaths due to illegal abortions, and the fact that it is poor women who suffer the most as a result of these laws, or else

they state that to deny a woman access to abortion is to deprive her of her right to control her own body. Unfortunately, however, the fact that restricting access to abortion has tragic side effects does not, in itself, show that the restrictions are unjustified, since murder is wrong regardless of the consequences of prohibiting it; and the appeal to the right to control one's body, which is generally construed as a property right, is at best a rather feeble argument for the permissibility of abortion. Mere ownership does not give me the right to kill innocent people whom I find on my property, and indeed I am apt to be held responsible if such people injure themselves while on my property. It is equally unclear that I have any moral right to expel an innocent person from my property when I know that doing so will result in his or her death.

Furthermore, it is probably inappropriate to describe a woman's body as her property, since it seems natural to hold that a person is something distinct from her property, but not from her body. Even those who would object to the identification of a person with her body, or with the conjunction of her body and her mind, must admit that it would be very odd to describe, say, breaking a leg, as damaging one's property, and much more appropriate to describe it as injuring one*self*. Thus it is probably a mistake to argue that the right to obtain an abortion is in any way derived from the right to own and regulate property.

But however we wish to construe the right to abortion, we cannot hope to convince those who consider abortion a form of murder of the existence of any such right unless we are able to produce a clear and convincing refutation of the traditional antiabortion argument, and this has not, to my knowledge, been done. With respect to the two most vital issues which that argument involves, i.e., the humanity of the fetus and its implication for the moral status of abortion, confusion has prevailed on both sides of the dispute. Thus, both proabortionists and antiabortionists have tended to abstract the question of whether abortion is wrong to that of whether it is wrong to destroy a fetus, just as though the rights of another person were

The Monist, Vol. 57, No. 1, January 1973, 43–61.

not necessarily involved. This mistaken abstraction has led to the almost universal assumption that if a fetus is a human being, with a right to life, then it follows immediately that abortion is wrong (except perhaps when necessary to save the woman's life), and that it ought to be prohibited. It has also been generally assumed that unless the question about the status of the fetus is answered, the moral status of abortion cannot possibly be determined.

Two recent papers, one by B. A. Brody,[2] and one by Judith Thomson,[3]* have attempted to settle the question of whether abortion ought to be prohibited apart from the question of whether or not the fetus is human. Brody examines the possibility that the following two statements are compatible: (I) that abortion is the taking of innocent human life, and therefore wrong; and (2) that nevertheless it ought not to be prohibited by law, at least under the present circumstances.[4] Not surprisingly, Brody finds it impossible to reconcile these two statements, since, as he rightly argues, none of the unfortunate side effects of the prohibition of abortion is bad enough to justify legalizing the *wrongful* taking of human life. He is mistaken, however, in concluding that the incompatibility of (1) and (2), in itself, shows that "the legal problem about abortion cannot be resolved independently of the status of the fetus problem" (p. 369).

What Brody fails to realize is that (1) embodies the questionable assumption that if a fetus is a human being, then of course abortion is morally wrong, and that an attack on *this* assumption is more promising, as a way of reconciling the humanity of the fetus with the claim that laws prohibiting abortion are unjustified, than is an attack on the assumption that if abortion is the wrongful killing of innocent human beings then it ought to be prohibited. He thus overlooks the possibility that a fetus may have a right to life and abortion still be morally permissible, in that the right of a woman to terminate an unwanted pregnancy might override the right of the fetus to be kept alive. The immorality of abortion is no more demonstrated by the humanity of the fetus, in itself, than the immorality of killing in self-defense is demonstrated by the fact that the assailant is a human being. Neither is it demonstrated by the *innocence* of the fetus, since there may be situations in which the killing of innocent human beings is justified.

*Editors' Note: See pp. 332–341 in this volume

It is perhaps not surprising that Brody fails to spot this assumption, since it has been accepted with little or no argument by nearly everyone who has written on the morality of abortion. John Noonan is correct in saying that "the fundamental question in the long history of abortion is, How do you determine the humanity of a being?"[5] He summarizes his own antiabortion argument, which is a version of the official position of the Catholic Church, as follows:

> . . . it is wrong to kill humans, however poor, weak, defenseless, and lacking in opportunity to develop their potential they may be. It is therefore morally wrong to kill Biafrans. Similarly, it is morally wrong to kill embryos.[6]

Noonan bases his claim that fetuses are human upon what he calls the theologians' criterion of humanity: that whoever is conceived of human beings is human. But although he argues at length for the appropriateness of this criterion, he never questions the assumption that if a fetus is human then abortion is wrong for exactly the same reason that murder is wrong.

Judith Thomson is, in fact, the only writer I am aware of who has seriously questioned this assumption; she has argued that, even if we grant the antiabortionist his claim that a fetus is a human being, with the same right to life as any other human being, we can still demonstrate that, in at least some and perhaps most cases, a woman is under no moral obligation to complete an unwanted pregnancy. Her argument is worth examining, since if it holds up it may enable us to establish the moral permissibility of abortion without becoming involved in problems about what entitles an entity to be considered human, and accorded full moral rights. To be able to do this would be a great gain in the power and simplicity of the proabortion position, since, although I will argue that these problems can be solved at least as decisively as can any other moral problem, we should certainly be pleased to be able to avoid having to solve them as part of the justification of abortion.

On the other hand, even if Thomson's argument does not hold up, her insight, i.e., that it requires *argument* to show that if fetuses are human then abortion is properly classified as murder, is an extremely valuable one. The assumption she attacks is particularly invidious, for it amounts to the decision that it is appropriate, in deciding the moral status of abortion, to leave the rights of the pregnant woman out of consideration entirely, except possibly when her life is threatened. Obviously, this will not do; determining what moral rights, if any, a fetus possesses is only the first step in determining the moral status of abortion. Step two, which is at least equally essential, is finding a just solution to the conflict between whatever rights the fetus may have, and the rights of the woman who is unwillingly pregnant. While the historical error has been to pay far too little attention to the second step, Ms. Thomson's suggestion is that if we look at the second step first we may find that a woman has a right to obtain an abortion *regardless* of what rights the fetus has.

Our own inquiry will also have two stages. In Section I, we will consider whether or not it is possible to establish that abortion is morally permissible even on the assumption that a fetus is an entity with a full-fledged right to life. I will argue that in fact this cannot be established, at least not with the conclusiveness which is essential to our hopes of convincing those who are skeptical about the morality of abortion, and that we therefore cannot avoid dealing with the question of whether or not a fetus really does have the same right to life as a (more fully developed) human being.

In Section II, I will propose an answer to this question, namely, that a fetus cannot be considered a member of the moral community, the set of beings with full and equal moral rights, for the simple reason that it is not a person, and that it is personhood, and not genetic humanity, i.e., humanity as defined by Noonan, which is the basis for membership in this community. I will argue that a fetus, whatever its stage of development, satisfies none of the basic criteria of personhood, and is not even enough *like* a person to be accorded even some of the same rights on the basis of this resemblance. Nor, as we will see, is a fetus's *potential* personhood a threat to the morality of abortion, since, whatever the rights of potential people may be, they are invariably overridden in any conflict with the moral rights of actual people.

I

We turn now to Professor Thomson's case for the claim that even if a fetus has full moral rights, abortion is still morally permissible, at least sometimes, and for some reasons other than to save the woman's life. Her argument is based upon a clever, but I think faulty, analogy. She asks us to picture ourselves waking up one day, in bed with a famous violinist. Imagine that you have been kidnapped, and your bloodstream hooked up to that of the violinist, who happens to have an ailment which will certainly kill him unless he is permitted to share your kidneys for a period of nine months. No one else can save him, since you alone have the right type of blood. He will be unconscious all that time, and you will have to stay in bed with him, but after the nine months are over he may be unplugged, completely cured, that is provided that you have cooperated.

Now then, she continues, what are your obligations in this situation? The antiabortionist, if he is consistent, will have to say that you are obligated to stay in bed with the violinist: for all people have a right to life, and violinists are people, and therefore it would be murder for you to disconnect yourself from him and let him die. But this is outrageous, and so there must be something wrong with the same argument when it is applied to abortion. It would certainly be commendable of you to agree to save the violinist, but it is absurd to suggest that your refusal to do so would be murder. His right to life does not obligate you to do whatever is required to keep him alive; nor does it justify anyone else in forcing you to do so. A law which required you to stay in bed with the violinist would clearly be an unjust law, since it is no proper function of the law to force unwilling people to make huge sacrifices for the sake of other people toward whom they have no such prior obligation.

Thomson concludes that, if this analogy be an apt one, then we can grant the antiabortionist his claim that a fetus is a human being, and still hold that it is at least sometimes the case that a pregnant woman has the right to refuse to be a Good Samaritan towards the fetus, i.e., to obtain an abortion. For there is a great gap between the claim that x has a right to life, and the claim that y is obligated to do whatever is necessary to keep x alive, let alone that she ought to be forced to do so. It is y's duty to keep x alive only if she has somehow contracted a *special* obligation to do so; and a woman who is unwillingly pregnant, e.g., who was raped, has done nothing which obligates her to make the enormous sacrifice which is necessary to preserve the conceptus.

This argument is initially quite plausible, and in the extreme case of pregnancy due to rape it is probably conclusive. Difficulties arise, however, when we try to specify more exactly the range of cases in which abortion is clearly justifiable even on the assumption that the fetus is human. Professor Thomson considers it a virtue of her argument that it does not enable us to conclude that abortion is *always* permissible. It would, she says, be "indecent" for a woman in her seventh month to obtain an abortion just to avoid having to postpone a trip to Europe. On the other hand, her argument enables us to see that "a sick and desperately frightened schoolgirl pregnant due to rape may *of course* choose abortion, and that any law which rules this out is an insane law." So far, so good; but what are we to say about the woman who becomes pregnant not through rape but as a result of her own carelessness, or because of contraceptive failure, or who gets pregnant intentionally and then changes her mind about wanting a child? With respect to such cases, the violinist analogy is of much less use to the defender of the woman's right to obtain an abortion.

Indeed, the choice of a pregnancy due to rape, as an example of a case in which abortion is permissible even if a fetus is considered a human being, is extremely significant; for it is only in the case of pregnancy due to rape that the woman's situation is adequately analogous to the violinist case for our intuitions about the latter to transfer convincingly. The crucial difference between a pregnancy due to rape and the normal case of an unwanted pregnancy is that in the *normal* case we cannot claim that the woman is in no way responsible for her predicament; she could have remained chaste, or taken her pills more faithfully, or abstained on dangerous days, and so on. If, on the other hand, you are kidnapped by strangers, and hooked up to a strange violinist, then you are free of any shred of responsibility for the situation, on the basis of which it could be argued that you are obligated to keep the violinist alive. Only when her pregnancy is due to rape is a woman clearly just as nonresponsible.[8]

Consequently, there is room for the antiabortionist to argue that in the normal case of unwanted pregnancy a woman has, by her own actions, assumed responsibility for the fetus. For if x

behaves in a way which she could have avoided, and which she knows involves, let us say, a 1 percent chance of bringing into existence a human being, with a right to life, and does so knowing that if this should happen then that human being will perish unless x does certain things to keep it alive, then it is by no means clear that when it does happen x is free of any obligation to what she knew in advance would be required to keep that human being alive.

The plausibility of such an argument is enough to show that the Thomson analogy can provide a clear and persuasive defense of a woman's right to obtain an abortion only with respect to those cases in which the woman is in no way responsible for her pregnancy, e.g., where it is due to rape. In all other cases, we would almost certainly conclude that it was necessary to look carefully at the particular circumstances in order to determine the extent of the woman's responsibility, and hence the extent of her obligation. This is an extremely unsatisfactory outcome, from the viewpoint of the opponents of restrictive abortion laws, most of whom are convinced that a woman has a right to obtain an abortion regardless of how and why she got pregnant.

Of course a supporter of the violinist analogy might point out that it is absurd to suggest that forgetting her pill one day might be sufficient to obligate a woman to complete an unwanted pregnancy. And indeed it *is* absurd to suggest this. As we will see, the moral right to obtain an abortion is not in the least dependent upon the extent to which the woman is responsible for her pregnancy. But unfortunately, once we allow the assumption that a fetus has full moral rights, we cannot avoid taking this absurd suggestion seriously. Perhaps we can make this point more clear by altering the violinist story just enough to make it more analogous to a normal unwanted pregnancy and less to a pregnancy due to rape, and then seeing whether it is still obvious that you are not obligated to stay in bed with the fellow.

Suppose, then, that violinists are peculiarly prone to the sort of illness the only cure for which is the use of someone else's bloodstream for nine months, and that because of this there has been formed a society of music lovers who agree that whenever a violinist is stricken they will draw lots and the loser will, by some means, be made the one and only person capable of saving him or her. Now then, would you be obligated to cooperate in curing the violinist if you had voluntarily joined this society, knowing the possible consequences, and then your name had been drawn and you had been kidnapped? Admittedly, you did not promise ahead of time that you would, but you did deliberately place yourself in a position in which it might happen that a human life would be lost if you did not. Surely this is at least a prima facie reason for supposing that you have an obligation to stay in bed with the violinist. Suppose that you had gotten your name drawn deliberately; surely that would be quite a strong reason for thinking that you have such an obligation.

It might be suggested that there is one important disanalogy between the modified violinist case and the case of an unwanted pregnancy, which makes the woman's responsibility significantly less, namely, the fact that the fetus *comes into existence* as the result of the woman's actions. This fact might give her a right to refuse to keep it alive, whereas she would not have had this right had it existed previously, independently, and then as a result of her actions become dependent upon her for its survival.

My own intuition, however, is that *x* has no more right to bring into existence, either deliberately or as a foreseeable result of actions she could have avoided, a being with full moral rights (*y*), and then refuse to do what she knew beforehand would be required to keep that being alive, than she has to enter into an agreement with an existing person, whereby she may be called upon to save that person's life, and then refuse to do so when so called upon. Thus, *x*'s responsibility for *y*'s existence does not seem to lessen her obligation to keep *y* alive, if she is also responsible for *y*'s being in a situation in which only she can save him or her.

Whether or not this intuition is entirely correct, it brings us back once again to the conclusion that once we allow the assumption that a fetus has full moral rights it becomes an extremely complex and difficult question whether and when abortion is justifiable. Thus the Thomson analogy cannot help us produce a clear and persuasive proof of the moral permissibility of abortion. Nor will the opponents of the restrictive laws thank us for anything less; for their conviction (for the most part) is that abortion is obviously *not* a morally serious

and extremely unfortunate, even though sometimes justified act, comparable to killing in self-defense or to letting the violinist die, but rather is closer to being a morally neutral act, like cutting one's hair.

The basis of this conviction, I believe, is the realization that a fetus is not a person, and thus does not have a full-fledged right to life. Perhaps the reason why this claim has been so inadequately defended is that it seems self-evident to those who accept it. And so it is, insofar as it follows from what I take to be perfectly obvious claims about the nature of personhood, and about the proper grounds for ascribing moral rights, claims which ought, indeed, to be obvious to both the friends and foes of abortion. Nevertheless, it is worth examining these claims, and showing how they demonstrate the moral innocuousness of abortion, since this apparently has not been adequately done before.

II

The question which we must answer in order to produce a satisfactory solution to the problem of the moral status of abortion is this: How are we to define the moral community, the set of beings with full and equal moral rights, such that we can decide whether a human fetus is a member of this community or not? What sort of entity, exactly, has the inalienable rights to life, liberty, and the pursuit of happiness? Jefferson attributed these rights to all *men*, and it may or may not be fair to suggest that he intended to attribute them *only* to men. Perhaps he ought to have attributed them to all human beings. If so, then we arrive, first, at Noonan's problem of defining what makes a being human, and, second, at the equally vital question which Noonan does not consider, namely, What reason is there for identifying the moral community with the set of all human beings, in whatever way we have chosen to define that term?

1. ON THE DEFINITION OF 'HUMAN'

One reason why this vital second question is so frequently overlooked in the debate over the moral status of abortion is that the term 'human' has two distinct, but not often distinguished, senses. This fact results in a slide of meaning, which serves to conceal the fallaciousness of the traditional argument that since (1) it is wrong to kill innocent human beings, and (2) fetuses are innocent human beings, then (3) it is wrong to kill fetuses. For if 'human' is used in the same sense in both (1) and (2) then, whichever of the two senses is meant, one of these premises is question-begging. And if it is used in two different senses then of course the conclusion doesn't follow.

Thus, (1) is a self-evident moral truth,[9] and avoids begging the question about abortion, only if 'human being' is used to mean something like 'a full-fledged member of the moral community.' (It may or may not also be meant to refer exclusively to members of the species *Homo sapiens*.) We may call this the *moral* sense of 'human.' It is not to be confused with what we will call the *genetic* sense, i.e., the sense in which *any* member of the species is a human being, and no member of any other species could be. If (1) is acceptable only if the moral sense is intended, (2) is non-question-begging only if what is intended is the genetic sense.

In "Deciding Who Is Human," Noonan argues for the classification of fetuses with human beings by pointing to the presence of the full genetic code, and the potential capacity for rational thought (p. 35). It is clear that what he needs to show, for his version of the traditional argument to be valid, is that fetuses are human in the moral sense, the sense in which it is analytically true that all human beings have full moral rights. But, in the absence of any argument showing that whatever is genetically human is also morally human, and he gives none, nothing more than genetic humanity can be demonstrated by the presence of the human genetic code. And, as we will see, the *potential* capacity for rational thought can at most show that an entity has the potential for *becoming* human in the moral sense.

2. DEFINING THE MORAL COMMUNITY

Can it be established that genetic humanity is sufficient for moral humanity? I think that there are very good reasons for not defining the moral community in this way. I would like to suggest an alternative way of defining the moral community, which I will argue for only to the extent of explaining why it is, or should be, self-evident. The suggestion is simply that the moral community consists of all and only *people*, rather than all and only human beings;[10] and probably the best way of demonstrating its self-evidence is by considering the concept of personhood, to see what sorts of entities are and are not persons, and what the decision that a being is or is not a person implies about its moral rights.

What characteristics entitle an entity to be considered a person? This is obviously not the place to attempt a complete analysis of the concept of personhood, but we do not need such a fully adequate analysis just to determine whether and why a fetus is or isn't a person. All we need is a rough and approximate list of the most basic criteria of personhood, and some idea of which, or how many, of these an entity must satisfy in order to properly be considered a person.

In searching for such criteria, it is useful to look beyond the set of people with whom we are acquainted, and ask how we would decide whether a totally alien being was a person or not. (For we have no right to assume that genetic humanity is necessary for personhood.) Imagine a space traveler who lands on an unknown planet and encounters a race of beings utterly unlike any she has ever seen or heard of. If she wants to be sure of behaving morally toward these beings, she has to somehow decide whether they are people, and hence have full moral rights, or whether they are the sort of thing which she need not feel guilty about treating as, for example, a source of food.

How should she go about making this decision? If she has some anthropological background, she might look for such things as religion, art, and the manufacturing of tools, weapons, or shelters, since these factors have been used to distinguish our human from our prehuman ancestors, in what seems to be closer to the moral than the genetic sense of 'human.' And no doubt she would be right to consider the presence of such factors as good evidence that the alien beings were people, and morally human. It would, however, be overly anthropocentric of her to take the absence of these things as adequate evidence that they were not, since we can imagine people who have progressed beyond, or evolved without ever developing, these cultural characteristics.

I suggest that the traits which are most central to the concept of personhood, or humanity in the moral sense, are, very roughly, the following:

1. consciousness (of objects and events external and/or internal to the being), and in particular the capacity to feel pain;
2. reasoning (the *developed* capacity to solve new and relatively complex problems);
3. self-motivated activity (activity which is relatively independent of either genetic or direct external control);
4. the capacity to communicate, by whatever means, messages of an indefinite variety of types, that is, not just with an indefinite number of possible contents, but on indefinitely many possible topics;
5. the presence of self-concepts, and self-awareness, either individual or racial, or both.

Admittedly, there are apt to be a great many problems involved in formulating precise definitions of these criteria, let alone in developing universally valid behavior criteria for deciding when they apply. But I will assume that both we and our explorer know approximately what (1)–(5) mean, and that she is also able to determine whether or not they apply. How, then, should she use her findings to decide whether or not the alien beings are people? We needn't suppose that an entity must have *all* of these attributes to be properly considered a person; (1) and (2) alone may well be sufficient for personhood, and quite probably (1)–(3) are sufficient. Neither do we need to insist that any one of these criteria is *necessary* for personhood, although once again (1) and (2) look like fairly good candidates for necessary conditions, as does (3), if 'activity' is construed so as to include the activity of reasoning.

All we need to claim, to demonstrate that a fetus is not a person, is that any being which satisfies *none* of (1)–(5) is certainly not a person. I consider this claim to be so obvious that I think anyone who denied it, and claimed that a being which satisfied none of (1)–(5) was a person all the same, would thereby demonstrate that she had no notion at all of what a person is—perhaps because she had confused the concept of a person with that of genetic humanity. If the opponents of abortion were to deny the appropriateness of these five criteria, I do not know what further arguments would convince them. We would probably have to admit that our conceptual schemes were indeed irreconcilably different, and that our dispute could not be settled objectively.

I do not expect this to happen, however, since I think that the concept of a person is one which is very nearly universal (to people), and that it is common to both proabortionists and antiabortionists, even though neither group has fully realized the relevance of this concept to the resolution of their dispute. Furthermore, I think that on reflection even the antiabortionists ought to agree not only that (1)–(5) are central to the concept of personhood, but also that it is a part of this concept that all and only people have full moral rights. The concept of a person is in part a moral concept; once we have admitted that x is a person we have recognized, even if we have not agreed to respect, x's right to be treated as a member of the moral community. It is true that the claim that x is a *human being* is more commonly voiced as part of an appeal to treat x decently than is the claim that x is a person, but this is either because 'human being' is here used in the sense which implies personhood, or because the genetic and moral senses of 'human' have been confused.

Now if (1)–(5) are indeed the primary criteria of personhood, then it is clear that genetic humanity is neither necessary nor sufficient for establishing that an entity is a person. Some human beings are not people, and there may well be people who are not human beings. A man or woman whose consciousness has been permanently obliterated but who remains alive is a human being which is no longer a person; defective human beings, with no appreciable mental capacity, are not and presumably never will be people; and a fetus is a human being which is not yet a person, and which therefore cannot coherently be said to have full moral rights. Citizens of the next century should be prepared to recognize highly advanced, self-aware robots or computers, should such be developed, and intelligent inhabitants of other worlds, should such be found, as people in the fullest sense, and to respect their moral rights. But to ascribe full moral rights to an entity which is not a person is as absurd as to ascribe moral obligations and responsibilities to such an entity.

3. FETAL DEVELOPMENT AND THE RIGHT TO LIFE

Two problems arise in the application of these suggestions for the definition of the moral community to the determination of the precise moral status of a human fetus. Given that the paradigm example of a person is a normal adult human being, then (1) How like this paradigm, in particular how far advanced since conception, does a human being need to be before it begins to have a right to life by virtue, not of being fully a person as of yet, but of being *like* a person? and (2) To what extent, if any, does the fact that a fetus has the *potential* for becoming a person endow it with some of the same rights? Each of these questions requires some comment.

In answering the first question, we need not attempt a detailed consideration of the moral rights of organisms which are not developed enough, aware enough, intelligent enough, etc., to be considered people, but which resemble people in some respects. It does seem reasonable to suggest that the more like a person, in the relevant respects, a being is, the stronger is the case for regarding it as having a right to life, and indeed the stronger its right to life is. Thus we ought to take seriously the suggestion that, insofar as "the human individual develops biologically in a continuous fashion. . . the rights of a human person might develop in the same way."[11] But we must keep in mind that the attributes which are relevant in determining whether or not an entity is enough like a person to be regarded as having some moral rights are no different from those which are relevant to determining whether or not it is fully a person—i.e., are no different from (1)–(5)—and that being genetically human, or having recognizably human facial and other physical features, or detectable brain activity, or the capacity to survive outside the uterus, are simply not among these relevant attributes.

Thus it is clear that even though a seven- or eight-month fetus has features which make it apt to arouse in us almost the same powerful protective instinct as is commonly aroused by a small infant, nevertheless it is not significantly more personlike than is a very small embryo. It is *somewhat* more personlike; it can apparently feel and respond to pain, and it may even have a rudimentary form of consciousness, insofar as its brain is quite active. Nevertheless, it seems safe to say that it is not fully conscious, in the way that an infant of a few months is, and that it cannot reason, or communicate messages of indefinitely many sorts, does not engage in self-motivated activity, and has no self-awareness. Thus, in the *relevant* respects, a fetus, even a fully developed one, is considerably less personlike than is the average mature mammal, indeed the average fish. And I think that a rational person must conclude that if the right to life of a fetus is to be based upon its resemblance to a person, then it cannot be said to have any more right to life than, let us say, a newborn guppy (which also seems to be capable of feeling pain), and that a right of that magnitude could never override a woman's right to obtain an abortion, at any stage of her pregnancy.

There may, of course, be other arguments in favor of placing legal limits upon the stage of pregnancy in which an abortion may be performed. Given the relative safety of the new techniques of artificially inducing labor during the third trimester, the danger to the woman's life or health is no longer such an argument. Neither is the fact that people tend to respond to the thought of abortion in the later stages of pregnancy with emotional repulsion, since mere emotional responses cannot take the place of moral reasoning in determining what ought to be permitted. Nor, finally, is the frequently heard argument that legalizing abortion, especially late in the pregnancy, may erode the level of respect for human life, leading, perhaps, to an increase in unjustified euthanasia and other crimes. For this threat, if it is a threat, can be better met by educating people to the kinds of moral distinctions which we are making here than by limiting access to abortion (which limitation may, in its disregard for the rights of women, be just as damaging to the level of respect for human rights).

Thus, since the fact that even a fully developed fetus is not personlike enough to have any significant right to life on the basis of its personlikeness shows that no legal restrictions upon the stage of pregnancy in which an abortion may be performed can be justified on the grounds that we should protect the rights of the older fetus; and since there is no other apparent justification for such restrictions, we may conclude that they are entirely unjustified. Whether or not it would be *indecent* (whatever that means) for a woman in her seventh month to obtain an abortion just to avoid having to postpone a trip to Europe, it would not, in itself, be *immoral*, and therefore it ought to be permitted.

4. POTENTIAL PERSONHOOD AND THE RIGHT TO LIFE

We have seen that a fetus does not resemble a person in any way which can support the claim that it has even some of the same rights. But what about its *potential*, the fact that if nurtured and allowed to develop naturally it will very probably become a person? Doesn't that alone give it at least some right to life? It is hard to deny that the fact that an entity is a potential person is a strong prima facie reason for not destroying it; but we need not conclude from this that a potential person has a right to life, by virtue of that potential. It may be that our feeling that it is better, other things being equal, not to destroy a potential person is better explained by the fact that potential people are still (felt to be) an invaluable resource, not to be lightly squandered. Surely, if every speck of dust were a potential person, we would be much less apt to conclude that every potential person has a right to become actual.

Still, we do not need to insist that a potential person has no right to life whatever. There may well be something immoral, and not just imprudent, about wantonly destroying potential people, when doing so isn't necessary to protect anyone's rights. But even if a potential person does have some prima facie right to life, such a right could not possibly outweigh the right of a woman to obtain an abortion, since the rights of any actual person invariably outweigh those of any potential person, whenever the two conflict. Since this may not be immediately obvious in the case of a human fetus, let us look at another case.

Suppose that our space explorer falls into the hands of an alien culture, whose scientists decide to create a few hundred thousand or more human beings, by breaking her body into its component cells, and using these to create fully developed human beings, with, of course, her genetic code. We may imagine that each of these newly created individuals will have all of the original individual's abilities, skills, knowledge, and so on, and

also have an individual self-concept, in short that each of them will be a bona fide (though hardly unique) person. Imagine that the whole project will take only seconds, and that its chances of success are extremely high, and that our explorer knows all of this, and also knows that these people will be treated fairly. I maintain that in such a situation she would have every right to escape if she could, and thus to deprive all of these potential people of their potential lives; for her right to life outweighs all of theirs together, in spite of the fact that they are all genetically human, all innocent, and all have a very high probability of becoming people very soon, if only she refrains from acting.

Indeed, I think she would have a right to escape even if it were not her life which the alien scientists planned to take, but only a year of her freedom, or, indeed, only a day. Nor would she be obligated to stay if she had gotten captured (thus bringing all these people-potentials into existence) because of her own carelessness, or even if she had done so deliberately, knowing the consequences. Regardless of how she got captured, she is not morally obligated to remain in captivity for *any* period of time for the sake of permitting any number of potential people to come into actuality, so great is the margin by which one actual person's right to liberty outweighs whatever right to life even a hundred thousand potential people have. And it seems reasonable to conclude that the rights of a woman will outweigh by a similar margin whatever right to life a fetus may have by virtue of its potential personhood.

Thus, neither a fetus's resemblance to a person, nor its potential for becoming a person provides any basis whatever for the claim that it has any significant right to life. Consequently, a woman's right to protect her health, happiness, freedom, and even her life,[12] by terminating an unwanted pregnancy, will always override whatever right to life it may be appropriate to ascribe to a fetus, even a fully developed one. And thus, in the absence of any overwhelming social need for every possible child, the laws which restrict the right to obtain an abortion, or limit the period of pregnancy during which an abortion may be performed, are a wholly unjustified violation of a woman's most basic moral and constitutional rights.[13]

POSTSCRIPT ON INFANTICIDE

Since the publication of this article, many people have written to point out that my argument appears to justify not only abortion, but infanticide as well. For a new-born infant is not significantly more personlike than an advanced fetus, and consequently it would seem that if the destruction of the latter is permissible so too must be that of the former. Inasmuch as most people, regardless of how they feel about the morality of abortion, consider infanticide a form of murder, this might appear to represent a serious flaw in my argument.

Now, if I am right in holding that it is only people who have a full-fledged right to life, and who can be murdered, and if the criteria of personhood are as I have described them, then it obviously follows that killing a new-born infant isn't murder. It does *not* follow, however, that infanticide is permissible, for two reasons. In the first place, it would be wrong, at least in this country and in this period of history, and other things being equal, to kill a new-born infant, because even if its parents do not want it and would not suffer from its destruction, there are other people who would like to have it, and would, in all probability, be deprived of a great deal of pleasure by its destruction. Thus, infanticide is wrong for reasons analogous to those which make it wrong to wantonly destroy natural resources, or great works of art.

Secondly, most people, at least in this country, value infants and would much prefer that they be preserved, even if foster parents are not immediately available. Most of us would rather be taxed to support orphanages than allow unwanted infants to be destroyed. So long as there are people who want an infant preserved, and who are willing and able to provide the means of caring for it, under reasonably humane conditions, it is, *ceteris parabis*, wrong to destroy it.

But, it might be replied, if this argument shows that infanticide is wrong, at least at this time and in this country, doesn't it also show that abortion is wrong? After all, many people value fetuses, and disturbed by their destruction, and would much prefer that they be preserved, even at some cost to themselves. Furthermore, as a potential source of pleasure to some foster family, a fetus is just as valuable as an infant. There is, however, a crucial difference between the two cases: so long as the fetus is unborn, its preservation, contrary to the wishes of the pregnant woman, violates her rights to freedom, happiness, and self-determination. Her rights override the rights of those who would like the fetus preserved, just as if someone's life or limb is threatened by a wild animal, his right to protect himself by destroying the animal overrides the rights of those who would prefer that the animal not be harmed.

The minute the infant is born, however, its preservation no longer violates any of its mother's rights, even if she wants it destroyed, because she is free to put it up for adoption. Consequently, while the moment of birth does not mark any sharp discontinuity in the degree to which an infant possesses the right to life, it does mark the end of its mother's right to determine its fate. Indeed, if abortion could be performed without killing the fetus, she would never possess the right to have the fetus destroyed, for the same reasons that she has no right to have an infant destroyed.

On the other hand, it follows from my argument that when an unwanted or defective infant is born into a society which cannot afford and/or is not willing to care for it, then its destruction is permissible. This conclusion will, no doubt, strike many people as heartless and immoral; but remember that the very existence of people who feel this way, and who are willing and able to provide care for unwanted infants, is reason enough to conclude that they should be preserved.

NOTES

1. For example, Roger Wertheimer, who in "Understanding the Abortion Argument" (*Philosophy and Public Affairs*, 1, No. 1 [Fall, 1971], 67–95), argues that the problem of the moral status of abortion is insoluble, in that the dispute over the status of the fetus is not a question of fact at all, but only a question of how one responds to the facts.
2. B. A. Brody, "Abortion and the Law," *The Journal of Philosophy*, 68, No.12 (June 17, 1971), 357–369.
3. Judith Thomson, "A Defense of Abortion," *Philosophy and Public Affairs*, 1, No. 1 (Fall, 1971), 47–66.
4. I have abbreviated these standards somewhat, but not in a way which affects the argument.
5. John Noonan, "Abortion and the Catholic Church: A Summary History," *Natural Law Forum*, 12 (1967), 125.

6. John Noonan, "Deciding Who Is Human," *Natural Law Forum,* 13 (1968), 134.

7. "A Defense of Abortion."

8. We may safely ignore the fact that she might have avoided getting raped, e.g., by carrying a gun, since by similar means you might likewise have avoided getting kidnapped, and in neither case does the victim's failure to take all possible precautions against a highly unlikely event (as opposed to reasonable precautions against a rather likely event) mean that she is morally responsible or what happens.

9. Of course, the principle that it is (always) wrong to kill innocent human beings is in need of many other modifications, e.g., that it may be permissible to do so to save a greater number of other innocent human beings, but we may safely ignore these complications here.

10. From here on, we will use 'human' to mean genetically human, since the moral sense seems closely connected to, and perhaps derived from, the assumption that genetic humanity is sufficient for membership in the moral community.

11. Thomas L. Hayes, "A Biological View," *Commonwealth* 85 (March 17, 1967), 677–78; quoted by Daniel Callahan, in *Abortion, Law, Choice, and Morality* (London: Macmillan & Co., 1970).

12. That is, insofar as the death rate, for the woman, is higher for childbirth than for early abortion.

13. My thanks to the following people, who were kind enough to read and criticize an earlier version of this paper: Herbert Gold, Gene Glass, Anne Lauterbach, Judith Thomson, Mary Mothersill, and Timothy Binkley.

Why Abortion Is Immoral

Don Marquis

I

. . . Consider the way a typical anti-abortionist argues. She will argue or assert that life is present from the moment of conception or that fetuses look like babies or that fetuses possess a characteristic such as a genetic code that is both necessary and sufficient for being human. Anti-abortionists seem to believe that (1) the truth of all of these claims is quite obvious, and (2) establishing any of these claims is sufficient to show that abortion is morally akin to murder.

A standard pro-choice strategy exhibits similarities. The pro-choicer will argue or assert that fetuses are not persons or that fetuses are not rational agents or that fetuses are not social beings. Pro-choicers seem to believe that (1) the truth of any of these claims is quite obvious, and (2) establishing any of these claims is sufficient to show that an abortion is not a wrongful killing.

In fact, both the pro-choice and the anti-abortion claims do seem to be true, although the "it looks like a baby" claim is more difficult to establish the earlier the pregnancy. We seem to have a standoff. How can it be resolved? . . .

Note what each partisan will say. The anti-abortionist will claim that her position is supported by such generally accepted moral principles as "It is always prima facie seriously wrong to take a human life" or "It is always prima facie seriously wrong to end the life of a baby." Since these are generally accepted moral principles, her position is certainly not obviously wrong. The pro-choicer will claim that her position is supported by such plausible moral principles as, "Being a person is what gives an individual intrinsic moral worth," or, "It is only seriously prima facie wrong to take the life of a member of the human community." Since these are generally accepted moral principles, the pro-choice position is certainly not obviously wrong. Unfortunately, we have again arrived at a standoff.

Now, how might one deal with this standoff? The standard approach is to try to show how the moral principles of one's opponent lose their plausibility under analysis. It is easy to see how this is possible. On the one hand, the anti-abortionist will defend a moral principle concerning the wrong-

Journal of Philosophy LXXXVI, No. 4, April 1989, 183–202. Reprinted by permission.

ness of killing which tends to be broad in scope in order that even fetuses at an early stage of pregnancy will fall under it. The problem with broad principles is that they often embrace too much. In this particular instance, the principle, "It is always prima facie wrong to take a human life," seems to entail that it is wrong to end the existence of a living human cancer-cell culture, on the grounds that the culture is both living and human. Therefore, it seems that the anti-abortionist's favored principle is too broad.

On the other hand, the pro-choicer wants to find a moral principle concerning the wrongness of killing which tends to be narrow in scope in order that fetuses will *not* fall under it. The problem with narrow principles is that they often do not embrace enough. Hence, the needed principles such as, "It is prima facie seriously wrong to kill only persons," or, "It is prima facie wrong to kill only rational agents," do not explain why it is wrong to kill infants or young children or the severely retarded or even perhaps the severely mentally ill. Therefore, we seem again to have a standoff. The anti-abortionist charges, not unreasonably, that pro-choice principles concerning killing are too narrow to be acceptable; the pro-choicer charges, not unreasonably, that anti-abortionist principles concerning killing are too broad to be acceptable.

Attempts by both sides to patch up the difficulties in their positions run into further difficulties. The anti-abortionist will try to remove the problem in her position by reformulating her principle concerning killing in terms of human beings. Now we end up with: "It is always prima facie seriously wrong to end the life of a human being." This principle has the advantage of avoiding the problem of the human cancer-cell culture counterexample. But this advantage is purchased at a high price. For although it is clear that a fetus is both human and alive, it is not at all clear that a fetus is a human *being*. There is at least something to be said for the view that something becomes a human being only after a process of development, and that, therefore, first trimester fetuses, and perhaps all fetuses, are not yet human beings. Hence, the anti-abortionist, by this move, has merely exchanged one problem for another.

The pro-choicer fares no better. She may attempt to find reasons why killing infants, young children, and the severely retarded is wrong which are independent of her major principle that is supposed to

explain the wrongness of taking human life, but which will not also make abortion immoral. This is no easy task. Appeals to social utility will seem satisfactory only to those who resolve not to think of the enormous difficulties with a utilitarian account of the wrongness of killing and the significant social costs of preserving the lives of the unproductive. A pro-choice strategy that extends the definition of 'person' to infants or even to young children seems just as arbitrary as an anti-abortion strategy that extends the definition of 'human being' to fetuses. Again, we find symmetries in the two positions and we arrive at a standoff.

There are even further problems that reflect symmetries in the two positions. In addition to counterexample problems, or the arbitrary application problems that can be exchanged for them, the standard anti-abortionist principle, "It is prima facie seriously wrong to kill a human being," or one of its variants, can be objected to on the grounds of ambiguity. If 'human being' is taken to be a *biological* category, then the anti-abortionist is left with the problem of explaining why a merely biological category should make a moral difference. Why, it is asked, is it any more reasonable to base a moral conclusion on the number of chromosomes in one's cells than on the color of one's skin? If 'human being', on the other hand, is taken to be a *moral* category, then the claim that a fetus is a human being cannot be taken to be a premise in the anti-abortion argument, for it is precisely what needs to be established. Hence, either the anti-abortionist's main category is a morally irrelevant, merely biological category, or it is of no use to the anti-abortionist in establishing (noncircularly, of course) that abortion is wrong.

Although this problem with the anti-abortionist position is often noticed, it is less often noticed that the pro-choice position suffers from an analogous problem. The principle, "Only persons have the right to life" also suffers from an ambiguity. The term 'person' is typically defined in terms of psychological characteristics, although there will certainly be disagreement concerning which characteristics are most important. Supposing that this matter can be settled, the pro-choicer is left with the problem of explaining why *psychological* characteristics should make a *moral* difference. If the pro-choicer should attempt to deal with this problem by claiming that an explanation is not necessary, that in fact we do treat such a cluster of psychological properties as having moral significance, the sharp-witted anti-abortionist should have a ready response. We do treat being both living and human as having moral significance. If it is legitimate for the pro-choicer to demand that the anti-abortionist provide an explanation of the connection between the biological character of being a human being and the wrongness of being killed (even though people accept this connection), then it is legitimate for the anti-abortionist to demand that the pro-choicer provide an explanation of the connection between psychological criteria for being a person and the wrongness of being killed (even though that connection is accepted).

[Joel] Feinberg has attempted to meet this objection (he calls psychological personhood "commonsense personhood"):

> The characteristics that confer commonsense personhood are not arbitrary bases for rights and duties, such as race, sex or species membership; rather they are traits that make sense out of rights and duties and without which those moral attributes would have no point or function. It is because people are conscious; have a sense of their personal identities; have plans, goals, and projects; experience emotions; are liable to pains, anxieties, and frustrations; can reason and bargain, and so on—it is because of these attributes that people have values and interests, desires and expectations of their own, including a stake in their own futures, and a personal well-being of a sort we cannot ascribe to unconscious or nonrational beings. Because of their developed capacities they can assume duties and responsibilities and can have and make claims on one another. Only because of their sense of self, their life plans, their value hierarchies, and their stakes in their own futures can they be ascribed fundamental rights. There is nothing arbitrary about these linkages.
> [Feinberg 1986]

The plausible aspects of this attempt should not be taken to obscure its implausible features. There is a great deal to be said for the view that being a psychological person under some description is a necessary condition for having duties. One cannot have a duty unless one is capable of behaving morally, and a being's capability of behaving morally will require having a certain psychology. It is far from obvious, however, that having rights entails consciousness or rationality, as Feinberg suggests. We

speak of the rights of the severely retarded or the severely mentally ill, yet some of these persons are not rational. We speak of the rights of the temporarily unconscious. The New Jersey Supreme Court based their decision in the Quinlan case on Karen Ann Quinlan's right to privacy, and she was known to be permanently unconscious at that time. Hence, Feinberg's claim that having rights entails being conscious is, on its face, obviously false. . . .

There is a way out of this apparent dialectical quandary. . . .

II

. . . We can start from the following unproblematic assumption concerning our own case: it is wrong to kill us. Why is it wrong? Some answers can be easily eliminated. It might be said that what makes killing us wrong is that a killing brutalizes the one who kills. But the brutalization consists of being inured to the performance of an act that is hideously immoral; hence, the brutalization does not explain the immorality. It might be said that what makes killing us wrong is the great loss others would experience due to our absence. Although such hubris is understandable, such an explanation does not account for the wrongness of killing hermits, or those whose lives are relatively independent and whose friends find it easy to make new friends.

A more obvious answer is better. What primarily makes killing wrong is neither its effect on the murderer nor its effect on the victim's friends and relatives, but its effect on the victim. The loss of one's life is one of the greatest losses one can suffer. The loss of one's life deprives one of all the experiences, activities, projects, and enjoyments that would otherwise have constituted one's future. Therefore, killing someone is wrong, primarily because the killing inflicts (one of) the greatest possible losses on the victim. . . . When I am killed, I am deprived both of what I now value which would have been part of my future personal life, but also what I would come to value. Therefore, when I die, I am deprived of all of the value of my future. Inflicting this loss on me is ultimately what makes killing me wrong. This being the case, it would seem that what makes killing *any* adult human being prima facie seriously wrong is the loss of his or her future. . . .

The claim that what makes killing wrong is the loss of the victim's future is directly supported by two considerations. In the first place, this theory explains why we regard killing as one of the worst of crimes. Killing is especially wrong, because it deprives the victim of more than perhaps any other crime. In the second place, people with AIDS or cancer who know they are dying believe, of course, that dying is a very bad thing for them. They believe that the loss of a future to them that they would otherwise have experienced is what makes their premature death a very bad thing for them. A better theory of the wrongness of killing would require a different natural property associated with killing which better fits with the attitudes of the dying. What could it be?

The view that what makes killing wrong is the loss to the victim of the value of the victim's future gains additional support when some of its implications are examined. In the first place, it is incompatible with the view that it is wrong to kill only beings who are biologically human. It is possible that there exists a different species from another planet whose members have a future like ours. Since having a future like that is what makes killing someone wrong, this theory entails that it would be wrong to kill members of such a species. Hence, this theory is opposed to the claim that only life that is biologically human has great moral worth, a claim which many anti-abortionists have seemed to adopt. This opposition, which this theory has in common with personhood theories, seems to be a merit of the theory.

In the second place, the claim that the loss of one's future is the wrong-making feature of one's being killed entails the possibility that the futures of some actual nonhuman mammals on our own planet are sufficiently like ours that it is seriously wrong to kill them also. Whether some animals do have the same right to life as human beings depends on adding to the account of the wrongness of killing some additional account of just what it is about my future or the futures of other adult human beings which makes it wrong to kill us. No such additional account will be offered in this essay. Undoubtedly, the provision of such an account would be a very difficult matter. Undoubtedly, any such account would be quite controversial. Hence, it surely should not reflect badly on this sketch of an elementary theory of the wrongness of killing that it is indeterminate with respect to some very difficult issues regarding animal rights.

In the third place, the claim that the loss of one's future is the wrong-making feature of one's being killed does not entail, as sanctity-of-human-life theories do, that active euthanasia is wrong. Persons who are severely and incurably ill, who face a future of pain and despair, and who wish to die will not have suffered a loss if they are killed. It is, strictly speaking, the value of a human's future which makes killing wrong in this theory. This being so, killing does not necessarily wrong some persons who are sick and dying. Of course, there may be other reasons for a prohibition of active euthanasia, but that is another matter. Sanctity-of-human-life theories seem to hold that active euthanasia is seriously wrong even in an individual case where there seems to be good reason for it independently of public policy considerations. This consequence is most implausible, and it is a plus for the claim that the loss of a future of value is what makes killing wrong that it does not share this consequence.

In the fourth place, the account of the wrongness of killing defended in this essay does straightforwardly entail that it is prima facie seriously wrong to kill children and infants, for we do presume that they have futures of value. Since we do believe that it is wrong to kill defenseless little babies, it is important that a theory of the wrongness of killing easily account for this. Personhood theories of the wrongness of killing, on the other hand, cannot straightforwardly account for the wrongness of killing infants and young children. Hence, such theories must add special ad hoc accounts of the wrongness of killing the young. The plausibility of such ad hoc theories seems to be a function of how desperately one wants such theories to work. The claim that the primary wrong-making feature of a killing is the loss to the victim of the value of its future accounts for the wrongness of killing young children and infants directly; it makes the wrongness of such acts as obvious as we actually think it is. This is a further merit of this theory. Accordingly, it seems that this value of a future-like-ours theory of the wrongness of killing shares strengths of both sanctity-of-life and personhood accounts while avoiding weaknesses of both. In addition, it meshes with a central intuition concerning what makes killing wrong.

The claim that the primary wrong-making feature of a killing is the loss to the victim of the value of its future has obvious consequences for the ethics of abortion. The future of a standard fetus includes a set of experiences, projects, activities, and such which are identical with the futures of adult human beings and are identical with the futures of young children. Since the reason that is sufficient to explain why it is wrong to kill human beings after the time of birth is a reason that also applies to fetuses, it follows that abortion is prima facie seriously morally wrong.

This argument does not rely on the invalid inference that, since it is wrong to kill persons, it is wrong to kill potential persons also. The category that is morally central to this analysis is the category of having a valuable future like ours; it is not the category of personhood. The argument that abortion is prima facie seriously morally wrong proceeded independently of the notion of person or potential person or any equivalent. Someone may wish to start with this analysis in terms of the value of a human future, conclude that abortion is, except perhaps in rare circumstances, seriously morally wrong, infer that fetuses have the right to life, and then call fetuses "persons" as a result of their having the right to life. Clearly, in this case, the category of person is being used to state the *conclusion* of the analysis rather than to generate the *argument* of the analysis. . . .

III

How complete an account of the wrongness of killing does the value of a future-like-ours account have to be in order that the wrongness of abortion is a consequence? This account does not have to be an account of the necessary conditions for the wrongness of killing. Some persons in nursing homes may lack valuable human futures, yet it may be wrong to kill them for other reasons. Furthermore, this account does not obviously have to be the sole reason killing is wrong where the victim did have a valuable future. This analysis claims only that, for any killing where the victim did have a valuable future like ours, having that future by itself is sufficient to create the strong presumption that the killing is seriously wrong.

One way to overturn the value of a future-like-ours argument would be to find some account of the wrongness of killing which is at least as intelligible and which has different implications for the ethics of abortion. Two rival accounts possess at least some degree of plausibility. One account is based on the obvious fact that people value the experience of living and wish for that valuable experience to continue. Therefore, it might be said, what makes killing wrong is the discontinuation of that experience for the victim. Let us call this the *discontinuation account*. Another rival account is based upon the obvious fact that people strongly desire to continue to live. This suggests that what makes killing us so wrong is that it interferes with the fulfillment of a strong and fundamental desire, the fulfillment of which is necessary for the fulfillment of any other desires we might have. Let us call this the *desire account*. . . .

One problem with the desire account is that we do regard it as seriously wrong to kill persons who have little desire to live or who have no desire to live or, indeed, have a desire not to live. We believe it is seriously wrong to kill the unconscious, the sleeping, those who are tired of life, and those who are suicidal. The value-of-a-human-future account renders standard morality intelligible in these cases; these cases appear to be incompatible with the desire account.

The desire account is subject to a deeper difficulty. We desire life, because we value the goods of this life. The goodness of life is not secondary to our desire for it. If this were not so, the pain of one's own premature death could be done away with merely by an appropriate alteration in the configuration of one's desires. This is absurd. Hence, it would seem that it is the loss of the goods of one's future, not the interference with the fulfillment of a strong desire to live, which accounts ultimately for the wrongness of killing.

It is worth noting that, if the desire account is modified so that it does not provide a necessary, but only a sufficient, condition for the wrongness of killing, the desire account is compatible with the value of a future-like-ours account. The combined accounts will yield an anti-abortion ethic. This suggests that one can retain what is intuitively plausible about the desire account without a challenge to the basic argument of this paper.

It is also worth noting that, if future desires have moral force in a modified desire account of the wrongness of killing, one can find support for an anti-abortion ethic even in the absence of a value of a future-like-ours account. If one decides that a morally relevant property, the possession of which is sufficient to make it wrong to kill some individual, is the desire at some future time to live—one might decide to justify one's refusal to kill suicidal teenagers on these grounds, for example—then, since typical fetuses will have the desire in the future to live, it is wrong to kill typical fetuses. Accordingly, it does not seem that a desire account of the wrongness of killing can provide a justification of a pro-choice ethic of abortion which is nearly as adequate as the value of a human-future justification on an anti-abortion ethic.

The discontinuation account looks more promising as an account of the wrongness of killing. It seems just as intelligible as the value of a future-like-ours account, but it does not justify an anti-abortion position. Obviously, if it is the continuation of one's activities, experiences, and projects, the loss of which makes killing wrong, then it is not wrong to kill fetuses for that reason, for fetuses do not have experiences, activities, and projects to be continued or discontinued. Accordingly, the discontinuation account does not have the anti-abortion consequences that the value of a future-like-ours account has. Yet, it seems as intelligible as the value of a future-like-ours account, for when we think of what would be wrong with our being killed, it does seem as if it is the discontinuation of what makes our lives worthwhile which makes killing us wrong.

Is the discontinuation account just as good an account as the value of a future-like-ours account? The discontinuation account will not be adequate at all, if it does not refer to the *value* of the experience that may be discontinued. One does not want the discontinuation account to make it wrong to kill a patient who begs for death and who is in severe pain that cannot be relieved short of killing. (I leave open the question of whether it is wrong for other reasons.) Accordingly, the discontinuation account must be more than a bare discontinuation account. It must make some reference to the positive value of the patient's experiences. But, by the same token, the value of a future-like-ours account cannot be a bare future account either. Just

having a future surely does not itself rule out killing the above patient. This account must make some reference to the value of the patient's future experiences and projects also. Hence, both accounts involve the value of experiences, projects, and activities. So far we still have symmetry between accounts.

The symmetry fades, however, when we focus on the time period of the value of the experiences, etc., which has moral consequences. Although both accounts leave open the possibility that the patient in our example may be killed, this possibility is left open only in virtue of the utterly bleak future for the patient. It makes no difference whether the patient's immediate past contains intolerable pain, or consists in being in a coma (which we can imagine is a situation of indifference), or consists in a life of value. If the patient's future is a future of value, we want our account to make it wrong to kill the patient. If the patient's future is intolerable, whatever his or her immediate past, we want our account to allow killing the patient. Obviously, then, it is the value of that patient's future which is doing the work in rendering the morality of killing the patient intelligible.

This being the case, it seems clear that whether one has immediate past experiences or not does no work in the explanation of what makes killing wrong. The addition the discontinuation account makes to the value of a human future account is otiose. Its addition to the value-of-a-future account plays no role at all in rendering intelligible the wrongness of killing. Therefore, it can be discarded with the discontinuation account of which it is a part.

IV

The analysis of the previous section suggests that alternative general accounts of the wrongness of killing are either inadequate or unsuccessful in getting around the anti-abortion consequences of the value of a future-like-ours argument. A different strategy for avoiding these anti-abortion consequences involves limiting the scope of the value of a future argument. More precisely, the strategy involves arguing that fetuses lack a property that is essential for the value-of-a-future argument (or for any anti-abortion argument) to apply to them.

One move of this sort is based upon the claim that a necessary condition of one's future being valuable is that one values it. Value implies a valuer. Given this one might argue that, since fetuses cannot value their futures, their futures are not valuable to them. Hence, it does not seriously wrong them deliberately to end their lives.

This move fails, however, because of some ambiguities. Let us assume that something cannot be of value unless it is valued by someone. This does not entail that my life is of no value unless it is valued by me. I may think, in a period of despair, that my future is of no worth whatsoever, but I may be wrong because others rightly see value—even great value—in it. Furthermore, my future can be valuable to me even if I do not value it. This is the case when a young person attempts suicide, but is rescued and goes on to significant human achievements. Such young people's futures are ultimately valuable to them, even though such futures do not seem to be valuable to them at the moment of attempted suicide. A fetus's future can be valuable to it in the same way. Accordingly, this attempt to limit the anti-abortion argument fails.

Another similar attempt to reject the anti-abortion position is based on [Michael] Tooley's claim that an entity cannot possess the right to life unless it has the capacity to desire its continued existence. It follows that, since fetuses lack the conceptual capacity to desire to continue to live, they lack the right to life. Accordingly, Tooley concludes that abortion cannot be seriously prima facie wrong. . . .

What could be the evidence for Tooley's basic claim? Tooley once argued that individuals have a prima facie right to what they desire and that the lack of the capacity to desire something undercuts the basis of one's right to it. . . . This argument plainly will not succeed in the context of the analysis of this essay, however, since the point here is to establish the fetus's right to life on other grounds. Tooley's argument assumes that the right to life cannot be established in general on some basis other than the desire for life. This position was considered and rejected in the preceding section of this paper.

One might attempt to defend Tooley's basic claim on the grounds that, because a fetus cannot apprehend continued life as a benefit, its continued life cannot be a benefit, or cannot be something it has a right to, or cannot be something that is in its interest. This might be defended in terms of the general proposition that, if an individual is literally incapable of caring about or taking an interest in some X, then one does not have a right to X, or X is not a benefit, or X is not something that is in one's interest.

Each member of this family of claims seems to be open to objections. As John C. Stevens has pointed out, one may have a right to be treated with a certain medical procedure (because of a health insurance policy one has purchased), even though one cannot conceive of the nature of the procedure. And, as Tooley himself has pointed out, persons who have been indoctrinated, or drugged, or rendered temporarily unconscious may be literally incapable of caring about or taking an interest in something that is in their interest, or is something to which they have a right, or is something that benefits them. Hence, the Tooley claim that would restrict the scope of the value of a future-like-ours argument is undermined by counterexamples.

Finally, Paul Bassen has argued that, even though the prospects of an embryo might seem to be a basis for the wrongness of abortion, an embryo cannot be a victim and therefore cannot be wronged [Bassen 1982, 332–326]. An embryo cannot be a victim, he says, because it lacks sentience. His central argument for this seems to be that, even though plants and the permanently unconscious are alive, they clearly cannot be victims. What is the explanation of this? Bassen claims that the explanation is that their lives consist of mere metabolism and mere metabolism is not enough to ground victimizability. Mentation is required.

The problem with this attempt to establish the absence of victimizability is that both plants and the permanently unconscious clearly lack what Bassen calls "prospects" or what I have called "a future life like ours." Hence, it is surely open to one to argue that the real reason we believe plants and the permanently unconscious cannot be victims is that killing them cannot deprive them of a future life like ours; the real reason is not their absence of present mentation.

Bassen recognizes that his view is subject to this difficulty, and he recognizes that the case of children seems to support this difficulty, for "much of what we do for children is based on prospects." He argues, however, that, in the case of children and in other such cases, "potentiality comes into play only where victimizability has been secured on other grounds" [Bassen 1982, 333]. . . .

Bassen's defense of his view is patently question-begging, since what is adequate to secure victimizability is exactly what is at issue. His examples do not support his own view against the thesis of this essay. Of course, embryos can be victims: when their lives are deliberately terminated, they are deprived of their futures of value, their prospects. This makes them victims, for it directly wrongs them.

The seeming plausibility of Bassen's view stems from the fact that paradigmatic cases of imagining someone as a victim involve empathy, and empathy requires mentation of the victim. The victims of flood, famine, rape, or child abuse are all persons with whom we can empathize. That empathy seems to be part of seeing them as victims.

In spite of the strength of these examples, the attractive intuition that a situation in which there is victimization requires the possibility of empathy is subject to counterexamples. Consider a case that Bassen himself offers: "Posthumous obliteration of an author's work constitutes a misfortune for him only if he had wished his work to endure" [Bassen 1982, 318]. . . . The conditions Bassen wishes to impose upon the possibility of being victimized here seem far too strong. Perhaps this author, due to his unrealistic standards of excellence and his low self-esteem, regarded his work as unworthy of survival, even though it possessed genuine literary merit. Destruction of such work would surely victimize its author. In such a case, empathy with the victim concerning the loss is clearly impossible.

Of course, Bassen does not make the possibility of empathy a necessary condition of victimizability; he requires only mentation. Hence, on Bassen's actual view, this author, as I have described him, can be a victim. The problem is that the basic intuition that renders Bassen's view plausible is missing in the author's case. In order to attempt to avoid counterexamples, Bassen has made his thesis too weak to be supported by the intuitions that suggested it.

Even so, the mentation requirement on victimizability is still subject to counterexamples. Suppose a severe accident renders me totally unconscious for a month, after which I recover. Surely killing me while I am unconscious victimizes me, even though I am incapable of mentation during that time. It thus follows that Bassen's thesis fails. Apparently, attempts to restrict the value of a future-like-ours argument so that fetuses do not fall within its scope do not succeed.

V

In this essay, it has been argued that the correct ethic of the wrongness of killing can be extended to fetal life and used to show that there is a strong presumption that any abortion is morally impermissible. If the ethic of killing adopted here entails, however, that contraception is also seriously immoral, then there would appear to be a difficulty with the analysis of this essay.

But this analysis does not entail that contraception is wrong. Of course, contraception prevents the actualization of a possible future of value. Hence, it follows from the claim that futures of value should be maximized that contraception is prima facie immoral. This obligation to maximize does not exist, however; furthermore, nothing in the ethics of killing in this paper entails that it does. The ethics of killing in this essay would entail that contraception is wrong only if something were denied a human future of value by contraception. Nothing at all is denied such a future by contraception, however.

Candidates for a subject of harm by contraception fall into four categories: (1) some sperm or other, (2) some ovum or other, (3) a sperm and an ovum separately, and (4) a sperm and an ovum together. Assigning the harm to some sperm is utterly arbitrary, for no reason can be given for making a sperm the subject of harm rather than an ovum. Assigning the harm to some ovum is utterly arbitrary, for no reason can be given for making an ovum the subject of harm rather than a sperm. One might attempt to avoid these problems by insisting that contraception deprives both the sperm and the ovum separately of a valuable future like ours. On this alternative, too many futures are lost. Contraception was supposed to be wrong, because it deprived us of one future of value, not two. One might attempt to avoid this problem by holding that contraception deprives the combination of sperm and ovum of a valuable future like ours. But here the definite article misleads. At the time of contraception, there are hundreds of millions of sperm, one (released) ovum and millions of possible combinations of all of these. There is no actual combination at all. Is the subject of the loss to be a merely possible combination? Which one? This alternative does not yield an actual subject of harm either. Accordingly, the immorality of contraception is not entailed by the loss of a future-like-ours argument simply because there is no nonarbitrarily identifiable subject of the loss in the case of contraception.

VI

The purpose of this essay has been to set out an argument for the serious presumptive wrongness of abortion subject to the assumption that the moral permissibility of abortion stands or falls on the moral status of the fetus. Since a fetus possesses a property, the possession of which in adult human beings is sufficient to make killing an adult human being wrong, abortion is wrong. This way of dealing with the problem of abortion seems superior to other approaches to the ethics of abortion, because it rests on an ethics of killing which is close to self-

evident, because the crucial morally relevant property clearly applies to fetuses, and because the argument avoids the usual equivocations on 'human life', 'human being', or 'person'. The argument rests neither on religious claims nor on papal dogma. It is not subject to the objection of "speciesism." Its soundness is compatible with the moral permissibility of euthanasia and contraception. It deals with our intuitions concerning young children.

Finally, this analysis can be viewed as resolving a standard problem—indeed, *the* standard problem—concerning the ethics of abortion. Clearly, it is wrong to kill adult human beings. Clearly, it is not wrong to end the life of some arbitrarily chosen single human cell. Fetuses seem to be like arbitrarily chosen human cells in some respects and like adult humans in other respects. The problem of the ethics of abortion is the problem of determining the fetal property that settles this moral controversy. The thesis of this essay is that the problem of the ethics of abortion, so understood, is solvable.

Abortion: A Feminist Perspective

Susan Sherwin

Feminist reasoning in support of women's right to choose abortion is significantly different from the reasoning used by nonfeminist supporters of similar positions. For instance, most feminist accounts evaluate abortion policy within a broader framework, according to its place among the social institutions that support the subordination of women. In contrast, most nonfeminist discussions of abortion consider the moral or legal permissibility of abortion in isolation; they ignore (and thereby

From *No Longer Patient* by Susan Sherwin, Temple University Press, 1992, pp. 99–116. Copyright © 1992 by Temple University. Reprinted by permission of The Publisher.

EDITOR'S NOTE: The notes and some of the references have been omitted; those wishing to follow up on sources should consult the original source.

obscure) relevant connections with other social practices, including the ongoing power struggle within sexist societies over the control of women and their reproduction. Feminist arguments take into account the actual concerns that particular women attend to in their decision-making on abortion, such as the nature of a woman's feelings about her fetus, her relationships with her partner, other children she may have, and her various obligations to herself and others. In contrast, most nonfeminist discussions evaluate abortion decisions in their most abstract form (for example, questioning what sort of being a fetus is); from this perspective, specific questions of context are deemed irrelevant. In addition, nonfeminist arguments in support of choice about abortion are generally grounded in masculinist conceptions of freedom (such as privacy, individual choice, and individuals' property rights with respect to their own bodies), which do not meet the needs, interests, and intuitions of many of the women concerned.

Feminists also differ from nonfeminists in their conception of what is morally at issue with abortion. Nonfeminists focus exclusively on the morality and legality of performing abortions, whereas feminists insist that other issues, including the accessibility and delivery of abortion services, must also be addressed. . . .

WOMEN AND ABORTION

The most obvious difference between feminist and nonfeminist approaches to abortion lies in the relative attention each gives in its analysis to the interests and experiences of women. Feminist analysis regards the effects of unwanted pregnancies on the lives of women individually and collectively as the central element in the moral examination of abortion; it is considered self-evident that the pregnant woman is the subject of principal concern in abortion decisions. In many nonfeminist accounts, however, not only is the pregnant woman not perceived as central, she is often rendered virtually invisible. Nonfeminist theorists, whether they support or oppose women's right to choose abortion, generally focus almost all their attention on the moral status of the fetus.

In pursuing a distinctively feminist ethics, it is appropriate to begin with a look at the role of abortion in women's lives. The need for abortion can be very intense; no matter how appalling and dangerous the conditions, women from widely diverse cultures and historical periods have pursued abortions. No one denies that if abortion is not made legal, safe, and accessible in our society, women will seek out illegal and life-threatening abortions to terminate pregnancies they cannot accept. Antiabortion activists seem willing to accept this cost, although liberals definitely are not; feminists, who explicitly value women, judge the inevitable loss of women's lives that results from restrictive abortion policies to be a matter of fundamental concern.

Antiabortion campaigners imagine that women often make frivolous and irresponsible decisions about abortion, but feminists recognize that women have abortions for a wide variety of com-

pelling reasons. Some women, for instance, find themselves seriously ill and incapacitated throughout pregnancy; they cannot continue in their jobs and may face insurmountable difficulties in fulfilling their responsibilities at home. Many employers and schools will not tolerate pregnancy in their employees or students, and not every woman is able to put her job, career, or studies on hold. Women of limited means may be unable to take adequate care of children they have already borne, and they may know that another mouth to feed will reduce their ability to provide for their existing children. Women who suffer from chronic disease, who believe themselves too young or too old to have children, or who are unable to maintain lasting relationships may recognize that they will not be able to care properly for a child when they face the decision. Some who are homeless, addicted to drugs, or diagnosed as carrying the AIDS virus may be unwilling to allow a child to enter the world with the handicaps that would result from the mother's condition. If the fetus is a result of rape or incest, then the psychological pain of carrying it may be unbearable, and the woman may recognize that her attitude to the child after birth will be tinged with bitterness. Some women learn that the fetuses that they carry have serious chromosomal anomalies and consider it best to prevent them from being born with a condition that is bound to cause them to suffer. Others, knowing the fathers to be brutal and violent, may be unwilling to subject a child to the beatings or incestuous attacks they anticipate; some may have no other realistic way to remove the child (or themselves) from the relationship.

Finally, a woman may simply believe that bearing a child is incompatible with her life plans at the time. Continuing a pregnancy may have devastating repercussions throughout a woman's life. If the woman is young, then a pregnancy will likely reduce her chances of pursuing an education and hence limit her career and life opportunities: "The earlier a woman has a baby, it seems, the more likely she is to drop out of school; the less education she gets, the more likely she is to remain poorly paid, peripheral to the labor market, or unemployed, and the more children she will have" (Petchesky 1985, 150). In many circumstances, having a child will exacerbate the social and economic forces already stacked against a woman by virtue of her sex (and her race, class, age, sexual orientation, disabilities, and so forth). Access to abortion is necessary for many women if they are to escape the oppressive conditions of poverty.

Whatever the specific reasons are for abortion, most feminists believe that the women concerned are in the best position to judge whether abortion is the appropriate response to a pregnancy. Because usually only the woman choosing abortion is properly situated to weigh all the relevant factors, most feminists resist attempts to offer general, abstract rules for determining when abortion is morally justified. Women's personal deliberations about abortion involve contextually defined considerations that reflect their commitments to the needs and interests of everyone concerned, including themselves, the fetuses they carry, other members of their household, and so forth. Because no single formula is available for balancing these complex factors through all possible cases, it is vital that feminists insist on protecting each woman's right to come to her own conclusions and resist the attempts of other philosophers and moralists to set the agenda for these considerations. Feminists stress that women must be acknowledged as full moral agents, responsible for making moral decisions about their own pregnancies. Women may sometimes make mistakes in their moral judgments, but no one else can be assumed to have the authority to evaluate and overrule their judgments.

. . . Because we live in a patriarchal society, it is especially important to ensure that women have the authority to control their own reproduction. Despite the diversity of opinion found among feminists on most other matters, most feminists agree that women must gain full control over their own reproductive lives if they are to free themselves from male dominance.

Moreover, women's freedom to choose abortion is linked to their ability to control their own sexuality. Women's subordinate status often prevents them from refusing men sexual access to their bodies. If women cannot end the unwanted pregnancies that result from male sexual dominance, then their sexual vulnerability to particular men may increase, because caring for an(other) infant involves greater financial needs and reduced economic opportunities for women. As a result, pregnancy often forces women to become dependent on

particular men. Because a woman's dependence on a man is assumed to entail her continued sexual loyalty to him, restriction of abortion serves to commit women to remaining sexually accessible to particular men and thus helps to perpetuate the cycle of oppression.

In contrast to most nonfeminist accounts, feminist analyses of abortion direct attention to how women get pregnant. Those who reject abortion seem to believe that women can avoid unwanted pregnancies "simply" by avoiding sexual intercourse. These views show little appreciation for the power of sexual politics in a culture that oppresses women. Existing patterns of sexual dominance mean that women often have little control over their sexual lives. They may be subject to rape by their husbands, boyfriends, colleagues, employers, customers, fathers, brothers, uncles, and dates, as well as by strangers. Often the sexual coercion is not even recognized as such by the participants but is the price of continued "good will"—popularity, economic survival, peace, or simple acceptance. Many women have found themselves in circumstances where they do not feel free to refuse a man's demands for intercourse, either because he is holding a gun to her head or because he threatens to be emotionally hurt if she refuses (or both). Women are socialized to be compliant and accommodating, sensitive to the feelings of others, and frightened of physical power; men are socialized to take advantage of every opportunity to engage in sexual intercourse and to use sex to express dominance and power. Under such circumstances, it is difficult to argue that women could simply "choose" to avoid heterosexual activity if they wish to avoid pregnancy. Catharine MacKinnon neatly sums it up: "The logic by which women are supposed to consent to sex [is]: preclude the alternatives, then call the remaining option 'her choice'" (MacKinnon 1989, 192).

Furthermore, women cannot rely on birth control to avoid pregnancy. No form of contraception that is fully safe and reliable is available, other than sterilization; because women may wish only to avoid pregnancy temporarily, not permanently, sterilization is not always an acceptable choice. The pill and the IUD are the most effective contraceptive means offered, but both involve significant health hazards to women and are quite dangerous for some. No woman should spend the thirty to forty years of her reproductive life on either form of birth control. Further, both have been associated with subsequent problems of involuntary infertility, so they are far from optimal for women who seek to control the timing of their pregnancies.

The safest form of birth control involves the use of barrier methods (condoms or diaphragms) in combination with spermicidal foams or jelly. But these methods also pose difficulties for women. They are sometimes socially awkward to use. Young women are discouraged from preparing for sexual activity that might never happen and are offered instead romantic models of spontaneous passion; few films or novels interrupt scenes of seduction for a partner to fetch contraceptives. Many women find their male partners unwilling to use barrier methods of contraception, and they often find themselves in no position to insist. Further, cost is a limiting factor for many women. Condoms and spermicides are expensive and are not covered under most health care plans. Only one contraceptive option offers women safe and fully effective birth control: barrier methods with the backup option of abortion.

From a feminist perspective, the central moral feature of pregnancy is that it takes place in women's bodies and has profound effects on women's lives. Gender-neutral accounts of pregnancy are not available; pregnancy is explicitly a condition associated with the female body. Because only women experience a need for abortion, policies about abortion affect women uniquely. Therefore, it is important to consider how proposed policies on abortion fit into general patterns of oppression for women. Unlike nonfeminist accounts, feminist ethics demands that the effects of abortion policies on the oppression of women be of principal consideration in our ethical evaluations.

THE FETUS

In contrast to feminist ethics, most nonfeminist analysts believe that the moral acceptability of abortion turns entirely on the question of the moral status of the fetus. Even those who support women's right to choose abortion tend to accept the premise of the antiabortion proponents that abortion can be tolerated only if we can first prove

that the fetus lacks full personhood. Opponents of abortion demand that we define the status of the fetus either as a being that is valued in the same way as other humans, and hence is entitled not to be killed, or as a being that lacks in all value. Rather than challenging the logic of this formulation, many defenders of abortion have concentrated on showing that the fetus is indeed without significant value; others offer a more subtle account that reflects the gradual development of fetuses and distinguishes between early fetal stages, where the relevant criterion for personhood is absent, and later stages, where it is present. Thus the debate often rages between abortion opponents, who describe the fetus as an "innocent," vulnerable, morally important, separate being whose life is threatened and who must be protected at all costs, and abortion supporters, who try to establish that fetuses are deficient in some critical respect and hence are outside the scope of the moral community. In both cases, however, the nature of the fetus as an independent being is said to determine the moral status of abortion.

The woman on whom the fetus depends for survival is considered as secondary (if she is considered at all) in these debates. The actual experiences and responsibilities of real women are not perceived as morally relevant to the debate, unless these women too, can be proved innocent by establishing that their pregnancies are a result of rape or incest. In some contexts, women's role in gestation is literally reduced to that of "fetal containers"; the individual women disappear or are perceived simply as mechanical life-support systems.

The current rhetoric against abortion stresses that the genetic makeup of the fetus is determined at conception and the genetic code is incontestably human. Lest there be any doubt about the humanity of the fetus, we are assailed with photographs of fetuses at various stages of development that demonstrate the early appearance of recognizably human characteristics, such as eyes, fingers, and toes. Modern ultrasound technology is used to obtain "baby's first picture" and stimulate bonding between pregnant women and their fetuses. That the fetus in its early stages is microscopic, virtually indistinguishable to the untrained eye from fetuses of other species, and lacking in the capacities that make human life meaningful and valuable is not deemed relevant by the self-appointed defenders of the fetus. The antiabortion campaign is directed at evoking sympathetic attitudes toward a tiny, helpless being whose life is threatened by its own mother; the fetus is characterized as a being entangled in an adversarial relationship with the (presumably irresponsible) woman who carries it. People are encouraged to identify with the "unborn child," not with the woman whose life is also at issue.

In the nonfeminist literature, both defenders and opponents of women's right to choose abortion agree that the difference between a late-term fetus and a newborn infant is "merely geographical" and cannot be considered morally significant. Daniel Callahan (1986), for instance, maintains a pro-choice stand but professes increasing uneasiness about this position in light of new medical and scientific developments that increase our knowledge of embryology and hasten the date of potential viability for fetuses; he insists that defenders of women's right to choose must come to terms with the question of the fetus and the effects of science on the fetus's prospects apart from the woman who carries it. Arguments that focus on the similarities between infants and fetuses, however, generally fail to acknowledge that a fetus inhabits a woman's body and is wholly dependent on her unique contribution to its maintenance, whereas a newborn is physically independent, although still in need of a lot of care. One can only view the distinction between being in or out of a woman's womb as morally irrelevant if one discounts the perspective of the pregnant woman; feminists seem to be alone in recognizing the woman's perspective as morally important to the distinction.

In antiabortion arguments, fetuses are identified as individuals; in our culture, which views the (abstract) individual as sacred, fetuses qua individuals are to be honored and preserved. Extraordinary claims are made to establish the individuality and moral agency of fetuses. At the same time, the women who carry these fetal individuals are viewed as passive hosts whose only significant role is to refrain from aborting or harming their fetuses. Because it is widely believed that a woman does not actually have to do anything to protect the life of her fetus, pregnancy is often considered (abstractly) to be a tolerable burden to protect the life of an individual so like us.

Medicine has played its part in supporting these attitudes. Fetal medicine is a rapidly expanding specialty, and it is commonplace in professional medical journals to find references to pregnant women as "the maternal environment." Fetal surgeons now have at their disposal a repertoire of sophisticated technology that can save the lives of dangerously ill fetuses; in light of the excitement of such heroic successes, it is perhaps understandable that women have disappeared from their view. These specialists see the fetuses as their patients, not the women who nurture the fetuses. As the "active" agents in saving fetal lives (unlike the pregnant women, whose role is seen as purely passive), doctors perceive themselves as developing independent relationships with the fetuses they treat. Barbara Katz Rothman observes: "The medical model of pregnancy, as an essentially parasitic and vaguely pathological relationship, encourages the physician to view the fetus and mother as two separate patients, and to see pregnancy as inherently a conflict of interests between the two" (Rothman 1986, 25). . . .

In other words, some physicians have joined antiabortion campaigners in fostering a cultural acceptance of the view that fetuses are distinct individuals who are physically, ontologically, and socially separate from the women whose bodies they inhabit and that they have their own distinct interests. In this picture, pregnant women are either ignored altogether or are viewed as deficient in some crucial respect, and hence they can be subject to coercion for the sake of their fetuses. In the former case, the interests of the women concerned are assumed to be identical with those of the fetus; in the latter, the women's interests are irrelevant, because they are perceived as immoral, unimportant, or unnatural. Focus on the fetus as an independent entity has led to presumptions that deny pregnant women their roles as active, independent, moral agents with a primary interest in what becomes of the fetuses they carry. The moral question of the fetus's status is quickly translated into a license to interfere with women's reproductive freedom.

On a feminist account fetal development is examined in the context in which it occurs, within women's bodies, rather than in the isolation of imagined abstraction. Fetuses develop in specific pregnancies that occur in the lives of particular women. They are not individuals housed in generic female wombs or full persons at risk only because they are small and subject to the whims of women. Their very existence is relationally defined, reflecting their development within particular women's bodies; that relationship gives those women reason to be concerned about them. Many feminists argue against a perspective that regards the fetus as an independent being and suggest that a more accurate and valuable understanding of pregnancy would involve regarding the pregnant woman "as a biological and social unit.". . . .

Most feminist views of what is valuable about persons reflect the social nature of individual existence. No human, especially no fetus, can exist apart from relationships; efforts to speak of the fetus itself, as if it were not inseparable from the woman in whom it develops, are distorting and dishonest. Fetuses have a unique physical status—within and dependent on particular women. That gives them also a unique social status. However much some might prefer it to be otherwise, no one other than the pregnant woman in question can do anything to support or harm a fetus without doing something to the woman who nurtures it. Because of this inexorable biological reality, the responsibility and privilege of determining a fetus's specific social status and value must rest with the woman carrying it. . . .

No absolute value attaches to fetuses apart from their relational status, which is determined in the context of their particular development. This is not the same, however, as saying that they have no value at all or that they have merely instrumental value, as some liberals suggest. The value that women place on their own fetuses is the sort of value that attaches to an emerging human relationship.

Nevertheless, fetuses are not persons, because they have not developed sufficiently in their capacity for social relationships to be persons in any morally significant sense (that is, they are not yet second persons). In this way they differ from newborns, who immediately begin to develop into persons by virtue of their place as subjects in human relationships; newborns are capable of some forms of communication and response. The moral status of fetuses is determined by the nature of their primary relationship and the value that is created

there. Therefore, feminist accounts of abortion emphasize the importance of protecting women's rights to continue or to terminate pregnancies as each sees fit.

THE POLITICS OF ABORTION

Feminist accounts explore the connections between particular social policies and the general patterns of power relationships in our society. . . . When we place abortion in the larger political context, we see that most of the groups active in the struggle to prohibit abortion also support other conservative measures to maintain the forms of dominance that characterize patriarchy (and often class and racial oppression as well). The movement against abortion is led by the Catholic church and other conservative religious institutions, which explicitly endorse not only fetal rights but also male dominance in the home and the church. Most opponents of abortion also oppose virtually all forms of birth control and all forms of sexuality other than monogamous, reproductive sex; usually, they also resist having women assume positions of authority in dominant public institutions. Typically, antiabortion activists support conservative economic measures that protect the interests of the privileged classes of society and ignore the needs of the oppressed and disadvantaged. Although they stress their commitment to preserving life, many systematically work to dismantle key social programs that provide life necessities to the underclass. Moreover, some current campaigns against abortion retain elements of the racism that dominated the North American abortion literature in the early years of the twentieth century, wherein abortion was opposed on the grounds that it amounted to racial suicide on the part of whites.

In the eyes of its principal opponents, then, abortion is not an isolated practice; their opposition to abortion is central to a set of social values that runs counter to feminism's objectives. Hence antiabortion activists generally do not offer alternatives to abortion that support feminist interests in overturning the patterns of oppression that confront women. Most deny that there are any legitimate grounds for abortion, short of the need to save a woman's life—and some are not even persuaded by this criterion. They believe that any pregnancy can and should be endured. If the mother is unable or unwilling to care for the child after birth, then they assume that adoption can be easily arranged.

It is doubtful, however, that adoptions are possible for every child whose mother cannot care for it. The world abounds with homeless orphans; even in the industrialized West, where there is a waiting list for adoption of healthy (white) babies, suitable homes cannot always be found for troubled adolescents; inner-city, AIDS babies, or many of the multiply handicapped children whose parents may have tried to care for them but whose marriages broke under the strain.

Furthermore, even if an infant were born healthy and could be readily adopted, we must recognize that surrendering one's child for adop-tion is an extremely difficult act for most women. The bond that commonly forms between women and their fetuses over the full term of pregnancy is intimate and often intense; many women find that it is not easily broken after birth. Psychologically, for many women adoption is a far more difficult response to unwanted pregnancies than abortion. Therefore, it is misleading to describe pregnancy as merely a nine-month commitment; for most women, seeing a pregnancy through to term involves a lifetime of responsibility and involvement with the resulting child and, in the overwhelming majority of cases, disproportionate burden on the woman through the child-rearing years. An ethics that cares about women would recognize that abortion is often the only acceptable recourse for them.

A Case for Pro-Life Feminism

Sidney Callahan

The abortion debate continues. In the latest and perhaps most crucial development, pro-life feminists are contesting pro-choice feminist claims that abortion rights are prerequisites for women's full development and social equality. The outcome of this debate may be decisive for the culture as a whole. Pro-life feminists, like myself, argue on good feminist principles that women can never achieve the fulfillment of feminist goals in a society permissive toward abortion.

These new arguments over abortion take place within liberal political circles. This round of intense intra-feminist conflict has spiraled beyond earlier right-versus-left abortion debates, which focused on 'tragic choices,'' medical judgments, and legal compromises. Feminist theorists of the pro-choice position now put forth the demand for unrestricted abortion rights as a moral imperative and insist upon women's right to complete reproductive freedom. They morally justify the present situation and current abortion practices. Thus it is all the more important that pro-life feminists articulate their different feminist perspective.

These opposing arguments can best be seen when presented in turn. Perhaps the most highly developed feminist arguments for the morality and legality of abortion can be found in Beverly Wildung Harrison's *Our Right to Choose* (Beacon Press, 1983) and Rosalind Pollack Petchesky's *Abortion and Woman's Choice* (Longman, 1984). Obviously it is difficult to do justice to these complex arguments, which draw on diverse strands of philosophy and social theory and are often interwoven in pro-choice feminists' own version of a "seamless garment." Yet the fundamental feminist case for the morality of abortion, encompassing the views of Harrison and Petchesky, can be analyzed in terms of four central moral claims: (1) the moral right to control one's own body; (2) the moral necessity of autonomy and choice in personal responsibility; (3) the moral claim for the

Commonweal Vol. 25, April 1986, pp. 232–238. Copyright © 1986 Commonweal Foundation. Reprinted by permission.

contingent value of fetal life; (4) the moral right of women to true social equality.

1. THE MORAL RIGHT TO CONTROL ONE'S OWN BODY

Pro-choice feminism argues that a woman choosing an abortion is exercising a basic right of bodily integrity granted in our common law tradition. If she does not choose to be physically involved in the demands of a pregnancy and birth, she should not be compelled to be so against her will. Just because it is her body which is involved, a woman should have the right to terminate any pregnancy, which at this point in medical history is tantamount to terminating fetal life. No one can be forced to donate an organ or submit to other invasive physical procedures for however good a cause. Thus no woman should be subjected to "compulsory pregnancy." And it should be noted that in pregnancy much more than a passive biological process is at stake.

From one perspective, the fetus is, as Petchesky says, a "biological parasite" taking resources from the woman's body. During pregnancy, a woman's whole life and energies will be actively involved in the nine-month process. Gestation and childbirth involve physical and psychological risks. After childbirth a woman will either be a mother who must undertake a twenty-year responsibility for childrearing, or face giving up her child for adoption or institutionalization. Since hers is the body, hers the risk, hers the burden, it is only just that she alone should be free to decide on pregnancy or abortion.

This moral claim to abortion, according to the pro-choice feminists, is especially valid in an individualistic society in which women cannot count on medical care or social support in pregnancy, childbirth, or childrearing. A moral abortion decision is never made in a social vacuum, but in the real life society which exists here and now.

2. THE MORAL NECESSITY OF AUTONOMY AND CHOICE IN PERSONAL RESPONSIBILITY

Beyond the claim for individual *bodily* integrity, the pro-choice feminists claim that to be a full adult *morally*, a woman must be able to make responsible life commitments. To plan, choose, and exercise personal responsibility, one must have control of reproduction. A woman must be able to make yes or no decisions about a specific pregnancy, according to her present situation, resources, prior commitments. and life plan. Only with such reproductive freedom can a woman have the moral autonomy necessary to make mature commitments, in the area of family, work, or education.

Contraception provides a measure of personal control, but contraceptive failure or other chance events can too easily result in involuntary pregnancy. Only free access to abortion can provide the necessary guarantee. The chance biological process of an involuntary pregnancy should not be allowed to override all the other personal commitments and responsibilities a woman has: to others, to family, to work, to education, to her future development, health, or well-being. Without reproductive freedom, women's personal moral agency and human consciousness are subjected to biology and chance.

3. THE MORAL CLAIM FOR THE CONTINGENT VALUE OF FETAL LIFE

Pro-choice feminist exponents like Harrison and Petchesky claim that the value of fetal life is contingent upon the woman's free consent and subjective acceptance. The fetus must be invested with maternal valuing in order to become human. This process of "humanization" through personal consciousness and "sociality" can only be bestowed by the woman in whose body and psychosocial system a new life must mature. The meaning and value of fetal life are constructed by the woman; without this personal conferral there only exists a biological, physiological process. Thus fetal interests or fetal rights can never outweigh the woman's prior interest and rights. If a woman does not consent to invest her pregnancy with meaning or value, then the merely biological process can be freely terminated. Prior to her own free choice and conscious investment, a woman cannot be described as a "mother" nor can a "child" be said to exist.

Moreover, in cases of voluntary pregnancy, a woman can withdraw consent if fetal genetic defects or some other problem emerges at any time before birth. Late abortion should thus be granted without legal restrictions. Even the minimal qualifications and limitations on women embedded in *Roe v. Wade* are unacceptable—repressive remnants of patriarchal unwillingness to give power to women.

4. THE MORAL RIGHT OF WOMEN TO FULL SOCIAL EQUALITY

Women have a moral right to full social equality. They should not be restricted or subordinated because of their sex. But this morally required equality cannot be realized without abortion's certain control of reproduction. Female social equality depends upon being able to compete and participate as freely as males can in the structures of educational and economic life. If a woman cannot control when and how she will be pregnant or rear children, she is at a distinct disadvantage, especially in our male-dominated world.

Psychological equality and well-being is also at stake. Women must enjoy the basic right of a person to the free exercise of heterosexual intercourse and full sexual expression, separated from procreation. No less than males, women should be able to be sexually active without the constantly inhibiting fear of pregnancy. Abortion is necessary for women's sexual fulfillment and the growth of uninhibited feminine self-confidence and ownership of their sexual powers.

But true sexual and reproductive freedom means freedom to procreate as well as to inhibit fertility. Pro-choice feminists are also worried that women's freedom to reproduce will be curtailed through the abuse of sterilization and needless hysterectomies. Besides the punitive tendencies of a male-dominated healthcare system, especially in response to repeated abortions or welfare pregnancies, there are other economic and social pressures inhibiting reproduction. Genuine reproductive freedom implies that day care, medical care, and financial support would be provided mothers, while fathers would take their full share in the burdens and delights of raising children.

Many pro-choice feminists identify feminist ideals with communitarian, ecologically sensitive approaches to reshaping society. Following theorists like Sara Ruddick and Carol Gilligan, they link abortion rights with the growth of "maternal thinking" in our heretofore patriarchal society. Maternal thinking is loosely defined as a responsible commitment to the loving nurture of specific human beings as they actually exist in socially embedded interpersonal contexts. It is a moral perspective very different from the abstract, competitive, isolated, and principled rigidity so characteristic of patriarchy.

How does a pro-life feminist respond to these arguments? Pro-life feminists grant the good intentions of their pro-choice counterparts but protest that the pro-choice position is flawed, morally inadequate, and inconsistent with feminism's basic demands for justice. Pro-life feminists champion a more encompassing moral ideal. They recognize the claims of fetal life and offer a different perspective on what is good for women. The feminist vision is expanded and refocused.

1. FROM THE MORAL RIGHT TO CONTROL ONE'S OWN BODY TO A MORE INCLUSIVE IDEAL OF JUSTICE

The moral right to control one's own body does apply to cases of organ transplants, mastectomies, contraception, and sterilization; but it is not a conceptualization adequate for abortion. The abortion dilemma is caused by the fact that 266 days following a conception in one body, another body will emerge. One's own body no longer exists as a single unit but is engendering another organism's life. This dynamic passage from conception to birth is genetically ordered and universally found in the human species. Pregnancy is not like the growth of cancer or infestation by a biological parasite: it is the way every human being enters the world. Strained philosophical analogies fail to apply: having a baby is not like rescuing a drowning person, being hooked up to a famous violinist's artificial life-support system, donating organs for transplant—or anything else.

As embryology and fetology advance, it becomes clear that human development is a continuum. Just as astronomers are studying the first three minutes in the genesis of the universe, so the first moments, days, and weeks at the beginning of human life are the subject of increasing scientific attention. While neonatology pushes the definition of viability ever earlier, ultrasound and fetology expand the concept of the patient in utero. Within such a continuous growth process, it is hard to defend logically any demarcation point after conception as the point at which an immature form of human life is so different from the day before or the day after, that it can be morally or legally discounted as a non-person. Even the moment of birth can hardly differentiate a nine-month fetus from a newborn. It is not surprising that those who countenance late abortions are logically led to endorse selective infanticide.

The same legal tradition which in our society guarantees the right to control one's own body firmly recognizes the wrongfulness of harming other bodies, however immature, dependent, different looking, or powerless. The handicapped, the retarded, and newborns are legally protected from deliberate harm. Pro-life feminists reject the suppositions that would except the unborn from this protection.

After all, debates similar to those about the fetus were once conducted about feminine personhood. Just as women, or blacks, were considered too different, too underdeveloped, too "biological," to have souls or to possess legal rights, so the fetus is now seen as "merely" biological life, subsidiary to a person. A woman was once viewed as incorporated into the "one flesh" of her husband's person; she too was a form of bodily property. In all patriarchal unjust systems, lesser orders of human life are granted rights only when wanted, chosen, or invested with value by the powerful.

Fortunately, in the course of civilization there has been a gradual realization that justice demands the powerless and dependent be protected against the uses of power wielded unilaterally. No human can be treated as a means to an end without consent. The fetus is an immature, dependent form of human life which only needs time and protection to develop. Surely, immaturity and dependence are not crimes.

In an effort to think about the essential requirements of a just society, philosophers like John Rawls recommend imagining yourself in an "original position," in which your position in the society to be created is hidden by a "veil of ignorance." You will have to weigh the possibility that any inequalities inherent in that society's practices may rebound upon you in the worst, as well as in the best, conceivable way. This thought experiment helps ensure justice for all.

Beverly Harrison argues that in such an envisioning of society everyone would institute abortion rights in order to guarantee that if one turned out to be a woman one would have reproductive freedom. But surely in the original position and behind the "veil of ignorance," you would have to contemplate the possibility of being the particular fetus to be aborted. Since everyone has passed through the fetal stage of development, it is false to refuse to imagine oneself in this state when thinking about a potential world in which justice would govern. Would it be just that an embryonic life—in half the cases, of course, a female life—be sacrificed to the right of a woman's control over her own body? A woman may be pregnant without consent and experience a great many penalties, but a fetus killed without consent pays the ultimate penalty.

It does not matter (*The Silent Scream* notwithstanding) whether the fetus being killed is fully conscious or feels pain. We do not sanction killing the innocent if it can be done painlessly or without the victim's awareness. Consciousness becomes important to the abortion debate because it is used as a criterion for the "personhood" so often seen as the prerequisite for legal protection. Yet certain philosophers set the standard of personhood so high that half the human race could not meet the criteria during most of their waking hours (let alone their sleeping ones). Sentience, self-consciousness, rational decision-making, social participation? Surely no infant, or child under two, could qualify. Either our idea of person must be expanded or another criterion, such as human life itself, be employed to protect the weak in a just society. Pro-life feminists who defend the fetus empathetically identify with an immature state of growth passed through by themselves, their children, and everyone now alive.

It also seems a travesty of just procedures that a pregnant woman now, in effect, acts as sole judge of her own case, under the most stressful conditions. Yes, one can acknowledge that the pregnant woman will be subject to the potential burdens arising from a pregnancy, but it has never been thought right to have an interested party, especially the more powerful party, decide his or her own case when there may be a conflict of interest. If one considers the matter as a case of a powerful versus a powerless, silenced claimant, the pro-choice feminist argument can rightly be inverted: since hers is the body, hers the risk, and hers the greater burden, then how in fairness can a woman be the sole judge of the fetal right to life?

Human ambivalence, a bias toward self-interest, and emotional stress have always been recognized as endangering judgment. Freud declared that love and hate are so entwined that if instant thoughts could kill, we would all be dead in the bosom of our families. In the case of a woman's involuntary pregnancy, a complex, long-term solution requiring effort and energy has to compete with the immediate solution offered by a morning's visit to an abortion clinic. On the simple, perceptual plane, with imagination and thinking curtailed, the speed, ease, and privacy of abortion, combined with the small size of the embryo, tend to make early abortions seem less morally serious—even though speed, size, technical ease, and the private nature of an act have no moral standing.

As the most recent immigrants from non-personhood, feminists have traditionally fought for justice for themselves and the world. Women rally to feminism as a new and better way to live. Rejecting male aggression and destruction, feminists seek alternative, peaceful, ecologically sensitive means to resolve conflicts while respecting human potentiality. It is a chilling inconsistency to see pro-choice feminists demanding continued access to assembly-line, technological methods of fetal killing—the vacuum aspirator, prostaglandins, and dilation and evacuation. It is a betrayal of feminism, which has built the struggle for justice on the bedrock of women's empathy. After all, "maternal thinking" receives its name from a mother's unconditional acceptance and nurture of dependent, immature life. It is difficult to develop concern for women, children, the poor and the dispossessed—and to care about peace—and at the same time ignore fetal life.

2. FROM THE NECESSITY OF AUTONOMY AND CHOICE IN PERSONAL RESPONSIBILITY TO AN EXPANDED SENSE OF RESPONSIBILITY

A distorted idea of morality overemphasizes individual autonomy and active choice. Morality has often been viewed too exclusively as a matter of human agency and decisive action. In moral behavior persons must explicitly choose and aggressively exert their wills to intervene in the natural and social environments. The human will dominates the body, overcomes the given, breaks out of the material limits of nature. Thus if one does not choose to be pregnant or cannot rear a child, who must be given up for adoption, then better to abort the pregnancy. Willing, planning, choosing one's moral commitments through the contracting of one's individual resources becomes the premier model of moral responsibility.

But morality also consists of the good and worthy acceptance of the unexpected events that life presents. Responsiveness and responsibility to things unchosen are also instances of the highest human moral capacity. Morality is not confined to contracted agreements of isolated individuals. Yes, one is obligated by explicit contracts freely initiated, but human beings are also obligated by implicit compacts and involuntary relationships in which persons simply find themselves. To be embedded in a family, a neighborhood, a social system, brings moral obligations which were never entered into with informed consent.

Parent-child relationships are one instance of implicit moral obligations arising by virtue of our being part of the interdependent human community. A woman, involuntarily pregnant, has a moral obligation to the now-existing dependent fetus whether she explicitly consented to its existence or not. No pro-life feminist would dispute the forceful observations of pro-choice feminists about the extreme difficulties that bearing an unwanted child in our society can entail. But the stronger force of the fetal claim presses a woman to accept these burdens; the fetus possesses rights arising from its extreme need and the interdependency and unity of humankind. The woman's moral obligation arises both from her status as a human being embedded in the interdependent human community and her unique life-giving female reproductive power. To follow the pro-choice feminist ideology of insistent individualistic autonomy and control is to betray a fundamental basis of the moral life.

3. FROM THE MORAL CLAIM OF THE CONTINGENT VALUE OF FETAL LIFE TO THE MORAL CLAIM FOR THE INTRINSIC VALUE OF HUMAN LIFE

The feminist pro-choice position which claims that the value of the fetus is contingent upon the pregnant woman's bestowal—or willed, conscious "construction"—of humanhood is seriously flawed. The inadequacies of this position flow from the erroneous premises (1) that human value and rights can be granted by individual will; (2) that the individual woman's consciousness can exist and operate in an *a priori* isolated fashion; and (3) that "mere" biological, genetic human life has little meaning. Pro-life feminism takes a very different stance to life and nature.

Human life from the beginning to the end of development *has* intrinsic value, which does not depend on meeting the selective criteria or tests set up by powerful others. A fundamental humanist assumption is at stake here. Either we are going to value embodied human life and humanity as a good thing, or take some variant of the nihilist position that assumes human life is just one more random occurrence in the universe such that each instance of human life must explicitly be justified to prove itself worthy to continue. When faced with a new life, or an involuntary pregnancy, there is a world of difference in whether one first asks, "Why continue?" or "Why not?" Where is the burden of proof going to rest? The concept of "compulsory pregnancy" is as distorted as labeling life "compulsory aging."

In a sound moral tradition, human rights arise from human needs, and it is the very nature of a right, or valid claim upon another, that it cannot be denied, conditionally delayed, or rescinded by more powerful others at their behest. It seems fallacious to hold that in the case of the fetus it is the pregnant woman alone who gives or removes its right to life and human status solely through her subjective conscious investment or "humanization." Surely no pregnant woman (or any other individual member of the species) has created her own human nature by an individually willed act of consciousness, nor for that matter been able to guarantee her own human rights. An individual woman and the unique individual embryonic life within her can only exist because of their participation in the genetic inheritance of the human species as a whole. Biological life should never be discounted. Membership in the species, or collective human family, is the basis for human solidarity, equality, and natural human rights.

4. THE MORAL RIGHT OF WOMEN TO FULL SOCIAL EQUALITY FROM A PRO-LIFE FEMINIST PERSPECTIVE

Pro-life feminists and pro-choice feminists are totally agreed on the moral right of women to the full social equality so far denied them. The disagreement between them concerns the definition of the desired goal and the best means to get there. Permissive abortion laws do not bring women reproductive freedom, social equality, sexual fulfillment, or full personal development.

Pragmatic failures of a pro-choice feminist position combined with a lack of moral vision are, in fact, causing disaffection among young women. Middle-aged pro-choice feminists blamed the "big chill" on the general conservative backlash. But they should look rather to their own elitist acceptance of male models of sex and to the sad picture they present of women's lives. Pitting women against their own offspring is not only morally offensive, it is psychologically and politically destructive. Women will never climb to equality and social empowerment over mounds of dead fetuses, numbering now in the millions. As long as most women choose to bear children, they stand to gain from the same constellation of attitudes and institutions that will also protect the fetus in the woman's womb—and they stand to lose from the cultural assumptions that support permissive abortion. Despite temporary conflicts of interest, feminine and fetal liberation are ultimately one and the same cause.

Women's rights and liberation are pragmatically linked to fetal rights because to obtain true equality, women need (1) more social support and changes in the structure of society, and (2) increased self-confidence, self-expectations, and self-esteem. Society in general, and men in particular, have to provide women more support in rearing the next generation, or our devastating feminization of poverty will continue. But if a woman claims the right to decide by herself whether the fetus becomes a child or not, what does this do to paternal and communal responsibility? Why should men share responsibility for child support or childrearing if they cannot share in what is asserted to be the woman's sole decision? Furthermore, if explicit intentions and consciously accepted contracts are necessary for moral obligations, why should men be held responsible for what *they* do not voluntarily choose to happen? By pro-choice reasoning, a man who does not want to have a child, or whose contraceptive fails, can be exempted from the responsibilities of fatherhood and child support. Traditionally, many men have been laggards in assuming parental responsibility and support for their children; ironically, ready abortion, often advocated as a response to male dereliction, legitimizes male irresponsibility and paves the way for even more male detachment and lack of commitment.

For that matter, why should the state provide a system of day-care or child support, or require workplaces to accommodate women's maternity and the needs of childrearing? Permissive abortion, granted in the name of women's privacy and reproductive freedom, ratifies the view that pregnancies and children are a woman's private individual responsibility. More and more frequently, we hear some versions of this old rationalization: if she refuses to get rid of it, it's her problem. A child becomes a product of the individual woman's freely chosen investment, a form of private property resulting from her own cost-benefit calculation. The larger community is relieved of moral responsibility.

With legal abortion freely available, a clear cultural message is given: conception and pregnancy are no longer serious moral matters. With abortion as an acceptable alternative, contraception is not as responsibly used; women take risks, often at the urging of male sexual partners. Repeat abortions increase, with all their psychological and medical repercussions. With more abortion there is more abortion. Behavior shapes thought as well as the other way round. One tends to justify morally what one has done; what becomes commonplace and institutionalized seems harmless. Habituation is a powerful psychological force. Psychologically it is also true that whatever is avoided becomes more threatening; in phobias it is the retreat from anxiety-producing events which reinforces future avoidance. Women begin to see themselves as too weak to cope with involuntary pregnancies. Finally, through the potency of social pressure and the force of inertia, it becomes more and more difficult, in fact almost unthinkable, not to use abortion to solve problem pregnancies. Abortion becomes no longer a choice but a "necessity."

But "necessity," beyond the organic failure and death of the body, is a dynamic social construction

open to interpretation. The thrust of present feminist pro-choice arguments can only increase the justifiable indications for "necessary" abortion; every unwanted fetal handicap becomes more and more unacceptable. Repeatedly assured that in the name of reproductive freedom, women have a right to specify which pregnancies and which children they will accept, women justify sex selection, and abort unwanted females. Female infanticide, after all, is probably as old a custom as the human species possesses. Indeed, all kinds of selection of the fit and the favored for the good of the family and the tribe have always existed. Selective extinction is no new program.

There are far better goals for feminists to pursue. Pro-life feminists seek to expand and deepen the more communitarian, maternal elements of feminism—and move society from its male-dominated course. First and foremost, women have to insist upon a different, woman-centered approach to sex and reproduction. While Margaret Mead stressed the "womb envy" of males in other societies, it has been more or less repressed in our own. In our male-dominated world, what men don't do, doesn't count. Pregnancy, childbirth, and nursing have been characterized as passive, debilitating, animal-like. The disease model of pregnancy and birth has been entrenched. This female disease or impairment, with its attendant "female troubles," naturally handicaps women in the "real" world of hunting, war, and the corporate fast track. Many pro-choice feminists, deliberately childless, adopt the male perspective when they cite the "basic injustice that women have to bear the babies," instead of seeing the injustice in the fact that men cannot. Women's biologically unique capacity and privilege has been denied, despised, and suppressed under male domination; unfortunately, many women have fallen for the phallic fallacy.

Childbirth often appears in pro-choice literature as a painful, traumatic, life-threatening experience. Yet giving birth is accurately seen as an arduous but normal exercise of life-giving power, a violent and ecstatic peak experience, which men can never know. Ironically, some pro-choice men and women think and talk of pregnancy and childbirth with the same repugnance that ancient ascetics displayed toward orgasms and sexual intercourse. The similarity may not be accidental. The obstetrician Niles Newton, herself a mother, has written of the extended threefold sexuality of women, who can experience orgasm, birth, and nursing as passionate pleasure-giving experiences. All of these are involuntary processes of the female body. Only orgasm, which males share, has been glorified as an involuntary function that is nature's great gift; the involuntary feminine processes of childbirth and nursing have been seen as bondage to biology.

Fully accepting our bodies as ourselves, what should women want? I think women will only flourish when there is a feminization of sexuality, very different from the current cultural trend toward masculinizing female sexuality. Women can never have the self-confidence and self-esteem they need to achieve feminist goals in society until a more holistic, feminine model of sexuality becomes the dominant cultural ethos. To say this affirms the view that men and women differ in the domain of sexual functioning, although they are more alike than different in other personality characteristics and competencies. For those of us committed to achieving sexual equality in the culture, it may be hard to accept the fact that sexual differences make it imperative to talk of distinct male and female models of sexuality. But if one wants to change sexual roles, one has to recognize preexisting conditions. A great deal of evidence is accumulating which points to biological pressures for different male and female sexual functioning.

Males always and everywhere have been more physically aggressive and more likely to fuse sexuality with aggression and dominance. Females may be more variable in their sexuality, but since Masters and Johnson, we know that women have a greater capacity than men for repeated orgasm and a more tenuous path to arousal and orgasmic release. Most obviously, women also have a far greater sociobiological investment in the act of human reproduction. On the whole, women as compared to men possess a sexuality which is more complex, more intense, more extended in time, involving higher investment, risks, and psychosocial involvement.

Considering the differences in sexual functioning, it is not surprising that men and women in the same culture have often constructed different sexual ideals. In Western culture, since the nineteenth century at least, most women have espoused a version of sexual functioning in which sex acts are embedded within deep emotional bonds and secure long-term commitments. Within these committed "pair bonds" males assume parental oblig-

ations. In the idealized Victorian version of the Christian sexual ethic, culturally endorsed and maintained by women, the double standard was not countenanced. Men and women did not need to marry to be whole persons, but if they did engage in sexual functioning, they were to be equally chaste, faithful, responsible, loving, and parentally concerned. Many of the most influential women in the nineteenth-century women's movement preached and lived this sexual ethic, often by the side of exemplary feminist men. While the ideal has never been universally obtained, a culturally dominant demand for monogamy, self-control, and emotionally bonded and committed sex works well for women in every stage of their sexual life cycles. When love, chastity, fidelity, and commitment for better or worse are the ascendant cultural prerequisites for sexual functioning, young girls and women expect protection from rape and seduction, adult women justifiably demand male support in childrearing, and older women are more protected from abandonment as their biological attractions wane.

Of course, these feminine sexual ideals always coexisted in competition with another view. A more male-oriented model of erotic or amative sexuality endorses sexual permissiveness without long-term commitment or reproductive focus. Erotic sexuality emphasizes pleasure, play, passion, individual self-expression, and romantic games of courtship and conquest. It is assumed that a variety of partners and sexual experiences are necessary to stimulate romantic passion. This erotic model of the sexual life has often worked satisfactorily for men, both heterosexual and gay, and for certain cultural elites. But for the average woman, it is quite destructive. Women can only play the erotic game successfully when like the "*Cosmopolitan* woman," they are young, physically attractive, economically powerful, and fulfilled enough in a career to be willing to sacrifice family life. Abortion is also required. As our society increasingly endorses this male-oriented, permissive view of sexuality, it is all too ready to give women abortion on demand. Abortion helps a woman's body be more like a man's. It has been observed that *Roe v. Wade* removed the last defense women possessed against male sexual demands.

Unfortunately, the modern feminist movement made a mistaken move at a critical juncture.

Rightly rebelling against patriarchy, unequal education, restricted work opportunities, and women's downtrodden political status, feminists also rejected the nineteenth-century feminine sexual ethic. Amative, erotic, permissive sexuality (along with abortion rights) became symbolically identified with other struggles for social equality in education, work, and politics. This feminist mistake also turned off many potential recruits among women who could not deny the positive dimensions of their own traditional feminine roles, nor their allegiance to the older feminine sexual ethic of love and fidelity.

An ironic situation then arose in which many pro-choice feminists preach their own double standard. In the world of work and career, women are urged to grow up, to display mature self-discipline and self-control; they are told to persevere in long-term commitments, to cope with unexpected obstacles by learning to tough out the inevitable sufferings and setbacks entailed in life and work. But this mature ethic of commitment and self-discipline, recommended as the only way to progress in the world of work and personal achievement, is discounted in the domain of sexuality.

In pro-choice feminism, a permissive, erotic view of sexuality is assumed to be the only option. Sexual intercourse with a variety of partners is seen as "inevitable" from a young age and as a positive growth experience to be managed by access to contraception and abortion. Unfortunately, the pervasive cultural conviction that adolescents, or their elders, cannot exercise sexual self-control, undermines the responsible use of contraception. When a pregnancy occurs, the first abortion is viewed in some pro-choice circles as a *rite de passage*. Responsibly choosing an abortion supposedly ensures that a young woman will take charge of her own life, make her own decisions, and carefully practice contraception. But the social dynamics of a permissive, erotic model of sexuality, coupled with permissive laws, work toward repeat abortions. Instead of being empowered by their abortion choices young women having abortions are confronting the debilitating reality of *not* bringing a baby into the world; *not* being able to count on a committed male partner; *not* accounting oneself strong enough, or the master of enough resources, to avoid killing the fetus. Young women are hardly going to develop the self-esteem, self-discipline,

and self-confidence necessary to confront a male-dominated society through abortion.

The male-oriented sexual orientation has been harmful to women and children. It has helped bring us epidemics of venereal disease, infertility, pornography, sexual abuse, adolescent pregnancy, divorce, displaced older women, and abortion. Will these signals of something amiss stimulate pro-choice feminists to rethink what kind of sex ideal really serves women's best interests? While the erotic model cannot encompass commitment, the committed model can—happily—encompass and encourage romance, passion, and playfulness. In fact, within the security of long-term commitments, women may be more likely to experience sexual pleasure and fulfillment.

The pro-life feminist position is not a return to the old feminine mystique. That espousal of "the eternal feminine" erred by viewing sexuality as so sacred that it cannot be humanly shaped at all. Woman's whole nature was supposed to be opposite to man's, necessitating complementary and radically different social roles. Followed to its logical conclusion, such a view presumes that reproductive and sexual experience is necessary for human fulfillment. But as the early feminists insisted, no woman has to marry or engage in sexual intercourse to be fulfilled, nor does a woman have to give birth and raise children to be complete, nor must she stay home and function as an earth mother. But female sexuality does need to be deeply respected as a unique potential and trust. Since most contraceptives and sterilization procedures really do involve only the woman's body rather than destroying new life, they can be an acceptable and responsible moral option.

With sterilization available to accelerate the inevitable natural ending of fertility and childbearing, a woman confronts only a limited number of years in which she exercises her reproductive trust and may have to respond to an unplanned pregnancy. Responsible use of contraception can lower the probabilities even more. Yet abortion is not decreasing. The reason is the current permissive attitude embodied in the law, not the "hard cases" which constitute 3 percent of today's abortions. Since attitudes, the law, and behavior interact, pro-life feminists conclude that unless there is an enforced limitation of abortion, which currently confirms the sexual and social status quo, alternatives will never be developed. For women to get what they need in order to combine childbearing, education, and careers, society has to recognize that female bodies come with wombs. Women and their reproductive power, and the children women have, must be supported in new ways. Another and different round of feminist consciousness-raising is needed in which all of women's potential is accorded respect. This time, instead of humbly buying entrée by conforming to male lifestyles, women will demand that society accommodate to them.

New feminist efforts to rethink the meaning of sexuality, femininity, and reproduction are all the more vital as new techniques for artificial repro-duction, surrogate motherhood, and the like present a whole new set of dilemmas. In the long run, the very long run, the abortion debate may be merely the opening round in a series of far-reaching struggles over the role of human sexuality and the ethics of reproduction. Significant changes in the culture, both positive and negative in outcome, may begin as local storms of controversy. We may be at one of those vaguely realized thresholds when we had best come to full attention. What kind of people are we going to be? Pro-life feminists pursue a vision for their sisters, daughters, and granddaughters. Will their great-granddaughters be grateful?

SECTION 3

Procreative Autonomy and Responsibility

The McCaughey Septuplets: Medical Miracle or Gambling with Fertility Drugs?

Bonnie Steinbock

On November 19, 1997, a 29-year-old woman from Carlisle, Iowa, made medical history by giving birth to seven babies, the first time in the United States, and only the second time anywhere, that so many infants have been born alive. (In September 1997, a Saudi Arabian woman became the first to deliver seven live babies, but three of them died one month after their birth.) A 66-member medical team at Iowa Methodist Medical Center delivered the four boys and three girls by cesarean section. They ranged in weight from 2.5 pounds to 3.4 pounds. As of this writing, all seven babies seem to be healthy, and all have left the hospital in late January 1998. Dr. Paula Mahone, a perinatologist who helped perform the delivery, was quoted as saying, "All the babies were so well-grown, so well-developed, it just strikes me as a miracle" (Pam Belluck, "Iowan Makes U.S. History, Giving Birth to 7 Live Babies," *The New York Times*, November 20, 1997, Al).

"Miracle" is how most newspaper headlines characterized the birth of the McCaughey septu-plets. Praise was heaped on Mrs. McCaughey for her grit and determination in continuing a very difficult pregnancy for more than 30 weeks. She had been confined to bed since her ninth week of pregnancy. The drugs administered toward the end to stop contractions had nasty side effects: headaches, hot flashes, a general feeling of being unwell. But even as the media featured pictures of the beaming parents and the cheering medical

---

EDITORS' NOTE: This case was written expressly for this volume.

team, and corporations showered the family with gifts (a new house, a 12-seat van, free diapers for life, car seats, strollers, even seven years of free cable), many fertility experts and ethicists expressed serious reservations.

Multiple births pose serious health risks, both for the pregnant woman and for the fetuses she carries. The health risks for women include anemia, hypertension and labor complications. The fetuses are typically premature and, as a result, have a significantly higher mortality risk than full-term babies. Even if they are born alive, "super-twins" (triplets, quadruplets and quintuplets) are 12 times more likely than other babies to die within a year. (Sextuplets and septuplets are so rare that there is no data on them.) Many will suffer from respiratory and digestive problems. They are also prone to a range of neurological disorders, including blindness, cerebral palsy and mental retardation. According to John P. Elliott, director of maternal-fetal medicine at Phoenix's Good Samaritan Medical Center, "When you look at the statistical chances that [Mrs. McCaughey] would be successful, you're literally talking about winning the lottery" (*Newsweek*, Dec. 1, 1997, p. 61).

Is taking such risks morally responsible? The answer does not depend on whether the harms actually occur. For example, it is irresponsible to leave young children unsupervised, because of what might happen, regardless of whether any harm in fact befalls them. It is irresponsible to leave loaded guns where children might get them, even if no child ever does. The fact that the McCaughey septuplets appear to be healthy does not settle the issue of whether the various decisions were responsible ones. In addition, it may be years before the children's full physical and mental potential is accurately assessed.

The issue of responsibility can be addressed from at least two different perspectives.

WERE THE PARENTS' DECISIONS MORALLY RESPONSIBLE?

Almost everyone would agree that Mrs. McCaughey had the right, based on autonomy and self-determination, to accept serious health risks for herself in her attempt to have a child. Did she also have the right to impose such risks on her offspring?

Up to 20 percent of pregnancies achieved with fertility drugs produce two or more babies. In light of this risk, some argue that fertility drugs should be used with caution and even reluctance. One issue is whether the McCaugheys were cautious enough. They already had one child, Mikayla, when they decided to have another. Mrs. McCaughey had had trouble conceiving Mikayla. She spent over a year on Clomiphene before finally switching to the more powerful Metrodin. According to a press release issued by her fertility doctor, Dr. Katherine Hauser, Mrs. McCaughey "did not want to repeat a therapy that had led to such frustration in the past," and so Mrs. McCaughey went right on Metrodin. But the decision to resort to fertility treatment when they already had one child, and that child was only 16 months old, might be questioned. Most obstetricians recommend a minimum of two years spacing between children. Nor was Bobbi McCaughey, at age 28, approaching the end of her fertility. That is, although she apparently could not ovulate without drugs, her eggs were youthful and viable. What, it may be asked, was the big rush?

The second decision that faced the parents occurred after the pregnancy was established, when they learned that Mrs. McCaughey was carrying seven fetuses. They were given the option of "selective reduction": the killing of some of the fetuses to give the remaining ones a better chance at healthy survival. This option was unacceptable to the McCaugheys, who are both devout Christians. Some commentators praised this decision, but others were critical. The McCaugheys' gamble paid off, but what if the babies had been stillborn, or had very serious medical problems? Is it fair to children to subject them to all the risks, emotional as well as physical that may be associated with being a "super-twin"? Barbara Luke, a perinatal epidemiologist at the University of Michigan, says, "It is an injustice to children to be born in litters" (*Time*, December 1, 1997, p. 37).

Other commentators reject the notion that imposing health or other risks can be unfair to the children, if the alternative is no life at all. Whatever problems the septuplets may face, their lives will probably be worth living. Life with problems, even serious problems, is better than no life at all. Therefore, they conclude, the septuplets were not harmed by being subjected to a risk of disability. For how can they be harmed if the outcome will invariably be in their own interest? And if the septuplets were not harmed, how can the decision to bring them into the world be irresponsible on grounds of being an injustice to them?

However, even if one accepts the view that procreation is not unfair to the child, if he or she has no other way to be born,* it is not clear that this is true in the case of the septuplets, since the parents could have improved the chances of healthy survival for some of the fetuses by sacrificing some of the others. Once again, the fact that all seven appear to be healthy, despite no reduction, does not determine the responsibility of the decision not to reduce. By refusing to reduce the pregnancy to the recommended twins or triplets, the McCaugheys took a risk with the health of the remaining fetuses. As it turned out, the gamble paid off. But if it had not, if some of the babies had died and others been neurologically impaired, the surviving children could claim that their impaired condition was a result of their parents' decision. If their parents had chosen reduction, they could have been born "healthy and whole." Therefore, their decision might be viewed as harmful (or potentially harmful) and thus irresponsible. However, from the McCaughey's perspective, it would be wrong to kill some of their children, even to give others a better chance at survival. And if this choice was morally impermissible, refusing to make it could never be irresponsible, whatever the consequences.

WHAT IS THE RESPONSIBILITY OF INFERTILITY SPECIALISTS TO PREVENT MULTIPLE BIRTHS?

A separate issue is how infertility specialists ought to approach the problem of multiples. Fertility drugs, like Pergonal or Metrodin can cause a woman's ovaries to release as many as 40 eggs in one cycle. In IVF, doctors can decide how many embryos to implant in the woman's uterus. With the use of fertility drugs, the number of eggs that get fertilized is not within medicine's control.

*EDITORS' NOTE: For more discussion of this question, see the articles by Adrienne Asch, Bonnie Steinbock and Ron McClamrock, and Dan Brock, which follow in this section.

Nevertheless, many fertility experts argue that multiple births can usually be prevented, in two ways. First, the dosage of the fertility drug can be regulated. Second, vaginal ultrasound can be used to monitor the number of eggs that has been produced. "If you see seven follicles about to erupt, you don't have to inseminate, you don't have to have intercourse," says Dr. Louis Keith, president of the Center for the Study of Multiple Birth and a professor of obstetrics and gynecology at Northwestern University. "The appropriate means to stop this is by canceling the entire cycle."

The daily doses of Metrodin Mrs. McCaughey received were identical to her first treatment, when she had Mikayla. Dr. Hauser's press release indicates that Bobbi McCaughey was monitored by vaginal ultrasound: "The estrogen levels achieved, and the number and size of follicles were all comparable [to her first treatment]." Based on this, Dr. Hauser probably expected that Mrs. McCaughey would have another singleton or at most twins. In eighteen years of practice, in which she has treated several hundred women, Dr. Hauser never had a pregnancy with more than triplets. Whether this time she discussed with the McCaugheys the number of follicles about to erupt, or whether she gave them the opportunity to stop the treatment cycle, is not known. According to *Newsweek,* during a press conference the day after the septuplets were born, Dr. Hauser bristled at the suggestion that seven fetuses might be too many, saying "Should we as a society dictate to individuals the size of their families or their choices of reproductive care?"

Apart from issues having to do with patient risk, there is the issue of cost. One maternal-fetal specialist estimates that it costs $1,000 a day just for a baby to lie in a bassinet in a neonatal intensive care unit (NICU). It costs a few thousand more a day for the ventilators, blood work and physician fees. Some question whether, in a time of limited health-care dollars, multiple births are an appropriate use of resources. Thus, physicians who specialize in infertility are faced with a barrage of questions: how should cost figure into their treatment of patients? To what extent should patient preference determine a treatment protocol? Is treatment which results in multiple pregnancies "good medicine"?

Prenatal Diagnosis

Barbara Katz Rothman

The typical medical ethics case, as it is standardly presented for discussion, involves Doctor Goodguy sitting at his desk, when in walks Patient Problem, presenting an ethical dilemma. In the area of prenatal diagnosis, the doctor is typically an obstetrician or a geneticist, the patient is a pregnant woman, and the dilemma is abortion. Very often, the case involves a woman who wants an abortion for a reason the doctor feels to be insufficient (with all the assumptions about sufficiency, abortion, fetuses, and women included). Occasionally, it involves a woman who refuses testing the doctor thinks necessary (again, with assumptions about necessity and all the rest included).

Example 1: Mrs. X (we are told) comes from a culture that strongly values sons. She is the mother of four daughters, and pregnant again at the age of 37. She requests amniocentesis, and since current medical thinking regards a woman over age 35 as "high risk" for Down's syndrome, she is considered to be "entitled" to this amnio. However, she makes it clear to the physician that a healthy girl would be just as unacceptable as would a child of either sex with Down's syndrome. Should Doctor Goodguy do the test? Can the doctor refuse to divulge information about fetal sex?

Example 2: Mrs. Y learns through a "routine" sonogram that her fetus has a limb deformity. She reacts with repulsion and horror, and wants the pregnancy aborted at once. Should Doctor Goodguy do the abortion?

Example 3: Miss Z (and this one is indeed most often presented as "miss") presents a different dilemma. She is not interested in the testing or the abortion being offered. Miss Z is a 22-year-old former or current user of IV drugs, and so, at risk for HIV infection. She either refuses HIV testing, or, if tested and found positive, she decides to continue the pregnancy and risk the

roughly one-in-three chance that her infant will develop AIDS.

First, it is important to note that each of these scenarios assumes that the dilemma arrives with the patient. That is probably because biomedical ethics as a field is often closely associated with hospitals, medical schools, and physicians. From the perspective of the patient, of course, the dilemma arrives with the doctor. A woman living in a culture that values sons over daughters is suddenly offered a test for fetal sex, creating an element of choice and responsibility, and thus, a dilemma. Or, in the second or third example, with much effort to "penetrate the maternal barrier" and "access the fetal patient," physicians developed, and then began to use routinely, ultrasonography. So, a woman arriving for routine prenatal care suddenly learns distressing things about her fetus—things she may not have asked to learn. Tests are developed for HIV status and then offered to women. With the offering of the test comes the dilemma for the woman.

There is, however, a more profound critique to make of these three examples and the assumptions that they embody. Each of these examples encourages us to focus on the level of individual decision making. We ask ourselves—and our students—what should Doctor Goodguy do? What should Patients X, Y, or Z decide? Often, the problem is presented to students with the five principles of autonomy, veracity, beneficence, nonmaleficence, and justice offered as guides to finding the best answer.

As a social scientist, I have a strong need to shift the focus. Dilemmas of this sort do not simply "arise" as if they were spontaneously generated, nor do they reside in either of the individuals, patient or doctor, presented as in conflict. These dilemmas are socially, politically, and economically constructed. This is particularly clear with the dilemmas presented by new technology. The institutionalization of new technologies does not occur on the individual level, and is not the work of individual inventors and consumers. We

Biomedical Ethics Reviews, J. Humber and R. Almeder, eds., 1991, 171–186. Used with permission of Humana Press.

must move considerably past questions of "choice" to understand the dilemmas that confront us.

The new reproductive technologies, including and perhaps especially, the technologies of prenatal diagnosis—amniocentesis, sonography, chorionic villus sampling, preimplantation diagnosis, and more to come—are offered to people in terms of expanding choices. However, it is always true that although new technology opens up some choices, it closes down others. The new choice is often greeted with such fanfare that the closing of the door on the old choice goes unheeded. To take a simple example, is there any meaningful way one could now choose horses over cars as a means of transportation? The new choice of a "horseless carriage" eventually left us "no choice" but to live with the pollution and dangers (as well as the convenience and speed, of course) of a car-based transportation system.

In the area of reproductive technologies, this closing down of choice happened first with the quantity of children. The oldest and most basic reproductive technology is the technology of fertility limitation. Self-imposed limits on fertility, through contraception, abortion, or a combination of the two, are the sine qua non of the reproductive rights movement, and yet, we must realize that the choice of contraception simultaneously closed down some of the choice for larger families. North American society is geared to small families, if indeed, to any children at all. Without the provision of good medical care, day care, decent housing, and schooling, children are luxury items; fine if you can afford them.

And so, it may be also with prenatal diagnosis, which serves as a technology of quality control, based on a given society's ideas about what constitutes "quality" in children. The ability to control the "quality" of our children may ultimately cost the choice of not controlling that quality. Individual families, but most especially individual mothers, bear the costs of children and the special costs of special children. How much any given child costs a mother is based not only on the condition of the child, but even more on the conditions of the mother's life. Any analysis of a woman's choice of any abortion, but most especially a selective abortion, has to recognize the context in which the decision to abort is made, and the circumstances in which

the woman is placed. As Rosalind Petchesky has stated:

> The "right to choose" means very little when women are powerless. . . .Women make their own reproductive choices, but they do not make them just as they please; they do not make them under conditions which they themselves create, but under social conditions and constraints which they, as mere individuals, are powerless to change.[1]

We live in a system in which women and children are both disvalued, an antichild-antiwoman society. It is women and children who are poor, whose needs are not being met. In this system, women and children are often pitted against each other, competing for scarce resources. The mother finds herself becoming a resource: Her own life (and specifically, her own time) is to be divided between herself and her children. Whatever the children get, it may very well be coming off the life of the mother—in time, in attention, in emotional support, sometimes in food and basic necessities. It is in this context that mothers are judged in terms of their willingness to sacrifice. The more she gives of herself to her children, the better a mother the society says she is. The more she holds back of herself, for herself, the more she runs the risk of being the "wicked stepmother," evil in her selfishness.

When women and children are both disvalued, to speak for the rights of either, to the needs of either to be met, is then to contribute to the disvaluation of the other. When one adds to the situation the virtually total disvaluation of the needs of the disabled, the "defective" or "invalid" people, the place of selective abortion in our society is highlighted. Women know that children with "special needs" make special demands. The society as a whole has shown itself unwilling to meet those demands—we are, as a society, unwilling to meet the ordinary needs of ordinary children. With wonderful and notable exceptions, fathers and other family members have not risen to the occasion. The burden of childrearing, of all childrearing, has fallen overwhelmingly on individual mothers. Although those in the disability rights movement rightly resent the use of the word "burden" to describe their lives, it is not a description unique to the disabled. Children, all children, can be described as burdensome when their needs fall almost exclusively on one person. Yes, they are also delightful, joyous, pleasures and treasures, whether able-bodied or disabled, but side-by-side with the pleasures come the sacrifices. The individual woman, or at the very best, the individual couple or family, can demand more and more from the society for the child, and, in fact, making such demands becomes one of the chief responsibilities of the parents of a disabled child. It is clear to us all, however, that the society will not respond with openness and generosity, and most assuredly cannot be depended on to continue responding to the child's needs when the mother is no longer there. Even if the woman were to be willing to sacrifice herself entirely to meet the needs of the child, it may still not be enough.

It is in this context that amniocentesis and the other technologies of prenatal diagnosis, permitting selective abortion, are introduced, giving an illusion of choice, allowing individuals to believe that they have gained control over the products of conception. However, the choices are made within an ever-narrowing structure. Issues of basic values, beliefs, and the larger moral questions will be lost in this narrowing of choices as decisions become pragmatic, often clinical, and always individual. Irving Kenneth Zola puts it this way:

> Bombarded on all sides by realistic concerns (the escalation of costs) and objective evidence (genetics) and techniques (genetic counseling), the basic value issues at stake will be obfuscated. The freedom to choose will be illusory. Someone will already have set the limits of choice (cuts in medical care and social benefits but not in defense spending), the dimensions of choice (if you do this then you will have an x probability of a defective child) and the outcomes of choice (you will have to endure the following social, political, legal and economic costs).[2]

Thus, the new technologies of prenatal diagnosis and selective abortion do, indeed, offer new choices, but they also create new structures and new limitations on choice. Because of the society in which we live, the choices are inevitably couched in terms of production and commodification, becoming matters of "quality control." The dilemmas then get seen in terms of choices about quality of life for the individuals and potential individuals involved.

It is with this context in mind that I turn now to the experiences of women with prenatal diagnosis and selective abortion. Because, whereas the social, economic, and political context is too often missing from discussions of biomedical ethics, so too is the voice of the lived experience.

Therefore, it is important to hear the actual words of women facing the decision to terminate a pregnancy following prenatal diagnosis. The women quoted below were interviewed as part of a larger study on women's experiences with prenatal diagnosis and selective abortion.[3] I will focus here on the issue of responsibility as experienced by women who had prenatal diagnosis and learned that there was a serious problem with the fetus. These women are in the nexus between the society that largely creates or structures the problem—the profound cutting of already limited services for disabled children and adults that we have seen over the decade; the deep stigma attached to disability; the privatized and relatively isolated nuclear family; the gender inequality that leaves women uniquely bearing the costs of their children's disabilities—and the technology that is supposed to solve the problem.

THE TENTATIVE PREGNANCY

How does anyone decide whether to continue or to terminate the pregnancy when given a bad diagnosis? The overwhelming majority of women who get a bad diagnosis do terminate. In part, that is because most of the women who would choose not to terminate sensibly avoid having the tests and facing their decisions. Even though the decision to have the amniocentesis implies, for most women, the willingness to abort for a bad diagnosis, the actuality of the diagnosis often requires that the decision be made anew. There are several reasons for this. Some women are pressured into the amniocentesis. They sometimes give in because the chances of a bad diagnosis are so remote that it is easier to go along with it than to argue with husband or doctor. Some women postpone the decision purposely, wanting to "get the information, and then decide." Some actively seek out amniocentesis, fully expecting to terminate for a bad diagnosis, but find themselves more deeply affected by the pregnancy itself than they had expected. The lateness of the results changes their readiness to abort, and they have to decide again. And some women get unexpected diagnoses, not the bad news for which they were prepared, but other, surprising bad news, requiring new decisions.

It is generally agreed that the most straightforward decision making occurs when the fetus is diagnosed as having a fatal condition. If the fetus is going to die at birth, then there is often understood to be "no point" in continuing the pregnancy. Six of the thirteen women I discuss in detail in this chapter were in, essentially, that position. Laura carried an anencephalic fetus, a fetus without sufficient brain development for it to survive more than days after birth. Laura herself, however, remains unsure that the condition was inevitably fatal. The rest of these six women were convinced that their fetus had no chance. Fern's fetus had a diagnosis of a genetic kidney disease and a 99 percent chance of dying even before the end of the pregnancy. Donna's fetus had a blood and bone disease in which the baby bleeds to death. Her third child had had the disease and died at five weeks. This was her fourth pregnancy. Shirley never got a clear diagnosis, but it was obvious that her fetus was dying and making her very sick as well. She aborted to save her own life. Denise carried a fetus with Trisomy 18 and spina bifida. She was told it had a small chance of survival and would lead only a minimal kind of existence at best. Andrea's fetus had Tay-Sachs disease, which kills not *in utero* or in infancy, but does invariably kill within the first years of life. The remaining seven women carried fetuses with the extra twenty-first chromosome that is Down's syndrome. Is it any easier for those women whose fetuses would die anyway? I am not sure. That knowledge does not take away the sense of responsibility the women feel. I specifically say responsibility, and not guilt. Some women express feelings of guilt, but all of them express "the inescapable sense of deep responsibility." Listen to Fern, who knew her fetus was dying of kidney disease:

> There are times that I really curse modern technology. No one should have to make these kinds of decisions. There are occasional flukes of nature where things don't work out, or at least they don't seem to, and yet I very firmly believe that there is always something good to be found

in every situation, no matter how grim. I also think that most women know in their hearts whether or not their baby is going to be normal, and that emotionally they are prepared for it before the baby's born.

Having articulately expressed the same feelings and beliefs held by so many of the women who refused amniocentesis, Fern, at this point, apologizes for "rambling" and being "not coherent." She goes on to say that it is an individual matter, and each time the decision needs to be made, all circumstances need to be evaluated. It is not that Fern feels she should not have done what she did. She is angry at the local hospital that refused her admission for what they called "abortion on demand," making her seek an outpatient facility:

> They were bound and determined for us to have this baby regardless of the pain and suffering he would have to endure prior to and after his birth.

Making the baby suffer would be wrong. The abortion had to be done, yet she wished that "the baby would just hurry up and die so that we wouldn't have to murder it first." She compared the abortion with a spontaneous miscarriage she had had, saying they are the same because "it is a life lost and with it all the hopes and dreams of that new being." However, the spontaneous miscarriage was different, "because I was not the one that actively murdered my baby." With the abortion, "I had good reason for doing it, but it was still a conscious decision to end that life."

Andrea, who terminated for Tay-Sachs disease, also expresses this sense of responsibility; not guilt, but certainly responsibility:

> This is your responsibility. You have to make the choice. No one makes that choice for you.

However, even believing that the fetus would die does not protect entirely from guilt. While all the women echo the theme of choice and responsibility, Denise remains the most troubled. Though she thought the amniocentesis was "a very intelligent thing," she says:

> In retrospect, I have wondered if it might have been easier on me just to carry the pregnancy to term and lose the child that way. I think emotionally it might have been—well, that's guessing. Maybe it would just have dragged it out for

a longer time and made it just as hard if not harder, for a longer period. Yeah, this was a real person to me, and all the rationalizing in the world is not going to change my feeling. But my husband doesn't consider that the baby was a person.

Denise comes back again and again to the ultimate responsibility in the decision: "An abortion is a choice that you make and despite what other people say to you, it's ultimately your own choice, it's something you do, and—I kind of feel like I committed a murder."

When the fetus will suffer and die, then the abortion can be seen as a painful obligation the mother has toward her fetus, toward her baby. Even Denise wonders only whether it might have been easier on herself had she continued the pregnancy "and lost the child that way." Fern, fighting her local hospital for admission for the abortion, is no different than the mothers of infants in neonatal intensive care units who fight to let their suffering babies die in peace. A sacrifice is occurring, suffering is happening, but in many ways it is the socially accepted sacrifice in mothering: The mother suffers to spare her child.

The question of responsibility and obligation, of choice and of sacrifice, becomes more complicated when the diagnosis is Down's syndrome. As Eleanor describes the dilemma:

> The baby can live to a mature age, and have a rather good life, so there's a tremendous amount of guilt involved—that you're getting rid of it because it is not a perfect human being—and it's your decision—it's not God's decision, or nature's decision, it's yours and yours alone, so it carries with it a heavy weight.

The responsibility, when the diagnosis is a fatal condition, is the responsibility for determining the timing and the mode of the baby's death. With Down's syndrome, the responsibility is more directly one of life and death.

No one can predict in detail the condition of the baby just by seeing the extra twenty-first chromosome. Some women are left wondering if the baby might have been only mildly retarded. One of the sadder ironies in the diagnostic process, however, is that some of the fetuses that are aborted would have miscarried shortly, and some would have died in infancy. The woman has the experience of shouldering responsibility for a decision that "God

or nature" might have made for her. Sondra had the comfort of learning that the fetus she carried did have many physical problems:

> It made me feel better in a sense, that it wasn't just Down's syndrome, but heart and lung damage. I never read the autopsy report; [the doctor] told us that, and it made me feel better.

It may have made her feel better but:

> The first few months were really horrible. . . . Guilt feelings, feelings of emptiness—it was terrible. My husband was really great—he had to drag me out of bed, I would just lie in bed. Didn't want to talk to anybody, didn't want to move, really didn't want to do anything.

Sondra did not know about the heart and lung problems before she aborted; she had to come to a decision based on only the information that the fetus had Down's syndrome. She thought about the kind of life the world would offer her baby:

> I have a handicapped sibling and I'm very conscious of how our society deals with the handicapped. I couldn't in right conscience at that time decide to bring a handicapped individual into the world. It's a tremendous decision.

Sondra is painfully aware of the seeming contradiction that exists between her commitment to the rights of the disabled, and the decision she made. "On the one hand you say the handicapped deserve all these rights and then on the other hand say that this child doesn't deserve to live." In addition to her experience with her sister, who had polio as a child, Sondra teaches emotionally disturbed children:

> I had trouble dealing with the kids, sort of like, "They're alive and they're going to go out and kill somebody one day, half of them, and Down's syndrome people don't. They're not doers, they just need a lot, they don't really take a lot." I was angry.

Even more than Sondra, Beryl understood what the world held in store for her fetus with Down's syndrome, should she have continued the pregnancy. Beryl has a Master's degree in special education, specializing in mental retardation, and worked for thirteen years teaching the moderately, severely, and profoundly retarded:

> How ironic to choose to terminate a pregnancy which, left to nature, I was thoroughly prepared

to cope with! . . . I told my geneticist I almost envied the relatively uninformed who could conjure up an image of the fat retardate on the street corner, mouth sagging, etcetera, and make their decision in the recoil. I think being aware of the tremendous steps which have been made with the retarded was less than an asset to me at times and merely introduced more irony into an already complex decision.

So, how did Beryl come to the decision to terminate a pregnancy for Down's syndrome? She does not "recoil" from the retarded; she clearly takes great satisfaction in her work and plans to continue in it. It seems, for Beryl as for Sondra, it is not what she knew about the fetus that determined the decision, but what she knows about our world:

> If all of society—including extended family—shared the enthusiasm and confidence in the retarded that we in my work field share, decisions such as ours would be fewer. . . . When I read accusations of being like the Nazis, having no room for anyone but the "perfect," etcetera, I sizzle. . . . Actually, if I were the only one involved, I would have kept the baby and used the best of my training to raise him. But to me the burden placed on the rest of the family, and on society, as I age or die, and the burden which in turn would fall upon the child, is too great to justify satisfying my ego.

Is this really any different than the decision that the other women faced, those whose fetuses were doing to die? There is going to be pain and suffering, there is going to be a sacrifice made. Once again, the woman chooses to take on the burden herself, to bear the responsibility for the choice. She lives with the pain of her choice, with her grief and loss, to spare her child.

However, it is not only their babies that they spare. Whereas the abortion calls forth pain and grief, so too does the experience of mothering a child with Down's syndrome. Knowing that the sacrifice of the fetus has not only cost the mother grief, but also spared her other grief, becomes a source of guilt. Since "goodness" for a woman is often measured by her willingness to give of herself,[4] can she be sure of her own motives in this complex decision? Sacrificing self for child is "good," sacrificing child for self, "wicked."

Guilt looms large for Anna. Months after her abortion, her car swerved as she and her husband drove in the rain. The thought flashed through her mind: "If we get killed, we deserve it." She sees what she avoided by aborting, and thinking about that, says she decided "for very selfish reasons . . . [to] take the choice encouragingly offered to me to abort the kid." Having made the choice, having terminated the pregnancy, "I felt sad but resigned, and a bitterness about these terrible choices set in that I'm still shrouded in. . . . I feel brittle, with an icy sheath around my heart. I'm on guard."

Elisabeth too speaks of guilt, and openly questions the rightness of her decision. She had the amniocentesis because:

> It seemed unkind to knowingly bring a Down's child into the world, and unkind to not find out if the possibility existed. There was no education for the hell of waiting for the results, or the excruciating continuing sadness and guilt at killing our child.

Elisabeth did what she did out of kindness, but now:

> The question I wonder about now is, is our assumption correct that it is unkind to knowingly bring a Down's child into the world. The Down's child can know and express love and joy and pain. Isn't this enough? By killing a Down's child I bow before the false god of intelligence. Isn't intelligence overvalued in our society at the expense of other values?

She remains isolated in her guilt and grief and she has never been able to talk with anyone who has made a similar decision. When I thank her for giving of herself to me, she says:

> I would talk with anyone, anytime, who has questions. It was the saddest, most guilt-producing anguish of my life.

Unlike those who seek comfort in another baby, Elisabeth and her husband "gave up our dream of a biological addition to our family." Her husband had a vasectomy. She did not want to face these choices again:

> I do not want to terminate the life of another child. I do not want to bring a Down's child into the world. I will not have another pregnancy.

It still seems wrong to Elisabeth to bring into the world a child the world so clearly does not want and will not care for. When both having the child and not having the child would be wrong, guilt is inescapable.

What does it do to a person to make a monumental decision, and not ever be able to be sure of its rightness? Heather says:

> I don't know what it is, but you lose a little bit of your beliefs—it changes you in many ways. Your outlook on life changes, the moral concept—I would say it affects everything. I'm not going to say what I would have been two years ago.

Heather had the abortion because it was the "mature" thing to do. She was visiting relatives when the results came:

> You go through all the stages, crying and resentment, it cannot be. . . . Some nights were sleepless, you toss and turn, angry, and then something tells you just be mature and approach it from the mature point of view. And so I just packed up my suitcase and went home. Sunday I flew in and Monday morning I was already in the hospital.

Maturity, morality, religion—all of her basic values were challenged:

> Morally, there is a question—you have to battle with yourself. . . . Here we talk about life, what is life, do we have a right—. . . [My religious beliefs] changed dramatically. In fact, I drew away from the church. Because how can I justify myself? . . . You never forget, your life is never the same, but it's still a life. Sometimes it seems like a movie, it just happened, it's not affecting you. My life is straightened out now.

With all of her own anguish, Heather still supports amniocentesis.

> I would only encourage the amniocentesis even though I do not think it is the most accurate test-

ing and there is a lot of pain involved too—and—the pain you cannot really describe. . . . It's a grieving process. . . . And emotional turmoil—there's a lot of whys asked, and questions asked. But I guess if you feel secure in your relationship and your environment, you can overcome it. You can cope with it, too. But you don't believe it's happened to you—it stays with you and you feel like you're a victim.

A victim. These women are not the villains some would have us believe, aborting fetuses it would be inconvenient to raise, searching for the "perfect" child. They are the victims. They are the victims of a social system that fails to take collective responsibility for the needs of its members, and leaves individual women to make impossible choices. We are spared collective responsibility because we individualize the problem. We make it the woman's own. She "chooses," and so we owe her nothing. Whatever the cost, she has chosen, and now it is her problem; not ours.

NOTES

1. Rosalyn Petchesky (1980) Reproductive freedom: Beyond a woman's right to choose. *Signs: Journal of Women in Culture and Society* 5, 661–685.
2. Irving Kenneth Zola (1983) *Socio-Medical Inquiries: Recollections, Reflections and Reconsiderations*, Temple University Press, Philadelphia, PA, p. 296.
3. Barbara Katz Rothman (1986) *The Tentative Pregnancy: Prenatal Diagnosis and the Future of Motherhood*, Viking Press, New York, NY.
4. Carol Gilligan (1982) *In a Different Voice: Psychological Theory and Women's Development*, Harvard University Press, Cambridge, MA.

Can Aborting "Imperfect" Children Be Immoral?

Adrienne Asch

Are there truly feminist criteria for abortion decision-making?

From Adrienne Asch, "Real Moral Dilemmas," *Christianity and Crisis*, vol. 46, no. 10, 237–240. Reprinted with permission.

. . .

Two preliminary points: First, the criteria advanced here are for this world, inegalitarian though it is. They recognize how inhospitable it can be to women, men, and children. Criteria might differ in a world with a host of social changes, or in a world with extrauterine means of reproduction. Second, these criteria grow out of the different weight I give to the major tenets of the feminist argument in support of a woman's right to reproductive choice. The feminist case can be summarized as follows: (1) Women have a substantial right to bodily integrity that is violated by involuntary pregnancy. So long as a fetus resides within her body, a woman may decide about whether she wishes her body to be used to support new life. (2) Women have a right to autonomy and choice in matters of responsibility. (3) The value of fetal life is contingent upon the decision of the woman in whose body it resides. (4) Women should not feel compelled to create new life. (5) Women's rights to full social and sexual equality with men are compromised without the option of abortion.

Primary for me is the last of these tenets. In order to participate in life, including sexual life, equally with men, women must feel that their bodies and lives will not be altered by involuntary pregnancy. Until a foolproof method of birth control exists, and as long as the only way for human life to develop is within women's bodies, women need the option of abortion in order to avoid being fettered by biology. Birth control and abortion offer women the opportunity to separate sexuality from parenthood, and thus enable us to undertake parenthood only when we feel it makes sense for our lives. As long as we accept the idea that sexuality is valuable for purposes other than reproduction, we can appreciate this means to separate sexual expression from procreation.

Much pro-choice writing moves from the evils of involuntary pregnancy to those of involuntary childrearing. Obviously, while pregnancy could and usually does lead to social parenthood, it need not. Those who question the morality of abortion and propose adoption as an alternative overlook the compromises pregnancy itself imposes on women's opportunities for equality. Because of these burdens pregnancy should not be compelled. The harm is not merely that one's body undergoes substantial change for nine months, some of which is irrevocable. In and of itself, pregnancy can impose financial, psychological, vocational, and social hardships. To *require* women to undertake these hardships constitutes a form of involuntary servitude. Until women are not censured for sexu-

ality and resulting pregnancy outside of marriage, and until women can count on unstigmatized adoption, a chance pregnancy punishes them for sexuality in a way that men escape, and threatens their equality in all spheres.

From the foregoing, I conclude that the involuntariness of a pregnancy is a sufficient criterion to justify an abortion. Pregnancy is itself so complex that any moral or social order compelling women to undertake it unwillingly violates any claim to promoting their full social and sexual equality with men.

Many Americans find poverty, unmarried status, young age of the woman, or her desire not to have more, or any, children "soft" reasons for abortion decisions and of dubious merit. I don't agree. Such reasons state facts or beliefs only about the woman's life and about the circumstances she chooses in which to become a mother. Birth control and abortion put her in a position comparable to her male counterpart who rejects fatherhood under the same life conditions yet sees value in engaging in sexual activity.

Moral dilemmas arise, however, when we consider the termination of a once-wanted pregnancy. Having consented to being pregnant, a woman knows that she plans to use her body to create new life and she has agreed to accept the manifold physical and social consequences entailed. She has thereby accorded the life process beginning within her some value as a potential human being. Suppose that during her fifth month of pregnancy, the husband she loves and with whom she had planned to share the parenting of the child dies or leaves her. Suddenly, totally unexpectedly, her circumstances and everything about the social context in which she conceived and dreamed of being a mother are radically altered. Are there any adverse moral or social consequences if the woman ends the pregnancy with a second-trimester abortion?

Although such a decision may be especially sad and stressful for the woman and for those close to her, it causes no moral qualms to say that she is caringly and responsibly deciding about the circumstances in her own life that no longer enable her to be the type of parent she wishes to be. Is there any sense in which she could be morally urged to go through with the pregnancy as she had planned and give up the child for adoption? She could, but she could counter such a request by the obvious answer that she would undergo extreme psychological stress in being forced to carry to term a pregnancy that now causes her only grief because of its link to the marriage or the husband that is no longer.

SELECTIVE ABORTION

Suppose now that a different woman in her fifth month of pregnancy receives the results of an amniocentesis and learns that she is carrying a girl and not the son she wanted. Or suppose she finds that the fetus is "the right sex" but is diagnosed as having Down's syndrome, spina bifida, cystic fibrosis, or muscular dystrophy. She had every reason to believe she was carrying a healthy child. She cannot imagine being the mother of a child with a disability.

I know of no feminist who countenances abortion for sex selection. An overwhelming number, along with at least 80 percent of the nation, condone abortion for fetal "deformities," "defects," or "abnormalities." Like other feminists, I deplore abortion as a means of sex selection. Unlike most others, I also question its use in the case of most of the impairments commonly tested for now and likely to be screened in the future. Ending pregnancies for reasons of sex selection or disability has serious moral and social consequences that go beyond an individual woman's reproductive decisions about her own life.

Why do people oppose abortion for sex selection? Because it violates our notion that we should not be allowed to end life because it does not meet our specifications. When we decide to be mothers, we should be open to the possibility that we will have children of either sex and should be prepared to welcome into the world and our lives either type of child. Furthermore, feminists argue, a society that condoned aborting fetuses after learning their sex would be communicating that gender alone is reason enough to make life-death decisions about one's potential or value. To say that it is acceptable to abort potential girls or boys (although probably it would most often be girls) sends a message to actual girls and boys about their worth.

The same argument can be applied with equal force to abortions after prenatal diagnoses of the four disabilities I've mentioned, and to any other diagnosed disability that would not result in protracted physical pain or death in infancy or early childhood. (I therefore exclude abortions for diagnoses of anencephaly, Tay-Sachs, Hunter's syndrome, and certain other conditions that cause degeneration and death within months or the first year or two of life.) Down's syndrome, spina bifida, cystic fibrosis, or muscular dystrophy cause degrees of impairment ranging from mild to severe, the degree indeterminable at the time of prenatal diagnosis. Most people with Down's syndrome are mildly or moderately mentally retarded and thus have the potential to interact with friends and family, to learn many skills, and to live as adults in the community in supported living arrangements or on their own. Spina bifida can cause intellectual impairment but often does not, and adults with this disability today can be found as social workers, lawyers, and parents themselves. Cystic fibrosis and muscular dystrophy entail no intellectual impairment, and although they are degenerative conditions that often bring death in childhood or adolescence, many people with the latter disability and some with the former live into adulthood, are self-supporting, and are themselves parents.

This brief account demonstrates the range, variety, and unpredictability of what life for anyone with a certain impairment will be like. Moreover, people with disabilities have grown up in an unwelcoming society that often failed to provide them and their families with the financial support, social services, and educational opportunities needed to maximize their potential. We can only wonder how many more people with these and other impairments might be leading rich, varied lives had they lived in a more supportive society.

The resurgence of feminism has meant major changes in the potential for women's lives. So, too, the creation of the disability rights movement of parents, advocates, and disabled people themselves has begun to change the social conditions under which disabled people live and to teach us that the major problems of disability are not biological but social—residing in individual attitudes and in institutional practices that prevent disabled people from having access to the services that those without impairments take for granted.

By contrast with the improvements of the past 15 years in education and employment for disabled people, prenatal diagnosis and selective abortion communicate that disability is so terrible it warrants not being alive. As prenatal diagnosis becomes more widespread, as the number of conditions that can be screened for increases, women will be forced to decide whether or not they want to carry their pregnancies to term knowing that their children are predisposed to cancer, heart disease, diabetes, or depression. As a society, do we wish to send the message to all such people now living that there should be "no more of your kind" in the future? If we use the technological solution of prenatal diagnosis to eliminate such people, what will become of our attitudes and practices toward any of those odd people who were missed by the technology and happened to be born? What will happen to our attitudes toward and services for the millions of people whose disabilities occur in childhood, adolescence, or later in life through accident, disease, or anything that could not be detected prenatally? What attention will we continue to give to the enforcement of civil rights or to the barely begun environmental and institutional changes that seek to remove barriers for disabled people and to encourage their full social, economic, and political participation?

Even if we grant the social consequences, we must relate them to the individual woman making individual decisions about her pregnancy, her possible child, her life. Many people who themselves use prenatal diagnosis also support disability rights but argue that the world is too unwelcoming toward disabled people for them to want to see their own child live through what is waiting. Alternatively, many people say that they cannot face being parents of a child with serious problems that will cause them pain, grief, frustration, disruption of other life commitments, or hardships to siblings or other family members. Feminists may argue that the woman who aborts a girl is misguided and acting on the legacy of sexism but that the woman who aborts a fetus diagnosed as having spina bifida is sparing her child and herself untold misery that reaps only pain and no reward.

How is an individual woman's act of abortion detrimental to herself, possible other children, or people with disabilities in the world? The consequences for the woman and for any other children she may bear and rear are at least as serious as those for current and future generations of people with disabilities. If women abort children for problems they can diagnose but feel they cannot cope with, what might happen when their children inevitably develop characteristics that women dislike or find overwhelming? Ruth Hubbard, a feminist biologist who writes about the new reproductive technologies, puts it well: ". . . even with all conceivable methods of prenatal screening and fetal therapy, having children and raising them will continue to be a gamble. And our decisions to have them will continue to need to be based on that peculiar mix of unpredictability and planning that makes childbearing and rearing often joyful, often painful, and always chancy" ("Personal Courage Is Not Enough," *Test-tube Women*, Pandora Press, 1984).

The woman who decides to abort for reasons of disability may be signaling an unwillingness or incapacity to recognize that not everything in life can be controlled and that parenthood is one of those things we should not undertake unless we are willing to face what we cannot control and to seek the resources in ourselves and the world to master it.

For all of these reasons, then, I question the wisdom of condoning or encouraging abortion for fetuses of the "wrong sex" or with most disabilities. Selective abortion differs from the decision to end a pregnancy because one's adult life has radically changed in that it is a statement not about the adult but about the value assigned to potential life that has characteristics we dislike. Aborting because of our own lives says something very different than aborting because we don't like what we find out about the potential life we carry. Support for women's equality with men should not be obtained by subverting other people's equality or potentiality—people with disabilities, or people of a certain sex—by the message we give of the rightness of selective abortion.

GET THE FACTS

All this being said, I support the feminist case for legal abortion. In particular, I do not support outlawing abortion after prenatal diagnosis. I remain firmly committed to the rights of women to decide about their own lives and about the uses made of their physical and psychological resources. Rather, I would urge women to obtain far more and very different information than they commonly get about people with disabilities, to examine what might lead them to abort for the "wrong sex," to consider whether they could imagine carrying the fetus to term and giving up the child for adoption if they cannot face raising it (since they voluntarily undertook pregnancy). More important, women should join this thinking with a process of examining *who* they are, what they want out of being parents, and whether an abortion decision makes a statement about the value of the potential life they carry or about aspects of themselves. We cannot outlaw any type of abortion without doing violence to the principles of women's autonomy and choice about their bodies and lives. We can only urge serious reevaluation of what aborting girls, boys, or less-than-perfect people will do to women, their children, and the society in which they want to live.

At the outset I suggested that my support for abortion rested primarily on my support for women's full social and sexual equality with men. Obviously, I also give weight to concerns of bodily integrity, to notions of opposing involuntary use of one's body, and to promoting women's autonomy and choice. I have always been less comfortable with the notion that fetal life is contingent on the value that is ascribed to it by an individual woman, preferring to acknowledge that intrauterine life exists even if it may not be as important as the lives of actual, born persons.

I am compelled to accord fetal life weight in my thinking. Although I have serious moral qualms about selective abortion for sex or disability, I do not have moral objections—albeit social and psychological ones—to deciding not to conceive if one knows that one's offspring will be of one sex or will have a certain disability. I consider women who refrain from childbearing and rearing for these reasons to be misguided, possibly depriving themselves of the joys of parenthood by their unthinking acceptance of the values of a society still deeply sexist and ambivalent about people with disabilities. Yet I would not consider such a decision immoral.

For me, then, fetuses are not babies, but they are more than ideas. Let us acknowledge that terminating a life process that has already begun is not like pulling an infected tooth. Let us continue this discussion about feminist criteria for abortion decisions, aware of the hard choices life brings us. If the protracted national struggle over abortion is of any value, perhaps it is that we will learn more about who we are, how we prize being parents, having children, and life itself.

When Is Birth Unfair to the Child?

Bonnie Steinbock and Ron McClamrock

Is it wrong to bring children who will have serious diseases and disabilities into the world? In particular, is it unfair to *them?* The notion that existence itself can be an injury is the basis for a recent new tort known as "wrongful life" (Steinbock, 1986). This paper considers Joel Feinberg's theory of harm as the basis for a claim of wrongful life, and concludes that rarely can the stringent conditions imposed by his analysis be met. Another basis for maintaining that it is morally wrong to have children under extremely adverse conditions is suggested: a principle of parental responsibility. We also argue that having children under such conditions may be *unfair* to the children, even if they have not been (in Feinberg's sense) *harmed*. Finally, we consider when conditions are sufficiently awful that having children might be viewed as incompatible with being a good parent and unfair to the child.

Hastings Center Report 24, No. 6, November 1994. Copyright © 1994 The Hastings Center.

1   MINIMAL BIRTHRIGHTS

On one very plausible conception of rights, the function of rights is to protect interests. To understand the claim that there can be a right not to be born, we must explain how someone can have an interest in not being born. *Born* children clearly have all kinds of interests, including an interest in healthy existence. A child who was injured *in utero*, and is subsequently born, has been harmed even if it is maintained that, at the time of the injury, there was no being with any interests at all. In fact, it is possible for a child to be harmed by negligence that occurs prior to that child's conception, when no being, not even an embryo, existed (although it must be admitted that courts have been extremely reluctant to acknowledge preconception torts).

By contrast, wrongful-life suits do not claim merely that the infant plaintiff was harmed before birth. They claim that the child was harmed by being born, implying an interest in not having been brought into existence. Someone can be said to have an interest in not being born if his or her existence is inexorably and irreparably such that life is not worth living. Feinberg explains the right not to be born this way:

> Talk of a "right not to be born" is a compendious way of referring to the plausible moral requirement that no child be brought into the world unless certain very minimal conditions of well-being are assured. When a child is brought into existence even though those requirements have not been observed, he has been wronged thereby . . . (Feinberg, 1984, p. 101).

Feinberg goes on to suggest that these "minimal conditions of well-being" amount to a requirement that we not doom the child's future interests to total defeat. The advance dooming of a child's most basic interests—those essential to the existence and advancement of any ulterior interests—deprives the child of what might be called his *birthrights*. And if you cannot have that to which you have a birthright, you are wronged if you are brought to birth.

Is the infant plaintiff in a wrongful-life suit also *harmed* by being born? In *Harm to Others* (Feinberg, 1984), Feinberg offers an analysis of harming as "the thwarting, setting back, or defeating of an interest." To have an interest in something is to have a "stake" in it: "In general, a person has a stake in X . . . when he stands to gain or lose depending on the nature or conditions of X":

> One's interests, then, taken as a miscellaneous collection, consist of all those things in which one has a stake. . . . [These] are distinguishable components of a person's well-being: he flourishes or languishes as they flourish or languish. What promotes them is to his advantage or *in his interest*; what thwarts them is to his detriment or *against his interest* (Feinberg, 1984, p. 34).

Applying this analysis to the case of prenatal harms, Feinberg concludes that harm can be caused to a person before his birth "in virtue of the later interests of the child that can already be anticipated" (Feinberg, 1984, p. 96). The pre-conscious, pre-sentient fetus has no actual interests, and therefore cannot be harmed (or benefited). But on the assumption that the fetus will be born, we can ascribe to it certain "future interests" which can be set back, thwarted, or defeated by actions done before the potential person becomes an actual person. For example, a negligent motorist who runs over a pregnant woman may cause damage to the fetus that causes it later to be born crippled. Sometime after birth the infant will have an actual welfare interest in self-locomotion. Feinberg writes:

> The child comes into existence in a harmed state caused by the earlier negligence of a motorist whose act initiated the causal sequence, at a point before actual personhood, that later resulted in the harm. The motorist's negligent driving made the actual person who came into existence months later worse off than she would otherwise have been. If the motorist had not been negligent, the child would have been born undamaged (Feinberg, 1984, p. 96).

Prenatal—and even preconception—torts can be explained and justified on Feinberg's analysis. But is it possible to explain how someone can be harmed or wronged by being born? The challenge is to explain what it means to say that someone is "worse-off" for coming into existence, or "better-off unborn."

It may help to start with the expression "better-off dead." To say that someone is better-off dead is not to compare his condition while alive with his condition after he is dead. That would be absurd, since after someone ceases to exist, he is in no condition at all. Instead, the phrase "better-off dead" simply means that life is so terrible that it is no longer a benefit or a good to the one who lives. In the case of a competent adult, a normal requirement for judging that a person is better-off dead is typically whether the person himself considers life not worth living.

This test, however, cannot be applied in the case of infants. It isn't just that infants cannot *express* their preferences; they do not yet have the intellectual equipment necessary for *having* the relevant preferences. Infants cannot understand the choice between severely handicapped existence and no existence at all. They cannot weigh up benefits and harms to reach a decision as to whether life is, on balance, worth living. Therefore, it doesn't make any sense to ask what the infant would want, if he could only tell us. The test of "substituted judgment" is simply inapplicable in the case of never-competent individuals (Buchanan, 1981).

What sense, then, can be given to the judgment that the infant would be better-off not existing? It might be thought that if we cannot consult the infant's own preferences, then life is necessarily a benefit and a good to the child. The implausibility of this is seen if we consider the example of an infant who is severely physically and mentally handicapped, and who suffers from chronic and unrelievable pain. The child's physical handicaps prevent him from the ordinary pleasures of infancy and childhood, while his mental handicaps prevent him from acquiring compensating interests. At the same time, he suffers without comprehension. Even if we cannot ascribe a *preference* for nonexistence to the child, surely we can say that this is a life so awful that *whatever* interests or preferences the child might come to acquire, they would be completely frustrated.

We do not then substitute a judgment based on some view about the child's *particular* interests. Instead, we offer the judgment of a "proxy chooser," who acts as the infant's advocate, concerned to promote his or her general welfare. Feinberg explains:

> [The proxy chooser] . . . exercises his judgment that *whatever* interests the impaired party might have, or come to have, they would already be doomed to defeat by his present incurable condition. Thus, it would be irrational—contrary to what reason decrees—for a representative and protector of those interests to prefer the continu-

ance of that condition to nonexistence (Feinberg, 1992, p. 22).

There are two important features of the proxy's choice. First, the choice of nonexistence is not merely rational in the weak sense of being in accordance with reason, but in the strong sense of being required by reason. Second, his nonexistence is rationally preferable in the strong sense if all of his interests, present and future, whatever they might be, are "doomed to defeat."

Although Feinberg's analysis may well give the correct answer in cases so dismal that *all* possible interests are *completely* "doomed to defeat," this will only cover a small fraction of the cases in which questions of wrongful life might seem to have at least some plausibility. The "doomed-to-defeat" test seems to apply only in cases so awful that the child faces chronic pain, combined with such severe mental retardation that developing any compensating interests is impossible. Such cases are (fortunately) quite rare. Relatively few impaired newborns, even those with the severest anomalies, have lives filled with severe, chronic, and intractable pain. Far more common are cases where the infant's condition precludes the ability to develop or to do any of the things that human beings characteristically develop (Arras, 1987). John Robertson considers the case of a profoundly retarded, nonambulatory, blind, and deaf infant who will spend his few years in a crib in the back wards of a state institution.

> One who has never known the pleasures of mental operation, ambulation, and social interaction surely does not suffer from the loss as much as one who has. While one who has known these capacities may prefer death to a life without them, we have no assurance that the handicapped person, with no point of comparison, would agree. Life and life alone, whatever its limitations, might be of sufficient worth to him (Robertson, 1974–75, p. 254).

If we confine ourselves to the infant's own perspective, it does not seem that we can say with confidence that the child is "better-off dead" or "better-off unborn." It is not clear that even the most radically impaired infant *suffers* from, or has interests *of his own* that are defeated by, his impaired condition.

Such examples emphasize the highly limited applicability of Feinberg's analysis. *Very* few lives meet the stringent conditions imposed by the wrongful life analysis outlined above. On this account, and strictly from the standpoint of the future child, it seems that we can very rarely say that it would be wrong to bring a child into existence. Even the most dismal sorts of circumstances of opportunity (including, for example, slavery, an extremely high chance of facing an agonizing death from starvation in the early years of life, severe retardation plus complete quadriplegia, etc.) are all cases which fail to be covered by this analysis.

2   OBLIGATIONS OF POTENTIAL PARENTS

Should we then conclude that it's acceptable to bring children into the world even when they are destined to have terrible lives? We find this implausible, and in this section we'll suggest how the decision to have children when a decent minimum cannot be provided *can* be criticized on moral grounds. Then in the following section, we'll turn to responding to what we see as the most important line of criticism against the general position we're taking—that is, a criticism coming from Feinberg and Parfit which claims that decisions to have children destined to terrible lives *cannot* be criticized on moral grounds if the children themselves are glad, on balance, that they were born.

Consider the case of a teenager who wants a baby (Parfit, 1984, pp. 357–361). Most people would agree that teenagers should not have babies. Teenagers who become mothers severely limit their own educational and job opportunities. They are more likely to be poor, and to raise families in poverty. In addition, teenage mothers tend to have babies who are low birth weight, a condition associated both with a significantly higher mortality rate than that of normal-sized babies, and with learning disabilities in the future. Children of teenagers are also unlikely to get adequate mothering, as their mothers are still children themselves. While there are no doubt exceptions, in general, young teenagers lack the maturity and stability necessary to be good parents. For all these

reasons, it would be better if teenagers did not have babies.

Notice that many of these reasons appeal to the harmful physical and psychological effects on the future children. A young girl who waits until she is older will give her child a better start in life. Therefore, even if she herself does not mind having fewer opportunities and living in poverty, she ought to wait, we might say, *for the sake of her child*. However, this claim bears closer examination. Derek Parfit points out that a young girl who is contemplating having a child cannot make *that child* better off by waiting. If she delays childbirth, she will give birth, not to that child, but to a *different* child, who will develop from a different egg and sperm. The child she will have if she becomes pregnant now cannot be born at a later time. It is either birth to a teenage mother, or no life at all.

This simple fact has provocative implications. If we maintain that it is for the sake of the child she would bear that she should avoid pregnancy, we seem to be committed to the view that it would be better never to be born at all than to be born to a very young mother. But this is surely implausible. Being born to a teenage mother isn't ideal, but neither can it be said to be so bad as to make nonexistence preferable. Despite the hardships they undergo, despite the fact that they might have preferred having an older mother, most children of very young mothers are probably glad they were born. If they were asked, "Would you prefer to have the life you have now, with a fourteen-year-old mother, or not to have been born at all?" they would choose this life.

What conclusions should we draw from this? We might conclude—implausibly—that it is *not* wrong for fourteen-year-olds to decide to have children. Or we might conclude that the reasons why it is wrong all have to do with the deleterious effects on the young girls themselves, on their parents, and on society in general. But to say this is to leave out the idea that having children under very adverse conditions is *unfair to them*. Can we make clear and coherent the *prima facie* plausible idea that it is unfair for parents to bring children into being without some reasonable prospects at a nonmiserable life?

The very particular and detailed ways such a *principle of parental responsibility* might be filled out will of course be very different given more globally differing metaethical perspectives. But the outlines of such a defense are not hard to see for the obvious mainstream possibilities. Whether utilitarian, virtue-based, deontological, or contractarian, it's not hard to see how the parents' special relationship to and control over the life and well-being of the child should be seen as giving them a special responsibility. So rather than spending time trying to fill that out in detail (and by so doing, making the appeal of the idea *less* rather than *more* general), we'll content ourselves here with spelling out some of the most general features such a principle might involve, and then in the next section turn to a very general criticism that any such principle must face.

A principle of parental responsibility should require of individuals that they attempt to refrain from having children, unless certain minimum conditions can be satisfied. This principle maintains that in deciding whether to have children, people should not be concerned only with their own interests in reproducing. They must think also, and perhaps primarily, of the welfare of the children they will bear. They should ask themselves, "What kind of life is my child likely to have?" Individuals who will make good parents—that is, loving, concerned parents—will want their children to have lives well worth living, and will strive to give them such lives. But what if the parents cannot give their children even a decent chance at a good life? The principle of parental responsibility maintains that under such conditions, it is better not to have children, and that it is in fact unfair to children to bring them into the world with "the deck stacked against them."

Although a principle of parental responsibility requires individuals to refrain (when possible) from having children if they cannot give them a decent chance of a happy life, this of course does not imply that responsible parents of born children should be willing to kill them if their lives fall below a certain standard. Given a child with severe handicaps and a very limited and considerably painful life (but still a life which the child finds worth living), parents should choose treatment that will allow their child to go on living, as he or she wants (*ceteris paribus*, of course; we're not assuming that issues about availability and cost of treatment or the like couldn't bear on the decision as well). Given a preference for life, it is not in general the parents' place to decide that the child would be better-off dead.

When the child is too young to have preferences, the parents will have to judge whether continued life is in the child's best interest. Depending on the prognosis, a reasonable judgment might be made either way (Steinbock, 1984). A decision to stop life-prolonging treatment could be consistent with, or possibly even required by, the special responsibility the parents have to the child.

But where there is no child at all, the question facing the prospective parents is not "what does my child want?" nor "what is best for my child?" It's rather a question of whether to create a child who is likely to have a life marked by pain and severe limitations. It seems to us that the answer to this question must be no. What reason could be offered in justification of an affirmative answer? That the child's life, while miserable, is not so awful that he or she will long for death? That is not the kind of answer that a loving parent could give. Anyone willing to subject a child to a miserable life when this could be avoided, would seem to fail to live up to a minimal ideal of parenting.

We've claimed that a child's being destined to a miserable life may well count strongly against having it. However, the fact that a child *would* have a happy life *if* brought into existence does *not* obligate its putative parents to having a child. If one decides not to have a child, one harms no one. It is not as if there are people in the wings, so to speak, hoping to get the gift of life. No one is injured or made unhappy or deprived by nonbirth (Brandt, 1974, p. 163). By contrast, if one decides to have a child, then there will exist a real person, with needs and interests that must be considered. Mary Anne Warren expresses the point this way:

> . . . failing to have a child, even when you could have had a happy one, is neither right nor wrong. . . . But the same cannot be said of *having* a child, since in this case the action results in the existence of a new person whose interests must be taken into account. Having a child under conditions which should enable one to predict that it will be very unhappy is morally objectionable, not because it violates the rights of a presently existing potential person, but because it results in the frustration of the interests of an actual person in the future (Warren, 1978, p. 25).

In this section, we've suggested some reasons for expanding the notion of parental responsibility for starting lives beyond the kind of minimal conditions suggested by Feinberg earlier. Any such expansion of this notion of parental responsibility must face a serious challenge: Is there any way to make a principle plausibly account for a kind of unfairness to the child from being born in very adverse conditions, even if the child itself prefers the dismal life it's been given to no life at all? In the next section, we'll consider an argument against any such expansions of parental responsibilities, and show why the argument fails.

3   BAD LIVES AND UNFAIR BIRTHS

Feinberg suggests a fundamental limitation on what sorts of unpromising births might reasonably be counted as bleak enough so as to be unfair to the child. This limitation comes out in the consideration of an example of Derek Parfit's: A woman is warned that if she becomes pregnant while she suffers from some temporary illness, the baby will be born in a defective condition. Whether through deliberate perversity or recklessness, the woman fails to take precautions and becomes pregnant during the dangerous period. She gives birth to a baby with a withered arm, a defect which is serious, but not totally incapacitating.

Has this child been harmed by the mother's act? We may suppose that while the child wishes he didn't have a withered arm, he does not regret being born. Given the choice between life with a withered arm and no life at all, he is glad to be alive. But if the child is glad to be alive, despite his or her suffering, then it would seem that the bad aspects have been outweighed by the good. He cannot therefore wish that his mother had followed her doctor's advice, for if she had, he would not have been born at all, which, as Feinberg says, "even the child acknowledges was the worse fate. Hence, she picked the option that had the best total consequences for the child that eventually emerged" (Feinberg, 1992, p. 27).

Feinberg concludes that the child's mother cannot be said to have harmed him, although she is responsible for his having come into existence in a harmed condition. And—importantly for our purposes—he further maintains that the mother has not *wronged* her child or been *unfair* to him by causing him to come into existence in a harmed (handicapped) existence. The reason:

> ... If he were to claim that she wronged him by doing what she did, that would commit him to the judgment that her duty to him had been to refrain from doing what she did; but if she had refrained, that would have led to his never having been born, an even worse result from his point of view. There is no doubt that the mother did act wrongly, but it does not follow that her wrongdoing wronged any particular person, or had any particular victim. She must be blamed for wantonly introducing a certain evil into the world, not for harming, or for violating the rights of, a person (Feinberg, 1992, p. 27).

Feinberg thus holds that when a child's existence is so miserable that he would have been better-off unborn, he has been both wronged and harmed; but when his condition is impaired, but not so seriously that nonexistence is preferable, he is neither wronged nor harmed. Of course, the person responsible for his harmed condition may still have acted wrongly. It might still be seen as wrong to have children under extremely adverse circumstances, as long as we reinterpret the wrongdoing so that it does not involve being unfair to anyone—and in particular, not to the child, so long as the child prefers existence to nonexistence.

This account of the ethical failure of the parents in terms of the wanton introduction of an evil into the world seems unsatisfactory. It suggests that the only thing wrong with having children likely to have very unhappy lives is that the *world* is thereby made a worse place. But surely this is not the whole story. Such an explanation leaves out our sense that the children whose lives fall below a decent minimum are *the victims* of their parents' decision to procreate. It leaves out the plausible and intuitive idea that bringing children into existence under very adverse conditions is unfair *to the children themselves.*

If Feinberg's position here is correct, he has effectively ruled out any claim by or on behalf of a child that he or she him/herself has been wronged or harmed by the action of being born as long as he/she prefers the state of having been born—as miserable as life is—to no life at all. What reason has Feinberg given for this? In the passage quoted above, he infers that the mother is not to be blamed for "harming or for violating the rights of" the child from the fact that not being born would be a "worse outcome from the child's point of view." Stated simply, it seems that something like the following principle underlies the inference here:

> If I prefer outcome A to outcome B, then I haven't been wronged or treated unfairly by your bringing about outcome A rather than outcome B.

But this principle is highly tendentious. If you act so as to utterly disregard my legitimate interests for your own (perhaps even minor) benefit, then you've wronged me by treating me unfairly, even if in the end (perhaps by some accident of chance) I end up in a situation preferable to the one I would have otherwise been in. Fairness of treatment is not necessarily determined by the end acceptance or approval of those receiving it with respect to the available alternatives.

Examples illustrating this are easy enough to produce. Suppose you, as District Attorney, frame me (just some random loser) for an unsolved crime to further your career. I then appeal my case and get my conviction overturned, and go on to write a book about the whole thing that makes me rich and famous. Or you hijack the plane I'm on and threaten to kill passengers until your demands are met. But I get the jump on you, save myself and the other passengers, become a big hero, write a book . . . (vamp till done). In each case, you wronged me and treated me unfairly by your disregard for my interests, even though the eventual outcome is one I'm delighted with.

Note that in such cases, it's not just that what was done overall was wrong, but that at least part of what was wrong was a matter of being unfair to *me*—even though the outcome is *better* in my view than the available alternatives. I may even be, in a certain odd sense, *glad* that things worked out the way they did; but that does not entail that your actions weren't unfair to me. Similarly then, the simple fact that I prefer the outcome of having been born severely handicapped to the available alternative (nonexistence) does not itself establish that I am not treated unfairly by my being born into dismal conditions of life.

These examples don't show that having a child destined for a bad (but not totally horrible) life

must be wrong. Real and concrete questions about this will turn on the kinds of details of opportunity and limitation considered in the next section. What they do show is how, *given* some principle of parental responsibility like that offered and motivated in the previous section, the fact that a child prefers the *outcome* of being born to the alternative does not make the claim of unfair treatment in any way inconsistent.

Without an answer of this sort to Feinberg's principle, any further considerations of detail would be constrained by the fundamental limitation that unless the child deems the life so bad as to be not worth living, there can be no claim of unfair treatment. Now having avoided this objection, we'll turn in conclusion to some discussion of the more concrete particulars that are faced in these decisions.

4   HOW BAD IS TOO BAD?

The principle of parental responsibility maintains that prospective parents are morally obligated to consider the kinds of lives their offspring are likely to have, and to refrain from having children if their lives will be sufficiently awful. But what is sufficiently awful? Laura Purdy considers the example of Huntington's disease (HD), a lethal genetic disorder (Purdy, 1989). Symptoms, which usually appear between ages 35 and 50, include spasmodic, involuntary movements, as well as personality changes (moodiness, paranoia, violent behavior, manic activity), memory loss, and chronic depression. The disease lasts approximately 15–20 years. At the end, the patient has degenerated to the point of being totally physically disabled and unable to communicate (Becker, 1988–89). HD inflicts severe and prolonged suffering on its victims. It is a horrible way to die. Purdy maintains that individuals at high risk of transmitting a serious disease to their offspring are unable to provide them with "at least a normal opportunity for a good life" and therefore such individuals should not reproduce.

However, judgments about the value of life are inescapably subjective. They vary depending on the individual's experience, personality, and general approach to life. Purdy acknowledges that not everyone will concur with her conclusion that individuals at risk of transmitting HD should refrain from procreating, because not everyone will share her pessimistic assessment of life with HD. She writes:

> Optimists argue that a child born into a family afflicted with Huntington's chorea has a reasonable chance of living a satisfactory life. . . . Even if it does have the illness, it will probably enjoy thirty years of healthy life before symptoms appear. . . . Optimists can list diseased or handicapped persons who have lived fruitful lives. They can also find individuals who seem genuinely glad to be alive (Purdy, 1989, p. 313).

Arlo Guthrie seems to have taken the optimistic point of view. His father, Woody Guthrie, died of HD, which means that Arlo has a 50 percent risk of developing the disease. Despite this, Arlo decided to have children, thereby imposing on each child a 25 percent chance of inheriting the disease. Of course, if Arlo did not have the disease, as now seems likely, then his children would not be affected. But he could not have known this at the time he decided to procreate. Therefore, he was taking a 25 percent chance that he would be passing on HD to his children. How could he justify this risk? Perhaps he reasoned as follows: "I haven't had a tragic life. I've had a very good life. The goodness of my life will not be destroyed if it turns out that I have Huntington's. I won't regret having been born, or resent my parents for having had me. So why is it wrong for me to have kids? I *can* give them a decent chance for a good life—as good a life as I had." If this is a good argument, then even if we accept Purdy's principle, that individuals who cannot give their potential offspring a reasonable chance at a satisfactory life should not reproduce, we might not accept HD as coming under Purdy's principle.

A stronger case for the moral obligation not to reproduce exists in the case of HIV-infected women, who run the risk of transmitting AIDS to their offspring. John Arras asks, "Ought such women to forgo childbearing for the sake of children who would have been born infected? If already pregnant, should they abort 'for the sake of the fetus'?" (Arras, 1990, p. 353)

AIDS is a painful and, so far as we know, invariably fatal disease. The aggregate median survival time for infected children is about 38 months from the time of diagnosis. The baby who develops AIDS does not get thirty (much less forty or fifty) healthy years, like the person with HD. Symptoms show up fairly early on, and for most afflicted children, their lives will be filled with considerable suffering. How, it may be asked, could someone aware of these facts even consider deliberately having a child?

The moral obligation of HIV-infected women to avoid conception is complicated by two factors. First, there is a pretty good chance that such women will *not* pass the virus on to their babies. Current studies indicate that the risk of actual perinatal HIV infection through any given pregnancy is somewhere between 20 and 30 percent (Arras, 1990, p. 355). Second, the severity of the disease varies widely. The most severely afflicted children present with adult-style opportunistic infections, such as *Pneumocystis carinii* pneumonia (PCP), during the first year of life. These children face painful death within a month or two after diagnosis. Such children have lives that clearly qualify as "wrongful." However, other children develop far milder manifestations, are diagnosed at a later date, and live much longer. Arras says:

> Only a relatively small percentage (say, 10 to 20 percent) of those born HIV infected actually fit the worst-case scenario of early infection, chronic hospitalization, and death before the age of two. The rest will develop different and often less lethal manifestations of AIDS later on and will live longer, perhaps to the age of ten or beyond. The longer these children live with a tolerable quality of life, the more their lives will be worth living. A child who lives at home, goes to school, and attends summer camp does not fall into the same category as a Tay-Sachs baby (Arras, 1990, p. 365).

Nevertheless, even the better-off AIDS babies have lives that are, in Arras's phrase, "decidedly grim." More than half will die before the age of seven, and the remainder must live under a cloud of impending death with progressively deteriorating immune systems. In addition, most HIV-infected babies are born to mothers (and fathers) who are themselves dying. Many of these parents are too sick to care for their own children, who are often abandoned in hospitals or put in foster care. When the medical and the social realities are considered, even an optimist should concede that it is very unlikely that an HIV-infected woman will be able to provide her baby with a reasonable (much less a normal) chance at a good life. Therefore knowingly to conceive a child under such conditions is morally wrong.

The basic idea is that before embarking on so serious an enterprise as parenthood, people should think about the consequences for their offspring. Some circumstances may be so awful that birth is unfair to the child. However, the principle of parental responsibility says only that it is wrong to bring children into the world when there is good reason to think that their lives will be terrible. It does not suggest that people should not have children unless conditions are ideal, still less that only conventional childrearing circumstances are morally permissible. Consider, for example, the enormous fuss raised recently by the story of a fifty-nine-year-old British woman who gave birth to twins on Christmas Day, 1993. The eggs, donated by a younger woman and fertilized *in vitro* by the older woman's husband, were implanted into her at a private fertility clinic in Rome. Doctors in London had earlier refused to perform the same procedure because they believed she was too old to face the emotional stress of being a mother. Virginia Bottomley, the British Secretary of Health, told the BBC, "Women do not have the right to have a child. The child has a right to a suitable home." But as the *New York Times* put it in an editorial:

> What makes Ms. Bottomley believe the twins won't have a suitable home? Youth is no guarantee of parenting skills: all too often the contrary is the case. And how would Ms. Bottomley define the homes in which parentless children are raised by grandmothers? Are they, *ipso facto*, unsuitable?

Undoubtedly, pregnancy poses special risks for many postmenopausal women, but most IVF programs carefully screen out candidates who are not in excellent condition. If society is going to decide which women are physically unsuited for pregnancy, it might start with young teenagers, as pregnancy in children who are not yet full-grown is risky both for the mother and the baby. And young teens are probably less emotionally equipped to be good parents than women in their fifties or sixties.

Another worry is that postmenopausal women won't live long enough to rear their children. According to Gail Sheehy, author of *Passages* and *The Silent Passage: Menopause*, "It's not a very nice prospect for a child of 10 or 12 to go to sleep every night, praying that his or her mother will live as long as he needs her." However, many women live into their eighties and nineties these days. The Italian doctor who helped the 59-year-old British woman give birth accepts only patients who have a life expectancy of at least 20 more years, based on their age and family history. They must be non-smokers and pass psychological and physical tests. These are conditions we do not require of any other mothers. Nor are they conditions imposed on fathers. Telly Savalas, the television star of "Kojak," died at the age of 70. The fact that he left behind school-age children was not even a subject of comment, much less outrage. It seems likely that the opposition to older women having babies expresses a prejudice against what is new or unconventional, rather than a position that can be rationally justified. So long as a woman is emotionally and physically equipped to be a reasonably good mother, there is no reason why age should be an absolute barrier for women, any more than it is for men.

Life is always a mixture of good and bad, pleasure and pain. We know that our children will have their share of suffering and adversity; that is the price of the ticket. This fact should stop no one who wants children from having them. At the same time, the judgment that the child you will conceive is likely to have a life that falls below a decent minimum provides a strong reason to avoid procreation. In some cases, all that is necessary is to postpone parenthood, as in the example of the young teenager who wants to have a child. The principle of parental responsibility tells her to wait, because if she does, she will be a much better parent to the child she eventually has. In other cases, where the risk is transmitting a disease, whether a genetic disease, such as sickle-cell anemia or cystic fibrosis, or a viral illness, such as AIDS, postponing pregnancy will not help. Prospective parents will have to base their decision on such factors as the risk of transmission, the nature and seriousness of the disease, the availability of ameliorative therapies, the possibility of a cure, and their ability to provide the child with a good life, despite the handicap. The principle of parental responsibility does not provide a formula for deciding such cases. Reasonable people can differ on what a decent chance at a happy life is, and what risks are worth taking.

Throughout this paper, we have been assuming that parenthood is deliberately chosen, something that is not always, perhaps not even typically, true. In many parts of the world, fertility is not so easily controlled, and becoming a parent is more of a *fait accompli* than a deliberate choice. The principle of parental responsibility is aimed only at those individuals who are capable of controlling their fertility, and of making a conscious decision whether to have children.

REFERENCES

Arras, J. D., "Quality of Life in Neonatal Ethics: Beyond Denial and Evasion," in W. B. Weil, Jr. and M. Benjamin (eds.), *Ethical Issues at the Outset of Life* (Blackwell Scientific Publications, 1987).

———, "AIDS and Reproductive Decisions: Having Children in Fear and Trembling," *The Milbank Quarterly* 68:3 (1990), 353–382.

Becker, C. L., "Legal Implications of the G-8 Huntington's Disease Genetic Marker," *Case Western Law Review* 39:273 (1988–89).

Brandt, R. B., "The Morality of Abortion," in R. L. Perkins (ed.), *Abortion: Pro and Con* (Cambridge, Mass.: Schenkman Publishing Company, 1974).

Buchanan, A. E., "The Limits of Proxy Decisionmaking for Incompetents," *UCLA Law Review* 29:386 (1981).

Feinberg, J., *Harm to Others* (New York: Oxford University Press, 1984).

———, "Wrongful Life and the Counterfactual Element in Harming," *Social Philosophy & Policy* 4 (1987). Reprinted in Feinberg, J., *Freedom and Fulfillment* (Princeton, 1992), pp. 3–36. References in this paper are to *Freedom and Fulfillment* (1992).

Harris, J., "The Wrong of Wrongful Life," *Journal of Law and Society* 17:1 (Spring 1990), 1–16.

Parfit, D., "On Doing the Best for Our Children," in M. D. Bayles (ed.), *Ethics and Population* (Cambridge, Mass.: Schenkman, 1976).

———, *Reasons and Persons*, Chapter 16. "The Non-Identity Problem," (Oxford: Clarendon Press, 1984).

Purdy, L. M., "Genetic Diseases: Can Having Children Be Immoral?" in John Arras and Nancy Rhoden (eds.), *Ethical Issues in Modern Medicine*, 3rd edition (Mountain View, California: Mayfield Publishing Company, 1989), pp. 311–317. Reprinted from John Buckley, Jr. (ed.) *Genetics Now: Ethical Issues in Genetic Research* (Washington, D.C.: University Press of America, 1978).

Robertson, J. A., "Involuntary Euthanasia of Defective Newborns: A Legal Analysis," *Stanford Law Review* 27:213 (1974–75).

Steinbock, B., "Baby Jane Doe in the Courts," *Hastings Center Report* 14:1 (1984), 13–19.

———, "The Logical Case for 'Wrongful Life'," *Hastings Center Report* 16:2 (1986), 15–20.

———, *Life Before Birth: The Moral and Legal Status of Embryos and Fetuses* (New York: Oxford University Press, 1992).

Warren, M. A., "Do Potential People Have Moral Rights?" in R. I. Sikora and B. Barry (eds.), *Obligations to Future Generations* (Philadelphia, Pa.: Temple University Press, 1978).

Working Group on HIV Testing of Pregnant Women and Newborns, "HIV Infection, Pregnant Women, and Newborns: A Policy Proposal for Information and Testing," *JAMA* 264:2416 (1990).

The Non-Identity Problem and Genetic Harms— The Case of Wrongful Handicaps

Dan W. Brock

The world-wide Human Genome Project (HGP) will produce information permitting genetic screening for an increasing number of genetic diseases and genetically based increased susceptibilities to

Bioethics, Vol. 9, No. 3/4, 289–275, 1995. Used with permission of the author.

diseases and other harmful conditions. In the foreseeable future, the capacities for preconception and prenatal screening for these diseases and conditions will almost certainly far outstrip our capacities for genetic therapy to correct for the harmful genes and their effects. The vast majority of decisions faced by prospective parents, consequently, will be whether to screen for particular genetic risks and/or conditions and when they are found to be present, whether to avoid conception or to terminate a pregnancy. Moreover, the vast majority of genetic risks that will be subject to screening will not be for diseases or conditions incompatible with life worth living—wrongful life cases—but rather for diseases and conditions sufficiently less severe or grave as to be compatible with having a life worth living. These genetic conditions and diseases will take different forms and many factors will affect the moral case for preventing them. But there is a systematic objection to all preconception wrongful handicap cases which must be resolved to clear the way for judgment about specific cases.

To fix attention on the general sort of case and problem in question, which is not restricted to the context of genetic disease, let us alter slightly a case of Derek Parfit's, call it case P1, in which a woman is told by her physician that she should not attempt to become pregnant now because she has a condition that would be highly likely to result in mild retardation in her child.[1] Her condition is easily and fully treatable by taking a quite safe medication for one month. If she takes the medication and delays becoming pregnant for two months there is every reason to expect that she will have a normal child. Because she is impatient to begin a family she refuses to wait, gets pregnant now, and gives birth to a child who is mildly retarded. In common sense moral views, the woman in case P1 acts wrongly, and in particular wrongs her child, by not preventing its handicap for such a morally trivial reason. Most people would likely say that her action in P1 is no different morally than if she failed to take the medicine in a case, P2, identical to P1 except that the condition is discovered, and so the medicine must be taken, after conception and when she is already pregnant, or if, in a case, P3, she failed to provide a similar medication to her born child, in each case necessary to prevent a comparable degree of mental retardation to her child. On what Derek Parfit has called the "no difference" view, the view of common sense morality that he endorses, her failure to employ the medication to prevent her child's mental retardation would be equally and seriously wrong in each of the three cases. But her action in P1, which is analogous in relevant respects to genetic screening to prevent handicaps, has a special feature that makes it not so easily

shown to be wrong as common sense morality might suppose.

In wrongful handicap cases such as this, the person's handicap leaves him with a worthwhile life, a life that is better than no life at all. The philosophical problem, as noted earlier, is how this judgment is compatible with the common view that it would be wrong not to prevent the handicap. The difficulty is that it would *not* be better for the person with the handicap to have had it prevented since that can only be done by preventing him from ever having existed at all; preventing the handicap would deny the individual a worthwhile, although handicapped, life. The handicap could be prevented either by conceiving at a different time and/or under different circumstances, in which case a different child would be conceived, or by terminating the pregnancy, in which case this child never comes into existence and a different child may or may not be conceived instead. None of these possible means of preventing the handicap would be better for the child with the handicap—all would deny him or her a worthwhile life. But if the mother's failing to prevent the handicap has not made her child worse off, then failing to prevent the handicap does not harm her child. And if she does not harm her child by not preventing its handicap, then why does she wrong her child morally by failing to do so? How could making her child better off by giving it a life worth living, albeit a life with a significant handicap, wrong it? A wrong action must be bad for someone, but her choice to create her child with its handicap is bad for no one. So actions with effects for a child that would constitute seriously wrongful child abuse if done to an existing child are no harm, and so no wrong, if done to a child when they are inextricable from the choice to bring that child into existence with a worthwhile life. This argument threatens to undermine common and firmly held moral judgments, as well as public policy measures, concerning prevention of such handicaps to children.

Some philosophers accept the implications of this argument and hold that in choices of whether a particular individual will be brought into existence, only the interests of actual persons, not the interests of possible persons, which here means the individual whose existence is in question, are relevant to the choice.[2] So in case P1 above, the effects on the parents and the broader society, such as the greater childrearing costs and difficulties of having the mildly retarded child instead of taking the medication and having a normal child two months later are relevant to the decision; but the effects on and interests of the child itself who would be mildly retarded are not relevant. In P2 and P3, on the other hand, the fundamental reason the woman's action would be wrong is the easily preventable harm that she causes her child, or allows it to suffer.

I share with Parfit the no difference view that the woman's action would be equally wrong in P1, P2, and P3. As Parfit notes, the difficulty is identifying and formulating the moral principle on the basis of which the woman's actions in all three cases are equally wrong, and which therefore remedies the limits of traditional ethical theories and their principles of beneficence—doing good—and non-maleficence—not causing or preventing harm. Perhaps the most natural way of trying to account for the moral wrong in wrongful handicap cases is to abandon the feature of the moral principles we appealed to above that generates the difficulty when we move from standard cases of prevention of harm to already existing persons, as in P3 above, to harm prevention in what David Heyd has called genesis cases like P1. That feature is what philosophers have called the person-affecting property of principles of beneficence and non-maleficence, such as principle M:

M: Those individuals responsible for a child's, or other dependent person's, welfare are morally required not to let it suffer a serious harm or handicap that they could have prevented without imposing substantial burdens or costs on themselves or others.

Since harms to persons must always be harms to some person, it may seem that there is no alternative to principles that are person-affecting, but that is not so. The alternative is clearest if we follow Derek Parfit by distinguishing "same person" from "same number" choices. In same person choices, the same persons exist in each of the different alternative courses of action from which an agent chooses. Cases P2 and P3 above were same person choices; the harm of mild retardation prevented is to the woman's fetus or born child. In same number choices, the same number of persons exist in each of the alternative courses of action from which an agent chooses, but the identities of some

of the persons who exist in those alternatives are affected by the choice. P1 is a same number, but not same person choice—the choice affects *who*, which child, will exist. If the woman does not take the medication nor wait to conceive, her child is born mildly retarded, whereas if she takes the medication and waits to conceive she gives birth to a different child who is not mildly retarded. Arguably, the concept of "harm" is necessarily comparative, and so the concept of "harm prevention" may seem necessarily person-affecting, which is why harm prevention principles seem not to apply to different person choices like P1. But it is a mistake to believe that non person-affecting principles, even harm prevention principles, are not possible. Suppose for simplicity that the harm in question in P1 from the mild retardation is suffering and limited opportunity. Then there would be suffering and limited opportunity in P1 if the woman were to choose to have the mildly retarded child which will not exist and so would be prevented if she made the other choice and took the medication while waiting to conceive a different normal child. An example of a non person-affecting principle that applies to P1 is:

N: Individuals are morally required not to let any possible child or other dependent person for whose welfare they are responsible experience serious suffering or limited opportunity if they can act so that, without imposing substantial burdens or costs on themselves or others, any alternative possible child or other dependent person for whose welfare they would be responsible will not experience serious suffering or limited opportunity.

Although, of course, suffering and limited opportunity must be experienced by some person—they cannot exist in disembodied form so in that sense N remains person-affecting, N does not require that the individuals who experience suffering and limited opportunity in one alternative exist without those effects in the other alternative; it is a same number, not same person principle. The non person-affecting nature of a moral principle concerning the evils of suffering and limited opportunity is clearer still in the following principle:

N': It is morally good to act in a way that results in less suffering and less limited opportunity in the world.

On N', the woman in P1 acts in a morally good way by taking the medication and waiting to conceive a normal child. In the genetic screening analog, a couple acts in a morally good way by taking steps not to have a child whom they learn from genetic screening will experience suffering and limited opportunity that another child they could have instead would not experience. On N', it is morally good to act in a way that makes the suffering and limited opportunity "avoidable by substitution," as Philip G. Peters, Jr. has put it.[3]

There is time to mention only one apparent difficulty with this way of avoiding the non-identity problem. It is that it does not account for the apparent aspect of the common sense moral judgment about P1 that the woman specifically wrongs her child by not preventing its handicap, that is, that her child is the victim of her wrong and so has a moral grievance against her. Her child is the person with the handicap which should have been prevented, but applying N or N' the handicap should not have been prevented for the sake of that child since doing so would have made that child worse off (it would never have had its worthwhile life). Rather, applying N or N', it should have been done only for the sake of less overall suffering and loss of opportunity.

This apparent difficulty with N and N' is that they fail to identify a victim of the harm done who as victim has a special moral complaint against its mother. But when we appeal to non person-affecting principles to criticize the failure of the mother to prevent harm in P1, her child who suffers the harm is not a victim who is worse-off and so does not have a special moral complaint against her for her failure which must be accounted for. Unlike the typical cases of harm and rights violations, her child *cannot* claim that *he* has a special complaint against her because he is better, not worse, off as a result of her not meeting her obligation. It is therefore unclear that our moral principles must account for any special wrong done the woman's child, as opposed to a non person-affecting wrong done. This suggests that non person-affecting principles like N or N' may not only be adequate for cases like P1, but that they are indeed preferable to person-affecting principles like M precisely because they do not direct us to the special standpoint and complaint of a victim who has been made worse-off; principles for P1 and other wrongful handicap cases

should not direct us to a victim in that way because there is no victim who has been made worse-off and so has a special complaint.

Abandoning person-affecting principles of beneficence and non-maleficence to account for wrongful handicap cases may thus be a promising approach to those cases, especially if reflection on them leaves us confident of our judgment that the woman in P1 acts wrongly, but weakens our earlier confidence that she wrongs her child in letting it be born handicapped. The latter confidence that she wrongs her child may be further weakened by reflection on wrongful life, not wrongful handicap, cases. Wrongful life cases arise only when the child has a life that is overall not worth living, a life that is worse than no life at all. That is the correct threshold for the claim that the mother acted wrongly in conceiving and/or carrying the child to term knowing how bad its quality of life would be. But since her child's handicap in P1 could also be prevented only by not conceiving it, or by terminating her pregnancy after it had been conceived, she would not wrong it by allowing it to be born unless its life is not worth living, which by definition in wrongful handicap cases like P1 it is not. If she does act wrongly, then perhaps it is correct to insist that she nevertheless wrongs no one, as N and N' imply, and that there is no wrong to her handicapped child for which our principles must account.

What principally explains resistance to this view, I believe, is the handicap that her child suffers, but if her child suffered a similar handicap as a result of an accident for which no one was at fault and which no one could have prevented, there would be no temptation to insist that it had been wronged. The difference, of course, is that she could, and I believe should, have prevented the handicap, but she could not have prevented this child from having the handicap except by never having conceived it, and so we should resist saying that she wrongs this child. In same number, but not same person, cases such as this, if anyone is wronged it is the class—her children—whom she permits without adequate reason or justification to be worse off than her children could have been.[4] But if this class—her children—has been wronged, it is in a sense from which it does not follow that any member of that class—that is, any one child—has been wronged. This is exactly the implication that N and N' have. I conclude that the apparent difficulty with abandoning person-affecting principles—that they fail to identify a victim of the wrong who has a special moral complaint—in favor of impersonal principles like N and N' in wrongful handicap cases is no difficulty after all.

It is worth pointing out one implication of my argument that any moral principle which best fits the features of wrongful handicap cases will be a non person-affecting principle. Others have attempted to solve Parfit's non-identity problem by seeking to show that person-affecting principles, such as appeal to moral rights, can be successfully applied to it.[5] But my argument has been that appeal to any person-affecting moral principles in cases of wrongful handicap like P1 will mischaracterize the wrong done. The very features of any appeal to person-affecting principles that are typically their advantage—that they make the wrong a wrong done *to the child* and the loss from the wrong a loss suffered *by the child*—mischaracterize wrongful handicap cases. Non person-affecting principles are correct for wrongful handicap cases because the non-identity problem at the heart of those cases makes the wrong that is done *not* done to the child and the handicap *not a loss* that is suffered by anyone. No person-affecting account of wrongful handicap cases will be correct. The general philosophical non-identity problem is not an obstacle to the position that a woman in cases like P1 is guilty of causing a wrongful handicap.

NOTES

1. Derek Parfit, *Reasons and Persons*, Oxford University Press, 1984, ch. 16.
2. David Heyd, *Genethics: Moral Issues in the Creation of People*, Berkeley, CA: University of California Press. 1992.
3. Philip G. Peters, "Protecting the Unconceived: Nonexistence, Avoidability, and Reproductive Technology." *Arizona Law Review* 31, 1989, 487–548.
4. Peters, *op cit.*; Michael D. Bayles, "Harm to the Unconceived", *Philosophy & Public Affairs* 5, 1976, 292–304.
5. James Woodward, "The NonIdentity Problem", *Ethics* 96, July 1986, 804–31; see also, Derek Parfit, "Comments", *Ethics* 96, July 1986, 854–62.

RECOMMENDED SUPPLEMENTARY READING

General Works

Beller, Fritz K., and Weir, Robert F., eds. *The Beginning of Human Life.* Dordrecht, Holland: Kluwer Academic Publishers, 1994.

Callahan, Joan C., ed. *Reproduction, Ethics, and the Law.* Bloomington: Indiana University Press, 1996.

Cohen, Sherrill, and Taub, Nadine, eds. *Reproductive Laws for the 1990s.* Clifton, NJ: Humana Press, 1989.

Evans, Donald, ed. *Conceiving the Embryo: Ethics, Law and Practice in Human Embryology.* Dordrecht, Holland: Kluwer Academic Publishers, 1996.

———— ed. *Creating the Child: The Ethics, Law and Practice of Assisted Procreation.* Dordrecht, Holland: Kluwer Academic Publishers, 1996.

Fotion, Nick, and Heller, Jan, eds. *Contingent Future Persons: On the Ethics of Deciding Who Will Live, or Not, in the Future.* Dordrecht, Holland: Kluwer Academic Publishers, 1997.

Goldworth, Amnon; Silverman, William; Stevenson, David K.; Young, Ernle W. D.; Rivers, Rodney. *Ethics and Perinatology.* New York: Oxford University Press, 1995.

Grobstein, Clifford. *Science and the Unborn.* New York: Basic Books, 1988.

Harris, John. *The Value of Life: An Introduction to Medical Ethics.* London: Routledge and Kegan Paul, 1985.

Mahowald, Mary Briody. *Women and Children in Health Care: An Unequal Majority.* Oxford: Oxford University Press, 1993.

McCullough, Laurence B., and Chervenak, Frank A. *Ethics in Obstetrics and Gynecology.* New York: Oxford University Press, 1994.

Rothman, Barbara Katz. *The Tentative Pregnancy: How Amniocentesis Changes the Experience of Motherhood.* New York: W. W. Norton, 1993.

Singer, Peter. *Animal Liberation.* New York: Avon Books, 1975.

"The Status of the Embryo and Policy Discourse." *The Journal of Medicine and Philosophy* 22, no. 5 (symposium, October 1997): 407ff.

Steinbock, Bonnie. *Life Before Birth: The Moral and Legal Status of Embryos and Fetuses.* New York: Oxford University Press, 1992.

Strong, Carson. *Ethics in Reproductive and Perinatal Medicine: A New Framework.* New Haven: Yale University Press, 1997.

Warren, Mary Anne. *Moral Status: Obligations to Persons and Other Living Things.* New York: Oxford University Press, 1997.

Wolf, Susan M., ed. *Feminism and Bioethics.* New York: Oxford University Press, 1996.

Controversies over Contraception

Alan Guttmacher Institute, "Facts in Brief: Teenage Sexual and Reproductive Behavior." November 1, 1992.

Arthur, Stacey L. "The Norplant Prescription: Birth Control, Woman Control, or Crime Control?" *UCLA Law Review* 40 (1992): 1–101.

Moskowitz, Ellen H., and Jennings, Bruce, eds. *Coerced Contraception? Moral and Policy Challenges of Long-Acting Birth Control.* Washington, DC: Georgetown University Press, 1996.

Noonan, John T., Jr. *Contraception: A History of Its Treatment by the Catholic Theologians and Canonists.* Cambridge, MA: Harvard University Press, 1965.

"Special Supplement: 'Long Acting Contraception: Moral Choices, Policy Dilemmas.'" *Hastings Center Report* (January–February, 1995). pp. S1–S32.

The Morality of Abortion

Bassen, Paul. "Present Stakes and Future Prospects: The Status of Early Abortion." *Philosophy and Public Affairs* 11: 4 (1982): 314–337.

Bayertz, Kurt, ed. *Sanctity of Life and Human Dignity.* Dordrecht, Holland: Kluwer Academic Publishers, 1996.

Callahan, Sidney, and Callahan, Daniel, eds. *Abortion: Understanding Differences.* New York: Plenum Press, 1984.

Davis, Nancy Ann. "The Abortion Debate: The Search for Common Ground." 2 parts. *Ethics* 103 (April/July 1993): 731–778.

———. "Abortion and Self-Defense." *Philosophy and Public Affairs* 13, no. 3 (Summer 1984): 516–539.

Dworkin, Ronald. *Life's Dominion: An Argument about Abortion, Euthanasia, and Individual Freedom.* New York: Alfred A. Knopf, 1993.

Dwyer, Susan, and Feinberg, Joel, eds. *The Problem of Abortion.* 3rd ed. Belmont, CA: Wadsworth Publishing Co., 1997.

Feinberg, Joel. "Abortion." In *Matters of Life and Death,* edited by Tom Regan. 2nd ed. New York: Random House, 1986.

Garrow, David J. *Liberty and Sexuality: The Right to Privacy and the Making of Roe v. Wade.* New York: Macmillan Publishing Company, 1994.

Gorney, Cynthia. *Articles of Faith: A Frontline History of the Abortion Wars.* New York: Simon & Schuster, 1998.

Graber, Mark A. *Rethinking Abortion: Equal Choice, the Constitution, and Reproductive Politics.* Princeton, NJ: Princeton University Press, 1996.

Hursthouse, Rosalind. *Beginning Lives.* Oxford: Basil Blackwell, 1987.

———. "Virtue Theory and Abortion." *Philosophy and Public Affairs* 20, no. 3 (Summer 1991): 223–246.

Kamm, Frances Myrna. *Creation and Abortion: A Study in Moral and Legal Philosophy.* New York: Oxford University Press, 1992.

Luker, Kristin. *Abortion and the Politics of Motherhood.* Berkeley: University of California Press, 1984.

Marquis, Don. "Justifying the Rights of Pregnancy: The Interest View." *Criminal Justice Ethics* (Winter/Spring 1994): 67–81.

McDonaugh, Eileen. *Breaking the Abortion Deadlock.* New York: Oxford University Press, 1996.

Norcross, Alastair. "Killing, Abortion, and Contraception: A Reply to Marquis." *Journal of Philosophy* (1990): 268–278.

Petchesky, Rosalind P. *Abortion and Woman's Choice: The State, Sexuality and Reproductive Freedom.* Revised ed. Boston, MA: Northeastern Press, 1990.

Regan, Donald. "Rewriting *Roe v. Wade.*" *Michigan Law Review* 77 (1979).

Robertson, John A. "*Casey* and the Resuscitation of *Roe v. Wade.*" *Hastings Center Report* 22, no. 5 (1992): 24–29.

Sumner, L. W. *Abortion and Moral Theory.* Princeton, NJ: Princeton University Press, 1981.

Tooley, Michael. *Abortion and Infanticide.* New York: Oxford University Press, 1983.

Tribe, Laurence. *Abortion: The Clash of Absolutes.* New York: W. W. Norton, 1990.

Procreative Autonomy and Responsibility

Arras, John D. "AIDS and Reproductive Decisions: Having Children in Fear and Trembling." *Milbank Quarterly* 68, no. 3 (1990): 353–382.

Astone, Nan Marie. "Thinking About Teenage Childbearing." *Report from the Institute for Philosophy and Public Policy* 13, no. 3 (1993): 8–13.

Bayer, Ronald. "AIDS and the Future of Reproductive Freedom." *Milbank Quarterly* 68 (supplement 2, 1990): 179–204.

Bayles, Michael D. "Limits to a Right to Procreate." In *Having Children: Philosophical and Legal Reflections on Parenthood,* edited by Onora O'Neill and William Ruddick. New York: Oxford University Press, 1979.

Faden, Ruth; Geller, Gail; and Powers, Madison. *AIDS, Women, and the Next Generation: Toward a Morally Acceptable Public Policy for HIV Testing of Pregnant Women and Newborns.* New York: Oxford University Press, 1991.

Faden, Ruth R., and Kass, Nancy E., eds. *HIV, AIDS, and Childbearing: Public Policy, Private Lives.* New York: Oxford University Press, 1996.

Feinberg, Joel. *Harm to Others.* New York: Oxford University Press, 1984.

Levine, Carol, and Dubler, Nancy N. "Uncertain Risks and Bitter Realities: The Reproductive Choices of HIV-Infected Women." *Milbank Quarterly* 68, no. 3 (1990): 321–352.

Luker, Kristin. *Dubious Conceptions: The Politics of Teenage Pregnancy.* Cambridge, MA: Harvard University Press, 1996.

Nelson, Hilde Lindemann. "Dethroning Choice: Analogy, Personhood, and the New Reproductive Technologies." *Journal of Law, Medicine and Ethics* 23, no. 2 (Summer 1995): 129–135.

Parfit, Derek. *Reasons and Persons.* New York: Oxford University Press, 1984, ch. 16.

Petchesky, Rosalind. "Reproductive Freedom: Beyond a Woman's Right to Choose." *Signs—Journal of Women in Culture and Society* 5 (1980): 661–685.

President's Commission for the Study of Ethical Problems in Medicine and Biomedical and Behavioral Research. *Screening and Counseling for Genetic Conditions: The Ethical, Social, and Legal Implications of Genetic Screening, Counseling, and Education Programs.* Washington, DC: U.S. Government Printing Office, 1983.

Robertson, John A. *Children of Choice: Freedom and the New Reproductive Technologies.* Princeton, NJ: Princeton University Press, 1994.

Rothman, Barbara Katz. *The Tentative Pregnancy: Prenatal Diagnosis and the Future of Motherhood.* New York: Penguin, 1987.

Warren, Mary Anne. *Gendercide: The Implications of Sex Selection.* Totowa, NJ: Rowman and Allenheld, 1985.

Wertheimer, Alan. "Two Questions about Surrogacy and Exploitation." *Philosophy and Public Affairs* 21, no. 3 (Summer 1992): 211–239.

"Symposium on 'Surrogate Motherhood.'" *Law, Medicine & Health Care* 16, nos. 1–2 (Spring/Summer 1988): 1–137.

Cloning

Allmers, H. and Kenwright, S. "Ethics of Cloning." *Lancet* 349 no. 9062 (May 10, 1997): 1401

Annas, George J. "Regulatory Models for Human Embryo Cloning: The Free Market, Professional Guidelines, and Government Restrictions." *Kennedy Institute of Ethics Journal* 4 (1994): 235–249.

Capron, Alexander Morgan. "Inside the Beltway Again: A Sheep of a Different Feather." *Kennedy Institute of Ethics Journal* 7 (1997): 171–179.

Carmen, Ira H. *Cloning & the Constitution: An Inquiry into Governmental Policy Making & Genetic Experimentation.* University of Wisconsin Press, 1986.

Chadwick, R. F. "Cloning," *Philosophy* 57 (1982): 201–209.

Cloning Human Beings: Report and Recommendations of the National Bioethics Advisory Commission. Rockville, MD, 1997.

"Cloning Human Beings: Responding to the National Bioethics Advisory Commission's Report." *Hastings Center Report* (September–October 1997).

Cloning Symposium, *Jurimetrics* 38, no. 1 (1997).

Hathout, M. "Cloning: Who Will Set the Limits." *The Minaret* 19, no. 3 (1997): 24–28.

Hefner, P. "Cloning as Quintessential Human Act." *Insights* (June 1997).

Kolata, Gina. *Clone.* New York: William Morrow & Co., 1998.

Lauritzen, Paul ed. *Cloning and the Future of Human Embryo Research* (forthcoming).

Lewontin, Richard. "The Confusion over Cloning." *New York Review of Books,* 44 (October 23, 1997):

Lewontin, Richard; with Harold T. Shapiro; James F. Childress; and Thomas H. Murray. "'The Confusion over Cloning': An Exchange." *New York Review of Books,* 45, no. 4 (March 5, 1998): 46–47.

Macklin, Ruth. "Splitting Embryos on the Slippery Slope: Ethics and Public Policy." *Kennedy Institute of Ethics Journal* 4, no. 3 (September 1994): 209–225.

McCormick, R. A. "Should We Clone Humans?" *The Christian Century* 17–24 (November 1993): 1148–1149.

Pence, Gregory. *Who's Afraid of Human Cloning?* Lanham, MD: Rowman & Littlefield, 1998.

Pizzulli, Francis C. "Asexual Reproduction and Genetic Engineering: A Constitutional Assessment of the Technology of Cloning." *Southern California Law Review* 47 (February 1974): 476–584.

Rhodes, R. "Clones, Harms, and Rights." *Cambridge Quarterly of Healthcare Ethics* 4 (1995): 285–290.

Robertson, J. A. "Liberty, Identity, and Human Cloning." *Texas Law Review* 76, no. 6 (1998).

Verhey, A. "Cloning: Revisiting an Old Debate." *Kennedy Institute of Ethics Journal* 4, no. 3 (September 1994): 227–234.

———. "Playing God and Invoking a Perspective." *Journal of Medicine and Philosophy* 20 (1995): 347–364.

Genetic Testing and Screening

Anderson, W. French. "Genetic Engineering and our Humanness." *Human Gene Therapy.* 5 (1994): 755–759.

Annas, George J., and Elias, Sherman, eds. *Gene Mapping: Using Law and Ethics as Guides.* New York: Oxford University Press, 1992.

Asch, Adrienne. "Reproductive Technology and Disability." In *Reproductive Laws for the 1990s,* edited by Sherill Cohen and Nadine Taub. Clifton, NJ: Humana Press, 1989.

Bartels, Dianne M., et al. *Prescribing Our Future: Ethical Challenges in Genetic Counseling.* New York: Aldine de Gruyter, 1993.

Bonnicksen, Andrea L. "National and International Approaches to Human Germ-Line Gene Therapy." *Politics and the Life Sciences* 13, no. 1 (1994): 39–49.

Botkin, Jeffrey R. "Fetal Privacy and Confidentiality." *Hastings Center Report* (September–October 1995): 32–39.

———. "Prenatal Screening: Professional Standards and the Limits of Parental Choice." *Obstetrics and Gynecology* 75, no. 5 (1990): 328–329.

Boyle, Philip. "Shaping Priorities in Genetic Medicine." *Hastings Center Report* 25, no. (special supplement, 1995): S2–S8.

Buchanan, Allen. "Choosing Who Will Be Disabled: Genetic Intervention and the Morality of Inclusion," *Social Philosophy & Policy,* 13, no. 2 (Summer 1996): 18–46.

Carson, Sandra A., and Buster, John E. "Diagnosis and Treatment before Implantation: The Ultimate Prenatal Medicine," *Contemporary OB/GYN* (December 1995): 71–85.

Davis, Dena. "Genetic Dilemmsa and the Child's Right to an Open Future." *Hastings Center Report* (March–April, 1997): 7–15.

DeCecco, John P., Parker, David Allen, eds. *Sex, Cells, and Same-Sex Desire: The Biology of Sexual Preference.* Haworth: New York, 1995.

"The Ethical Use of Technology in Genetics." *Journal of Clinical Ethics* 2, no. 4 (special section, 1991): 259–281.

Fletcher, John C. "Moral Problems and Ethical Guidance in Prenatal Diagnosis." In *Genetic Disorders and the Fetus,* edited by A. Milunsky, 2nd ed. New York: Plenum Press, 1986.

Fletcher, John C., and Anderson, W. French. "Germ-Line Gene Therapy: A New Stage of Debate." *Law, Medicine & Health Care* 20, nos. 1–2 (Spring/Summer 1992): 26–39.

Fost, Norman. "Ethical Issues in Genetics." *Pediatric Clinics of North America* 39, no. 1 (February 1992): 79–89.

Fost, Norman. "Genetic Diagnosis and Treatment," *AJDC* 147 (November 1993): 1190–1195.

Gardner, William. "Can Human Genetic Enhancement Be Prohibited?" *Journal of Medicine and Philosophy* 20, no. 1 (February 1995): 65–84.

"Genetic Grammar: 'Health,' 'Illness,' and the Human Genome Project." *Hastings Center Report* 22, no. 4 (special supplement, 1992): S1–S20.

"The Genome Imperative." *Journal of Law, Medicine and Ethics.* 23 no. 4 (symposium, Winter 1995): 309ff.

Green, Ronald M. "Paternal Autonomy and the Obligation Not to Harm One's Child Genetically," *Journal of Law, Medicine and Ethics* 25 (1997): 5–15.

Gustafson, James M. "Genetic Therapy: Ethical and Religious Reflections." *Journal of Contemporary Health Law and Policy* 8 (Spring 1992): 183–200.

Halley, Janet. "Sexual Orientation and the Politics of Biology: A Critique of the New Argument from Immutability." *Stanford Law Review* 46 (1994): 503–568.

Heyd, David. *Genethics: Moral Issues in the Creation of People.* Berkeley: University of California Press, 1992.

"The Human Genome Initiative and the Impact of Genetic Testing and Screening Technologies." *American Journal of Law and Medicine* 17, nos. 1–2 (symposium, 1991).

Juengst, Eric T., ed. "Human Germ-Line Engineering." *Journal of Medicine and Philosophy* 16, no. 6 (December 1991): 587–694.

———. "'Prevention' and the Goals of Genetic Medicine." *Human Gene Therapy* 6 (December 1995): 1595–1605.

Kelves, Daniel J. *In the Name of Eugenics: Genetics and the Uses of Human Heredity.* New York: Alfred A. Knopf, 1985.

Kusum. "The Use of Prenatal Diagnostic Techniques for Sex Selection: The Indian Scene." *Bioethics* 7 (1993): 149–165.

McGee, Glenn. *The Perfect Baby: A Pragmatic Approach to Genetics.* New York: Rowan and Littlefield, 1997.

Munson, Ronald, and Davis, Lawrence H. "Germ-Line Gene Therapy and the Medical Imperative." *Kennedy Institute of Ethics Journal* 2, no. 2 (June 1992): 137–158.

Murphy, Timothy F. *Gay Science: The Ethics of Sexual Orientation Research.* Columbia UP: New York, 1998.

Murray, Thomas H. "Genetics and the Moral Mission of Health Insurance." *Hastings Center Report* 22, no. 6 (1992): 12–17.

———. "The Growing Danger from Gene-Spliced Hormones." *Discover* (February 1987): 88–92.

National Institutes of Health (NIH) Consensus Development Conference Statement. "Genetic Testing for Cystic Fibrosis." April 14–16, 1997.

Parens, Erik. "The Goodness of Fragility: On the Prospect of Genetic Technologies Aimed at the Enhancement of Human Capacities." *Kennedy Institute of Ethics Journal* (1996).

————. "Should We Hold the (Germ) Line?" *Journal of Law, Medicine and Ethics* 23, no. 2 (Summer 1995): 173–176.

————. "Taking Behavioral Genetics Seriously." *Hastings Center Report* (July–August 1996): 13–22.

President's Commission for the Study of Ethical Problems in Medicine and Biomedical and Behavioral Research. *Screening and Counseling for Genetic Conditions: A Report on the Ethical, Social, and Legal Implications of Genetic Screening, Counseling, and Education Programs.* Washington, DC: U. S. Government Printing Office, 1983.

————. *Splicing Life: A Report on the Social and Ethical Issues of Genetic Engineering with Human Beings.* Washington, DC: U. S. Government Printing Office, 1982.

Rosario, Vernon A. ed. *Science and Homosexualities.* Routledge: New York, 1997.

Rothenberg, Karen H., and Thomson, Elizabeth J., eds. *Women & Prenatal Testing: Facing the Challenges of Genetic Technology.* Columbus, Ohio: Ohio State University Press, 1994.

Rothman, Barbara Katz. *The Tentative Pregnancy: Prenatal Diagnosis and the Future of Motherhood.* New York: Viking Press, 1986.

Snowden, C. and Green, J. "Preimplantation Diagnosis and Other Reproductive Options: Attitudes of Male and Female Carriers of Recessive Disorders." *Human Reproduction* 12, no. 2 (1997): 341–350.

Suzuki, David, and Knudtson, Peter. *Genethics: The Clash between the New Genetics and Human Values.* Cambridge, MA: Harvard University Press, 1990.

"Symposium on Genetics and the Law." *Emory Law Journal* 39, no. 3 (Summer 1990): 619–936.

Walters, Leroy. "Human Gene Therapy: Ethics and Public Policy." *Human Gene Therapy* 2 (1991): 115–122.

Walters, Leroy, and Palmer, Julie Gage. *The Ethics of Human Gene Therapy.* New York: Oxford University Press, 1996.

Wertz, Dorothy C. "Society and the Not-So-New Genetics: What Are We Afraid Of? Some Future Predictions from a Social Scientist," *Journal of Contemporary Health Law and Policy* 13 (1997): 299–346.

Wertz, Dorothy C., and Fletcher, John C., eds. *Ethics and Human Genetics: A Cross-Cultural Perspective.* New York: Springer-Verlag, 1989.

Wivel, Nelson A., and Walters, LeRoy. "Germ-Line Gene Modification and Disease Prevention: Some Medical and Ethical Perspectives." *Science* 262 (October 22, 1993): 533–538.

Wolf, Susan M. "Beyond 'Genetic Discrimination' toward the Broader Harm of Geneticism," *Journal of Law, Medicine and Ethics* 23 (1995): 345–353.

PART FOUR

ASSISTED REPRODUCTIVE TECHNOLOGIES AND GENETICS

Of all the recent changes that have occurred in bioethics, none has been more rapid, more dramatic, and more sweeping than those in assisted reproductive technologies (ART) and genetics. In the last few years, the world has witnessed a 63-year-old woman bearing a healthy baby, the ability to freeze human eggs, the live birth of septuplets, and cloning. Should we regard these developments as advances in reproductive medicine, or as reproductive technology gone mad? The need for in-depth ethical reflection has never been more apparent.

What, for example, are the implications of freezing ova? It has long been possible to freeze sperm, giving men the option of storing healthy sperm before undergoing procedures such as chemotherapy that might render them sterile. Some men have even attempted to bequeath their sperm for posthumous reproduction (Robertson 1994, Steinbock 1995). In 1997, scientists were able, for the first time, to freeze human ova, after years of unsuccessful attempts. A few women have given birth to healthy babies from frozen (donated) eggs. Fertility experts say that the age of the uterus is not the prime consideration in a successful pregnancy. As long as donor eggs from younger women are used, women—like men—could theoretically be "of childbearing age" their entire lives. This has given rise to speculation that women might choose to freeze their eggs in their twenties, at the height of their fertility, for childbearing in their thirties, forties, or even fifties, after they had established careers. Although some women might wish to avail themselves of this option as a hedge against later infertility, the idea that reproduction by ART might become the norm ignores the physical and emotional burdens of the treatment, its cost, and its relatively high failure rate of 70 to 80 percent.

Fertility treatment has enabled thousands of infertile couples to have families, but a side effect is multiple births. Most fertility experts view multiple births as something to be avoided at all costs, saying that women's bodies were not intended to carry more than one or two babies. Yet fertility treatment continues to "push the envelope," and 1997 saw the birth of the first set of septuplets to survive the neonatal period (see "The McCaughey Septuplets: Medical Miracle or Gambling with Fertility Drugs?" in Part Three, Section Three). Will seven be the maximum, or will we see live births of eight or more babies? And what will be the impact on the lives of the children, their families, and society as a whole?

Finally, and most dramatically, 1997 saw the birth of Dolly the lamb, the first mammal cloned from a cell taken from an adult, in a technique known as "somatic cell nuclear transfer" (SCNT) cloning. The initial reaction of the public to cloning was revulsion and fear, a sense that mad scientists were attempting to play God. The initial, nearly hysterical, reaction was replaced by a more objective and cautious attitude. The real concern may not be cloning itself, but rather the opportunity it provides to intervene in an individual's genome. Ultimately, scientists expect cloning to be combined with genetic enhancement, adding genes to give desired traits; this was the fundamental reason cloning was studied in animal research. Some people fear we have taken the first step on a very slippery slope to a world in which parents "design" their children. They worry that the ability to enhance offspring genetically will further widen the gap in opportunities between rich and poor. In addition, some fear that if parents can choose their children's traits, they will be unable or unwilling to accept children who turn out contrary to specification, with detrimental effects on the relations between parents and children. How, then, should we view the developments in reproductive medicine? As advances that enable infertile people to have much-desired children, thus furthering "family values"? Or as harbingers of a world in which women and children are commodities and products, and human relations are destroyed?

ADVOCATES AND CRITICS OF ASSISTED REPRODUCTIVE TECHNOLOGIES (ART)

Assisted reproductive technologies run the gamut from the low-tech (though not without risk) administration of fertility drugs to more high-tech procedures, such as *in vitro* fertilization (IVF) and cryopreservation of embryos for later implantation. In addition to IVF, gamete intrafallopian transfer (GIFT), zygote intrafallopian transfer (ZIFT), and a slew of other acronyms identify each new procedure. A procedure known as intracytoplasmic sperm injection (ICSI) involves injecting a single sperm by pipette into an egg, thus enabling men who have a very low sperm count to procreate. Many new techniques are improvements of earlier techniques, although many fertility experts in the United States complain that restrictions on federal funding for embryo research hamper progress in fertility treatments.

All of these procedures are incredibly expensive. A single attempt at IVF may cost anywhere from $5,000 to $12,000. GIFT and ZIFT may be even more expensive. All of these techniques have discouragingly low "take-home baby" rates. Even the best clinics treating the least-impaired couples report success rates only in the mid-30-percent range. Physical and emotional risks are always involved. All of these procedures raise questions of medical, legal, and social ethics (Robin 1993).

John Robertson is perhaps the most prominent defender of procreative liberty. The first article in Section One is a selection from his book, *Children of Choice*. Robertson supports allowing individuals to make their own reproductive decisions, including decisions about fertility treatments and collaborative reproduction. He believes that attempts to ban or restrict reproductive techniques violate the reproductive rights of infertile people, in the absence of demonstrable proof that such techniques would cause tangible harm to existing people. By contrast, the Catholic Church opposes virtually every assisted reproductive technique, including artificial insemination by husband (AIH), also known as homologous artificial fertilization, at least where AIH is a substitute for, as opposed to a facilitator of, the conjugal act, or sexual intercourse within marriage. The usual objections to ART (discussed further in Section Two), such as commercialization and the introduction of a "third party" into the marital relationship and subsequent confusion about lineage, are not present in AIH. Nevertheless, the Church objects to AIH for the same reason it objects to contraception: Both are seen as severing the connection between procreation and the conjugal act.

Mary Anne Warren addresses specifically feminist concerns about IVF. She argues that although the new reproductive technologies pose some significant dangers for women, it would be wrong for women to demand an end to IVF and other reproductive research. In particular, she rejects the argument that because women are conditioned to desire motherhood in patriarchal society, they are therefore incapable of giving free and informed consent to infertility treatment. Rather, Warren thinks that women must take into account the social pressures to have children before they decide whether to use IVF. Some women will undoubtedly make mistakes, but this does not necessarily mean that they would benefit from paternalistic constraints. At the same time, Warren agrees with the feminist objection to male domination over women's reproductive abilities, and calls for greater participation by women in all areas of medicine and biomedical research. She also notes that it would be better to prevent infertility in the first place, rather than rely on expensive, high-tech cures, and she calls for greater societal attention to this issue.

CONTRACT PREGNANCY, COMMODIFICATION, AND THE FAMILY

Section Two deals with perhaps the most controversial of the new reproductive modalities, and the one that most clearly raises concerns about commercialization and commodification, namely contract pregnancy, or "surrogate motherhood." Typically, a woman is hired to bear a child for a couple in which the wife is infertile or incapable of a safe pregnancy. Sometimes a surrogate is hired to bear a child for a single person, a homosexual couple, or a woman who, for reasons of her own, does not want to go through pregnancy. Surrogate motherhood itself is neither new nor high-tech; in the Bible, the infertile Sarah has her servant Hagar

bear a child by Abraham. Various commentators have pointed out that in a standard contract pregnancy, the woman who bears a child for someone else is not a surrogate mother, but actually the child's genetic and gestational mother. She is more appropriately called a surrogate wife, since she takes over one of a wife's functions (having a child). Nevertheless, the term "surrogate mother" has stuck and is used here.

In biblical times, the surrogate became pregnant the old-fashioned way, through sexual intercourse. Today, the surrogate is usually artificially inseminated. Artificial insemination is not a high-tech procedure; it can be performed with a turkey baster. However, sometimes surrogacy is combined with IVF so that the embryo implanted in the surrogate's womb has no genetic relationship to her. If a dispute then arises regarding custody of the resulting child, who is the mother? The woman who provided the egg or the woman who gestated the fetus?

The courts have confronted conflicts between a genetic and a gestational mother only twice, both times favoring the genetic over the gestational mother. In *Johnson* v. *Calvert*, the California appellate court characterized the woman who gave birth as merely a "foster parent" for the "natural" mother whose egg had been used. As Alta Charo points out in the last selection in Section Two, the court "never confronted the implications of its ruling for California's flourishing egg donation practices, in which genetic mothers expect to be treated as legal strangers from their genetic offspring, while birth mothers using purchased eggs expect to be treated as legal parents of their offspring." Can there be a consistent definition of parenthood that responds to the wide variety of reproductive technologies and practices, respects the procreative interests of the various parties, and protects of the best interests of the child?

Feminist Barbara Katz Rothman opts for a gestational definition of motherhood: The woman who gives birth is the child's mother. As Charo points out, this is the solution adopted by virtually every other country that has examined the problem (Israel being a notable exception). In effect, this means a rejection of commercial surrogacy. According to Rothman, a woman is never pregnant with someone else's baby; the idea is repugnant, and reduces the woman to a container. "In that sense, surrogacy is the reductio ad absurdum of technological, patriarchal capitalism."

Bonnie Steinbock discusses surrogate motherhood in the context of the notorious case of "Baby M," in which Mary Beth Whitehead, a surrogate mother, decided that she wanted to keep the biological child of William Stern and his wife Elizabeth. Thus ensued a lengthy and highly publicized custody battle between the Whiteheads and the Sterns. George Annas (1987) has argued that the temporary custody order imposed by Judge Sorkow evidenced the judge's "overt contempt" for the lower-middle-class Whiteheads and "obsequiousness" toward the upper-middle-class Sterns. He also maintains that the contract Mrs. Whitehead signed was totally one-sided and violated her constitutional rights. Individuals can waive their parental rights, but not prospectively. Finally, the contract was against New Jersey law in that it clearly provided not for gestational services, but for the sale of a child; Mrs. Whitehead was to be paid $10,000 to deliver a live child, but would receive only $1,000 if she had a miscarriage after the fifth month, and nothing in the event of a miscarriage prior to the fifth month (Annas 1987).

Bonnie Steinbock agrees with Annas that the contract between Mrs. Whitehead and the Stems provided for the sale of a child. However, Steinbock does not think that surrogacy necessarily involves baby-selling, instead suggesting that it can be regarded as a form of "prenatal adoption" in which the surrogate agrees to give the biological father sole custody of the child after birth. The payment should be seen as compensation for the risk, sacrifice, loss of income, and discomfort the surrogate undergoes during pregnancy. If the baby is stillborn, through no fault of the surrogate's, the woman should still be paid in full, since she has fulfilled her part of the bargain. If, however, she changes her mind and decides to keep the child, she breaks the agreement and relinquishes any compensation. While legislative efforts should be directed toward preventing fiascoes like the Baby M case, Steinbock finds none of the arguments against surrogacy (such as that it exploits disadvantaged women and/or causes psychological harm to children who learn that they were bartered before birth) convincing enough to justify state intervention as substantial as complete prohibition. She favors state regulation, but only to min-

imize potential harms without infringing on personal liberty.

Thomas Murray acknowledges both the profound longing for children that leads people to undergo fertility treatments, and the charges of exploitation and commodification made by critics of ART. He suggests that discomfort with ART stems from a sense that they threaten to undermine the very values that prompted their creation in the first place. The problem with ART is not that it is artificial, but rather that it often brings the values of the marketplace into the sphere of the family. This is particularly so in the case of commercial surrogacy, but it is also a danger when gametes are bought and sold. Murray criticizes John Robertson, who defends commercial surrogacy as protected by the right to reproduce. Objecting to the language of individual rights as ill-suited to the sphere of the family, Murray asks us to consider instead whether children are likely to flourish in a society that permits commercial surrogacy and gamete donation. According to Murray, the burden of proof is on the proponents of marketplace values to show that the practices they advocate do not threaten what we value about family life.

Murray's rejection of individual rights as the fundamental element in an analysis of assisted reproduction, and his critique of marketplace values, are likely to resonate with many readers. At the same time, it is not clear why paying gamete donors or surrogates is necessarily detrimental to the "family values" he identifies, such as love, nurturing, loyalty, trust, and maturation. A variety of professionals—therapists, teachers, childcare workers, pediatricians—work intimately with family members and expect to be paid for doing so. If financial compensation does not threaten family values in these contexts, why is it objectionable in the context of reproduction?

Like Murray, Alta Charo is also concerned with the effects on children of assisted reproduction. However, rather than rejecting the new arrangements that ART makes possible, she views it as an opportunity to rethink the definition of family. Why must we determine who the "real" parents are, and whether genetic ties are more important than gestational ones or whether the intent to rear trumps genetic heritage? Instead, Charo argues, courts should recognize that children can have more than two parents, and that they need not always be of different genders. The best interests of the child, she suggests, may be promoted if we recognize that "you can never have too many parents to love you."

CLONING

Section Three is devoted to the newest technique of possible application to reproductive medicine—cloning, or more precisely, somatic cell nuclear transfer (SCNT) cloning. In July 1997, Dr. Ian Wilmut announced that he had successfully cloned a lamb, Dolly, using SCNT cloning. Wilmut's team took the DNA from a somatic cell (in this case, a mammary cell) of an adult ewe and placed it in an egg cell from another ewe, from which the nucleus had been removed. The resulting embryo was carried to term by yet a third sheep. Thus, Dolly was a (nearly) identical genetic copy of one sheep ("nearly" because a small amount of mitochondrial DNA remained in the enucleated egg cell), or a "delayed" genetic twin of an adult sheep.

President Clinton immediately imposed a temporary ban on federal funding of human cloning research. He directed the National Bioethics Advisory Commission (NBAC) to undertake a thorough review of the legal and ethical issues and to report back to him within ninety days with recommendations on possible federal actions to prevent the abuse of this new technology. To no one's surprise, the NBAC report recommended that the President's moratorium be continued. It held, almost exclusively on the basis of safety considerations, that it was morally unacceptable at this time for anyone, privately or publicly funded, to engage in SCNT cloning research aimed at creating a child. The report stressed the medical and scientific potential of cloning, such as the creation of tissue for burn victims or bone marrow for transplantation, and it emphasized the need to make a distinction between "human cloning" and "cloning a human being" so as not to hinder important, and morally noncontroversial, areas of scientific research. As for the use of SCNT cloning to create human beings, the report recommended further dialogue on the nonsafety objections (ethical, religious, and policy), and suggested that the issue be revisited in three to five years.

NBAC's sober presentation of the scientific facts, and in particular its attack on "genetic determin-

ism" (the view that everything about us is determined by our genetic makeup) undoubtedly prevented a total ban on research that might yield important scientific and medical results. However, this reasonable and cautious approach may have been undercut by the announcement on January 7, 1998, by physicist Richard Seed of his intention to begin working on human cloning using a newly developed technique. Many commentators expressed skepticism regarding Seed's technical credibility. Although he and his brother, a medical doctor, were involved in fertility research in the 1980s, critics maintain that he lacks expertise in the latest advances. Nevertheless, in response to his announcement, at the urging of President Clinton, Congress banned the cloning of human beings. On January 12, nineteen European nations signed an agreement banning any intervention seeking to create a human being genetically identical to another human being, whether living or dead, calling this a misuse of science.

In a carefully balanced article, Dan Brock examines the main moral arguments for and against cloning human beings. Brock argues that the moral right to reproductive freedom creates a presumption that individuals should be free to choose the means of reproduction that bests serves their interests and desires. The question is whether the potential benefits of SCNT cloning outweigh its potential dangers. Brock first examines the possible uses of SCNT. To take just one example, suppose a couple has male-factor infertility, that is, the man has no viable sperm. Rather than resort to donor insemination, which brings a third party into their reproduction, such a couple might prefer to extract the DNA from a cell of the husband, put it in an enucleated egg cell of the wife, and implant the resulting embryo in her uterus. Both parents would have a biological connection with the resulting child, although the child would be (nearly) genetically identical to the husband. The motivation in this case would be the same as that of other infertile couples: to have a child of their own. Would cloning in these circumstances be morally objectionable? After examining possible objections, Brock concludes that the ethical pros and cons are "sufficiently balanced and uncertain that there is not an ethically decisive case either for or against" cloning human beings. He urges careful public oversight of research and wider public debate before the technique is used on human beings.

In sharp contrast to Brock, Leon Kass offers an impassioned plea for an international legal ban on research on cloning humans. Cloning is one more example of how we have been led astray by technology; it reflects our narcissism, obsession with control, and loss of the capacity for awe at the mysteries of nature and life. Noting a widespread visceral reaction to cloning, Kass suggests that this repugnance, while not an argument, is "the emotional expression of deep wisdom, beyond reason's power fully to articulate it." We experience such repugnance at incest, bestiality, and cannibalism even though we may not be able to give completely rational explanations of what is morally wrong with these practices. Yet we would be less than fully human, Kass maintains, if we were not repulsed by them. "Shallow are the souls that have forgotten how to shudder."

Kass also objects to cloning because it permits the creation of offspring who do not have two biological progenitors. As "a radical departure from the natural human way" of having children, asexual reproduction threatens both identity and family relationships. Moreover, he regards the severing of procreation from sex, love, and intimacy as "inherently dehumanizing," echoing the objections of the Catholic Church to ART (see "Instruction on Respect for Human Life in Its Origin and on the Dignity of Procreation" in Section One). In addition, engaging in cloning humans "would be taking a major step into making man himself simply another one of the man-made things," further dehumanizing procreation. Finally, cloning is "inherently despotic" in that it imposes excessive expectations on offspring to resemble their genetic originals. Kass believes our response to human cloning will determine whether we become slaves of unregulated progress or remain free human beings who use technology to enhance human dignity. His article can be used not only to consider the morality of cloning, but also to consider the degree to which ethical judgments should be based on feelings. In his testimony before NBAC, Senator Bill Frist, himself a heart and lung transplant surgeon, pointed out that heart transplants occasioned the same initial reaction of shock and horror as cloning, but transplants have now become an accepted part of medicine. Readers will have to decide for themselves whether revulsion to cloning embodies, as Kass maintains, "the wisdom of repugnance" or whether it reflects merely fear in the face of something completely new.

GENETIC SCREENING AND TESTING

The amount of available genetic information has increased astronomically in the late 1990s. The opportunities to predict, cure, and prevent disease using genetic technology seem limitless. According to one commentator,

> Thanks to rapid private-sector advances in molecular biology and a $3 billion federal Human Genome Project that will map and sequence the genetic makeup of humans, a plethora of population screens, diagnostic tests, and therapies will be available—perhaps commonplace—in the next decade. Conservative estimates are that some 50,000 gene markers will be developed as a result of molecular biology and translated into easy-to-employ biochemical assays, genetic tests, new drugs, and genetic therapies. (Boyle 1995, p. S2.)

As we learn more about genetic disorders, there is increased pressure for genetic testing. In part, this is due to the emergence of a biotechnology industry that profits financially from testing. Using the example of cystic fibrosis (CF), Wilfond and Fost provide several reasons for being cautious about instituting screening programs, especially mass screening programs.

About 30,000 Americans have cystic fibrosis. The disease is far more prevalent among whites; as many as one in twenty Caucasians carries a gene with a cystic fibrosis defect. When both members of a couple carry such a gene, their children have one chance in four of inheriting the disease. Although severity varies greatly and the life span of CF patients is increasing, most of them do not live beyond their twenties. In 1989, when scientists isolated the gene that causes CF, many of them believed that screening for the gene would provide the prototype for national screening programs to combat other dread diseases, in addition to providing widespread prenatal diagnosis for couples who are found to carry the defective CF gene. However, the issue has proven to be more complex than originally thought. The most common genetic mutation responsible for CF is called the ΔF508 mutation. Since the gene and the major mutation responsible for CF were identified, more than 600 additional mutations and DNA sequence variations have been identified in the CF transmembrane conductance regulator (CFTR) gene. But the test for CF picks out only the most common mutation, the delta ΔF508 mutation. Since one or both partners might have one of the rarer mutations, a negative test can not assure couples that they will not have a baby with CF. At the same time the CF test has a high degree of sensitivity. "In Caucasians in the United States, it is feasible to approach 90 percent sensitivity at the current time" (NIH 1997, p. 5).

In addition to testing individuals to discover their carrier status, prenatal testing can be performed on fetuses. However, a positive result does not invariably signify that the child, if born, would develop CF. Even people who inherit mutated genes from both parents do not necessarily develop cystic fibrosis. They may instead have less serious disorders, such as infertility, asthma, or chronic bronchitis. Many couples who would abort a pregnancy if the fetus were affected with CF probably would not abort for these less serious disorders.

Some geneticists think that since the test can pick up the majority of carriers, it is better to offer it than to wait for a more accurate test, and they argue that it should be up to patients to decide whether they want to be tested. Others say that it is pointless, even harmful, to offer testing to individuals without a family history of the disease, since it would offer uncertainty rather than reassurance or guidance to most of them. In 1997, a panel of experts from the National Institutes of Health recommended that genetic testing for CF should be offered to all couples currently planning a pregnancy and to couples seeking prenatal testing, whether or not they have a family history of CF. The panel did not recommend offering CF genetic testing to the general public or newborn infants (NIH 1997).

 The NIH consensus statement does not speculate on the number of people who would be offered CF genetic testing if its recommendation were followed, but presumably the number would be very high. One of the issues Wilfond and Fost address is whether adequate genetic counseling will be available for a group of this size. According to the NIH consensus statement, there are only approximately 2,000 genetic professionals nationally, so implementation of widespread genetic testing would have to rely heavily on primary care providers and prenatal providers, who may lack both expertise and interest in providing this service.

Another issue is cost-effectiveness. Wilfond and Fost suggest that it might cost as much as 2.4 million dollars to avoid one CF birth, although some studies estimate a considerably lower cost (NIH 1997, p. 8). Aside from the issue of cost, there is a question about the desirability of terminating a pregnancy when the baby that would be born may later develop CF. Disability advocates view prenatal screening in general with disfavor, because they believe it reflects prejudiced and inaccurate views about the lives of people who have disabilities (see Asch, "Prenatal Screening" in Part Three, Section Three). Even if we accept the value of prenatal screening in general, it seems clear that potential parents' decisions about testing and selective abortion can be influenced in one direction or another, depending how the information is presented; therefore it is imperative that information about CF and other genetic disorders be presented in a balanced fashion.

If genetic screening is to be done at all, its use seems most clearly justified in preventing the births of people with serious, life-threatening, genetic diseases. However, researchers have become interested in the genetic components of diseases that do not (directly) shorten lifespan (such as bipolar disorder and schizophrenia) and of nondisease behaviors, such as shyness and sexual orientation. In "The Ethics of Genetic Research on Sexual Orientation," Schüklenk, Stein, Kerin, and Byne first warn against a simplistic understanding of genetic inheritance. It is highly unlikely, for example, that a gene could cause a person to be sexually attracted to a member of the same sex. "No one has, however, presented evidence in support of such a simple and direct link between genes and sexual orientation." An "indirect effect model" is more plausible (though currently unsupported by scientific evidence). That is, genes might be responsible for temperamental factors that influence how one interacts with and shapes one's environment and formative experiences. On this model, genes alone are not responsible for sexual orientation—environment would also play a role. In some environments, one's genetic make-up might predispose one to become homosexual, in others, heterosexual, or bisexual, and in still others, might have no influence on sexuality at all.

The problem, the authors argue, is not simply a misunderstanding of the workings of genetics. A genetic screening test based on "good science" might be developed that could pick out a predisposition for homosexuality. Prospective parents opposed to homosexuality might opt to have such testing and choose to abort the fetus identified as being homosexually predisposed. In fact, they might opt for such tests even if the tests were based on bad science, and did not work. Parents who used such a procedure might believe it had worked even if it had not: The child might not have discovered his or her sexual orientation, or might hide homosexuality from his or her parents. Regardless of their effectiveness, the use of tests to identify fetuses as homosexually predisposed would likely "engender and perpetuate attitudes that lesbians and gay men are undesirable and not valuable. . . ." For these reasons, the authors main-

tain that biological research into sexual orientation should not be done.

The same argument is made by those who oppose prenatal testing for disabilities. They believe it sends a message that disabled individuals are undesirable. If this is a legitimate argument against prenatal testing for sexual orientation, is it equally legitimate against prenatal testing for disability? Some maintain there is no difference, but argue that prospective parents are the ones to decide what they will test for and why, whether they want to test for disability, sexual orientation, or sex. Disability rights advocates agree that there is no difference between testing for sex and testing for disability, but most reject both kinds of prenatal diagnosis. Those in the middle attempt to distinguish between testing for disability and testing for sex or sexual orientation. They are faced with the challenge of justifying this distinction, in light of persuasive arguments made by the disability community that prenatal testing is often motivated by ignorance and prejudice, which is as offensive when it is directed against disabled people as when it is directed against homosexuals and lesbians.

SECTION 1

Advocates and Critics of Assisted Reproductive Technologies

The Presumptive Primacy of Procreative Liberty

John Robertson

Procreative liberty has wide appeal but its scope has never been fully elaborated and often is contested. The concept has several meanings that must be clarified if it is to serve as a reliable guide for moral debate and public policy regarding new reproductive technologies.

WHAT IS PROCREATIVE LIBERTY?

At the most general level, procreative liberty is the freedom either to have children or to avoid having them. Although often expressed or realized in the context of a couple, it is first and foremost an individual interest. It is to be distinguished from freedom in the ancillary aspects of reproduction, such as liberty in the conduct of pregnancy or choice of place or mode of childbirth.

The concept of reproduction, however, has a certain ambiguity contained within it. In a strict sense, reproduction is always genetic. It occurs by provision of one's gametes to a new person, and thus includes having or producing offspring. While female reproduction has traditionally included gestation, in vitro fertilization (IVF) now allows female genetic and gestational reproduction to be separated. Thus a woman who has provided the egg that is carried by another has reproduced, even if she has not gestated and does not rear resulting offspring. Because of the close link between gestation and female reproduction, a woman who gestates the embryo of another may also reasonably be viewed as having a reproductive experience, even though she does not reproduce genetically.[1]

In any case, reproduction in the genetic or gestational sense is to be distinguished from child rearing. Although reproduction is highly valued in part because it usually leads to child rearing, one can produce offspring without rearing them and rear children without reproduction. One who rears an adopted child has not reproduced, while one who has genetic progeny but does not rear them has.

In this book the terms "procreative liberty" and "reproductive freedom" will mean the freedom to reproduce or not to reproduce in the genetic sense, which may also include rearing or not, as intended by the parties. Those terms will also include female gestation whether or not there is a genetic connection to the resulting child.

Often the reproduction at issue will be important because it is intended to lead to child rearing. In cases where rearing is not intended, the value to be assigned to reproduction *tout court* will have to be determined. Similarly, when there is rearing without genetic or gestational involvement, the value of nonreproductive child rearing will also have to be assessed. In both cases the value assigned may depend on the proximity to reproduction where rearing is intended.

Two further qualifications on the meaning of procreative liberty should be noted. One is that "liberty" as used in procreative liberty is a negative right. It means that a person violates no moral duty in making a procreative choice, and that

From *Children of Choice: Freedom and the New Reproductive Technologies* by John Robertson, Princeton University Press, 1994. Copyright © 1994 Princeton University Press. Reprinted by permission of the publisher.

EDITORS' NOTE: Many of the notes in this chapter have been omitted; those wishing to follow up on sources should consult the original.

other persons have a duty not to interfere with that choice. However, the negative right to procreate or not does not imply the duty of others to provide the resources or services necessary to exercise one's procreative liberty despite plausible moral arguments for governmental assistance.

As a matter of constitutional law, procreative liberty is a negative right against state interference with choices to procreate or to avoid procreation. It is not a right against private interference, though other laws might provide that protection. Nor is it a positive right to have the state or particular persons providing the means or resources necessary to have or avoid having children. The exercise of procreative liberty may be severely constrained by social and economic circumstances. Access to medical care, child care, employment, housing, and other services may significantly affect whether one is able to exercise procreative liberty. However, the state presently has no constitutional obligation to provide those services. Whether the state should alleviate those conditions is a separate issue of social justice.

The second qualification is that not everything that occurs in and around procreation falls within liberty interests that are distinctively procreative. Thus whether the father may be present during childbirth, whether midwives may assist birth, or whether childbirth may occur at home rather than in a hospital may be important for the parties involved, but they do not implicate the freedom to reproduce (unless one could show that the place or mode of birth would determine whether birth occurs at all). Similarly, questions about a pregnant woman's drug use or other conduct during pregnancy . . . implicates liberty in the course of reproduction but not procreative liberty in the basic sense. Questions about whether the use of a technology is distinctively procreative recur throughout this book.

THE IMPORTANCE OF PROCREATIVE LIBERTY

Procreative liberty should enjoy presumptive primacy when conflicts about its exercise arise because control over whether one reproduces or not is central to personal identity, to dignity, and to the meaning of one's life. For example, deprivation of the ability to avoid reproduction determines one's self-definition in the most basic sense. It affects women's bodies in a direct and substantial way. It also centrally affects one's psychological and social identity and one's social and moral responsibilities. The resulting burdens are especially onerous for women, but they affect men in significant ways as well.

On the other hand, being deprived of the ability to reproduce prevents one from an experience that is central to individual identity and meaning in life. Although the desire to reproduce is in part socially constructed, at the most basic level transmission of one's genes through reproduction is an animal or species urge closely linked to the sex drive. In connecting us with nature and future generations, reproduction gives solace in the face of death. As Shakespeare noted, "nothing 'gainst Time's scythe can make defense/save breed."[2] For many people "breed"—reproduction and the parenting that usually accompanies it—is a central part of their life plan, and the most satisfying and meaningful experience they have. It also has primary importance as an expression of a couple's love or unity. For many persons, reproduction also has religious significance and is experienced as a "gift from God." Its denial—through infertility or governmental restriction—is experienced as a great loss, even if one has already had children or will have little or no rearing role with them.

Decisions to have or to avoid having children are thus personal decisions of great import that determine the shape and meaning of one's life. The person directly involved is best situated to determine whether that meaning should or should not occur. An ethic of personal autonomy as well as ethics of community or family should then recognize a presumption in favor of most personal reproductive choices. Such a presumption does not mean that reproductive choices are without consequence to others, nor that they should never be limited. Rather, it means that those who would limit procreative choice have the burden of showing that the reproductive actions at issue would create such substantial harm that they could justifiably be limited. Of course, what counts as the "substantial harm" that justifies interference with procreative choice may often be contested, as the discussion of reproductive technologies in this book will show.

A closely related reason for protecting reproductive choice is to avoid the highly intrusive measures that governmental control of reproduction usually entails. State interference with reproductive choice may extend beyond exhortation and penalties to gestapo and police state tactics. Margaret Atwood's powerful futuristic novel *The Handmaid's Tale* expresses this danger by creating a world where fertile women are forcibly impregnated by the ruling powers and their pregnancies monitored to replenish a decimated population.[3]

Equally frightening scenarios have occurred in recent years when repressive governments have interfered with reproductive choice. In Romania and China, men and women have had their most private activities scrutinized in the service of state reproductive goals. In Ceaușescu's Romania, where contraception and abortion were strictly forbidden, women's menstrual cycles were routinely monitored to see if they were pregnant. Women who did not become pregnant or who had abortions were severely punished. Many women nevertheless sought illegal abortions and died, leaving their children orphaned and subject to sale to Westerners seeking children for adoption.

In China, forcible abortion and sterilization have occurred in the service of a one-child-per-family population policy. Village cadres have seized pregnant women in their homes and forced them to have abortions. A campaign of forcible sterilization in India in 1977 was seen as an "attack on women and children" and brought Indira Gandhi's government down. In the United States, state-imposed sterilization of "mental defectives," sanctioned in 1927 by the United States Supreme Court in *Buck* v. *Bell*, resulted in 60,000 sterilizations over a forty-year period. Many mentally normal people were sterilized by mistake, and mentally retarded persons who posed little risk of harm to others were subjected to surgery. It is no surprise that current proposals for compulsory use of contraceptives such as Norplant are viewed with great suspicion.

TWO TYPES OF PROCREATIVE LIBERTY

To see how values of procreative liberty affect the ethical and public policy evaluation of new reproductive technologies, we must determine whether the interests that underlie the high value accorded procreative liberty are implicated in their use. This is not a simple task because procreative liberty is not unitary, but consists of strands of varying interests in the conception and gestation of offspring. The different strands implicate different interests, have different legal and constitutional status, and are differently affected by technology.

An essential distinction is between the freedom to avoid reproduction and the freedom to reproduce. When people talk of reproductive rights, they usually have one or the other aspect in mind. Because different interests and justifications underlie each and countervailing interests for limiting each aspect vary, recognition of one aspect does not necessarily mean that the other will also be respected; nor does limitation of one mean that the other can also be denied.

However, there is a mirroring or reciprocal relationship here. Denial of one type of reproductive liberty necessarily implicates the other. If a woman is not able to avoid reproduction through contraception or abortion, she may end up reproducing, with all the burdens that unwanted reproduction entails. Similarly, if one is denied the liberty to reproduce through forcible sterilization, one is forced to avoid reproduction, thus experiencing the loss that absence of progeny brings. By extending reproductive options, new reproductive technologies present challenges to both aspects of procreative choice.

AVOIDING REPRODUCTION: THE LIBERTY NOT TO REPRODUCE

One sense in which people commonly understand procreative liberty is as the freedom to avoid reproduction—to avoid begetting or bearing offspring and the rearing demands they make. Procreative liberty in this sense could involve several different choices, because decisions to avoid procreation arise at several different stages. A decision not to procreate could occur prior to conception through sexual abstinence, contraceptive use, or refusal to seek treatment for infertility. At this stage, the main issues concern freedom to refrain from sexual intercourse, the freedom to use contraceptives, and the freedom to withhold gametes for use in noncoital conception. Countervailing interests concern societal interests in increasing population, a partner's interest in sexual intimacy and progeny, and moral views about the unity of sex and reproduction.

Once pregnancy has occurred, reproduction can be avoided only by termination of pregnancy. Procreative freedom here would involve the freedom to abort the pregnancy. Competing interests are protection of embryos and fetuses and respect for human life generally, the most heated issue of reproductive rights. They may also include moral or social beliefs about the connectedness of sex and reproduction, or views about a woman's reproductive and work roles.

Once a child is born, procreation has occurred, and the procreators ordinarily have parenting obligations. Freeing oneself from rearing obligations is not strictly speaking a matter of procreative liberty, though it is an important personal interest. Even if parents relinquish the child for adoption, the psychological reality that one has reproduced remains. Opposing interests at this stage involve the need to provide parenting, nurturing, and financial support to offspring. The right to be free of those obligations, as well as the right to assume them after birth occurs, is not directly addressed in this book except to the extent that those rights affect reproductive decisions.

TECHNOLOGY AND THE AVOIDANCE OF REPRODUCTION

Many reproductive technologies raise questions about the scope of the liberty interest in avoiding reproduction. New contraceptive, contragestive, and abortion technologies raise avoidance issues directly, though the issues raised are not always novel. For example, an important issue in voluntary use of long-lasting contraceptives concerns access by minors and the poor, an issue of justice in the distribution of medical resources that currently exists with other contraceptives. The more publicized issue of whether the state may require child abusers or women on welfare to use Norplant implicates the target group's right to procreate, not their liberty interest in avoiding reproduction.

Contragestive agents such as RU486, which prevent reproduction after conception has occurred, raise many of the current issues of the abortion debate. Because RU486 operates so early in pregnancy, however, it focuses attention on the moral status of very early abortions and the moral differences, if any, between postcoital contraceptives and abortifacients. Ethical assessment and legal rights to use contragestives will depend on the ethical and legal status of early prenatal stages of human life.

More novel avoidance issues will arise with IVF and embryo cryopreservation technology. IVF often produces more embryos than can be safely implanted in the uterus. If couples must donate rather than discard unwanted embryos, they will become biologic parents against their will. This prospect raises the question of whether the liberty interest in avoiding reproduction includes avoiding genetic offspring when no rearing obligations will attach—reproduction *tout court*. Is one's fundamental interest in avoiding reproduction seriously implicated if one will never know or have contact with one's offspring? The resulting moral and policy issue is how to balance the interest in avoiding genetic offspring *tout court* with respect for preimplantation stages of human life.

Technologies of quality control and selection through genetic screening and manipulation will also raise novel questions about the right to avoid reproduction. Prenatal screening enables couples to avoid reproduction because of the genetic characteristics of expected offspring. Are the interests that support protecting the freedom to avoid reproduction present when that freedom is exercised selectively? Because some reasons for rejecting fetuses are more appealing than others, would devising criteria for such choices violate the right not to procreate? For example, should law or morality permit abortion of a fetus with Tay-Sachs disease or Down's syndrome but not female fetuses or fetuses with a disease of varying expressivity such as cystic fibrosis?

LEGAL STATUS OF AVOIDING REPRODUCTION

Legally, the negative freedom to avoid reproduction is widely recognized, though great controversy over abortion persists, and there is no positive constitutional right to contraception and abortion. The freedom to avoid reproduction is clearest for men and women prior to conception. In the United States and most developed countries, marriage and sexual intercourse are a matter of choice. However, rape laws do not always effectively protect women, and some jurisdictions do not criminalize marital rape. Legal access to contraception and sterilization is firmly established, though controversy exists over providing contraception to adolescents because of fears that it would encourage nonmarital sexual intercourse.

Constitutional recognition of the right to use contraceptives—to have sex and not reproduce—occurred in the 1965 landmark case of *Griswold* v. *Connecticut*. The executive director of Planned Parenthood and its medical director, a licensed physician, challenged a Connecticut law that made it a crime to use or distribute contraceptives. The United States Supreme Court found that the law violated a fundamental liberty right of married couples, which it later extended to unmarried persons, to use contraceptives as a matter of personal liberty or privacy. Although the Court alluded to the unsavory prospect of police searching the marital bedroom for evidence of the crime as a reason for invalidating the law, it is clear that the Court was protecting the right of persons who engage in sexual intimacy to avoid unwanted reproduction. The right to avoid reproduction through contraception is thus firmly protected, even where fornication laws remain in effect.

Legal protection also exists for other activities tied to avoiding reproduction prior to pregnancy. Thus both men and women are deemed owners of gametes within or outside their bodies, so that they may prevent them from being used for reproduction without their permission. Men and women also have rights to prevent extracorporeal embryos formed from their gametes from being placed in women and brought to term without their consent.

Once conception has occurred, the right to avoid reproduction differs for the woman and man involved. In the United States and most of Western Europe, abortion in early stages of the pregnancy is widely permitted. Under *Roe* v. *Wade,* whose central holding was reaffirmed in 1992 in *Planned Parenthood* v. *Casey,* women, whether single or married, adult or minor, have a right to terminate pregnancy up to viability. However, the state may inform them of its views concerning the worth of the fetus and require them to wait 24 hours before obtaining an abortion. Parental consent or notification requirements can be imposed

on minors, as long as a judicial bypass is provided in cases in which the minor does not wish to inform her parents. Also, because the right to abortion is a negative right, the state has no obligation to fund abortions for indigent women.

Although pregnancy termination usually kills the fetus, the right to end pregnancy does not protect the right to cause the death of a fetus that has emerged alive from the abortion process, or even to choose a method of abortion that is most likely to cause fetal demise. Nor does it give a woman the right to engage in prenatal conduct that poses unreasonable risks to the health of future offspring when she is choosing to go to term. After birth occurs, the mother and father have obligations to the child until custody is formally relinquished or transferred to others.

The father, once conception through sexual intercourse has occurred, has no right to require or prevent abortion, and cannot avoid rearing duties of financial support once birth occurs. This is true even if the woman has lied to him about her fertility or her use of contraceptives. However, he is free to relinquish custody and give up for adoption. He is also free to determine whether IVF embryos formed from his sperm should be implanted in the uterus.

The law's recognition of a right to avoid reproduction both prior to and after conception provides the legal framework for resolving conflicts presented by new reproductive technologies that affect interests in avoiding reproduction. While many technologies raise the same issues confronted in *Griswold* and *Roe,* new twists will arise that directly challenge the scope of that right. To resolve those conflicts, the separate elements that comprise the interest in avoiding reproduction must be analyzed and evaluated against the competing interests affected by those technologies.

THE FREEDOM TO PROCREATE

In addition to freedom to avoid procreation, procreative liberty also includes the freedom to procreate—the freedom to beget and bear children if one chooses. As with avoiding reproduction, the right to reproduce is a negative right against public or private interference, not a positive right to the services or the resources needed to reproduce.

It is an important freedom that is widely accepted as a basic, human right. But its various components and dimensions have never been fully analyzed, as technologies of conception and selection now force us to do.

As with avoiding reproduction, the freedom to procreate involves the freedom to engage in a series of actions that eventuate in reproduction and usually in child rearing. One must be free to marry or find a willing partner, engage in sexual intercourse, achieve conception and pregnancy, carry a pregnancy to term, and rear offspring. Social and natural barriers to reproduction would involve the unavailability of willing or suitable partners, impotence or infertility, and lack of medical and child-care resources. State barriers to marriage, to sexual intercourse, to conception, to infertility treatment, to carrying pregnancies to term, and to certain child-rearing arrangements would also limit the freedom to procreate. The most commonly asserted reasons for limiting coital reproduction are overpopulation, unfitness of parents, harm to offspring, and costs to the state or others. Technologies that treat infertility raise additional concerns that are discussed below.

The moral right to reproduce is respected because of the centrality of reproduction to personal identity, meaning, and dignity. This importance makes the liberty to procreate an important moral right, both for an ethic of individual autonomy and for ethics of community or family that view the purpose of marriage and sexual union as the reproduction and rearing of offspring. Because of this importance, the right to reproduce is widely recognized as a prima facie moral right that cannot be limited except for very good reason.

Recognition of the primacy of procreation does not mean that all reproduction is morally blameless, much less that reproduction is always responsible and praiseworthy and can never be limited. However, the presumptive primacy of procreative liberty sets a very high standard for limiting those rights, tilting the balance in favor of reproducing but not totally determining its acceptability. A two-step process of analysis is envisaged here. The first question is whether a distinctively procreative interest is involved. If so, the question then is whether the harm threatened by reproduction satisfies the strict standard for overriding this liberty interest.

The personal importance of procreation helps answer questions about who holds procreative rights and about the circumstances under which the right to reproduce may be limited. A person's capacity to find significance in reproduction should determine whether one holds the presumptive right, though this question is often discussed in terms of whether persons with such a capacity are fit parents. To have a liberty interest in procreating, one should at a minimum have the mental capacity to understand or appreciate the meanings associated with reproduction. This minimum would exclude severely retarded persons from having reproductive interests, though it would not remove their right to bodily integrity. However, being unmarried, homosexual, physically disabled, infected with HIV, or imprisoned would not disqualify one from having reproductive interests, though they might affect one's ability to rear offspring. Whether those characteristics justify limitations on reproduction is discussed later. Nor would already having reproduced negate a person's interest in reproducing again, though at a certain point the marginal value to a person of additional offspring diminishes.

What kinds of interests or harms make reproduction unduly selfish or irresponsible and thus could justifiably limit the presumptive right to procreate? To answer this question, we must distinguish coital and noncoital reproduction. Surprisingly, there is a widespread reluctance to speak of coital reproduction as irresponsible, much less to urge public action to prevent irresponsible coital reproduction from occurring. If such a conversation did occur, reasons for limiting coital reproduction would involve the heavy costs that it imposed on others—costs that outweighed whatever personal meaning or satisfaction the person(s) reproducing experienced. With coital reproduction, such costs might arise if there were severe overpopulation, if the persons reproducing were unfit parents, if reproduction would harm offspring, or if significant medical or social costs were imposed on others.

Because the United States does not face the severe overpopulation of some countries, the main grounds for claiming that reproduction is irresponsible is where the person(s) reproducing lack the financial means to raise offspring or will otherwise harm their children. As later discussions will show, both grounds are seriously inadequate as justifications for interfering with procreative choice. Imposing rearing costs on others may not rise to the level of harm that justifies depriving a person of a fundamental moral right. Moreover, protection of offspring from unfit parenting requires that unfit parents not rear, not that they not reproduce. Offspring could be protected by having others rear them without interfering with parental reproduction.

A further problem, if coital reproduction were found to be unjustified, concerns what action should then be taken. Exhortation or moral condemnation might be acceptable, but more stringent or coercive measures would act on the body of the person deemed irresponsible. Past experience with forced sterilization of retarded persons and the inevitable focus on the poor and minorities as targets of coercive policies make such proposals highly unappealing. Because of these doubts, there have been surprisingly few attempts to restrict coital reproduction in the United States since the era of eugenic sterilization, even though some instances of reproduction—for example, teenage pregnancy, inability to care for offspring—appear to be socially irresponsible.

An entirely different set of concerns arises with noncoital reproductive techniques. Charges that noncoital reproduction is unethical or irresponsible arise because of its expense, its highly technological character, its decomposition of parenthood into genetic, gestational, and social components, and its potential effects on women and offspring. To assess whether these effects justify moral condemnation or public limitation, we must first determine whether noncoital reproduction implicates important aspects of procreative liberty.

THE RIGHT TO REPRODUCE AND NONCOITAL TECHNOLOGY

If the moral right to reproduce presumptively protects coital reproduction, then it should protect noncoital reproduction as well. The moral right of the coitally infertile to reproduce is based on the same desire for offspring that the coitally fertile have. They too wish to replicate themselves, transmit genes, gestate, and rear children biologically related to them. Their infertility should no more disqualify them from reproductive experiences

than physical disability should disqualify persons from walking with mechanical assistance. The unique risks posed by noncoital reproduction may provide independent justifications for limiting its use, but neither the noncoital nature of the means used nor the infertility of their beneficiaries means that the presumptively protected moral interest in reproduction is not present.

A major question about this position, however, is whether the noncoital or collaborative nature of the means used truly implicates reproductive interests. For example, what if only one aspect of reproduction—genetic transfer, gestation, or rearing—occurs, as happens with gamete donors or surrogates who play no rearing role? Is a person's procreative liberty substantially implicated in such partial reproductive roles? The answer will depend on the value attributed to the particular collaborative contribution and on whether the collaborative enterprise is viewed from the donor's or recipient's perspective.

Gamete donors and surrogates are clearly reproducing even though they have no intention to rear. Because reproduction *tout court* may seem less important than reproduction with intent to rear, the donor's reproductive interest may appear less important. However, more experience with these practices is needed to determine the inherent value of "partial" reproductive experiences to donors and surrogates. Experience may show that it is independently meaningful, regardless of their contact with offspring. If not, then countervailing interests would more easily override their right to enter these roles.

Viewed from the recipient's perspective, however, the donor or surrogate's reproduction *tout court* does not lessen the reproductive importance of her contribution. A woman who receives an egg or embryo donation has no genetic connection with offspring but has a gestational relation of great personal significance. In addition, gamete donors and surrogates enable one or both rearing partners to have a biological relation with offspring. If one of them has no biological connection at all, they will still have a strong interest in rearing their partner's biologic offspring. Whether viewed singly through the eyes of the partner who is reproducing, or jointly as an endeavor of a couple seeking to rear children who are biologically related to at least one of the two, a significant reproductive interest is at stake. If so, noncoital, collaborative treatments for infertility should be respected to the same extent as coital reproduction is.

Questions about the core meaning of reproduction will also arise in the temporal dislocations that cryopreservation of sperm and embryos make possible. For example, embryo freezing allows siblings to be conceived at the same time, but born years apart and to different gestational mothers. Twins could be created by splitting one embryo into two. If one half is frozen for later use, identical twins could be born at widely different times. Sperm, egg, and embryo freezing also make posthumous reproduction possible.

Such temporally dislocative practices clearly implicate core reproductive interests when the ultimate recipient has no alternative means of reproduction. However, if the procreative interests of the recipient couple are not directly implicated, we must ask whether those whose gametes are used have an independent procreative interest, as might occur if they directed that gametes or embryos be thawed after their death for purposes of posthumous reproduction. In that case the question is whether the expectancy of posthumous reproduction is so central to an individual's procreative identity or life-plan that it should receive the same respect that one's reproduction when alive receives. The answer to such a question will be important in devising policy for storing and posthumously disposing of gametes and embryos. The answer will also affect inheritance questions and have implications for management of pregnant women who are irreversibly comatose or brain dead.

The problem of determining whether technology implicates a major reproductive interest also arises with technologies that select offspring characteristics. Some degree of quality control would seem logically to fall within the realm of procreative liberty. For many couples the decision whether to procreate depends on the ability to have healthy children. Without some guarantee or protection against the risk of handicapped children, they might not reproduce at all.

Thus viewed, quality control devices become part of the liberty interest in procreating or in avoiding procreation, and arguably should receive the same degree of protection. If so, genetic screening and selective abortion, as well as the right to select a mate or a source for donated eggs, sperm, or embryos should be protected as part of procreative liberty. The same arguments would apply to positive interventions to cure disease at the fetal or embryo stage. However, futuristic practices such as non-therapeutic enhancement, cloning, or intentional diminishment of offspring characteristics may so deviate from the core interests that make reproduction meaningful as to fall outside the protective canopy of procreative liberty.

Finally, technology will present questions of whether one may use one's reproductive capacity to produce gametes, embryos, and fetuses for nonreproductive uses in research or therapy. Here the purpose is not to have children to rear, but to get material for research or transplant. Are such uses of reproductive capacity tied closely enough to the values and interests that underlie procreative freedom to warrant similar respect? Even if procreative choice is not directly involved, other liberties may protect the activity.

ARE NONCOITAL TECHNOLOGIES UNETHICAL?

If this analysis is accepted, then procreative liberty would include the right to use noncoital and other technologies to form a family and shape the characteristics of offspring. Neither infertility nor the fact that one will only partially reproduce eliminates the existence of a prima facie reproductive experience for someone. However, judgments about the proximity of these partial reproductive experiences to the core meanings of reproduction will be required in balancing those claims against competing moral concerns.

Judgment about the reproductive importance of noncoital technologies is crucial because many people have serious ethical reservations about them, and are more than willing to restrict their use. The concerns here are not the fears of overpopulation, parental unfitness, and societal costs that arise with allegedly irresponsible coital reproduction. Instead, they include reduction of demand for hard-to-adopt children, the coercive or exploitive bargains that will be offered to poor women, the commodification of both children and reproductive collaborators, the objectification of women as reproductive vessels, and the undermining of the nuclear family.

However, often the harms feared are deontological in character. In some cases they stem from a religious or moral conception of the unity of sex and reproduction or the definition of family. Such a view characterizes the Vatican's strong opposition to IVF, donor sperm, and other noncoital and collaborative techniques. Other deontological concerns derive from a particular conception of the proper reproductive role of women. Many persons, for example, oppose paid surrogate motherhood because of a judgment about the wrongness of a woman's willingness to sever the mother-child bond for the sake of money. They also insist that the gestational mother is always morally entitled to rear, despite her preconception promise to the contrary. Closely related are dignitary objections to allowing any reproductive factors to be purchased, or to having offspring selected on the basis of their genes.

Finally, there is a broader concern that noncoital reproduction will undermine the deeper community interest in having a clear social framework to define boundaries of families, sexuality, and reproduction. The traditional family provides a container for the narcissism and irrationality that often drives human reproduction. This container assures commitments to the identifications and taboos that protect children from various types of abuse. The technical ability to disaggregate and recombine genetic, gestational, and rearing connections and to control the genes of offspring may thus undermine essential protections for offspring, couples, families, and society.

These criticisms are powerful ones that explain much of the ambivalence that surrounds the use of certain reproductive technologies. They call into question the wisdom of individual decisions to use them, and the willingness of society to promote or facilitate their use. Unless one is operating out of a specific religious or deontological ethic, however, they do not show that all individual uses of these techniques are immoral, much less that public policy should restrict or discourage their use.

These criticisms seldom meet the high standard necessary to limit procreative choice. Many of them are mere hypothetical or speculative possibilities. Others reflect moralisms concerning a "right" view of reproduction, which individuals in a pluralistic society hold or reject to varying degrees. In any event, without a clear showing of substantial harm to the tangible interests of others, speculation or mere moral objections alone should not override the moral right of infertile couples to use those techniques to form families. Given the primacy of procreative liberty, the use of these techniques should be accorded the same high protection granted to coital reproduction.

RESOLVING DISPUTES OVER PROCREATIVE LIBERTY

As this brief survey shows, new reproductive technologies will generate ethical and legal disputes about the meaning and scope of procreative liberty. Because procreative liberty has never been fully elaborated, the importance of procreative choice in many novel settings will be a question of first impression. The ultimate decision reached will reflect the value assigned to the procreative interest at stake in light of the effects causing concern. In an important sense, the meaning of procreative liberty will be created or constituted for society in the process of resolving such disputes.

If procreative liberty is taken seriously, a strong presumption in favor of using technologies that centrally implicate reproductive interests should be recognized. Although procreative rights are not absolute, those who would limit procreative choice should have the burden of establishing substantial harm. This is the standard used in ethical and legal analyses of restrictions on traditional reproductive decisions. Because the same procreative goals are involved, the same standard of scrutiny should be used for assessing moral or governmental restrictions on novel reproductive techniques.

In arbitrating these disputes, one has to come to terms with the importance of procreative interests relative to other concerns. The precise procreative interest at stake must be identified and weighed against the core values of reproduction. As noted, this will raise novel and unique questions when the technology deviates from the model of two-person coital reproduction, or otherwise disaggregates or alters ordinary reproductive practices.

However, if an important reproductive interest exists, then use of the technology should be presumptively permitted. Only substantial harm to tangible interests of others should then justify restriction.

In determining whether such harm exists, it will be necessary to distinguish between harms to individuals and harms to personal conceptions of morality, right order, or offense, discounted by their probability of occurrence. As previously noted, many objections to reproductive technology rest on differing views of what "proper" or "right" reproduction is aside from tangible effects on others. For example, concerns about the decomposition of parenthood through the use of donors and surrogates, about the temporal alteration of conception, gestation and birth, about the alienation or commercialization of gestational capacity, and about selection and control of offspring characteristics do not directly affect persons so much as they affect notions of right behavior. Disputes over early abortion and discard or manipulation of IVF-created embryos also exemplify this distinction, if we grant that the embryo/previable fetus is not a person or entity with rights in itself.

At issue in these cases is the symbolic or constitutive meaning of actions regarding prenatal life, family, maternal gestation, and respect for persons over which people in a secular, pluralistic society often differ. A majoritarian view of "right" reproduction or "right" valuation of prenatal life, family, or the role of women should not suffice to restrict actions based on differing individual views of such preeminently personal issues. At a certain point, however, a practice such as cloning, enhancement, or intentional diminishment of offspring may be so far removed from even pluralistic notions of reproductive meaning that they leave the realm of protected reproductive choice. People may differ over where that point is, but it will not easily exclude most reproductive technologies of current interest.

To take procreative liberty seriously, then, is to allow it to have presumptive priority in an individual's life. This will give persons directly involved the final say about use of a particular technology, unless tangible harm to the interests of others can be shown. Of course, people may differ over whether an important procreative interest is at stake or over how serious the harm posed from use of the reproductive technology is. Such a focused debate, however, is legitimate and ultimately essential in developing ethical standards and public policy for use of new reproductive technologies.

THE LIMITS OF PROCREATIVE LIBERTY

The emphasis on procreative liberty that informs this book provides a useful but by no means complete or final perspective on the technologies in question. Theological, social, psychological, economic, and feminist perspectives would emphasize different aspects of reproductive technology, and might be much less sanguine about potential benefits and risks. Such perspectives might also offer better guidance in how to use these technologies to protect offspring, respect women, and maintain other important values.

A strong rights perspective has other limitations as well. Recognition of procreative liberty, whether in traditional or in new technological settings, does not guarantee that people will achieve their reproductive goals, much less that they will be happy with what they do achieve. Nature may be recalcitrant to the latest technology. Individuals may lack the will, the perseverance, or the resources to use effective technologies. Even if they do succeed, the results may be less satisfying than envisaged. In addition, many individual instances of procreative choice may cumulate into larger social changes that from our current vantage point seem highly undesirable. But these are the hazards and limitations of any scheme of individual rights.

Recognition of procreative liberty will protect the right of persons to use technology in pursuing their reproductive goals, but it will not eliminate the ambivalence that such technologies engender. Societal ambivalence about reproductive technology is recapitulated at the individual level, as individuals and couples struggle with whether to use the technologies in question. Thus recognition of procreative liberty will not eliminate the dilemmas of personal choice and responsibility that reproductive choice entails. The freedom to act does not mean that we will act wisely, yet denying that freedom may be even more unwise, for it denies individuals' respect in the most fundamental choices of their lives.

NOTES

1. Whether labeled reproductive or not, gestation is a central experience for women and should enjoy the special respect or protected status accorded reproductive activities. On this view, a woman who receives an embryo donation or who serves as a gestational surrogate is having a reproductive experience, whether or not she also rears.

2. Sonnet 12 ("When I do count the clock that tells the time/And see the brave day sunk in hideous night"). Sonnet 2 ("When forty winters shall besiege thy brow/And dig deep trenches in thy beauty's field") also sings the praises of reproduction as an answer to death and old age.
3. Margaret Atwood, *The Handmaid's Tale* (Boston: Houghton Mifflin, 1986).

Instruction on Respect for Human Life in Its Origin and on the Dignity of Procreation

Vatican, Congregation for the Doctrine of the Faith

BIOMEDICAL RESEARCH AND THE TEACHING OF THE CHURCH

The gift of life which God the Creator and Father has entrusted to man calls him to appreciate the inestimable value of what he has been given and to take responsibility for it: This fundamental principle must be placed at the center of one's reflection in order to clarify and solve the moral problems raised by artificial interventions on life as it originates and on the processes of procreation.

Thanks to the progress of the biological and medical sciences, man has at his disposal ever more effective therapeutic resources; but he can also acquire new powers, with unforeseeable consequences, over human life at its very beginning and in its first stages. Various procedures now make it possible to intervene not only in order to assist, but also to dominate the processes of procreation. These techniques can enable man to "take in hand his own destiny," but they also expose him "to the temptation to go beyond the limits of a reasonable dominion over nature." They might constitute progress in the service of man, but they also involve serious risks. Many people are therefore expressing an urgent appeal

that in interventions on procreation the values and rights of the human person be safeguarded. Requests for clarification and guidance are coming not only from the faithful, but also from those who recognize the church as "an expert in humanity" with a mission to serve the "civilization of love" and of life.

The church's magisterium [asserts] . . . the criteria of moral judgment as regards the applications of scientific research and technology, especially in relation to human life and its beginnings . . . to be the respect, defense and promotion of man, his "primary and fundamental right" to life, his dignity as a person who is endowed with a spiritual soul and with moral responsibility and who is called to beatific communion with God. . . .

ANTHROPOLOGY AND PROCEDURES IN THE BIOMEDICAL FIELD

Which moral criteria must be applied in order to clarify the problems posed today in the field of biomedicine? The answer to this question presupposes a proper idea of the nature of the human person in his bodily dimension.

For it is only in keeping with his true nature that the human person can achieve self-realization as a "unified totality"; and this nature is at the same time corporal and spiritual. By virtue of its substantial union with a spiritual soul, the human body

---

Origins 16, No. 40, March 19, 1987. Abridged.
EDITORS' NOTE: The notes have been omitted; those wishing to follow up on sources should consult the original.

cannot be considered as a mere complex of tissues, organs and functions, nor can it be evaluated in the same way as the body of animals; rather, it is a constitutive part of the person who manifests and expresses himself through it.

The natural moral law expresses and lays down the purposes, rights and duties which are based upon the bodily and spiritual nature of the human person. Therefore this law cannot be thought of as simply a set of norms on the biological level; rather, it must be defined as the rational order whereby man is called by the Creator to direct and regulate his life and actions and in particular to make use of his own body.

A first consequence can be deduced from these principles: An intervention on the human body affects not only the tissues, the organs and their functions, but also involves the person himself on different levels. It involves, therefore, perhaps in an implicit but nonetheless real way, a moral significance and responsibility. . . .

Applied biology and medicine work together for the integral good of human life when they come to the aid of a person stricken by illness and infirmity and when they respect his or her dignity as a creature of God. No biologist or doctor can reasonably claim, by virtue of his scientific competence, to be able to decide on people's origin and destiny. This norm must be applied in a particular way in the field of sexuality and procreation, in which man and woman actualize the fundamental values of love and life.

God, who is love and life, has inscribed in man and woman the vocation to share in a special way in his mystery of personal communion and in his work as Creator and Father. For this reason marriage possesses specific goods and values in its union and in procreation which cannot be likened to those existing in lower forms of life. Such values and meanings are of the personal order and determine from the moral point of view the meaning and limits of artificial interventions on procreation and on the origin of human life. These interventions are not to be rejected on the grounds that they are artificial. As such, they bear witness to the possibilities of the art of medicine. But they must be given a moral evaluation in reference to the dignity of the human person, who is called to realize his vocation from God to the gift of love and the gift of life.

FUNDAMENTAL CRITERIA FOR A MORAL JUDGMENT

The fundamental values connected with the techniques of artificial human procreation are two: the life of the human being called into existence and the special nature of the transmission of human life in marriage. The moral judgment on such methods of artificial procreation must therefore be formulated in reference to these values.

Physical life, with which the course of human life in the world begins, certainly does not itself contain the whole of a person's value, nor does it represent the supreme good of man, who is called to eternal life. However it does constitute in a certain way the "fundamental" value of life precisely because upon this physical life all the other values of the person are based and developed. The inviolability of the innocent human being's right to life "from the moment of conception until death" is a sign and requirement of the very inviolability of the person to whom the Creator has given the gift of life.

By comparison with the transmission of other forms of life in the universe, the transmission of human life has a special character of its own, which derives from the special nature of the human person. "The transmission of human life is entrusted by nature to a personal and conscious act and as such is subject to the all-holy laws of God: immutable and inviolable laws which must be recognized and observed. For this reason one cannot use means and follow methods which could be licit in the transmission of the life of plants and animals."

Advances in technology have now made it possible to procreate apart from sexual relations through the meeting *in vitro* of the germ cells previously taken from the man and the woman. But what is technically possible is not for that very reason morally admissible. Rational reflection on the fundamental values of life and of human procreation is therefore indispensable for formulating a moral evaluation of such technological interventions on a human being from the first stages of his development. . . .

I. RESPECT FOR HUMAN EMBRYOS

What respect is due to the human embryo, taking into account his nature and identity?

The human being must be respected—as a person—from the very first instant of his existence. . . .

This congregation is aware of the current debates concerning the beginning of human life, concerning the individuality of the human being and concerning the identity of the human person. The congregation recalls the teachings found in the Declaration on Procured Abortion:

"From the time that the ovum is fertilized, a new life is begun which is neither that of the father nor of the mother; it is rather the life of a new human being with his own growth. It would never be made human if it were not human already. To this perpetual evidence . . . modern genetic science brings valuable confirmation. It has demonstrated that, from the first instant, the program is fixed as to what this living being will be: a man, this individual man with his characteristic aspects already well determined. Right from fertilization is begun the adventure of a human life, and each of its great capacities requires time . . . to find its place and to be in a position to act."

This teaching remains valid and is further confirmed, if confirmation were needed, by recent findings of human biological science which recognize that in the zygote (the cell produced when the nuclei of the two gametes have fused) resulting from fertilization the biological identity of a new human individual is already constituted.

Certainly no experimental datum can be in itself sufficient to bring us to the recognition of a spiritual soul; nevertheless, the conclusions of science regarding the human embryo provide a valuable indication for discerning by the use of reason a personal presence at the moment of this first appearance of a human life: How could a human individual not be a human person? The magisterium has not expressly committed itself to an affirmation of a philosophical nature, but it constantly reaffirms the moral condemnation of any kind of procured abortion. This teaching has not been changed and is unchangeable.

Thus the fruit of human generation from the first moment of its existence, that is to say, from the moment the zygote has formed, demands the unconditional respect that is morally due to the human being in his bodily and spiritual totality. The human being is to be respected and treated as a person from the moment of conception and therefore from that same moment his rights as a person must be recognized, among which in the first place is the inviolable right of every innocent human being to life.

This doctrinal reminder provides the fundamental criterion for the solution of the various problems posed by the development of the biomedical sciences in this field: Since the embryo must be treated as a person, it must also be defended in its integrity, tended and cared for, to the extent possible, in the same way as any other human being as far as medical assistance is concerned. . . .

How is one to evaluate morally research and experimentation on human embryos and fetuses?
Medical research must refrain from operations on live embryos, unless there is a moral certainty of not causing harm to the life or integrity of the unborn child and the mother, and on condition that the parents have given their free and informed consent to the procedure. It follows that all research, even when limited to the simple observation of the embryo, would become illicit were it to involve risk to the embryo's physical integrity or life by reason of the methods used or the effects induced.

As regards experimentation, and presupposing the general distinction between experimentation for purposes which are not directly therapeutic and experimentation which is clearly therapeutic for the subject himself, in the case in point one must also distinguish between experimentation carried out on embryos which are still alive and experimentation carried out on embryos which are dead. *If the embryos are living, whether viable or not, they must be respected just like any other human person; experimentation on embryos which is not directly therapeutic is illicit.*

No objective, even though noble in itself such as a foreseeable advantage to science, to other human beings or to society, can in any way justify experimentation on living human embryos or fetuses, whether viable or not, either inside or outside the mother's womb. The informed consent ordinarily required for clinical experimentation on adults cannot be granted by the parents, who may not freely dispose of the physical integrity or life of the unborn child. Moreover, experimentation on embryos and fetuses always involves risk, and indeed in most cases it involves the certain expectation of harm to their physical integrity or even their death.

To use human embryos or fetuses as the object or instrument of experimentation constitutes a crime against their dignity as human beings having a right to the same respect that is due to the child already born and to every human person. . . .

In the case of experimentation that is clearly therapeutic, namely, when it is a matter of experimental forms of therapy used for the benefit of the embryo itself in a final attempt to save its life and in the absence of other reliable forms of therapy, recourse to drugs or procedures not yet fully tested can be licit.

The corpses of human embryos and fetuses, whether they have been deliberately aborted or not, must be respected just as the remains of other human beings. In particular, they cannot be subjected to mutilation or to autopsies if their death has not yet been verified and without the consent of the parents or of the mother. Furthermore, the moral requirements must be safeguarded that there be no complicity in deliberate abortion and that the risk of scandal be avoided. Also, in the case of dead fetuses, as for the corpses of adult persons, all commercial trafficking must be considered illicit and should be prohibited.

How is one to evaluate morally the use for research purposes of embryos obtained by fertilization "in vitro?"
Human embryos obtained *in vitro* are human beings and subjects with rights: Their dignity and right to life must be respected from the first moment of their existence. *It is immoral to produce human embryos destined to be exploited as disposable "biological material."*

In the usual practice of *in vitro* fertilization, not all of the embryos are transferred to the woman's body; some are destroyed. Just as the church condemns induced abortion, so she also forbids acts against the life of these human beings. *It is a duty to condemn the particular gravity of the voluntary destruction of human embryos obtained "in vitro" for the sole purpose of research, either by means of artificial insemination or by means of "twin fission." By acting in this way the researcher usurps the place of God; and, even though he may be unaware of this, he sets himself up as the master of the destiny of others inasmuch as he arbitrarily chooses whom he will allow to live and whom he will send to death and kills defenseless human beings.*

Methods of observation or experimentation which damage or impose grave and disproportionate risks upon embryos obtained *in vitro* are morally illicit for the same reasons. Every human being is to be respected for himself and cannot be reduced in worth to a pure and simple instrument for the advantage of others. *It is therefore not in conformity with the moral law deliberately to expose to death human embryos obtained "in vitro."* In consequence of the fact that they have been produced *in vitro*, those embryos which are not transferred into the body of the mother and are called "spare" are exposed to an absurd fate, with no possibility of their being offered safe means of survival which can be licitly pursued.

What judgment should be made on other procedures of manipulating embryos connected with the "techniques of human reproduction?"
Techniques of fertilization *in vitro* can open the way to other forms of biological and genetic manipulation of human embryos, such as attempts or plans for fertilization between human and animal gametes and the gestation of human embryos in the uterus of animals, or the hypothesis or project of constructing artificial uteruses for the human embryo. *These procedures are contrary to the human dignity proper to the embryo, and at the same time they are contrary to the right of every person to be conceived and to be born within marriage and from marriage. Also, attempts or hypotheses for obtaining a human being without any connection with sexuality through "twin fission," cloning or parthenogenesis are to be considered contrary to the moral law, since they are in opposition to the dignity both of human procreation and of the conjugal union.*

The freezing of embryos, even when carried out in order to preserve the life of an embryo—cryopreservation—*constitutes an offense against the respect due to human beings* by exposing them to grave risks of death or harm to their physical integrity and depriving them, at least temporarily, of maternal shelter and gestation, thus placing them in a situation in which further offenses and manipulation are possible.

Certain attempts to influence chromosomic or genetic inheritance are not therapeutic, but are aimed at producing human beings selected according to sex or other predetermined qualities. These manipulations are contrary to the personal dignity of the human being and his or her integrity and identity. . . .

II. INTERVENTIONS UPON HUMAN PROCREATION

. . . A preliminary point for the moral evaluation of [*in vitro* fertilization and artificial insemination] is constituted by the consideration of the circumstances and consequences which those procedures involve in relation to the respect due the human embryo. Development of the practice of *in vitro* fertilization has required innumerable fertilizations and destructions of human embryos. Even today, the usual practice presupposes a hyperovulation on the part of the woman: A number of ova are withdrawn, fertilized and then cultivated *in vitro* for some days. Usually not all are transferred into the genital tracts of the woman; some embryos, generally called "spare," are destroyed or frozen. On occasion, some of the implanted embryos are sacrificed for various eugenic, economic or psychological reasons. Such deliberate destruction of human beings or their utilization for different purposes to the detriment of their integrity and life is contrary to the doctrine on procured abortion already recalled.

The connection between *in vitro* fertilization and the voluntary destruction of human embryos occurs too often. This is significant: Through these procedures, with apparently contrary purposes, life and death are subjected to the decision of man, who thus sets himself up as the giver of life and death by decree. This dynamic of violence and domination may remain unnoticed by those very individuals who, in wishing to utilize this procedure, become subject to it themselves. The facts recorded and the cold logic which links them must be taken into consideration for a moral judgment on *in vitro* fertilization and embryo transfer: The abortion mentality which has made this procedure possible thus leads, whether one wants it or not, to man's domination over the life and death of his fellow human beings and can lead to a system of radical eugenics. . . .

A.   Heterologous* artificial fertilization
Why must human procreation take place in marriage?
Every human being is always to be accepted as a gift and blessing of God. However, from the moral point of

*[Heterologous: involving sperm and egg from a man and woman who are not married to each other.]

view a truly responsible procreation vis-a-vis the unborn child must be the fruit of marriage.

For human procreation has specific characteristics by virtue of the personal dignity of the parents and of the children: The procreation of a new person, whereby the man and the woman collaborate with the power of the Creator, must be the fruit and the sign of the mutual self-giving of the spouses, of their love and of their fidelity. *The fidelity of the spouses in the unity of marriage involves reciprocal respect of their right to become a father and a mother only through each other.*

The child has the right to be conceived, carried in the womb, brought into the world and brought up within marriage: It is through the secure and recognized relationship to his own parents that the child can discover his own identity and achieve his own proper human development.

The parents find in their child a confirmation and completion of their reciprocal self-giving: The child is the living image of their love, the permanent sign of their conjugal union, the living and indissoluble concrete expression of their paternity and maternity.

By reason of the vocation and social responsibilities of the person, the good of the children and of the parents contributes to the good of civil society; the vitality and stability of society require that children come into the world within a family and that the family be firmly based on marriage.

The tradition of the church and anthropological reflection recognize in marriage and in its indissoluble unity the only setting worthy of truly responsible procreation.

Does heterologous artificial fertilization conform to the dignity of the couple and to the truth of marriage?
Through *in vitro* fertilization and embryo transfer and heterologous artificial insemination, human conception is achieved through the fusion of gametes of at least one donor other than the spouses who are united in marriage. *Heterologous artificial fertilization is contrary to the unity of marriage, to the dignity of the spouses, to the vocation proper to parents, and to the child's right to be conceived and brought into the world in marriage and from marriage.*

Respect for the unity of marriage and for conjugal fidelity demands that the child be conceived in marriage; the bond existing between husband and wife accords the spouses, in an objective and inalienable manner, the exclusive right to become father and mother solely through each other. Recourse to the gametes of a third person in order to have sperm or ovum available constitutes a violation of the reciprocal commitment of the spouses and a grave lack in regard to that essential property of marriage which is its unity.

Heterologous artificial fertilization violates the rights of the child; it deprives him of his filial relationship with his parental origins and can hinder the maturing of his personal identity. Furthermore, it offends the common vocation of the spouses who are called to fatherhood and motherhood: It objectively deprives conjugal fruitfulness of its unity and integrity; it brings about and manifests a rupture between genetic parenthood, gestational parenthood and responsibility for upbringing. Such damage to the personal relationships within the family has repercussions on civil society: What threatens the unity and stability of the family is a source of dissension, disorder and injustice in the whole of social life.

These reasons lead to a negative moral judgment concerning heterologous artificial fertilization: Consequently, fertilization of a married woman with the sperm of a donor different from her husband and fertilization with the husband's sperm of an ovum not coming from his wife are morally illicit. Furthermore, the artificial fertilization of a woman who is unmarried or a widow, whoever the donor may be, cannot be morally justified.

The desire to have a child and the love between spouses who long to obviate a sterility which cannot be overcome in any other way constitute understandable motivations; but subjectively good intentions do not render heterologous artificial fertilization conformable to the objective and inalienable properties of marriage or respectful of the rights of the child and of the spouses.

Is "surrogate" motherhood morally licit?
No, for the same reasons which lead one to reject heterologous artificial fertilization: For it is contrary to the unity of marriage and to the dignity of the procreation of the human person. . . .

B.   Homologous* artificial fertilization
Since heterologous artificial fertilization has been declared unacceptable, the question arises of how to evaluate morally the process of homologous artificial fertilization: *in vitro* fertilization and embryo transfer and artificial insemination between husband and wife. First a question of principle must be clarified.

What connection is required from the moral point of view between procreation and the conjugal act?
a) The church's teaching on marriage and human procreation affirms the "inseparable connection, willed by God and unable to be broken by man on his own initiative, between the two meanings of the conjugal act: the unitive meaning and the procreative meaning. Indeed, by its intimate structure the conjugal act, while most closely uniting husband and wife, capacitates them for the generation of new lives according to laws inscribed in the very being of man and of woman." . . . "By safeguarding both these essential aspects, the unitive and the procreative, the conjugal act preserves in its fullness the sense of true mutual love and its ordination toward man's exalted vocation to parenthood."

The same doctrine concerning the link between the meanings of the conjugal act and between the goods of marriage throws light on the moral problem of homologous artificial fertilization, since "it is never permitted to separate these different aspects to such a degree as positively to exclude either the procreative intention or the conjugal relation."

Contraception deliberately deprives the conjugal act of its openness to procreation and in this way brings about a voluntary dissociation of the ends of marriage. Homologous artificial fertilization, in seeking a procreation which is not the fruit of a specific act of conjugal union, objectively effects an analogous separation between the goods and the meanings of marriage.

Thus . . . *from the moral point of view procreation is deprived of its proper perfection when it is not desired as the fruit of the conjugal act, that is to say, of the specific act of the spouses' union.*

b) The moral value of the intimate link between the goods of marriage and between the meanings of the conjugal act is based upon the unity of the human being, a unity involving body and spiritual soul. Spouses mutually express their personal love in the "language of the body," which clearly involves both "spousal meanings" and parental

---

*[Homologous: involving sperm and egg from a man and woman who are married to each other.]

ones. The conjugal act by which the couple mutually express their self-gift at the same time expresses openness to the gift of life. It is an act that is inseparably corporal and spiritual. It is in their bodies and through their bodies that the spouses consummate their marriage and are able to become father and mother. In order to respect the language of their bodies and their natural generosity, the conjugal union must take place with respect for its openness to procreation; and the procreation of a person must be the fruit and the result of married love. The origin of the human being thus follows from a procreation that is "linked to the union, not only biological but also spiritual, of the parents, made one by the bond of marriage." Fertilization achieved outside the bodies of the couple remains by this very fact deprived of the meanings and the values which are expressed in the language of the body and in the union of human persons.

c) Only respect for the link between the meanings of the conjugal act and respect for the unity of the human being make possible procreation in conformity with the dignity of the person. In his unique and irrepeatable origin, the child must be respected and recognized as equal in personal dignity to those who give him life. The human person must be accepted in his parents' act of union and love; the generation of a child must therefore be the fruit of that mutual giving which is realized in the conjugal act wherein the spouses cooperate as servants and not as masters in the work of the Creator, who is love.

In reality, the origin of a human person is the result of an act of giving. The one conceived must be the fruit of his parents' love. He cannot be desired or conceived as the product of an intervention of medical or biological techniques; that would be equivalent to reducing him to an object of scientific technology. No one may subject the coming of a child into the world to conditions of technical efficiency which are to be evaluated according to standards of control and dominion.

The moral relevance of the link between the meanings of the conjugal act and between the goods of marriage, as well as the unity of the human being and the dignity of his origin, demand that the procreation of a human person be brought about as the fruit of the conjugal act specific to the love between spouses. . . .

Is homologous "in vitro" fertilization morally licit?

The answer to this question is strictly dependent on the principles just mentioned. Certainly one cannot ignore the legitimate aspirations of sterile couples. For some, recourse to homologous *in vitro* fertilization and embryo transfer appears to be the only way of fulfilling their sincere desire for a child. The question is asked whether the totality of conjugal life in such situations is not sufficient to ensure the dignity proper to human procreation. It is acknowledged that *in vitro* fertilization and embryo transfer certainly cannot supply for the absence of sexual relations and cannot be preferred to the specific acts of conjugal union, given the risks involved for the child and the difficulties of the procedure. But it is asked whether, when there is no other way of overcoming the sterility which is a source of suffering, homologous *in vitro* fertilization may not constitute an aid, if not a form of therapy, whereby its moral licitness could be admitted.

The desire for a child—or at the very least an openness to the transmission of life—is a necessary prerequisite from the moral point of view for responsible human procreation. But this good intention is not sufficient for making a positive moral evaluation of *in vitro* fertilization between spouses. The process of *in vitro* fertilization and embryo transfer must be judged in itself and cannot borrow its definitive moral quality from the totality of conjugal life of which it becomes part nor from the conjugal acts which may precede or follow it. . . .

[E]ven in a situation in which every precaution were taken to avoid the death of human embryos, homologous *in vitro* fertilization and embryo transfer dissociates from the conjugal act the actions which are directed to human fertilization. For this reason the very nature of homologous *in vitro* fertilization and embryo transfer also must be taken into account, even abstracting from the link with procured abortion.

Homologous *in vitro* fertilization and embryo transfer is brought about outside the bodies of the couple through actions of third parties whose competence and technical activity determine the success of the procedure. Such fertilization entrusts the life and identity of the embryo into the power of doctors and biologists and establishes the domination of technology over the origin and destiny of the human person. Such a relationship of domination is in itself contrary to the dignity and equality that must be common to parents and children.

Conception *in vitro* is the result of the technical action which presides over fertilization. *Such fertilization is neither in fact achieved nor positively willed as the expression and fruit of a specific act of the conjugal union. In homologous "in vitro " fertilization and embryo transfer, therefore, even if it is considered in the context of de facto existing sexual relations, the generation of the human person is objectively deprived of its proper perfection: namely, that of being the result and fruit of a conjugal act* in which the spouses can become "cooperators with God for giving life to a new person." . . .

Although the manner in which human conception is achieved with *in vitro* fertilization and embryo transfer cannot be approved, every child which comes into the world must in any case be accepted as a living gift of the divine Goodness and must be brought up with love.

How is homologous artificial insemination to be evaluated from the moral point of view?

Homologous artificial insemination within marriage cannot be admitted except for those cases in which the technical means is not a substitute for the conjugal act but serves to facilitate and to help so that the act attains its natural purpose. . . .

"In its natural structure, the conjugal act is a personal action, a simultaneous and immediate cooperation on the part of the husband and wife, which by the very nature of the agents and the proper nature of the act is the expression of the mutual gift which, according to the words of Scripture, brings about union 'in one flesh.'" Thus moral conscience "does not necessarily proscribe the use of certain artificial means destined solely either to the facilitating of the natural act or to ensuring that the natural act normally performed achieves its proper end." If the technical means facilitates the conjugal act or helps it to reach its natural objectives, it can be morally acceptable. If, on the other hand, the procedure were to replace the conjugal act, it is morally illicit.

Artificial insemination as a substitute for the conjugal act is prohibited by reason of the voluntarily achieved dissociation of the two meanings of the conjugal act. Masturbation, through which the sperm is normally obtained, is another sign of this dissociation: Even when it is done for the purpose of procreation the act remains deprived of its unitive meaning: "It lacks the sexual relationship called for by the moral order, namely the relationship which realizes 'the full sense of mutual self-giving and human procreation in the context of true love.'" . . .

What moral criterion can be proposed with regard to medical intervention in human procreation?

The medical act must be evaluated not only with reference to its technical dimension, but also and above all in relation to its goal, which is the good of persons and their bodily and psychological health. The moral criteria for medical intervention in procreation are deduced from the dignity of human persons, of their sexuality and of their origin.

Medicine which seeks to be ordered to the integral good of the person must respect the specifically human values of sexuality. The doctor is at the service of persons and of human procreation. He does not have the authority to dispose of them or to decide their fate. A medical intervention respects the dignity of persons when it seeks to assist the conjugal act either in order to facilitate its performance or in order to enable it to achieve its objective once it has been normally performed.

On the other hand, it sometimes happens that a medical procedure technologically replaces the conjugal act in order to obtain a procreation which is neither its result nor its fruit. In this case the medical act is not, as it should be, at the service of conjugal union, but rather appropriates to itself the procreative function and thus contradicts the dignity and the inalienable rights of the spouses and of the child to be born.

The humanization of medicine, which is insisted upon today by everyone, requires respect for the integral dignity of the human person first of all in the act and at the moment in which the spouses transmit life to a new person. It is only logical therefore to address an urgent appeal to Catholic doctors and scientists that they bear exemplary witness to the respect due to the human embryo and to the dignity of procreation. The medical and nursing staff of Catholic hospitals and clinics are in a special way urged to do justice to the moral obligations which they have assumed, frequently also, as part of their contract. Those who are in charge of Catholic hospitals and clinics and who are often religious will take special care to safeguard and promote a diligent observance of the moral norms recalled in the present instruction.

The suffering caused by infertility in marriage.

The suffering of spouses who cannot have children or who are afraid of bringing a handicapped child into the world is a suffering that everyone must understand and properly evaluate.

On the part of the spouses, the desire for a child is natural: It expresses the vocation to fatherhood and motherhood inscribed in conjugal love. This desire can be even stronger if the couple is affected by sterility which appears incurable. Nevertheless, marriage does not confer upon the spouses the right to have a child, but only the right to perform those natural acts which are per se ordered to procreation.

A true and proper right to a child would be contrary to the child's dignity and nature. The child is not an object to which one has a right nor can he be considered as an object of ownership: Rather, a child is a gift, "the supreme gift" and the most gratuitous gift of marriage, and is a living testimony of the mutual giving of his parents. For this reason, the child has the right as already mentioned, to be the fruit of the specific act of the conjugal love of his parents; and he also has the right to be respected as a person from the moment of his conception.

Nevertheless, whatever its cause or prognosis, sterility is certainly a difficult trial. The community of believers is called to shed light upon and support the suffering of those who are unable to fulfill their legitimate aspiration to motherhood and fatherhood. Spouses who find themselves in this sad situation are called to find in it an opportunity for sharing in a particular way in the Lord's cross, the source of spiritual fruitfulness. Sterile couples must not forget that "even when procreation is not possible, conjugal life does not for this reason lose its value. Physical sterility in fact can be for spouses the occasion for other important services to the life of the human person, for example, adoption, various forms of educational work and assistance to other families and to poor or handicapped children."...

III. MORAL AND CIVIL LAW

The Values and Moral Obligations That Civil Legislation Must Respect and Sanction in This Matter

The inviolable right to life of every innocent human individual and the rights of the family and of the institution of marriage constitute fundamental moral values because they concern the natural condition and integral vocation of the human person; at the same time they are constitutive elements of civil society and its order.

For this reason the new technological possibilities which have opened up in the field of biomedicine require the intervention of the political authorities and of the legislator, since an uncontrolled application of such techniques could lead to unforeseeable and damaging consequences for civil society. Recourse to the conscience of each individual and to the self-regulation of researchers cannot be sufficient for ensuring respect for personal rights and public order....

The intervention of the public authority must be inspired by the rational principles which regulate the relationships between civil law and moral law. The task of the civil law is to ensure the common good of people through the recognition of and the defense of fundamental rights and through the promotion of peace and of public morality....

As a consequence of the respect and protection which must be ensured for the unborn child from the moment of his conception, the law must provide appropriate penal sanctions for every deliberate violation of the child's rights. The law cannot tolerate—indeed it must expressly forbid—that human beings, even at the embryonic stage, should be treated as objects of experimentation, be mutilated or destroyed with the excuse that they are superfluous or incapable of developing normally.

The political authority is bound to guarantee to the institution of the family, upon which society is based, the juridical protection to which it has a right. From the very fact that it is at the service of people, the political authority must also be at the service of the family. Civil law cannot grant approval to techniques of artificial procreation which, for the benefit of third parties (doctors, biologists, economic or governmental powers), take away what is a right inherent in the relationship between spouses; and therefore civil law cannot legalize the donation of gametes between persons who are not legitimately united in marriage.

Legislation must also prohibit, by virtue of the support which is due to the family, embryo banks, post-mortem insemination and "surrogate motherhood." . . .

IVF and Women's Interests: An Analysis of Feminist Concerns

Mary Anne Warren

Thus far, little of the public and professional debate about the ethics of *in vitro* fertilization (IVF) and other new reproductive technologies (NRTs) has focused upon the possible negative effects of these technologies on women. There is endless discussion of the moral status of the fertilized ovum or pre-embryo, and its possible moral rights. Theologians and nonreligious critics debate the propriety of conceiving human beings "artificially," that is, without heterosexual intercourse. Concern is also voiced—and appropriately so—about the possible physical or mental effects of technologically assisted reproduction upon the resulting children. But with the exception of a small group of feminist critics, few have paid much attention to the dangers to the women who serve as experimental subjects in reproductive research and, indirectly, to all women.

In what follows, I will examine some of the feminist objections to IVF and other NRTs. I will argue that, although the NRTs pose some significant dangers for women, it would be wrong to conclude that women's interests demand an end to IVF and other reproductive research. But if we are to understand the ethics of IVF, we must ask not only whether it is in itself morally objectionable, but also whether it is (part of) an adequate societal response to the problem of involuntary infertility among women. IVF is at best a small part of a

solution to that problem; it can help only a small minority of infertile women, and does nothing to address the underlying social causes which contribute to the problem. Moreover, the publicity surrounding IVF and other NRTs may deflect attention and resources from the potentially more important tasks of understanding and counteracting the preventable causes of infertility.

1. FEMINIST CRITICISMS: THE MICROLEVEL

Feminist critiques of the NRTs operate in part on the microlevel, that is, the level of individual behavior, individual rights and wrongs; and in part on the macrolevel, the level of historical context and social implications. I will begin with the microlevel criticisms.

At the microlevel, the primary issue is whether IVF is sufficiently beneficial to IVF patients to justify the commercial marketing of the procedure, or even continued research and development. IVF is usually depicted as an astonishing success story: infertile women are enabled to have beautiful, healthy children. We hear far less about the associated dangers. We do not yet know the long-term side effects of the use of drugs and hormones to induce superovulation. The collection of ova through abdominal surgery, usually under general anaesthesia, carries a significant risk of mortality or morbidity. The replacement of the fertilized ovum in the uterus may cause infection, physical damage, or ectopic pregnancy. An abnormally high percentage of IVF pregnancies end in sponta-

Bioethics 2, No. 1, 1988, 37–57. Used with permission of Blackwell Publishers.

EDITORS' NOTE: Most notes have been omitted, and the remaining renumbered. Readers wishing to follow up sources should consult the original.

neous abortion or stillbirth. There are additional risks to mother and infant, associated not with the IVF procedure itself but with the ways in which IVF pregnancies are generally monitored (e.g., through ultrasound, amniocentesis, and endometrial biopsy), and with the exceptionally high rate of cesarean section which is typical of IVF births.

In addition to these physical risks, women who undergo IVF bear personal and psychological burdens. These include the emotional ups and downs inherent in the cycle of hope and disappointment; the disruption of work and, often, personal relationships; and the humiliation and depersonalization that may result from the submission to painful and embarrassing invasions of their bodies. When these costs are considered in conjunction with the fact that only a small minority of women who undergo IVF treatments will give birth to a viable infant, it is far from clear that IVF provides a net benefit to participating patients.

2. IVF AND INFORMED CONSENT

Whether or not the benefits of IVF treatment will outweigh its costs and risks to female patients depends in part upon just how severe these costs and risks turn out to be, and in part upon whether success rates can be improved in existing programs and high standards maintained in new ones. It also depends upon just how great a boon motherhood is to those women for whom IVF leads to a successful pregnancy. Those who regard motherhood as the greatest pleasure or achievement of which (some) women are capable will be prepared to tolerate greater risks and uncertainties than those who see motherhood—or, rather, the way it is institutionalized—as a significant burden.

In spite of these uncertainties—indeed, precisely because of them—it may be argued that women have the right to undertake the risks associated with IVF if *they* judge those risks to be worth taking. If women's right to reproductive autonomy means anything, it must mean that we are entitled to take some risks with our physical and psychological health, in the attempt to either have or not have children. Neither abortion nor many forms of contraception are entirely safe, but women sometimes reasonably judge that the alternatives are even less desirable. Having a wanted child can be

as important a goal as avoiding an unwanted birth. If the costs and dangers of IVF to individual women and children were so great that no informed and responsible person would attempt that route to parenthood, then perhaps the paternalistic protection of women through the prohibition of IVF would be appropriate. But if these costs and dangers are not, so far as we can now determine, so great as to *clearly* outweigh the possible benefits, then the matter is properly left to individual choice.

Of course, the right to the voluntary use of contraception, abortion, or the newer reproductive technologies is meaningless unless the requirements are met for informed and voluntary consent. Informed consent requires, among other things, an understanding of the medical and psychological risks, and the probability of success. There are troubling questions about whether all of the women who have been patients and experimental subjects in IVF programs have fully understood the risks to which they were being exposed and the often slight chances that they themselves would benefit from the research done. Debate continues about the adequacy of the counselling and information received by women in current IVF programs. However, many of these women are very well-informed, not only through counselling but through their own reading and investigation. For them, at least, participation in an IVF program would seem to be an exercise of the right to reproductive autonomy.

Some of the feminist critics of IVF accept this argument for reproductive autonomy, arguing only for the kinds of legal regulation and ethical supervision necessary to ensure that women's consent to IVF treatments is adequately informed and voluntary, and that necessary precautions are taken to make the procedure as safe as possible. Others, however, reject this argument as superficial. In their view, women cannot give truly voluntary consent to IVF treatments, regardless of how well-informed they may be about the risks, costs, and odds of success. They argue that women's reproductive "choices" are conditioned by the patriarchal power structure and the pronatalist ideology with which it is associated. Having children is still commonly regarded as a duty or a prerequisite for adult status, especially for women. This pronatalist ideology makes it difficult for women to make genuinely free choices about reproduction in general, or IVF in particular. Gena Corea says,

> The propaganda . . . that women are nothing unless they bear children, that if they are infertile, they lose their most basic identity as women . . . has a coercive power. It conditions a woman's choices as well as her *motivations* to choose. Her most heartfelt desire, the pregnancy for which she so desperately yearns, has been— to varying degrees—conditioned.[1]

There is surely some truth in this response. The "desperation of women who cannot meet the cultural definition of womanhood by becoming mothers"[2] is, to some extent, a cultural artifact. We hear far less about the plight of infertile men. There are, in all probability, infertile men who are equally "desperate" to have children; some even undergo painful surgical procedures (e.g., vasectomy reversal) in the pursuit of that goal. But we do not often see photographs in the newspaper of smiling fathers, proudly displaying infants that they have conceived with the help of such surgery.

It is true that female infertility is, in some respects, a more severe problem for a heterosexual couple than male infertility. Male infertility, though no easier to cure, is more easily circumvented: it is much easier for the couple to use AID (artificial insemination with donated sperm) than to obtain a donor egg or to "rent" another woman's womb, if the infertility is on the female side—and much less legally and morally problematic. Nevertheless, the apparently greater desperation of many infertile women, and the attention paid to that supposed desperation, probably also reflect the degree to which the perception of women's social worth is still tied to their function as childbearers.

The question is whether or not these points demonstrate that the opportunity to make their own choices about IVF and other NRTs is of no value to women. I think that they do not. Freedom is not an all-or-nothing affair. We can rarely be completely free of unjust or inappropriate social and economic pressures, but we can sometimes make sound and appropriate decisions, in the light of our own circumstances.

Neither the patriarchal power structure nor pronatalist ideology makes women incapable of reasoned choice about childbearing. Rather, the social pressures upon some women to have children—and the pressures upon others not to have children—are circumstances which we must take into account in our deliberations. Either having children or not having them can be socially (and financially) expensive. Motherhood is apt to interfere with other life goals to a degree that fatherhood usually does not. This is not so much because of female biology as because of the social expectation that mothers will also be the primary childrearers, and the shortage of adequate childcare facilities and flexible working arrangements which would enable women to combine parenting and paid working without heroic effort. Yet childlessness, especially when it is involuntary, can be a great and lasting grief. This is particularly true in a society like our own, in which most people who are not parents have little opportunity to have long-term nurturing relationships with children.

Women are not unaware of these social realities. In deliberating about either "natural" motherhood or the use of IVF, we may sometimes be wrong about what is in our own interests, and perhaps some of us are excessively influenced by pronatalist ideology. But it does not follow that we would benefit from additional paternalistic constraints. Autonomy necessarily implies the right to make our own mistakes.

Unfortunately, not all infertile women have the opportunity to make use of IVF. Some causes of infertility (e.g., some anatomical or hormonal abnormalities) cannot be circumvented by external fertilization. Worse, IVF—like AID—is often restricted, either by law or by medical practice, to married heterosexual women. It is often argued that this discrimination is pragmatically necessary, since making IVF available to all infertile women who can afford it might provoke so much conservative opposition that IVF programs would be eliminated altogether. It is nevertheless an injustice. Such discrimination could be justified only if there were some evidence that women who are single or lesbian are more likely to be inadequate parents than are married and heterosexual women; and there is no such evidence. It is also arguably unjust —and certainly unfortunate—that the high cost of IVF treatments effectively excludes many women. But denying IVF to all women, for paternalistic reasons, would also be an injustice. To be subject to inappropriate social pressures is not necessarily to be deprived of either judgment or will. We need to be suspicious of analyses which "deny our power and our ability to make choices, even within the constraints of patriarchy."[3]

Of course, the right of individuals to make their own choices must sometimes be constrained for the sake of the general welfare. If the advent of IVF and other NRTs can be proved detrimental to women or to society as a whole, then we shall have to regard women who serve as researchers or clinicians, patients or experimental subjects in IVF programs, as unwittingly working against women's larger interests. Their choices may be individually rational, but collectively harmful. Arguments to this effect are what I call macrolevel arguments.

3. THE MACROLEVEL CRITIQUE

Some feminist critics have sought to place the NRTs in their social and historical context, by looking at the history of iatrogenic harms to women caused by male-dominated medicine, and at the possible future abuses of reproductive technologies. Mary O'Brien and others have argued that men suffer from an envy of the larger role that women play in human procreation, and from their own natural inability to know with certainty which children are genetically their own. On this view, men have long sought to control women and women's reproductive processes, in order to assure themselves biological as well as social heirs. Patriarchal marriage, the sexual double standard, the confinement and legal disenfranchisement of women, the massacre of women healers and wise women during the witch-craze era, and the subsequent ascendancy of male-dominated obstetrics and gynecology, are all seen as part of this male project of control.

It would be difficult to deny that women have suffered from the male domination of medicine, not only in the loss of control over their own reproductive processes, but in iatrogenic illness and death. The entry of male physicians into obstetric practice in the seventeenth century led to a centuries-long plague of puerperal fever. Male physicians in the nineteenth century campaigned successfully for the prohibition of abortion and contra-

ception, and castrated thousands of women for supposed psychological problems. In this century, the DES, thalidomide, and Dalkon Shield disasters, the overuse of hysterectomy and other gynecological surgery, and the over-technologization of birth, all illustrate the same tendency to intervene in women's reproductive processes without good evidence of the safety and/or necessity of the intervention. Needless to say, modern obstetrics and gynecology have also produced some benefits for women. Many of the physical problems associated with pregnancy and birth can be more effectively treated than in the past. But we cannot know how much greater these benefits might have been had the medical profession not excluded women for many generations.

Given this history of iatrogenic harm to women, it is not surprising that many women regard the advent of IVF and other NRTs with suspicion. They fear that the new reproductive technologies will not only intensify male control of female reproductive processes, but may eventually remove women from the process of reproduction altogether. Irene Elia warns that,

> If men ever controlled parthenogenesis, using sperm nuclei placed in thawed or simulated egg cytoplasm and gestated in artificial or non-human wombs, they could enjoy total domination. With their gametes, they could produce either males or females—motherless all![4]

(There does, however, seem to be a biological problem here which Elia has overlooked: parthenogenesis using a sperm with a Y nucleus would produce a nonviable YY embryo; while the use of an X sperm would produce an XX—or female—offspring.)

Another cause for concern, not only among feminists, is that the NRTs are providing a means for the possible implementation of repressive eugenics programs. Many fear that the new methods for controlling the quality of our offspring, e.g., by embryo screening, prenatal diagnosis and selective abortion, or the use of donor gametes, will eventually become socially and/or legally mandatory. Corea asks, "Will those searching for perfect babies begin first by socially outlawing major . . . birth defects . . . and then . . . move on to ever lesser defects like asthma?"[5] Perhaps in the future women who try to reproduce without such eugenic interventions will be accused of child abuse, as are women today who give birth at home with the help of a midwife, rather than in a hospital setting.

4. THE SHAPE OF THE FUTURE

The dangers of male control of women's reproductive processes, and of the implementation of repressive eugenics programs, are real. There are, however, ways of resisting these dangers without calling for the termination of IVF and other reproductive research. None are simple, but all are morally essential for independent reasons.

Perhaps the most essential need is for more equal participation by women in all areas of medicine and biomedical research. It is difficult for any male-dominated profession either to understand women's needs or to serve them effectively. The new reproductive technologies should not be primarily in the hands of male physicians and researchers, but neither should any other form of medical treatment. It is equally essential that women (and men) from the various racial and ethnic groups and socioeconomic classes have a voice in determining the kinds of reproductive technologies that are developed and the ways in which they are used; for each of these groups may also be especially vulnerable to possible misuses of these technologies.

Many members of the medical professions would deny that the lesser participation of women in these fields is due to any remaining discrimination. The legal barriers to women's entry to medical studies and practice have been largely removed, and more or less nondiscriminatory criteria are increasingly used in the selection of medical students. But this is not enough. It would not even be enough if 50 percent of all medical *students* were women; for there are still powerful social and structural barriers to women's entry and success in such medical and scientific specialities as gynecology, obstetrics, embryology, neonatology, and endocrinology. These barriers include simple prejudice, as well as the excessively long hours required during the years of training and apprenticeship, and the difficulty of resuming that training after an extended break. All medical specializations need to be made more compatible with the needs of many women (and many men as well) for flexible working hours and interruptible career schedules. Otherwise, women in medicine will continue to be forced either to curtail their professional aspirations, or to forgo childbearing, or postpone it beyond the biologically optimal years.

Opening the medical and research professions to greater participation by women and other underrepresented groups is a long-term goal. In the meantime, it is essential that every government body with responsibility for the regulation of the NRTs, every ethical oversight committee, and every public agency which funds reproductive research be at least 50 percent composed of women. Among these, there should be some who have been on the receiving end of the new reproductive technologies—and some who have chosen not to be. An effort should also be made to include (proportionate numbers of) individuals from diverse racial, ethnic, and socioeconomic groups. This is probably the best immediate way of improving the likelihood that the interests of the consumers of reproductive technologies will be fairly represented in making of policy decisions.

But will this be enough to prevent the NRTs from being used coercively? Will women in the future be *required* to submit to IVF treatments, in order that their embryos may be screened for imperfections, genetically engineered, or replaced with embryos derived from "superior" individuals? This could happen only if our most basic civil liberties were lost. However, basic civil liberties, especially those affecting reproductive rights, are still far from adequate, and could easily be lost. In Australia, the legal status of abortion is still somewhat ambiguous. And in the United States, the right to legal abortion may stand or fall upon the confirmation or rejection by the Senate of a single Supreme Court nominee.

This fact provides reason for continued feminist struggle; but it does not provide support for the suppression of all reproductive technologies that can be used coercively. Women's reproductive autonomy cannot be secured through such suppression. The history of coercive population control programs, e.g., in India and China, amply demonstrates that even the older—but still most important—reproductive technologies of contraception and abortion can be coercively used. Yet it is also clear that the *suppression* of contraception and abortion could virtually ensure the reproductive enslavement of women, as it has in the past. Nor do coercive eugenics programs require new reproductive technologies. The Nazi genocides of World War II, which are often cited as grounds for rejecting new technologies that could be used to implement immoral eugenics programs, clearly demonstrate that innovative biotechnology is not essential for the commission of atrocities in the name of eugenics. For these reasons, the defense of basic civil rights seems to be a more promising way of preventing the implementation of immoral eugenics programs than the suppression of reproductive technologies.

More to be feared, perhaps, is the covertly coercive force of social expectation. New technologies often have a momentum of their own; once they exist, they are likely to be seen as pragmatically and morally superior to any less highly technological option, even when the reverse may be the case. Some feminists argue that the very existence of IVF as a treatment for female infertility increases the pressures on infertile women to keep on trying until they have exhausted every possible treatment for their infertility. The prevailing pronatalist ideology may thereby be strengthened, and the social stigma and suffering of all infertile women increased.

This is a realistic concern. The possibility of an IVF baby, however slight, may make it harder for infertile women to accept their condition and get on with their lives, or to defend the childlessness they may prefer. So too, the new methods for the prenatal diagnosis and selective abortion of defective fetuses may be eroding women's freedom *not* to try to control the quality of their children, but simply to accept them as they are. But this subtle erosion of freedom is not inevitable. Women can learn to exercise the legal right to refuse medical interventions that they do not need or want. We shall also have to work to retain that legal right, and to extend it in some areas. These are difficult tasks, but they are tasks that would be no less essential if there were no *new* reproductive technologies.

5. THE FINAL SOLUTION?

Perhaps the most alarming scenario suggested by some critics of the NRTs is that women may be altogether eliminated from the reproductive process. Once ectogenesis is perfected, natural pregnancy may come to be seen as dangerous and irresponsible; it may even be outlawed. Some speculate further, that once men have ectogenesis they will see no reason for women to exist at all, and consequently will create an all-male world.

But neither of these scenarios is likely to come about. Even if there were a realistic prospect for the achievement of total (i.e., conception-to-birth) ectogenesis in the nonremote future—which there is not—there would be little danger that ectogenesis will replace uterine gestation as the usual way of making babies. It will almost certainly be economically impossible to replace natural wombs with artificial ones. Extrauterine gestation, should it become possible, could hardly be much less expensive than contemporary neonatal intensive care. Thus, it would be beyond the reach of all but the very wealthy. This is an excellent reason for not devoting massive public resources to the attempt to develop methods of total ectogenesis. But it also shows that even if ectogenesis were perfected tomorrow, the elimination of natural pregnancy would remain a remote possibility.

It is still less likely that artificial gestation would threaten women's continued existence. Robyn Rowland asks, as man gets closer to reproducing himself, what forces can possibly stop him? . . . Will this last act of power make women obsolete; permanently unemployed; disposable?[6] Ectogenesis would likely lead to women's perceived obsolescence only if women were valued exclusively or primarily for our reproductive function. But that is clearly false, even in the most highly patriarchal societies. There are, no doubt, many men who agree in principle with Thomas Aquinas's dictum that women were created to help men in the work of reproduction, and *only* in that work "since [a] man can be more efficiently helped by another man in other works."[7] There is, and perhaps has always been, a strong current of misogyny in much male culture. Yet most men still regard heterosexual practices as preferable to the alternatives—and not just because of the reproductive function of these practices. More importantly, perhaps, women's paid and unpaid labor is essential to the functioning of virtually every social and economic institution throughout the world. Few men are willing to undertake the tasks of homemaking and childrearing without female assistance. If there has been a central patriarchal project, it has been to control women and channel their energies into the service of male needs—not to eliminate women, which would be self-defeating.

6. THE MYSTIQUE OF MOTHERHOOD

There is a deeper reason why some women are angered and alarmed by the NRTs. Some have argued the increased control of the female reproductive process which the NRTs give (certain) men will be detrimental to women's social status and sense of personal agency. These feminist critics maintain that women's procreativity has long been a source of social power, but that the NRTs are progressively robbing us of that power. Corea deplores the way that, "Woman, once deified as the life-creating Goddess, is now lying on a table with her mouth taped shut, having the eggs sucked out of her body."[8] Rowland says,

> How powerful we have always seemed; we who can bleed regularly and not die; we who can grow another human being inside our own bodies. Dubious though it has been in real terms, this has since "primitive" times been a source of mythical power for women when all else was kept from them. For many women it is the only experience of power they will ever have.[9]

Despite these eloquent pleas, I doubt that the NRTs are depriving women of any important source of social power which we now enjoy, or once enjoyed. The contrast between the hypothetical days when women were worshipped as the sole givers of life, and the new age in which some women need medical assistance in order to conceive, is probably less great than is sometimes supposed. Women may have sought supernatural or "professional" help in conceiving since prehistoric times. Neolithic images of fecund women predate the written word by tens of thousands of years. These images seem to express an awe of female procreativity; but they may have also had a practical use, e.g., as fertility charms. There is little reason to believe that early fertility magic was entirely in the hands of women—though it may have

been. In any case, the essential role of the male in conception has been known in most societies for at least several millennia. Thus, if the resort to male assistance inevitably undermines the awe of female fertility, then women in earlier times may have derived less social power from this source than is sometimes assumed.

There are other reasons for doubting the practical value of whatever mystical power may be ascribed to the female role in procreation. The power that supposedly flows from motherhood is often cited by apologists for patriarchy, as a reason why women have no need for other forms of power or even for personal autonomy. These apologists would have us believe that the hand that rocks the cradle rules the world—even if the hand's owner is deprived of the most basic civil liberties. But such "power" is a poor substitute for social, economic, and political equality. It may even make life worse for women. The suspicion of mystical or supernatural power, especially when associated with women, inspires not just respect, but fear and hostility. The women who were burned as witches at the dawn of the so-called age of reason had good reason to wish that they had not been credited with supernatural agency.

What feminists want, or should want, for women is not the largely symbolic power that comes from the awe of female procreativity, but respect for women as persons. Persons are due respect, not primarily because of the mystical powers that may act in or through them, but because of their capacity to think, feel, and act. The power to act effectively is achieved through the use of "our intellects, our imaginations, and our capacity for collective action."[10] The mystification of motherhood can do little to enhance that power. On the contrary, it would seem more apt to encourage the notion that women's "natural task . . . [is] accomplished by being rather than doing."[11] It may also reinforce the tendency to view women less as persons than as parts of "alien Nature," vessels of a force that is awesome but not entirely human. If the new reproductive technologies, by subjecting some female reproductive processes to apparently greater control, serve to undermine that mystification, then the appropriate feminist reaction may be, "So much the better."

7. THE SOCIAL CAUSES OF FEMALE INFERTILITY

I have saved for last what may be the most important feminist objection to IVF. It is an objection not to the continuation of IVF programs at some level of funding, but rather to the relative neglect of potentially more effective ways of approaching the problem.

Involuntary infertility has always been a problem for some women, and (though this was less often recognized) some men. Whether it currently affects a larger proportion of women than in previous generations is unclear, though many believe that it does. The causes of human infertility are not well understood, but neither are they entirely mysterious. A study of 708 couples attending fertility clinics in one part of England found that in 28 percent of cases the cause of the failure to conceive could not be identified, while in 26 percent, the problem was on the male side. The most common cause of female infertility was ovulatory failure, which apparently responded very well to treatment; the pregnancy rate after two years was approximately 96 percent. The next most common cause was infective damage to the fallopian tubes; here, the outlook was much poorer, with only about 19 percent conceiving after two years, despite surgery and other treatments. IVF was originally developed primarily for the treatment of this kind of female infertility, though it is now also used in some cases where the cause of the woman's infertility is unclear, or where the problem is due to some defect in the male's sperm.

For some infertile women or couples, for whom other treatments have failed, IVF probably offers the best remaining hope of biological parenthood—though it is often a rather slim hope. But it would obviously be better to prevent infertility in the first place, if this were possible. Much female infertility is socially caused, and probably could have been prevented. Prevention and cure are obviously not mutually exclusive approaches. But feminist critics have argued that the primary focus of the medical profession and the society as a whole has been too much on the treatment of infertility and too little on its prevention, and that the publicity given to IVF is symptomatic of this imbalance. In Heather Dietrich's words,

> IVF is valenced towards a medical, high-tech solution rather than the prevention of infertility. . . . It will emphasize and extend the isolation and analysis of fertility, as a discrete process, rather than [contributing to] a holistic approach to fertility within a woman's body and life.[12]

A more holistic approach to the problem of infertility would include an investigation of the social, as well as the physiological, causes of involuntary infertility. One group of social causes comprises a large range of sexual and contraceptive practices. As noted above, much female infertility is caused by infective damage to the fallopian tubes. Such infections are, in the majority of cases, sexually transmitted; and sexual practices and modes of contraception can affect the likelihood of contracting such sexually transmitted diseases (STDs).

Other things being equal, the more sexual partners a woman has, and the more partners each of them has had, the greater her risk of contracting an infection which will eventually damage her fertility. Thus, some might be tempted simply to blame the apparent increase in this form of female infertility on the so-called sexual revolution, which has meant that more women have become sexually active earlier, and have had, on the average, more sexual partners. But this would be a mistake. The sexual revolution need not have led to an increase in the incidence of STDs, or in consequent infertility. If it has, this is due in part to the kinds of contraceptives and prophylactics that have—or have not—been used. Some contraceptives are known to increase the danger of pelvic inflammatory disease (PID). IUDs, for instance, can cause acute or chronic inflammation, and are associated with a 600 percent increase in PID. Hormone-based contraceptives also appear, at least in some cases, to increase susceptibility to PID. In contrast, barrier methods, particularly condoms, and particularly when used in combination with spermicides, provide a fair degree of protection against most STDs—although they also tend to be somewhat less effective in preventing pregnancy. For maximum protection against both unwanted pregnancy and the transmission of infection, heterosexual couples who have not practiced long-term monogamy probably should use both condoms and some female contraceptive. But, for a variety of reasons, most do not.

The particular sexual activities in which people commonly engage may also increase the risk of infertility. Heterosexual intercourse, of the kind usually described as "normal" or "ordinary" is much more likely to transmit infection than either oral sex or masturbation (mutual or solitary). If the orientation of the majority of adults towards such "normal" sexual practice is an inalterable result of human biology, as most assume, then social mores can make little difference to this particular cause of infertility. But if, as some have argued, heterosexuality and the ways in which it is commonly expressed are social institutions rather than strictly natural phenomena, then some of these institutions must be included among the social causes of infertility.

There are many other social causes of infertility. Exposure to toxic substances, in the workplace and the general environment, is certainly involved in some cases. Among the poor, inadequate nutrition, generally poor health, and limited access to health care are often contributing factors. Where abortion is illegal or beyond the reach of many women, improperly performed abortions are a common cause of infertility—and often death. Poor women are sometimes surgically sterilized against their will, or without an understanding of the permanence of the procedure. Because their other options are likely to be more limited, poor women are also more likely to choose surgical sterilization, and some of them may later regret that decision. Unnecessary hysterectomies and other surgical procedures are another cause of involuntary infertility. In parts of Africa and the Middle East, the complications of genital mutilation ("female circumcision") undoubtedly cause much infertility.

While this is not a complete list of the social causes of female infertility, it is enough to show that they are many and varied. Some, such as involuntary sterilization and unnecessary surgery, are clear abuses. Few would dispute the need to prevent such abuses, though there is much debate about just how commonly they occur. Some, such as the lack of legal, safe, and affordable abortion in much of the world, could readily be remedied through changes in the law, but there is bitter controversy about the morality of such changes. And some, such as the relative frequency of "ordinary" heterosexual intercourse, would probably be extremely resistant to change, even if we could

agree that such change would be desirable.

Thus, there can be no simple solution to the problem of socially caused involuntary infertility. Yet there is room for a wider societal response to that problem. That response should include a more concerted effort to develop safer new contraceptives and to improve the older barrier methods. Often, it will need to include a more equitable distribution of medical resources, and better access to contraception and abortion—and to some of the NRTs. But the first step should be the better dissemination of information about ways of protecting oneself and others from the more common and preventable causes of infertility.

The international AIDS epidemic has led to a widespread recognition of a distinction between "safe" and "unsafe" sex. Although AIDS can be transmitted in many ways besides sexual contact, that mode of transmission is common, and some sexual practices are evidently more dangerous than others in this regard. Thus, in many parts of the world, public information campaigns and school sex education programs are being created or supplemented to teach basic facts about AIDS, how it is transmitted, and how the danger of transmission can be minimized.

A skeptical feminist might wonder whether it is coincidental that this public concern with safer sexual practices has arisen only when—perhaps for the first time ever—more men than women are suffering some of the most lethal consequences of unsafe sexual practices. On the other hand, gay rights advocates may be correct in their suspicion that more might have been done to help the victims of AIDS and to stop the spread of the illness, had not so many of these victims been homosexual males. Yet, however belated or inadequate, the new openness to the dissemination of information about relatively safe and unsafe sexual practices, prophylactics, and the like, is surely a positive development. This new openness may facilitate the prevention of other STDs as well, including those that—though not usually fatal—can lead to infertility.

But the idea that making sex safer is a legitimate public goal meets strong opposition from sexual and religious conservatives. Right-wing groups have long opposed attempts to ameliorate the harmful consequences of sexual activity, e.g., through the legalization of contraception and abortion, sex education in schools, or the public advertising of condoms and other contraceptives. They believe that women who do not want to have children should either avoid heterosexual intercourse altogether, or "accept the consequences," and that anyone who wants to avoid contracting a sexually transmitted disease should either remain celibate or practice lifelong monogamy with a partner who does likewise.

These attitudes have had a considerable influence, particularly in societies strongly influenced by Christianity. In effect, both "Pregnancy and disease have been pervasively and systematically used to inhibit sexual activity."[13] This punitive attitude is often based upon the distinctively—though not universally—Christian idea that all sexual activity is inherently sinful, except that which is apt for the production of children within a monogamous marriage. (This exception is only partial, since some Christian authorities have held that even procreative marital sexual intercourse can be sinful, if it is motivated by lust.) From this perspective, it can seem entirely appropriate, a kind of natural justice, that those who engage in nonmonogamous or nonprocreative sexual activities should be penalized by unwanted pregnancies, sexually transmitted diseases, and perhaps infertility. Attempts to prevent these harmful consequences of unsafe sex will therefore be seen as encouraging immoral sexual behavior.

Far from receding into the past, this punitive attitude towards much human sexual activity may currently be gaining strength, at least in some parts of the world. In this social context, it is doubly unrealistic to approach involuntary female infertility as though it were basically a medical problem. Improving IVF and other medical treatments for infertility would remain an important goal even if all of the social causes of infertility were eliminated, since not all infertility is socially caused. But there is some danger that the enormous publicity attendant upon the development of IVF and other NRTs will foster the illusion that the problem of involuntary infertility is being largely solved, when it is not.

8. CONCLUSION

Taken together, these objections are sufficient to cast some doubt upon the net value of IVF to women. They do not, however, support the conclusion that a just concern for women's interests demands the elimination of IVF and other NRTs. The costs and risks of IVF treatments to the female patient are substantial, but they are not known to be so great as to clearly outweigh the potential benefits in every case. Pronatalist ideology may put undue pressure upon infertile women to submit to IVF, but so long as potential IVF patients are adequately informed about the costs, risks, and odds of success, such covert social pressures need not make valid consent impossible.

Feminists are rightly concerned that if the NRTs continue to be developed and delivered by largely male teams, women's interests will not be as well served as they ought to be. The interests of women and men will be affected in different ways by the development of these technologies. Insofar as it is women who more often undergo invasive and/or potentially dangerous medical procedures associated with the NRTs, their interests are somewhat more centrally affected. Women should, therefore, be at least equally represented in the development of these technologies. Members of various racial, ethnic, or socioeconomic groups may also have special needs, or be especially vulnerable to harmful uses or abuses of the NRTs, and they too should be represented.

There is a need for more participation by women in all aspects of the practice, funding, and supervision of such biomedical research, as well as in the provision of medical care. Some of the ways in which the medical and research professions have been structured have served, perhaps inadvertently, as barriers to women, and other "minority" groups in these professions. The members of those professions have an obligation to remove those barriers—not by lowering standards, but by altering institutions and practices that discriminate needlessly against some competent individuals.

Even with greater participation by women in the development of the NRTs, there will remain some danger that the NRTs will contribute to the subtle erosion of women's reproductive autonomy. The use of new reproductive technologies might in time become legally or socially mandatory even for (some) fertile women, e.g., as a way of implementing eugenic goals. But this danger can better be counteracted by protecting individual civil rights than by seeking to eliminate the new reproductive technologies.

If these conclusions are correct, then IVF is probably a justifiable means of attempting to overcome infertility. But IVF can help only a small proportion of infertile women and men, and it inflicts heavy costs and risks on all who undergo it. It can, therefore, be only a small part of an adequate societal response to the problem of involuntary infertility.

One major element of a more adequate societal response to that problem is the better dissemination of knowledge about the preventable causes of infertility, e.g., those associated with particular sexual practices and contraceptive methods. A more concerted effort should also be made to develop safer (and cheaper) contraceptives and prophylactics, especially of the kinds that protect against both pregnancy and the transmission of STDs. Contraceptives, safe abortion, and other kinds of medical care need to be available to all women, including those who are underage or unable to pay. These are practical goals, which need not be prohibitively expensive, and which have already been at least partially achieved in some places.

If more is done to counteract the social causes of infertility, there may eventually be less need for IVF. Yet IVF may remain the best (medical) approach to the treatment of some forms of infertility. Thus, it is too soon to conclude that this new reproductive technology will not serve women's interests. If women and other underrepresented groups can gain a larger presence in the medical and research professions, and if suitable modes of regulation can be implemented, then the NRTs may provide more benefits than dangers. If not, then feminists may be right to remain somewhat skeptical about the long-term value of these new technologies for women.

NOTES

1. Gena Corea, *The Mother Machine: Reproductive Technologies from Artificial Insemination to Artificial Wombs* (New York: Harper and Row, 1985), pp. 149–59, at p. 170.
2. Rebecca Albury, "Who Owns the Embryo?" in *Test-Tube Women: What Future for Motherhood?* edited by Rita Arditti, Renate Duelli Klein, and Shelly Minden (London: Pandora Press, 1984), p. 57.
3. Lynne M. Paltrow, review of *Test-Tube Women*, in *Women's Rights Law Reporter* 8:4 (1985), p. 307.
4. Irene Elia, *The Female Animal* (New York: Oxford University Press, 1985), p. 280.
5. Corea, p. 93.
6. Robyn Rowland, "Reproductive Technologies: The Final Solution to the Woman Question?" in *Test-Tube Women*, p. 365–69, at p. 365.
7. Thomas Aquinas, *Summa Theologica*, Vol. I, Part 1, Question 92, Article 1 (New York: Benziger Brothers, 1947, p. 466).
8. Corea, p. 176.
9. Rowland, "Reproductive Technologies," p. 363.
10. Paltrow, p. 304.
11. John Stuart Mill, "Early Essays on Marriage and Divorce," in *Essays on Sex Equality*, edited by Alice Rossi (Chicago: University of Chicago Press, 1979), p. 77.
12. Heather Dietrich, "IVF: What Can We Do?" A paper presented at the National Conference on Reproductive Technologies, sponsored by the National Feminist Network on Reproductive Technology, Canberra, Australia, May 1986 p. 8.
13. Cindy Patton, *Sex and Germs: The Politics of AIDS* (Boston: South End Press, 1985), p. 10.

SECTION 2

Contract Pregnancy, Commodification, and the Family

On "Surrogacy"[1]

Barbara Katz Rothman

A QUESTION OF POLICY

The first thing to bear in mind is that surrogate motherhood is not a new procreative technology. The business of "surrogacy" has nothing to do with scientific progress, and everything to do with marketing. The procreative technology used is artificial insemination. Artificial insemination with donor sperm has been used in human beings for over a hundred years. The "technologies" involved are the technology of masturbation, and of the turkey baster or its equivalent.

It is important to remember that is the case, because we are sometimes overwhelmed with the developments of the new procreative technology, as with our other technologies. Sometimes we think—and sometimes we are encouraged to think—that there is nothing we can do to halt "progress." If science can produce "test-tube babies," how can we ever stop it? And if our new knowledge gives us these new powers, should we even want to stop it?

These are important questions. But they are not the questions of surrogate motherhood. Surrogate motherhood was not brought to us by the march of scientific progress. It was brought to us by brokers, by people who saw a new market and went after it. And the market is something we know we *can* control, and often *should* control.

When artificial insemination was introduced, it was used to support the traditional family structure, husbands and wives having and raising babies. In earlier times, when couples were unable to start a pregnancy, it was most often assumed to be the fault of the wife, and in some cultures husbands had the recourse of divorce. With expanding knowledge, infertility was shown to be sometimes a problem in the husband's body. Wives were not given the recourse of divorce under these circumstances, and artificial insemination became a way of maintaining the intact husband-wife unit. Wives were not encouraged to take a "surrogate," a substitute lover, but rather doctors used semen, given anonymously, to impregnate wives.

The process was undertaken with the greatest of secrecy. According to some accounts, the wife herself was not told what was done to her in the first American use of artificial insemination.[2] Certainly, no one outside of the couple and the doctor were told—artificial insemination was shrouded in silence. This enabled men to be the social fathers of the children their wives bore.

Social fatherhood is the key issue here. What makes a woman a mother has always been quite obvious. But what makes a man a father has been subject to some question. The formula our society (along with many others) has arrived at is that fatherhood is determined by the man's relationship to the child's mother. A man married to a woman is the recognized father of her children. This way of reckoning fatherhood builds on two things: the obvious and unquestioned nature of biological motherhood, and the traditional patriarchal relationship of men and their wives. This is a way of acknowledging parenthood that is based on relationships: the relationship of the woman to her baby as it grows within, and the relationship of the man to the woman.

From *Recreating Motherhood: Ideology and Technology in a Patriarchal Society* by Barbara Katz Rothman. Copyright © 1989 by Barbara Katz Rothman. Reprinted with permission of W. W. Norton & Company, Inc.

And so it stood for over a hundred years: artificial insemination was a way of managing male infertility that kept the patriarchal family intact, that allowed children to be born to a couple, children who would be truly theirs, to bring into the world together, to raise and to cherish together.

So what changed? For one thing, infertility appears to be more of a social problem: the actual rates of infertility may or may not be rising, but societal concern certainly is. For another, the supply of babies available for adoption has dropped dramatically. Young women, faced with unwanted pregnancies, have been given choices: the choice of abortion and the choice of raising a child without a husband. Infertile couples can no longer benefit, no matter how innocently, from the tragedies of young mothers. Our attitude toward infertility has also changed—and this may indeed be an indirect result of scientific progress. Progress against infertility has become a newspaper and television staple. Remember the excitement that surrounded the first in vitro baby, the first American in vitro baby, the first in vitro twins, and so on. The first in vitro quints were the cover story of *People* magazine in 1988.[3] The idea began to be generated that infertility was curable, if only a couple tried hard enough, saw enough doctors, went through enough procedures. The reality is something quite different. Only 10 percent of those couples attempting in vitro fertilization will have a baby. There is a 90 percent failure rate with that technology.

What we have done is to create a population of desperate, heartbroken infertile people: people who cannot find babies to adopt, who have "tried everything" and cannot get pregnant, people who have devoted years of their lives to trying, one way or another, to get a baby.

The medical technology has enabled the couple to sort out "whose fault" the infertility is. When it is the husband who is infertile, the use of insemination with donor sperm remains a solution, enabling the couple to have a pregnancy and the much-wanted baby. When it is the wife who is infertile, the pressures mount on the woman to feel guilt at not being able to "give her husband" a child. A baby is what they want more than anything. And he could have one, if not for her.

It is in this context that the marketing of "surrogate" motherhood developed. Brokers entered the scene, telling the couple that they can indeed have a baby, and it will be "his" baby. "Surrogate motherhood" was sold as a solution to the tragedy of infertility and a way of resolving women's guilt at their own infertility. For couples who had spent untold thousands of dollars on medical treatments, the thousands more for surrogacy contracts may have seemed a bargain. For people living without these many thousands of dollars, infertility remains unsolved.

With this new use of artificial insemination, the relationships of the parties involved changed totally. The relationship of the mother to her baby within her no longer counts. The baby has become a commodity, something a woman can produce and sell. She is encouraged to think of the baby as no more hers than a factory worker thinks of the car he works on as his. The relationship of the father to the mother no longer counts: it will cease to exist as motherhood is made anonymous, handled by brokers and doctors. The relationships that will count are that of the father to his sperm donation and that of the market: the contracts and the fees. What makes a man a father is not his relationship to the mother, we are told, but that it is his sperm and his money.

The brokers tell us that this is not baby selling: how can a man buy his own baby? they ask. And true enough, how can someone buy something which is already his? But what makes the baby his? If the sperm donor in more traditional artificial insemination came up to the couple a year later, said he had had an accident and was now infertile, and would like to have their baby, he would have no right to it. If he offered them money, he would not be buying that which is his, but that which is theirs: producing a semen sample does not make a man a social father, does not make that his baby. Is it then his intention that makes the child his? The fathers in the surrogacy cases do not donate their sperm. They are not donating or giving or selling. They are buying. Then how is this different from any other example of baby buying and selling? The answer is it is not.

If we legalize surrogacy arrangements, then to buy a baby one will need sperm and money. Couples—or just men—who have both can buy babies. But what of lesbian couples? And what of men without adequate sperm? Many cases of infertility involve both partners. What of a couple desperate to have a baby in which the wife cannot carry a pregnancy and the husband has insufficient sperm, or carries a deadly disease? Sperm, too, is for sale: we literally have sperm banks. If we permit surrogate motherhood for the situation of men who produce their "own" sperm, then what of the men who must buy sperm? Broker Noel Keane says he is prepared to make such arrangements.[4] Once sperm is purchased, the owners of the sperm can use that sperm as their "own" to make their "own" baby with a surrogate. We are going to find ourselves selling babies in "kit" form, purchasing the pieces and services separately: sperm here, an egg there, a rented uterus somewhere else. This is of course a "slippery slope" kind of argument—once you permit some people to buy some babies under some conditions, it is very hard to justify any given person not being allowed to purchase a baby under other circumstances.

So surrogacy is baby selling. As Angela Holder has said, "If I order a widget from a widget maker, and I pay cash money for that widget, and a widget is delivered to me, I defy you to tell me I have not bought a widget."[5]

And what would be wrong with simply opening up a market economy in babies? Others have argued eloquently what the problems are with baby selling, and we have as a society accepted those arguments. Some things, we have felt, should simply not be sold—and certainly not people. One of the strongest arguments against baby selling is that we know that if we allowed babies to be sold, some people would be put under great pressure to sell their babies. This is the same reason that we do not allow organs to be sold from living people, even when we know that lives might actually be saved. If we allowed some people to sell, say, a kidney, we know that some might feel forced to do so. And so now and again someone with much money dies for lack of an organ that he or she was willing to buy and someone else was willing to sell because such a sale, such a contract, even if arguably in the best interests of the parties involved, would be against the best interests of the society as a whole. I believe that "surrogacy" presents a situation parallel to organ selling, and that the same arguments apply.

I began by saying that surrogacy is not a result of new procreative technology, but must be understood entirely as a marketing strategy. Let me now amend that slightly. Most of the surrogate motherhood cases that reach the courts and the media are based on the old technology of artificial insemination. But some are using a newer technology. We must consider what these new developments in procreative technology will mean for the future of surrogacy contracts.

The new technologies are varied, but share in common the use of genetic material from one woman to create a pregnancy in the body of another woman. There are several ways this can be done. An egg from one woman can be removed, fertilized in vitro (in glass), and put into the body of another woman. Some in vitro fertilization clinics are doing this for women who want to become mothers but cannot produce eggs. Other women, who produce "extra" eggs, donate those eggs for the use of infertile women who cannot produce their own eggs. Sometimes the donors are other women in the program who are ovulating well, sometimes they are hired egg donors, and sometimes they are friends or relatives of the infertile woman. Whether donated or purchased, genetic material from outside of the couple is used to enable a woman and her husband to have a pregnancy and share in the birthing and rearing of a baby. The situation is most closely analogous to artificial insemination with donated or purchased sperm.

Another way that this same thing can be accomplished is by allowing fertilization to take place within the body of the woman who is donating the egg. A fertilized egg, what some call a pre-embryo or pre-implantation embryo, is moved from the donor and placed within the body of the woman who will be the mother. This, too, is much like artificial insemination. Some months later we look at a pregnant woman and her husband expecting their child. In these situations of embryo transfer or egg donation, like the situation of artificial insemination with donor sperm, genetic material from outside the couple is used to create the pregnancy, but social parenthood, from the point of early pregnancy on, is shared within the couple.

That then is the technology. And what of the marketing? Like the marketing of artificial insemination, egg donations can also be turned around and used to create a pregnancy not within the family, but in a hired woman, leading to the ultimate purchase of a baby.

With this technology, it is not necessary for the "surrogate" to be genetically related to the baby she bears. So one marketing strategy is to hire a woman to carry a pregnancy for a woman who can produce eggs but not carry a pregnancy for herself. Now something challenging happens to our thinking: we are forced to confront the question of what makes a woman a mother. Is it the egg, or is it the pregnancy? In the cases mentioned above, where a woman is unable to create an egg, the transfer of the egg or embryo left the pregnant woman the social mother: it was the pregnant woman who intended to be the mother, who not only intended to bear and birth the child, but to raise the child as well. But if we hire a woman to carry the pregnancy, who then is the mother? Is it the egg donor, or the pregnant woman?

In one court decision involving such a case, the egg donor was named as the mother, and the name of the pregnant woman—the gestational mother—was not put on the birth certificate. This is of course analogous to the marketing of surrogate motherhood with the old technology of artificial insemination. Relationships are discounted, and the genetic tie as well as the exchange of money are given primacy. We are asked to accept the idea that the mother is the person who owned the egg and paid for the service, just as we are asked to accept the man who owned the sperm and paid for the services as the father.

This opens up an enormous new profit potential for the brokers in the surrogacy market. The technologies of egg and embryo transfer, were surrogate motherhood contracts made enforceable, could be used to drive costs down and keep profits up for the baby brokers. As it stands now, the brokers are limited in their use of surrogate mothers. Because the women are genetically related to the babies they produce, the father-purchasers want only certain kinds of women: intelligent, attractive, and most assuredly of the same race as the couple. Since it is predominantly white couples who have the $25,000 and up that the brokers charge, and since it is particularly white babies that are in scarce supply for adoption, what brokers need are intelligent, attractive, healthy white women to act as surrogates. In our society, such women can command some money for their services, not enormous sums compared, say, to what corporate executives—or for that matter truck dri-

vers—get, but at this moment the going rate is $10,000 to the mother.

But what will happen if the new technology allows brokers to hire women who are not related genetically to the babies that are to be sold? Like the poor and non-white women who are hired to do other kinds of nurturing and caretaking work, these mothers can be paid very little, with few benefits, and no long-term commitment. The same women who are pushing white babies in strollers, white old folks in wheelchairs, can be carrying white babies in their bellies. Poor, uneducated third-world women and women of color from the United States and elsewhere, with fewer economic alternatives, can be hired more cheaply. They can also be controlled more tightly. With a legally supported surrogate motherhood contract, and with the new technology, the marketing possibilities are enormous—and terrifying. Just as Perdue and Holly Farms advertise their chickens based on superior breeding and feeding, the baby brokers could begin to advertise their babies: brand name, state-of-the-art babies produced from the "finest" of genetic materials and an all-natural, vitamin-enriched diet.

I used to envision such "baby farms" located in third-world countries, supplying babies to American purchasers. But now I wonder: most European countries have outlawed surrogacy-for-hire. In the United States, as long as one state permits it, if we have no national legislation barring it, the business can be legally established. Remember, in the most famous surrogacy case to date, that of Baby M, both the Sterns and the Whiteheads lived in New Jersey, the broker lived in Michigan, the clinic was located in New York, and the adoption was slated to go through Florida. If just one state exists for the legal paperwork, it may be the third-world women of America—the women of our inner-city ghettos—who grow babies for "export." It is in the United States that the rights of rich people to buy are most deeply held.

The time to stop such nightmare visions is now. We stop it by not acknowledging the underlying principle of surrogate contracts, by not accepting the very concept of "surrogacy" for motherhood. A surrogate is a substitute. In some human relations, we can accept no substitutes. Any pregnant woman is the mother of the child she bears. Her gestational relationship establishes her motherhood. We will not accept the idea that we can look at a woman, heavy with child, and say the child is not hers. The fetus is part of the woman's body, regardless of the source of the egg and sperm. Biological motherhood is not a service, not a commodity, but a relationship. Motherhood can remain obvious. If a woman is carrying a baby, then it is her baby and she is its mother. Of course it is true that a mother, any mother, can abdicate her motherhood, can give away a baby. But it is hers to give. And if we were to allow the selling of babies, then it is hers to sell, or refuse to sell.

And what can we do with fatherhood? How can we protect the relationship between a father and his child? What will make a man a father? One possibility is to stay with the model that we had: a father can continue to take his fatherhood from his relationship with the mother of the child. In a married couple, the father can continue to be, as hitherto, the husband of the mother.

That is not a perfect solution to the troubling question of fatherhood. It gives, in some ways, too much power to women over men's procreation. And it gives, in other ways, too much power to men over women's procreation. But this is not a new problem. We are not struggling here with questions of science and new technology. Here we are struggling with age-old questions of relationships, of family, of how we are bound together. We have not found perfect ways of dealing with these issues in all of history. But we have, in this society, been clear in rejecting the use of money in these relationships. We have said that in our society husbands and wives, mothers and fathers, and babies are not for sale. Nothing in the new procreative technology need change that.

Those engaged in surrogacy brokering tell us that if we do not bring surrogacy into the open market, it, like adoption, will continue to exist in "gray-" or black-market forms. And they are probably right. Preventing the open sale of babies has not prevented couples from having to spend much money on getting babies, nor has it prevented brokers from making money out of matching babies to adopters.

I do not disagree with the brokers over acknowledging the problem, but over choosing the solution. There are grave costs to any form of open market in baby selling. If we wish to legalize baby selling, let us acknowledge what we are doing, and offer the appropriate protections to the parties involved. If we choose to allow a woman to sell her baby, so be it. But let us recognize that it is indeed her baby that she is selling. And if we do not wish to permit baby selling, then there is nothing in the new procreative technology that forces us to do so. We do not have to give the support of the state and of the courts to a view of babies as purchasable commodities or motherhood as a salable service.

In sum, the legislation I feel we need to develop as national policy in the United States would recognize that *the gestational mother is the mother.* Any pregnant woman is the mother of the child she bears, regardless of the source of the egg or the sperm. The rights and the responsibilities of motherhood are the same for all gestational mothers, regardless of the source of the egg and the sperm.

Therefore, *purchasing a baby from its mother, regardless of the source of the egg and the sperm, is purchasing a baby.* Until or unless we legalize baby selling, the law cannot acknowledge paid surrogacy contracts. Surrogacy is not to be used as a way around the laws against the sale of babies: it is itself a variation of baby selling.

Further, *accepting a baby as a gift from its mother, regardless of the source of the egg and the sperm, is a form of adoption.* The laws that govern the rights and responsibilities of all parties to an adoption must apply to so-called surrogate arrangements as well.

A QUESTION OF VALUES

People—friends, colleagues, maybe especially family—keep pointing out to me, with a bemused air, how strange it is to find me arguing on the same side as religious leaders in the debate on surrogacy arrangements. And I, too, occasionally find some amusement in the "strange bedfellows" phenomenon. Indeed, with carefully groomed "happy surrogates" and their equally well-groomed brokers placed on a TV or radio show by a professional public relations firm, I often find myself, side-by-side with some priest or rabbi, brought in by a producer to give a "balanced" view. And so we argue out the problems of surrogacy, sandwiched between car commercials, wine cooler ads, and other signs of the times.

The "tag" they use to identify me on television—the white line of print that shows up on the screen but which I never get to see in the studio—sometimes reads *author,* rarely reads *sociologist,* but most often they seem to use *feminist.* And so there we are, "feminist" and "priest" or "rabbi" arguing the same, anti-surrogacy side.

But it is only on the very surface that I am on the same side as these religious leaders. We may have landed on the same side of this particular fence, but we've taken very different paths to get there, and we are headed in very different directions. The values that I use in my opposition to surrogacy are fundamentally different from those the religious leaders are using, and the goals I seek are just as different. And strangely enough, in many ways my values and goals are much the same as those used by those of my feminist colleagues who have come to an opposite conclusion.

The arguments against surrogacy that come out of traditional religious context most often rest on two basic principles: first that surrogacy is "unnatural," because it goes against the nature of women and especially of mothers; second, that it violates the sanctity of the family.

Feminists are a lot less sure about just what is "natural" for women, but on the whole we've concluded that the institution of motherhood as it exists in our society is pretty far from any natural state. Neither I nor my feminist colleagues are about to get caught up in any "maternal instincts" arguments. Women end pregnancies with abortions, or end their motherhood by giving a baby up for adoption, when that is what they feel they need to do. Being pregnant does not necessarily mean a woman is going to mother, to raise the child that might be born of that pregnancy. Nor are we going to claim that only a birth mother can mother, can nurture a baby. We know that loving people, men as well as women, can provide all the warm, caring, loving nurturance a baby needs.

Feminists are also not concerned with maintaining the "sanctity of the family," a pleasant enough phrase that has been used to cover an awful lot of damage. That was the argument used to stop funding day-care centers, the argument offered to allow men to beat their wives and children, the argument most generally used to stop women from controlling their own lives and their own bodies. The "family" whose "sanctity" is being maintained is the patriarchal, male-dominated family. Feminists have a different sense of family—

we need to protect the single young mother and her child, the lesbian couple and their children, the gay man's family. As feminists, we are concerned not with the control and ownership and kinship issues of the traditional family, but with the *relationships* people establish with one another, with adults and with children.

So why then, as a feminist, do I oppose the surrogacy relationship? The "liberal" wing of feminism does not necessarily oppose those contracts. As long as the women entering them do so of their own volition, with fully informed consent, and as long as they maintain their control over their own bodies throughout the pregnancies, some feminists have said that surrogacy contracts should be supported by the state. Some even go as far as Lori Andrews, for instance, a noted feminist attorney, who says that these contracts should be binding with absolutely no opportunity for the mother to change her mind.

What then are the objections that I, out of my vision of feminism, raise to surrogacy? And more important, on what values am I basing my objections?

My values place relationships as central. Rather than the ownership or kinship ties that appear to epitomize the "traditional" or patriarchal family, I value the interpersonal relations people establish. A man does not own his wife, nor does he have ownership rights over the child she produces of her body. Men may own their sperm, but children are not sperm grown up. Children are not "owned," and they are not available for sale. On the other hand, children do not enter the world from Mars, or out of a black box. Children, as it says in the books for children, come from mothers. They enter the world in a relationship, a physical and social and emotional relationship with the woman in whose body they have been nurtured. The nurturance of pregnancy is a relationship, one that develops as a fetus becomes more and more a baby.

That does not mean that the maternal relationship cannot be ended. Nor does it mean that the relationship is the most overwhelming, all-powerful relationship on earth. In fact, we know it to be a fairly fragile relationship. The intimacy that a mother and her baby experience can be easily lost if they are separated. If a woman chooses to end this relationship, so be it. When a mother chooses to give a baby up to others who want to raise that baby as their own, she is doing what we have all done sometime in our lives—ending a relationship. Sometimes this is done with less and sometimes with more pain, but rarely is it an easy thing for a mother to do.

The relationship that a woman has established by the time she births her baby has more weight, in my value system, than claims of genetic ties, of contracts signed, or of down payments made.

When I make this argument with traditionally oriented people, I am often asked if this doesn't contradict my ideas about a woman's right to abort an unwanted pregnancy. Not at all, I think. When a woman chooses an abortion, she is choosing not to enter into a maternal relationship. Women want access to safe abortions as quickly as possible, before quickening, before a relationship can begin.

In sum, in my value system, I am placing the woman, her experiences and her relationships, at the very heart of my understanding of all pregnancies.

The second value I bring as a feminist to my understanding of surrogacy contracts is the value of women's bodily autonomy, our control over our own bodies. And I see the fetus as part of a woman's body. Traditional patriarchal values would see the fetus as part of its father's body, his "seed" planted in a woman's body. In a patriarchal system, the father—or the state or the church—is held to have special control over a woman's body and life because of that fetus she can bear. As a feminist, I reject that. The fetus is *hers*. Women never bear anybody else's baby: not their husband's, not the state's, and not the purchaser's in a surrogacy contract. Every woman bears her *own* baby. I believe that is true regardless of the source of the sperm, and regardless also of the source of the egg.

As I said earlier, most of the surrogacy arrangements we have seen so far, like the Stern-Whitehead case, were done not with elaborate new technology, but with the very old and very simple technology of artificial insemination. The "surrogate" has been in every possible way the mother to the baby she bore. But some newer technology will allow eggs to be transferred from woman to woman, allowing a woman to be pregnant with fetus grown of another woman's egg.

The Catholic Church and some other religious groups reject that technology. I do not. When that technology is used to enable a woman to enter motherhood with a pregnancy, in just the way that artificial insemination has been used to allow an infertile man to become a social father beginning with pregnancy, I have no problem with it. My concern is when that technology is used in a so-called surrogacy arrangement—when the birth mother, the pregnant woman, is declared to be only a "rented womb," a "surrogate," and the *real* mother is declared to be the woman who produced the egg.

The church and other conservative forces object to the technology because they value the fertilized egg itself as an object believed to be human. I object when women are "used," when parts of women are put up for sale or hire, when our relationships are discounted in favor of genetic and monetary ties.

Those feminists, like Lori Andrews, who would allow surrogacy contracts still demand rights of bodily autonomy for the pregnant woman. The compromise position they maintain is that it is indeed her body, and she must have all decision-making control over her pregnancy—but it is not her baby in her body, not if she has contracted it away. I feel that kind of "compromise" does a profound disservice to women. I cannot ever believe that a woman is pregnant with someone else's baby. The idea is repugnant—it reduces the woman to a container. Nor do I think that that kind of compromise, saying the pregnancy is indeed hers, but the fetus/baby theirs, the purchasers', can be workable. The "preciousness" of the very wanted, very expensive baby will far outweigh the value given to the "cheap labor" of the surrogate.

This is the inevitable result of thinking of pregnancy not as a relationship between a woman and her fetus but as a service she provides for others, and of thinking of the woman herself not as a person but as the container for another, often more valued, person. In that sense, surrogacy is the reductio ad absurdum of technological, patriarchal capitalism.

The values that I bring to motherhood, the values that I take from my feminism, all the values that I've tried to express in this book, all come together in my opposition to surrogacy. And this, to answer a question I began this book with, is what I think feminism has to offer the Mary Beth Whiteheads of the world.

NOTES

1. Portions of this chapter were presented as testimony to the Judiciary Committee of the New York State Senate hearings on "Surrogate Parenthood and New Reproductive Technology," October 16, 1986, and portions appear in *Conscience,* May 1987, pp. 1–4.
2. Gena Corea, 1985, *The Mother Machine: Reproductive Technologies from Artificial Insemination to Artificial Wombs* (New York: Harper and Row).

3. *People,* February 15, 1988.
4. Noel Keane and I discussed this on the "MacNeil, Leher Newshour," March 31, 1987.
5. Angela Holder, 1984, presentation to the American Society of Law and Medicine conference, "What About the Children?" An International Conference on the Legal, Social, and Ethical Implications of New Reproductive and Prenatal Technologies," Boston, Massachusetts, October 29, 1984.

Surrogate Motherhood as Prenatal Adoption

Bonnie Steinbock

The recent case of "Baby M" has brought surrogate motherhood to the forefront of American attention. Ultimately, whether we permit or prohibit surrogacy depends on what we take to be good reasons for preventing people from acting as they wish. A growing number of people want to be, or hire, surrogates; are there legitimate reasons to prevent them? Apart from its intrinsic interest, the issue of surrogate motherhood provides us with an opportunity to examine different justifications for limiting individual freedom.

In the first section, I examine the Baby M case, and the lessons it offers. In the second section, I examine claims that surrogacy is ethically unacceptable because it is exploitive, inconsistent with human dignity, or harmful to the children born of such arrangements. I conclude that these reasons justify restrictions on surrogate contracts, rather than an outright ban.

From *Law, Medicine & Health Care* 16, Spring/Summer 1988:40–50. Reprinted with the permission of the American Society of Law, Medicine & Ethics.

I. BABY M

Mary Beth Whitehead, a married mother of two, agreed to be inseminated with the sperm of William Stern, and to give up the child to him for a fee of $10,000. The baby (whom Mrs. Whitehead named Sara, and the Sterns named Melissa) was born on March 27, 1986. Three days later, Mrs. Whitehead took her home from the hospital, and turned her over to the Sterns.

Then Mrs. Whitehead changed her mind. She went to the Sterns' home, distraught, and pleaded to have the baby temporarily. Afraid that she would kill herself, the Sterns agreed. The next week, Mrs. Whitehead informed the Sterns that she had decided to keep the child, and threatened to leave the country if court action was taken.

At that point, the situation deteriorated into a cross between the Keystone Kops and Nazi storm troopers. Accompanied by five policemen, the Sterns went to the Whitehead residence armed with a court order giving them temporary custody of the child. Mrs. Whitehead managed to slip the baby out of a window to her husband, and the following morning the Whiteheads fled with the child to Florida, where Mrs. Whitehead's parents lived. During the next three months, the Whiteheads lived in roughly twenty different hotels, motels, and homes to avoid apprehension. From time to time, Mrs. Whitehead telephoned Mr. Stern to discuss the matter: He taped these conversations on the advice of his counsel. Mrs. Whitehead threatened to kill herself, to kill the child, and falsely to accuse Mr. Stern of sexually molesting her older daughter.

At the end of July 1986, while Mrs. Whitehead was hospitalized with a kidney infection, Florida police raided her mother's home, knocking her down, and seized the child. Baby M was placed in the custody of Mr. Stern, and the Whiteheads returned to New Jersey, where they attempted to regain custody. After a long and emotional court battle, Judge Harvey R. Sorkow ruled on March 31, 1987, that the surrogacy contract was valid, and that specific performance was justified in the best interests of the child. Immediately after reading his decision, he called the Sterns into his chambers so that Mr. Stern's wife, Dr. Elizabeth Stern, could legally adopt the child.

This outcome was unexpected and unprecedented. Most commentators had thought that a court would be unlikely to order a reluctant surrogate to give up an infant merely on the basis of a contract. Indeed, if Mrs. Whitehead had never surrendered the child to the Sterns, but had simply taken her home and kept her there, the outcome undoubtedly would have been different. It is also likely that Mrs. Whitehead's failure to obey the initial custody order angered Judge Sorkow, and affected his decision.

The decision was appealed to the New Jersey Supreme Court, which issued its decision on February 3, 1988. Writing for a unanimous court, Chief Justice Wilentz reversed the lower court's ruling that the surrogacy contract was valid. The court held that a surrogacy contract which provides money for the surrogate mother, and which includes her irrevocable agreement to surrender her child at birth, is invalid and unenforceable. Since the contract was invalid, Mrs. Whitehead did not relinquish, nor were there any other grounds for terminating, her parental rights. Therefore, the adoption of Baby M by Mrs. Stern was improperly granted, and Mrs. Whitehead remains the child's legal mother.

The Court further held that the issue of custody is determined solely by the child's best interests,

and it agreed with the lower court that it was in Melissa's best interests to remain with the Sterns. However, Mrs. Whitehead, as Baby M's legal as well as natural mother, is entitled to have her own interest in visitation considered. The determination of what kind of visitation rights should be granted to her, and under what conditions, was remanded to the trial court.

The distressing details of this case have led many people to reject surrogacy altogether. Do we really want police officers wrenching infants from their mothers' arms, and prolonged custody battles when surrogates find they are unable to surrender their children, as agreed? Advocates of surrogacy say that to reject the practice wholesale, because of one unfortunate instance, is an example of a "hard case" making bad policy. Opponents reply that it is entirely reasonable to focus on the worst potential outcomes when deciding public policy. Everyone can agree on at least one thing: This particular case seems to have been mismanaged from start to finish, and could serve as a manual of how not to arrange a surrogate birth.

First, it is now clear that Mary Beth Whitehead was not a suitable candidate for surrogate motherhood. Her ambivalence about giving up the child was recognized early on, although this information was not passed on to the Sterns.[1] Second, she had contact with the baby after birth, which is usually avoided in "successful" cases. Typically, the adoptive mother is actively involved in the pregnancy, often serving as the pregnant woman's coach in labor. At birth, the baby is given to the adoptive, not the biological, mother. The joy of the adoptive parents in holding their child serves both to promote their bonding, and to lessen the pain of separation of the biological mother.

At Mrs. Whitehead's request, no one at the hospital was aware of the surrogacy arrangement. She and her husband appeared as the proud parents of "Sara Elizabeth Whitehead," the name on her birth certificate. Mrs. Whitehead held her baby, nursed her, and took her home from the hospital—just as she would have done in a normal pregnancy and birth. Not surprisingly, she thought of Sara as her child, and she fought with every weapon at her disposal, honorable and dishonorable, to prevent her being taken away. She can hardly be blamed for doing so.[2]

Why did Dr. Stern, who supposedly had a very good relationship with Mrs. Whitehead before the birth, not act as her labor coach? One possibility is that Mrs. Whitehead, ambivalent about giving up her baby, did not want Dr. Stern involved. At her request, the Sterns' visits to the hospital to see the newborn baby were unobtrusive. It is also possible that Dr. Stern was ambivalent about having a child. The original idea of hiring a surrogate was not hers, but her husband's. It was Mr. Stern who felt a "compelling" need to have a child related to him by blood, having lost all his relatives to the Nazis.

Furthermore, Dr. Stern was not infertile, as was stated in the surrogacy agreement. Rather, in 1979 she was diagnosed by two eye specialists as suffering from optic neuritis, which meant that she "probably" had multiple sclerosis. (This was confirmed by all four experts who testified.) Normal conception was ruled out by the Sterns in late 1982, when a medical colleague told Dr. Stern that his wife, a victim of multiple sclerosis, had suffered a temporary paralysis during pregnancy. "We decided the risk wasn't worth it," Mr. Stern said.[3]

Mrs. Whitehead's lawyer, Harold J. Cassidy, dismissed the suggestion that Dr. Stern's "mildest case" of multiple sclerosis determined their decision to seek a surrogate. He noted that she was not even treated for multiple sclerosis until after the Baby M dispute had started. "It's almost as though it's an afterthought," he said.[4]

Judge Sorkow deemed the decision to avoid conception "medically reasonable and understandable." The Supreme Court did not go so far, noting that "her anxiety appears to have exceeded the actual risk, which current medical authorities assess as minimal."[5] Nonetheless the court acknowledged that her anxiety, including fears that pregnancy might precipitate blindness and paraplegia, was "quite real." Certainly, even a woman who wants a child very much may reasonably wish to avoid becoming blind and paralyzed as a result of pregnancy. Yet is it believable that a woman who really wanted a child would decide against pregnancy *solely* on the basis of *someone else's* medical experience? Would she not consult at least one specialist on her *own* medical condition before deciding it wasn't worth the risk? The conclusion that she was

at best ambivalent about bearing a child seems irresistible.

This possibility conjures up many people's worst fears about surrogacy: That prosperous women, who do not want to interrupt their careers, will use poor and educationally disadvantaged women to bear their children. I will return shortly to the question of whether this is exploitive. The issue here is psychological: What kind of mother is Dr. Stern likely to be? If she is unwilling to undergo pregnancy, with its discomforts, inconveniences, and risks, will she be willing to make the considerable sacrifices which good parenting requires? Mrs. Whitehead's ability to be a good mother was repeatedly questioned during the trial. She was portrayed as immature, untruthful, hysterical, overly identified with her children, and prone to smothering their independence. Even if all this description is true—and I think that Mrs. Whitehead's inadequacies were exaggerated—Dr. Stern may not be such a prize either. The choice for Baby M may have been between a highly strung, emotional, over-involved mother, and a remote, detached, even cold one.

The assessment of Mrs. Whitehead's ability to be a good mother was biased by the middle-class prejudices of the judge and the mental health officials who testified. Mrs. Whitehead left school at 15, and is not conversant with the latest theories on child rearing: She made the egregious error of giving Sara teddy bears to play with, instead of the more "age-appropriate," expert-approved pans and spoons. She proved to be a total failure at patty-cake. If this is evidence of parental inadequacy, we're all in danger of losing our children.

The Supreme Court felt that Mrs. Whitehead was "rather harshly judged" and acknowledged the possibility that the trial court was wrong in its initial award of custody. Nevertheless, it affirmed Judge Sorkow's decision to allow the Sterns to retain custody, as being in Melissa's best interests. George Annas disagrees with the "best interests" approach. He points out that Judge Sorkow awarded temporary custody of Baby M to the Sterns in May 1986 without giving the Whiteheads notice or an opportunity to obtain legal representation. That was a serious wrong and injustice to the Whiteheads. To allow the Sterns to keep the child compounds the original unfairness: ". . . justice requires that reasonable consideration be given to returning Baby M to the permanent custody of the Whiteheads."[6]

But a child is not a possession, to be returned to the rightful owner. It is not fairness to all parties that should determine a child's fate, but what is best for her. As Chief Justice Wilentz rightly stated, "The child's interests come first: We will not punish it for judicial errors, assuming any were made."[7]

Subsequent events have substantiated the claim that giving custody to the Sterns was in Melissa's best interests. After losing custody of Melissa, Mrs. Whitehead, whose husband had undergone a vasectomy, became pregnant by another man. She divorced her husband and married Dean R. Gould last November. These developments indicate that the Whiteheads were not able to offer a stable home, although the argument can be made that their marriage might have survived, but for the strains introduced by the court battle, and the loss of Baby M. But even if Judge Sorkow had no reason to prefer the Sterns to the Whiteheads back in May 1986, he was still right to give the Sterns custody in March 1987. To take her away then, at nearly eighteen months of age, from the only parents she had ever known, would have been disruptive, cruel, and unfair to her.

Annas's preference for a just solution is premised partly on his belief that there *is* no "best interest" solution to this "tragic custody case." I take it that he means that however custody is resolved, Baby M is the loser. Either way, she will be deprived of one parent. However, a best interests solution is not a perfect solution. It is simply the solution which is on balance best for the child, given the realities of the situation. Applying this standard, Judge Sorkow was right to give the Sterns custody, and the Supreme Court was right to uphold the decision.

The best interests argument is based on the assumption that Mr. Stern has at least a *prima facie* claim to Baby M. We certainly would not consider allowing a stranger who kidnapped a baby, and managed to elude the police for a year, to retain custody on the grounds that he was providing a good home to a child who had known no other parent. However, the Baby M case is not analogous. First, Mr. Stern is Baby M's biological father

and, as such, has at least some claim to raise her, which no non-parental kidnapper has. Second, Mary Beth Whitehead *agreed* to give him their baby at birth. Unlike the miller's daughter in *Rumpelstiltskin*, the fairy tale to which the Baby M case is sometimes compared, she was not forced into the agreement. Because both Mary Beth Whitehead and Mr. Stern have *prima facie* claims to Baby M, the decision as to who should raise her should be based on her present best interests. Therefore we must, regretfully, tolerate the injustice to Mrs. Whitehead, and try to avoid such problems in the future.

It is unfortunate that the Court did not decide the issue of visitation on the same basis as custody. By declaring Mrs. Whitehead Gould the legal mother, and maintaining that she is entitled to visitation, the Court has prolonged the fight over Baby M. It is hard to see how this can be in her best interests. This is no ordinary divorce case, where the child has a relation with both parents which it is desirable to maintain. As Mr. Stern said at the start of the court hearing to determine visitation, "Melissa has a right to grow and be happy and not be torn between two parents."[8]

The court's decision was well-meaning but internally inconsistent. Out of concern for the best interests of the child, it granted the Sterns custody. At the same time, by holding Mrs. Whitehead Gould to be the legal mother, with visitation rights, it precluded precisely what is most in Melissa's interest, a resolution of the situation. Further, the decision leaves open the distressing possibility that a Baby M situation could happen again. Legislative efforts should be directed toward ensuring that this worst-case scenario never occurs.

II. SHOULD SURROGACY BE PROHIBITED?

On June 27, 1988, Michigan became the first state to outlaw commercial contracts for women to bear children for others. Yet making a practice illegal does not necessarily make it go away: Witness black market adoption. The legitimate concerns which support a ban on surrogacy might be better served by careful regulation. However, some practices, such as slavery, are ethically unaccept-able, regardless of how carefully regulated they are. Let us consider the arguments that surrogacy is intrinsically unacceptable.

A. PATERNALISTIC ARGUMENTS

These arguments against surrogacy take the form of protecting a potential surrogate from a choice she may later regret. As an argument for banning surrogacy, as opposed to providing safeguards to ensure that contracts are freely and knowledge-ably undertaken, this is a form of paternalism.

At one time, the characterization of a prohibition as paternalistic was a sufficient reason to reject it. The pendulum has swung back, and many people are willing to accept at least some paternalistic restrictions on freedom. Gerald Dworkin points out that even Mill made one exception to his other-wise absolute rejection of paternalism: He thought that no one should be allowed to sell himself into slavery, because to do so would be to destroy his future autonomy.

This provides a narrow principle to justify some paternalistic interventions. To preserve freedom in the long run, we give up the freedom to make cer-tain choices, those which have results which are "far-reaching, potentially dangerous and irre-versible."[9] An example would be a ban on the sale of crack. Virtually everyone who uses crack becomes addicted and, once addicted, a slave to its use. We reasonably and willingly give up our free-dom to buy the drug, to protect our ability to make free decisions in the future.

Can a Dworkinian argument be made to rule out surrogacy agreements? Admittedly, the deci-sion to give up a child is permanent, and may have disastrous effects on the surrogate mother. However, many decisions may have long-term, disastrous effects (e.g., postponing childbirth for a career, having an abortion, giving a child up for adoption). Clearly we do not want the state to make decisions for us in all these matters. Dworkin's argument is rightly restricted to pater-nalistic interferences which protect the individ-ual's autonomy or ability to make decisions in the future. Surrogacy does not involve giving up one's autonomy, which distinguishes it from both the crack and selling-oneself-into-slavery examples. Respect for individual freedom requires us to per-mit people to make choices which they may later regret.

B. MORAL OBJECTIONS

Four main moral objections to surrogacy were out-lined in the Warnock Report.[10]

1. It is inconsistent with human dignity that a woman should use her uterus for financial profit.
2. To deliberately become pregnant with the intention of giving up the child distorts the relationship between mother and child.
3. Surrogacy is degrading because it amounts to child-selling.
4. Since there are some risks attached to preg-nancy, no woman ought to be asked to undertake pregnancy for another in order to earn money.

We must all agree that a practice which exploits people or violates human dignity is immoral. However, it is not clear that surrogacy is guilty on either count.

1. Exploitation   The mere fact that pregnancy is *risky* does not make surrogate agreements exploitive, and therefore morally wrong. People often do risky things for money; why should the line be drawn at undergoing pregnancy? The usual response is to compare surrogacy and kid-ney-selling. The selling of organs is prohibited because of the potential for coercion and exploita-tion. But why should kidney-selling be viewed as intrinsically coercive? A possible explanation is that no one would do it, unless driven by poverty. The choice is both forced and dangerous, and hence coercive.

The situation is quite different in the case of the race car driver or stunt performer. We do not think that they are *forced* to perform risky activities for money: They freely choose to do so. Unlike selling one's kidneys, these are activities which we can understand (intellectually, anyway) someone choosing to do. Movie stuntmen and women, for example, often enjoy their work, and derive satis-faction from doing it well. Of course they "do it for the money," in the sense that they would not do it without compensation; few people are willing to work "for free." The element of coercion is missing, however, because they enjoy the job, despite the risks, and could do something else if they chose.

The same is apparently true of most surrogates. "They choose the surrogate role primarily because the fee provides a better economic opportunity than alternative occupations, but also because they enjoy being pregnant and the respect and attention that it draws."[11] Some may derive a feeling of self-worth from an act they regard as highly altruistic: providing a couple with a child they could not otherwise have. If these motives are present, it is far from clear that the surrogate is being exploited. Indeed, it seems objectionably paternalistic to insist that she is.

2. Human Dignity   It may be argued that even if womb-leasing is not necessarily exploitive, it should still be rejected as inconsistent with human dignity. But why? As John Harris points out, hair, blood, and other tissue is often donated or sold; what is so special about the uterus?[12]

Human dignity is more plausibly invoked in the strongest argument against surrogacy, namely, that it is the sale of a child. Children are not property, nor can they be bought or sold. It could be argued that surrogacy is wrong because it is analogous to slavery, and so is inconsistent with human dignity.

However, there are clearly important differences between slavery and a surrogate agreement. The child born of a surrogate is not treated cruelly or deprived of freedom or resold; none of the things which make slavery so awful are part of surrogacy. Still, it may be thought that simply putting a market value on a child is wrong. Human life has its own intrinsic value; it is literally priceless. Arrangements which ignore this belief violate our deepest notions of the value of human life. It is profoundly disturbing to hear the boyfriend of a surrogate say, quite candidly in a television documentary on surrogacy, "We're in it for the money."

Judge Sorkow accepted the premise that producing a child for money denigrates human dignity, but he denied that this happens in a surrogate agreement. Mrs. Whitehead was not paid for the surrender of the child to the father: She was paid for her willingness to be impregnated and carry Mr. Stern's child to term. The child, once born, is his biological child. "He cannot purchase what is already his."

This is misleading, and not merely because Baby M is as much Mrs. Whitehead's child as Mr. Stern's. It is misleading because it glosses over the fact that the surrender of the child was part—indeed, the whole point—of the agreement. If the surrogate were paid merely for being willing to be impregnated and carrying the child to term, then she would fulfill the contract upon giving birth. She could take the money *and* the child. Mr. Stern did not agree to pay Mrs. Whitehead merely to *have* his child, but to provide him with a child. The New Jersey Supreme Court held that this violated New Jersey's laws prohibiting the payment or acceptance of money in connection with adoption.

One way to remove the taint of baby-selling would be to limit payment to medical expenses associated with the birth or incurred by the surrogate during pregnancy (as is allowed in many jurisdictions, including New Jersey, in ordinary adoptions). Surrogacy could be seen not as baby-selling, but as a form of adoption. Nowhere did the Supreme Court find any legal prohibition against surrogacy when there is no payment, and when the surrogate has the right to change her mind and keep the child. However, this solution effectively prohibits surrogacy, since few women would become surrogates solely for self-fulfillment or reasons of altruism.

The question, then, is whether we can reconcile paying the surrogate, beyond her medical expenses, with the idea of surrogacy as prenatal adoption. We can do this by separating the terms of the agreement, which include surrendering the infant at birth to the biological father, from the justification for payment. The payment should be seen as compensation for the risks, sacrifice, and discomfort the surrogate undergoes during pregnancy. This means that if, through no fault on the part of the surrogate, the baby is stillborn, she should still be paid in full, since she has kept her part of the bargain. (By contrast, in the Stern-Whitehead agreement, Mrs. Whitehead was to receive only $1,000 for a stillbirth.) If, on the other hand, the surrogate changes her mind and decides to keep the child, she would break the agreement, and would not be entitled to any fee, or compensation for expenses incurred during pregnancy.

C. THE RIGHT OF PRIVACY

Most commentators who invoke the right of privacy do so in support of surrogacy. However, George Annas makes the novel argument that the right to rear a child you have borne is also a privacy right, which cannot be prospectively waived. He says:

> [Judge Sorkow] grudgingly concedes that [Mrs. Whitehead] could not prospectively give up her right to have an abortion during pregnancy. . . . This would be an intolerable restriction on her liberty and under *Roe* v. *Wade*, the state has no constitutional authority to enforce a contract that prohibits her from terminating her pregnancy.
>
> But why isn't the same logic applicable to the right to rear a child you have given birth to? Her constitutional rights to rear the child she has given birth to are even stronger since they involve even more intimately, and over a lifetime, her privacy rights to reproduce and rear a child in a family setting.[13]

Absent a compelling state interest (such as protecting a child from unfit parents), it certainly would be an intolerable invasion of privacy for the state to take children from their parents. But Baby M has two parents, both of whom now want her. It is not clear why only people who can give birth (i.e., women) should enjoy the right to rear their children.

Moreover, we do allow women to give their children up for adoption after birth. The state enforces those agreements, even if the natural mother, after the prescribed waiting period, changes her mind. Why should the right to rear a child be unwaivable before, but not after, birth? Why should the state have the constitutional authority to uphold postnatal, but not prenatal, adoption agreements? It is not clear why birth should affect the waivability of this right, or have the constitutional significance which Annas attributes to it.

Nevertheless, there are sound moral and policy, if not constitutional, reasons to provide a postnatal waiting period in surrogate agreements. As the Baby M case makes painfully clear, the surrogate may underestimate the bond created by gestation, and the emotional trauma caused by relinquishing the baby. Compassion requires that we acknowledge these feelings, and not deprive a woman of the baby she has carried because, before conception, she underestimated the strength of her feelings for it. Providing a waiting period, as in ordinary postnatal adoptions, will help protect women from making irrevocable mistakes, without banning the practice.

Some may object that this gives too little protection to the prospective adoptive parents. They cannot be sure that the baby is theirs until the waiting period is over. While this is hard on them, a similar burden is placed on other adoptive parents. If the absence of a guarantee serves to discourage people from entering surrogacy agreements, that is not necessarily a bad thing, given all the risks inherent in such contracts. In addition, this requirement would make stricter screening and counselling of surrogates essential, a desirable side effect.

D. HARM TO OTHERS

Paternalistic and moral objections to surrogacy do not seem to justify an outright ban. What about the effect on the offspring of such contracts? We do not yet have solid data on the effects of being a "surrogate child." Any claim that surrogacy creates psychological problems in the children is purely speculative. But what if we did discover that such children have deep feelings of worthlessness from learning that their natural mothers deliberately created them with the intention of giving them away? Might we ban surrogacy as posing an unacceptable risk of psychological harm to the resulting children?

Feelings of worthlessness are harmful. They can prevent people from living happy, fulfilling lives. However, a surrogate child, even one whose life is miserable because of these feelings, cannot claim to have been harmed by the surrogate agreement. Without the agreement, the child would never have existed. Unless she is willing to say that her life is not worth living because of these feelings, that she would be better-off never having been born, she cannot claim to have been harmed by being born of a surrogate mother.

Children can be *wronged* by being brought into existence, even if they are not, strictly speaking, *harmed*. They are wronged if they are deprived of the minimally decent existence to which all citizens are entitled. We owe it to our children to see that they are not born with such serious impairments that their most basic interests will be doomed in advance. If being born to a surrogate is a handicap of this magnitude, comparable to being born blind or deaf or severely mentally retarded, then surrogacy can be seen as wronging the offspring. This would be a strong reason against permitting such contracts. However, it does not seem likely. Probably the problems arising from surrogacy will be like those faced by adopted children and children whose parents divorce. Such problems are not trivial, but neither are they so serious that the child's very existence can be seen as wrongful.

If surrogate children are neither harmed nor wronged by surrogacy, it may seem that the argument for banning surrogacy on grounds of its harmfulness to the offspring evaporates. After all, if the children themselves have no cause for complaint, how can anyone else claim to reject it on their behalf? Yet it seems extremely counterintuitive to suggest that the risk of emotional damage to the children born of such arrangements is not even relevant to our deliberations. It seems quite reasonable and proper—even morally obligatory—for policymakers to think about the possible detrimental effects of new reproductive technologies, and to reject those likely to create physically or emotionally damaged people. The explanation for this must involve the idea that it is wrong to bring people into the world in a harmful condition, even if they are not, strictly speaking, harmed by having been brought into existence. Should evidence emerge that surrogacy produces children with serious psychological problems, that would be a strong reason for banning the practice.

There is some evidence on the effect of surrogacy on the other children of the surrogate mother. One woman reported that her daughter, now 17, who was 11 at the time of the surrogate birth, "is still having problems with what I did, and as a result she is still angry with me." She explains, "Nobody told me that a child could bond with a baby while you're still pregnant. I didn't realize then that all the times she listened to his heartbeat and felt his legs kick that she was becoming attached to him."[14]

A less sentimental explanation is possible. It seems likely that her daughter, seeing one child given away, was fearful that the same might be done to her. We can expect anxiety and resentment on the part of children whose mothers give away a brother or sister. The psychological harm to these children is clearly relevant to a determination of whether surrogacy is contrary to public policy. At the same time, it should be remembered that many things, including divorce, remarriage, and even moving to a new neighborhood, create anxiety and resentment in children. We should not use the effect on children as an excuse for banning a practice we find bizarre or offensive.

CONCLUSION

There are many reasons to be extremely cautious of surrogacy. I cannot imagine becoming a surrogate, nor would I advise anyone else to enter into a contract so fraught with peril. But the fact that a practice is risky, foolish, or even morally distasteful is not sufficient reason to outlaw it. It would be better for the state to regulate the practice, and minimize the potential for harm, without infringing on the liberty of citizens.

NOTES

1. Had the Sterns been informed of the psychologist's concerns as to Mrs. Whitehead's suitability to be a surrogate, they might have ended the arrangement, costing the Infertility Center its fee. As Chief Justice Wilentz said, "It is apparent that the profit motive got the better of the Infertility Center." In the matter of Baby M, Supreme Court of New Jersey, A-39, at 45.
2. "[W]e think it is expecting something well beyond normal human capabilities to suggest that this mother should have parted with her newly born infant without a struggle. . . . We . . . cannot conceive of any other case where a perfectly fit mother was expected to surrender her newly born infant, perhaps forever, and was then told she was a bad mother because she did not." *Id.* at 79.
3. Father recalls surrogate was "perfect." *New York Times*, January 6, 1987, B2.
4. *Id.*
5. In the matter of Baby M, *supra* note 1 at 8.
6. Annas GJ: Baby M: babies (and justice) for sale. *Hastings Center Report* 17 (3): 15, June 1987.
7. In the matter of Baby M, *supra* note 1, at 75.
8. Anger and anguish at Baby M visitation hearing. *New York Times*, March 29, 1988, 17.
9. Dworkin G: Paternalism. In Wasserstrom RA, ed., *Morality and the Law.* Belmont, Cal: Wadsworth, 1971;

reprinted in Feinberg J, Gross H, eds., *Philosophy of Law*, 3rd ed. Wadsworth, 1986, p. 265.

10. Warnock M, chair: *Report of the committee of inquiry into human fertilisation and embryology*. London: Her Majesty's Stationery Office, 1984.

11. Robertson JA: Surrogate mothers: not so novel after all. *Hastings Center Report* 13 (5): 29, 1983. Citing Parker

P: Surrogate mother's motivations: initial findings. *American Journal of Psychiatry* (140): 1, 1983.

12. Harris J: *The Value of Life*. London: Routledge & Kegan Paul, 1985, p. 144.

13. Annas, *supra* note 6.

14. Baby M case stirs feelings of surrogate mothers. *New York Times*, March 2, 1987, B1.

Families, the Marketplace, and Values

Thomas H. Murray

If collaborative reproduction is viewed positively, reproduction contracts become the instruments of reproductive freedom....In liberal society, the invisible hand of productive preference must be allowed to flourish, despite the qualms of those who think it debases our humanity.

—JOHN A. ROBERTSON, "Embryos, Families and Procreative Liberty"

Surrogacy is like slavery in the absence of reciprocity, in the fact that one person becomes what Aristotle called an "animated tool" of another, serving simply as a means to another's end.

—DAVID H. SMITH, "Wombs for Rent, Selves for Sale?"

There are times when adults hunger for children. *Hunger* is the right word, for it can be felt as a need, a profound longing, not a mere appetite for something pleasant. When we speak of the suffering of people who want to have children but cannot, "suffering" is neither metaphor nor hyperbole: people who crave children to raise and love but cannot have them suffer because, for many of us, our children are a vital part of our own flourishing. The chief moral impetus behind alternative reproductive practices—from medical interventions to surrogacy contracts—is the desire to ease the suffering of infertility.[1]

Despite this worthy purpose, these new arrangements inspire wariness. They are accused of intensifying medical, especially male, control over reproduction; of treating women as nothing more than vehicles for reproduction; of treating children as commodities or products; and of threatening the intimacy of natural reproduction. The uneasiness lingers despite responses that can be given to each of the particular complaints.

Rather than rehearse these arguments, I want to see if it is possible to uncover the root of our discomfort. Could our uneasiness with certain alternative reproductive practices stem from a sense that they threaten to undermine the very values that prompted us to create these alternatives in the first place? In particular, do the values of the marketplace, with their exaltation of individual liberty, control, and choice, endanger what we value in family life?

Suppose the answer to this question is yes. How could such self-defeating practices have emerged? In brief, the story is this: Proponents of alternative reproductive practices defend them as expressions of procreative liberty. This is not surprising. Liberty is a powerful principle with great resonance in our political and moral traditions. We rely heavily on liberty to defend the option *not* to reproduce by using contraceptives or abortion. If we are free to avoid having children, shouldn't we have equal freedom to pursue parenthood? The fallacy here is a presumption that the choice *to have* a child is morally parallel to the choice *not to have* a child. The former is a choice to initiate a very special human relationship; the latter is a choice to decline such a relationship. The values at the core of the parent-child relationship constrain the former in ways they do not affect the latter.

The story also concerns the tapestry in which negative liberty is such a prominent strand. Negative liberty is freedom *from*, the liberty to do as one wishes without the interference of others. Great principles like liberty do not stand in isolation. They draw their strength from a culture's traditions; those same traditions link liberty so closely with other values that they become a kind of web, each strand supporting and supported by the other strands. In the web of values supporting alternative reproductive practices, liberty is interwoven with an emphasis on the individual who bears rights in sometimes isolated splendor. The web also contains strong threads representing the value we place on choice and control. The model of human relationship favored in this web is the contract, the free agreement of independent, autonomous actors. The social institution that best fits with these strands—liberty, individualism, choice, control, contract—is the market. If you frame your response to the needs of the infertile and childless in terms of procreative liberty, you will find yourself in the web that includes these other values. Buying and selling reproductive products and services—sperm, ova, embryos, and gestation—will appear as straightforward expressions of that liberty. It will become difficult to see why we should be more wary of choice and control here than in other spheres of life.

I want to try to understand the ethics of alternative reproductive practices by reflecting on what we value about having children and living in families. What we discover there will give us a different perspective on those practices. It will allow us to distinguish morally permissible arrangements from those that threaten to undermine what we value about families and parent-child relationships. It will also help us to make sense of our often inchoate fears about the excesses committed in the pursuit of parenthood. . . .

RETHINKING PROCREATIVE LIBERTY

Alternative reproductive practices challenge our notions of family because they expose what has been at the core of the family—creating and raising children—to values more at home in the mar-

ketplace. To some champions of new reproductive arrangements, a set of values fits neatly together. Respecting liberty and privacy means that people in pursuit of their reproductive goals may make agreements with other people to help them reach those goals. In this line of reasoning the fees we pay to purchase gametes or embryos or the services of a gestational mother are no different from the fees we pay physicians and laboratories. Liberty and privacy mesh neatly with concepts of contract and property. Crudely put, in this way of thinking about human reproduction, if people desire to obtain a child, they have a right to pursue that goal, just as they have a right to fulfill their desire for fresh bread by buying a bread machine. We put stricter boundaries on the pursuit of babies than on the pursuit of bread machines. In neither case do we think it is permissible to walk into a place where the desired items lie (respectively, a newborn nursery and an appliance store), slip one under your coat and walk out with it. At a minimum, we insist on a mutually voluntary transfer. The two kinds of goods—bread machines and babies—do differ. We forbid the sale of used versions of the one type (three-year-old children) while feeling completely comfortable with a market in used versions of the other (that is, three-year-old bread machines).

By now, this discussion will strike some readers as utterly bizarre—because it is.[2] Something is out of joint here. Babies are not bread machines. Both can smell very good in the morning (though the baby may need a change and bath first). But the person who supplies the genetic material or gestation for a baby has a different relationship to that infant than the manufacturer or seller of a bread machine has to that appliance.

In the realm of commerce, moral relationships are relatively simple. These are owners and property and prospective buyers. The property has no independent moral significance. Its "worth" is measured fully by the price agreed upon by buyer and seller. The relationship of buyer and seller is governed by contract, an agreement that specifies in often precise detail what each party expects from the other. The relationship between buyer and seller is merely instrumental to the exchange of goods. I give you, the store owner, $150; you give me the bread machine. In the realm of parents and children, of family, the new additions—that is, children—have a more complex moral status than mere property (though children have been so regarded at times). And the relationships among the various parties who may be involved in providing babies—suppliers of gametes, gestational services, and those who wish to rear the children—are more complex as well, to say nothing of the relationships between each of those parties and the children they create. Indeed, it could be said that the main point in having a child is to initiate the relationships that will develop between that child, its siblings, and the adults in its life.

Proponents of strong individual rights in reproductive technology generally acknowledge the great moral importance of children. The importance, for advocates, helps explain why the liberty to pursue parenthood is even more important than the liberty to pursue more prosaic commercial transactions. A fundamental problem remains: We recognize that thinking of children as property, and of family life as essentially a series of commercial transactions, is a grievous distortion. We know of cultures that have treated children as a form of property; indeed, there are practices in our society, in our adoption laws, for example, that appear to be surviving remnants of that idea.[3] It is also possible to analyze family relationships in economic terms. Economic analysis may help us understand how families interact with the larger world of markets. But it remains a fiction, not an insightful description of how families function or, more important, why people live in families. We probably all know families in which relationships have deteriorated so badly that the individuals in them treat each other like untrustworthy business associates. But we recognize those as failed families that could not achieve the abiding relationships of trust, equity, and love to which families aspire, and so had either to split apart or to fall back on relationships based more on contracts than on loyalty and affection. . . .

. . . One of the most touching ironies in the debate over the ethical limits of reproductive technologies is that ideas about individual liberty and property rights are being advanced in the service of a desire to transcend individualism, constrain liberty (in at least one important sense), and nurture a sphere of human relationship in which property has no place. . . .

. . . Contemporary Americans overwhelmingly identify their family as the primary source of

meaning in their lives.[4] In a culture that celebrates autonomy and individualism, this may seem surprising. But our freedom is the liberty to seek or create meaning in our lives; it does not itself provide that meaning. We are deeply sociable creatures who find much of what gives our lives meaning in our enduring, intimate relationships. We share the most intimate and enduring ties within our families. . . .

"FAMILY VALUES" AND THE VALUES FAMILIES SERVE

It is important to head off one important potential source of misunderstanding. To understand the impact of new reproductive practices on the family, we will need to talk about the values integral to family life and the larger social values served by having families. Here is the problem: the phrase "family values" has become a political slogan, a shorthand for a lengthy catalog of political views, ranging from an affirmation that families are important to advocacy of narrowly limited roles for women, attitudes toward corporal punishment and prayer in school, condemnations of homosexuality, and a host of other moral and political positions.

"Family values" in contemporary American politics has become synonymous with the views of a narrow portion of the political Right. However, both Right and Left in American politics share the blame for the sorry recent history of discussions of values and the family. The Right has promoted its particular roster of positions as *the* only legitimate values associated with family life. At the same time it implied that those who disagree have *no* values worth mentioning. The Left, for its part, did virtually nothing to challenge the Right's claim to a monopoly on values. This was due in part to a greater tolerance for diversity, but also, I believe, to the suspicion that to affirm any set of substantive values was inherently oppressive. The characteristic view seemed to be that we should throw all questions back to what each individual would freely choose, on the assumption that this would be wholly liberating. Individuals, that is, should be free to do anything—except talk seriously about what might be good for themselves and others that people would *not* always freely choose.

Rather than attack the Right for promoting a narrow and occasionally mean-spirited set of values for the family, the Left effectively ceded the entire issue of values and the family to the far Right. The great bulk of the American public, however uncomfortable they might be with portions of the Right's agenda, knew that values and families were important, but got mostly an embarrassed silence from the Left. Other than an espousal of liberty and justice, and a defense of diversity, the Left was reluctant to talk about values. This, I believe, was one of the great failures of American political life in the 1970s and 1980s. The only way I know to reinvigorate that political and moral debate is to call us back to the reasons why people make families—to the crucial values served by families. But to do that requires first taking a closer look at the way the debate over the ethics of new reproductive technologies typically has been framed—as a weighing of fundamental individual rights against an array of vague concerns.

Advocates of alternative reproductive practices tend to dismiss the misgivings people express as misunderstandings, superstitions, or concern about mere "symbolic harm."[5] But I want to take seriously the possibility that the discomfort people feel at a practice such as commercial surrogacy has legitimate concerns at its root. Intellectuals may be overly eager to reject such concerns. When the culture's ideology supports values that exclude, or are incongruous with, the sources of misgiving— when the language of individual rights, property, consent, and contract disguises what is morally significant about families—it becomes difficult to take seriously or to give effective voice to what is genuinely valuable in family life.

We should not overemphasize the distinction between the sphere of the family and the spheres of the market and politics. Family life intersects with these other spheres in countless ways. But it would also be a mistake to collapse the distinction, to see family life as essentially the same as life in these other spheres. Collapsing the distinction ignores what is obvious to anyone who has lived within a modestly well-functioning family: that families serve very important values, values not served at all well by the marketplace or the public forum. For one thing, well-functioning families are the locus for the development of emotionally and physically healthy children. Families are also a principal site

for the emotional and moral development of adults. Families provide the setting for nurturing relationships characterized at their best by love, loyalty, and a healthy measure of forgiveness.

Of course, even in the best of families not all things go well. And many families are riven by anger, cruelty, and bitterness. When we think about families we must avoid the temptation to romanticize, to picture only one type of family as the ideal, to deny the ambivalence that infuses even the best of family relationships. Nevertheless, even in troubled families children can experience love, learn that some people are trustworthy, and develop a sense of their own worth and efficacy. We need to be realistic about the many difficulties families encounter or cause, about the rich varieties of ways in which people make families. But we must not allow cynicism, which is sometimes justified, to blind us to what is valuable in families.

Love. Loyalty. Affection. Forgiveness. Trust. Care. Nurturing. Maturation. This is a partial list of the values families serve. But I believe that it will be a recognizable list to most late-twentieth-century Americans. For that matter, it should not have seemed strange to a literate American in the mid-1800s. The ideal of companionate marriage and the view that children are creatures to be nurtured and loved, rather than little demons to be broken, were already a part of American popular culture nearly one hundred fifty years ago.[6] Nor would it surprise me to learn that many of these values were present in far distant times and cultures. John Boswell's study of child abandonment in ancient Rome and medieval Europe suggests that some parents were at least as fond of their children as contemporary Americans fancy themselves to be.[7] A study of eighteenth-century families in the Chesapeake region of Virginia and Maryland likewise found abundant evidence for great affection between parents and children—and great grief when, as often happened, the child died.[8] Thomas Jefferson, probably the best-known resident of that place and time, wrote to his daughter about his hope that his granddaughter "will make us all, and long, happy as the centre of our common love"[9]

Families, although they constitute a distinctive sphere of human life, do not and cannot exist in isolation. Just as children need families and many adults need children, so do families need supportive social institutions and communities. Without a web of support in the wider culture, individual families may collapse under the weight of external blows and the inevitable injuries that even the best of families inflict on themselves.

The values we think of as crucial to family life tend either to be found only in the context of relationships—love, loyalty, affection, trust, care—or, given our social natures, to depend utterly on a foundation of good, enduring relationships—identity, self-confidence, maturation. The centrality of relationships in the values important to families points up another contrast with the spheres of the market and politics. In the market, relationships are secondary to the fair and efficient exchange of goods and services: I deal with you not because I prize the intrinsic value of our relationship but because you have something I want, and vice versa. The relationship exists primarily to promote the exchange of goods. . . .

THINKING ABOUT VALUES AND THE FAMILY: JUSTICE AND INDIVIDUAL RIGHTS IN FAMILY LIFE

. . . Justice is important in families. Attentiveness to justice is necessary to prevent the wounds that family members habitually inflict on each other from becoming persistent, suppurating sores that drain moral and emotional strength and ultimately sicken the family. Justice is a kind of maintenance value in family life. If you don't keep it fresh and vigorous, then you will find it impossible to achieve the values families make possible. When some members of a family oppress and exploit other members, injustice corrodes that family from within. Families poisoned with injustice are poor soil for the growth of enduring love, loyalty, and intimacy.

In families we learn what it means to be just, and what it means to suffer the sting of injustice. I suspect we also learn, at a deep, nonrational level, that it is important to seek justice and to avoid injustice. Or, sadly, that it is fruitless to be just and that what really matters is becoming the oppressor, not the oppressed.[10]

Insisting, though, that justice be the predominant value in family life is a mistake. It's a very understandable mistake when we consider how readily injustice can seep into our lives as spouse,

parent, or offspring, and how pernicious it can be. The mistake is in forgetting why we make families. We enter families not to seek justice but to seek other values—love, learning to care for other people, enjoying the mutual affection and interdependence of parents and children. Justice is not the reason we make families, but it is crucial to any chance we have for achieving those values.

Like justice, the concept of individual rights has shortcomings in this sphere. Individual rights are blunt and clumsy instruments with which to understand the ethics of family life. Suppose you knocked on the door of all of the houses in your neighborhood with young children in them and asked the parents in each house why they feed their children. What sort of answers would you get? Most parents would think it was a very strange question. But I expect that they would usually mention two sorts of reasons: that children need to be fed and that making certain your child is well nourished is just one of those things that a good parent does. One answer I do not expect to hear is that they feed their children because they have a right to be fed.

Does this mean that these parents believe that their own children, or other parents' children, have no right to be fed? Hardly that. There are times when it seems appropriate—indeed necessary—to assert that a child's right is being ignored. If parents persistently fail to feed their child, then government child welfare agencies may intervene. The state's intrusion becomes necessary because of a grave breakdown within the family, a failure, for whatever reason, to provide one of the essential elements of child nurture. The language of rights, here, serves to justify state intervention into the sphere of the family.

Talk about "rights" works best when it is doing one of two things. First, we invoke rights when we want to erect boundaries against interference by others. The "others" may be the government, an institution or a corporation, or individuals. This sort of claim against interference by others is often called a negative right—for example, the right to be left alone or the right to privacy. Second, we sometimes use the language of rights to state a positive claim—a claim *to* something, such as a claim to be fed by you. One way of thinking is to presume that all cases in which you have a duty to provide me with certain goods or services are best expressed in terms of rights. But there are many circumstances in which the language of rights seems awkward and second best—for example, when talking about why parents feed their children. Perhaps it is more useful to see claims about positive rights as fallbacks—efforts to obtain something that could not be better assured by ties of affection or loyalty or by moral duties deeply ingrained into complex social practices, like parenting.

Understanding the moral intricacies of family relationships through a concept like individual rights is like opening a beautifully carved front door with an ax. It is undeniably effective; it thrusts the state into the middle of family life; it leaves a heavy toll of destruction in its path; and it is justified only by an emergency such as a fire. A fireman's ax, of course, is not the preferred way of opening your front door. Similarly, asserting that someone rights are being violated within a family may be necessary; it inflicts its own kind of violence; and it is wise to limit it to occasions when great harm would otherwise be caused.

The language of rights is a language most at home in the spheres of public life, government, and commerce. I have a right to keep you from trespassing on my land; I have rights of free speech and freedom from governmental interference into my political and religious activities; I have a right to go to court to ask that you fulfill the terms of the contract we both signed. In these spheres, the concept of a right is powerful and important and represents a great moral and political advance. The concept of universal human rights is a growing bulwark against oppression by governments that succumb to the temptation to abuse their own citizens.

Even outside the sphere of the family, however, talk about rights expresses only a small part of what is important in our moral relationships with one another. We do many things out of friendship, kindness, sympathy, and solidarity—not because you have a "right" to our friendship, kindness, sympathy, or solidarity. Indeed these sound like oxymorons: a "right" to my friendship? to my sympathy? If someone insisted that she or he had a right to my friendship, I might feel pity or annoyance; I would certainly feel that they failed to grasp something very important about the nature of friendship. The same is true of

efforts to understand the ethics of family life in terms of rights.

Because the decision whether to make a family, especially whether to have children, may be the most profoundly important life decision most individuals face, we are inclined to the language of rights in thinking about the ethics of such choices. But perhaps a moral concept most helpful for understanding our moral relationships with the state and with strangers in the marketplace is not as helpful in understanding family life. Especially a language that carries with it powerful connotations of property and that elevates choice to a position of near-supreme moral importance. Asserting a right to unlimited choice without regard for its meaning and impact in this sphere could threaten what we value about families. The language of rights with its close affinities for property and contract is an ill-fitting ethic for the family.

FINDING AN ETHIC THAT FITS

The values embedded in certain alternative reproductive practices form a constellation that aligns poorly with other values at the heart of family life. Two contrasting images of values and relationships within families illustrate the point.

The champion of procreative liberty celebrates control and choice and portrays decisions about whether and how to acquire children as similar to decisions to acquire other new entities, only more important than most. If choice is valued in selecting a new appliance, all the more should it be valued in selecting a new child. If we are permitted to make voluntary agreements to spend our money to obtain new objects, all the more important to allow us similar freedom of contract and commerce to obtain new children, with one caveat: the children should not be harmed.

The other image is harder to label. It sees a role for values like control and choice within families but insists that these are not the principal values for which we make families; it is aware of the tension between unbridled liberty and control, on the one hand, and the values at the core of family life, on the other. It is vigilant against the encroachment of marketplace values into the family sphere because it recognizes that in commercial relationships the goal is to purchase a good or service, not to deepen the relationship, whereas all that is most valuable in family life centers on nurturing relationships.[11] Potential ways of adding children to the family must be scrutinized to assure that they will not undermine the values sought in family life, now or in the long run. . . .[12]

The difference between the two images is clearest in their responses to surrogate motherhood for pay. How does a paid surrogate childbearer explain to her other children what has happened? Does she say, "Mommy loves her children so much that she wants to give another woman a chance to have her own children to love"? Does she add, "Oh, by the way, it also lets us buy groceries/pay off the mortgage/go to Disney World/finish the third floor"? What do her children think about their own security? Their relationship with their parents? What have they learned about the nature of the parent-child relationship? Have they learned that it is subject to the same harsh rules of supply and demand as any other commodity? Will such doubts make them more secure, contribute to their emotional development?

What of the surrogate herself? David H. Smith observes that the surrogate contract signed by Mary Beth Whitehead, biological mother of the famous Baby M, gave striking power over Mrs. Whitehead to William Stern, her fetus's biological father. Indeed, the contract gave Mr. Stern "rights Whitehead's husband would not have had if he and Whitehead had engendered a child." Smith grants the appeal of such control to the Sterns, but he worries about the "status they impose upon the surrogate, whose entire life is subordinated to 'the delivery of a product' for another."[13] He considers the analogy of surrogacy to slavery, admitting that there are important dissimilarities but insisting that "surrogacy is like slavery in the absence of reciprocity, in the fact that one person becomes what Aristotle called an 'animated tool' of another, serving simply as a means to another's end."[14]

We need to think not only about the impact on those directly and immediately involved but also about the values, practices, and institutions that affect families now and in the future. Are children likely to flourish in a culture where making children is governed by the same rules that govern the making of automobiles or VCRs? Or is their flourishing more assured in a culture where making children, and matching children with nurturing

adults, is treated as a sphere separate from the marketplace, a sphere governed by the ethics of gift and relationship, not contract and commerce?

My claim is not that a market in children, embryos, or gametes violates some abstract principle in the noumenal realm. Rather, it is that given the sort of creatures we humans are, our patterns of psychosocial development, our needs at different stages of our lives—given these facts, certain values, institutions, and practices support our mutual flourishing better than others. Specifically, the values of the marketplace are ill suited for nurturing the values, institutions, and practices that support the flourishing of children and adults within families. . . .

WHAT DIFFERENCE DOES IT MAKE?

If we set aside the moral framework of contract and market in favor of one more in tune with what we value about families, how would we regard alternative methods of reproduction? Most significant would be a shift in how we frame the moral question. The currently fashionable way to think about such matters is to place individual liberty and choice on one side of the balance and the harms caused on the other side. Robertson uses this strategy frequently and skillfully. His analysis of surrogacy provides a typical example.[15] Robertson emphasizes the voluntary nature of the agreement between the paying couple and the paid surrogate. He looks at potential harms to the couple and the surrogate as unlikely, not that different from other things we already tolerate, and in any event a consequence of their own free choice.

The child-product of the surrogacy contract is a more difficult story. But not much more difficult. The prospect of harms to such children could be dismissed as implausible or unproved, or as not so different from other practices we tolerate anyway, especially adoption. The parallel with harms to the adults involved in surrogacy ends there. Robertson, like other defenders of commercial surrogacy, cannot use the child's fictitious "consent" to justify any harms that might come to it. But he has another strategy. The child, he argues, benefits because "but for the surrogacy contract, this child would not exist at all. . . [E]ven if the child does suffer identity problems, as adopted children often do . . . this child has benefited, or at least has not been wronged, for without the surrogate arrangement, she would not have been born at all."[16]

Try now to imagine some novel method of bringing children into the world which this way of framing the issues would condemn, as long as the adults participating did so freely. Cloning human embryos? No problem. Cloning embryos, freezing some and thawing them out later for implantation in someone else? Still no problem. Implanting an aborted fetus's ovary, with its millions of yet-unripe eggs, into a woman's body, so that she might become pregnant with that fetus's ova? It is difficult to see how anyone who frames the argument as Robertson and other enthusiasts do could make a strong objection to the practice. Who is harmed? Not the woman who chose to abort the fetus and gave her consent to using its ovaries. Certainly not the woman or her spouse who wants this supply of healthy ova. As for any children born from these eggs, who could prove they would have been better off never existing?

Would it matter if the reason the woman desired the fetal ovary was her own infertility, or because she is thirty-five and wanted to avoid the increased risk of birth defects that comes from older eggs? Or that she and her spouse wanted children with blue eyes, or some other genetically linked characteristics? I doubt that Robertson or most other supporters of reproductive alternatives would embrace such bizarre practices. But, it is also hard to see how, given the way they structure the ethical balancing, they could argue persuasively against them. You would have to demonstrate harms of such magnitude and certainty to individuals who have not, by their own choice, accepted the risks, that they overwhelm the powerful presumption in favor of liberty. Robertson, for one, looks with favor on doing genetic screening on and then freezing embryos while a woman is young, "until education, career, or relationship goals are worked out. They can then be transferred to the woman when there is a lower risk of a handicapped birth than if fertilization occurred shortly before implantation."[17]

What of healthy fertile women, who want to have their own genetic child, but do not want to go through pregnancy? Robertson believes that "surrogacy for convenience . . . may turn out to be more acceptable if it proves to be an effective way for women to combine work and reproduction. . . . As long as surrogate interests are protected, an optimal situation for all might result from surrogacy for convenience, if one accepts the change in the concept of mother that it would appear to entail."[18] This is precisely the inexorable moral logic of the marketplace, a logic that sweeps everything before it, deterred only by compelling evidence of serious, direct harm to those who have not consented by virtue of their own participation. As for the children thus created, we would have to prove that they would have been better off never being born.

New York State's Task Force on Life and the Law argues that the way the question is framed essentially dictates the answer because it presupposes that the children in question already exist. The task force suggests an alternative framing: whether, given the disadvantages of commercial surrogacy for future children, the practice should be permitted in the first place.[19] We should extend the task force's question and ask if these alternative means of creating children support or interfere with what we value in family and parenthood. Would they, on balance, create not just individual parent-child relationships but the kind of relationships that foster mutuality, loyalty, and love; relationships that endure, that survive the inevitable occasions when the relationship is causing a great deal more pain than pleasure? Beyond individual relationships, would they help build social attitudes and institutions that support the flourishing of children and adults within families?

I am suspicious of practices such as paying gamete suppliers or surrogate child-bearers that thrust the values of the market into the heart of the family. It would be ridiculous to argue that all children born of such arrangements are irreparably damaged, or their relationships with their rearing parents warped. But I do not think it is silly to worry about the effect such practices have on our intimate relationships more generally and on parent-child relationships in particular. Unreflective ideological commitments can and do lead us astray, away from what we genuinely and deeply value. The attitudes and institutions that provide the absolutely necessary cultural support for what we value can be eroded, so gradually that we scarcely notice.

I agree with Robertson and other proponents of new reproductive arrangements about the enormous importance of children in the lives of adults. We both want to promote social practices that match children with nurturing adults. But where he regards contract and commercialization as "the instruments of reproductive freedom," I view them as, at best, threats and, at worst, inimical to the values families are meant to promote. They should be our culture's last resort, if we allow resort to them at all. Cultural meanings are shared creations, and their protection, or change, a shared project.

There is enough reason for concern to throw the burden of proof back onto the shoulders of proponents of marketplace values in reproduction. Show us that the practices you advocate do not threaten what we value about family life and that reasonable alternatives are lacking. Artificial insemination by vendor, for example, would not be justifiable because a nonmarket alternative exists—genuine donors.

To protect the few against the tyranny of the majority, the law may have to permit in the name of liberty some practices that we believe are unwise. But our moral vision must remain clear. If commercializing reproductive practices threatens cultural meanings and institutions, then our respect for political liberty does not require us to welcome such practices. Some commentators argue that procreative liberty is a fundamental constitutional right. Under our Constitution, the government must have a compelling purpose to justify interfering with a fundamental constitutional right. But other experts disagree with the claim that our reproductive rights encompass practices such as gestation for pay. Alex Capron and Margaret Radin conclude that the "claim that the right to privacy protects surrogacy may be more plausible for noncommercial than for commercial surrogacy; even if the Constitution should be understood as including a right to bear a child for someone else, it should not be interpreted as including a right to be paid for it."[20] They argue that there is no obstacle in the Constitution to prevent a community from banning commercial surrogacy agencies, brokers, or advertising. I believe that we should prohibit commercial surrogacy.

There is another kind of surrogacy—gift surrogacy. A woman who is willing to bear her sister's or best friend's child out of loyalty and affection is acting in harmony with the values we prize in families. I would urge caution on the part of everyone involved, but I see what she is doing as an act of generosity, an extraordinary gift. Despite the outward physiological similarity between surrogacy-for-love and surrogacy-for-pay, the meanings of the two acts could not be more different. The former builds on a relationship of affection to create new affectionate relationships. The latter transmutes the creation of a child into a commercial transaction—a sort of reverse alchemy, turning gold into dross.

I began this chapter with the vague uneasiness many people feel about some of the new reproductive alternatives, wondering if the qualms were the product of mere habit and superstition or if they sprang from well-founded concerns. I looked at the terms in which the public debate has been conducted, and found them severely wanting. Finally, I tried to recast that debate in terms more faithful to what we value about families and the relationships families make possible, in the hope that this recasting could help us make moral sense out of the proliferation of new ways to make children

Our concerns, I believe, were well founded. The uncritical celebration of procreative liberty and other marketplace values in reproduction is indeed a threat to what we value about families. Reproductive alternatives need to be examined in the light of those same values.

NOTES

1. It is difficult to find or invent a phrase that captures concisely and accurately the range of practices included in discussions about what are typically dubbed "new reproductive technologies." Not all are new, for example, artificial insemination, and not all of them involve sophisticated technology. One of the most controversial practices, surrogacy for pay, is notable primarily for its legal rather than its technological novelty. To avoid tedious repetition, I will use several variants including the old standby new reproductive technologies. They are meant to be taken as synonyms for alternative reproductive practices.

2. In an extraordinary article, Margaret Jane Radin considers the appropriate scope and limits of markets in human affairs. Responding to an economic analysis of rape, she notes that "for all but the deepest enthusiast, market rhetoric seems intuitively out of place here, so inappropriate that it is either silly or somehow insulting

to the value being discussed." Radin, "Market-Inalienability," *Harvard Law Review* 100 (1987): 1849, 1880. Radin and I agree on several points:

(1) that a market in surrogacy is problematic;

(2) that the dominant moral language in which the debate is conducted emphasizes a conception of liberty as negative liberty, a conception of the person that disguises the significance of nonmarket realms and leads readily to acceptance of the market as a central expression of human freedom;

(3) that a preferable alternative exists which emphasizes human moral development as essential to the growth of positive liberty and accepts certain limitations on negative liberty as they contribute to that development;

(4) that, as Radin puts it, "the rhetoric of the market . . . foster(s) an inferior conception of human flourishing" (pp. 1885–1886); and

(5) that a proper understanding of new reproductive arrangements requires the best understanding of human flourishing we can achieve.

3. See chapter 3, *The Worth of a Child*, "Adoption and the Meanings of Parenthood."

4. B. Berger and P. L. Berger, *The War over the Family: Capturing the Middle Ground* (New York: Anchor/Doubleday, 1983).

5. See any of the articles about reproduction by the distinguished legal scholar John A. Robertson, e.g., "Embryos, Families and Procreative Liberty: The Legal Structure of the New Reproduction," *Southern California Law Review* 59, no.5 (1986): 939. For a rejoinder, see Maura A. Ryan, "The Argument for Unlimited Procreative Liberty: A Feminist Critique," *Hastings Center Report* (July-August 1990): 6–12. Ryan writes, "attention to women's experience has taught feminists that there are no 'merely symbolic' harms; we interpret and shape experience through our symbols and therefore how we think about persons, events, and biological processes has a great deal to do with how we behave toward them" (p. 12).

6. See Bernard Wishy, *The Child and the Republic: The Dawn of Modern American Child Nurture* (Philadelphia: University of Pennsylvania Press, 1968), for an analysis of how children were portrayed in American popular culture. For a description of the rise of companionate marriage and the changes in family relations in the first century and a quarter after the Revolutionary War, see Michael Grossberg, *Governing the Hearth: Law and Family in Nineteenth-Century America* (Chapel Hill: University of North Carolina Press, 1985).

7. John Boswell, *The Kindness of Strangers: The Abandonment of Children in Western Europe from Late Antiquity to the Renaissance* (New York: Pantheon Press, 1988).

8. Daniel Blake Smith, "Autonomy and Affection: Parents and Children in Chesapeake Families," in Gordon, *The American Family in Social-Historical Perspective*, 209–228.

9. Letter from Thomas Jefferson to Mary Jefferson Randolph, 31 May 1791, in Sarah N. Randolph, *The Domestic Life of Thomas Jefferson* (New York: Frederick Ungar, 1958), 202.

10. See Susan Moller Okin for an occasionally scathing view of injustice in family relationships and the failure of moral theorists to confront it effectively. Okin, *Justice, Gender, and the Family* (New York: Basic Books, 1989).

11. Even incursions of the market as simple as children's allowances must be handled carefully. See Viviana Zelizer, *Pricing the Priceless Child* (New York: Basic Books, 1985).

12. David H. Smith makes a related distinction. In a discussion of surrogacy, he describes alternative "ways of thinking about a woman's relationship to a child she bears and indeed to her own reproductive processes. In one of these perspectives the relationship between self and reproductive involvement is extrinsic and contingent. Pregnancy is viewed externally and objectively as a temporary state one is in for any one of a number of reasons. The self calculates its reasons for pregnancy, mode and form of personal involvement . . . . Another perspective on body is also possible: I identify with my body. I not only control it, but I have to listen to it . . . . I have embodied involvements with others, involvements that are constitutive of me as a self. These constitutive, involving embodiments are clearest in our relations with our parents and our children." Smith, "Wombs for Rent, Selves for Sale?" *Journal of Contemporary Health Law and Policy* 4 (1988): 30–31.

13. Smith, "Wombs for Rent, Selves for Sale?" 33.

14. Ibid, 34.

15. John A. Robertson, "Surrogate Mothers: Not So Novel After All," *Hastings Center Report* 13, no. 5 (1983): 28–34.

16. Ibid., 29.

17. Robertson, "Embryos, Families and Procreative Liberty," 1030.

18. Ibid.

19. New York State Task Force on Life and the Law, *Surrogate Parenting: Analysis and Recommendations for Public Policy* (1988). The task force concluded unanimously that public policy ought to discourage surrogate parenting and proposed legislation to ban fees to surrogates or brokers and to void surrogacy contracts. Their response to the argument that children born under surrogacy arrangements are better off because otherwise they would not have been born at all is as follows:

But this argument assumes the very factor under deliberation—the child's conception and birth. The assessment for public policy occurs prior to conception when the surrogate arrangements are made. The issue then is not whether a particular child should be denied life, but whether children should be conceived in circumstances that would place them at risk. The notion that children have an interest in being born prior to their conception and birth is not embraced in other public policies and should not be assumed in the debate on surrogate parenting. (p. 120)

I am grateful to John Arras for pointing out this argument to me.

20. Alexander M. Capron and Margaret J. Radin, "Choosing Family Law over Contract Law as a Paradigm for Surrogate Motherhood," *Law, Medicine & Health Care* 16, nos. 1–2 (1988): 34, 40.

And Baby Makes Three—or Four, or Five, or Six: Redefining the Family After the Reprotech Revolution

R. Alta Charo

Biology employs definitions in a way that is useful to the study of *biology*, not law. Thus, the definition of "father" is that of male progenitor. This helps biologists to trace genetic inheritance patterns. The legal category of "father," however, is similar but not entirely co-incident. Indeed, the law recognizes this fact when it presumes the husband of a married woman to be the "legal father" of the children she conceives during the marriage, even though a "biological" father may exist elsewhere.

Still, the *impulse* to equate legal parentage with biological parentage is present. By and large, U.S. law gives preferential legal status to the biological mother and father of a child. And this accounts for the judicial panic that took place when the biological definition of "mother" suddenly became ambiguous with the advent of gestational surrogacy and egg donation, techniques that separate genetic from gestational maternity. Suddenly, in order to identify the woman with legal priority, courts had to either twist biological definitions to suit social needs (such as defining a gestational

surrogate as a "human incubator") or to re-examine the reasons *why* biological parents are given preference, in order to determine which form of biological maternity most closely served those social goals.

The latter exercise, in turn, opened up for question the entire presumption in favor of biological parents, as courts were asked to consider, at base, the values to be protected by choosing specific individuals to be the preferred legal parents. Indeed, the unreflective use of biological definitions of mother and father to assign priorities in legal rights has been attacked by many for unnecessarily barring polygamous, polyandrous, and homosexual parenting groups that offer every prospect of providing loving and stable care to their children.

Our emotional attachment to a definition of family based on blood, our modern tendency toward a definition based on contract, and our legal definitions based on fictional re-creations of the biological nuclear family are all ripe for reform and integration. The result could be an expansion in the number of adults recognized as having parental ties to a particular child, an end to unthinking opposition to gay and lesbian or group marriage, and a flowering of classical liberal theory, in which the role of government is to facilitate individual choice rather than shape it.

This redefinition of "family" is timely for many reasons. First, the increased frequency of divorce

Wisconsin Women's Law Journal, Vol. VII: 1, 1992–1993. Reprinted with permission of the *Wisconsin Women's Law Journal*.

EDITOR'S NOTE: This article has been edited, and most of the notes have been omitted. Readers wishing to follow up on sources should consult the original.

and step-parenting has made traditional allocations of parental rights and responsibilities unworkable in light of the day to day experience of children living with "step-parents." Second, the frequency of single persons and gay and lesbian couples seeking to parent has strained the two-person, two-gender model of parenthood. Third, the advent of so-called "gestational surrogacy" has clouded identification of "biological" maternity, thus for the first time opening the door to an examination of just what it is about biological parenthood that entitles it to such extraordinary respect.

Finally, the human genome project promises to usher in an era of genetic exploration and invention. As with nineteenth-century advances, this knowledge may well become the basis for profound shifts in public thinking and public policy, just as Darwinian evolutionary theory became the basis of Spencerian libertarian theory and subsequent eugenic social policy. With increasing understanding of genetic influences on physical and psychological phenotypical expression comes the temptation to identify genetic coding as the ultimate expression of personal identity, and genetic linkages as the fundamental expression of human relationships. But such a development would be overly reductionist and lead to unfortunate public policy.

Indeed, the tragic stories of Baby Jessica, Kimberly Mays, and Baby Pete, which captivated the American public in 1993, demonstrate beyond question that simplistic and reductionist approaches fail to capture the emotional complications and the public attitudes toward parenting. In those three cases, a child ended up with her biological parents (Jessica), rearing parent (Kimberly), and both (Pete). These three cases tested the sympathies of the American public, which wavered wildly among preferring biology over adoption, intention over genetics, and happiness over everything. They demonstrated that the law's attempt to make biology (read: genetics and gestation) and contract (read: adoption and surrogacy) yield to public policy (read: heterosexual, marital families that resemble biological families in the wild) is flawed, because no one of these factors can easily and consistently outweigh all the others.

The essay will review the inconsistencies in European and American legal definitions of the family. Following a description of the competing claims of gestational, genetic, and contractual relationships to preferential treatment in cases of contested parenthood, the paper concludes that each type of relationship has been made to yield to significant nonbiological concerns. Thus, over time, biology and intent to parent have been sacrificed to the need for orderly transmission of property between generations, stability of marital units as the fundamental structure of social organization, and finally, protection of children's perceived best interests.

As it appears that social policy provides an acceptable reason to violate the integrity of parent-child relationships, this paper argues that social policy could similarly be used to maintain that integrity. While eschewing empirical arguments on the administrability or psychological superiority of expanded family definitions as beyond the scope of this paper, the paper does maintain that the compartmentalization, commercialization, and contractualization of reproductive materials and relationships offers an intriguing opportunity to re-examine some of the assumptions of current family law.

Specifically, the paper argues that the preference for heterosexual couples as parents is unwarranted, and that single persons, gay and lesbian couples, and larger groups of adults may serve equally well as parents. Furthermore, expanding the definition of parenthood to permit all genetic, gestational, and contractual parents to be recognized permanently and simultaneously could spare courts the task of identifying which adults to discard from the child's life. This abandonment of legal fictions—which maintain that a child has at most two parents of different gender, regardless of biological and psychological reality—is a recognition that law need not slavishly follow cramped visions of nature but could instead facilitate broad visions of justice.

THE GENETIC MODEL OF THE FAMILY

The blood ties between parent and child have almost mythological significance in every culture. They represent both the act of procreation and the physical reflection of the parent's body in the body of the child. The importance of genetic ties is confirmed by research suggesting that many psychological attributes may also be influenced by genetic heritage, although environmental influences may swamp these effects. "In sum," states one commentator, "it is only natural that our sublime and complex feelings regarding this issue reflect precisely the sentiment that law should preserve as a family unit that which nature has rendered genetically similar."[1]

The emotional significance of that biological link became enshrined in religious traditions that grappled with death and the finiteness of humankind. Many cultures and religious traditions, such as Judaism, hold that there is no formal "afterlife." Rather, we live on through our children, a kind of limited, genetic immortality. Their memories of us continue our existence. And when the memories fail, a small part of ourselves, our genes and our traits, still persist. It is no coincidence, then, that Jewish tradition dictates that a man marry his brother's widow if the brother should die childless. To do less would be to allow the brother's genes to go untransmitted, surely condemning him to true death.

"The significance of the genetic connection between parent and child," writes one commentator, "undoubtedly is part of what makes infertility a painful experience. While adoption may satisfy one's desire to nurture for a child, adoption cannot satisfy the yearning to create the child and to watch as a version of oneself unfolds and develops."[2] And it is the very fact that many reproductive technologies involve relinquishing access to children who are one's genetic progeny that has led some to condemn the practice as "unnatural" or "immoral."

But it is easy to place too much mystical importance on genetic connections. After all, there is no statistically significant genetic difference between a genetic parent and child and the genetic relationship between full siblings. It is the added psychological aspects of parenting that give the parental genetic connection such an entitlement to legal recognition. Nor should the fact that one's child shares one's genes become the basis for a property rights argument, in which the child is in some sense "owned" by the parent. Not only is this a dangerous doctrine that long led to child abuse and child labor, it fails to distinguish between owning the raw materials and owning the creation arising from them.

Thus, the emphasis on biological formation of families may overvalue the significance of genetic linkages. Further, it marginalizes some children and adults with a significant involvement in the family. It ignores, for example, the frequent presence in nonadoptive families of children with biological ties to only one of the parents. Such children, when unrelated to the *marital* partner of the mother, were until recently deemed illegitimate, severely disadvantaging them and their mothers.

The biological model of the family, with this overlay of insistence upon expressing biological relationships within a socially sanctioned, heterosexual marriage, has resulted in the creation of a grand presumption, to wit, that all "real" families follow this biological model.

But the reality has always been that some families have more than two parents. Some became parents by virtue of biology, a bond that cannot be broken no matter how many legal proceedings are used to push the biological parents out of the child's life. Others became parents by contract, and by virtue of marriage to the child's mother or contract with the state created a psychological, economic, and legal relationship with the child. But the legal fiction that there can only be two parents was always maintained, possibly due to the fear that non-exclusivity of parental status would lead to hampered decisionmaking among the adults and thus thwart state efforts to make parents the primary providers of services and discipline to minors.

Developments in foster parenting and the explosion of step-parenting continued this trend of parental exclusivity. No third party could gain a permanent, legally recognized relationship with a child absent an extraordinary intervention by the courts or by the permanent withdrawal of the natural parents from the child's life. These biological, or "real," parents were given an almost unbeatable presumption in their favor when it came to contested custody and parenting cases, and when supplanted by nonbiological parents, they were made to disappear in order to recreate the illusion of a "biological" family. Thus this western tradition dictated that there could be only one of each type of parent, although other societies freely experimented with polygyny.

DISCARDING BIOLOGICAL RELATIONSHIPS TO FURTHER THE CONTRACTUAL MODEL OF THE FAMILY

At the same time, though, this seeming fascination with biology had a strong competitor—the need to find substitute parents when genetic linkages were missing or inconvenient. Adoption, a statutory creation not existing at common law though long taking place informally or with private legislation, is evidence of a strong social tradition that recognizes the purely social and psychological dimensions of parenting, even where these occur in the absence of biological ties. Yet even with adoption, adoptive parents may acquire parental status with respect to a particular child only after termination of the parental rights of the child's biological parents, particularly those of the natural mother. The "presumption of biology" serves as an irrebuttable legal presumption that the birth mother of the child is its legal mother and that adoption can take place only consequent to a termination of the parental rights of the birth mother.

In early Rome and in other ancient cultures adoption served a primarily religious function associated with ensuring a legitimate male heir to carry out sacred obligations. Even after the religious overtones vanished, civil law countries viewed adoption principally as a vehicle for perpetuating the adoptive parent's name and property rather than as a means of benefiting the adoptee. A more cynical explanation, therefore, of the romanticization of genetic linkages between father and child, and the degree to which adoption is structured to re-create families with clear lines of succession from a single father, rests on the needs of men to conserve their property for the benefit of only a few children, those to whom they are truly related by blood and whom they have, in a sense, contracted to sire.

In the United States, adoption began as a means for privatizing the cost of maintaining orphans. Although some attention was paid to the child's well-being, placement mainly served to privatize the cost of the child's education and care, while providing inexpensive labor to the adults taking in the child. It only later became grounded in child welfare, and that welfare was generally defined as re-creation of a biological-style family unit for the child to enter. Adoption statutes soon followed

suit, reflecting a slow shift in public attitudes from the notions of apprenticeship and service to the notion that child placement should primarily serve the welfare of the dependent child.

Modern adoption statutes are replete with statements that make it clear that the primary focus of today's adoption laws is the well-being of the adopted child. The requirement of many modern adoption statutes that prospective adoptive parents pass a rigorous screening process before the adoption is finalized illustrates this concern. In the case of the out-of-wedlock infant given to strangers for adoption, society generally deems it in the adoptee's best interests to make him a full-fledged member of his adoptive family, as though he had been born into his adoptive family.

Furthermore, it is widely believed that an adoptee's retention of ties with his biological family can undermine the psychological aspect of this assimilation. Thus, courts have described adoption statutes as "giving the adopted child a 'fresh start' by treating him as the natural child of the adoptive parent,"[3] in essence a "substitution of the adoptive in place of the natural family and severance of legal ties with the child's natural family."[4] And in the 1993 gestational surrogacy case *Johnson* v. *Calvert*,[5] which will be discussed more extensively *infra* the California Supreme Court wrote that:

> We decline to accept the contention of amicus curiae the American Civil Liberties Union (ACLU) that we should find the child has two mothers. Even though rising divorce rates have made multiple parent arrangements common in our society, we see no compelling reason to recognize such a situation here. The Calverts are the genetic and intending parents of their son and have provided him, by all accounts, with a stable, intact, and nurturing home. To recognize parental rights in a third party with whom the Calvert family has had little contact since shortly after the child's birth would diminish Crispina's role as mother.[6]

Thus, once created by statute, adoption was designed to use law to recreate the image of biological family unit. It required that the biological parents be permanently removed from the child's life and the adoptive parents substituted for them, a policy that would be followed in the 1990s by the permanent removal of inconvenient genetic or gestational parents. It was not possible for the child to be adopted without the natural parents relinquishing all parental rights and responsibilities. Under law, they became legal strangers.

DISCARDING BIOLOGICAL RELATIONSHIPS TO FURTHER MARITAL STABILITY AND MAINTAIN BIOLOGICAL APPEARANCES

The other important purpose to be served whenever deviating from biological definitions of the family was the preservation of the heterosexual marital unit. Thus, many states preserved English tradition and passed laws that created a presumption of paternity on the part of a mother's husband. Indeed, the husband did not have to be physically present at the time of conception. The Supreme Court recognized the importance of this policy by pointing out in *Michael H.* v. *Gerald D.* that if a husband, not physically incapable, was within 'the four seas of England' during the period of gestation, the court would not listen to evidence casting doubt on his paternity.

Common law went so far as to deny the biological father the opportunity to assert his own paternity of a child born to a woman married to another man, although it could be asserted *against* him by the mother or her husband. This generally remains true today, even though forensic uses of DNA testing now enable paternity determinations to be made with great accuracy.

Thus, the biological progenitor of a child does not enjoy a constitutional right to establish paternity for his own pleasure or to seek any form of legal recognition of the relationship if the mother of the child is married to another man, even where he has actively sought to establish a relationship with the child. In *Michael H.* v. *Gerald D.,*[7] a plurality of the Supreme Court held that a state may constitutionally deny a man parental rights with respect to a child he fathered during a liaison with the wife of another man, since it is the marital family that traditionally has been accorded a protected liberty interest, as reflected in the historic presumption of legitimacy of a child born into such a family. In this way, biological reality gives way to strong public policy considerations: that a child not be stigmatized by illegitimacy; that a husband should not be cuckolded against his will; that an adulterer not enjoy the

fruits of his sin; and that the appearance of a biological family unit be maintained whenever possible.

The conflicting interests here—the child's interest in having a recognized mother and father, men's interests in avoiding unwanted responsibility for non-biological children, and men's interests in having access to biological children—are difficult to reconcile in a coherent fashion. Neither biology nor contractual relationship is the clear trump. What *is* clear, however, is that these interests must be sorted out within the paradigm of a two-parent, heterosexual marital parenting unit. The solution of declaring both the husband and the progenitor as fathers is simply not available. The Uniform Parentage Act makes these policy considerations quite evident.

Thus, the genetic relationship between father and child is considered secondary to the public policy of maintaining the integrity of "traditional" marriage and of rearing children, as often as possible, within such confines. Where no such "traditional" family is available, however, for example when the child is born to a mother who is single or part of a lesbian couple, the law *does* permit the biological father to assert his paternal rights, *even* if he clearly stated his intention prior to conception to have no relationship to the child. This has been the case, for example, with sperm donors. The Supreme Court has elevated this principle to a constitutional level. Thus, a man achieves constitutional protection as parent of his child by virtue of the genetic relationship alone *if* there is no substitute male parent and he does not otherwise appear to waive the right.

With the advent of artificial insemination by donor (AID) services, courts and legislatures faced a fresh challenge. The procedure posed squarely the problem of determining whether genetic mixing without sexual intercourse constituted an affront to the marriage. Early on, courts held that it did, likening AID to adultery, although that trend was later reversed. Second, courts were called on to determine whether genetic parentage, by itself, would be recognized under law as equivalent to legal parentage. As in non-adulterous situations of nonmarital sexual intercourse, the answer generally was "yes." Without a husband available to substitute for the genetic father, biological linkage created legal parenthood.

But where the recipient of the donor semen is married, the presumption of spousal paternity comes into play, just as it does in situations of true adultery. Over half the states have passed laws specifically stating that a donor is not to be considered the legal father of a child conceived by a married woman. But if the woman is not married, she is either denied access to the service entirely, or the donor is potentially considered the legal father, despite the fact that she is resorting to AID specifically because she does not want the genetic father to have a legal status vis-a-vis the child. The hope is illusory that the magical desexualization of conception by using a syringe rather than intercourse will yield the protection of the law against unwanted intrusions by the genetic father.

THE PROBLEM OF DECEPTIVE APPEARANCES

At least with ordinary AID by married women, appearances of a typical, biologically related family can be maintained by discarding the inconvenient genetic parent. Not so with contract motherhood (more commonly known as surrogate motherhood). The wife of the genetic father, who intends to rear the child, is visibly un-pregnant. Therefore, she is disfavored as compared to the biological mother. For example, the New Jersey Supreme Court held that Mary Beth Whitehead (now Gould), the genetic and gestational mother of a child conceived with semen from Bill Stern, was still the legal mother of the child, the surrogacy contract notwithstanding. Bill Stern was the legal father, based on his biological relationship, despite the existence of Mary Beth's husband as a potential competitor for the title based on presumptions of husband paternity. And Mrs. Stern was left without any legal relationship to the child, despite the fact that she would be the child's custodial maternal figure. The result was prescient as well as self-fulfilling; in disputed cases, contract mothers generally retain parental status but lose custody.

DEFINING BIOLOGICAL RELATIONSHIPS

The effort to give biological relationships precedence over contractual and intention-based relationships (outside of a few special instances) is probably based on administrative considerations as much as on philosophical ones. A biological delineation of family seems to provide a bright-line definition, and presumably offers history and common sense as its policy underpinnings without any further explanation. But biology is not nearly as clearly defined as the law imagines; the recent separation of biological motherhood into its genetic and gestational components demonstrates the point. And when commentators begin to argue whether the genetic mother or the gestational mother should be granted the title "biological," it is usually argued in terms of which one fulfills the relevant "biological" function. But the "relevant" function here is the one which gives biology its entitlement to primacy, thus forcing a more explicit discussion of exactly what emotional or psychological or administrative goals are being furthered and exalted by current family law. This exercise is precisely why the advent of compartmentalized reproduction has led to the opportunity to re-examine assumptions, values, and the very definition of "family" to be used by American law.

The courts have confronted conflicts between a genetic mother and a gestational mother only twice, both times favoring the genetic over the gestational mother. In the first case, *Smith* v. *Jones*,[8] the proceeding was a "set-up" to allow the egg donor to adopt the child, and in accordance with the surrogate agreement, the surrogate did not contest the ruling. In the second, *Johnson* v. *Calvert,* the trial and appellate courts found that the definition of a "biological" relationship is that of genetic linkage.[9]

The reasons for favoring a genetic model of the family have already been discussed. But there are arguments to be made that where a conflict arises between genetic and gestational relationships for women, gestation should prevail. These include arguments based on prenatal and postnatal bonding, the harmful effects to the birth mother of forcibly removing the child, the physical involvement of the birth mother in bringing the child to term, and the administrative difficulties presented by a world in which no hospital and no physician can securely hand a newborn up from the birth mother's loins to her arms.

It would be simple enough, then, to state that the woman giving birth is the sole biological, and therefore legal, mother. This maintains appearances.

And it would effectively protect the egg donation programs that are beginning to flourish in states such as California, where women seek to use substituted gametes in the same way that men have done since the advent of AID. Those programs require that, as with sperm donation, the female gamete donor vanish into the mists of legal fictions.

But it would appear that this is not the approach of the California courts. In the *Johnson* case, the California appellate court held that a woman giving birth may be nothing more than a glorified wet nurse, and the child's real mother is the woman whose egg was used for the conception.

The attorney for the gestational contract mother, Anna Johnson, said his client wanted only "a profound parental relationship" with the boy she gave birth to more than two years ago. Sensing that his best chance was to argue that his client was the "natural" mother, who is given preference under California law in cases of disputed custody, Johnson's attorney argued that "the term 'natural mother' means the woman who gave birth. Crispina [Calvert, the female progenitor] is not the mother."

A lawyer for the Calverts argued that state statutory guidelines for determining parentage in the context of paternity suits clearly mandate that the genetic parents be declared legal parents. "We can't deny that Anna Johnson had an important role, but does that confer a legal prescription that she is a parent?" asked the lawyer; "I think not." But Johnson's lawyer responded by arguing that "[i]t is the relationship between the birth mother and her baby that is legally protected. It tortures the English language to say that a woman (like Mrs. Calvert) who was never pregnant and never gave birth meets the traditional definition of the term mother."

Nonetheless, the California appellate court upheld the trial court's conclusions, characterizing the woman who gave birth as merely a "foster parent" for the "natural" mother whose egg had been used. It never confronted the implications of its ruling for California's flourishing egg donation practices, in which genetic mothers expect to be treated as legal strangers from their genetic offspring, while birth mothers using purchased eggs expect to be treated as legal parents of their offspring.

The continued viability of the "traditional" family unit, one that mimics what happens in nature, was very much on the minds of the California Supreme Court justices when they heard oral argument on the case. Several seemed leery of the child ending up with a father and two legally recognized mothers. "Here we could have a genetic parent . . . and a gestational parent," said Justice Panelli. "Is that the traditional family unit?" Chief Justice Malcolm Lucas deplored the prospect of growing up with both a "mother" and a "genetic progenitor." And the court-appointed lawyer for the child argued: "The minor in this case can be served only by being raised in the traditional, two-parent family. To declare (Johnson) a parent would complicate the child's life—and has never been recognized under law."

One justice, however, did seem intent on examining the broader issues, asking whether it is possible to have two biological mothers. She also suggested during oral argument that one thing "seems to be forgotten in this tug-of-war. . . . What importance should be given to the child's best interests?" But the Calverts' attorney responded that the language of the Uniform Parentage Act, which defines a parent in terms of genetic linkages, already incorporates a child's best interests, i.e., that it is in a child's best interest to be considered the child of his or her genetic parents. The attorney did not comment, however, on the degree to which spousal paternity presumptions and adoption would therefore presumably not serve a child's best interests.

SO WHAT IS A "NATURAL" PARENT AFTER ALL?

The dilemma faced by the California appellate court, who insisted upon a single definition of "natural" mother but found that none will fit the needs of both egg donation programs and gestational surrogacy programs, is that it tried to move toward a contractual model of the family without having fully abandoned the old biological models. In fact, it is the very power of genetic relationships that is driving infertile people and the courts to find ways to regularize surrogacy and AID.

One of the reasons given by Bill Stern in the *Baby M* case for his decision to hire a contract mother was that his family had been wiped out in the Holocaust, and he wished to have blood relations with someone, somewhere. Egg donation is sought by women who want desperately to have the experience of being pregnant and giving birth to the child whom they will raise. AID is used so that women with infertile husbands can nonetheless have children to whom they are genetically related.

But in order to make this possible within the strait-jacketed confines of the western, heterosexual marriage, it is necessary that we simultaneously devalue the genetic and gestational relationships of the men and women who give or sell their gametes or their capability for gestation. Those biological connections must be considered less valuable than the contract these people signed when they became donors or surrogates. Unfortunately, the very fact that the infertile persons or couples who sought their services did not seek adoption to begin with testifies to the enormous significance of that biological tie. And the agreement the infertile partners of these biological parents have made to raise these children as their own testifies to the parallel significance of contractual agreements to take on these children as their own.

So if we insist upon a preference for "natural" parents, perhaps the definition of "natural" mother depends not upon biology but upon psychology —the intent to take the baby home. After all, what could be more "unnatural" than a woman who denies her own child? Consider two stories from Australia. In the first, Linda K. agreed to give a child to her sister. She gestated and gave birth to a child conceived with her infertile sister's egg. As she, the gestational mother, relinquished the child to the infertile sister who was the child's genetic mother, she denied feeling as if she was giving up her own baby girl: "I always considered myself her aunt." By contrast, Carol C. donated eggs to her infertile sister so the sister could become pregnant and give birth to a child of whom the infertile sister would be the gestational and rearing mother. Reflecting on her relationship with the resulting children, who were her genetic offspring, Carol said "I could never regard the twins as anything but my nephews." The two births occurred in Melbourne within weeks of each other.

But if the definition of the natural mother depends primarily upon the intention to take care of the resulting child, then another California court decision, in the Moschetta case, makes no sense. Cynthia and Robert Moschetta hired a woman to act as a contract mother because Mrs. Moschetta was infertile. The contract mother, Elvira Jordan, was impregnated with Mr. Moschetta's semen, and relinquished the child at birth to the hiring couple. Mrs. Moschetta cared for the baby at home for seven months, until the day Mr. Moschetta walked out on the marriage, taking the baby with him. In a three-way custody battle between Mr. Moschetta, Mrs. Moschetta, and the "surrogate," the California court promptly threw out the application of the one parent who had actually taken care of the child, day in and day out, for over half a year. Mrs. Moschetta, the court explained, was not the child's natural or (yet) adoptive parent, and therefore had no rights at all. An argument can be made for the moral priority of this intended mother; but for her and her husband, and their desire to have a child, there would be no infant and no need for Solomonic decisions.

The Moschetta case is reminiscent of controversies concerning foster care, where the Supreme Court has said: "[n]o one would seriously dispute that a deeply loving and interdependent relationship between an adult and a child in his or her care may exist even in the absence of blood relationship." Nevertheless, "the usual understanding of 'family' implies biological relationships, and most decisions treating the relation between parent and child have stressed this element." "In the end," states one commentator,

> the Court appeared to create a distinction based on natural law, arguing that the relationship between foster parent and child is a creation of the state, whereas the biological relationship between parent and child is grounded in a "liberty interest in family privacy [which] has its source, and its contours not in state law, but in intrinsic human rights, as they have been understood in 'this Nation's history and tradition.'" While marriage traditionally has been the most important type of relationship, ascription of paternal rights also may depend upon the type of nonmarital relationship.[10]

SHAPING THE FAMILY TO CONFORM TO PUBLIC POLICY NEEDS

Another possible explanation of all these seemingly inconsistent precedents is that courts are assigning parental status primarily to protect societal or child interests. Thus, the genetic father in the *Michael H.* case, who is both a psychological and biological father, is denied parental status because the mother's husband provides a substitute who fills important policy needs. Single women who become pregnant via intercourse or AID, regardless of the original intentions of the genetic father, are faced with court decisions declaring the donors to be the legal fathers. If such women are married, however, their husbands can substitute for the genetic father and provide the necessary camouflage. Egg donation poses no problem, as the egg donor simply vanishes in the face of the gestational mother who uses the egg to create a child for herself to rear. But where there are competing claims made to motherhood, based on psychological, gestational, and genetic factors, the maternal status seems to be assigned to the woman who has two out of three characteristics, a kind of "2/3" rule.

Carol C. from Australia, for example, may be genetically a mother, but she is not the "natural" (i.e. "legal") mother because it was her sister who wanted children and brought the twins to term.

"[U]nder our analysis," stated the California Supreme Court, "in a true 'egg donation' situation, where a woman gestates and gives birth to a child formed from the egg of another woman with the intent to raise the child as her own, the birth mother is the natural mother under California law.[11] And Mrs. Calvert in the *Johnson* case is the "natural" mother because she is genetically linked and she was the first one who wanted the child, thus having a "2/3" claim on the baby:

> Because two women each have presented acceptable proof of maternity, we do not believe this case can be decided without enquiring into the parties' intentions as manifested in the surrogacy agreement. . . . We conclude that although the [California legislation based upon the Uniform Parentage] Act recognizes both genetic consanguinity and giving birth as means of establishing a mother and child relationship, when the two means do not coincide in one woman, she who intended to procreate the child —that is, she who intended to bring about the birth of a child that she intended to raise as her own—is the natural mother under California law."[12]

Finally, the *Baby M* and *Moschetta* cases demonstrate that where there is a woman who has a genetic and gestational relationship to a child, another woman's intentions and desires will be irrelevant, even if it was those desires that initiated the sequence of events leading to conception and birth.

Looked at this way, it is evident that there is nothing sacred about either genetic *or* gestational linkages, or, for that matter, about psychological linkages. All are accommodated only to the extent that they are consistent with an overriding public policy in favor of placing children in homes with two parents, of different gender, and married to one another if at all possible.

This, then, opens the door to an explicit examination of *which* forms of biological relationship define "natural" parenting, *which* public policies are important enough to supplant our innate preference for favoring biological definitions of parenthood, and *why* we prefer when possible to place children in "traditional" homes, even at the expense of the interests of their genetic and gestational parents. Justice Kennard, dissenting in the *Johnson* case, argued:

> For each child, California law accords the legal rights and responsibilities of parenthood to only one "natural mother." When, as here, the female reproductive role is divided between two women, California law requires courts to make a decision as to which woman is the child's natural mother, but provides no standards by which to make that decision. The majority's resort to "intent" to break the "tie" between the genetic and gestational mothers is unsupported by statute, and in the absence of appropriate protections in the law to guard against abuse of surrogacy arrangements, it is ill-advised. To determine who is the legal mother of a child born of a gestational surrogacy arrangement, I would apply the standard most protective of child welfare—the best interests of the child.[13]

But while courts hold that primary custody should be granted to the parent who would best serve the interests of the child, these principles are not supposed to operate to remove a child from a fit parent merely to enhance the child's life chances. So if both of the biological mothers, one genetic and one gestational, are fit mothers, then deciding between them based on the best interests of the child is to deny that *either* woman should be treated as a biological mother, from whom no child could be taken unless she was shown to be unfit.

This then returns us to the question of biological primacy in gestational surrogacy. If one and only one woman must be chosen to be the "natural" parent, whom should it be? A majority of American courts, newspapers, and academic commentators have already adopted the term "natural" or "biological" mother to mean "genetic" mother, and write of conflicts between genetic and gestational mothers as that of "nature versus nurture." And perhaps it shouldn't surprise us, since many of these judges and commentators are men whose only possible biological links are genetic. They can never have "morning" sickness in the afternoon or swollen ankles in the eighth month, and so may find it difficult to relate to the physiological (read: biological) phenomena that are solely related to the fact of the pregnancy, not the genetic link between parent and child. In a man's world, biology begins and ends with the DNA chains that link one generation to another.

In a woman's world, however, pregnancy is indisputably a biological fusing of fetal and maternal bodies, health, and well-being. The imposition of a male definition on a uniquely female biological experience would almost be a bad feminist joke if it didn't have such potentially troubling consequences for women's liberties. Names are a form of classification that shape substantive rights. When Mary Beth Whitehead, a genetic and gestational parent, was called a "surrogate" instead of a "mother," the infamous *Baby M* case was already halfway decided, regardless of whether a preconception parenting contract should be enforceable. In the words of courts and commentators, a pregnant woman may be no more than a walking womb, a human incubator working on behalf of a future child. A month before the birth, one Michigan court declared that "plaintiff Mary Smith is the mother of the child to be born to defendant Jane Jones on or about July 1987.[14] In other words, a woman can be pregnant and already a legal stranger to the unborn child within her.

In a country that has seen prosecutors, hospital lawyers, and judges use court orders to stop pregnant women from smoking or to force them to undergo caesarean sections, it is frightening to imagine what could happen when it's not strangers but the "natural" and "legal" parents of an unborn child still in another's womb who are trying to ensure the gestational mother, this "foster parent," does everything the way they would have done it. A pregnant woman's sense of fused biological well-being may stand little chance against a legal property interest that others have in the fetus still within her body.

Thus, there are strong public policy arguments to be made in favor of a gestational definition of motherhood. And just as genetic parenthood has yielded to public policy in the cases of illegitimacy, AID, and adoption, so too could genetic maternity yield to gestational maternity. California's *Johnson* decision that a gestational mother can be no more than a foster parent to her own child is almost without precedent in the world. Only Israel, bound by unique aspects of religious identity law, has adopted a genetic definition of motherhood. Every other country that has examined the problem—including the United Kingdom, Germany, Switzerland, Bulgaria, and even South Africa with its race-conscious legal structure—has concluded for historical, ethical, or administrative reasons that the woman who gives birth is the child's mother.

MAKE ROOM FOR DADDY . . . AND PAPA, AND MOMMY, AND MAMA . . .

But in fact, there is a better solution than choosing between competing biological mothers, or between genetic and social fathers. We've already entered an era of "crazy making," where courts are re-examining the prejudice against polygamy when reviewing adoption requests by certain Mormon families, and are granting visitation rights to step-parents and the gay and lesbian partners of biological parents. The next step would be to toss out legal fictions altogether and recognize in court what has already happened in the physical world. Some children have three biological parents, not two. Some children have two biological mothers, not one. Acknowledging that two women are biologically related to the same child, that both women are "natural" mothers, does not necessarily determine which will have superior claims to raise the child. As every divorced parent in America knows, biology alone does not dictate custody.

Hundreds of children, most in San Francisco, New York, and other urban centers, grow up with multiple parents, usually due to arrangements among gay and lesbian couples and their friends of the opposite sex who were involved in the conception and birth. The lovers of the biological mother and father frequently take an active role in rearing children. Private contracts attempt to spell out relative degrees of involvement. Such co-parents argue that their children, far from being confused by the unusual circumstances, actually benefit from being exposed to a wider range of adult influences. These families are more significant than their numbers suggest because they challenge the foundation of laws based on the heterosexual, nuclear-family model.

Although the logistics can be complicated, co-parents reportedly say that their real problems stem from a legal system that fails to certify their families. As a result, the nonbiological parents in co-parenting arrangements often worry about their legal relationship to the child, and may even resort to judicial efforts to cement their relationships in situations where more legally secure parties would negotiate.

Thus, resolutions of cases concerning the opportunity of a lesbian woman to adopt her lover's biological child and thereby become a second, legally recognized mother are of great importance. A probate judge ruled in June 1992, for example, that Vermont's adoption law does not allow someone who is not married to a legal, custodial parent to become a second, adoptive parent of the legal parent's children. Despite this obstacle, though, family law is yielding. As of September 1993, California, the District of Columbia, Alaska, Vermont, New York, Texas, and Washington have taken the radical step of approving homosexual adoption in a manner that creates two parents of the same sex.

Perhaps it is time to take a great leap in family law. We could recognize that all biological relationships—genetic and gestational—are irrevocable. The emotional and medical significance of the bonds cannot be undone by signing a contract or adoption papers. The thousands of children who have wondered about the biological parents who gave them up for adoption or the sperm donors used to conceive them already know this. The numerous possibilities the Human Genome Initiative has identified for using a biological parent's medical history to help in the diagnosis or treatment of even late-onset disorders in the adopted-out children also testifies to this.

At the same time, the voluntary social responsibilities we take on when we adopt children are equally permanent, and no less profound. That is why so many adopted children, though they may wonder about their biological parents, take no action to find them. Forced by society to choose among various adults, these adopted children understand that the most important parent is the one who tries to stay around.

Why not give these children a break? Once a parent enters into a child's life, whether by virtue of genes, gestation, or declaration, there is an unbreakable bond of psychology and history between the two. Crispina Calvert, Anna Johnson, Elvira Jordan, Cynthia Moschetta, Linda K., Carol C., and Mary Beth Whitehead are all mothers to their children, just as Robert Moschetta, Michael H., and Bill Stern are fathers to their children. Even for those whose parents are absent due to contract, abandonment, or involuntary events there is a mutual tie of emotion, of wondering how the other is doing, and of moral responsibility.

In an age when courts have been forced to manage the untidy families created by divorce and remarriage, it is simply not enough to argue that it will be difficult to organize a regime of family law that accommodates the permanency of both contractual and biological (both genetic and gestational) ties. And having admitted already that stepparents and grandparents are indeed real family members, what legitimate obstacle remains to accepting the adults who enter family arrangements via group marriage or homosexual marriage? Surely we can be creative enough to create a new category, somewhere between custodial parent and legal stranger, that captures these relationships.

Certainly the administrative and emotional complications of recognizing as permanent all biological and contractual ties are daunting. Nothing better demonstrates this point than the case of

Kimberly Mays, whose biological parents were unwittingly separated from her, and whose attempts to form a relationship fourteen years later were eventually rebuffed by both their biological daughter and her rearing father. But this case is, thankfully, rare and unusual in its details. Empirical research on polygamous families, families with homosexual parents, and other nontraditional families may yet demonstrate that it *is* possible to recognize more than two adults, while also maintaining clear lines of authority and responsibility. While courts and legislatures may see the need to determine who has a primary role in raising the child, there may well be no need to cut these other people out entirely. Indeed, from the child's point of view, it may simply be wrong to do so.

It has been said that you can never be too rich or too thin. Shall we add, perhaps, that you can never have too many parents to love you?

NOTES

1. John L. Hill, *What Does It Mean to Be a "Parent"? The Claims of Biology as the Basis for Parental Rights*, 66 N.Y.U.L. REV. 353, 390 (1991).
2. Hill, *supra* note 1, at 389.
3. In re Estates of Donnelly, 81 Wash. 2d 430, 436 (1972).
4. *Crumpton* v. *Mitchell*, 303 N.C. 657, 664 (1981).
5. *Johnson* v. *Calvert*, 19 Cal. Rptr. 2d 494 (1993).
6. *Id* at 499 n. 8.
7. 491 U.S. 110 (1989).
8. *Smith* v. *Jones*, No. 85-532014 DZ (Mich. Cir. Ct. Mar. 14, 1986).
9. *Johnson*, 19 Cal. Rptr. 2d, 494.
10. Hill, *supra* note 1, at 381 (quoting *Smith*, 431 U.S. at 845 and *Moore* v. *City of E. Cleveland*, 431 U.S. 494, 503 (1977)).
11. *Johnson*, 19 Cal. Rptr. 2d at 500, n. 10.
12. *Id.*
13. *Johnson*, 19 Cal. Rptr. 2d at 507 (Kennard, J., dissenting).
14. *Smith* v. *Jones*, No. 85-532014 DZ (Mich. Cir. Ct. Mar.14, 1986).

SECTION 3

Cloning

Executive Summary: Cloning Human Beings

The National Bioethics Advisory Commission (NBAC)

The idea that humans might someday be cloned—created from a single somatic cell without sexual reproduction—moved further away from science fiction and closer to a genuine scientific possibility on February 23, 1997. On that date, *The Observer* broke the news that Ian Wilmut, a Scottish scientist*, and his colleagues at the Roslin Institute were about to announce the successful cloning of a sheep by a new technique which had never before been fully successful in mammals. The technique involved transplanting the genetic material of an adult sheep, apparently obtained from a differentiated somatic cell, into an egg from which the nucleus had been removed. The resulting birth of the sheep, named Dolly, on July 5, 1996, was different from prior attempts to create identical offspring since Dolly contained the genetic material of only one parent, and was, therefore, a "delayed" genetic twin of a single adult sheep.

This cloning technique is an extension of research that had been ongoing for over 40 years using nuclei derived from non-human embryonic and fetal cells. The demonstration that nuclei from cells

This is the Executive Summary of the report of the National Bioethics Advisory Commission: Cloning Human Beings.

*EDITORS' NOTE: Ian Wilmut is an Englishman working in Scotland.

derived from an adult animal could be "reprogrammed," or that the full genetic complement of such a cell could be reactivated well into the chronological life of the cell, is what sets the results of this experiment apart from prior work. In this report we refer to the technique, first described by Wilmut, of nuclear transplantation using nuclei derived from somatic cells other than those of an embryo or fetus as "somatic cell nuclear transfer."

Within days of the published report of Dolly, President Clinton instituted a ban on federal funding related to attempts to clone human beings in this manner. In addition, the President asked the recently appointed National Bioethics Advisory Commission (NBAC) to address within ninety days the ethical and legal issues that surround the subject of cloning human beings. This provided a welcome opportunity for initiating a thoughtful analysis of the many dimensions of the issue, including a careful consideration of the potential risks and benefits. It also presented an occasion to review the current legal status of cloning and the potential constitutional challenges that might be raised if new legislation were enacted to restrict the creation of a child through somatic cell nuclear transfer cloning.

The Commission began its discussions fully recognizing that any effort in humans to transfer a somatic cell nucleus into an enucleated egg involves the creation of an embryo, with the apparent potential to be implanted in utero and developed to term. Ethical concerns surrounding issues of embryo research have recently received extensive analysis and deliberation in our country. Indeed, federal funding for human embryo research is severely restricted, although there are few restrictions on human embryo research carried out in the private sector. Thus, under current law, the use of somatic cell nuclear transfer to create an embryo solely for research purposes is already restricted in cases involving federal funds. There are, however, no current federal regulations on the use of private funds for this purpose.

The unique prospect, vividly raised by Dolly, is the creation of a new individual genetically identical to an existing (or previously existing) person—a "delayed" genetic twin. This prospect has been the source of the overwhelming public concern about such cloning. While the creation of embryos for research purposes alone always raises serious ethical questions, the use of somatic cell nuclear transfer to create embryos raises no new issues in this respect. The unique and distinctive ethical issues raised by the use of somatic cell nuclear transfer to create children relate to, for example, serious safety concerns, individuality, family integrity, and treating children as objects. Consequently, the Commission focused its attention on the use of such techniques for the purpose of creating an embryo which would then be implanted in a woman's uterus and brought to term. It also expanded its analysis of this particular issue to encompass activities in both the public and private sector.

In its deliberations, NBAC reviewed the scientific developments which preceded the Roslin announcement, as well as those likely to follow in its path. It also considered the many moral concerns raised by the possibility that this technique could be used to clone human beings. Much of the initial reaction to this possibility was negative. Careful assessment of that response revealed fears about harms to the children who may be created in this manner, particularly psychological harms associated with a possibly diminished sense of individuality and personal autonomy. Others expressed concern about a degradation in the quality of parenting and family life.

In addition to concerns about specific harms to children, people have frequently expressed fears that the widespread practice of somatic cell nuclear transfer cloning would undermine important social values by opening the door to a form of eugenics or by tempting some to manipulate others as if they were objects instead of persons. Arrayed against these concerns are other important social values, such as protecting the widest possible sphere of personal choice, particularly in matters pertaining to procreation and child rearing, maintaining privacy and the freedom of scientific inquiry, and encouraging the possible development of new biomedical breakthroughs.

To arrive at its recommendations concerning the use of somatic cell nuclear transfer techniques to create children, NBAC also examined long-standing religious traditions that guide many citizens' responses to new technologies and found that religious positions on human cloning are pluralistic in their premises, modes of argument, and conclusions. Some religious thinkers argue that the use of somatic cell nuclear transfer cloning to create a child would be intrinsically immoral and thus could never be morally justified. Other religious thinkers contend that human cloning to create a child could be morally justified under some circumstances, but hold that it should be strictly regulated in order to prevent abuses.

The public policies recommended with respect to the creation of a child using somatic cell nuclear transfer reflect the Commission's best judgments about both the ethics of attempting such an experiment and our view of traditions regarding limitations on individual actions in the name of the common good. At present, the use of this technique to create a child would be a premature experiment that would expose the fetus and the developing child to unacceptable risks. This in itself might be sufficient to justify a prohibition on cloning human beings at this time, even if such efforts were to be characterized as the exercise of a fundamental right to attempt to procreate.

Beyond the issue of the safety of the procedure, however, NBAC found that concerns relating to the potential psychological harms to children and effects on the moral, religious, and cultural values of society merited further reflection and deliberation. Whether upon such further deliberation our nation will conclude that the use of cloning techniques to create children should be allowed or permanently banned is, for the moment, an open question. Time is an ally in this regard, allowing for the accrual of further data from animal experimentation, enabling an assessment of the prospective safety and efficacy of the procedure in humans, as well as granting a period of fuller national debate on ethical and social concerns. The Commission therefore concluded that there should be imposed a period of time in which no attempt is made to create a child using somatic cell nuclear transfer.[1]

Within this overall framework the Commission came to the following conclusions and recommendations:

I. The Commission concludes that at this time it is morally unacceptable for anyone in the public or private sector, whether in a research or clinical setting, to attempt to create a child using somatic cell nuclear transfer cloning. We have reached a consensus on this point because current scientific information indicates that this technique is not safe to use in humans at this time. Indeed, we believe it would violate important ethical obligations were clinicians or researchers to attempt to create a child using these particular technologies, which are likely to involve unacceptable risks to

the fetus and/or potential child. Moreover, in addition to safety concerns, many other serious ethical concerns have been identified, which require much more widespread and careful public deliberation before this technology may be used.

The Commission, therefore, recommends the following for immediate action:

- A continuation of the current moratorium on the use of federal funding in support of any attempt to create a child by somatic cell nuclear transfer.

- An immediate request to all firms, clinicians, investigators, and professional societies in the private and non-federally funded sectors to comply voluntarily with the intent of the federal moratorium. Professional and scientific societies should make clear that any attempt to create a child by somatic cell nuclear transfer and implantation into a woman's body would at this time be an irresponsible, unethical, and unprofessional act.

II. The Commission further recommends that:

- Federal legislation should be enacted to prohibit anyone from attempting, whether in a research or clinical setting, to create a child through somatic cell nuclear transfer cloning. It is critical, however, that such legislation include a sunset clause to ensure that Congress will review the issue after a specified time period (three to five years) in order to decide whether the prohibition continues to be needed. If state legislation is enacted, it should also contain such a sunset provision. Any such legislation or associated regulation also ought to require that at some point prior to the expiration of the sunset period, an appropriate oversight body will evaluate and report on the current status of somatic cell nuclear transfer technology and on the ethical and social issues that its potential use to create human beings would raise in light of public understandings at that time.

III. The Commission also concludes that:

- Any regulatory or legislative actions undertaken to effect the foregoing prohibition on creating a child by somatic cell nuclear transfer should be carefully written so as not to interfere with other important areas of scientific research. In particular, no new regulations are required regarding the cloning of human DNA sequences and cell lines, since neither activity raises the scientific and ethical issues that arise from the attempt to create children through somatic cell nuclear transfer, and these fields of research have already provided important scientific and biomedical advances. Likewise, research on cloning animals by somatic cell nuclear transfer does not raise the issues implicated in attempting to use this technique for human cloning, and its continuation should only be subject to existing regulations regarding the humane use of animals and review by institution-based animal protection committees.

- If a legislative ban is not enacted, or if a legislative ban is ever lifted, clinical use of somatic cell nuclear transfer techniques to create a child should be preceded by research trials that are governed by the twin protections of independent review and informed consent, consistent with existing norms of human subjects protection.

- The United States Government should cooperate with other nations and international organizations to enforce any common aspects of their respective policies on the cloning of human beings.

IV. The Commission also concludes that different ethical and religious perspectives and traditions are divided on many of the important moral issues that surround any attempt to create a child using somatic cell nuclear transfer techniques. Therefore, we recommend that:

- The federal government, and all interested and concerned parties, encourage widespread and continuing deliberation on these issues in order to further our understanding of the ethical and social implications of this technology and to enable society to produce appropriate long-term policies regarding this technology should the time come when present concerns about safety have been addressed.

V. Finally, because scientific knowledge is essential for all citizens to participate in a full and informed fashion in the governance of our complex society, the Commission recommends that:

- Federal departments and agencies concerned with science should cooperate in seeking out and supporting opportunities to provide information and education to the public in the area of genetics, and on other developments in the biomedical sciences, especially where these affect important cultural practices, values, and beliefs.

NOTES

1. The Commission also observes that the use of any other technique to create a child genetically identical to an existing (or previously existing) individual would raise many, if not all, of the same non-safety-related ethical concerns raised by the creation of a child by somatic cell nuclear transfer.

Cloning Human Beings: An Assessment of the Ethical Issues Pro and Con

Dan W. Brock

INTRODUCTION

The world of science and the public at large were both shocked and fascinated by the announcement in the journal *Nature* by Ian Wilmut and his colleagues that they had successfully cloned a sheep from a single cell of an adult sheep. Scientists were in part surprised because many had believed that after the very early stage of embryo development at which differentiation of cell function begins to take

Commissioned by the National Bioethics Advisory Commission.

EDITORS' NOTE: This article has been edited and most of the notes omitted. Readers who wish to follow up on sources should consult the original.

place it would not be possible to achieve cloning of an adult mammal by nuclear transfer. In this process the nucleus from the cell of an adult mammal is inserted into an enucleated ovum, and the resulting embryo develops following the complete genetic code of the mammal from which the inserted nucleus was obtained. But some scientists and much of the public were troubled or apparently even horrified at the prospect that if adult mammals such as sheep could be cloned, then cloning of adult humans by the same process would likely be possible as well. Of course, the process is far from perfected even with sheep—it took 276 failures by Wilmut and his colleagues to produce Dolly, their one success, and whether the process can be successfully replicated in other mammals, much less in humans, is not now known. But those who were horrified at the prospect of human cloning were not assuaged by the fact that the science with humans is not yet there, for it looked to them now perilously close.

The response of most scientific and political leaders to the prospect of human cloning, indeed of Dr. Wilmut as well, was of immediate and strong condemnation. In the United States President Clinton immediately banned federal financing of human cloning research and asked privately funded scientists to halt such work until the newly formed National Bioethics Advisory Commission could review the "troubling" ethical and legal implications. The Director-General of the World Health Organization characterized human cloning as "ethically unacceptable as it would violate some of the basic principles which govern medically assisted reproduction. These include respect for the dignity of the human being and the protection of the security of human genetic material." Around the world similar immediate condemnation was heard as human cloning was called a violation of human rights and human dignity. Even before Wilmut's announcement, human cloning had been made illegal in nearly all countries in Europe and had been condemned by the Council of Europe.

A few more cautious voices were heard both suggesting some possible benefits from the use of human cloning in limited circumstances and questioning its too quick prohibition, but they were a clear minority. In the popular media, nightmare scenarios of laboratory mistakes resulting in monsters, the cloning of armies of Hitlers, the exploitative use of cloning for totalitarian ends as in Huxley's *Brave New World*, and the murderous replicas of the film *Blade Runner*, all fed the public controversy and uneasiness. A striking feature of these early responses was that their strength and intensity seemed far to outrun the arguments and reasons offered in support of them—they seemed often to be "gut level" emotional reactions rather than considered reflections on the issues. Such reactions should not be simply dismissed, both because they may point us to important considerations otherwise missed and not easily articulated, and because they often have a major impact on public policy. But the formation of public policy should not ignore the moral reasons and arguments that bear on the practice of human cloning—these must be articulated in order to understand and inform people's more immediate emotional responses. This paper is an effort to articulate, and to evaluate critically, the main moral considerations and arguments for and against human cloning. Though many people's religious beliefs inform their views on human cloning, and it is often difficult to separate religious from secular positions, I shall restrict myself to arguments and reasons that can be given a clear secular formulation and will ignore explicitly religious positions and arguments pro or con. I shall also be concerned principally with cloning by nuclear transfer, which permits cloning of an adult, not cloning by embryo splitting, although some of the issues apply to both.

I begin by noting that on each side of the issue there are two distinct kinds of moral arguments brought forward. On the one hand, some opponents claim that human cloning would violate fundamental moral or human rights; while some proponents argue that its prohibition would violate such rights. On the other hand, both opponents and proponents also cite the likely harms and benefits, both to individuals and to society, of the practice. While moral and even human rights need not be understood as absolute, that is, as morally requiring people to respect them no matter how great the costs or bad consequences of doing so, they do place moral restrictions on permissible actions that an appeal to a mere balance of benefits over harms cannot justify overriding. For example, the rights of human subjects in research must be respected even if the result is that some potentially beneficial research is more difficult or cannot be done, and the right of free expression prohibits the silencing of unpopular or even abhorrent views; in Ronald Dworkin's striking formulation, rights trump utility (Dworkin 1978). I shall take up both the moral rights implicated in human cloning, as well as its more likely significant benefits and harms, because none of the rights as applied to human cloning is sufficiently uncontroversial and strong to settle decisively the morality of the practice one way or the other. But because of their strong moral force, the assessment of the moral rights putatively at stake is especially important. A further complexity here is that it is sometimes controversial whether a particular consideration is merely a matter of benefits and harms, or is instead a matter of moral or human rights. I shall begin with the arguments in support of permitting human cloning, although with no implication that it is the stronger or weaker position.

MORAL ARGUMENTS IN SUPPORT OF HUMAN CLONING

A. IS THERE A MORAL RIGHT TO USE HUMAN CLONING?

What moral right might protect at least some access to the use of human cloning? Some commentators have argued that a commitment to individual liberty, as defended by J.S. Mill, requires that individuals be left free to use human cloning if they so choose and if their doing so does not cause significant harms to others, but liberty is too broad in scope to be an uncontroversial moral right. Human cloning is a means of reproduction (in the most literal sense) and so the most plausible moral right at stake in its use is a right to reproductive freedom or procreative liberty. Reproductive freedom includes not only the familiar right to choose not to reproduce, for example, by means of contraception or abortion, but also the right to reproduce. The right to reproductive freedom is properly understood to include as well the use of various artificial reproductive technologies, such as in vitro fertilization (IVF), oocyte donation, and so forth. The reproductive right relevant to human cloning is a negative right, that is, a right to use assisted reproduc-

tive technologies without interference by the government or others when made available by a willing provider. The choice of an assisted means of reproduction, such as surrogacy, can be defended as included within reproductive freedom even when it is not the only means for individuals to reproduce, just as the choice among different means of preventing conception is protected by reproductive freedom. However, the case for permitting the use of a particular means of reproduction is strongest when that means is necessary for particular individuals to be able to procreate at all. Sometimes human cloning could be the only means for individuals to procreate while retaining a biological tie to the child created, but in other cases different means of procreating would also be possible.

It could be argued that human cloning is not covered by the right to reproductive freedom because whereas current assisted reproductive technologies and practices covered by that right are remedies for inabilities to reproduce sexually, human cloning is an entirely new means of reproduction; indeed, its critics see it as more a means of manufacturing humans than of reproduction. Human cloning is a different means of reproduction than sexual reproduction, but it is a means that can serve individuals' interest in reproducing. If it is not covered by the moral right to reproductive freedom, I believe that must be not because it is a new means of reproducing, but instead because it has other objectionable moral features, such as eroding human dignity or uniqueness; we shall evaluate these other ethical objections to it below.

When individuals have alternative means of procreating, human cloning typically would be chosen because it replicates a particular individual's genome. The reproductive interest in question then is not simply reproduction itself, but a more specific interest in choosing what kind of children to have. The right to reproductive freedom is usually understood to cover at least some choice about the kind of children one will have; for example, genetic testing of an embryo or fetus for genetic disease or abnormality, together with abortion of an affected embryo or fetus, is now used to avoid having a child with that disease or abnormality. Genetic testing of prospective parents before conception to determine the risk of transmitting a genetic disease is also intended to avoid having children with particular diseases. Prospective parents' moral interest in self-determination, which is one of the grounds of a moral right to reproductive freedom, includes the choice about whether to have a child with a condition that is likely to place severe burdens on them, and to cause severe burdens to the child itself.

The more a reproductive choice is not simply the determination of oneself and one's own life but the determination of the nature of another, as in the case of human cloning, the more moral weight the interests of that other person, that is, the cloned child, should have in decisions that determine its nature. But even then parents are typically taken properly to have substantial, but not unlimited, discretion in shaping the persons their children will become, for example, through education and other childrearing decisions. Even if not part of reproductive freedom, the right to raise one's children as one sees fit, within limits mostly determined by the interests of the children, is also a right to determine within limits what kinds of persons one's children will become. This right includes not just preventing certain diseases or harms to children, but selecting and shaping desirable features and traits in one's children. The use of human cloning is one way to exercise that right.

It is worth pointing out that current public and legal policy permits prospective parents to conceive, or to carry a conception to term, when there is a significant risk, or even certainty that the child will suffer from a serious genetic disease. Even when others think the risk or presence of genetic disease makes it morally wrong to conceive, or to carry a fetus to term, the parents' right to reproductive freedom permits them to do so. Most possible harms to a cloned child that I shall consider below are less serious than the genetic harms with which parents can now permit their offspring to be conceived or born.

I conclude that there is good reason to accept that a right to reproductive freedom presumptively includes both a right to select the means of reproduction, as well as a right to determine what kind of children to have, by use of human cloning. However, the particular reproductive interest of determining what kind of children to have is less weighty than other reproductive interests and

choices whose impact falls more directly and exclusively on the parents rather than the child. Accepting a moral right to reproductive freedom that includes the use of human cloning does not settle the moral issue about human cloning, however, since there may be other moral rights in conflict with this right, or serious enough harms from human cloning to override the right to use it; this right can be thought of as establishing a serious moral presumption supporting access to human cloning. . . .

B. WHAT INDIVIDUAL OR SOCIAL BENEFITS MIGHT HUMAN CLONING PRODUCE?

Largely Individual Benefits

The literature on human cloning by nuclear transfer, as well as the literature on embryo splitting where it is relevant to the nuclear transfer case, contain a few examples of circumstances in which individuals might have good reasons to want to use human cloning. However, a survey of that literature strongly suggests that human cloning is not the unique answer to any great or pressing human need and that its benefits would at most be limited. What are the principal benefits of human cloning that might give persons good reasons to want to use it?

1. Human cloning would be a new means to relieve the infertility some persons now experience. Human cloning would allow women who have no ova or men who have no sperm to produce an offspring that is biologically related to them. Embryos might also be cloned, either by nuclear transfer or embryo splitting, in order to increase the number of embryos for implantation and improve the chances of successful conception. While the moral right to reproductive freedom creates a presumption that individuals should be free to choose the means of reproduction that best serves their interests and desires, the benefits from human cloning to relieve infertility are greater the more persons there are who cannot overcome their infertility by any other means acceptable to them. I do not know of data on this point, but they should be possible to obtain or gather from national associations concerned with infertility.

It is not enough to point to the large number of children throughout the world possibly available for adoption as a solution to infertility, unless we are prepared to discount as illegitimate the strong desire many persons, fertile and infertile, have for the experience of pregnancy and for having and raising a child biologically related to them. While not important to all infertile (or fertile) individuals, it is important to many and is respected and met through other forms of assisted reproduction that maintain a biological connection when that is possible; there seems no good reason to refuse to respect and respond to it when human cloning would be the best or only means of overcoming individuals' infertility.

2. Human cloning would enable couples in which one party risks transmitting a serious hereditary disease, a serious risk of disease, or an otherwise harmful condition to an offspring, to reproduce without doing so. Of course, by using donor sperm or egg donation, such hereditary risks can generally be avoided now without the use of human cloning. These procedures may be unacceptable to some couples, however, or at least considered less desirable than human cloning because they introduce a third party's genes into their reproduction, instead of giving their offspring only the genes of one of them. Thus, in some cases human cloning would be a means of preventing genetically transmitted harms to offspring. Here too, there are not data on the likely number of persons who would wish to use human cloning for this purpose instead of either using other available means of avoiding the risk of genetic transmission of the harmful condition or accepting the risk of transmitting the harmful condition.

3. Human cloning a later twin would enable a person to obtain needed organs or tissues for transplantation. Human cloning would solve the problem of finding a transplant donor who is an acceptable organ or tissue match and would eliminate, or drastically reduce, the risk of transplant rejection by the host. The availability of human cloning for this purpose would amount to a form of insurance policy to enable treatment of certain kinds of medical needs. Of course, sometimes the medical need would be too urgent to permit waiting for the cloning, gestation and development of the later twin necessary before tissues or organs for transplant could be obtained. In other cases, the need for an organ that the later twin would

him- or herself need to maintain life, such as a heart or a liver, would preclude cloning and then taking the organ from the later twin.

Such a practice has been criticized on the ground that it treats the later twin not as a person valued and loved for his or her own sake, as an end in itself in Kantian terms, but simply as a means for benefiting another. This criticism assumes, however, that only this one motive would determine the relation of the person to his or her later twin. The well-known case some years ago in California of the Ayalas, who conceived in the hopes of obtaining a source for a bone marrow transplant for their teenage daughter suffering from leukemia illustrates the mistake in this assumption. They argued that whether or not the child they conceived turned out to be a possible donor for their daughter, they would value and love the child for itself, and treat it as they would treat any other member of their family. That one reason it was wanted was as a means to saving their daughter's life did not preclude its also being loved and valued for its own sake; in Kantian terms, it was treated as a possible means to saving their daughter, but not *solely as a means,* which is what the Kantian view proscribes.

Indeed, when people have children, whether by sexual means or with the aid of assisted reproductive technologies, their motives and reasons for doing so are typically many and complex, and include reasons less laudable than obtaining life-saving medical treatment, such as having a companion like a doll to play with, enabling one to live on one's own, qualifying for public or government benefit programs, and so forth. While these other motives for having children sometimes may not bode well for the child's upbringing and future, public policy does not assess prospective parents motives and reasons for procreating as a condition of their doing so.

One commentator has proposed human cloning for obtaining even lifesaving organs. After cell differentiation some of the brain cells of the embryo or fetus would be removed so that it could then be grown as a brain dead body for spare parts for its earlier twin. This body clone would be like an anencephalic newborn or presentient fetus, neither of whom arguably can be harmed because of their lack of capacity for consciousness. Most people would likely find this practice appalling and immoral, in part because here the cloned later twin's capacity for conscious life is destroyed *solely as a means* for the benefit of another. Yet if one pushes what is already science fiction quite a bit further in the direction of science fantasy, and imagines the ability to clone and grow in an artificial environment only the particular lifesaving organ a person needed for transplantation, then it is far from clear that it would be morally impermissible to do so.

4. Human cloning would enable individuals to clone someone who had special meaning to them, such as a child who had died. There is no denying that if human cloning were available, some individuals would want to use it in order to clone someone who had special meaning to them, such as a child who had died, but that desire usually would be based on a deep confusion. Cloning such a child would not replace the child the parents had loved and lost, but rather would create a new different child with the same genes. The child they loved and lost was a unique individual who had been shaped by his or her environment and choices, not just his or her genes, and more importantly who had experienced a particular relationship with them. Even if the later cloned child could have not only the same genes but also be subjected to the same environment, which of course is in fact impossible, it would remain a different child than the one they had loved and lost because it would share a different history with them. Cloning the lost child might help the parents accept and move on from their loss, but another already existing sibling or another new child that was not a clone might do this equally well; indeed, it might do so better since the appearance of the cloned later twin would be a constant reminder of the child they had lost. Nevertheless, if human cloning enabled some individuals to clone a person who had special meaning to them and doing so gave them deep satisfaction, that would be a benefit to them even if their reasons for wanting to do so, and the satisfaction they in turn received, were based on a confusion.

Largely Social Benefits

5. Human cloning would enable the duplication of individuals of great talent, genius, character, or other exemplary qualities. The first four reasons for human cloning considered above all looked to benefits to specific individuals, usually parents, from being able to reproduce by means of human cloning. This reason looks to benefits to the broader society from being able to replicate extraordinary individuals—a Mozart, Einstein, Gandhi, or Schweitzer. Much of the appeal of this reason, like much thinking both in support of and in opposition to human cloning, rests on a confused and mistaken assumption of genetic determinism, that is, that one's genes fully determine what one will become, do, and accomplish. What made Mozart, Einstein, Gandhi, and Schweitzer the extraordinary individuals they were was the confluence of their particular genetic endowments with the environments in which they were raised and lived and the particular historical moments they in different ways seized. Cloning them would produce individuals with the same genetic inheritances (nuclear transfer does not even produce 100% genetic identity, although for the sake of exploring the moral issues I have followed the common assumption that it does), but neither by cloning, nor by any other means, would it be possible to replicate their environments or the historical contexts in which they lived and their greatness flourished. We do not know, either in general or with any particular individual, the degree or specific respects in which their greatness depended on their "nature" or their "nurture," but we do know in all cases that it depended on an interaction of them both. Thus, human cloning could never replicate the extraordinary accomplishments for which we admire individuals like Mozart, Einstein, Gandhi, and Schweitzer.

If we make a rough distinction between the extraordinary capabilities of a Mozart or an Einstein and how they used those capabilities in the particular environments and historical settings in which they lived, it would also be a mistake to assume that human cloning could at least replicate their extraordinary capabilities, if not the accomplishments they achieved with them. Their capabilities too were the product of their inherited genes and their environments, not of their genes alone, and so it would be a mistake to think that cloning them would produce individuals with the same capabilities, even if they would exercise those capabilities at different times and in different ways. In the case of Gandhi and Schweitzer, whose extraordinary greatness lies more in their moral character and commitments, we understand even less well the extent to which their moral character and greatness was produced by their genes.

None of this is to deny that Mozart's and Einstein's extraordinary musical and intellectual capabilities, nor even Gandhi's and Schweitzer's extraordinary moral greatness, were produced in part by their unique genetic inheritances. Cloning them might well produce individuals with exceptional capacities, but we simply do not know how close their clones would be in capacities or accomplishments to the great individuals from whom they were cloned. Even so, the hope for exceptional, even if less and different, accomplishment from cloning such extraordinary individuals might be a reasonable ground for doing so.

I have used examples above of individuals whose greatness is widely appreciated and largely uncontroversial, but if we move away from such cases we encounter the problem of whose standards of greatness would be used to select individuals to be cloned for the benefit of society or mankind at large. This problem inevitably connects with the important issue of who would control access to and use of the technology of human cloning, since those who controlled its use would be in a position to impose their standards of exceptional individuals to be cloned. This issue is especially worrisome if particular groups or segments of society, or if government, controlled the technology for we would then risk its use for the benefit of those groups, segments of society, or governments under the cover of benefiting society or even mankind at large.

6. Human cloning and research on human cloning might make possible important advances in scientific knowledge, for example about human development. While important potential advances in scientific or medical knowledge from human cloning or human cloning research have frequently been cited in some media responses to Dolly's cloning there are at least three reasons why these possible benefits are highly uncertain. First, there is always considerable uncertainty about the nature and importance of the new scientific or medical knowledge that a dramatic new technology like human cloning will lead to; the road to that new knowledge is never mapped in advance and takes many unexpected turns. Second, we also do not know what new knowledge from human cloning or human cloning research could also be gained by other methods and research that do not have the problematic moral features of human cloning to which its opponents object. Third, what human cloning research would be compatible with ethical and legal requirements for the use of human subjects in research is complex, controversial, and largely unexplored. For example, in what contexts and from whom would it be necessary, and how would it be possible, to secure the informed consent of parties involved in human cloning? No human cloning should ever take place without the consent of the person cloned and the woman receiving a cloned embryo, if they are different. But we could never obtain the consent of the cloned later twin to being cloned, so research on human cloning that produces a cloned individual might be barred by ethical and legal regulations for the use of human subjects in research. Moreover, creating human clones solely for the purpose of research would be to use them solely for the benefit of others without their consent, and so unethical. Of course, once human cloning was established to be safe and effective, then new scientific knowledge might be obtained from its use for legitimate, non-research reasons. How human subjects regulations would apply to research on human cloning, needs much more exploration than I can give it here in order to help clarify how significant and likely the potential gains are in scientific and medical knowledge from human cloning research and human cloning.

Although there is considerable uncertainty concerning most of the possible individual and social benefits of human cloning that I have discussed above, and although no doubt it may have other benefits or uses that we cannot yet envisage, I believe it is reasonable to conclude that human cloning at this time does not seem to promise great benefits or uniquely to meet great human needs. Nevertheless, a case can be made that scientific freedom supports permitting research on human cloning to go forward and that freedom to use human cloning is protected by the important moral right to reproductive freedom. We must therefore assess what moral rights might be violated, or harms produced, by research on or use of human cloning.

MORAL ARGUMENTS AGAINST HUMAN CLONING

A. WOULD THE USE OF HUMAN CLONING VIOLATE IMPORTANT MORAL RIGHTS?

Many of the immediate condemnations of any possible human cloning following Wilmut's cloning of an adult sheep claimed that it would violate moral or human rights, but it was usually not specified precisely, or often even at all, what the rights were that would be violated. I shall consider two possible candidates for such a right: a right to have a unique identity and a right to ignorance about one's future or to an open future. The former right is cited by many commentators, but I believe even if any such a right exists, it is not violated by human cloning. The latter right has only been explicitly defended to my knowledge by two commentators, and in the context of human cloning, only by Hans Jonas; it supports a more promising, even if in my view ultimately unsuccessful, argument that human cloning would violate an important moral or human right. . . .

We need not pursue what the basis or argument in support of a moral or human right to a unique identity might be—such a right is not found among typical accounts and enumerations of moral or human rights—because even if we grant that there is such a right, sharing a genome with another individual as a result of human cloning would not violate it. The idea of the uniqueness, or unique identity, of each person historically predates the development of modern genetics and the knowledge that except in the case of homozygous twins each individual has a unique genome. A unique genome thus could not be the ground of this long-standing belief in the unique human identity of each person.

I turn now to whether human cloning would violate what Hans Jonas called a right to ignorance, or what Joel Feinberg called a right to an open future (Feinberg 1980). Jonas argued that human cloning in which there is a substantial time gap between the beginning of the lives of the earlier and later twin is fundamentally different from the simultaneous beginning of the lives of homozygous twins that occur in nature. Although contemporaneous twins begin their lives with the same genetic inheritance, they also begin their lives or biographies at the same time, and so in ignorance of what the other who shares the same genome will by his or her choices make of his or her life. To whatever extent one's genome determines one's future, each begins ignorant of what that determination will be and so remains as free to choose a future, to construct a particular future from among open alternatives, as are individuals who do not have a twin. Ignorance of the effect of one's genome on one's future is necessary for the spontaneous, free, and authentic construction of a life and self.

A later twin created by human cloning, Jonas argues, knows, or at least believes he or she knows, too much about him- or herself. For there is already in the world another person, one's earlier twin, who from the same genetic starting point has made the life choices that are still in the later twin's future. It will seem that one's life has already been lived and played out by another, that one's fate is already determined, and so the later twin will lose the spontaneity of authentically creating and becoming his or her own self. One will lose the sense of human possibility in freely creating one's own future. It is tyrannical, Jonas claims, for the earlier twin to try to determine another's fate in this way. And even if it is a mistake to believe the crude genetic determinism according to which one's genes determine one's fate, what is important for one's experience of freedom and ability to create a life for oneself is whether one thinks one's future is open and undetermined, and so still to be determined by one's own choices. . . .

In a different context, and without applying it to human cloning, Joel Feinberg has argued for a child's right to an open future. This requires that others raising a child not so close off the future possibilities that the child would otherwise have as to eliminate a reasonable range of opportunities for the child to choose autonomously and construct his or her own life. One way this right to an open future would be violated is to deny even a basic education to a child, and another way might be to create it as a later twin so that it will believe its future has already been set for it by the choices made and the life lived by its earlier twin.

A central difficulty in evaluating the implications for human cloning of a right either to ignorance or to an open future, is whether the right is violated merely because the later twin may be likely to *believe* that its future is already determined, even if that belief is clearly false and supported only by the crudest genetic determinism. I believe that if the twin's future in reality remains open and his to freely choose, then someone's acting in a way that unintentionally leads him to believe that his future is closed and determined has not violated his right to ignorance or to an open future. Likewise, suppose I drive down the twin's street in my new car that is just like his knowing that when he sees me he is likely to believe that I have stolen his car, and therefore to abandon his driving plans for the day. I have not violated his property right to his car even though he may feel the same loss of opportunity to drive that day as if I had in fact stolen his car. In each case he is mistaken that his open future or car has been taken from him, and so no right of his to them has been violated. If we know that the twin will believe that his open future has been taken from him as a result of being cloned, even though in reality it has not, then we know that cloning will cause him psychological distress, but not that it will violate his right. Thus, I believe Jonas' right to ignorance, and our employment of Feinberg's analogous right of a child to an open future, turns out not to be violated by human cloning, though they do point to psychological harms that a later twin may be likely to experience and that I will take up below.

The upshot of our consideration of a moral or human right either to a unique identity or to ignorance and an open future, is that neither would be violated by human cloning. Perhaps there are other possible rights that would make good the charge that human cloning is a violation of moral or human rights, but I am unsure what they might be. I turn now to consideration of the harms that human cloning might produce.

B. WHAT INDIVIDUAL OR SOCIAL HARMS MIGHT HUMAN CLONING PRODUCE?

There are many possible individual or social harms that have been posited by one or another commentator and I shall only try to cover the more plausible and significant of them.

Largely Individual Harms
1. Human cloning would produce psychological distress and harm in the later twin. This is per-

haps the most serious individual harm that opponents of human cloning foresee, and we have just seen that even if human cloning is no violation of rights, it may nevertheless cause psychological distress or harm. No doubt knowing the path in life taken by one's earlier twin may in many cases have several bad psychological effects. The later twin may feel, even if mistakenly, that his or her fate has already been substantially laid out, and so have difficulty freely and spontaneously taking responsibility for and making his or her own fate and life. The later twin's experience or sense of autonomy and freedom may be substantially diminished, even if in actual fact they are diminished much less than it seems to him or her. Together with this might be a diminished sense of one's own uniqueness and individuality, even if once again these are in fact diminished little or not at all by having an earlier twin with the same genome. If the later twin is the clone of a particularly exemplary individual, perhaps with some special capabilities and accomplishments, he or she may experience excessive pressure to reach the very high standards of ability and accomplishment of the earlier twin. All of these psychological effects may take a heavy toll on the later twin and be serious burdens under which he or she would live. One commentator has also cited special psychological harms to the first, or first few, human clones from the great publicity that would attend their creation. While public interest in the first clones would no doubt be enormous, medical confidentiality should protect their identity. Even if their identity became public knowledge, this would be a temporary effect only on the first few clones and the experience of Louise Brown, the first child conceived by IVF, suggests this publicity could be managed to limit its harmful effects.

While psychological harms of these kinds from human cloning are certainly possible, and perhaps even likely, they do remain at this point only speculative since we have no experience with human cloning and the creation of earlier and later twins. With naturally occurring identical twins, while they sometimes struggle to achieve their own identity, a struggle shared by many people without a twin, there is typically a very strong emotional bond between the twins and such twins are, if anything, generally psychologically stronger and better adjusted than non-twins (Robertson 1994b).

Scenarios are even possible in which being a later twin confers a psychological benefit on the twin; for example, having been deliberately cloned with the specific genes the later twin has might make the later twin feel especially wanted for the kind of person he or she is. Nevertheless, if experience with human cloning confirmed that serious and unavoidable psychological harms typically occurred to the later twin, that would be a serious moral reason to avoid the practice.

In the discussion above of potential psychological harms to a later twin, I have been assuming that one later twin is cloned from an already existing adult individual. Cloning by means of embryo splitting, as carried out and reported by Hall and colleagues at George Washington University in 1993, has limits on the number of genetically identical twins that can be cloned. Nuclear transfer, however, has no limits to the number of genetically identical individuals who might be cloned. Intuitively, many of the psychological burdens and harms noted above seem more likely and serious for a clone who is only one of many identical later twins from one original source, so that the clone might run into another identical twin around every street corner. This prospect could be a good reason to place sharp limits on the number of twins that could be cloned from any one source. . . .

2. Human cloning procedures would carry unacceptable risks to the clone. One version of this objection to human cloning concerns the research necessary to perfect the procedure, the other version concerns the later risks from its use. Wilmut's group had 276 failures before their success with Dolly, indicating that the procedure is far from perfected even with sheep. Further research on the procedure with animals is clearly necessary before it would be ethical to use the procedure on humans. But even assuming that cloning's safety and effectiveness is established with animals, research would need to be done to establish its safety and effectiveness for humans. Could this research be ethically done? There would be little or no risk to the donor of the cell nucleus to be transferred, and his or her informed consent could and must always be obtained. There might be greater risks for the woman to whom a cloned embryo is transferred, but these should be comparable to those associated with IVF procedures and the woman's informed consent too could and must be obtained.

What of the risks to the cloned embryo itself? Judging by the experience of Wilmut's group in their work on cloning a sheep, the principal risk to the embryos cloned was their failure successfully to implant, grow, and develop. Comparable risks to cloned human embryos would apparently be their death or destruction long before most people or the law consider it to be a person with moral or legal protections of its life. Moreover, artificial reproductive technologies now in use, such as IVF, have a known risk that some embryos will be destroyed or will not successfully implant and will die. It is premature to make a confident assessment of what the risks to human subjects would be of establishing the safety and effectiveness of human cloning procedures, but there are no unavoidable risks apparent at this time that would make the necessary research clearly ethically impermissible.

Could human cloning procedures meet ethical standards of safety and efficacy? Risks to an ovum donor (if any), a nucleus donor, and a woman who receives the embryo for implantation would likely be ethically acceptable with the informed consent of the involved parties. But what of the risks to the human clone if the procedure in some way goes wrong, or unanticipated harms come to the clone; for example, Harold Varmus, director of the National Institutes of Health, has raised the concern that a cell many years old from which a person is cloned could have accumulated genetic mutations during its years in another adult that could give the resulting clone a predisposition to cancer or other diseases of aging. Moreover, it is impossible to obtain the informed consent of the clone to his or her own creation but, of course no one else is able to give informed consent for their creation either.

I believe it is too soon to say whether unavoidable risks to the clone would make human cloning unethical. At a minimum, further research on cloning animals, as well as research to better define the potential risks to humans, is needed. For the reasons given above, we should not set aside risks to the clone on the grounds that the clone would not be harmed by them since its only alternative is not to exist at all; I have suggested that is a bad argument. But we should not insist on a standard that requires risks to be lower than those we accept in sexual reproduction, or in other forms of assisted reproduction. It is not possible now to know when, if ever, human cloning will satisfy an appropriate standard limiting risks to the clone.

Largely Social Harms
3. Human cloning would lessen the worth of individuals and diminish respect for human life. Unelaborated claims to this effect in the media were common after the announcement of the cloning of Dolly. Ruth Macklin has explored and criticized the claim that human cloning would diminish the value we place on, and our respect for, human life because it would lead to persons being viewed as replaceable (Macklin 1994). As I argued above concerning a right to a unique identity, only on a confused and indefensible notion of human identity is a person's identity determined solely by their genes. Instead, an individual's identity is determined by the interaction of his or her genes over time with his or her environment, including the choices the individual makes and the important relations he or she forms with other persons. This means in turn that no individual could be fully replaced by a later clone possessing the same genes. Ordinary people recognize this clearly. For example, parents of a 12-year-old child dying of a fatal disease would consider it insensitive and ludicrous if someone told them they should not grieve for their coming loss because it is possible to replace him by cloning him; it is *their child who is dying* whom they love and value, and that child and his importance to them could never be replaced by a cloned later twin. Even if they would also come to love and value a later twin as much as their child who is dying, that would be to love and value that *different child* who could never replace the child they lost. Ordinary people are typically quite clear about the importance of the relations they have to distinct, historically situated individuals with whom over time they have shared experiences and their lives, and whose loss to them would therefore be irreplaceable.

A different version of this worry is that human cloning would result in persons' worth or value seeming diminished because we would now see humans as able to be manufactured or "handmade." This demystification of the creation of human life would reduce our appreciation and awe of it and of its natural creation. It would be a mistake, however, to conclude that a human being created by human cloning is of less value or is less worthy of respect than one created by sexual reproduction. It is the nature of a being, not how it is created, that is the source of its value and makes it worthy of respect. Moreover, for many people gaining a scientific understanding of the extraordinary complexity of human reproduction and development increases, instead of decreases, their awe of the process and its product.

A more subtle route by which the value we place on each individual human life might be diminished could come from the use of human cloning with the aim of creating a child with a particular genome, either the genome of another individual especially meaningful to those doing the cloning or an individual with exceptional talents, abilities, and accomplishments. The child might then be valued only for its genome, or at least for its genome's expected phenotypic expression, and no longer be recognized as having the intrinsic equal moral value of all persons, simply as persons. For the moral value and respect due all persons to come to be seen as resting only on the instrumental value of individuals, or of individuals' particular qualities, to others would be to fundamentally change the moral status accorded to persons. Everyone would lose their moral standing as full and equal members of the moral community, replaced by the different instrumental value each of us has to others.

Such a change in the equal moral value and worth accorded to persons should be avoided at all costs, but it is far from clear that such a change would take place from permitting human cloning. Parents, for example, are quite capable of distinguishing their children's intrinsic value, just as individual persons, from their instrumental value based on their particular qualities or properties. The equal moral value and respect due all persons just as persons is not incompatible with the different instrumental value of people's particular qualities or properties; Einstein and an untalented physics graduate student have vastly different value as scientists, but share and are entitled to equal moral value and respect as persons. It would be a mistake and a confusion to conflate the two kinds of value and respect. Making a large number of clones from one original person might be more likely to foster this mistake and confusion in the public, and if so that would be a further reason to limit the number of clones that could be made from one individual.

4. Human cloning would divert resources from other more important social and medical needs. As we saw in considering the reasons for, and potential benefits from, human cloning, in only a limited number of uses would it uniquely meet important human needs. There is little doubt that in the United States, and certainly elsewhere, there are more pressing unmet human needs, both medical or health needs and other social or individual needs. This is a reason for not using public funds to support human cloning, at least if the funds actually are redirected to more important ends and needs. It is not a reason, however, either to prohibit other private individuals or institutions from using their own resources for research on human cloning or for human cloning itself, or to prohibit human cloning or research on human cloning.

The other important point about resource use is that it is not now clear how expensive human cloning would ultimately be, for example, in comparison with other means of relieving infertility. The procedure itself is not scientifically or technologically extremely complex and might prove not to require a significant commitment of resources.

5. Human cloning might be used by commercial interests for financial gain. Both opponents and proponents of human cloning agree that cloned embryos should not be able to be bought and sold. In a science fiction frame of mind, one can imagine commercial interests offering genetically certified and guaranteed embryos for sale, perhaps offering a catalogue of different embryos cloned from individuals with a variety of talents, capacities, and other desirable properties. This would be a fundamental violation of the equal moral respect and dignity owed to all persons, treating them instead as objects to be differentially valued, bought, and sold in the marketplace. Even if embryos are not yet persons at the time they would be purchased or sold, they would be being valued, bought, and sold for the persons they will become. The moral consensus against any commercial market in embryos, cloned or otherwise, should be enforced by law whatever public policy ultimately is on human cloning. It has been argued that the law may already forbid markets in embryos on grounds that they would violate the thirteenth amendment prohibiting slavery and involuntary servitude (Turner 1981).

6. Human cloning might be used by governments or other groups for immoral and exploitative purposes. In *Brave New World*, Aldous Huxley imagined cloning individuals who have been engineered with limited abilities and conditioned to do, and to be happy doing, the menial work that society needed done. Selection and control in the creation of people was exercised not in the interests of the persons created, but in the interests of the society and at the expense of the persons created. Any use of human cloning for such purposes would exploit the clones solely as means for the benefit of others, and would violate the equal moral respect and dignity they are owed as full moral persons. If human cloning is permitted to go forward, it should be with regulations that would clearly prohibit such immoral exploitation.

Fiction contains even more disturbing and bizarre uses of human cloning, such as Mengele's creation of many clones of Hitler in Ira Levin's *The Boys from Brazil*, Woody Allen's science fiction cinematic spoof *Sleeper* in which a dictator's only remaining part, his nose, must be destroyed to keep it from being cloned, and the contemporary science fiction film *Blade Runner*. Nightmare scenarios like Huxley's or Levin's may be quite improbable, but their impact should not be underestimated on public concern with technologies like human cloning. Regulation of human cloning must assure the public that even such farfetched abuses will not take place.

7. Human cloning used on a very widespread basis would have a disastrous effect on the human gene pool by reducing genetic diversity and our capacity to adapt to new conditions. This is not a realistic concern since human cloning would not be used on a wide enough scale, substantially replacing sexual reproduction, to have the feared effect on the gene pool. The vast majority of humans seem quite satisfied with sexual means of reproduction; if anything, from the standpoint of worldwide population, we could do with a bit less enthusiasm for it. Programs of eugenicists like Herman Mueller earlier in the century to impregnate thousands of women with the sperm of exceptional men, as well as the more recent establishment of sperm banks of Nobel laureates, have met with little or no public interest or success. People prefer sexual means of reproduction and they prefer to keep their own biological ties to their offspring.

CONCLUSION

Human cloning has until now received little serious and careful ethical attention because it was typically dismissed as science fiction, and it stirs deep, but difficult to articulate, uneasiness and even revulsion in many people. Any ethical assessment of human cloning at this point must be tentative and provisional. Fortunately, the science and technology of human cloning are not yet in hand, and so a public and professional debate is possible without the need for a hasty, precipitate policy response.

The ethical pros and cons of human cloning, as I see them at this time, are sufficiently balanced and uncertain that there is not an ethically decisive case either for or against permitting it or doing it. Access to human cloning can plausibly be brought within a moral right to reproductive freedom, but the circumstances in which its use would have significant benefits appear at this time to be few and infrequent. It is not a central component of a moral right to reproductive freedom and it serves no major or pressing individual or social needs. On the other hand, contrary to the pronouncements of many of its opponents, human cloning seems not to be a violation of moral or human rights. But it does risk some significant individual or social harms, although most are based on common public confusions about genetic determinism, human identity, and the effects of human cloning. Because most moral reasons against doing human cloning remain speculative they seem insufficient to warrant at this time a complete legal prohibition of either research on or later use of human cloning. Legitimate moral concerns about the use and effects of human cloning, however, underline the need for careful public oversight of research on its development, together with a wider public debate and review before cloning is used on human beings.

REFERENCES

Dworkin, R. (1978). *Taking Rights Seriously*. London: Duckworth.

Feinberg, J. (1980). "The Child's Right to an Open Future," in *Whose Child? Children's Rights, Parental Authority, and State Power*, ed. W. Aiken and H. LaFollette. Totowa, NJ: Rowman and Littlefield.

Macklin, R. (1994). "Splitting Embryos on the Slippery Slope: Ethics and Public Policy." *Kennedy Institute of Ethics Journal* 4: 209–226.

The Wisdom of Repugnance

Leon R. Kass

Our habit of delighting in news of scientific and technological breakthroughs has been sorely challenged by the birth announcement of a sheep named Dolly. Though Dolly shares with previous sheep the "softest clothing, woolly, bright," William Blake's question, "Little Lamb, who made thee?" has for her a radically different answer: Dolly was, quite literally, made. She is the work not of nature or nature's God but of man, an Englishman, Ian Wilmut, and his fellow scientists. What's more, Dolly came into being not only asexually—ironically, just like "He [who] calls Himself a Lamb"—but also as the genetically identical copy (and the perfect incarnation of the form or blueprint) of a mature ewe, of whom she is a clone. This long-awaited yet not quite expected success in cloning a mammal raised immediately the prospect—and the specter—of cloning human beings: "I a child and Thou a lamb," despite our

Excerpted, with consent of the author, from "The Wisdom of Repugnance: Why We Should Ban the Cloning of Humans," *The New Republic*, June 2, 1997.

differences, have always been equal candidates for creative making, only now, by means of cloning, we may both spring from the hand of man playing at being God.

After an initial flurry of expert comment and public consternation, with opinion polls showing overwhelming opposition to cloning human beings, President Clinton ordered a ban on all federal support for human cloning research (even though none was being supported) and charged the National Bioethics Advisory Commission to report in ninety days on the ethics of human cloning research. The commission (an eighteen-member panel, evenly balanced between scientists and non-scientists, appointed by the president and reporting to the National Science and Technology Council) invited testimony from scientists, religious thinkers and bioethicists, as well as from the general public. It is now deliberating about what it should recommend, both as a matter of ethics and as a matter of public policy.

Congress is awaiting the commission's report, and is poised to act. Bills to prohibit the use of federal funds for human cloning research have been introduced in the House of Representatives and the Senate; and another bill, in the House, would make it illegal "for any person to use a human somatic cell for the process of producing a human clone." A fateful decision is at hand. To clone or not to clone a human being is no longer an academic question.

TAKING CLONING SERIOUSLY, THEN AND NOW

Cloning first came to public attention roughly thirty years ago, following the successful asexual production, in England, of a clutch of tadpole clones by the technique of nuclear transplantation. The individual largely responsible for bringing the prospect and promise of human cloning to public notice was Joshua Lederberg, a Nobel Laureate geneticist and a man of large vision. In 1966, Lederberg wrote a remarkable article in *The American Naturalist* detailing the eugenic advantages of human cloning and other forms of genetic engineering, and the following year he devoted a column in *The Washington Post*, where he wrote regularly on science and society, to the prospect of human cloning. He suggested that cloning could help us overcome the unpredictable variety that still rules human reproduction, and allow us to benefit from perpetuating superior genetic endowments. These writings sparked a small public debate in which I became a participant. At the time a young researcher in molecular biology at the National Institutes of Health (NIH), I wrote a reply to the *Post*, arguing against Lederberg's amoral treatment of this morally weighty subject and insisting on the urgency of confronting a series of questions and objections, culminating in the suggestion that "the programmed reproduction of man will, in fact, dehumanize him."

Over the last 30 years, it has become harder, not easier, to discern the true meaning of human cloning. We have in some sense been softened up to the idea—through movies, cartoons, jokes and intermittent commentary in the mass media, some serious, most lighthearted. We have become accustomed to new practices in human reproduction: not just in vitro fertilization, but also embryo manipulation, embryo donation and surrogate pregnancy. Animal biotechnology has yielded transgenic animals and a burgeoning science of genetic engineering, easily and soon to be transferable to humans.

Even more important, changes in the broader culture make it now vastly more difficult to express a common and respectful understanding of sexuality, procreation, nascent life, family, and the meaning of motherhood, fatherhood and the links between the generations. Twenty-five years ago, abortion was still largely illegal and thought to be immoral, the sexual revolution (made possible by the extramarital use of the pill) was still in its infancy, and few had yet heard about the reproductive rights of single women, homosexual men and lesbians. (Never mind shameless memoirs about one's own incest!) Then one could argue, without embarrassment, that the new technologies of human reproduction—babies without sex—and their confounding of normal kin relations—who's the mother: the egg donor; the surrogate who carries and delivers, or the one who rears?—would "undermine the justification and support that biological parenthood gives to the monogamous marriage." Today, defenders of stable, monogamous marriage risk charges of giving offense to those adults who are living in "new family forms" or to those children who, even without the benefit of assisted reproduction, have acquired either three or four parents or one or none at all. Today, one must even apologize for voicing opinions that twenty-five years ago were nearly universally regarded as the core of our culture's wisdom on these matters. In a world whose once-given natural boundaries are blurred by technological change and whose moral boundaries are seemingly up for grabs, it is much more difficult to make persuasive the still compelling case against cloning human beings. As Raskolnikov put it "man gets used to everything—the beast!"

Indeed, perhaps the most depressing feature of the discussions that immediately followed the news about Dolly was their ironical tone, their genial cynicism, their moral fatigue: "AN UDDER WAY OF MAKING LAMBS" *(Nature)*, "WHO WILL CASH IN ON BREAKTHROUGH IN CLONING?" *(The Wall Street Journal)*, "IS CLONING BAAAAAAAAD?" *(The Chicago Tribune)*. Gone from the scene are the wise and courageous voices of Theodosius Dobzhansky (genetics), Hans Jonas (philosophy) and Paul Ramsey (theology) who, only twenty-five years ago, all made powerful moral arguments against ever cloning a human being. We are now too sophisticated for such argumentation; we wouldn't be caught in public with a strong moral stance, never mind an absolutist one. We are all, or almost all, post-modernists now.

Cloning turns out to be the perfect embodiment of the ruling opinions of our new age. Thanks to the sexual revolution, we are able to deny in practice, and increasingly in thought, the inherent procreative teleology of sexuality itself. But, if sex has no intrinsic connection to generating babies, babies need have no necessary connection to sex. Thanks to feminism and the gay rights movement, we are increasingly encouraged to treat the natural heterosexual difference and its preeminence as a matter of "cultural construction." But if male and female are not normatively complementary and generatively significant, babies need not come from male and female complementarity. Thanks to the prominence and the acceptability of divorce and out-of-wedlock births, stable, monogamous marriage as the ideal home for procreation is no longer the agreed-upon cultural norm. For this new dispensation, the clone is the ideal emblem: the ultimate "single-parent child."

Thanks to our belief that all children should be *wanted* children (the more high-minded principle we use to justify contraception and abortion), sooner or later only those children who fulfill our wants will be fully acceptable. Through cloning, we can work our wants and wills on the very identity of our children, exercising control as never before. Thanks to modern notions of individualism and the rate of cultural change, we see ourselves not as linked to ancestors and defined by traditions, but as projects for our own self-creation, not only as self-made men but also man-made selves; and self-cloning is simply an extension of such rootless and narcissistic self-re-creation.

Unwilling to acknowledge our debt to the past and unwilling to embrace the uncertainties and the limitations of the future, we have a false relation to both: cloning personifies our desire fully to control the future, while being subject to no controls ourselves. Enchanted and enslaved by the glamour of technology, we have lost our awe and wonder before the deep mysteries of nature and of life. We cheerfully take our own beginnings in our hands and, like the last man, we blink.

Part of the blame for our complacency lies, sadly, with the field of bioethics itself, and its claim to expertise in these moral matters. Bioethics was founded by people who understood that the new biology touched and threatened the deepest matters of our humanity: bodily integrity, identity and individuality, lineage and kinship, freedom and self-command, eros and aspiration, and the relations and strivings of body and soul. With its capture by analytic philosophy, however, and its inevitable routinization and professionalization, the field has by and large come to content itself with analyzing moral arguments, reacting to new technological developments and taking on emerging issues of public policy, all performed with a naive faith that the evils we fear can all be avoided by compassion, regulation and a respect for autonomy. Bioethics has made some major contributions in the protection of human subjects and in other areas where personal freedom is threatened; but its practitioners, with few exceptions, have turned the big human questions into pretty thin gruel.

One reason for this is that the piecemeal formation of public policy tends to grind down large questions of morals into small questions of procedure. Many of the country's leading bioethicists have served on national commissions or state task forces and advisory boards, where, understandably, they have found utilitarianism to be the only ethical vocabulary acceptable to all participants in discussing issues of law, regulation and public policy. As many of these commissions have been either officially under the aegis of NIH or the Health and Human Services Department, or otherwise dominated by powerful voices for scientific progress, the ethicists have for the most part been content, after some "values clarification" and wringing of hands, to pronounce their blessings upon the inevitable. Indeed, it is the bioethicists, not the scientists, who are now the most articulate defenders of human cloning: the two witnesses testifying before the National Bioethics Advisory Commission in favor of cloning human beings were bioethicists, eager to rebut what they regard as the irrational concerns of those of us in opposition. We have come to expect from the "experts" an accomodationist ethic that will rubber-stamp all technical innovation, in the mistaken belief that all other goods must bow down before the gods of better health and scientific advance.

If we are to correct our moral myopia, we must first of all persuade ourselves not to be complacent about what is at issue here. Human cloning, though it is in some respects continuous with previous reproductive technologies, also represents something radically new, in itself and in its easily foreseeable consequences. The stakes are very high indeed. I exaggerate, but in the direction of the truth, when I insist that we are faced with having to decide nothing less than whether human procreation is going to remain human, whether children are going to be made rather than begotten, whether it is a good thing, humanly speaking, to say yes in principle to the road which leads (at best) to the dehumanized rationality of *Brave New World*. This is not business as usual, to be fretted about for a while but finally to be given our seal of approval. We must rise to the occasion and make our judgments as if the future of our humanity hangs in the balance. For so it does.

THE STATE OF THE ART

If we should not underestimate the significance of human cloning, neither should we exaggerate its imminence or misunderstand just what is involved. The procedure is conceptually simple. The nucleus of a mature but unfertilized egg is removed and replaced with a nucleus obtained from a specialized cell of an adult (or fetal) organism (in Dolly's case, the donor nucleus came from mammary gland epithelium). Since almost all the hereditary material of a cell is contained within its nucleus, the renucleated egg and the individual into which this egg develops are genetically identical to the organism that was the source of the transferred nucleus. An unlimited number of genetically identical individuals—clones—could be produced by nuclear transfer. In principle, any person, male or female, newborn or adult, could be cloned, and in any quantity. With laboratory cultivation and storage of tissues, cells outliving their sources make it possible even to clone the dead.

The technical stumbling block, overcome by Wilmut and his colleagues, was to find a means of reprogramming the state of the DNA in the donor cells, reversing its differentiated expression and restoring its full totipotency, so that it could again direct the entire process of producing a mature organism. Now that this problem has been solved, we should expect a rush to develop cloning for other animals, especially livestock, in order to propagate in perpetuity the champion meat or milk producers. Though exactly how soon someone will succeed in cloning a human being is anybody's guess, Wilmut's technique, almost certainly applicable to humans, makes *attempting* the feat an imminent possibility.

Yet some cautions are in order and some possible misconceptions need correcting. For a start, cloning is not Xeroxing. As has been reassuringly reiterated, the clone of Mel Gibson, though his genetic double, would enter the world hairless, toothless and peeing in his diapers, just like any other human infant. Moreover, the success rate, at least at first, will probably not be very high: the British transferred 277 adult nuclei into enucleated sheep eggs, and implanted twenty-nine clonal embryos, but they achieved the birth of only one live lamb clone. For this reason, among others, it is unlikely that, at least for now, the practice would be very popular, and there is no immediate worry of mass-scale production of multicopies. The need of repeated surgery to obtain eggs and, more crucially, of numerous borrowed wombs for implantation will surely limit use, as will the expense; besides, almost everyone who is able will doubtless prefer nature's sexier way of conceiving.

Still, for the tens of thousands of people already sustaining over 200 assisted-reproduction clinics in the United States and already availing themselves of in vitro fertilization, intracytoplasmic sperm injection and other techniques of assisted reproduction, cloning would be an option with virtually no added fuss (especially when the success rate improves). Should commercial interests develop in "nucleus-banking," as they have in sperm-banking; should famous athletes or other celebrities decide to market their DNA the way they now market their autographs and just about everything else; should techniques of embryo and germline genetic testing and manipulation arrive as anticipated, increasing the use of laboratory assistance in order to obtain "better" babies—should all this come to pass, then cloning, if it is permitted, could become more than a marginal practice simply on the basis of free reproductive choice, even without any social encouragement to upgrade the gene pool or to replicate superior types. Moreover, if laboratory research on human cloning proceeds, even without any intention to produce cloned humans, the existence of cloned human embryos in the laboratory, created to begin with only for research purposes, would surely pave the way for later baby-making implantations.

In anticipation of human cloning, apologists and proponents have already made clear possible uses of the perfected technology, ranging from the sentimental and compassionate to the grandiose. They include: providing a child for an infertile couple; "replacing" a beloved spouse or child who is dying or has died; avoiding the risk of genetic disease; permitting reproduction for homosexual men and lesbians who want nothing sexual to do with the opposite sex; securing a genetically identical source of organs or tissues perfectly suitable for transplantation; getting a child with a genotype of one's own choosing, not excluding oneself; replicating individuals of great genius, talent or beauty—having a child who really could "be like Mike"; and creating large sets of genetically identical humans suitable for research on, for instance, the question of nature versus nurture, or for special missions in peace and war (not excluding espionage), in which using

identical humans would be an advantage. Most people who envision the cloning of human beings, of course, want none of these scenarios. That they cannot say why is not surprising. What is surprising, and welcome, is that, in our cynical age, they are saying anything at all.

THE WISDOM OF REPUGNANCE

"Offensive." "Grotesque." "Revolting." "Repugnant." "Repulsive." These are the words most commonly heard regarding the prospect of human cloning. Such reactions come both from the man or woman in the street and from the intellectuals, from believers and atheists, from humanists and scientists. Even Dolly's creator has said he "would find it offensive" to clone a human being.

People are repelled by many aspects of human cloning. They recoil from the prospect of mass production of human beings, with large clones of look-alikes, compromised in their individuality; the idea of father-son or mother-daughter twins; the bizarre prospects of a woman giving birth to and rearing a genetic copy of herself, her spouse or even her deceased father or mother; the grotesqueness of conceiving a child as an exact replacement for another who has died; the utilitarianism creation of embryonic genetic duplicates of oneself, to be frozen away or created when necessary, in case of need for homologous tissues or organs for transplantation; the narcissism of those who would clone themselves and the arrogance of others who think they know who deserves to be cloned or which genotype any child-to-be should be thrilled to receive; the Frankensteinian hubris to create human life and increasingly to control its destiny; man playing God. Almost no one finds any of the suggested reasons for human cloning compelling; almost everyone anticipates its possible misuses and abuses. Moreover, many people feel oppressed by the sense that there is probably nothing we can do to prevent it from happening. This makes the prospect all the more revolting.

Revulsion is not an argument; and some of yesterday's repugnances are today calmly accepted—though one must add, not always for the better. In crucial cases, however, repugnance is the emotional expression of deep wisdom, beyond reason's power fully to articulate it. Can anyone really give an argument fully adequate to the horror which is father-daughter incest (even with consent), or having sex with animals, or mutilating a corpse, or eating human flesh, or even just (just!) raping or murdering another human being? Would anybody's failure to give full rational justification for his or her revulsion at these practices make that revulsion ethically suspect? Not at all. On the contrary, we are suspicious of those who think that they can rationalize away our horror, say, by trying to explain the enormity of incest with arguments only about the genetic risks of inbreeding.

The repugnance at human cloning belongs in this category. We are repelled by the prospect of cloning human beings not because of the strangeness or novelty of the undertaking, but because we intuit and feel, immediately and without argument, the violation of things that we rightfully hold dear. Repugnance, here as elsewhere, revolts against the excesses of human willfulness, warning us not to transgress what is unspeakably profound. Indeed, in this age in which everything is held to be permissible so long as it is freely done, in which our given human nature no longer commands respect, in which our bodies are regarded as mere instruments of our autonomous rational wills, repugnance may be the only voice left that speaks up to defend the central core of our humanity. Shallow are the souls that have forgotten how to shudder.

The goods protected by repugnance are generally overlooked by our customary ways of approaching all new biomedical technologies. The way we evaluate cloning ethically will in fact be shaped by how we characterize it descriptively, by the context into which we place it, and by the perspective from which we view it. The first task for ethics is proper description. And here is where our failure begins.

Typically, cloning is discussed in one or more of three familiar contexts, which one might call the technological, the liberal and the meliorist. Under the first, cloning will be seen as an extension of existing techniques for assisting reproduction and determining the genetic makeup of children. Like them, cloning is to be regarded as a neutral technique, with no inherent meaning or goodness, but subject to multiple uses, some good, some bad. The morality of cloning thus depends absolutely on the goodness or badness of the motives and intentions of the cloners: as one bioethicist defender of cloning puts it, "the ethics must be judged [only] by the way the parents nurture and rear their resulting child and whether they bestow the same love and affection on a child brought into existence by a technique of assisted reproduction as they would on a child born in the usual way."

The liberal (or libertarian or liberationist) perspective sets cloning in the context of rights, freedoms and personal empowerment. Cloning is just a new option for exercising an individual's right to reproduce or to have the kind of child that he or she wants. Alternatively, cloning enhances our liberation (especially women's liberation) from the confines of nature, the vagaries of chance, or the necessity for sexual mating. Indeed, it liberates women from the need for men altogether, for the process requires only eggs, nuclei and (for the time being) uteri—plus, of course, a healthy dose of our (allegedly "masculine") manipulative science that likes to do all these things to mother nature and nature's mothers. For those who hold this outlook, the only moral restraints on cloning are adequately informed consent and the avoidance of bodily harm. If no one is cloned without her consent, and if the clonant is not physically damaged, then the liberal conditions for licit, hence moral, conduct are met. Worries that go beyond violating the will or maiming the body are dismissed as "symbolic"—which is to say, unreal.

The meliorist perspective embraces valetudinarians and also eugenicists. The latter were formerly more vocal in these discussions, but they are now generally happy to see their goals advanced under the less threatening banners of freedom and technological growth. These people see in cloning a new prospect for improving human beings—minimally, by ensuring the perpetuation of healthy individuals by avoiding the risks of genetic disease inherent in the lottery of sex, and maximally, by producing "optimum babies," preserving outstanding genetic material, and (with the help of soon-to-come techniques for precise genetic engineering) enhancing inborn human capacities on many fronts. Here the morality of cloning as a means is justified solely by the excellence of the end, that is, by the outstanding traits or individuals cloned—beauty, or brawn, or brains.

These three approaches, all quintessentially American and all perfectly fine in their places, are sorely wanting as approaches to human procreation. It is, to say the least, grossly distorting to view the wondrous mysteries of birth, renewal and individuality, and the deep meaning of parent-child relations, largely through the lens of our reductive science and its potent technologies. Similarly, considering reproduction (and the intimate relations of family life!) primarily under the political-legal, adversarial and individualistic notion of rights can only undermine the private yet fundamentally social, cooperative and duty-laden character of child-bearing, child-rearing and their bond to the covenant of marriage. Seeking to escape entirely from nature (in order to satisfy a natural desire or a natural right to reproduce!) is self-contradictory in theory and self-alienating in practice. For we are erotic beings only because we are embodied beings, and not merely intellects and wills unfortunately imprisoned in our bodies. And, though health and fitness are clearly great goods, there is something deeply disquieting in looking on our prospective children as artful products perfectible by genetic engineering, increasingly held to our willfully imposed designs, specifications and margins of tolerable error.

The technical, liberal and meliorist approaches all ignore the deeper anthropological, social and, indeed, ontological meanings of bringing forth new life. To this more fitting and profound point of view, cloning shows itself to be a major alteration, indeed, a major violation, of our given nature as embodied, gendered and engendering beings—and of the social relations built on this natural ground. Once this perspective is recognized, the ethical judgment on cloning can no longer be reduced to a matter of motives and intentions, rights and freedoms, benefits and harms, or even means and ends. It must be regarded primarily as a matter of meaning: Is cloning a fulfillment of human begetting and belonging? Or is cloning rather, as I contend, their pollution and perversion? To pollution and perversion, the fitting response can only be horror and revulsion; and conversely, generalized horror and revulsion are prima facie evidence of foulness and violation. The burden of moral argument must fall entirely on those who want to declare the widespread repugnances of humankind to be mere timidity or superstition.

Yet repugnance need not stand naked before the bar of reason. The wisdom of our horror at human cloning can be partially articulated, even if this is finally one of those instances about which the heart has its reasons that reason cannot entirely know.

THE PROFUNDITY OF SEX

To see cloning in its proper context, we must begin not, as I did before, with laboratory technique, but with the anthropology—natural and social—of sexual reproduction.

Sexual reproduction—by which I mean the generation of new life from (exactly) two complementary elements, one female, one male, (usually) through coitus—is established (if that is the right term) not by human decision, culture or tradition, but by nature; it is the natural way of all mammalian reproduction. By nature, each child has two complementary biological progenitors. Each child thus stems from and unites exactly two lineages. In natural generation, moreover, the precise genetic constitution of the resulting offspring is determined by a combination of nature and chance, not by human design: each human child shares the common natural human species genotype, each child is genetically (equally) kin to each (both) parent(s), yet each child is also genetically unique.

These biological truths about our origins foretell deep truths about our identity and about our human condition altogether. Every one of us is at once equally human, equally enmeshed in a particular familial nexus of origin, and equally individuated in our trajectory from birth to death—and, if all goes well, equally capable (despite our mortality) of participating, with a complimentary other, in the very same renewal of such human possibility through procreation. Though less momentous than our common humanity, our genetic individuality is not humanly trivial. It shows itself forth in our distinctive appearance through which we are everywhere recognized; it is revealed in our "signature" marks of fingerprints and our self-recognizing immune system; it symbolizes and foreshadows exactly the unique, never-to-be-repeated character of each human life.

Human societies virtually everywhere have structured child-rearing responsibilities and systems of identity and relationship on the bases of these deep natural facts of begetting. The mysterious yet ubiquitous "love of one's own" is everywhere culturally exploited, to make sure that children are not just produced but well cared for and to create for everyone clear ties of meaning, belonging and obligation. But it is wrong to treat such naturally rooted social practices as mere cultural constructs (like left- or right-driving, or like burying or cremating the dead) that we can alter with little human cost. What would kinship be without its clear natural grounding? And what would identity be without kinship? We must resist those who have begun to refer to sexual reproduction as the "traditional method of reproduction," who would have us regard as merely traditional, and by implication arbitrary, what is in truth not only natural but most certainly profound.

Asexual reproduction, which produces "single-parent" offspring, is a radical departure from the natural human way, confounding all normal understandings of father, mother, sibling, grandparent, etc., and all moral relations tied thereto. It becomes even more of a radical departure when the resulting offspring is a clone derived not from an embryo, but from a mature adult to whom the clone would be an identical twin; and when the process occurs not by natural accident (as in natural twinning), but by deliberate human design and manipulation; and when the child's (or children's) genetic constitution is preselected by the parent(s) (or scientists). Accordingly, as we will see, cloning is vulnerable to three kinds of concerns and objections, related to these three points: cloning threatens confusion of identity and individuality, even in small-scale cloning; cloning represents a giant step (though not the first one) toward transforming procreation into manufacture, that is, toward the increasing depersonalization of the process of generation and, increasingly, toward the "production" of human children as artifacts, products of human will and design (what others have called the problem of "commodification" of new life); and cloning—like other forms of eugenic engineering of the next generation—represents a form of despotism of the cloners over the cloned, and thus (even in benevolent cases) represents a blatant violation of the inner meaning of parent-child relations, of what it means to have a child, of what it means to say "yes" to our own demise and "replacement."

Before turning to these specific ethical objections, let me test my claim of the profundity of the natural way by taking up a challenge recently posed by a friend. What if the given natural human way of reproduction were asexual, and we now had to deal with a new technological innovation—artificially induced sexual dimorphism and the fusing of complementary gametes—whose inventors argued that sexual reproduction promised all sorts of advantages, including hybrid vigor and the creation of greatly increased individuality? Would one then be forced to defend natural asexuality because it was natural? Could one claim that it carried deep human meaning?

The response to this challenge broaches the ontological meaning of sexual reproduction. For it is impossible, I submit, for there to have been human life—or even higher forms of animal life—in the absence of sexuality and sexual reproduction. We find asexual reproduction only in the lowest forms of life: bacteria, algae, fungi, some lower invertebrates. Sexuality brings with it a new and enriched relationship to the world. Only sexual animals can seek and find complementary others with whom to pursue a goal that transcends their own existence. For a sexual being, the world is no longer an indifferent and largely homogeneous *otherness*, in part edible, in part dangerous. It also contains some very special and related and complementary beings, of the same kind but of opposite sex, toward whom one reaches out with special interest and intensity. In higher birds and mammals, the outward gaze keeps a lookout not only for food and predators, but also for prospective mates; the beholding of the many splendored world is suffused with desire for union, the animal antecedent of human eros and the germ of sociality. Not by accident is the human animal both the sexiest animal—whose females do not go into heat but are receptive throughout the estrous cycle and whose males must therefore have greater sexual appetite and energy in order to reproduce successfully—and also the most aspiring, the most social, the most open and the most intelligent animal.

The soul-elevating power of sexuality is, at bottom, rooted in its strange connection to mortality, which it simultaneously accepts and tries to overcome. Asexual reproduction may be seen as a continuation of the activity of self-preservation. When one organism buds or divides to become two, the original being is (doubly) preserved, and nothing dies. Sexuality, by contrast, means perishability and serves replacement; the two that come together to generate one soon will die. Sexual desire, in human beings as in animals, thus serves an end that is partly hidden from, and finally at odds with, the self-serving individual. Whether we know it or not, when we are sexually active we are voting with our genitalia for our own demise. The salmon swimming upstream to spawn and die tell the universal story: sex is bound up with death, to which it holds a partial answer in procreation.

The salmon and the other animals evince this truth blindly. Only the human being can understand what it means. As we learn so powerfully from the story of the Garden of Eden, our humanization is coincident with sexual self-consciousness, with the recognition of our sexual nakedness and all that it implies: shame at our needy incompleteness, unruly self-division and finitude; awe before the eternal; hope in the self-transcending possibilities of children and a relationship to the divine. In the sexually self-conscious animal, sexual desire can become eros, lust can become love. Sexual desire humanly regarded is thus sublimated into erotic longing for wholeness, completion and immortality, which drives us knowingly into the embrace and its generative fruit—as well as into all the higher human possibilities of deed, speech and song.

Through children, a good common to both husband and wife, male and female achieve some genuine unification (beyond the mere sexual "union," which fails to do so). The two become one through sharing generous (not needy) love for this third being as good. Flesh of their flesh, the child is the parents' own commingled being externalized, and given a separate and persisting existence. Unification is enhanced also by their commingled work of rearing. Providing an opening to the future beyond the grave, carrying not only our seed but also our names, our ways and our hopes that they will surpass us in goodness and happiness, children are a testament to the possibility of transcendence. Gender duality and sexual desire, which first draws our love upward and outside of ourselves, finally provide for the partial overcoming of the confinement and limitation of perishable embodiment altogether.

Human procreation, in sum, is not simply an activity of our rational wills. It is a more complete activity precisely because it engages us bodily, erotically and spiritually, as well as rationally. There is wisdom in the mystery of nature that has joined the pleasure of sex, the inarticulate longing for union, the communication of the loving embrace and the deep-seated and only partly articulate desire for children in the very activity by which we continue the chain of human existence and participate in the renewal of human possibility. Whether or not we know it, the severing of procreation from sex, love and intimacy is inherently dehumanizing, no matter how good the product.

We are now ready for the more specific objections to cloning.

THE PERVERSITIES OF CLONING

First, an important if formal objection: any attempt to clone a human being would constitute an unethical experiment upon the resulting child-to-be. As the animal experiments (frog and sheep) indicate, there are grave risks of mishaps and deformities. Moreover, because of what cloning means, one cannot presume a future cloned child's consent to be a clone, even a healthy one. Thus, ethically speaking, we cannot even get to know whether or not human cloning is feasible.

I understand, of course, the philosophical difficulty of trying to compare a life with defects against nonexistence. Several bioethicists, proud of their philosophical cleverness, use this conundrum to embarrass claims that one can injure a child in its conception, precisely because it is only thanks to that complained-of conception that the child is alive to complain. But common sense tells us that we have no reason to fear such philosophisms. For we surely know that people can harm and even maim children in the very act of conceiving them, say, by paternal transmission of the AIDS virus, maternal transmission of heroin dependence or, arguably, even by bringing them into being as bastards or with no capacity or willingness to look after them properly. And we believe that to do this intentionally, or even negligently, is inexcusable and clearly unethical. . . .

Cloning creates serious issues of identity and individuality. The cloned person may experience concerns about his distinctive identity not only because he will be in genotype and appearance identical to another human being, but, in this case, because he may also be twin to the person who is his "father" or "mother"—if one can still call them that. What would be the psychic burdens of being the "child" or "parent" of your twin? The cloned individual, moreover, will be saddled with a genotype that has already lived. He will not be fully a surprise to the world. People are likely always to compare his performances in life with that of his alter ego. True, his nurture and his circumstance in life will be different; genotype is not exactly destiny. Still, one must also expect parental and other efforts to shape this new life after the original—or at least to view the child with the original version always firmly in mind. Why else did they clone from the star basketball player, mathematician and beauty queen—or even dear old dad—in the first place?

Since the birth of Dolly, there has been a fair amount of doublespeak on this matter of genetic identity. Experts have rushed in to reassure the public that the clone would in no way be the same person, or have any confusions about his or her identity: as previously noted, they are pleased to point out that the clone of Mel Gibson would not be Mel Gibson. Fair enough. But one is short-changing the truth by emphasizing the additional importance of the intrauterine environment, rearing and social setting: genotype obviously matters plenty. That, after all, is the only reason to clone, whether human beings or sheep. The odds that clones of Wilt Chamberlain will play in the NBA are, I submit, infinitely greater than they are for clones of Robert Reich.

Curiously, this conclusion is supported, inadvertently, by the one ethical sticking point insisted on by friends of cloning: no cloning without the donor's consent. Though an orthodox liberal objection, it is in fact quite puzzling when it comes from people (such as Ruth Macklin) who also insist that genotype is not identity or individuality, and who deny that a child could reasonably complain about being made a genetic copy. If the clone of Mel Gibson would not be Mel Gibson, why should Mel Gibson have grounds to object that someone had been made his clone? We already allow researchers to use blood and tissue samples for research purposes of no benefit to their sources: my falling hair, my expectorations, my urine and even my biopsied tissues are "not me" and not mine. Courts have

held that the profit gained from uses to which scientists put my discarded tissues do not legally belong to me. Why, then, no cloning without consent—including, I assume, no cloning from the body of someone who just died? What harm is done the donor, if genotype is "not me"? Truth to tell, the only powerful justification for objecting is that genotype really does have something to do with identity, and everybody knows it. If not, on what basis could Michael Jordan object that someone cloned "him," say, from cells taken from a "lost" scraped-off piece of his skin? The insistence on donor consent unwittingly reveals the problem of identity in all cloning.

Genetic distinctiveness not only symbolizes the uniqueness of each human life and the independence of its parents that each human child rightfully attains. It can also be an important support for living a worthy and dignified life. Such arguments apply with great force to any large-scale replication of human individuals. But they are sufficient, in my view, to rebut even the first attempts to clone a human being. One must never forget that these are human beings upon whom our eugenic or merely playful fantasies are to be enacted.

Troubled psychic identity (distinctiveness), based on all-too-evident genetic identity (sameness), will be made much worse by the utter confusion of social identity and kinship ties. For, as already noted, cloning radically confounds lineage and social relations, for "offspring" as for "parents." As bioethicist James Nelson has pointed out, a female child cloned from her "mother" might develop a desire for a relationship to her "father," and might understandably seek out the father of her "mother" who is after all also her biological twin sister. Would "grandpa," who thought his paternal duties concluded, be pleased to discover that the clonant looked to him for paternal attention and support?

Social identity, and social ties of relationship and responsibility are widely connected to, and supported by, biological kinship. Social taboos on incest (and adultery) everywhere serve to keep clear who is related to whom (and especially which child belongs to which parents), as well as to avoid confounding the social identity of parent-and-child (or brother-and-sister) with the social identity of lovers, spouses and co-parents. True, social identity is altered by adoption (but as a matter of the best interest of already living children: we do not deliberately produce children for adoption). True, artificial insemination and in vitro fertilization with donor sperm, or whole embryo donation, are in some way forms of "prenatal adoption"—a not altogether unproblematic practice. Even here, though, there is in each case (as in all sexual reproduction) a known male source of sperm and a known single female source of egg—a genetic father and a genetic mother—should anyone care to know (as adopted children often do) who is genetically related to whom.

In the case of cloning, however, there is but one "parent." The usually sad situation of the "single-parent child" is here deliberately planned, and with a vengeance. In the case of self-cloning, the "offspring" is, in addition, one's twin; and so the dreaded result of incest—to be parent to one's sibling—is here brought about deliberately, albeit without any act of coitus. Moreover, all other relationships will be confounded. What will father, grandfather, aunt, cousin, sister mean? Who will bear what ties and what burdens? What sort of social identity will someone have with one whole side—"father's" or "mother's"—necessarily excluded? It is no answer to say that our society, with its high incidence of divorce, remarriage, adoption, extramarital child-bearing and the rest, already confounds lineage and confuses kinship and responsibility for children (and everyone else), unless one also wants to argue that this is, for children, a preferable state of affairs.

Human cloning would also represent a giant step toward turning begetting into making, procreation into manufacture (literally, something "handmade"), a process already begun with in vitro fertilization and genetic testing of embryos. With cloning, not only is the process in hand, but the total genetic blueprint of the cloned individual is selected and determined by the human artisans. To be sure, subsequent development will take place according to natural processes; and the resulting children will still be recognizably human. But we here would be taking a major step into making man himself simply another one of the man-made things. Human nature becomes merely the last part of nature to succumb to the technological project, which turns all of nature into raw material at human disposal, to be homogenized by our rationalized technique according to the subjective prejudices of the day.

How does begetting differ from making? In natural procreation, human beings come together, complementarily male and female, to give existence to another being who is formed, exactly as we were, *by what we are*: living, hence perishable, hence aspiringly erotic, human beings. In clonal reproduction, by contrast, and in the more advanced forms of manufacture to which it leads, we give existence to a being not by what we are but by what we intend and design. As with any product of our making, no matter how excellent, the artificer stands above it, not as an equal but as a superior, transcending it by his will and creative prowess. Scientists who clone animals make it perfectly clear that they are engaged in instrumental making; the animals are, from the start, designed as means to serve rational human purposes. In human cloning, scientists and prospective "parents" would be adopting the same technocratic mentality to human children: human children would be their artifacts.

Such an arrangement is profoundly dehumanizing, no matter how good the product. Mass-scale cloning of the same individual makes the point vividly; but the violation of human equality, freedom and dignity are present even in a single planned clone. And procreation dehumanized into manufacture is further degraded by commodification, a virtually inescapable result of allowing baby-making to proceed under the banner of commerce. Genetic and reproductive biotechnology companies are already growth industries, but they will go into commercial orbit once the Human Genome Project nears completion. Supply will create enormous demand. Even before the capacity for human cloning arrives, established companies will have invested in the harvesting of eggs from ovaries obtained at autopsy or through ovarian surgery, practiced embryonic genetic alteration, and initiated the stockpiling of prospective donor tissues. Through the rental of surrogate-womb services, and through the buying and selling of tissues and embryos, priced according to the merit of the donor, the commodification of nascent human life will be unstoppable.

Finally, and perhaps most important, the practice of human cloning by nuclear transfer—like other anticipated forms of genetic engineering of the next generation—would enshrine and aggravate a profound and mischievous misunderstanding of the meaning of having children and of the parent-child relationship. When a couple now chooses to procreate, the partners are saying yes to the emergence of new life in its novelty, saying yes not only to having a child but also, tacitly, to having whatever child this child turns out to be. In accepting our finitude and opening ourselves to our replacement, we are tacitly confessing the limits of our control. In this ubiquitous way of nature, embracing the future by procreating means precisely that we are relinquishing our grip, in the very activity of taking up our own share in what we hope will be the immortality of human life and the human species. This means that our children are not *our* children: they are not our property, not our possessions. Neither are they supposed to live our lives for us, or anyone else's life but their own. To be sure, we seek to guide them on their way, imparting to them not just life but nurturing, love, and a way of life; to be sure, they bear our hopes that they will live fine and flourishing lives, enabling us in small measure to transcend our own limitations. Still, their genetic distinctiveness and independence are the natural foreshadowing of the deep truth that they have their own and never-before-enacted life to live. They are sprung from a past, but they take an uncharted course into the future.

Much harm is already done by parents who try to live vicariously through their children. Children are sometimes compelled to fulfill the broken dreams of unhappy parents: John Doe Jr. or the III is under the burden of having to live up to his forebear's name. Still, if most parents have hopes for their children, cloning parents will have expectations. In cloning, such overbearing parents take at the start a decisive step which contradicts the entire meaning of the open and forward-looking nature of parent-child relations. The child is given a genotype that has already lived, with full expectation that this blueprint of a past life ought to be controlling of the life that is to come. Cloning is inherently despotic, for it seeks to make one's children (or someone else's children) after one's own image (or an image of one's choosing) and their future according to one's will. In some cases, the despotism may be mild and benevolent. In other cases, it will be mischievous and downright tyrannical. But despotism—the control of another through one's will—it inevitably will be.

MEETING SOME OBJECTIONS

The defenders of cloning, of course, are not wittingly friends of despotism. Indeed, they regard themselves mainly as friends of freedom: the freedom of individuals to reproduce, the freedom of scientists and inventors to discover and devise and to foster "progress" in genetic knowledge and technique. They want large-scale cloning only for animals, but they wish to preserve cloning as a human option for exercising our "right to reproduce"—our right to have children, and children with "desirable genes." As law professor John Robertson points out, under our "right to reproduce" we already practice early forms of unnatural, artificial and extramarital reproduction, and we already practice early forms of eugenic choice. For this reason, he argues, cloning is no big deal.

We have here a perfect example of the logic of the slippery slope, and the slippery way in which it already works in this area. Only a few years ago, slippery slope arguments were used to oppose artificial insemination and in vitro fertilization using unrelated sperm donors. Principles used to justify these practices, it was said, will be used to justify more artificial and more eugenic practices, including cloning. Not so, the defenders retorted, since we can make the necessary distinctions. And now, without even a gesture at making the necessary distinctions, the continuity of practice is held by itself to be justificatory.

The principle of reproductive freedom as currently enunciated by the proponents of cloning logically embraces the ethical acceptability of sliding down the entire rest of the slope—to producing children ectogenetically from sperm to term (should it become feasible) and to producing children whose entire genetic makeup will be the product of parental eugenic planning and choice. If reproductive freedom means the right to have a child of one's own choosing, by whatever means, it knows and accepts no limits.

But, far from being legitimated by a "right to reproduce," the emergence of techniques of assisted reproduction and genetic engineering should compel us to reconsider the meaning and limits of such a putative right. In truth, a "right to reproduce" has always been a peculiar and problematic notion. Rights generally belong to individuals, but this is a right which (before cloning) no one can exercise alone. Does the right then inhere only in couples? Only in married couples? Is it a (woman's) right to carry or deliver or a right (of one or more parents) to nurture and rear? Is it a right to have your own biological child? Is it a right only to attempt reproduction, or a right also to succeed? Is it a right to acquire the baby of one's choice?

The assertion of a negative "right to reproduce" certainly makes sense when it claims protection against state interference with procreative liberty, say, through a program of compulsory sterilization. But surely it cannot be the basis of a tort claim against nature, to be made good by technology, should free efforts at natural procreation fail. Some insist that the right to reproduce embraces also the right against state interference with the free use of all technological means to obtain a child. Yet such a position cannot be sustained: for reasons having to do with the means employed, any community may rightfully prohibit surrogate pregnancy, or polygamy, or the sale of babies to infertile couples, without violating anyone's basic human "right to reproduce." When the exercise of a previously innocuous freedom now involves or impinges on troublesome practices that the original freedom never was intended to reach, the general presumption of liberty needs to be reconsidered.

We do indeed already practice negative eugenic selection, through genetic screening and prenatal diagnosis. Yet our practices are governed by a norm of health. We seek to prevent the birth of children who suffer from known (serious) genetic diseases. When and if gene therapy becomes possible, such diseases could then be treated, in utero or even before implantation—I have no ethical objection in principle to such a practice (though I have some practical worries), precisely because it serves the medical goal of healing existing individuals. But therapy, to be therapy, implies not only an existing "patient." It also implies a norm of health. In this respect, even germline gene "therapy," though practiced not on a human being but on egg and sperm, is less radical than cloning, which is in no way therapeutic. But once one blurs the distinction between health promotion and genetic enhancement, between so-called negative and positive eugenics, one opens the door to all future eugenic designs. "To make sure that a child will be healthy and have good chances in life": this is Robertson's principle, and owing to its latter clause it is an utterly elastic principle, with no

boundaries. Being over eight feet tall will likely produce some very good chances in life, and so will having the looks of Marilyn Monroe, and so will a genius-level intelligence.

Proponents want us to believe that there are legitimate uses of cloning that can be distinguished from illegitimate uses, but by their own principles no such limits can be found. (Nor could any such limits be enforced in practice.) Reproductive freedom, as they understand it, is governed solely by the subjective wishes of the parents-to-be (plus the avoidance of bodily harm to the child). The sentimentally appealing case of the childless married couple is, on these grounds, indistinguishable from the case of an individual (married or not) who would like to clone someone famous or talented, living or dead. Further, the principle here endorsed justifies not only cloning but, indeed, all future artificial attempts to create (manufacture) "perfect" babies.

A concrete example will show how, in practice no less than in principle, the so-called innocent case will merge with, or even turn into, the more troubling ones. In practice, the eager parents-to-be will necessarily be subject to the tyranny of expertise. Consider an infertile married couple, she lacking eggs or he lacking sperm, that wants a child of their (genetic) own, and propose to clone either husband or wife. The scientist-physician (who is also co-owner of the cloning company) points out the likely difficulties—a cloned child is not really their (genetic) child, but the child of only *one* of them; this imbalance may produce strains on the marriage; the child might suffer identity confusion; there is a risk of perpetuating the cause of sterility; and so on—and he also points out the advantages of choosing a donor nucleus. Far better than a child of their own would be a child of their own choosing. Touting his own expertise in selecting healthy and talented donors, the doctor presents the couple with his latest catalog containing the pictures, the health records and the accomplishments of his stable of cloning donors, samples of whose tissues are in his deep freeze. Why not, dearly beloved, a more perfect baby?

The "perfect baby," of course, is the project not of the infertility doctors, but of the eugenic scientists and their supporters. For them, the paramount right is not the so-called right to reproduce but what biologist Bentley Glass called, a quarter of a century ago, "the right of every child to be born with a sound physical and mental constitution, based on a sound genotype . . . the inalienable right to a sound heritage." But to secure this right, and to achieve the requisite quality control over new human life, human conception and gestation will need to be brought fully into the bright light of the laboratory, beneath which it can be fertilized, nourished, pruned, weeded, watched, inspected, prodded, pinched, cajoled, injected, tested, rated, graded, approved, stamped, wrapped, sealed and delivered. There is no other way to produce the perfect baby.

Yet we are urged by proponents of cloning to forget about the science fiction scenarios of laboratory manufacture and multiple-copied clones, and to focus only on the homely cases of infertile couples exercising their reproductive rights. But why, if the single cases are so innocent, should multiplying their performance be so off-putting? (Similarly, why do others object to people making money off this practice, if the practice itself is perfectly acceptable?) When we follow the sound ethical principle of universalizing our choice—"would it be right if everyone cloned a Wilt Chamberlain (with his consent, of course)? Would it be right if everyone decided to practice asexual reproduction?"—we discover what is wrong with these seemingly innocent cases. The so-called science fiction cases make vivid the meaning of what looks to us, mistakenly, to be benign.

Though I recognize certain continuities between cloning and, say, in vitro fertilization, I believe that cloning differs in essential and important ways. Yet those who disagree should be reminded that the "continuity" argument cuts both ways. Sometimes we establish bad precedents, and discover that they were bad only when we follow their inexorable logic to places we never meant to go. Can the defenders of cloning show us today how, on their principles, we will be able to see producing babies ("perfect babies") entirely in the laboratory or exercising full control over their genotypes (including so-called enhancement) as ethically different, in any essential way, from present forms of assisted reproduction? Or are they willing to admit, despite their attachment to the principle of continuity, that the complete obliteration of "mother" or "father," the complete depersonalization of procreation, the complete manufacture of human beings and the complete genetic control of one

generation over the next would be ethically problematic and essentially different from current forms of assisted reproduction? If so, where and how will they draw the line, and why? I draw it at cloning, for all the reasons given.

BAN THE CLONING OF HUMANS

What, then, should we do? We should declare that human cloning is unethical in itself and dangerous in its likely consequences. In so doing, we shall have the backing of the overwhelming majority of our fellow Americans, and of the human race, and (I believe) of most practicing scientists. Next, we should do all that we can to prevent the cloning of human beings. We should do this by means of an international legal ban if possible, and by a unilateral national ban, at a minimum. Scientists may secretly undertake to violate such a law, but they will be deterred by not being able to stand up proudly to claim the credit for their technological bravado and success. Such a ban on clonal baby-making, moreover, will not harm the progress of basic genetic science and technology. On the contrary, it will reassure the public that scientists are happy to proceed without violating the deep ethical norms and intuitions of the human community.

This still leaves the vexed question about laboratory research using early embryonic human clones, specially created only for such research purposes, with no intention to implant them into a uterus. There is no question that such research holds great promise for gaining fundamental knowledge about normal (and abnormal) differentiation, and for developing tissue lines for transplantation that might be used, say, in treating leukemia or in repairing brain or spinal cord injuries—to mention just a few of the conceivable benefits. Still, unrestricted clonal embryo research will surely make the production of living human clones much more likely. Once the genies put the cloned embryos into the bottles, who can strictly control where they go (especially in the absence of legal prohibitions against implanting them to produce a child)? . . .

The president's call for a moratorium on human cloning has given us an important opportunity. In a truly unprecedented way, we can strike a blow for the human control of the technological project, for wisdom, prudence and human dignity. The prospect of human cloning, so repulsive to contemplate, is the occasion for deciding whether we shall be slaves of unregulated progress, and ultimately its artifacts, or whether we shall remain free human beings who guide our technique toward the enhancement of human dignity. If we are to seize the occasion, we must, as the late Paul Ramsey wrote,

> raise the ethical questions with a serious and not a frivolous conscience. A man of frivolous conscience announces that there are ethical quandaries ahead that we must urgently consider before the future catches up with us. By this he often means that we need to devise a new ethics that will provide the rationalization for doing in the future what men are bound to do because of new actions and interventions science will have made possible. In contrast a man of serious conscience means to say in raising urgent ethical questions that there may be some things that men should never do. The good things that men do can be made complete only by the things they refuse to do.

SECTION 4

Genetic Screening and Testing

The Introduction of Cystic Fibrosis Carrier Screening into Clinical Practice : Policy Considerations

Benjamin S. Wilfond and Norman Fost

Since the identification of the gene associated with cystic fibrosis (CF), interest in general population CF carrier screening has been growing. Screening has the potential to allow individuals to make more informed reproductive decisions and to increase the choices available to them for avoiding the birth of a child with CF while offering society the potential public health benefit of a reduced incidence of individuals with CF. With the anticipated expansion of genetic knowledge resulting from the Human Genome Initiative, the experience of providing CF screening to the general population may become a model for developing new genetic tests and subsequently integrating them into clinical medical practice. More important, the potential magnitude of CF carrier testing in the reproductive-aged population gives this issue immediate relevance.

Soon after the CF gene mutation sequence was published, several biotechnology companies offered this service to physicians. However, enthusiasm for screening has been tempered by two policy statements, one issued by the American Society of Human Genetics (ASHG) in November 1989, and the other by the National Institutes of Health (NIH) during a workshop on population screening for the CF gene held in March 1990, both recommending a moratorium on routine screening. The statements concur on several key points:

1. Routine screening should be delayed until pilot studies are completed, as "there is little experience in the delivery of such complex information to large populations." The com-

Milbank Quarterly, Vol. 70, No. 4, 1992, 629–659. Used with permission.

EDITORS' NOTE: References have been omitted; those wishing to follow up on sources should consult the original article.

plexity of the information derives from the ambiguity of negative test results and the variable prognosis for CF, complicating the education and counseling process, which would be formidable for a large population even with a simpler test.

2. If the test had a greater detection rate, then it might be appropriate to consider mass population screening. The NIH workshop report recommends that "screening could be offered to all persons of reproductive age if a 95 [percent] level of carrier detection were achieved," but only if additional conditions were met.

3. "Carrier testing should be offered couples in which either partner has a close relative affected with CF."

4. The "optimal setting for carrier testing is through primary health care providers."

Although these recommendations have dampened the initial drive for screening while articulating the current consensus on practice recommendations, they have not been analyzed in detail. Our purpose in this article is to review critically the ASHG and the NIH workshop recommendations, to evaluate some of the legal and ethical issues that will influence physicians' screening practices for cystic fibrosis, and to propose guidelines for their screening practices to primary care physicians and genetics services providers.

CLINICAL BACKGROUND

Cystic fibrosis is one of the most common significant autosomal recessive diseases affecting the white population. The median life expectancy of about 28 years has been steadily rising for more than two decades. The median survival of patients born in 1990 has been estimated to be 40 years, based on an observed decline in infant mortality of CF patients. Current investigational therapies, such as DNase, offer the potential for even longer survival. Patients are variably affected, dying in infancy from meconium ileus, a neonatal intestinal obstruction, some severely disabled with chronic obstructive pulmonary disease (COPD) as children, whereas others are rarely hospitalized, play competitive sports, and may not even develop symptoms until adulthood. However, most people with CF develop moderate lung disease by adolescence or early adulthood.

The CF incidence in whites ranges from 1 in 1,700 to 1 in 6,500 in various populations, but is generally estimated to be 1 in 2,500 live births. Assuming this incidence, approximately 1 in 25 white individuals (4 percent) are heterozygotes—asymptomatic carriers with a 1 in 4 chance of having a child with CF if their partners are also carriers. Recent newborn screening data from Colorado and Wisconsin suggest that the incidence of CF in whites may be the range of from 1 in 3,000 to 1 in 3,500. The Cystic Fibrosis Patient Registry estimates the incidence to be 1 in 3,400 in whites and 1 in 15,000 in blacks, with a corresponding carrier frequency of 1 in 30 for whites and 1 in 62 for blacks. Risk calculations in this article will be based on the most current data.

Cystic fibrosis results from mutations in a gene mapped to chromosome 7 that codes for a protein, the cystic fibrosis transmembrane conductance regulator (CFTR), which facilitates chloride transport. In the United States, the most common CFTR mutation, ΔF508, a three-base pair deletion, has been found on approximately 75 percent of chromosomes from CF patients. Over 175 additional mutations have been identified, most of them rare, but analysis of from four to seven of the most common mutations, using polymerase chain reaction (PCR) amplification and gel electrophoresis, could increase the carrier detection rate in the U.S. population to about 85 percent. With this detection rate, 72 percent (85 x 85) of at-risk couples will be identifiable. For varying ethnic and geographic groups, different mutations occur more commonly, which may require individualizing the testing protocol. Although the charge for the test is currently between $150 and $200, if screening is done on a mass scale, and with improved technology, the charge may be reduced to a range of from $30 to $50.

DEFERMENT OF POPULATION SCREENING UNTIL PILOT STUDIES DEMONSTRATE ITS SAFETY AND EFFECTIVENESS

The ASHG and the NIH workshop statements advocate that mass CF carrier-screening programs should only be implemented after pilot studies are completed. Pilot studies prior to mass genetic testing have been recommended by reports from the Hastings Center, the National Academy of Sciences, and the President's Commission for the Study of

Ethical Problems in Medicine and Biomedical and Behavioral Research. The rationale for pilot testing is that previous experiences with genetic testing have demonstrated serious problems such as confusion, stigmatization, and discrimination when no comprehensive infrastructure was in place to provide education, informed consent, and counseling. The primary purpose of pilot studies is to establish effective educational methods, to determine interest in testing, to evaluate the influence of test results on reproductive behavior, and to document the occurrence of adverse psychological and social effects.

Support for pilot studies of CF carrier screening has been articulated in the medical literature by ethicists, geneticists, obstetricians, pediatricians, and pulmonologists. Recently, the American Medical Association adopted a report affirming the same position, as did the American College of Obstetrics and Gynecology. As a result of the professional consensus for pilot studies, the NIH Ethical, Legal, and Social Implications Program of the National Center for Human Genome Research funded seven pilot programs for CF screening in October 1991.

However, many individuals with a commercial interest suggest that mass screening should be instituted without prior pilot studies. In 1989, Keith Brown, president of Gene Screen, a biotechnology company that markets the test, suggested that pilot studies were not reasonable and that mass screening was inevitable: "to [expect us to] wait until we get 99 percent of the mutations and a national program is defined in 2½ years, that's kind of dreaming. The genetics community is thinking about how to make it happen ideally. Forget it, that game is already lost". Others believe the potential benefits of testing sufficiently outweigh the possible risks and suggest that empirical verification of benefit is not necessary. For example, Schulman et al., writing for the Genetics and IVF [In Vitro Fertilization] Institute, a private laboratory and clinic in Virginia, argue that it is "neither necessary nor desirable to delay access to a test now capable of detecting the large majority of CF carriers and families [and that the] benefits to the general public must take priority over possible perturbations within the healthcare delivery system (expanded education and counseling efforts) if CF screenings were implemented without delay."

The central ethical dilemma is how to balance the benefit to persons who may wish to avoid the birth of a child with CF against the potential harm that would result from the confusion, stigmatization, and discrimination associated with testing. Although the rationale for pilot studies prior to population testing is based on the duty to avoid harm, it does not mean that interventions must carry no risks because this requirement would preclude most medical care. Rather, risks are expected to have at least the potential of compensating benefits: in this ease, that patients have sufficient information to allow an informed choice. The problem with Schulman's argument is that weighing the potential benefits and harms of mass screening cannot be performed without the empirical evidence from pilot studies.

Brock, who runs a pilot screening program in Scotland, puts forth a different argument in favor of screening, focusing on the autonomy of the patient. He asks "whether we have the right to withhold, largely because of our own unresolved worries about the capacity to provide adequate counseling, screening from those who request it." He implies that patients' requests for testing should outweigh paternalistic actions to withhold testing. However, such paternalism is consistent with long-standing policies that limit the use of experimental drugs and devices unless there has been institutional review and patient consent after being informed about the experimental nature of the medical intervention. There is no clear obligation to provide experimental interventions to persons who request them. However, what is actually experimental in CF carrier testing is not the test itself, but the mechanism to provide the test to large groups of people.

The mechanism to provide education, consent, and counseling should be evaluated because these activities will determine the balance between benefits and harms. Before deciding whether the benefits of screening are worth the risks, potential screenees must be educated so they can make a preliminary judgement about their reproductive options. In CF carrier testing, the major benefit is the opportunity to avoid the birth of an affected child, but this benefit disappears if test results would not affect a couple's reproductive plans. Unless the person identified another potential benefit, there would be no reason to conduct the tests. Other benefits of testing would include reassurance that a fetus does not have CF or emotional preparation for the birth of an affected child. The knowledge of an affected fetus may offer families the following practical benefits:

1. arranging for adequate medical insurance
2. providing for perinatal assessment
3. moving closer to a CF center that provides medical care
4. moving closer to family or other support networks
5. changing employment for the purpose of providing home care

Whether such potential benefits will be sufficient motivators to obtain testing is unknown.

In deciding whether to be tested, an individual would also need accurate, balanced information about the medical aspects of cystic fibrosis and, in order to comprehend their reproductive options, about the potential risks of being identified as a carrier and the implications of a negative test. Using current standards, such informed consent may require one to two hours of a genetic counselor's time. The use of alternative delivery systems, including pamphlets, videos, computers, or group sessions, will reduce personnel time, but these, too, need to be studied. The results of the NIH-funded pilot studies, which may not be avail-

able for at least two years, may not answer these questions sufficiently. Further studies may be required before population testing can be adequately assessed.

THE LIMITED RELEVANCE OF THE DETECTION RATE

Both documents cite the limited sensitivity of the tests as a major impediment to mass screening. Several biotechnology companies also acknowledge this factor, but their opinions vary as to what degree of sensitivity would justify mass screening. One commercial brochure states: "We would like the test to detect at least 90 [percent] of CF carriers before advising routine screening." Others claim that, at 75 percent, the necessary threshold had been reached. In fact, as early as February 1990, the Genetics and IVF Institute began offering prenatal ΔF508 screening of fetuses to all white couples undergoing amniocentesis or chorionic villus sampling (CVS) (Bick et al. 1990)

The NIH workshop noted the 95 percent threshold because of a concern for couples in which one partner is a carrier while the other has a negative test (table 1). Approximately 5 percent (1 in 18) of the couples in the general population would fall into this category (table 2). These couples cannot

Table 1. Cystic Fibrosis Carrier Testing—Changes After Mutation Analysis[a]

Percent of cystic fibrosis mutations detectable	Chance of being a carrier risk for person after a negative test	Chance of cystic fibrosis in offspring		
		One partner tested	Both partners tested	
		Negative	Both negative	One positive/ one negative
0	1 in 30	1 in 3,400	1 in 3,400	1 in 3,400
55	1 in 66	1 in 7,900	1 in 17,400	1 in 264
75	1 in 118	1 in 14,200	1 in 55,700	1 in 472
85	1 in 196	1 in 23,500	1 in 154,000	1 in 784
90	1 in 294	1 in 35,300	1 in 346,000	1 in 1,180
95	1 in 587	1 in 70,400	1 in 1,380,000	1 in 2,350
96	1 in 838	1 in 101,000	1 in 2,810,000	1 in 3,350

[a]Calculations described in Lemna et al. (1990). The chance of being a carrier (assuming an incidence of 1 in 3,400) after a negative test (assuming a detection rate [d]) is obtained by calculating the joint probability that a person is a carrier and has a negative test (.033 × [1 − d]) divided by the sum of the joint probabilities that a person is a carrier and has a negative test plus that of a person being a noncarrier and having a negative test (.097 × 1).

Table 2. Genetic Counseling Hours for 3 Million Couples

Carrier status	Frequency (%)[a]	Total couples	Minutes per couple	Hours
No carriers	94.47	2,834,100	10	472,400
One carrier	5.45	163,500	60	163,500
Two carriers	.08	2,400	60	2,400
Total	—	—	—	638,300

[a]Calculated given a carrier frequency $q = .033$ and detection rate $d = .85$; $(1 - dq)^2 + 2\,dq(1 - dq) + (dq)^2 = 1$.

be reassured that they are not at risk. The complexities associated with an imperfect CF test will be difficult to convey and understand, as evidenced by this confusing excerpt from the consent form of one commercial company:

> Due to the present inability to detect all CYSTIC FIBROSIS CARRIERS, if I am a carrier of the cystic fibrosis gene, and if the other parent of any child I may have is also a carrier of the cystic fibrosis gene, and if either of us are [sic] not detected to be carriers of the CYSTIC FIBROSIS GENE using the test presently available, then a child born to us may be affected with CYSTIC FIBROSIS.

The challenge for education and consent posed by these complexities has been a deterrent to mass screening. Ten-Kate has argued that once the detection rate is greater than 95 percent, the major barrier to mass population screening will have been removed because the risk to couples with only one detected carrier of having a child with CF will be no greater than the a priori risk in the general population (table 1). Although an improved detection rate is necessary, it is not sufficient, as indicated in the NIH workshop statement:

> These difficulties would be substantially reduced if testing could detect at least 90 to 95 percent of carriers. There is a consensus that population-based screening for carriers could be offered to all persons of reproductive age if a 95 percent level of carrier detection were achieved. The offering of population-based screening would still require that substantial educational and counselling guidelines be satisfied.

However, the NIH workshop statement has been misrepresented by at least one commercial company, whose brochure implies that a 90 percent detection rate would be sufficient:

> The members of that workshop also suggested that testing of individuals with no family history of the disease should not begin until, among other things, the test could detect "at least 90-95 [percent] of carriers". *This new CF carrier test satisfies that requirement* for Caucasians of northern European ancestry.
>
> For those individuals who are found not to carry any of these ten mutations, the negative results will, in effect, reduce their chance of being a CF carrier to only about 1 in 250. Thus, this new test may be of interest to ANYONE who has not yet completed their reproductive plans. (emphasis in original)

The brochure creates the impression that the NIH workshop would endorse screening for "anyone" because 90 percent of carriers are detectable. However, the consensus was 95 percent, not 90 percent. More important, the counseling and educational guidelines for population testing have not been sufficiently developed because the necessary research is still in progress.

CONCERN ABOUT PERSISTENT UNCERTAINTY

Although a higher detection rate will simplify the information, a detection rate of 93 percent is not sufficient justification for mass screening. It is still possible that families with one positive and one negative test will be left with uncertainty and a sense of increased risk. Basic concepts of probability and risk are not easily understood. A study of middle-class, pregnant women found that 25 percent interpreted a 1 in 1,000 chance to mean 10 percent or greater. People also tend to translate uncertainty into a binary form that focuses on the numerator of one, projecting from it that the event either will occur or not. Even though the majority of couples is not at risk of having a child with CF, some might alter their reproductive plans (including the abortion of healthy fetuses) because they are confused about the impression of risk created by testing results.

Even with a 95 percent rate, as a result of the testing process, a couple with one positive test may falsely *perceive* their risk for having an affected child to be higher than before testing. Without testing, the couple may have given little thought to CF, unaware of the baseline risk. The process of carrier testing may heighten a couple's concern about CF, causing anxiety or irrational changes in reproductive plans, particularly if genetic counseling is inadequate. For example, although few couples' reproductive plans are influenced by the theoretical 2 percent risk of serious congenital problems, a couple that was informed about a "test" result showing a 2 percent chance of their child having a major birth defect may become anxious or change their reproductive plans. An effective, research-based counseling program for avoiding these problems and the practical ability to provide such a system are necessary criteria for population testing.

THE NEED FOR AN EFFECTIVE INFRASTRUCTURE

Even with 100 percent sensitivity, an effective program to provide education, consent, and counseling is still necessary. This lesson was demonstrated by the experience of the sickle cell screening programs of the early 1970s. Even though the sickle cell tests had a specificity and sensitivity of virtually 100 percent, the early programs generally did not adequately provide for education. Misunderstanding about the difference between being a sickle cell carrier and having the disease, sickle cell anemia, led to persons being stigmatized and experiencing discrimination in their access to employment and ability to obtain life insurance.

In contrast, Kaback and Zeiger established an effective pretesting education program for the voluntary Tay–Sachs screening program piloted in the Baltimore and Washington Jewish community in the early 1970s. In addition to informed consent,

Kaback emphasized community support and multimedia educational information; more than one year was devoted to educating the community before the first person was tested. The program was well received by the community and there was an effective transfer of information with minimal adverse psychological effects. This program differed from the sickle cell program in that there were no racial issues involved in the screening, prenatal diagnosis was available, and the population was better educated.

Public education will be important in shaping attitudes toward genetic disorders and genetic testing to avoid stigmatization. Genetic counseling is necessary, but not sufficient, to prevent problems of stigmatization. A study of the long-term effects of a screening program for Tay–Sachs disease among high school students in Montreal revealed that, eight years later, 19 percent of carriers still attached some anxiety to being a carrier. A seven-year follow-up study of the sickle cell carrier screening program in Orchomenos, Greece revealed that 34 percent of couples perceived the trait as a mild disease. Twenty percent of these families felt that sickle cell trait meant a restriction of freedom and a risk of social stigmatization. Frequently, carrier status was concealed at the time of marriage arrangements, and engagements between carriers and unaffected individuals were broken once carrier status was disclosed. Furthermore, the study found no reduction in sickle cell births. However, experiences with heterozygote detection for other diseases have fared better than those with sickle cell anemia. For example, screening for β–thalassemia in Sardinia resulted in a decline in incidence from 1 in 250 to 1 in 1,200.

Genetic counseling for CF will require extensive explanation about CF and the potential risks associated with screening, particularly the possibility of insurance or employment discrimination (Billings et al. 1992). Medical insurers may attempt to coerce reproductive decisions. For example, a Los Angeles couple who already had a child with CF was informed that their health maintenance organization (HMO) would cover either prenatal diagnosis or the medical care of an affected child, but not both. The fetus was diagnosed with CF and the couple elected to continue the pregnancy. The HMO told the family that they would not cover the medical expenses of the child. When challenged, the HMO reversed its decision, but the case demonstrates the potential for coercion. Potential screenees will at least need to be aware of these risks before they consent to testing. Recently, Wisconsin enacted legislation to prevent medical insurers either from requiring individuals to reveal whether a genetic test has been obtained, and, if so, the results, or from requesting genetic tests as a condition of coverage or in order to set rates.[1] The impact of this legislation is unclear, as the subsequent regulations are still being developed.

Given the complexities of genetic counseling for CF carrier testing, the development of an effective mass population screening program will be challenging because of its potential to screen the entire childbearing population. Pilot studies will be needed to determine the amount of personnel time required and whether there are sufficient resources to provide effective counseling. Even if ten minutes of direct personnel time were devoted to pre-screening consent and education, an annual screening program for three million couples (an estimate of the potential magnitude if screening was provided to 75 percent of the four million women who become pregnant annually) would require at least 638,000 hours (table 2). Counseling provided by the approximately 1,000 certified clinical geneticists and genetic counselors would require each provider to spend 16 weeks every year on CF testing. Therefore, a mass screening program would require a tremendous increase in trained personnel to achieve only a minimum standard of consent and counseling. The only current alternative is to assign this very complex counseling task to persons not trained in genetics or genetic counseling, and unlikely to be informed about the rapidly changing complexities of CF testing. Alternative mechanisms for counseling, including multimedia resources (such as interactive computers and video), community-based programs, and improved training of primary care providers, especially nurses, need to be developed and assessed.

COST-EFFECTIVENESS CONSIDERATIONS

Even if a safe and effective delivery infrastructure were developed, policy makers will need to look carefully at the program costs per case of CF prevented. Commonly the public health goal of

reducing disease as the raison d'être of genetic counseling is disavowed; the purpose instead is generally described as one of allowing more informed reproductive decisions by individuals. Policy makers must consider whether it would be a fair or prudent use of resources to spend money on this arguably discretionary program at a time when approximately 33 million Americans are without basic health insurance. It is not enough to point out that most of the money for screening would be spent in the private sector because this does not address the question of whether such services should be available to Medicaid recipients or persons with no third-party coverage. Moreover, dollars spent for CF screening are unavailable for other social needs. If costs incurred through population screening did not avert a single case of cystic fibrosis, it would be difficult to defend the expenditure for the sole benefit of providing more informed decisions. Evidence that testing does result in the reduction of disease, and at what cost, will be needed before funding of such a program could be justified from a public health perspective.

The impact of a screening program on the incidence of CF is uncertain, but preliminary evidence suggests that many people may not be interested in undergoing testing, prenatal diagnosis, or aborting a fetus with CF. CF differs from many other diseases for which there is interest in prenatal diagnosis because the severity of symptoms in a particular individual is unpredictable, there is the potential for survival into middle age, and normal intelligence is preserved. In a survey of parents of children with CF, Wertz et al. found that only 20 percent indicated a willingness to abort a fetus with CF, compared with 79 percent of this group who indicated a willingness to abort a pregnancy to save the mother's life, 75 percent for rape, and 58 percent for severe mental retardation. In another study, 214 pregnant women in the general population were surveyed after reading educational materials on CF. Although 98 percent believed carrier testing should be available, only 84 percent would have taken the test prior to pregnancy. If found to be at risk, 67 percent would be interested in prenatal diagnosis, whereas only 29 percent indicated a willingness to abort an affected fetus.

If these preliminary findings reflect actual practices, the direct costs to avoid one CF birth could be close to 2.4 million dollars and might involve

Table 3. Cost of General Population CF Carrier Testing to Avoid One CF Birth[a]

Number of families		Services	Costs ($)
Total couples approached	27,010	Education and consent @ $10	270,100
Couples tested (.8)	21,607	Testing and counseling @ $100	2,160,700
Couples at risk (.033 x .85)^2	17	Counseling @ $100	1,700
Prenatal diagnosis (.7)	12	CVS and CF testing @ $1,200	14,400
Affected fetuses (.25)	3	Counseling @ $100	300
Abortions (.33)	1	Abortion @ $2,000	2,000
		Total	$2,449,200

[a]Based on estimates of utilization and direct costs. Abbreviation: CVS, chorionic villus sampling.

screening as many as 27,000 couples (table 3). An accurate cost-effective analysis will require further empiric assessment of behaviors. However, there may be less test-seeking behavior than these studies suggest because responses in questionnaires do not always translate to behavior. For example, although approximately 70 percent of at-risk people for Huntington disease indicated an interest in being tested, when the test was offered fewer than 15 percent actually responded. In fact, in one of the few reports of CF testing, from a self-paying CF screening program, only 43 percent of CVS patients and 19 percent of amniocentesis patients agreed also to have their fetus tested for CF.

THE ROLE OF PRIMARY HEALTH CARE PROVIDERS

The NIH workshop statement concluded that the "optimal setting for carrier testing is through primary health care providers." Involvement of primary care providers is attractive for mass population genetic testing because of the apparent logistical advantage of using a large personnel reservoir. However, the primary care setting may not be ideal for population carrier screening. Primary health care providers may not have the time, information, training, experience, or interest to provide this service well.

Physicians may not be sufficiently informed about the genetic testing and reproductive counseling to provide the necessary information. For example, a study involving pediatricians found that 54 percent could not accurately state the risk of phenylketonuria (PKU) in a neonate with a moderately elevated test result. In another study, Holtzman found that only 22 percent of a sample of obstetricians could describe the recommended clinical course of action following an elevated maternal serum alpha fetoprotein (MSAFP). Some respondents may have recommended abortion instead of first repeating the test or obtaining sonography, as recommended by the American College of Obstetrics and Gynecology.

The NIH workshop statement on CF states: "Providers of screening services have an obligation to ensure [that] adequate education and counseling are included in the program." The National Academy of Sciences report recommended that a comprehensive program include an ongoing assessment of patients' comprehension of information. Such standards would be difficult for most primary care providers to fulfill. It is not clear whether primary care providers will be willing or able to spend the time for education, consent, test interpretation, counseling, and assessment that is necessary in a CF screening program. However, it may be feasible to train primary care nurses, perhaps under the supervision of genetic counselors, to provide at least such services as prescreening education and consent.

Some primary care settings may pose additional problems. For example, prenatal visits appear to be an efficient setting for population CF carrier testing. However, the NIH workshop concluded that, ideally, population screening should be done prior to conception so that patients could avail themselves of preconception alternatives such as adoption or artificial insemination, and decisions would not be complicated by the urgency and emotional burden of an existing pregnancy.

Carrier screening during pregnancy is also likely initially to involve testing only women, which is not desirable for several reasons. First, any adverse effects of carrier identification would fall disproportionately on women. Second, testing both partners together would reduce the anxiety associated with the time delay in obtaining the partner's results after the woman has a positive test. Finally, the test results of the partner would greatly alter the risk assessment. For example, at an 85 percent detection rate, a person with a negative test has an apparent risk of 1 in 23,500 of having a child with CF (table 1). If the partner was negative, the risk would be reduced to 1 in 154,000; if the partner was positive, the risk would be 1 in 784. Testing the partner is desirable because these results could alter the apparent risk by close to 200-fold.

RELEVANCE OF A FAMILY HISTORY OF CF

The ASHG and the NIH workshop statements acknowledged that people with a family history of CF should be offered testing. Testing of family members has been available since the late 1980s, using linkage analysis. Combining this with mutation analysis could allow carrier testing of blood relatives to be informative at close to 100 percent, provided that a proband's chromosomes were available. The chance of a relative of a CF patient being a carrier is 67 percent for a sibling, 50 percent in an aunt or uncle, 33 percent in a niece or nephew, and 25 percent in a first cousin. Relatives of identified carriers are also at increased risk.

Testing a population whose a priori chance of being a carrier is higher will result in proportionately fewer false positives for a given specificity, increasing the positive predictive value of the test. Although the specificity of mutation analysis is unknown, false positives should be uncommon. However, laboratory or clerical errors will still cause a low proportion of false positive results and even this will become a finite number if screening is done on a mass scale.

The potential benefits of testing individuals with a positive family history are greater than for the general population. Some may already be anxious about their uncertain carrier status. Couples may otherwise have chosen not to bear children. High-risk couples with negative results could be reassured; the knowledge may allow some to bear children without fear. A couple found to be at a one in four risk prior to conception would be able to apply that knowledge to a full range of reproductive options. These families should be easier to counsel than the general population, as they are more likely to be familiar with the clinical course of CF and the associated burden of care. However, because more than 85 percent of CF patients are born to families without a prior family history, testing this high-risk population is not likely to result in substantial reduction in CF incidence.

A screening program directed toward relatives of CF patients would limit the size and cost of the program. Cystic fibrosis centers could facilitate such a program by informing their patients that carrier testing is available for interested family members. Interested persons could be referred to genetic counseling programs, or counseled directly in centers that have genetic counselors or other clinicians competent in genetic counseling. Physicians and other health professionals in the CF centers would be able to play a substantial role in providing education and counseling. The CF Foundation could establish criteria for quality control of the test, as is currently done for the diagnostic test for CF known as the "sweat test". The resources for counseling and quality control of testing even within such a limited program remain to be organized, but an infrastructure using existing resources has a greater potential of being developed to meet these needs. . . .

GUIDELINES FOR PRIMARY CARE PHYSICIANS

Physicians could fulfill the potential legal and ethical duty to inform all patients about test availability without necessarily being prepared to provide testing. However, they must recognize the potential for this information to influence behavior, depending on what information is given and how it is framed and delivered. Although the goal of disclosure should be to provide nondirective information, how the information is presented may motivate people to be tested. For example, Goodman and Goodman have commented that some of the brochures used in Tay–Sachs screening programs successfully promoted screening because they generated anxiety. Private companies with financial interests in promoting screening are also likely to present information in a potentially misleading fashion. A brochure from the Genetics and IVF Institute states: "Could I have a child with CF? The answer is probably yes. Almost any couple is at risk for having children with CF". In fact, fewer than 1 in 900 couples are at risk, but information presented in this way may be a strong motivation for screening.

Decisions to be tested for CF may also be influenced by how information about the disease is presented. An illustration of the possible impact of an arguably biased presentation is provided by the following excerpt from a consent form used in a pilot study from Denmark:

> Cystic fibrosis is a serious disease that causes a marked tendency to pneumonia and a reduced function of the pancreas. Today, the disease is incurable and, if untreated, it leads to death in childhood as a result of increasing damage to the lung tissue. A very intensive lifelong treatment of the lung disease now enables many patients to reach adulthood, but many still risk acquiring some degree of lung disablement at an early stage. At present, most patients are hospitalized every three months for two weeks of intensive treatment of infections; they also are treated daily for several hours in their homes.

Not surprisingly, more than 90 percent of clients who read this description accepted testing. Consider the difference in a client's reaction to the following alternative hypothetical version:

> CF is an inherited disease which used to be fatal, but now half of all patients will live into their fourth decade. CF does not affect intelligence; many people with CF go to college, enter professional occupations, get married, and have children. CF affects the respiratory and digestive systems, but symptoms can be controlled by taking enzyme capsules to help digestion, as well as antibiotics to fight off lung infections.
> Average life expectancy is steadily increasing, with rapidly advancing research producing the potential for better controls in the near future, and perhaps even a cure.

Both descriptions provide accurate, but limited, information. The second version, if read and understood, would almost certainly lead to a lower interest in testing than the Danish model. The point is not that either description is better, but only that the information sent by the counselor and the way it is sent, or more important, the way it is received by the client, will have a profound impact on what reproductive decisions are made.

Therefore, CF testing will need to be presented in a balanced fashion. If, once informed, patients then want to learn more about the test, they could be referred to a genetics counseling program. A proposal for a more balanced disclosure follows:

> There is now a blood test to identify carriers of the cystic fibrosis gene. Carriers are healthy but may be at risk for having a child with CF. CF occurs in about 1 in 3,400 births, but it is more likely to happen if there is a history of CF in your family. People with CF have chronic lung disease, but normal intelligence, and usually live into early adulthood. Testing is done in conjunction with genetic counseling, which may require one to two hours of your time before you would be in a position to know whether you would want to be tested. If you are interested in hearing more about this, please let your doctor know.

One argument for mentioning CF testing to all white patients, not just those with a family history, is because CF is a relatively common genetic disease in that population. However, what counts as common is arbitrary. Because the CF carrier frequency in blacks is close to half that of whites, some might suggest that blacks also be tested. Others might claim that CF is a relatively infrequent occurrence, even in whites. These potentially conflicting interpretations suggest that the frequency of the disease is not itself the central issue, but one of several that must be considered.

As physicians become more oriented to initiating discussions about reproductive health issues with their patients, information about CF testing, and genetic testing in general, should be discussed with patients along with such issues as family planning and contraception. However, there are over a hundred conditions for which carrier detection and prenatal diagnosis are potentially available and the Human Genome Initiative will increase this number. Primary care physicians are not likely to have the time to inquire about a family history, ethnic background, or interest in testing for each of these diseases. The patient's genuine interest in being informed of available tests could be supported by a checklist to be completed in the physician's waiting room and reviewed during the visit. The checklist might include a list of genetic diseases with brief descriptions, as well as a list of symptoms suggestive of genetic disease. If the patient is interested in further testing, the primary care practitioner could provide it if he or she is prepared also to provide genetics counseling; if not, the patient could be referred to a genetics counselor. This approach has been implemented in family planning clinics in New England.

GUIDELINES FOR GENETICISTS AND GENETIC COUNSELORS

Geneticists and genetic counselors are more likely to have the time and training to provide the education, consent, and counseling needed for CF screening. However, because providing CF testing to all genetics clients who are seen for other reasons would place a great strain on these counseling programs, an additional hour might be required for each visit. Like primary care physicians, clinicians could acknowledge the availability of the CF test during a visit by asking patients to review a checklist and arranging an additional appointment for those interested in further testing. A generic list of testable genetic disorders may be less likely to raise anxiety about CF than a brochure specifically about CF. Persons interested in CF testing should be informed that the test is not yet routine, and may not be covered by insurance. Finally, the patient should be aware that pre-screening counseling, ideally for both partners, is necessary, and this may take up to an hour. Unless the interest in CF testing exceeds the resources of a particular genetics clinic, counseling and testing should be provided to anyone who requests it. It is possible that referrals from primary care physicians and interest among existing genetics counseling clients still could exceed the resources of a particular clinic, in which case the clinic might

consider giving priority to patients who have a relative with a CF mutation.

The distinction between informing and providing draws attention to the ethical obligation to inform patients about the test. Although this distinction is valuable in determining the extent of a physician's obligation toward patients, it may be lost on other practicing clinicians whose manner of informing may motivate patients to be tested, but who do not provide adequate education, consent, and counseling. Geneticists' practice of informing patients about CF testing might result in other less qualified practitioners informing, offering, and providing testing to their patients. This might result in de facto mass testing with a great potential to cause harm. Thus a geneticist's decision of whether to inform patients about CF testing must not only include an evaluation of his or her obligation to promote the autonomy of the patient at hand, but must also account for the social consequences of this action on other patients, who may be harmed by an unevaluated mass testing program. Because providing specific information about CF is more likely than mentioning CF as one of many potentially available tests to result in the rapid diffusion of testing, we recommend that genetics providers meet their ethical obligation to inform patients by providing a generic checklist.

CONCLUSION

The ASHG and NIH workshop reports concluded that mass population CF screening should be deferred until pilot studies demonstrating effective mechanisms for delivery of these services are completed. The NIH statement emphasized the importance of a 95 percent detection rate in deciding whether population screening should be initiated. We have argued that a high detection rate is not the central issue. It is a necessary, but not sufficient, reason for population screening. Even with 100 percent detection of carriers, the personnel and logistical resources needed to meet education and counseling needs must be developed and evaluated. Furthermore, policy makers must determine whether the goals of a population program—prevention of CF or informed reproductive decision making—warrant public funding or private reimbursement preferentially over other urgent health care needs of the American public.

Primary care physicians may not be the ideal providers of mass population carrier screening programs. Alternative mechanisms of community-organized programs with trained providers and multimedia educational resources should be developed and evaluated. There is no clear legal duty for primary care physicians to provide patients who have no family history with direct access to the test. Primary care physicians who are concerned about liability may discharge their ethical and legal duty by *informing* patients that CF carrier testing is available. *Providing* testing requires adherence to strict standards of education and consent. This should include information about CF, reproductive options, the meaning of a negative test, and the risks of testing. Providers may be liable if information is not communicated accurately or clearly. Therefore, primary care physicians who are not equipped to provide such services should refer interested patients to qualified genetics counseling programs. Ideally, geneticists and genetics counselors should inform patients about the availability of CF carrier testing. However, because this might result in de facto mass testing, as the distinction between informing and providing is easily blurred, geneticists should exercise restraint in informing patients about CF testing except in the context of a general description of potentially available tests.

In response to the ASHG and NIH workshop statements, most physicians have not provided CF screening to patients. Biotechnology companies have backed off from initial marketing positions. The NIH has funded pilot studies. In one to two years, we will have more data from which to develop a rational screening policy for CF. The initial experience with CF carrier testing indicates that it is possible to learn from past mistakes. This is encouraging, in light of the anticipated mapping and sequencing of the human genome, which will continue to raise the question of whether or not to screen.

ACKNOWLEDGMENTS

Some of this work was part of a report prepared for the National Institutes of Health–Department of Energy Working Group on Ethical, Legal, and Social Implications (ELSI) of Human Genome Research. We thank John Robertson, JD, and Ellen Wright Clayton, JD, MD, for their criticism and suggestions on the report submitted to ELSI.

NOTES

1. Wis. Stat. § 631.89.

AUTHORS' NOTE: Between 1991 and 1994, there were eight studies of CF carrier testing in the United States funded by the Ethical, Legal, and Social Implications Program (ELSI) at the National Institutes of Health. Some studies, in the general population, found a minimal level of interest in the general population, from 4 to 20 percent. However, prenatal studies demonstrated a level of interest between 50 and 70 percent. There have been similar results in the United Kingdom, and one study in particular suggested that even in the general population, the level of interest in testing is influenced by active versus passive presentation of information, convenience of testing, and whether the information is presented by a health care professional. The results of these studies raise questions about how decisions regarding the structure of the screening program could influence the interest rate.

In 1997, a Consensus Development Conference sponsored by the NIH recommended that CF testing be offered to the prenatal population but not to the general population. The report seemed to assume that programs with higher interest rates should be supported more than those with lower interest rates. However, the report never explicitly considered the malleability of interest rates and did not seem to give much weight to the complexities of effectively educating people. Professional organizations have not adopted these recommendations, in part because the Consensus Development Conference did not adequately address these issues. Thus in 1998, CF carrier testing is not yet the standard of care.

The Ethics of Genetic Research on Sexual Orientation

Udo Schüklenk, Edward Stein, Jacinta Kerin, and William Byne

Research on the origins of sexual orientation has received much public attention in recent years, especially findings consistent with the notion of relatively simple links between genes and sexual orientation. Investigation into the causes of same-sex attraction has, however, been ongoing for more than one hundred years. Claims that such inquiry is dangerous, especially in certain social and political climates, are as old as the research itself. In this paper, we show that such genetic research in particular gives rise to serious ethical issues.

GENETIC RESEARCH

Scientific research on sexual orientation has taken many forms. One early idea was to find evidence of a person's sexual orientation in such bodily features as amount of facial hair, size of external genitalia, and the ratio of shoulder width to hip width. Today's seemingly more sophisticated morphological research looks instead at neuroanatomical structures. Such inquiry usually assumes sexual orientation is a trait with two forms, one typically associated with males and the other typically associated with females. Researchers who accept this assumption expect particular aspects of an individual's brain or physiology to conform to either a male type that causes sexual attraction to women (shared by heterosexual men and lesbians) or a female type that causes sexual attraction to men (shared by heterosexual women and gay men). This assumption is scientifically unsupported and there are alternatives to it.

Hastings Center Report, vol. 27, No. 4, July/August 1997, 6–13. Copyright © The Hasting Center. Used with permission.
EDITORS' NOTE: The notes have been omitted. Readers wishing to follow up on sources should consult the original. All sources are listed in the Recommended Supplementary Reading of Part Four.

Another early approach was to find evidence of a person's sexual orientation in his or her endocrine system. The idea was that gay men would have less androgenic hormones (the so-called male-typical hormones) or more estrogenic hormones (the so-called female-typical sex hormones) than straight men and that lesbians would have more androgynic and less estrogenic sex hormones than straight women. However, an overwhelming majority of studies failed to demonstrate any correlation between sexual orientation and adult hormonal constitution. According to current hormonal theories of sexual orientation, lesbians and gay men were exposed to atypical hormone levels early in their development. Such theories draw heavily on the observation that, in rodents, hormonal exposure in early development exerts organizational influences on the brain that determine the balance between male and female patterns of mating behaviors in adulthood. Extrapolating from behaviors in rodents to psychological phenomena in humans is, however, quite problematic. In rodents, a male who allows himself to be mounted by another male is counted as homosexual, while a male that mounts another male is considered heterosexual. This model defines sexual orientation in terms of specific postures and behaviors. In contrast, in the human case, sexual orientation is defined not by what "position" one takes in sexual intercourse but by one's pattern of erotic responsiveness and the sex of one's preferred sex partner.

Although early sex researchers reported that homosexuality runs in families, careful studies of this hypothesis are only beginning to be done. Several studies suggest that male homosexuality runs in families, but they are not helpful in distinguishing between genetic and environmental influences because most related individuals share both genes and environmental variables. Further disentanglement of genetic and environmental influences requires adoption studies.

The only heritability study of male homosexuality that includes an adoption component is the highly publicized study of Bailey and Pillard. The study suggests a significant environmental contribution to the development of sexual orientation in men in addition to a moderate genetic influence. This study assessed sexual orientation not only in the identical and fraternal twins, but also in the nontwin biological brothers and the unrelated adopted brothers of the gay men who volunteered for the study. The concordance rate for identical twins (52 percent) was much higher than the concordance rate for the fraternal twins (22 percent). These concordance rates show that the environment must play a significant role in sex orientation because approximately half of the monozygotic twin pairs were discordant for sexual orientation despite sharing both their genes and familial environments. The higher concordance rate in the identical twins is *consistent* with a genetic effect because identical twins share all of their genes while fraternal twins, on average, share only half. Genes cannot, however, explain the remaining results of this study. In the absence of a significant environmental influence, the incidence of homosexuality among the adopted brothers of gay men should be equal to the rate of homosexuality in the general population, which recent studies place at somewhere between 2 and 5 percent. The observed concordance rate was 11 percent (two and five times higher than expected given the estimates); this suggests a major environmental contribution. Further, no genetic explanation can account for the fact that the concordance rate for homosexuality among nontwin brothers was about the same whether or not they were genetically related (the rate for homosexuality among nontwin biological brothers was 9 percent; among adopted brothers it was 11 percent).

When all the data from the twin study are considered, it appears that sexual orientation is the result of a combination of both genetic and environmental influences. Further, the combined effect of genetic and environmental influences might not simply be their sum; these factors could interact in a nonadditive or synergistic manner. In fact, recent heritability studies consistently find that almost half of the identical twin pairs are discordant for sexual orientations even though they share the same genes and similar familial environments. This finding underscores how little we know about the origins of sexual orientation.

Of all the recent biological studies, the genetic linkage study by Dean Hamer's group is the most conceptually complex. This study presents statistical evidence that genes influencing sexual orientation may reside in the q28 region of the X chromosome. Females have two X chromosomes, but they pass a copy of only one to a son. The theoretical probability of two sons receiving a copy of the same Xq28 from their mother is thus 50 percent. Hamer found that of forty pairs of gay siblings, thirty-three instead of the expected twenty had received the same Xq28 region from their mother. Hamer's finding is often misinterpreted as showing that all sixty-six men from these thirty-three pairs shared the same Xq28 sequence. In fact, all he showed was that each member of the thirty-three concordant pairs shared his Xq28 region with his brother but not with any of the other sixty-four men. No single specific Xq28 sequence was common to all sixty-six men.

There are several problems with Hamer's study. First, a Canadian research team has been unable to duplicate the finding using a comparable experimental design. Second, Hamer confined his search to the X-chromosome on the basis of family interviews, which seems to reveal a disproportionately high number of male homosexuals on the mothers' side of the family. Women might, however, be more likely to know details of family medical history, rendering these interviews less than objective in terms of directing experimental design. Third, one of Hamer's coauthors has expressed serious concerns about the methodology of the study. Fourth, there is some question about whether Hamer's results, correctly interpreted, are statistically significant. His conclusions rest on the assumption that the rate of homosexuality in the population at large (the base rate of homosexuality) is two percent. If the base rate is actually four percent or higher, then Hamer's results are not statistically significant. A leading geneticist argues that Hamer's own data support the four percent estimate.

To understand what is at issue here, it is useful to contrast three models of the role genes might play in sexual orientation. According to the "permissive effect model," genes or other biological factors influence the neural substrate on which sexual orientation is inscribed by formative experience. On this view, genetic factors might also delimit the period during which experience can affect a person's sexual orientation. According to the "indirect effect model," genes code for (or other biological factors influence) temperamental or personality factors that influence how one interacts with and shapes one's environment and formative experiences. On this view, the same gene (or set of genes) might predispose to homosexuality in some environments, to heterosexuality in others, and have no effect on sexual orientation in others. Finally, according to the "direct effect model," genes (or other biological factors) influence the brain structures that mediate sexual orientation. Hamer, LeVay, and most other researchers seem to favor the direct model.

One version of the direct model involves talk of "gay genes." It is important to remember that genes in themselves cannot directly specify any behaviors or psychological phenomena; rather, a gene directs a particular pattern of RNA synthesis that in turn specifies the amino acid sequence of a particular protein that may influence behavior. There are necessarily many intervening pathways between a gene and a behavior and even more between a gene and a pattern that involves both thinking and behaving. For the term "gay gene" to have a clear meaning, one needs to propose that a particular gene, perhaps through a hormonal mechanism, organizes the brain specifically to support the desire to have sex with people of the same sex. No one has, however, presented evidence in support of such a simple and direct link between genes and sexual orientation.

Importantly, "gay genes" are not required for homosexuality to be heritable. This is because heritability has a precise technical meaning; it refers to the ratio of genetic variation to total (phenotypic) variation. As such, heritability merely reflects the degree to which a given outcome is linked to genetic factors; it says nothing about the nature of those factors nor about their mechanism of action. Homosexuality would be heritable if genes worked through a very indirect mechanism. For example, if the indirect model is right and genes act on temperamental variables that influence how we perceive and interact with our environment, then temperament could play an important role from the moment of birth in shaping the relationships and experience that influence how sexual orientation develops. The moral is that any genetic

influence on sexual orientation might prove to be very indirect. In general, there is no convincing evidence to support the direct model; current biological evidence is equally compatible with both the direct and the indirect model.

ETHICAL CONCERNS

We have several ethical concerns about genetic research on sexual orientation. Underlying these concerns is the fact that even in our contemporary societies, lesbians, gay men, and bisexuals are subject to widespread discrimination and social disapprobation. Against this background, we are concerned about the particularly gruesome history of the use of such research. Many homosexual people have been forced to undergo "treatments" to change their sexual orientation, while others have "chosen" to undergo them in order to escape societal homophobia. All too often, scientifically questionable "therapeutic" approaches destroyed the lives of perfectly healthy people. "Conversion therapies" have included electroshock treatment, hormonal therapies, genital mutilation, and brain surgery. We are concerned about the negative ramifications of biological research on sexual orientation, especially in homophobic societies. In Germany, some scholars have warned of the potential for abuse of such genetic research, while others have called for a moratorium on such research to prevent the possible abuse of its results in homophobic societies. These warnings should be taken seriously.

We are concerned that people conducting research on sexual orientation work within homophobic frameworks, despite their occasional claims to the contrary. A prime example is the German obstetrician Günter Dörner, whose descriptions of homosexuality ill-conceal his heterosexism. Dörner writes about homosexuality as a "dysfunction" or "disease" based on "abnormal brain development." He postulates that it can be prevented by *"optimizing"* natural conditions or by *"correcting* abnormal hormonal concentrations prenatally"(emphasis added). Another example is provided by psychoanalyst Richard Friedman, who engages in speculation about nongay outcome given proper therapeutic intervention. Research influenced by homophobia is likely to result in significantly biased accounts of human sexuality; further, such work is more likely to strengthen and perpetuate the homophobic attitudes on which it is based.

SEXUAL ORIENTATION RESEARCH IS NOT VALUE NEUTRAL

Furthermore, we question whether those who research sexual orientation can ever conduct their work in a value-neutral manner. One might think that the majority of American sex researchers treats homosexuality not as a disease, but rather as a variation analogous to a neutral polymorphism. To consider whether or not this is the case, one must look at the context in which interest in sexual orientation arises. Homophobia still exists to some degree in all societies within which sexual orientation research is conducted. The cultures in which scientists live and work influence both the questions they ask and the hypotheses they imagine and explore. Given this, we believe it is unlikely that the sexual orientation research of any scientist (even one who is homosexual) will escape some taint of homophobia. This argument is importantly different from one which claims that objective research can be used unethically in discriminatory societies. The latter logic implies that what should be questioned is the regulation of the application of technology, not the development of the technology in the first place. While we do provide arguments for questioning the efficacy of such regulations should they be developed, our deeper concerns are directed toward the institutional and social structures that constrain sex research. Attention to these contextual details shows that research into sexual orientation is different from research into most other physical/behavioral variations. Since sexual orientation is the focus of intense private and public interest, relevant inquiry cannot be studied independently of societal investment. It is naive to suggest that individual researchers might suddenly find themselves in the position of neutral inquirers. Social mores both constrain and enable the ways in which an individual's research is focused.

We are not claiming that all researchers are homophobic to some degree whether or not they are aware of it. Nor are we talking about the implicit or explicit intentions of individual sexual orientation researchers. Rather we are seeking to highlight that the very motivation for seeking the "origin" of homosexuality has its source within social frameworks that are pervasively homophobic. Recog-nition that scientific projects are constituted by, and to some degree complicit in, social structures does not necessarily entail that all such science should cease. At the very least, however, it follows that sexual orientation research and its use should be subject to critique. Such a critique will call into question the claim that, by treating homosexuality as a mere variation of human behavior, researchers are conducting neutral investigations into sexual orientation.

PREDICTING SEXUAL ORIENTATION IN UTERO

We are also worried that an amniocentesis-like test will be developed that claims to detect genes or hormonal levels that might predispose for homosexuality. This concern may seem paradoxical, since the development of such a test seems to rely on the truth of the direct model of sexual orientation, which we describe as scientifically unsupported. Yet the development of such a test is, in principle, compatible with either the direct or indirect genetic model of sexual orientation. While current scientific results favor neither model, it is conceivable that future studies might clarify this impasse. Even evidence for the indirect model might inform the creation of a genetic screening technique that purports to influence sexual orientation in a given environment. Thus we are concerned that tests which do no more than suggest a predisposition for homosexuality would be favorably received in homophobic societies. If prospective parents believe they are able to predict the sexual orientation of a fetus by using a prenatal screening technique, it is possible that they would choose to abort a fetus that seemed to be "homosexually predisposed." In many countries, the preference for male versus female offspring leads to the abortion of female fetuses. This preference is clearly connected to sexism operating at a societal level. In such instances, science is subverted to serve the interests of discriminatory societies. Thus, discrimination can be institutionalized through genetic screening techniques.

Moreover, tests can be both developed and well received even if they are based on bad science. People might make use of genetic screening procedures that are supposed to select for heterosexual children even if such procedures did not work. This is partly for the general reason that the public can, in various ways, be lead to accept unsound scientific procedures. More specifically, potential users of sexual-orientation-selection procedures will have a difficult time assessing the efficacy of such procedures for at least three reasons. First, since some children turn out to be heterosexual even without the use of such a procedure, many parents who make use of it will believe that the procedure has worked, even though the procedure has done nothing. Second, many people take a long time to come to grips with their sexual orientation. Parents who made use of such a procedure might think that it had been successful, but only because their child had not yet figured out her or his sexual orientation. Third, because some lesbians, gay men, and bisexuals hide their sexual orientation, many parents will think that their attempt at selecting their child's sexual orientation has worked when in fact it has not. Further, if a lesbian, gay man, or bisexual knows that his or her parents used such a procedure, this would increase the likelihood that the person would hide his or her sexual orientation from them. For these reasons, such a procedure is likely to appear to work even if it does not. Given the appearance that such procedures work, as well as the widespread prejudice and discrimination against lesbians, gay men, and bisexuals, some people will attempt to select the sexual orientation of their children. This would likely engender and perpetuate attitudes that lesbians and gay men are undesirable and not valuable, policies that discriminate against lesbians and gay men, and the very conditions that give rise to such attitudes and policies.

REPLIES TO THESE CONCERNS

Given the wide-ranging abuse of the results of biological research on sexual orientation in the past, it is not surprising that people realize that ethical justifications for this work are needed. Some researchers say their work can provide answers to century old questions surrounding religious propo-

sitions that homosexuality is abnormal or unnatural. However, biological research on the causes of sexual orientation cannot possibly provide answers to questions concerning the nature and normality of homosexuality. As we will go on to illustrate, the only senses in which homosexuality can be said to be, or fail to be, natural or normal are of no ethical relevance. Given that some scientists claim their *empirical* research can provide answers to *normative* questions, the danger of committing a naturalistic fallacy in this context is very real.

NORMATIVITY OF NATURALNESS AND NORMALITY

Why is there a dispute as to whether homosexuality is natural or normal? We suggest it is because many people seem to think that nature has a prescriptive normative force such that what is deemed natural or normal is necessarily good and therefore *ought* to be. Everything that falls outside these terms is constructed as unnatural and abnormal, and it has been argued that this constitutes sufficient reason to consider homosexuality worth avoiding. Arguments that appeal to "normality" to provide us with moral guidelines also risk committing the naturalistic fallacy. The naturalistic fallacy is committed when one mistakenly deduces from the way things are to the way they ought to be. For instance, Dean Hamer and colleagues commit this error in their *Science* article when they state that "it would be fundamentally unethical to use such information to try to assess or alter a person's current or future sexual orientation, either heterosexual or homosexual, or other normal attributes of human behavior." Hamer and colleagues believe that there is a major genetic factor contributing to sexual orientation. From this they think it follows that homosexuality is normal, and thus worthy of preservation. Thus they believe that genetics can tell us what is normal, and that the content of what is normal tells us what ought to be. This is a typical example of a naturalistic fallacy.

Normality can be defined in a number of ways, but none of them direct us in the making of moral judgments. First, normality can be reasonably defined in a *descriptive* sense as a statistical average. Appeals to what is usual, regular, and/or conforming to existing standards ultimately collapse into statistical statements. For an ethical evaluation of homosexuality, it is irrelevant whether homosexuality is normal or abnormal in this sense. All sorts of human traits and behaviors are abnormal in a statistical sense, but this is not a sufficient justification for a negative ethical judgment about them. Second, "normality" might be defined in a functional sense, where what is normal is something that has served an adaptive function from an evolutionary perspective. This definition of normality can be found in sociobiology, which seeks biological explanations for social behavior. There are a number of serious problems with the sociobiological project. For the purposes of this argument, however, suffice it to say that even if sociobiology could establish that certain behavioral traits were the direct result of biological evolution, no moral assessment of these traits would follow. To illustrate our point, suppose any trait that can be reasonably believed to have served an adaptive function at some evolutionary stage is normal. Some questions arise that exemplify the problems with deriving normative conclusions from descriptive science. Are traits that are perpetuated simply through linkage to selectively advantageous loci less "normal" than those for which selection was direct? Given that social contexts now exert "selective pressure" in a way that nature once did, how are we to decide which traits are to be intentionally fostered?

Positions holding the view that homosexuality is unnatural, and therefore wrong, also inevitably develop incoherencies. They often fail to explicate the basis upon which the line between natural and unnatural is drawn. More importantly, they fail to explain why we should consider all human-made or artificial things as immoral or wrong. These views are usually firmly based in a nonempirical, *prescriptive* interpretation of nature rather than a scientific *descriptive* approach. They define arbitrarily what is natural and have to import other normative assumptions and premises to build a basis for their conclusions. For instance, they often claim that an entity called "God" has declared homosexuality to be unnatural and sinful. Unfortunately, these analyses have real-world consequences. In Singapore, "unnatural acts" are considered a criminal offense, and "natural intercourse" is arbitrarily defined as "the coitus of the male and female organs." A recent High Court decision there declared oral sex "unnatural," and therefore a criminal offense, unless it leads to subsequent reproductive intercourse.

HISTORICAL EVIDENCE

In response to some of the ethical concerns about biological research on sexual orientation, some people have appealed to previous research on homosexuality that has *not* been used to the detriment of homosexuals. For example, Timothy Murphy invokes the work of Evelyn Hooker, which arguably provided evidence for the "normality" of homosexuals. However, historical examples are often disanalogous to present-day biological research. Hooker's small-scale study, in fact, had nothing to do with the origins of sexual orientation. Rather, she sought to discover whether or not homosexual people were "well-adapted" (by assessing the degree to which their daily practices conformed with that of "normal" Americans). Showing that nonbiological research has not been used unethically does not show that biological research will be used ethically. It is important to discern which *sorts* of historical events can be considered relevant to the debate concerning the implications and applications of research on sexual orientation.

Another defense of genetic research on sexual orientation, offered by Simon LeVay, suggests that psychological and sociological research is even more dangerous. LeVay bases his argument on the assertion that, for ideological reasons, the Nazis did not generally consider homosexuality to be innate or a sign of degeneracy, but rather that they thought homosexuality was spread by seduction. This is historically not true. The Nazis were as supportive of genetic research as they were of any other type of research designed to support the elimination of homosexuality. Even if LeVay's assertions were historically correct, however, they would not provide any support (ethical or otherwise) for genetic research. Arguing that one type of research is ethically problematic does not legitimize the other; indeed, it only provides further reason to question the whole enterprise.

U.S.-SPECIFIC ARGUMENTS

In the United States, several scholars and lesbian and gay activists have argued that establishing a genetic basis for sexual orientation will help make the case for lesbian and gay rights. The idea is that scientific research will show that people do not choose their sexual orientations and therefore they should not be punished or discriminated against in virtue of them. This general argument is flawed in several ways. First, we do not need to show that a trait is genetically determined to argue that it is not amenable to change at will. This is clearly shown by the failure rates of conversion "therapies." These failures establish that sexual orientation is resistant to change, but they do not say anything about its ontogeny or etiology. Sexual orientation can be unchangeable without being genetically determined. There is strong observational evidence to support the claim that sexual orientation is difficult to change, but this evidence is perfectly compatible with nongenetic accounts of the origins of sexual orientations. More importantly, we should not embrace arguments that seek to legitimate homosexuality by denying that there is any choice in sexual preference because the implicit premise of such arguments is that if there *was* a choice, then homosexuals would be blameworthy.

Relatedly, arguments for lesbian and gay rights based on scientific evidence run the risk of leading to impoverished forms of lesbian and gay rights. Regardless of what causes homosexuality, a person has to decide to publicly identify as a lesbian, to engage in sexual acts with another woman, to raise children with her same-sex lover, or to be active in the lesbian and gay community. It is when people make such decisions that they are likely to face discrimination, arrest, or physical violence. It is decisions like these that need legal protection. An argument for lesbian and gay rights based on genetic evidence is impotent with respect to protecting such decisions because it focuses exclusively on the very aspects of sexuality that might not involve choices.

Another version of this argument focuses on the specifics of U.S. law. According to this version, scientific evidence will establish the immutability of sexual orientation, which, according to one current interpretation of the Equal Protection Clause of the Fourteenth Amendment of the U.S. Constitution, is one of three criteria required of a classification if it is to evoke heightened judicial scrutiny. While this line of argument has serious internal problems, such an argument, like a good deal of American bioethical reasoning, has limited or no

relevance to the global context. Since the results of the scientific research are not confined within American borders, justifications that go beyond U.S. legislation are required.

The same sort of problem occurs in other defenses of sexual orientation research that discuss possible ramifications in U.S.-specific legislative terms. For instance, Timothy Murphy claims that, even if a genetic probe predictive of sexual orientation were available, mandatory testing would be unlikely. He bases this claim on the fact that in some states employment and housing discrimination against homosexual people is illegal. In many countries, however, the political climate is vastly different, and legal anti-gay discrimination is widespread. And there is evidence that scientific research would be used in a manner that discriminates against homosexuals. As already mentioned, in Singapore, homosexual sex acts are a criminal offense. The Singapore Penal Code sections 377 and 377A threaten sentences ranging from two years to life imprisonment for homosexual people engaging in same-sex acts. Not coincidentally, in light of our concerns, a National University of Singapore psychiatrist recently implied that "pre-symptomatic testing for homosexuality should be offered in the absence of treatment," thereby accepting the idea that homosexuality is something in need of a cure.

GENETIC SCREENING

Several attempts to defend sexual orientation research against ethical concerns related to the selective abortion of "pre-homosexual" fetuses have been made. It has been claimed that this sort of genetic screening will not become commonplace because "diagnostic genetic testing is at present the exception rather than the rule." While this may indeed be true in the U.S., it has far more to do with the types of tests currently offered than with a reluctance on the part of either the medical profession or the reproducing public to partake of such technology. For example, the types of tests available are diagnostic for diseases and are offered on the basis of family history or specific risk factors. The possibility of tests that are supposed to be (however vaguely) predictive of behavioral traits opens genetic technology to a far greater population, especially when the traits in question are undesired by a largely prejudiced society.

Furthermore, it has been claimed that the medical profession would not advocate such a test that does not serve "important state interests." This argument not only ignores the existence of homophobia among individuals within medicine, it assumes also that public demand for genetic testing varies predominantly according to medical advice. However, should such a test become available, the media hype surrounding its market arrival would render its existence common knowledge, which, coupled with homophobic bias, would create a demand for the test irrespective of its accuracy and of any kind of state interest. Furthermore, this argument ignores the fact that genetic screening for a socially undesirable characteristic has already been greeted with great public demand in countries such as India, where abortion on the basis of female sex is commonplace, irrespective of its legality. Techniques to select the sexual orientation of children, if made available, might well be widely utilized.

Some have argued that orientation-selection techniques involving genetic screening will not succeed because environmental factors influencing sexual orientation would elude genetic screening. While there are such environmental factors, we are still concerned about the potential effects of the availability of orientation-selection techniques, even if they fail to work. Further, if environmental factors are identified, their modification could be defended on the same grounds as the elimination of "gay genes." In fact, behavior modification techniques have been, and continue to be, used to prevent homosexuality in children with "gender identity disorder" (that is, "sissies" and "tomboys").

It has also been claimed that if homosexual people themselves made use of orientation-selection techniques (whether to ensure homosexual or heterosexual offspring), the charge that such testing is inherently homophobic becomes "paradoxical." However, just as the fact that homosexual people conduct scientific research on sexual orientation does not show that such research is ethically justifiable, the fact that some homosexuals might use such techniques would not prove that the technology does not serve to discriminate. To illustrate this point, consider that in a society like India in which wide-spread discrimination against women exists, there are many pragmatic reasons why one might prefer a male child. We would not argue, however, that prenatal sex selection is no longer discriminatory against females because women sometimes seek abortions for the purpose of having male offspring. Similarly, in societies with entrenched homophobia, a heterosexual child might be preferable for reasons that might appear most salient to homosexuals themselves in lieu of the discrimination they have encountered. The use of a technology by people against whom it may discriminate (even if they attempt to use it to their benefit) does not establish its neutrality. It does, however, highlight the pervasive biases within a given society that should be addressed directly rather than be fostered with enabling technology. Discriminated-against users of discriminatory technology might have a variety of motives, none of which necessarily diffuse the charge of bias.

THE VALUE OF KNOWING THE TRUTH

Finally, various scholars appeal to the value of the truth to defend research on sexual orientation in the face of ethical concerns. Scientific research does, however, have its costs and not every research program is of equal importance. Even granting that, in general, knowledge is better than ignorance, not all risks for the sake of knowledge are worth taking. With respect to sexual orientation, historically, almost every hypothesis about the causes of homosexuality led to attempts to "cure" healthy people. History indicates that current genetic research is likely to have negative effects on lesbians and gay men, particularly those living in homophobic societies.

A GLOBAL PERSPECTIVE

Homosexual people have in the past suffered greatly from societal discrimination. Historically, the results of biological research on sexual orientation have been used against them. We have analyzed the arguments offered by well-intentioned defenders of such work and concluded that none survive philosophical scrutiny. It is true that in some countries in Scandinavia, North America, and most parts of Western Europe, the legal situation of homosexual people has improved, but an adequate ethical analysis of the implications of genetic inquiry into the causes of sexual orientation must operate from a global perspective. Sexual orientation researchers should be aware that their work may harm homosexuals in countries other than their own. It is difficult to imagine any good that could come of genetic research on sexual orientation in homophobic societies. Such work faces serious ethical concerns so long as homophobic societies continue to exist. Insofar as socially responsible genetic research on sexual orientation is possible, it must begin with the awareness that it will not be a cure for homophobia and that the ethical status of lesbians and gay men does not in any way hinge on its results.

RECOMMENDED SUPPLEMENTARY READING

General Works

Alpern, Kenneth D., ed. *The Ethics of Reproductive Technology.* New York: Oxford University Press, 1992.

Asch, Adrienne. "Reproductive Technology and Disability." In *Reproductive Laws for the 1990s,* edited by Sherill Cohen and Nadine Taub. Clifton, NJ: Humana Press, 1989.

Bartels, Dianne M., et al., eds. *Beyond Baby M: Ethical Issues in the New Reproductive Technologies.* Clifton, NJ: Humana Press, 1990.

Brock, Dan; Buchanan, Allan; Daniels, Norman; Wikler, Daniel. *Genes and the Just Society: Genetic Intervention in the Shadow of Eugenics.* Forthcoming.

Callahan, Joan C., ed. *Reproduction, Ethics, and the Law.* Bloomington: Indiana University Press, 1995.

Congregation for the Doctrine of the Faith. "Instruction on Respect for Human Life in Its Origin and on the Dignity of Procreation: Replies to Certain Questions of the Day." Rome, Italy: The Vatican, March 10, 1987.

Dyson, Anthony, and Harris, John, eds. *Ethics and Biotechnology.* London: Routledge, 1994.

Elias, Sherman, and Annas, George J. *Reproductive Genetics and the Law.* Chicago: Year Book Medical Publishers, 1987.

Glover, Jonathan. *What Sort of People Should There Be?* New York: Random House, 1977.

Harris, John. *Wonderwoman and Superman: The Ethics of Human Biotechnology.* Oxford: Oxford University Press, 1992.

Holmes, Helen Bequaert, and Purdy, Laura M. *Feminist Perspectives in Medical Ethics.* Bloomington: Indiana University Press, 1992.

Kass, Leon R. *Toward a More Natural Science.* New York: Free Press, 1985.

Murray, Thomas. *The Worth of a Child.* Berkeley: University of California Press, 1996.

Purdy, Laura. *Reproducing Persons: Issues in Feminist Bioethics.* Ithaca, New York: Cornell University Press, 1996.

Ramsey, Paul. *Fabricated Man: The Ethics of Genetic Control.* New Haven, CT: Yale University Press, 1970.

Robertson, John A. *Children of Choice: Freedom and the New Reproductive Technologies.* Princeton: Princeton University Press, 1994.

Rothman, Barbara Katz. *Recreating Motherhood: Ideology and Technology in a Patriarchal Society.* New York: W. W. Norton, 1989.

Singer, Peter, and Wells, Deane. *Making Babies: The New Science and Ethics of Conception.* New York: Charles Scribner's Sons, 1985.

Symposium: "Reproductive Technologies." *Journal of Medicine and Philosophy* 21, no.5 (October 1996): 471ff.

Advocates and Critics of Assisted Reproductive Technologies

Bonnicksen, Andrea L. *In Vitro Fertilization: Building Policy from Laboratories to Legislatures.* New York: Columbia University Press, 1989.

Capron, Alexander Morgan. "Grandma! No, I'm the Mother!" *Hastings Center Report* 24, no.2 (1994): 24–25.

Cohen, Cynthia B. " 'Give Me Children or I Shall Die!' New Reproductive Technologies and Harm to Children." *Hastings Center Report* (March–April 1996): 19–29.

———. ed. *New Ways of Making Babies.* Bloomington: Indiana University Press, 1996.

Corea, Gena. *The Mother Machine: Reproductive Technologies from Artificial Insemination to Artificial Wombs.* New York: Harper, 1985.

"From Cells to Selves: Ethics at the Beginning of Life." *Cambridge Quarterly of Healthcare Ethics* 2, no.3 (special section, 1993): 259–326.

Glover, Jonathan. *Ethics of New Reproductive Technologies: The Glover Report to the European Commission.* DeKalb, IL: Northern Illinois University Press, 1989.

Gorovitz, Samuel. "Progeny, Progress and Primrose Paths." In *Doctors' Dilemmas: Moral Conflict and Medical Care.* New York: Oxford University Press, 1982.

Hanscombe, Gillian. "The Right to Lesbian Parenthood." *Journal of Medical Ethics* 9 (1983): 133–135.

Hull, Richard T., ed. *Ethical Issues in the New Reproductive Technologies.* Belmont, CA: Wadsworth Publishing Company, 1990.

Lauritzen, Paul. *Pursuing Parenthood: Ethical Issues in Assisted Reproduction.* Bloomington: Indiana University Press, 1993.

Macklin, Ruth. "Artificial Means of Reproduction and Our Understanding of the Family." *Hastings Center Report* 21, no. 1 (1991): 5–11.

McCormick, Richard A. "Who or What Is a Preembryo?" *Kennedy Institute of Ethics Journal* 1, no. 1 (1991): 1–15.

Neumann, Peter J. "Should Health Insurance Cover IVF? Issues and Options." *Journal of Health Politics, Policy and Law* 22, no. 5 (October 1997): 1215–1240.

Robertson, John A. *Children of Choice: Freedom and the New Reproductive Technologies.* Princeton, NJ: Princeton University Press 1994.

———— "Posthumous Reproduction," *Indiana Law Journal* 69, no. 4 (1994): 1027–1065.

Robin, Peggy. *How to Be a Successful Fertility Patient.* New York: William Morrow and Company, 1993.

Seibel, Michelle M., and Crockin, Susan, eds. *Family Building through Egg and Sperm Donation: Medical, Legal and Ethical Issues.* Sudbury, MA: Jones and Bartlett, 1996.

Steinbock, Bonnie. "The Moral Status of Extracorporeal Embryos: Pre-Born Children, Property, or Something Else?" In *Ethics and Biotechnology,* edited by Anthony Dyson and John Harris. London: Routledge, 1994.

————. "Sperm as Property," *Stanford Law & Policy Review* 6, no. 2 (1995): 57–71.

Warnock, Mary. *A Question of Life: The Warnock Report on Human Fertilization and Embryology.* Oxford: Basil Blackwell, 1985.

Zaner, Richard M. "A Criticism of Moral Conservatism's View of In Vitro Fertilization and Embryo Transfer." *Perspectives in Biology and Medicine* 27, no. 2 (Winter 1984).

Contract Pregnancy, Commodification, and the Family

Anderson, Elizabeth S. "Is Women's Labor a Commodity?" *Philosophy and Public Affairs* 19, no. 1 (Winter 1990).

Annas, George J. "Baby M: Babies (and Justice) for Sale." *Hastings Center Report* 17, no. 3 (1987).

Arneson, Richard J. "Commodification and Commercial Surrogacy." *Philosophy and Public Affairs* 21, no. 2 (Spring 1992).

Field, Martha A. *Surrogate Motherhood: The Legal and Human Issues.* Cambridge, MA: Harvard University Press, 1988.

Gostin, Larry O., ed. *Surrogate Motherhood: Politics and Privacy.* Bloomington: Indiana University Press, 1990.

Ketchum, Sara Ann. "Selling Babies and Selling Bodies." *Hypatia* 4, no. 3 (Fall 1989): 116–127.

Krimmel, Herbert T. "The Case against Surrogate Parenting." *Hastings Center Report* (October 1983).

Nelson, Hilde Lindemann, and Nelson, James Lindemann. "Cutting Motherhood in Two: Suspicions Concerning Surrogacy." *Hypatia* 4, no. 3 (Fall 1989): 84–94.

New Jersey Commission on Legal and Ethical Problems in the Delivery of Health Care. *After Baby M: The Legal, Ethical and Social Dimensions of Surrogacy.* Trenton: 1992.

New York State Task Force on Life and the Law. *Surrogate Parenting* 1988.

Radin, Margaret Jane. "Market-Inalienability." *Harvard Law Review* 100 (1987): 1839–1947.

Satz, Debra. "Markets in Women's Reproductive Labor." *Philosophy and Public Affairs* 21, no. 2 (Spring 1992).

"Symposium on 'Surrogate Motherhood.'" *Law, Medicine & Health Care* 16, nos. 1–2 (Spring/Summer 1988): 1–137.

Wertheimer, Alan. "Two Questions about Surrogacy and Exploitation." *Philosophy and Public Affairs* 21, no. 3 (Summer 1992).

Cloning

Allmers, H. and Kenwright, S. "Ethics of Cloning." *Lancet* 349 no. 9062 (May 10, 1997): 1401

Annas, George J. "Regulatory Models for Human Embryo Cloning: The Free Market, Professional Guidelines, and Government Restrictions." *Kennedy Institute of Ethics Journal* 4 (1994): 235–249.

Capron, Alexander Morgan. "Inside the Beltway Again: A Sheep of a Different Feather." *Kennedy Institute of Ethics Journal* 7 (1997): 171–179

Carmen, Ira H. *Cloning & the Constitution: An Inquiry into Governmental Policy Making & Genetic Experimentation.* University of Wisconsin Press, 1986.

Chadwick, R. F. "Cloning." *Philosophy* 57 (1982): 201–209.

Cloning Human Beings: Report and Recommendations of the National Bioethics Advisory Commission. Rockville, MD, 1997.

"Cloning Human Beings: Responding to the National Bioethics Advisory Commission's Report." *Hastings Center Report* (September–October 1997).

Cloning Symposium, *Jurimetrics* 38, no. 1(1997).

Gregory E. Pence, *Who's Afraid of Human Cloning?* Lanhan, MD: Rowman & Littlefield, 1998.

Hathout, M. "Cloning: Who Will Set the Limits." *The Minaret* 19, no. 3 (March 199): 8.

Hefner, P. "Cloning as Quintessential Human Act." *Insights* (June 1997).

Kolata, Gina. *Clone.* New York: William Morrow & Co., 1998.

Lauritzen, Paul ed. *Cloning and the Future of Human Embryo Research* (forthcoming).

Lewontin, Richard. "The Confusion over Cloning." *New York Review of Books,* 44 (October 23, 1997):

Lewontin, Richard; with Harold T. Shapiro; James F. Childress; and Thomas H. Murray. " 'The Confusion over Cloning': An Exchange." *New York Review of Books,* 45, no. 4 (March 5, 1998): 46–47.

Macklin, Ruth. "Splitting Embryos on the Slippery Slope: Ethics and Public Policy." *Kennedy Institute of Ethics Journal* 4 no. 3 (September 1994): 209–225.

McCormick, R. A. "Should We Clone Humans?" *The Christian Century* 17–24 (November 1993): 1148–1149.

Pizzulli, Francis C. "Asexual Reproduction and Genetic Engineering: A Constitutional Assessment of the Technology of Cloning." *Southern California Law Review* 47 (February 1974): 476–584.

Rhodes, R. "Clones, Harms, and Rights." *Cambridge Quarterly of Healthcare Ethics* 4 (1995): 285–290.

Robertson, J. A. "Liberty, Identity, and Human Cloning." *Texas Law Review* 76, no. 6 (1998):

Special issue on cloning. *Cambridge Quarterly of Healthcare Ethics* 7, no. 2 (Spring 1998): 115ff.

Verhey, A. "Cloning: Revisiting an Old Debate." *Kennedy Institute of Ethics Journal* 4, no. 3 (September 1994): 227–234.

———. "Playing God and Invoking a Perspective." *Journal of Medicine and Philosophy* 20 (1995): 347–364.

Genetic Testing and Screening

Anderson, W. French. "Genetic Engineering and our Humanness." *Human Gene Therapy.* 5 (1994): 755–759.

Annas, George J., and Elias, Sherman, eds. *Gene Mapping: Using Law and Ethics as Guides.* New York: Oxford University Press, 1992.

Asch, Adrienne. "Reproductive Technology and Disability." In *Reproductive Laws for the 1990s,* edited by Sherill Cohen and Nadine Taub. Clifton, NJ: Humana Press, 1989.

Bailey, J. Michael, and Pillard, Richard. "A Genetic Study of Male Sexual Orientation." *Archives of General Psychiatry* 48 (1991): 1089–1096.

Bartels, Dianne M., et al. *Prescribing Our Future: Ethical Challenges in Genetic Counseling.* New York: Aldine de Gruyter, 1993.

Billings, Paul. "Genetic Discrimination and Behavioural Genetics: The Analysis of Sexual Orientation." In *Intractable Neurological Disorders, Human Genome, Research and Society,* edited by Norio Fujiki and Darryl Macer. Christchurch and Tsukuba: Eubios Ethics Institute, 1993.

——— "International Aspects of Genetic Discrimination." In *Human Genome Research and Society,* ed. Norio Fujiki and Darryl Macer (Christchurch and Tsukuba: Eubios Ethics Institute, 1992), pp. 114–17.

Bonnicksen, Andrea L. "National and International Approaches to Human Germ-Line Gene Therapy." *Politics and the Life Sciences* 13, no. 1(1994): 39–49.

Botkin, Jeffrey R. "Fetal Privacy and Confidentiality." *Hastings Center Report* (September–October 1995): 32–39.

———. "Prenatal Screening: Professional Standards and the Limits of Parental Choice." *Obstetrics and Gynecology* 75, no. 5 (1990): 328–329.

Boyle, Philip. "Shaping Priorities in Genetic Medicine." *Hastings Center Report* 25, no. (special supplement, 1995): S2–S8.

Buchanan, Allen. "Choosing Who Will Be Disabled: Genetic Intervention and the Morality of Inclusion," *Social Philosophy & Policy,* Vol. 13, no. 2 (Summer 1996): 18–46.

Bullough, Vern. *Science in the Bedroom: The History of Sex Research* (Basic Books: New York, 1994).

Burke, Phyllis. *Gender Shock: Exploding the Myths of Male and Female.* New York: Anchor Books, 1996.

Byne, William. "Biology and Sexual Orientation: Implications of Endocronological and Neuroanatomical Research." In *Comprehensive Textbook of Homosexuality,* edited by R. Labaj and T. Stein. Washington, D.C.: American Psychiatric Press, 1996.

Carson, Sandra A., and Buster, John E. "Diagnosis and Treatment before Implantation: The Ultimate Prenatal Medicine," *Contemporary OB/GYN* (December 1995): 71–85.

D'Alessio, V. "Born to be Gay?" *New Scientist* (28 September 1996): 32–35.

Davis, Dena. "Genetic Dilemmas and the Child's Right to an Open Future." *Hastings Center Report* (March–April, 1997): 7–15.

Deussen, Julius. "Sexualpathologie." In *Fortschritte der Erbpathologie, Rassenhygiene und ihrer Grenzgebiete* 2 (1939): 67–102.

Dörner, Günter. "Hormone-Dependent Brain Development and Neuroendocrine Prophylaxis." *Experimental and Clinical Endocrinology* 94 (1989): 4–22.

"The Ethical Use of Technology in Genetics." *Journal of Clinical Ethics* 2, no. 4 (special section, 1991): 259–281.

Fletcher, John C. "Moral Problems and Ethical Guidance in Prenatal Diagnosis." In *Genetic Disorders and the Fetus,* edited by A. Milunsky, 2nd ed. New York: Plenum Press, 1986.

Fletcher, John C., and Anderson, W. French. "Germ-Line Gene Therapy: A New Stage of Debate." *Law, Medicine & Health Care* 20, nos. 1–2 (Spring/Summer 1992): 26–39.

Fost, Norman. "'Ethical Issues in Genetics." *Pediatric Clinics of North America* 39, no. 1 (February 1992): 79–89.

Fost, Norman. "Genetic Diagnosis and Treatment," *AJDC* 147 (November 1993): 1190–1195.

Friedman, Richard C. *Male Homosexuality: A Contemporary Psychoanalytic Perspective.* New Haven: Yale University Press, 1988.

Gardner, William. "Can Human Genetic Enhancement be Prohibited?" *The Journal of Medicine and Philosophy* 20, no. 1 (February 1995): 65–84.

"Genetic Grammar: 'Health,' 'Illness,' and the Human Genome Project." *Hastings Center Report* 22, no. 4 (special supplement, 1992): S1–S20.

Green, Ronald M. "Paternal Autonomy and the Obligation Not to Harm One's Child Genetically," *Journal of Law, Medicine and Ethics* 25 (1997): 5–15.

Green, Richard. *The 'Sissy Boy' Syndrome and the Development of Homosexuality.* New Haven: Yale University Press, 1987.

Gustafson, James M. "Genetic Therapy: Ethical and Religious Reflections." *Journal of Contemporary Health Law and Policy* 8 (Spring 1992): 183–200.

Halley, Janet. "Sexual Orientation and the Politics of Biology: A Critique of the New Argument from Immutability." *Stanford Law Review* 46 (1994): 503–568.

Hamer, Dean, et al. "A Linkage Between DNA Markers on the X Chromosome and Male Sexual Orientation." *Science* 261 (1993): 321–327.

Heyd, David. *Genethics: Moral Issues in the Creation of People.* Berkeley: University of California Press, 1992.

"The Human Genome Initiative and the Impact of Genetic Testing and Screening Technologies." *American Journal of Law and Medicine* 17, nos. 1–2 (symposium, 1991).

Juengst, Eric T., ed. "Human Germ-Line Engineering." *Journal of Medicine and Philosophy* 16, no. 6 (December 1991): 587–694.

———. '"Prevention' and the Goals of Genetic Medicine." *Human Gene Therapy* 6 (December 1995): 1595–1605.

Katz, Jonathan Ned. *Gay American History.* New York: Thomas Crowell, 1976.

Kelves, Daniel J. *In the Name of Eugenics: Genetics and the Uses of Human Heredity.* New York: Alfred A. Knopf, 1985.

Kitcher, Philip. *Vaulting Ambition: Sociobiology and the Quest for Human Nature.* Cambridge, MA: MIT Press, 1985.

Kusum, "The Use of Prenatal Diagnostic Techniques for Sex Selection: The Indian Scene." *Bioethics* 7 (1993): 149–165.

Lautmann, Rüdiger, ed., *Homosexualität: Handbuch der Theorie und Forschungsgeschichte.* Campus Verlag: Frankfurt am Main, 1993.

LeVay, Simon. *Queer Science: The Use and Abuse of Research on Homosexuality.* Cambridge, MA: MIT Press, 1996.

Levin, Michael. "Why Homosexuality Is Abnormal," *Monist* 67 (1984): 251–283.

Lim, L. C. C. "Present Controversies in the Genetics of Male Homosexuality." *Annals of the Academy of Medicine Singapore* 24 (1995): 759–762.

Marshall, E. "NIH 'Gay Gene' Study Questioned," *Science* 268 (1995): 1841.

Mazumdar, Pauline M. H. *Eugenics, Human Genetics and Human Failings: The Eugenics Society, Its Sources and Its Critics in Britain.* London: Routledge, 1992.

McGee, Glenn. *The Perfect Baby: A Pragmatic Approach to Genetics.* New York: Rowan and Littlefield, 1997.

Meyer-Bahlburg, Heino. "Psychoendocrine Research on Sexual Orientation: Current Status and Future Options." *Progress in Brain Research* 71 (1984): 375–397.

Munson, Ronald, and Davis, Lawrence H. "Germ-Line Gene Therapy and the Medical Imperative." *Kennedy Institute of Ethics Journal* 2, no. 2 (June 1992): 137–158.

Murphy, Timothy. "Abortion and the Ethics of Genetic Sexual Orientation Research." *Cambridge Quarterly of Healthcare Ethics* 4 (1995): 340–350.

Murray, Thomas H. "Genetics and the Moral Mission of Health Insurance." *Hastings Center Report* 22, no. 6 (1992): 12–17.

———. "The Growing Danger from Gene-Spliced Hormones." *Discover* (February 1987): 88–92.

National Institutes of Health (NIH) Consensus Development Conference Statement. "Genetic Testing for Cystic Fibrosis." April 14–16, 1997.

Parens, Erik. "The Goodness of Fragility: On the Prospect of Genetic Technologies Aimed at the Enhancement of Human Capacities." *Kennedy Institute of Ethics Journal* (1996):

———. "Should We Hold the (Germ) Line?" *Journal of Law, Medicine and Ethics* 23, no. 2 (Summer 1995): 173–176.

———. "Taking Behavioral Genetics Seriously." *Hastings Center Report* (July- August, 1996): 13–22.

Pillard, Richard, and Weinrich, James. "Evidence for a Familial Nature of Male Homosexuality." *Archives of General Psychiatry* 43 (1986): 808–812.

Posner, Richard. *Sex and Reason.* Cambridge, MA: Harvard University Press, 1992.

President's Commission for the Study of Ethical Problems in Medicine and Biomedical and Behavioral Research. *Screening and Counseling for Genetic Conditions: A Report on the Ethical, Social, and Legal Implications of Genetic Screening, Counseling, and Education Programs.* Washington, DC: U.S. Government Printing Office, 1983.

———. *Splicing Life: A Report on the Social and Ethical Issues of Genetic Engineering with Human Beings.* Washington, DC: U.S. Government Printing Office, 1982.

Rice, G., et al. "Male Homosexuality: Absence of Linkage to Microsatellite Markers on the X Chromosome in a Canadian Study," presented at the 21st Annual Meeting of the International Academy of Sex Research, 1995, Provincetown. MA.

Risch, Neil, Squires-Wheeler, Elizabeth, and Keats, Bronya. "Male Sexual Orientation and Genetic Evidence," *Science* 262 (1993): 2063–2065.

Rothenberg, Karen H., and Thomson, Elizabeth J., eds. *Women & Prenatal Testing: Facing the Challenges of Genetic Technology.* Columbus, Ohio: Ohio State University Press, 1994.

Rothman, Barbara Katz. *The Tentative Pregnancy: Prenatal Diagnosis and the Future Of Motherhood.* New York: Viking Press, 1986.

Schüklenk, Udo, and Mertz, David. "Christliche Kirchen und AIDS." In *Die Lehre des Unheils* edited by Edgar Dahl. Hamburg: Carlsen, 1993.

Schüklenk, Udo, and Ristow, Michael. "The Ethics of Research into the Causes of Homosexuality." *Journal of Homosexuality* 31, nos. 3, 4 (1996): 5–30.

Silverstein, Charles. "Psychological and Medical Treatments of Homosexuality." In *Homosexuality: Research Implications for Public Policy,* edited by J. C. Gonsiorek and J. D. Weinrich. Newbury Park. CA: Sage. 1991.

Snowden, C. and Green, J. "Preimplantation Diagnosis and Other Reproductive Options: Attitudes of Male and Female Carriers of Recessive Disorders." *Human Reproduction* 12, no. 2 (1997): 341–350.

Speight, Kevin. "Homophobia Is a Health Issue." *Health Care Analysis* 3 (1995): 143–148.

Stein, Edward. "Choosing the Sexual Orientation of Children." *Bioethics* 12, no. 1 (January 1998).

————. "The Relevance of Scientific Research Concerning Sexual Orientation to Lesbian and Gay Rights." *Journal of Homosexuality* 27 (1994): 269–308.

Stein, Edward, Schüklenk, Udo, and Kerin, Jacinta. "Scientific Research on Sexual Orientation." In *Encyclopedia of Applied Ethics,* edited by Ruth Chadwick. San Diego: Academic Press, 1997.

Suzuki, David, and Knudtson, Peter. *Genethics: The Clash between the New Genetics and Human Values.* Cambridge, MA: Harvard University Press, 1990.

"Symposium on Genetics and the Law." *Emory Law Journal* 39, no. 3 (Summer 1990): 619–936.

"The Genome Imperative." *Journal of Law, Medicine and Ethics* 23, no. 4 (Symposium, Winter 1995):

"The Genetic Privacy Act Roundtable Commentary." *Journal of Law, Medicine and Ethics* 23, no. 4 (Symposium, Winter 1995):

Walters, LeRoy. "Human Gene Therapy: Ethics and Public Policy." *Human Gene Therapy* 2 (1991): 115–122.

Walters, Leroy, and Palmer, Julie Gage. *The Ethics of Human Gene Therapy.* New York: Oxford University Press, 1996.

Weber, Matthias. *Ernst Rüdin. Eine kritische Biographie.* Berlin: Springer, 1993.

Wertz, Dorthy C. "Society and the Not-So-New Genetics: What Are We Afraid Of? Some Future Predictions from a Social Scientist," *The Journal of Contemporary Health Law and Policy* 13 (1997): 299–346.

Wertz, Dorothy C., and Fletcher, John C., eds. *Ethics and Human Genetics: A Cross-Cultural Perspective.* New York: Springer-Verlag, 1989.

Wilfond, Benjamin S., and Nolan, Kathleen. "National Policy Development for the Clinical Application of Genetic Diagnostic Technologies: Lessons from Cystic Fibrosis," *Journal of the American Medical Association* 270 (1993): 2948–2954.

Wivel, Nelson A., and Walters, LeRoy. "Germ-Line Gene Modification and Disease Prevention: Some Medical and Ethical Perspectives." *Science* 262 (October 22, 1993).

Wolf, Susan M. "Beyond 'Genetic Discrimination' toward the Broader Harm of Geneticism," *Journal of Law, Medicine and Ethics* 23 (1995): 345–353.

PART FIVE

EXPERIMENTATION ON HUMAN SUBJECTS

Self-conscious scientific experimentation is a relatively new phenomenon in the long history of medicine. For centuries, the introduction of innovative medical procedures was regarded with suspicion; the upstart medical heretic could even be charged with the tort of negligence, or "malpractice," for having deviated from the established standard of care. But the advent of properly scientific medicine in the nineteenth and twentieth centuries transformed controlled scientific investigation into the driving force behind the spectacular successes of modern medicine. What previous centuries had labeled assault and battery has now become a scientific, and even ethical, imperative.

But here, as elsewhere in the field of biomedicine, success has not been unalloyed: Ethical problems of the greatest magnitude have been posed by the methods of scientific medicine. The most gruesomely spectacular of these problems were showcased at the trials of Nazi doctors at Nuremberg and in the tragic forty-year history of our own Tuskegee syphilis experiment. The latter study was designed to measure the ravages of untreated syphilis in black males, 400 of whom were systematically deceived about the nature of their condition and were given aspirin instead of proven treatments. Those subjects "lucky" enough to endure twenty-five years were rewarded a $50 bonus for funeral payments in exchange for their written consent to autopsy. At both Nuremberg and Tuskegee, the hallmarks of unethical medical experimentation were exposed to an aggrieved and shocked public: (1) The experiments were scientifically pointless or redundant, (2) their design was shoddy, precluding meaningful results, (3) subjects were either coerced or deceived into participating, (4) research subjects were drawn from socially deprived groups (captive Jews, prisoners of war, poor and uneducated sharecroppers), and (5) apart from the aforementioned burial fees, the subjects were not compensated for injuries (or death) sustained in the course of experimentation.

The ethics of human experimentation has come a long way in the decade following the denouement at Tuskegee. Local and national rules and regulations have been promulgated; institutional review boards (IRBs) routinely scrutinize new experimental protocols at most hospitals and research centers; and a Presidential Commission has recommended federal policies for the protection of human subjects in research involving children, fetuses, and prisoners. Nevertheless, many of the basic issues surrounding human experimentation remain controversial and have thus far evaded definitive resolution. Is informed consent really necessary in all experimental procedures, including research in the social sciences? How informed must consent be to be truly valid? Should special groups—such as fetuses, children, the mentally incompetent, the senile elderly, and prisoners—be allowed to participate in experiments not directly addressed to their own welfare? These seemingly narrow questions lead us to reflect more profoundly upon the moral bond uniting physician-researchers with their patient-subjects and also upon the moral limits of the relationship between individuals and the larger social groups to which they belong.

SOCIAL WELFARE AND INFORMED CONSENT

Part Five, Section One, begins with a case—"'Experimental' Pregnancy," presented by Robert M. Veatch—that raises many troubling questions surrounding the use of human subjects. In order to determine whether some of the unpleasant side effects of the birth control pill were psychologically induced, investigators designed an experiment in which several women were assigned randomly to a control group that received a placebo (or "sugar pill") instead of the (real) Pill. A number of these women, all of whom were poor Mexican-Americans, predictably became pregnant. Was the goal sufficiently important to put these women at risk? Who approved and funded the experiment? Does anyone have a moral or legal responsibility to compensate these "unexpectant" mothers? Should

the findings of unethical research be published in scientific journals? Should the poor and underprivileged bear the brunt of experimental risk taking for the rest of our society? And, perhaps most importantly, is it ever morally justifiable to coerce or deceive subjects into participating in experimental trials? In other words, is the subject's "informed consent" a necessary condition of ethical research on humans?

As we saw in Part One, the requirement of informed consent is designed to protect the right of the patient-subject to the inviolability of his or her person; the moral content of this requirement is perhaps best described by the Kantian principle of treating other persons as ends in themselves and never simply as means to ends that they do not share. For example, when an investigator fails to mention the risks inherent in the trial of a new drug, it could be said that the patient-subject's status as a person is debased to that of a mere thing. Thus, the informed consent requirement can be seen as protecting the moral status of persons who also happen to be experimental subjects.

The insistence upon informed consent as a moral prerequisite of biomedical research is a relatively new phenomenon. Prior to the advent of World War II, medical research tended to be small-scale and animated primarily by therapeutic motives. Research during this "premodern" period raised few ethical difficulties and attracted even less public attention and controversy. During and immediately after the war, however, medical research became a large-scale, highly organized, and well-funded effort harnessed to military objectives and the national interest. In this climate, Rothman contends, the use of our most vulnerable citizens—institutionalized children, the mentally retarded, and prisoners—came to be seen a a sacrifice entirely justified by the national interest in the "war" against disease (Rothman, 1991).

Just how easily such sacrifices could be justified is perhaps most shockingly illustrated by the Tuskegee study, recounted by historian Allan Brandt in "Racism and Research: The Case of the Tuskegee Syphilis Study." This project involved the systematic deception and abuse of poor African American men, incredibly, from 1936 to 1972. Undertaken in part to determine the effects of untreated syphilis in this population, the researchers recruited subjects by lying to them outright, saying they would *treat* the men for "bad blood." As Brandt observes, "deceit was integral to the study." In addition to this flagrant disregard for the principles of veracity and informed consent, the Tuskegee researchers, drawn largely from the U.S. Public Health Service, also withheld all medical treatments that were considered standard therapy for syphilis at the time, including penicillin when it became available during World War II. There can be no doubt that this failure to treat led to the suffering and premature deaths of many study subjects, their spouses and sexual partners, and their children.

Brandt concludes that "the Tuskegee study revealed more about the pathology of racism than it did about the pathology of syphilis; more about the nature of scientific inquiry than the nature of the disease process." It was not until the summer of 1997 that President Clinton finally apologized on behalf of the United States to a handful of aged survivors and their relatives. In spite of this long-overdue gesture of repentance and reconciliation, much damage had already been done both to the human beings involved in the study and to the fabric of trust between the enterprise of medical science and the African-American community.

When challenged by reformers in the late 1960s and early 1970s, many researchers resorted to frankly utilitarian arguments against increased ethical and legal regulation of biomedical research. Walsh McDermott provides a good example of this utilitarian defense in his 1967 "Opening Comments on the Changing Mores of Biomedical Research." McDermott contends that medical research has bestowed great benefits on society and in so doing created a kind of societal expectation—indeed a societal right—to the fruits of further research. This premise then engendered a painful moral dilemma for morally sensitive researchers such as McDermott: What should be done when this societal right to miracle cures conflicts with the rights of individuals as potential research subjects? According to McDermott, there may well be times, hopefully few, when the good of society must take precedence over the good of the individual; indeed, he notes that our society often calls for such sacrifices outside the sphere of medicine, such as in capital punishment and the military draft. At such times, he concludes, researchers must, in effect, play God by arbitrarily singling out certain luckless individuals for participation in research. Rather than rigidly codifying the proper relations between physician-researchers and their subjects; rather than officially stating, as did the Declaration of Helsinki (included at the end of Section One) that the good of individual patients must *always* take precedence over the good of society; McDermott concludes that society must simply continue to trust the research community to do the right thing, and this community will, on occasion, call for individual sacrifice. Given the basic tension he perceived between individual and social rights, McDermott firmly believed that high-sounding declarations and regulations could not resolve the moral dilemma and, in fact, only made it more public and therefore more acute.

McDermott's utilitarian defense of the prerogatives of researchers may have represented a broad spectrum of opinion within organized medicine at the time it was written, but a mere five years later, with the shocking revelations of the Tuskegee experiment, the trust he had called for had been effectively shattered, and increased public regulation of biomedical research had become inevitable. The philosophical case for increased regulation and a strong consent requirement is nicely summarized by Alan Donagan in "Informed Consent to Experimentation." Donagan argues that attempts to sidestep the informed consent requirement represent a sanitized version of the defense proffered by Nazi physicians at Nuremberg. Couching his accusation in less inflammatory language, Donagan asserts that such attempts to dispense with the requirement of consent are based on the moral theory of utilitarianism. From the perspective of this theory, even the "experimental pregnancy" case mentioned earlier could be justified on the grounds that the harm of ten unwanted pregnancies in the control group is outweighed by thousands of women switching to the more effective Pill once their fears of side effects are allayed. Donagan responds by noting that utilitarianism isn't the only available theory. According to the tradition of Judeo-Christian morality—ably represented by such writers as Kant, Hans Jonas, Paul Ramsey, and Donagan himself—the future of medical progress cannot be purchased at the expense of the autonomy of present patient-subjects.

THE ETHICS OF RANDOMIZED CLINICAL TRIALS

The Hippocratic tradition and recent codes of medical ethics speak clearly and emphatically concerning the physician's duty to individual patients. The tradition has emphasized the physician's covenantal duty of undivided loyalty to the patient, as opposed to what Paul Ramsey has called "that celebrated non-patient—the future of medical science." This traditional duty of exclusive personal care for the individual patient is expressed in a number of applicable codes. For example, the AMA Principles of Medical Ethics state, "Physicians should merit the confidence of patients entrusted to their care, rendering to each a full measure of service and devotion . . . "while the AMA's Ethical Guidelines for Clinical Investigation declare, "In conducting clinical investigation, the investigator should demonstrate the same concern and caution for the welfare, safety, and comfort of the person involved as is required of a physician who is furnishing medical care to a patient independent of any clinical investigation."

This traditional posture of undivided loyalty to the patient-subject was easy to maintain when clear-cut distinctions could be made between "therapeutic" and "nontherapeutic" experimentation—that is, between trials performed primarily for the benefit of patient-subjects and those designed primarily for the purpose of gaining valuable knowledge for future patients. Although this distinction is still useful in some contexts, the boundaries between these different kinds of experimentation have become blurred in the conduct of modern biomedical research.

Physicians plausibly maintain that they have a *moral obligation* to employ the most effective means for combatting disease and disability, regardless of the time-honored status of standard procedures, many of which often turn out to be quite useless or even harmful. The duty, grounded in the physician's Hippocratic commitment to "do no harm," is expressed in Section 3 of the AMA Principles of Medical Ethics, which states that "a physician should practice a method of healing founded on a scientific basis. . . ." The vexing ethical problem posed by this kind of clinical research is that it places the physician's traditional duty of personal care in direct opposition to his or her duty to practice scientific medicine. Whereas the horrors of Nuremberg and Tuskeegee invited spontaneous moral outrage, the dilemmas posed by research today demand nuanced ethical reflection and creative thinking about experimental design.

One of the most problematic features of scientific research design is the common practice of "randomizing" patients—i.e., assigning them by chance—to one of several competing treatments or to a control group receiving no treatment. Section Two begins with three case studies of morally troubling randomizations, presented by Maurie Markham, a prominent cancer researcher. According to the advocates of so-called "randomized clinical trials" (RCTs), there are both scientific and ethical advantages to assigning research subjects to treatment groups by chance. By eliminating bias in the selection and care of patient-subjects, randomization helps generate scientifically reliable data that will enable future patients to receive better care. Indeed, some defenders of RCTs claim that this disciplined procedure is *more ethical* than introducing new procedures on the informal basis of clinical impressions and historical comparisons.

The critics of RCTs, including Dr. Markham, are less sanguine about the prospects of reconciling the imperatives of hard science with the physician's duty to provide personal care. Samuel and Deborah Hellman, in "Of Mice but Not Men," object to the fact that in an RCT, the individual's therapy is determined not simply by an investigation into his or her physical needs and personal values, but also by consideration of the needs of the experimental design. Randomization for the sake of future patients, they claim, thus supersedes the individualized treatment of present patients. Does this not amount to a sacrifice of the individual for the sake of society at large? Samuel and Deborah Hellman conclude that it does, and they therefore condemn RCTs for violating the central tenet of Kantian ethics: that the personhood of the individual should not be submerged in utilitarian calculations of social benefit. The Hellmans urge the medical community to develop and use less morally problematic techniques for gaining reliable knowledge.

Defenders of RCTs attempt to counter these objections by noting that in order to be ethically justified, the two (or more) arms of study—e.g., comparing two different drugs, or one drug against a placebo—must be in "equipoise." That is, the researchers must not have any scientifically sound reason for preferring one arm to another. But what is to count as "scientific soundness" here?

Some critics of RTCs argue that such studies are problematic if the researchers have formed a "treatment preference" either before or after the initiation of the trial. In one of his case studies, for example, Markham contends that a physician who has a strong opinion in favor of a new cancer drug, taxol, cannot ethically advise his or her patients about a trial comparing taxol to the standard treatment. According to this view, if researchers develop a "strong hunch" about the comparative effectiveness of a new drug, either at the beginning or in the midst of a trial, it is unethical to continue an RCT.

Benjamin Freedman, in his "Response" to Markham, claims that such worries are based on a flawed conception of equipoise. Instead of insisting that the evidence on behalf of two treatments be exactly balanced and that the researchers develop no treatment preferences throughout the duration of the trial—both seemingly impossible requirements—Freedman argues for a concept of equipoise based on the existence of honest, professional disagreement within the scientific community. So long as there exists a genuine dispute among clinicians, Freedman contends, RCTs are ethically permissible even if a particular physician has a decided preference for one treatment over others. Indeed, he adds, the original and overriding purpose of RCTs is to dispel precisely this kind of professional disagreement. Many a strong hunch has become standard practice in medicine, not by virtue of meeting rigorous scientific standards, but rather by dint of the investigator's passionate commitment, charisma, or professional standing. When this has happened, patients have often been subjected to unnecessary risk and harm for extended periods of time.

ACCESS TO EXPERIMENTAL THERAPIES AND EXPERIMENTATION ON "VULNERABLE POPULATIONS"

As we saw in Section One, the uproar over flagrant abuses of the rights of human subjects both abroad and at home led to the establishment of serious protections both at the national level, through the

Food and Drug Administration, and at the local level, through institutional review boards (IRBs). This new era in biomedical research was defined by several assumptions. It was assumed, for example, that participation in research was both risky and burdensome; that the maintenance of high ethical standards justified a slower rate of progress in finding medical cures; and that populations that may be more vulnerable to exploitation—such as the minority group at Tuskeegee and the institutionalized children at Willowbrook—should be either shielded or excluded altogether from participation in research studies.

By far the most dramatic development in debates over the ethics of human experimentation has been the direct challenge that the AIDS epidemic and AIDS activists pose to all of these assumptions. Watching their family and friends die of AIDS while the nation's government and research establishment respond at glacial speed, a new generation of activists claim that participation in research is a *benefit*; that unproven medications are actually a form of *treatment* to which AIDS patients have a *right*; that the pace of scientific progress has to accelerate, even at the expense of various "ethical" constraints; and, finally, that various groups of "vulnerable" patient-subjects need increased access to, not increased protection from, experimental treatment. Indeed, to many activists, the entire edifice of measures designed to protect patients from undue risk and abuse constitutes the worst kind of paternalism. "It's my life and my body," they argue. "Who are you [the government or research establishment] to tell me, a dying patient, what risks I am allowed to run?"

As Carol Levine points out in "Changing Views of Justice after Belmont: AIDS and the Inclusion of 'Vulnerable' Subjects," paternalism wasn't the only problem. During this era of protectionism, researchers systematically excluded women of childbearing age in order to prevent possible harm to future offspring (and the subsequent lawsuits they might engender). This often worked to the disadvantage of women as a class because researchers, working only with male subjects, could only extrapolate their findings to women on the basis of what they knew of a drug's effect on men. This policy of exclusion disadvantaged women suffering from diseases such as AIDS. By excluding them in principle, researchers were in effect saying that it was more important to protect fetuses and future children from possible harm than it was to offer these women beneficial treatment. The first article in Section Three is a sensitive discussion of this issue, in which Carol Levine attempts to strike a sensible moral balance between the rights and interests of women and those of their future children.

This moral tension between protectionism and access is nicely illustrated in two case studies. First, we present the moral dilemmas encountered by international researchers studying treatments for the AIDS virus in underdeveloped nations in Africa and Asia. Recent research in the U.S. has demonstrated that the rate of HIV infection from mothers to children can be dramatically reduced (from roughly 30 to 8 percent) by giving pregnant women several doses of the drug AZT during pregnancy and at birth, followed by administering the drug to the infants themselves after delivery. This particular regimen (called the 076 protocol) was immediately hailed as a major breakthrough and soon became the accepted standard of medical practice throughout the U.S. But what of the millions of HIV-infected women in foreign countries too poor to afford AZT for everyone? What can and should be done for them?

This question led health officials in Africa and Asia to join forces with researchers at the U.S. National Institutes of Health (NIH) and Centers for Disease Control (CDC) in an effort to test a lower and less expensive dose of AZT in pregnant women. A wide variety of studies, examining a wide variety of doses and drugs, have subsequently been initiated throughout Africa. With few exceptions, however, these studies exhibit a very controversial design element: Almost all of them compare the new, less expensive drug regimens with a placebo group. In effect, a set proportion of the women in each study intentionally receives nothing, while their more fortunate counterparts receive a lesser (experimental) amount of the active drug; meanwhile, the truly fortunate inhabitants of Europe and North America receive a standard dose that is known to effect a dramatic reduction in the rate of infection from mothers to children.

Although they agree that the discovery of a less expensive preventive treatment for HIV-infected pregnant women is an important goal, critics have charged researchers and their spon-soring institutions with exploiting the vulnerable people of impoverished, postcolonial societies in a manner reminiscent of the infamous Tuskegee study (Angell 1997). Peter Lurie and Sidney Wolfe in "Unethical Trials of Interventions to Reduce Perinatal Transmission of the Human Immunodeficiency Virus in Developing Countries," charge that the use of placebo controls following the discovery of an effective treatment constitutes a blatant violation of human rights and of codes of research ethics that would never have been contemplated, let alone implemented, in developed countries. They contend that researchers from developed countries should apply the same high ethical standards and norms of appropriate treatment that they observe at home while collaborating with their counterparts in poorer nations. If, as Benjamin Freedman would put it, protocol 076 has upset "clinical equipoise" in Boston, researchers in Zaire cannot pretend clinical equipoise exists in Zaire merely because governments and drug companies have decided not to make an effective drug available. Lurie and Wolfe conclude that sufficient information about these new drugs and doses may be obtained by pitting them in trials against the standard dose of the 076 protocol.

In defense of these trials, Harold Varmus and David Satcher, in "Ethical Complexities of Conducting Research in Developing Countries", point to many medical and social factors prevalent in underdeveloped countries that make the implementation of the 076 protocol both impractical and unwise. Most importantly, they note that placebo-controlled trials of alternative treatments may well be the only way to obtain answers that are useful to people in societies very different from our own. Unless these alternatives are compared with placebos, they claim, we will never learn just how much better than nothing they are; and without that crucial piece of information, responsible health officials in developing countries will be unable to make sound medical and financial judgments regarding the implementation of the new treatments. According to Varmus and Satcher, these new studies thus represent neither the exploitation of vulnerable, post-colonial populations, nor a callous Tuskegee-like refusal of beneficial treatment; rather, they represent a reasoned and collaborative attempt to provide urgently needed answers to questions that can be readily answered in no other way.

We close this section with a case study and critical reflections on a persistent problem in research with psychiatric patients. The problem concerns the fate of severely schizophrenic patients who are taking powerful drugs to control such symptoms as hallucinations, delusions, disorganized thinking, social withdrawal, and, most seriously, suicide. Current antipsychotic medications generally work well, but at the cost of serious side-effects, such as tardive dyskinesia, a syndrome characterized by involuntary muscle ticks. Researchers are thus keenly interested in learning which patients might be able to quit taking these drugs without suffering a relapse of their psychotic symptoms. To answer this important question, researchers at UCLA designed a controversial protocol described by psychiatrist Paul Appelbaum in "Drug-Free Research in Schizophrenia." The UCLA study called for a period of withdrawal from all drugs; a standard dose of a standard drug for all patients, instead of individualized treatment; and for the use of placebo controls at various phases of the experiment. Some of the test subjects relapsed with very disconcerting results, and one committed suicide; charges of unethical research and calls for federal investigation followed shortly thereafter.

In his comprehensive and thoughtful assessment, Paul Appelbaum notes that many schizophrenics are at elevated risk of having impaired capacity for giving informed consent. Although he is sensitive to the many risks and ethical difficulties surrounding such research, Appelbaum suggests several ways in which such clearly important and desirable research might be carried out with increased protections for such a vulnerable position. In his case commentary, Jay Katz notes several shortcomings in the informed consent form used in the UCLA study, including the understatement of some serious risks involved with schizophrenic relapse. Katz also observes that many patients in this study had difficulty understanding the difference between clinical treatment and research designed primarily to gain generalizable knowledge, and he criticizes the UCLA team for their apparent reluctance to emphasize their research orientation in discussions with potential subjects. This so-called "therapeutic misconception" is widespread in the area of clinical research (Appelbaum 1987) and is particularly problematic when dealing with patients who are mentally ill.

We are thus confronted with the essential tension haunting all research with so-called vulnerable populations. In spite of recent crusades for increased access to the fruits of research to benefit HIV-infected patients, women, and others, some groups of patients, such as the schizophrenics enrolled in the UCLA study, remain particularly vulnerable to abuse and/or neglect and may well require an enhanced level of protection in the design and conduct of medical research. On the other hand, such enhanced protection always carries the potential for excessive and misguided paternalism. As we protect such patients from overreaching on the part of researchers, we must guard against a failure to acknowledge their capacity, when present, for meaningful participation in, and consent to, research of the utmost importance.

SECTION 1

Social Welfare and Informed Consent

"Experimental" Pregnancy

Robert M. Veatch

Whether it achieved its original purpose or not, a recent experiment with birth control pills proved conclusively that (a) placebos don't prevent pregnancy, and (b) the issues raised in biomedical research are complex and tricky. The experiment, conducted mostly upon poor, multiparous, Mexican-American women who had come to a San Antonio clinic for contraceptives, raises dozens of medical, ethical, and social questions.

According to Dr. Joseph Goldzieher of the Southwest Foundation for Research and Education, who conducted the experiment, its purpose was to find out whether some of the reported side effects of the Pill were physiological or psychological. In a double-blind experiment, 76 of the women received dummy pills while another group got various hormone contraceptives. All had come not to assist in research, but to prevent further pregnancies. None were told they were receiving placebos, or even that they were partici-pating in research, but they were instructed to use a vaginal cream in addition since the pill might not be "completely effective."*

The results, reported to the American Fertility Society in New Orleans and described in *Medical World News:* the women on placebos had many of the same side effects—nervousness, depression, breast tenderness, and headaches—as those on the Pill. But 10 of the 76 women on placebos became pregnant.

Some of the more obvious ethical questions were raised in the *Medical World News* report. Dr. Christopher Tietze of the Population Council was quoted as saying that "No responsible investigator would take it upon himself to expose women seeking protection to the risk of pregnancy by ostensibly giving them . . . mere glucose or at best some vitamins." But there are many other questions worth asking. Here are some of them.

Hastings Center Report, No. 1, June 1971, 2–3. Copyright © 1971 The Hastings Center. Used with permission.

*EDITORS' NOTE: In subsequent reviews of the Goldzieher experiment, conducted by the Economic Opportunities Development Corporation of San Antonio and by an ad-hoc committee of the Bexar County Medical Society, it was determined that precautions were taken to ensure that participants understood that they were involved in a research project; that each participant signed an informed-consent release; and that six of the seven pregnancies were due to admitted carelessness on the part of patients. Nevertheless, the records furnished to us by Dr. Goldzieher do not indicate that the women knew they might be receiving placebos or that they were made aware of the *significantly increased* risk of pregnancy posed by reliance on vaginal cream alone. If such omissions were in fact made, serious questions would remain concerning the validity of the consent obtained.

IMPORTANCE OF THE RESEARCH

It is clear that at least some people thought this research was important. Certainly there is considerable confusion about the side effects of oral contraceptives. It would indeed be helpful to know more. More than that, many unwanted pregnancies and a statistically measurable number of maternal deaths could be prevented if it could be shown that side effects were a figment of the imagination and because of this, women returned to the Pill.

On the other hand, one critic was quoted as saying that "[t]he thing that bothers me most about this study is that the results weren't worth it." Who is to decide whether the results of an experimental procedure are even potentially "worth it"? If scientists have more than typical commitment to the value of knowledge, are they the ones to decide? Or are government policy makers? What is the experimental subject's role in that decision?

INSTITUTIONAL CONTROLS AND REVIEW PROCEDURES

This experiment raises serious questions about the present levels of control over experimental procedure. Informed consent is a classic ethical norm of experimentation on human subjects. Anyone who thinks he can get "fully" informed consent is naive, but was there even any semblance of consent to this experiment? Why could patient subjects not be told, as one critic suggests, that there is a placebo group in the experimental design? If patient/subjects then knowledgeably refuse to participate, the message should be clear.

In many research institutions and funding agencies, review procedures are now established. What are the procedures in effect at the Southwest Foundation for Research and Education? The study was funded by Syntex Labs, a manufacturer of oral contraceptives, and the federal government Agency for International Development—an agency with primary interests in an area other than biomedical research. What was Syntex's interest in this project, and what review and control procedures do they use? Would the experiment have been approved for funding by the National Institutes of Health? If not, is the moral that if one wants to conduct questionable research, he should seek out research facilities and funding where fewer questions will be asked? And can a study funded in large part by the drug manufacturer be expected to be as impartial as one funded without a vested interest?

PUBLICATION

Responsibility for ethically acceptable research goes beyond funder, institution, and researcher. Should publishers accept reports of research where consent procedures are not clearly specified? By providing a public forum for the research, a publication or a learned society shares responsibility for the research. Should *Medical World News*

have transmitted the findings of this work to the nation's medical community? Should the American Fertility Society have provided a forum for the dissemination of the findings? We are well beyond the day when professional journals and professional scientists can plead value-free scientific objectivity. Whether or not they finally decide to participate in the research by providing a public forum, they cannot avoid facing the hard ethical questions. . . .

DESIGN OF THE EXPERIMENT

Almost certainly if this Goldzieher experiment does receive attention, the focus will be on the use of the placebo. But what about the rest of the design? The four other groups in the experimental design received either high-estrogen sequential, high-estrogen combination, low-estrogen combination, or chlormadinone acetate. Of these, sequentials are well-known to have substantially higher failure rates. High-estrogen combinations are being used less frequently because of often-documented higher incidence of side effects.

Chlormadinone acetate is a research progestin which has since been banned from all further human investigation because of reported side effects observed in beagles. The experimental design, even without the placebo group, raises all of the same questions about consent and review. If it is wrong to expose women unknowingly to pregnancy risk from placebos, is it right to expose them to smaller, but already documented risks from sequentials?

The research design included the use of vaginal cream to give additional contraceptive protection. Leaving aside the questions raised by the use of an admittedly poor backup contraceptive agent, does not the introduction of the vaginal cream necessarily convey to the patient that she is getting something other than routine oral contraceptive agents? (In Dr. Goldzieher's words vaginal cream "just doesn't work all that well.")

ABORTION AS A BACKUP

Dr. Goldzieher is quoted as saying that "we could have aborted them if the abortion statute here in Texas weren't in limbo right now." (An appeal of the Texas law is before the Supreme Court.*) Certainly he doesn't mean that the law's being in limbo put greater restrictions on him than a firmly established anti-abortion law would.

But there is an even more fundamental ethical question raised with the suggestion that abortion should be a backup for pregnancies induced for the good of scientific experiment in the face of the explicitly expressed wishes of the individual woman not to become pregnant. Is abortion ethically such a trivial procedure that it can be casually introduced in this way? Should not one at least consider the physical and psychological consequences to the woman, if not to the conceptus? It could reasonably be predicted that several of the women who conceived in the experiment would be morally opposed to abortion under these circumstances. Would this have been taken into account if backup abortion were incorporated into the research design?

THE RESEARCHER'S RESPONSIBILITY

But what were the limitations the researcher was under? A researcher conducting experiments on human beings must assume responsibility for the harmful effects of the experimental procedure on the subjects. Were the experimenters and funders of the research in this case willing to make this ultimate commitment? If so, was it really the case that no abortions were available to the women who conceived? This seems unlikely in light of the millions of abortions being performed yearly throughout the world. Even more fundamentally, are the researchers and the funders of the research now prepared to provide financial and other support for the products of their experiment? The patient/subjects seem to have a just claim not only for full support for the children produced, but for the psychological and social burdens placed on

*EDITORS' NOTE: The appeal was successful. See *Roe* v. *Wade*, 410 U.S. 113 (1973).

them as parents. Will the researcher offer such assistance? Will legal aid be available for the parents who may have to bring suit?

WHY CLINIC PATIENTS?

This case makes clear that the ethical implications of biomedical research are usually social and rarely merely personal. Why is it that the subjects for the experiment are "almost all of them Mexican-American and poor"? Will the astute scientist now ask whether the same results would be obtained among upper-middle class women—say researchers' wives? Why is it that clinic patients— that is, people too poor to pay for medical care— are the subjects for so much of the biomedical research conducted?

DETERIORATION OF TRUST

Finally, the clinical and the scientific community also have a stake in the ethical execution of each individual research project. Even if this particular act of deception could be defended on the basis of the utility of the knowledge to be gained, what is its effect upon the clinical institution involved, upon clinical institutions generally, and upon the scientists who are attempting to carry out morally acceptable research? Trust is a central value in the patient-physician relationship. Does not each such violation challenge that trust in a very realistic way? Does not each researcher, when evaluating his experimental design, have an obligation to protect that trust and confidence along with his primary obligation to protect the interests and well-being of the subject?

The case of the placebo for contraception raises even more ethical questions than are at first apparent. The question now is: What steps are now being taken to prepare the scientific community and the society at large to cope with these questions and protect themselves against potential future ethical abuses?

Racism and Research: The Case of the Tuskegee Syphilis Study

Allan M. Brandt

In 1932 the U.S. Public Health Service (USPHS) initiated an experiment in Macon County, Alabama, to determine the natural course of untreated, latent syphilis in black males. The test comprised 400 syphilitic men, as well as 200 uninfected men who served as controls. The first published report of the study appeared in 1936 with subsequent papers issued every four to six years, through the 1960s. When penicillin became widely available by the early 1950s as the preferred treatment for syphilis, the men did not receive therapy. In fact on several occasions, the USPHS actually sought to prevent treatment. Moreover, a committee at the federally operated Center for Disease Control decided in 1969 that the study should be continued. Only in 1972, when accounts of the study first appeared in the national press, did the Department of Health, Education and Welfare halt the experiment. At that time seventy-four of the test subjects were still alive; at least twenty-eight, but perhaps more than 100, had died directly from advanced syphilitic lesions.[1] In August 1972, HEW appointed an investigatory panel which issued a report the following year. The panel found the study to have been "ethically unjustified," and argued that penicillin should have been provided to the men.[2]

This article attempts to place the Tuskegee Study in a historical context and to assess its ethical implications. Despite the media attention which the study received, the HEW *Final Report,* and the criticism expressed by several professional organizations, the experiment has been largely misunderstood. The most basic questions of *how* the study was undertaken in the first place and *why* it continued for forty years were never addressed by the HEW investigation. Moreover, the panel misconstrued the nature of the

experiment, failing to consult important documents available at the National Archives which bear significantly on its ethical assessment. Only by examining the specific ways in which values are engaged in scientific research can the study be understood.

RACISM AND MEDICAL OPINION

A brief review of the prevailing scientific thought regarding race and heredity in the early twentieth century is fundamental for an understanding of the Tuskegee Study. By the turn of the century, Darwinism had provided a new rationale for American racism. Essentially primitive peoples, it was argued, could not be assimilated into a complex, white civilization. Scientists speculated that in the struggle for survival the Negro in America was doomed. Particularly prone to disease, vice, and crime, black Americans could not be helped by education or philanthropy. Social Darwinists analyzed census data to predict the virtual extinction of the Negro in the twentieth century, for they believed the Negro race in America was in the throes of a degenerative evolutionary process.

The medical profession supported these findings of late nineteenth- and early twentieth-century anthropologists, ethnologists, and biologists. Physicians studying the effects of emancipation on health concluded almost universally that freedom had caused the mental, moral, and physical deterioration of the black population. They substantiated this argument by citing examples in the comparitive anatomy of the black and white races. As Dr. W. T. English wrote: "A careful inspection reveals the body of the negro a mass of minor defects and imperfections from the crown of the head to the soles of the feet. . . ."[3] Cranial structures, wide nasal apertures, receding chins, projecting jaws, all typed the Negro as the lowest species in the Darwinian hierarchy.

Interest in racial differences centered on the sexual nature of blacks. The Negro, doctors explained,

Hastings Center Report, December 1978, pp. 21–29. Copyright © 1978 The Hastings Center. Used with permission.

EDITORS' NOTE: Many notes have been omitted. Readers who wish to follow up on sources should consult the original article.

possessed an excessive sexual desire, which threatened the very foundations of white society. As one physician noted in the *Journal of the American Medical Association*, "The negro springs from a southern race, and as such his sexual appetite is strong; all of his environments stimulate this appetite, and as a general rule his emotional type of religion certainly does not decrease it." Doctors reported a complete lack of morality on the part of blacks:

Virtue in the negro race is like angels' visits— few and far between. In a practice of sixteen years I have never examined a virgin negro over fourteen years of age.[4]

A particularly ominous feature of this overzealous sexuality, doctors argued, was the black males' desire for white women. "A perversion from which most races are exempt," wrote Dr. English, "prompts the negro's inclination towards white women, whereas other races incline towards females of their own."[5] Though English estimated the "gray matter of the negro brain" to be at least a thousand years behind that of the white races, his genital organs were overdeveloped. As Dr. William Lee Howard noted:

The attacks on defenseless white women are evidences of racial instincts that are about as amenable to ethical culture as is the inherent odor of the race. . . . When education will reduce the size of the negro's penis as well as bring about the sensitiveness of the terminal fibers which exist in the Caucasian, then will it also be able to prevent the African's birthright to sexual madness and excess.[6]

One southern medical journal proposed "Castration Instead of Lynching," as retribution for black sexual crimes. "An impressive trial by a ghost-like kuklux klan [sic] and a 'ghost' physician or surgeon to perform the operation would make it an event the 'patient' would never forget," noted the editorial.[7]

According to these physicians, lust and immorality, unstable families, and reversion to barbaric tendencies made blacks especially prone to venereal diseases. One doctor estimated that over 50 percent of all Negroes over the age of twenty-five were syphilitic.[8] Virtually free of disease as slaves, they were now overwhelmed by it, according to informed medical opinion. Moreover, doctors believed that treatment for venereal disease among blacks was impossible, particularly because

in its latent stage the symptoms of syphilis become quiescent. As Dr. Thomas W. Murrell wrote:

They come for treatment at the beginning and at the end. When there are visible manifestations or when they are harried by pain, they readily come, for as a race they are not averse to physic; but tell them not, though they look well and feel well, that they are still diseased. Here ignorance rates science a fool. . . .[9]

Even the best educated black, according to Murrell, could not be convinced to seek treatment for syphilis. Venereal disease, according to some doctors, threatened the future of the race. The medical profession attributed the low birth rate among blacks to the high prevalence of venereal disease which caused stillbirths and miscarriages. Moreover, the high rates of syphilis were thought to lead to increased insanity and crime. One doctor writing at the turn of the century estimated that the number of insane Negroes had increased thirteenfold since the end of the Civil War. Dr. Murrell's conclusion echoed the most informed anthropological and ethnological data:

So the scourge sweeps among them. Those that are treated are only half cured and the effort to assimilate a complex civilization driving their diseased minds until the results are criminal records. Perhaps here, in conjunction with tuberculosis, will be the end of the negro problem. Disease will accomplish what man cannot do.[10]

This particular configuration of ideas formed the core of medical opinion concerning blacks, sex, and disease in the early twentieth century. Doctors generally discounted socioeconomic explanations of the state of black health, arguing that better medical care could not alter the evolutionary scheme. These assumptions provide the backdrop for examining the Tuskegee Syphilis Study.

THE ORIGINS OF THE EXPERIMENT

In 1929, under a grant from the Julius Rosenwald Fund, the USPHS conducted studies in the rural South to determine the prevalence of syphilis among blacks and explore the possibilities for mass treatment. The USPHS found Macon County, Alabama, in which the town of Tuskegee is located, to have the highest syphilis rate of the six counties surveyed. The Rosenwald Study concluded that mass treatment could be successfully implemented among rural blacks.[11] Although it is doubtful that the necessary funds would have been allocated even in the best economic conditions, after the economy collapsed in 1929, the findings were ignored. It is, however, ironic that the Tuskegee Study came to be based on findings of the Rosenwald Study that demonstrated the possibilities of mass treatment.

Three years later, in 1932, Dr. Taliaferro Clark, Chief of the USPHS Venereal Disease Division and author of the Rosenwald Study report, decided that conditions in Macon County merited renewed attention. Clark believed the high prevalence of syphilis offered an "unusual opportunity" for observation. From its inception, the USPHS regarded the Tuskegee Study as a classic "study in nature,"* rather than an experiment.[12] As long as syphilis was so prevalent in Macon and most of the blacks went untreated throughout life, it seemed only natural to Clark that it would be valuable to observe the consequences. He described it as a "ready-made situation." Surgeon General H. S. Cumming wrote to R. R. Moton, Director of the Tuskegee Institute:

> The recent syphilis control demonstration carried out in Macon County, with the financial assistance of the Julius Rosenwald Fund, revealed the presence of an unusually high rate in this county and, what is more remarkable, the fact that 99 per cent of this group was entirely without previous treatment. This combination, together with the expected cooperation of your hospital, offers an unparalleled opportunity for carrying on this piece of scientific research which probably cannot be duplicated anywhere else in the world.

Although no formal protocol appears to have been written, several letters of Clark and

Cumming suggest what the USPHS hoped to find. Clark indicated that it would be important to see how disease affected the daily lives of the men:

> The results of these studies of case records suggest the desirability of making a further study of the effect of untreated syphilis on the human economy among people now living and engaged in their daily pursuits.

It also seems that the USPHS believed the experiment might demonstrate that antisyphilitic treatment was unnecessary. As Cumming noted: "It is expected the results of this study may have a marked bearing on the treatment, or conversely the non-necessity of treatment, of cases of latent syphilis."

The immediate source of Cumming's hypothesis appears to have been the famous Oslo Study of untreated syphilis. Between 1890 and 1910, Professor C. Boeck, the chief of the Oslo Venereal Clinic, withheld treatment from almost two thousand patients infected with syphilis. He was convinced that therapies then available, primarily mercurial ointment, were of no value. When arsenic therapy became widely available by 1910, after Paul Ehrlich's historic discovery of "606," the study was abandoned. E. Bruusgaard, Boeck's successor, conducted a follow-up study of 473 of the untreated patients from 1925 to 1927. He found that 27.9 percent of these patients had undergone a "spontaneous cure," and now manifested no symptoms of the disease. Moreover, he estimated that as many as 70 percent of all syphilitics went through life without inconvenience from the disease.[13] His study, however, clearly acknowledged the dangers of untreated syphilis for the remaining 30 percent.

Thus every major textbook of syphilis at the time of the Tuskegee Study's inception strongly advocated treating syphilis even in its latent stages, which follow the initial inflammatory reaction. In discussing the Oslo Study, Dr. J. E. Moore, one of the nation's leading venereologists wrote, "This summary of Bruusgaard's study is by no means intended to suggest that syphilis be allowed to pass untreated."[14] If a complete cure could not be effected, at least the most devastating effects of the disease could be avoided. Although the standard therapies of the time, arsenical compounds and bismuth injection, involved certain

---

*In 1865, Claude Bernard, the famous French physiologist, outlined the distinction between a "study in nature" and experimentation. A study in nature required simple observation, an essentially passive act, while experimentation demanded intervention which altered the original condition. The Tuskegee Study was thus clearly not a study in nature. The very act of diagnosis altered the original conditions. "It is on this very possibility of acting or not acting on a body," wrote Bernard, "that the distinction will exclusively rest between sciences called sciences of observation and sciences called experimental."

dangers because of their toxicity, the alternatives were much worse. As the Oslo Study had shown, untreated syphilis could lead to cardiovascular disease, insanity, and premature death.[15] Moore wrote in his 1933 textbook:

> Though it imposes a slight though measurable risk of its own, treatment markedly diminishes the risk from syphilis. In latent syphilis, as I shall show, the probability of progression, relapse, or death is reduced from a probable 25-30 percent without treatment to about 5 percent with it; and the gravity of the relapse if it occurs, is markedly diminished.[16]

"Another compelling reason for treatment," noted Moore, "exists in the fact that every patient with latent syphilis may be, and perhaps is, infectious for others."[17] In 1932, the year in which the Tuskegee Study began, the USPHS sponsored and published a paper by Moore and six other syphilis experts that strongly argued for treating latent syphilis.

The Oslo Study, therefore, could not have provided justification for the USPHS to undertake a study that did not entail treatment. Rather, the suppositions that conditions in Tuskegee existed "naturally" and that the men would not be treated anyway provided the experiment's rationale. In turn, these two assumptions rested on the prevailing medical attitudes concerning blacks, sex, and disease. For example, Clark explained the prevalence of venereal disease in Macon County by emphasizing promiscuity among blacks:

> This state of affairs is due to the paucity of doctors, rather low intelligence of the Negro population in this section, depressed economic conditions, and the very common promiscuous sex relations of this population group which not only contribute to the spread of syphilis but also contribute to the prevailing indifference with regard to treatment.

In fact, Moore, who had written so persuasively in favor of treating latent syphilis, suggested that existing knowledge did not apply to Negroes. Although he had called the Oslo Study "a never-to-be-repeated human experiment," he served as an expert consultant to the Tuskegee Study:

> I think that such a study as you have contemplated would be of immense value. It will be necessary of course in the consideration of the results to evaluate the special factors introduced by a selection of the material from negro males. Syphilis in the negro is in many respects almost a different disease from syphilis in the white.

Dr. O. C. Wenger, chief of the federally operated venereal disease clinic at Hot Springs, Arkansas, praised Moore's judgment, adding, "This study will emphasize those differences." On another occasion he advised Clark, "We must remember we are dealing with a group of people who are illiterate, have no conception of time, and whose personal history is always indefinite."

The doctors who devised and directed the Tuskegee Study accepted the mainstream assumptions regarding blacks and venereal disease. The premise that blacks, promiscuous and lustful, would not seek or continue treatment, shaped the study. A test of untreated syphilis seemed "natural" because the USPHS presumed the men would never be treated; the Tuskegee Study made that a self-fulfilling prophecy.

SELECTING THE SUBJECTS

Clark sent Dr. Raymond Vonderlehr to Tuskegee in September 1932 to assemble a sample of men with latent syphilis for the experiment. The basic design of the study called for the selection of syphilitic black males between the ages of twenty-five and sixty, a thorough physical examination including x-rays, and finally, a spinal tap to determine the incidence of neuro-syphilis. They had no intention of providing any treatment for the infected men.[18] The USPHS originally scheduled the whole experiment to last six months; it seemed to be both a simple and inexpensive project.

The task of collecting the sample, however, proved to be more difficult than the USPHS had supposed. Vonderlehr canvassed the largely illiterate, poverty-stricken population of sharecroppers and tenant farmers in search of test subjects. If his circulars requested only men over twenty-five to attend his clinics, none would appear, suspecting he was conducting draft physicals. Therefore, he was forced to test large numbers of women and men who did not fit the experiment's specifications. This involved considerable expense since the USPHS had promised the Macon County Board of Health that it would treat those who were infected, but not included in the study. Clark wrote to

Vonderlehr about the situation: "It never once occured to me that we would be called upon to treat a large part of the county as return for the privilege of making this study. . . . I am anxious to keep the expenditures for treatment down to the lowest possible point because it is the one item of expenditure in connection with the study most difficult to defend despite our knowledge of the need therefor." Vonderlehr responded: "If we could find from 100 to 200 cases . . . we would not have to do another Wassermann on useless individuals . . ."

Significantly, the attempt to develop the sample contradicted the prediction the USPHS had made initially regarding the prevalence of the disease in Macon County. Overall rates of syphilis fell well below expectations; as opposed to the USPHS projection of 35 percent, 20 percent of those tested were actually diseased. Moreover, those who had sought and received previous treatment far exceeded the expectations of the USPHS. Clark noted in a letter to Vonderlehr:

I find your report of March 6th quite interesting but regret the necessity of Wassermanning [sic] . . . such a large number of individuals in order to uncover this relatively limited number of untreated cases.

Further difficulties arose in enlisting the subjects to participate in the experiment, to be "Wassermanned," and to return for a subsequent series of examinations. Vonderlehr found that only the offer of treatment elicited the cooperation of the men. They were told they were ill and were promised free care. Offered therapy, they became willing subjects.[19] The USPHS did not tell the men that they were participants in an experiment; on the contrary, the subjects believed they were being treated for "bad blood"—the rural South's colloquialism for syphilis. They thought they were participating in a public health demonstration similar to the one that had been conducted by the Julius Rosenwald Fund in Tuskegee several years earlier. In the end, the men were so eager for medical care that the number of defaulters in the experiment proved to be insignificant.

To preserve the subjects' interest, Vonderlehr gave most of the men mercurial ointment, a noneffective drug, while some of the younger men apparently received inadequate dosages of neoarsphenamine. This required Vonderlehr to write

frequently to Clark requesting supplies. He feared the experiment would fail if the men were not offered treatment.

It is desirable and essential if the study is to be a success to maintain the interest of each of the cases examined by me through to the time when the spinal puncture can be completed. Expenditure of several hundred dollars for drugs for these men would be well worth while if their interest and cooperation would be maintained in so doing. . . . It is my desire to keep the main purpose of the work from the negroes in the county and continue their interest in treatment. That is what the vast majority wants and the examination seems relatively unimportant to them in comparison. It would probably cause the entire experiment to collapse if the clinics were stopped before the work is completed.

On another occasion he explained:

Dozens of patients have been sent away without treatment during the past two weeks and it would have been impossible to continue without the free distribution of drugs because of the unfavorable impression made on the negro.

The readiness of the test subjects to participate of course contradicted the notion that blacks would not seek or continue therapy.

The final procedure of the experiment was to be a spinal tap to test for neuro-syphilis. The USPHS presented this purely diagnostic exam, which often entails considerable pain and complications, to the men as a "special treatment." Clark explained to Moore:

We have not yet commenced the spinal punctures. This operation will be deferred to the last in order not to unduly disturb our field work by any adverse reports by the patients subjected to spinal puncture because of some disagreeable sensations following this procedure. These negroes are very ignorant and easily influenced by things that would be of minor significance in a more intelligent group.

The letter to the subjects announcing the spinal tap read:

Some time ago you were given a thorough examination and since that time we hope you have gotten a great deal of treatment for bad blood. You will now be given your last chance to get a second examination. This examination is a very special one and after it is finished you will be given a special treatment if it is believed you are in a condition to stand it. . . .

REMEMBER THIS IS YOUR LAST CHANCE FOR SPECIAL FREE TREATMENT. BE SURE TO MEET THE NURSE.[20]

The HEW investigation did not uncover this crucial fact: the men participated in the study under the guise of treatment.

Despite the fact that their assumption regarding prevalence and black attitudes toward treatment had proved wrong, the USPHS decided in the summer of 1933 to continue the study. Once again, it seemed only "natural" to pursue the research since the sample already existed, and with a depressed economy, the cost of treatment appeared prohibitive—although there is no indication it was ever considered. Vonderlehr first suggested extending the study in letters to Clark and Wenger:

At the end of this project we shall have a considerable number of cases presenting various complications of syphilis, who have received only mercury and may still be considered untreated in the modern sense of therapy. Should these cases be followed over a period of from five to ten years many interesting facts could be learned regarding the course and complications of untreated syphilis.

"As I see it," responded Wenger, "we have no further interest in these patients *until they die.*" Apparently, the physicians engaged in the experiment believed that only autopsies could scientifically confirm the findings of the study. Surgeon General Cumming explained this in a letter to R. R. Moton, requesting the continued cooperation of the Tuskegee Institute Hospital:

This study which was predominantly clinical in character points to the frequent occurrence of severe complications involving the various vital organs of the body and indicates that syphilis as a disease does a great deal of damage. Since clinical observations are not considered final in the medical world, it is our desire to continue observation on the cases selected for the recent study and if possible to bring a percentage of these cases to autopsy so that pathological confirmation may be made of the disease processes.

Bringing the men to autopsy required the USPHS to devise a further series of deceptions and inducements. Wenger warned Vonderlehr that the men must not realize that they would be autopsied:

There is one danger in the latter plan and that is if the colored population become aware that accepting free hospital care means a post-mortem, every darkey will leave Macon County and it will hurt [Dr. Eugene] Dibble's hospital.

"Naturally," responded Vonderlehr, "it is not my intention to let it be generally known that the main object of the present activities is the bringing of the men to necropsy." The subjects' trust in the USPHS made the plan viable. The USPHS gave Dr. Dibble, the Director of the Tuskegee Institute Hospital, an interim appointment to the Public Health Service. As Wenger noted:

One thing is certain. The only way we are going to get post-mortems is to have the demise take place in Dibble's hospital and when these colored folks are told that Doctor Dibble is now a Government doctor too they will have more confidence.*

After the USPHS approved the continuation of the experiment in 1933, Vonderlehr decided that it would be necessary to select a group of healthy, uninfected men to serve as controls. Vonderlehr, who had succeeded Clark as Chief of the Venereal Disease Division, sent Dr. J. R. Heller to Tuskegee to gather the control group. Heller distributed

---

*The degree of black cooperation in conducting the study remains unclear and would be impossible to properly assess in an article of this length. It seems certain that some members of the Tuskegee Institute staff such as R. R. Moton and Eugene Dibble understood the nature of the experiment and gave their support to it. There is, however, evidence that some blacks who assisted the USPHS physicians were not aware of the deceptive nature of the experiment. Dr. Joshua Williams, an intern at the John A. Andrew Memorial Hospital (Tuskegee Institute) in 1932, assisted Vonderlehr in taking blood samples of the test subjects. In 1973 he told the HEW panel: "I know we thought it was merely a service group organized to help the people in the area. We didn't know it was a research project at all at the time." (See, "Transcript of Proceedings," Tuskegee Syphilis Study Ad Hoc Advisory Panel, February 23, 1973, Unpublished typescript. National Library of Medicine, Bethesda, Maryland.) It is also apparent that Eunice Rivers, the black nurse who had primary responsibility for maintaining contact with the men over the forty years, did not fully understand the dangers of the experiment. In any event, black involvement in the study in no way mitigates the racial assumptions of the experiment, but rather, demonstrates their power.

drugs (noneffective) to these men, which suggests that they also believed they were undergoing treatment. Control subjects who became syphilitic were simply transferred to the test group—a strikingly inept violation of standard research procedure.[21]

The USPHS offered several inducements to maintain contact and to procure the continued co-operation of the men. Eunice Rivers, a black nurse, was hired to follow their health and to secure approval for autopsies. She gave the men noneffective medicines—"spring tonic" and aspirin—as well as transportation and hot meals on the days of their examinations.[22] More important, Nurse Rivers provided continuity to the project over the entire forty-year period. By supplying "medicinals," the USPHS was able to continue to deceive the participants, who believed that they were receiving therapy from the government doctors. Deceit was integral to the study. When the test subjects complained about spinal taps one doctor wrote:

> They simply do not like spinal punctures. A few of those who were tapped are enthusiastic over the results but to most, the suggestion causes violent shaking of the head; others claim they were robbed of their procreative powers (regardless of the fact that I claim it stimulates them).

Letters to the subjects announcing an impending USPHS visit to Tuskegee explained: "[The doctor] wants to make a special examination to find out how you have been feeling and whether the treatment has improved your health." In fact, after the first six months of the study, the USPHS had furnished no treatment whatsoever.

Finally, because it proved difficult to persuade the men to come to the hospital when they became severely ill, the USPHS promised to cover their burial expenses. The Milbank Memorial Fund provided approximately $50 per man for this purpose beginning in 1935. This was a particularly strong inducement as funeral rites constituted an important component of the cultural life of rural blacks. One report of the study concluded, "Without this suasion it would, we believe, have been impossible to secure the cooperation of the group and their families."

Reports of the study's findings, which appeared regularly in the medical press beginning in 1936, consistently cited the ravages of untreated syphilis. The first paper, read at the 1936 American Medical Association annual meeting, found "that syphilis in this period [latency] tends to greatly increase the frequency of manifestations of cardiovascular disease." Only 16 percent of the subjects gave no sign of morbidity as opposed to 61 percent of the controls. Ten years later, a report noted coldly, "The fact that nearly twice as large a proportion of the syphilitic individuals as of the control group has died is a very striking one." Life expectancy, concluded the doctors, is reduced by about 20 percent.

A 1955 article found that slightly more than 30 percent of the test group autopsied had died *directly* from advanced syphilitic lesions of either the cardiovascular or the central nervous system.[23] Another published account stated, "Review of those still living reveals that an appreciable number have late complications of syphilis which probably will result, for some at least, in contributing materially to the ultimate cause of death."[24] In 1950, Dr. Wenger had concluded, "We now know, where we could only surmise before, that we have contributed to their ailments and shortened their lives." As black physician Vernal Cave, a member of the HEW panel, later wrote, "They proved a point, then proved a point, then proved a point."

During the forty years of the experiment the USPHS had sought on several occasions to ensure that the subjects did not receive treatment from other sources. To this end, Vonderlehr met with groups of local black doctors in 1934, to ask their cooperation in not treating the men. Lists of subjects were distributed to Macon County physicians along with letters requesting them to refer these men back to the USPHS if they sought care. The USPHS warned the Alabama Health Department not to treat the test subjects when they took a mobile VD unit into Tuskegee in the early 1940s. In 1941, the Army drafted several subjects and told them to begin antisyphilitic treatment immediately. The USPHS supplied the draft board with a list of 256 names they desired to have excluded from treatment, and the board complied.

In spite of these efforts, by the early 1950s many of the men had secured some treatment on their own. By 1952, almost 30 percent of the test subjects had received some penicillin, although only 7.5 percent had received what could be considered adequate doses.[25] Vonderlehr wrote to one of the participating physicians, "I hope that the availability of antibiotics has not interfered too much with this project." A report published in 1955 considered whether the treatment that some of the men had obtained had "defeated" the study. The article attempted to explain the relatively low exposure to penicillin in an age of antibiotics, suggesting as a reason: "the stoicism of these men as a group; they still regard hospitals and medicines with suspicion and prefer an occasional dose of time-honored herbs or tonics to modern drugs." The authors failed to note that the men believed they were already under the care of the government doctors and thus saw no need to seek treatment elsewhere. Any treatment which the men might have received, concluded the report, had been insufficient to compromise the experiment.

When the USPHS evaluated the status of the study in the 1960s they continued to rationalize the racial aspects of the experiment. For example, the minutes of a 1965 meeting at the Center for Disease Control recorded:

> Racial issue was mentioned briefly. Will not affect the study. Any questions can be handled by saying these people were at the point that therapy would no longer help them. They are getting better medical care than they would under any other circumstances.

A group of physicians met again at the CDC in 1969 to decide whether or not to terminate the study. Although one doctor argued that the study should be stopped and the men treated, the consensus was to continue. Dr. J. Lawton Smith remarked, "You will never have another study like this; take advantage of it." A memo prepared by Dr. James B. Lucas, Assistant Chief of the Venereal Disease Branch, stated: "Nothing learned will prevent, find, or cure a single case of infectious syphilis or bring us closer to our basic mission of controlling venereal disease in the United States." He concluded, however, that the study should be continued "along its present lines." When the first accounts of the experiment appeared in the national press in July 1972, data were still being collected and autopsies performed.

THE HEW FINAL REPORT

HEW finally formed the Tuskegee Syphilis Study Ad Hoc Advisory Panel on August 28, 1972, in response to criticism that the press descriptions of the experiment had triggered. The panel, composed of nine members, five of them black, concentrated on two issues. First, was the study justified in 1932 and had the men given their informed consent? Second, should penicillin have been provided when it became available in the early 1950s? The panel was also charged with determining if the study should be terminated and assessing current policies regarding experimentation with human subjects. The group issued their report in June 1973.

FROM THE HEW FINAL REPORT (1973)

1. In retrospect, the Public Health Service Study of Untreated Syphilis in the Male Negro in Macon County, Alabama, was ethically unjustified in 1932. The judgement made in 1973 about the conduct of the study in 1932 is made with the advantage of hindsight acutely sharpened over some forty years, concerning an activity in a different age with different social standards. Nevertheless, one fundamental ethical rule is that a person should not be subjected to avoidable risk of death or physical harm unless he freely and intelligently consents. There is no evidence that such consent was obtained from the participants in this study.

2. Because of the paucity of information available today on the manner in which the study was conceived, designed and sustained, a scientific justification for a short term demonstration study cannot be ruled out. However, the conduct of the longitudinal study as initially reported in 1936 and through the years is judged to be scientifically unsound and its results are disproportionately meager compared with known risk to human subjects involved. . . .

By focusing on the issues of penicillin therapy and informed consent, the *Final Report* and the investigation betrayed a basic misunderstanding of the experiment's purposes and design. The HEW report implied that the failure to provide penicillin constituted the study's major ethical misjudgment; implicit was the assumption that no adequate therapy existed prior to penicillin. Nonetheless medical authorities firmly believed in the efficacy of arsenotherapy for treating syphilis at the time of the experiment's inception in 1932. The panel further failed to recognize that the entire study had been predicated on nontreatment. Provision of effective medication would have violated the rationale of the experiment—to study the natural course of the disease until death. On several occasions, in fact, the USPHS had prevented the men from receiving proper treatment. Indeed, there is no evidence that the USPHS ever considered providing penicillin.

The other focus of the *Final Report*—informed consent—also served to obscure the historical facts of the experiment. In light of the deceptions and exploitations which the experiment perpetrated, it is an understatement to declare, as the *Report* did, that the experiment was "ethically unjustified," because it failed to obtain informed consent from the subjects. The *Final Report's* statement, "Submitting voluntarily is not informed consent," indicated that the panel believed that the men had volunteered *for the experiment*.[26] The records in the National Archives make clear that the men did not submit voluntarily to an experiment; they were told and they believed that they were getting free treatment from expert government doctors for a serious disease. The failure of the HEW *Final Report* to expose this critical fact—that the USPHS lied to the subjects—calls into question the thoroughness and credibility of their investigation.

Failure to place the study in a historical context also made it impossible for the investigation to deal with the essentially racist nature of the experiment. The panel treated the study as an aberration, well-intentioned but misguided.[27] Moreover, concern that the *Final Report* might be viewed as a critique of human experimentation in general seems to have severely limited the scope of the inquiry. The *Final Report* is quick to remind the reader on two occasions: "The position of the Panel must not be construed to be a general repudiation of scientific research with human subjects."[28] The *Report* assures us that a better designed experiment could have been justified:

> It is possible that a scientific study in 1932 of untreated syphilis, properly conceived with a clear protocol and conducted with suitable subjects who fully understood the implications of their involvement, might have been justified in the prepenicillin era. This is especially true when one considers the uncertain nature of the results of treatment of late latent syphilis and the highly toxic nature of therapeutic agents then available.[29]

This statement is questionable in view of the proven dangers of untreated syphilis known in 1932.

Since the publication of the HEW *Final Report*, a defense of the Tuskegee Study has emerged. These arguments, most clearly articulated by Dr. R. H. Kampmeier in the *Southern Medical Journal*, center on the limited knowledge of effective therapy for latent syphilis when the experiment began. Kampmeier argues that by 1950, penicillin would have been of no value for these men.[30] Others have suggested that the men were fortunate to have been spared the highly toxic treatments of the earlier period. Moreover, even these contemporary defenses assume that the men never would have been treated anyway. As Dr. Charles Barnett of Stanford University wrote in 1974, "The lack of treatment was not contrived by the USPHS but was an established fact of which they proposed to take advantage."[31] Several doctors who participated in the study continued to justify the experiment. Dr. J. R. Heller, who on one occasion had referred to the test subjects as the "Ethiopian population," told reporters in 1972:

> I don't see why they should be shocked or horrified. There was no racial side to this. It just happened to be in a black community. I feel this was a perfectly straightforward study, perfectly ethical, with controls. Part of our mission as physicians is to find out what happens to individuals with disease and without disease.[32]

These apologies, as well as the HEW *Final Report*, ignore many of the essential ethical issues which the study poses. The Tuskegee Study reveals the persistence of beliefs within the medical profession about the nature of blacks, sex, and disease—beliefs that had tragic repercussions long after their alleged "scientific" bases were known to be incorrect. Most strikingly, the entire health of a community was jeopardized by leaving a communicable disease untreated.[33] There can be little doubt that the Tuskegee researchers regarded their subjects as less than human.[34] As a result, the ethical canons of experimenting on human subjects were completely disregarded.

The study also raises significant questions about professional self-regulation and scientific bureaucracy. Once the USPHS decided to extend the experiment in the summer of 1933, it was unlikely that the test would be halted short of the men's deaths. The experiment was widely reported for forty years without evoking any significant protest within the medical community. Nor did any bureaucratic mechanism exist within the government for the periodic reassessment of the Tuskegee experiment's ethics and scientific value. The USPHS sent physicians to Tuskegee every several years to check on the study's progress, but never subjected the morality or usefulness of the experiment to serious scrutiny. Only the press accounts of 1972 finally punctured the continued rationalizations of the USPHS and brought the study to an end. Even the HEW investigation was compromised by fear that it would be considered a threat to future human experimentation.

In retrospect the Tuskegee Study revealed more about the pathology of racism than it did about the pathology of syphilis; more about the nature of scientific inquiry than the nature of the disease process. The injustice committed by the experiment went well beyond the facts outlined in the press and the HEW *Final Report*. The degree of deception and damages have been seriously underestimated. As this history of the study suggests, the notion that science is a value-free discipline must be rejected. The need for greater vigilance in assessing the specific ways in which social values and attitudes affect professional behavior is clearly indicated.

NOTES

1. The best general account of the study is James Jones, *Bad Blood*, 2nd ed. (New York: The Free Press, 1993).

2. *Final Report* of the Tuskegee Syphilis Study Ad Hoc Advisory Panel, Department of Health, Education, and Welfare (Washington, D.C.: GPO, 1973). (Hereafter, HEW *Final Report*).

3. W. T. English, "The Negro Problem from the Physician's Point of View," *Atlanta Journal-Record of Medicine* 5 (October 1903), 461.

4. Daniel David Quillian. "Racial Peculiarities: A Cause of the Prevalence of Syphilis in Negroes," *American Journal of Dermatology and Genito-Urinary Diseases* 10 (July 1906), p. 277.

5. English, p. 463.

6. William Lee Howard. "The Negro as a Distinct Ethnic Factor in Civilization," *Medicine* (Detroit) 9 (June 1903), 424.

7. "Castration Instead of Lynching," *Atlanta Journal-Record of Medicine* 8 (October 1906), 457.

8. Searle Harris, "The Future of the Negro from the Standpoint of the Southern Physician." *Alabama Medical Journal* 14 (January 1902), 62.

9. Thomas W. Murrell, "Syphilis in the Negro: Its Bearing on the Race Problem," *American Journal of Dermatology and Genito-Urinary Diseases* 10 (August 1906), 307.

10. Murrell, "Syphilis in the Negro; Its Bearing on the Race Problem," p. 307

11. Taliaferro Clark, *The Control of Syphilis in Southern Rural Areas* (Chicago: Julius Rosenwald Fund, 1932), 53-58. Approximately 35 percent of the inhabitants of Macon County who were examined were found to be syphilitic.

12. See Claude Bernard, *An Introduction to the Study of Experimental Medicine* (New York: Dover, 1865, 1957), pp. 5-26.

13. The best discussion of the Boeck-Bruusgaard data is E. Gurney Clark and Niels Danbolt, "The Oslo Study of the Natural History of Untreated Syphilis," *Journal of Chronic Diseases* 2 (September 1955), 311-44.

14. Joseph Earl Moore, *The Modern Treatment of Syphilis* (Baltimore: Charles C. Thomas, 1933), p. 24.

15. Moore, pp. 231-47.

16. Moore, p. 237.

17. Moore, p. 236.

18. As Clark wrote: "You will observe that our plan has nothing to do with treatment. It is purely a diagnostic procedure carried out to determine what has happened to the syphilitic Negro who has had no treatment." Clark to Paul A. O'Leary, September 27, 1932, NA-WNRC.

19. Vonderlehr later explained: The reason treatment was given to many of these men was twofold: First, when the study was started in the fall of 1932, no plans had been made for its continuation and a few of the patients were treated before we fully realized the need for continuing the project on a permanent basis. Second it was difficult to hold the interest of the group of Negroes in Macon County unless some treatment was given." Vonderlehr to Austin V. Diebert, December 5, 1938, Tuskegee Syphilis Study Ad Hoc Advisory Panel Papers, Box 1, National Library of Medicine, Bethesda, Maryland (Hereafter, TSS-NLM). This collection contains the materials assembled by the HEW investigation in 1972.

20. Macon County Health Department, "Letter to Subjects," n.d., NA-WNRC.

21. Austin V. Diebert and Martha C. Bruyere, "Untreated Syphilis in the Male Negro, III." *Venereal Disease Information* 27 (December 1946), 301-14.

22. Eunice Rivers, Stanley Schuman, Lloyd Simpson, Sidney Olansky, "Twenty-Years of Followup Experience In a Long-Range Medical Study," *Public Health Reports* 68 (April 1953), 391-95. In this article Nurse Rivers explains her role in the experiment. She

wrote: "Because of the low educational status of the majority of the patients, it was impossible to appeal to them from a purely scientific approach. Therefore, various methods were used to maintain their interest. Free medicines, burial assistance or insurance (the project being referred to as 'Miss Rivers' Lodge'), free hot meals on the days of examination, transportation to and from the hospital, and an opportunity to stop in town on the return trip to shop or visit with friends on the streets all helped. In spite of these attractions, there were some who refused their examinations because they were not sick and did not see that they were being benefitted." (p. 393).

23. Jesse J. Peters, James H. Peers, Sidney Olansky, John C. Cutler, and Geraldine Gleeson, "Untreated Syphilis in the Male Negro: Pathologic Findings in Syphilitic and Non-Syphilitic Patients," *Journal of Chronic Diseases* 1 (February 1955), 127-48.

24. Sidney Olansky, Stanley H. Schuman, Jesse J. Peters, C. A. Smith, and Dorothy S. Rambo, "Untreated Syphilis in the Male Negro, X. Twenty Years of Clinical Observation of Untreated Syphilitic and Presumably Nonsyphilitic Groups," *Journal of Chronic Diseases* 4 (August 1956), 184.

25. Stanley H. Schuman, Sidney Olansky, Eunice Rivers, C. A. Smith, and Dorothy S. Rambo, "Untreated Syphilis in the Male Negro: Background and Current Status of Patients in the Tuskegee Study," *Journal of Chronic Diseases* 2 (November 1955), 550-53.

26. HEW *Final Report*, p. 7.

27. The notable exception is Jay Katz's eloquent "Reservations About the Panel Report on Charge 1," HEW *Final Report*, pp. 14-15.

28. HEW *Final Report*, pp. 8, 12.

29. HEW *Final Report*, pp. 8, 12.

30. See R. H. Kampmeier, "The Tuskegee Study of Untreated Syphilis," *Southern Medical Journal* 65 (October 1972), 1247-51; and "'Final Report on the 'Tuskegee Syphilis Study,'" *Southern Medical Journal* 67 (November 1974), 1349-53.

31. Quoted in "Debate Revives on the PHS Study," *Medical World News* (April 19, 1974), p. 37.

32. Heller to Vonderlehr, November 28, 1933, quoted in *Medical Tribune* (August 23, 1972), p. 14.

33. Although it is now known that syphilis is rarely infectious after its early phase, at the time of the study's inception latent syphilis was thought to be communicable. The fact that members of the control group were placed in the test group when they became syphilitic proves that at least some infectious men were denied treatment.

34. When the subjects are drawn from minority groups, especially those with which the researcher cannot identify, basic human rights may be compromised. Hans Jonas has clearly explicated the problem in his "Philosophical Reflections on Experimentation," *Daedalus* 98 (Spring 1969), 234-37. As Jonas writes: "If the properties we adduced as the particular qualifications of the members of the scientific fraternity itself are taken as general criteria of selection, then one should look for additional subjects where a maximum of identification, understanding, and spontaneity can be expected—that is, among the most highly motivated, the most highly educated, and the least 'captive' members of the community."

Opening Comments on the Changing Mores of Biomedical Research

Walsh McDermott

When the needs of society come in head-on conflict with the rights of an individual, someone has to play God. We can avoid this responsibility so long as the power to decide the particular case-in-point

Annals of Internal Medicine 1967; 67 (sup 7), 39–42. Used with permission from the American College of Physicians.

is clearly vested in someone else, for example, a duly elected governmental official. But in clinical investigation, the power to determine this issue of "the individual versus society" is clearly vested in the physician. Both the power itself and, above all, *our awareness that we are wielding it* are increasing every day and can be expected to increase much further. It is this inescapable *awareness* that we are wielding power that has us so deeply troubled, for we are a generation nurtured on the slogan "the end does not justify the means" in matters concerning the individual and his society. Yet as a society we enforce the social good over the individual good across a whole spectrum of nonmedical activities every day, and many of these activities ultimately affect the health or the life of an individual.

Traditionally in our Judeo-Christian culture we have handled this issue by one of two mechanisms. When, as in our racial problem for example, the conflict contains no built-in contradiction, we publicly and officially subscribe to a set of ideals. We can work privately and publicly toward the attainment of these ideals, and with their attainment would come the solution of the problem. This mechanism works when the forces in conflict are intrinsically reconcilable even though the reconciliation might take many decades or a century. But we use another mechanism when the conflict is head on, when the group interest and the individual interest are basically irreconcilable.

In circumstances like these, such as the decision to impose capital punishment or the selection of only a minority of our young men to become soldiers, the issue is decided by a judgment that is arbitrary as it affects the individual. In short, we play God. When we take away an individual's life or liberty by one of these arbitrary judgments we try to depersonalize the process by spreading responsibility for the decision throughout a framework of legal institutions. Thus, it is usually a jury, not a judge, that determines the death penalty: a local draft board, not a bureaucrat, that decides who goes to Vietnam. This second type of mechanism works only because there is widespread public acceptance that society has rights too, and that it is preferable that the power to enforce these rights over the rights of the individual be institutionalized.

I submit that the core of this ethical issue as it arises in clinical investigation lies in this second category—the one wherein, to ensure the rights of society, an arbitrary judgment must be made against an individual.

This is not to say that all ethical problems in clinical investigation fall into the irreconcilable category. On the contrary, in numerical terms most of them probably do not.

Without question, a considerable portion of the lapses in fully protecting individual rights in clinical investigation can be avoided by more careful and open attention to the subject and by our ingenuity in developing new practices to attain some of the same old ends. This will prove quite costly in financial terms, but what is being accomplished in this way is very much to the good and is to be strongly encouraged. But there remains that hard core of the problem: the kind of situation in which it clearly seems to be in the best interests of society that the information be obtained. It can be obtained only from studies on certain already unlucky individuals, and no convincing case can be made that they can expect much in the way of benefits except those accruing to them as members of society.

Clearly there are three questions here: (1) From where does society get its right or interest that makes it imperative to perform biomedical studies on an individual? (2) how is the individual subject selected? and (3) how are the social priorities decided?

The social priorities are easy; any small group of certified medical statesmen can settle them in one afternoon. As we all know, however, it is the other two questions that are so thorny.

Without too deep reflection it seems to me that society's actually having a right here is a relatively new phenomenon that is chiefly derived from the demonstration that knowledge gained by studies in a few humans can show us how to operate programs of great practical benefit to the group. Until the late nineteenth century, as I understand it, most human experimentation expanded knowledge but did not increase the power to control disease. The physicians of that day thus had no problem in maintaining the double ethical charge still preserved in the Helsinki Declaration: to "safeguard the health of the people," on the one hand, and to make the health of "my patient" the first consideration, on the other hand. But starting, I suppose, with the yellow fever studies in Havana, we have seen large social payoffs from certain experiments in humans, and there is no reason to doubt that the process could continue. It is by this demonstration, analogous to the great "invention of invention" of Newton's era, that medicine has given to society the case for its rights in the continuation of clinical investigation. Once this demonstration was made, we could no longer maintain, in strict honesty, that in the study of disease the interests of the individual are invariably paramount.

Yet we are temperamentally incapable of leaving it at that. Our reflex action here is to try to imitate what we do when the same conflict arises in irreconcilable form elsewhere in our society. That is to say, we are willing to concede that some judgments must be arbitrary, but we attempt to clothe them with institutional forms so that at least the judgments are not made solely by one person. We will play God, but we would like to do it by group effort.

I am deeply convinced that such efforts provide no real solution because our culture has not yet faced up to the irreconcilable nature of the conflict at the heart of this particular issue. And until it does so, there exists no recognized consensus or article in the "social contract," if you will, to provide that base on which any law or regulation must rest if it is to be viable.

Conventional juridical procedures including the traditional jury system are too slow to fit the urgent nature of many clinical decisions. [B]y the terms of our culture, as may be seen in the Declaration of Helsinki, no matter who the investigator takes into partnership when he acts, he acts alone.

What can we do to solve this agonizing dilemma? Obviously we cannot convene a constitutional convention of the Judeo-Christian culture and add a few amendments to it. Yet, in a figurative sense, until we can do something very much like that, I believe deeply that the problem, at its roots, is unsolvable and that we must continue to live with it.

To be sure, by careful attention we can cut down the number of instances in which the problem presents itself to us in its starkest form. But there is no escape from the fact that, if the future good of society is to be served, there will be times when the clinical investigator must make an arbitrary judgment with respect to an individual. The necessity for such arbitrary judgments has had *tacit* social recognition and approval for some time. Because the approval *was* tacit, however, there was an imbalance of actions and words, in effect, a hypocrisy, that marvelous human invention by which we are enabled to adapt to problems judged to be not yet ripe for solution. By this hypocrisy

society had its future medical interests fully protected. At the same time the attitude could be maintained that in medical matters, *as contrasted with those in many other walks of life*, the sole public interest was in the inviolability of the individual.

Now, most unfortunately, these essentially harmless hypocrisies of our culture have been codified. For the Helsinki Declaration . . . if . . . followed to the letter . . . would produce the curious situation in which the only stated public interest is that of the individual. The future interest of society and its sometime conflict with the interest of the individual, in effect, are ignored. I believe it has been most unwise to try to extend the principle of "a government of laws and not men" into areas of such great ethical subtlety as clinical investigation.

When in our cultural evolution it has not yet been possible to develop an institutional framework for a particular kind of arbitrary decision that may affect an individual, there is only one basis on which to proceed, and that is on the basis of trust. My position may sound paternalistic, as indeed it is. Making arbitrary decisions concerning an individual in conflicts as yet unsolved by our society is one of the major responsibilities of a parent.

Society may not have given us a clear blueprint for clinical investigation, but it has long since given us immense trust to handle moral dilemmas of other sorts, including many in which, in effect, we have to play God. Thus, the moral dilemma of clinical investigation is not something new; what is new about the problem is its rapid increase in size. This rapid increase in size is no help to us now, but it may hasten the day, still far off, when in medical investigations we can institutionalize this making of arbitrary decisions between an individual and his society.

In the meantime we can do no more than carry on under the mantle of the trust we now possess. To continue to receive that trust we must be ever conscious that the issue of the individual vis-à-vis society is always *there*, and we can try our best to create an environment of awareness of it on our clinical services. For once a moral dilemma has become clearly recognized; whenever each person acts within that dilemma, his act can be seen for what it is, and the extent to which he has seemed to act with acceptable propriety can be judged.

But the hard core of our moral dilemma will not yield to the approaches of "Declarations" or

"Regulations"; for as things stand today such statements must completely ignore the fact that society, too, has rights in human experimentation. Somehow, somewhere, in this question of human experimentation, as in so many other aspects of our society, we will have to learn how to institutionalize "playing God" while still maintaining the key elements of a free society.

Informed Consent to Experimentation

Alan Donagan

Therapeutic medicine is inescapably experimental; for, since no two patients are medically identical, even in a case in which prognosis after treatment is regarded as unproblematic, every physician ought to be alert should *this* one, after all, turn out to be exceptional. However, even when, with his informed consent, a highly risky treatment is administered to a patient, in therapeutic experimentation the end that determines whether or not that treatment is administered is the patient's good. That, incidentally, it may advance medical science, and so presumably benefit many human beings in the future, is a secondary and nondetermining consideration.

Medical science advanced rapidly in the past century because the haphazard experimentation inseparable from any intelligently administered medical treatment was supplemented by systematic experimentation, more or less well designed. Some of it was abhorrent. For example, valuable results on the transmission of venereal diseases were obtained by methods differing from the abominations punished at Nuremberg only in scale and in that the wretched subjects were procured by deceit rather than by force. But such cases were a minority. The great nineteenth-century authority, Claude Bernard, both preached and practiced, as "the principle of medical moral-ity," that one is "never to carry out on a human being an experiment that cannot but be injurious to him in some degree, even if the outcome could be of great interest to science, that is to say, the health of other human beings." However, in Walter Reed's classic experimental investigation at Havana in 1900 of how yellow fever is transmitted, and in subsequent experiments by Richard P. Strong in the Philippines on plague and beriberi, it was held permissible to carry out procedures that could be nothing but harmful, provided that the subjects were volunteers. In these experiments there was no question of carrying out any procedure known to be gravely harmful or lethal; but procedures were permitted that could not but be harmful to some degree, and that could have been gravely harmful or lethal, and sometimes were.

In this paper, it is assumed that a human being is entitled to volunteer the use of his body for at least some risky experiments. . . . Hence it will also be assumed that the genuine consent of human subjects to risky experiments for which they are entitled to volunteer is a sufficient condition of the moral permissibility of those experiments. But whether it is also a necessary condition has been questioned, in view of the magnitude of the benefits to mankind at large of the experiments of Reed, Strong, and others. Is it wrong to sacrifice the health of a few, or even their lives, for the sake of the lives and health of the many, both now and in the future?

At the Nuremberg trials, the defense recognized that if the voluntary consent of the human subjects to an experiment is essential to its legal permissibility, as the tribunal ultimately ruled that it is,

Journal of Medicine and Philosophy, 1977, 2, pp. 318–329. Copyright © Swets & Zeitlinger Publishers. Used with permission.

EDITORS' NOTE: All references have been deleted. Readers who wish to follow up on sources should consult the original article.

then the case for the defendants was hopeless. And so it had no choice but to argue that such consent is not legally essential. The argument for this position by Dr. Robert Servatius, on behalf of Dr. Karl Brandt, although primarily legal, is of very great ethical interest. Its cardinal points were three. (1) A state may demand a sacrifice from an individual on behalf of the community; and decisions as to what the interests of the community are, what those interests require, and how great a sacrifice may be demanded are all to be made by the state alone. (2) There are no pertinent valid distinctions to be drawn between conscripting somebody for military service, ordering somebody to drop an atomic bomb, and requiring somebody to submit to medical experimentation. (3) In the history of medicine, numerous experiments have been carried out on human beings without their informed consent; and "looking through the medical literature, one cannot escape the growing conviction that the word 'volunteer,' where it appears at all, is used only as a word of protection and camouflage."

The most embarrassing of Servatius's three points, namely, [point] 3, morally tended to support the prosecution. It is true that numerous experiments have been carried out by physicians on unconsenting human beings, but for most of the present century at least, they have been the shame of medicine. And even if the word "volunteer" in the report of an experiment is for protection and camouflage, that only shows that camouflage was thought necessary—and why should it have been, unless it was acknowledged that to experiment on a human being without his consent is wrong? It should be added that Servatius seems to have been mistaken as to the facts. Although there are strong objections to some of the kinds of volunteers that have been used as subjects in the United States— for example, imprisoned or condemned criminals—there is also good evidence that most of them have genuinely been volunteers.

Servatius's first two points, however, are in no way weakened by the failure of his third. Yet they are formulated in terms of a political theory that is anathema to those who uphold classical Western, that is, nonstatist, political theories, and the conceptions of the human good that go with them. But it is plain that his first point would be unaffected as an argument against the requirement of consent

had he spoken of a genuinely democratic society instead of *a* state, and of the institutions of a genuinely democratic society instead of *the* state. Genuinely democratic societies have been known to compel unwelcome actions in the name of social goods, although not always the same goods as those in the name of which undemocratic societies have acted.

A second adjustment that must be made in order fairly to appraise Servatius's arguments is to separate their appraisal from all the circumstances of the Nuremberg medical case not directly relevant to them. As I read the published volumes, most, if not all, the accused would justly have been condemned even had the necessity of consent not been affirmed by the tribunal, on the ground that the scientific incompetence of some of the experimental designs, and the nonmedical purposes of others, would have left no choice but to pronounce the experimenters guilty of gratuitous killing, mutilating, and other forms of injury. There is every reason to suppose that, even if the first two points in Servatius's argument were to be accepted, modifying them according to a less obnoxious political theory, the number of sanctioned dangerous experiments would be comparatively few, as would the number of deaths and serious injuries caused by them.

Once they have been sanitized in this way, Servatius's two points are not shocking at all, academically at least: they are straightforward applications of a disputed but academically respectable doctrine, namely, utilitarianism in its generalized form, according to which what is right is defined as what is for the greatest *good* of the greatest number. (Its most familiar specific form is the hedonistic one of Bentham and Mill, in which good is identified with happiness.) Hence it is not surprising that, during the very period in which the organized medical profession was preparing to reaffirm at Helsinki the Nuremberg principle of informed consent, many individual physicians were concluding that the principle need not be observed in responsibly conducted scientific experimentation. What the Nuremberg tribunal really condemned, they appear to have thought, was not experimentation without informed consent, but only atrocious experimentation. Indeed, in 1962, in a passage endorsed by Beecher himself, Walter Modell wrote: "I . . . think that when society confers the degree of physician on a man it instructs him to experiment on his fellow. I think that when a patient goes to a physician for treatment, regardless of whether he consents to it, he is also unconsciously presenting himself for the purpose of experimentation."

What happens when those who thus unconsciously present themselves for experimentation become conscious of it was demonstrated in the Jewish Chronic Diseases Hospital case, which began less than two years after Modell wrote. That case is particularly important, because the experiment involved was perfectly harmless and was, from a scientific point of view, admirably conducted. The facts of the case pertinent to the present study are as follows. In the summer of 1963, at the request of an outside cancer research institute, the medical director of the hospital agreed to permit physicians from the institute to inject into twenty-two patients suspensions of cells obtained from cultures of human cancer tissue, in order to determine the mechanism and rate of rejection of the injected material by debilitated but noncancerous subjects. It was asserted by the experimenters that spoken consent was obtained from the subjects, but it was not disputed that the subjects were not told that what was to be injected contained cancer cells. The reason given for this reticence was that, although the experiment was neither harmful nor hazardous, if the dread word "cancer" had been used the subjects would have been misled and unnecessarily distressed. Ultimately, the medical director of the hospital and the principal investigator were found by the Board of Regents of the University of the State of New York (which has jurisdiction over all licensed professions excluding that of law) to be guilty of fraud and deceit in the practice of medicine.

Much sympathy was rightly expressed for the physicians thus censured. For they had acted in good conscience, even if erroneously; and they had done nothing different in kind from what many others had done or advocated. And some sympathizers went further. Had the censured physicians not achieved a significant if modest scientific result, at the cost of no harm to anybody beyond a temporary mild discomfort? Why then should the attorney general for New York, in a memorandum to the Board of Regents, have written as though he was addressing the Nuremberg tribunal?

The answer emerges from what the defenders of experimentation without informed consent wrote in the years that followed; for it became evident that, if from excusing what was done in the Jewish Chronic Diseases Hospital case (which they seldom mentioned, although they cannot but have had it in mind) they were to pass on to justifying it, they would have no option but to present a sanitized version of the defense offered by Servatius at Nuremberg.

With exemplary courage, a number of them did so. The most forthright was Walsh McDermott, in some "Opening Comments" that have already outlived the 1967 Colloquium they introduced. He put forward a democratic version of Servatius's first point in these words: " . . . as a society we enforce the social good over the individual good across a whole spectrum of nonmedical activities every day, and many of these activities ultimately affect the health or the life of an individual. . . . [W]hen the conflict is head on, when the group interest and the individual interest are basically irreconcilable . . . we try to depersonalize the process by spreading responsibility for decision throughout a framework of legal institutions." It should be noticed that McDermott acknowledged that "we" only "try to depersonalize" this process, without noting that those societies that have succeeded are unappealing as models.

He also enriched Servatius's second point with an additional example of a head-on conflict between individual interest and social interest that is resolved according to the latter, namely, "the decision to impose capital punishment." But, in declaring that situations in clinical medicine "in which it clearly seems to be in the best interests of society that [certain scientific] information be obtained . . . [which] can be obtained only from studies on certain already unlucky individuals" belong to the same "hard core" of cases as situations requiring military conscription or capital punishment, he did not substantially differ from Servatius .

The same two points recur in papers by Guido Calabresi, Louis L. Jaffe, and Louis Lasagna, which arose out of conferences arranged by the American Academy of Arts and Sciences, and were published in *Daedalus* for Spring 1969. Calabresi, indeed, furnished yet another example of Servatius's second point: "Many activities are permitted, even though *statistically* we know they will lose lives, since it costs too much to engage in these activities more safely, or to abstain from them altogether." All three followed McDermott in concluding that, in the Helsinki Declaration, and in subsequent promulgations by such bodies as the U.S. Food and Drug Administration and the National Institutes of Health, our society either has mistaken the nature of its own morality, as evidenced by the practices it sanctions, or is hypocritical. Its error or hypocrisy ought to be corrected by repudiating the requirement of informed consent. But even when that correction has been made, the problem will remain of how nonvolunteer research subjects are to be obtained. At this point Jaffe assured his readers that his argument was not "the ominous prolegomenon to a program for conscripting human guinea pigs," and those who accept the utilitarian argument would probably do the same. Calabresi, for example, declared that right-minded scholars "ought to be devoting themselves to the development of a workable but not too obvious control system. . . ." Jaffe himself looked to developments in the common law. Lasagna appeared to imagine that all would be well if physicians and public alike would only embrace situation ethics.[1] None made any significant advance upon McDermott's ironical conclusion: "Obviously we cannot convene a constitutional convention of the Judeo-Christian culture and add a few amendments to it. Yet, in a figurative sense, unless we can do something very much like that . . . the problem, at its roots, is unsolvable and we must continue to live with it."

1. That there can be such a thing as "situation ethics" as opposed to "rule ethics" is a gross error, which has a common ancestry with the discredited educational fallacy that there is such a thing as "teaching children" as opposed to "teaching subjects." Any rational system of moral rules has to do with how human beings ought to act in different situations, and, when from a moral point of view situations differ relevantly, it must treat them differently. But this in no way entails that there are not kinds of action that are wrong in all situations, e.g., murder—accurately defined to exclude such justifiable forms of homicide as self-defense. The contention that experimenting on a responsible adult human being without his consent is wrong in all situations entails neither that all situations should be treated in the same way nor that there are no situations in which it is permissible to experiment on a human being without his consent—e.g., certain kinds of situations, not discussed in this paper, in which responsibility is impaired.

It is regrettable that these distinguished physicians and lawyers should have assumed that generalized utilitarianism is the only moral position pertinent to examining the cases which, according to their second point, are of the same kind as the "hard core" ones in medical experimentation. It is true by definition that, from the point of view of generalized utilitarianism, the only thing that counts in settling any moral question is what would be for the greatest good of the greatest number. But there are other moral positions, among them the Judeo-Christian one, according to which a variety of nonutilitarian considerations may count.

Setting aside Servatius's case of dropping an atomic bomb on a city, on the ground that it is dubious whether that is permissible on either utilitarian or Judeo-Christian grounds, let us consider the cases offered by Servatius, McDermott, and Calabresi. In the Judeo-Christian moral tradition, it is held permissible for a civil society to attach penal sanctions to its laws, in extreme cases even the sanction of death, without ceasing to treat the persons so punished as ends; for when laws themselves have a moral sanction, to punish those who break them in itself treats them as genuinely responsible for their deeds. Punishment is not inflicted primarily for deterrence or reformation, but as what the criminal deserves. Again, in compelling citizens to serve in a just war on threat of punishment, a civil society only compels them to uphold a good common to them all, and not primarily the good of others. The very concept of a common good has fallen into disrepute partly because it has become confounded with the idea of the good of the many as opposed to that of the few. Even though the Judeo-Christian tradition applauds a sacrifice by one man for his fellows, it utterly denies the right of his fellows, no matter how many, to compel that sacrifice. Finally, while certain kinds of laxity in safety regulations are morally objectionable, for example, allowing a machine tended by human beings to be used when it is only a question of time when it will blow up, other kinds are not; for example, allowing the use of a machine that would be dangerous in the hands of an unskilled operator. Laxities of the latter kind, even when it is statistically predictable that some injuries will result, and not necessarily to the negligent operator, do not sacrifice the few to the many: they merely allow, without compelling, many to risk being among the few. Hence, from a Judeo-Christian point of view, securing nonvolunteer subjects for medical research is *not* an action of the same kind as conscripting for military service, imposing capital punishment, or tolerating certain kinds of risky activities: they have nonutilitarian justifications, it does not.

And so we come to the first point. If a piece of medical research would be for the greatest good of the greatest number, then according to generalized utilitarianism, nonvolunteer subjects may be procured for it by one or other of the only two possible methods: lawful compulsion as in the Nuremberg case, or deception as in the Jewish Chronic Diseases Hospital case. Is this justification of those methods acceptable?

The consensus reached by the organized medical profession is that it is not acceptable. And, in a case study such as this, that is the principal thing to be said. Among physicians, "there is essentially no valid argument about the basic principle that informed consent—or whatever may be its legal equivalent in a specialized situation—is a prerequisite for human experimentation." They recognize that they have neither legal nor moral authority to compel nonvolunteers to be experimental subjects; and the great majority of them would repudiate, as unprofessional, any suggestion that they experiment on conscripts provided by the state. And most of them now agree that it is equally inadmissible to procure experimental subjects by deception, whether by misrepresentation or by withholding information those subjects would consider material.

It is not disputed that observing the requirement of informed consent may delay otherwise desirable scientific progress. But David D. Rutstein's doctrine is now widely accepted, that "ethical constraints that prohibit certain human experiments are similar in their effects as are scientific constraints on the design of experiments." To use his example, in research on infectious hepatitis, it is a scientific constraint that no laboratory animal has been found that is susceptible to hepatitis, in which the large quantities of the virus needed for vaccine manufacture can be grown, and it is an ethical constraint that "it is not ethical to use human subjects for the growth of a virus for any purpose."

Hermann L. Blumgart has succinctly formulated the accepted reason why the requirement of informed consent must be satisfied, and it is the familiar Judeo-Christian one: "To use a person for an experiment without his consent is untenable; the advance of science may be retarded, but more important values are at stake." Preeminent among those values is respecting the autonomy of potential experimental subjects. The decision whether or not they are to participate can only be theirs. Admittedly, invading their autonomy may be good for science and good for most people. But, in Beecher's words, "a particularly pernicious myth is the one that depends on the view that ends justify means. A study is ethical or not at its inception. It does not become ethical merely because it turned up valuable data. Sometimes such a view is rationalized by the investigator as having produced the most good for the most people. This is blatant statism. Whoever gave the investigator the god-like right to choose martyrs?" He might have added that those who fancy they are playing God are nearly always possessed by devils.

RETROSPECT

The history has been outlined of two cases in which the medical profession confronted a conflict between a supposed moral constraint on professional practice and the attainment of two of its supposed ends—the health of each patient,* and the health of the community at large. In both, the issue was between conceptions of moral duty, that on the one side being based on unconditional respect for persons as ends, each of those on the other alleging a requirement that a certain producible good be maximized: in the first, an individual good; in the second, a universal or "utilitarian" one. For both of the latter "consequentialist" positions, appeal was made to ends that have important places in the practice of medicine. Hence, both were perceived at once to have serious claims to acceptance, and were ably defended.

---

*EDITORS' NOTE: Donagan's discussion of informed consent to therapy has been omitted.

The history of how the conflict between the anti-consequentialist position and its consequentialist rivals was resolved is of the greatest interest to moral philosophy. From the beginning, physicians were forced to consider what is implicit in the traditional—and imperfectly understood—relation between physician and patient on which medical morality ultimately depends, and to investigate whether what on the surface seem plainly to be ultimate ends of medicine—in therapy, the health of the individual patient, and in experimentation, the health of the community at large—can justify weakening the commitment to respect for human beings that was more and more seen to underlie the traditional physician-patient relation. The result, as we have seen, was the reaffirmation of the less obvious position. The doctrine was repudiated that admittedly good consequences can justify attaining them by means in which the respect owed to human beings as such is violated. And in the process, the "common moral knowledge" implicit in the best traditional medical practice was consciously formulated as a general truth. There was a transition from common moral knowledge to knowledge of the kind Kant called "philosophical."

As Kant recognized, any such transition raises further philosophical problems. Having identified the ethical principles that are the foundation of a certain part of our common moral knowledge, we must go on to investigate the nature of those principles and how they are justified—to construct what he called a "metaphysic of morals," that is, a philosophical theory of morality.

And a further problem can be discerned. The moral principle implicit in the traditional conception of the physician-patient relationship rests on the conception of all human beings as autonomous ends in themselves, whose existence is beyond price. But do the theoretical medical sciences regard human beings in that way? Do they not rather lead to the concept of man which William James called "medical materialism"? If so, can these two points of view be reconciled? Or is medicine afflicted with multiple personalities? But that is for another study.

The Nuremberg Code

1. The voluntary consent of the human subject is absolutely essential.

This means that the person involved should have legal capacity to give consent; should be so situated as to be able to exercise free power of choice, without the intervention of any element of force, fraud, deceit, duress, over-reaching, or other ulterior form of constraint or coercion; and should have sufficient knowledge and comprehension of the elements of the subject matter involved as to enable him to make an understanding and enlightened decision. This latter element requires that before the acceptance of an affirmative decision by the experimental subject there should be made known to him the nature, duration, and purpose of the experiment; the method and means by which it is to be conducted; all inconveniences and hazards reasonably to be expected; and the effects upon his health or person which may possibly come from his participation in the experiment.

The duty and responsibility for ascertaining the quality of the consent rests upon each individual who initiates, directs or engages in the experiment. It is a personal duty and responsibility which may not be delegated to another with impunity.

2. The experiment should be such as to yield fruitful results for the good of society, unprocurable by other methods or means of study, and not random and unnecessary in nature.

3. The experiment should be so designed and based on the results of animal experimentation and a knowledge of the natural history of the disease or other problem under study that the

From "Permissible Medical Experiments," *Trials of War Criminals before the Nuernberg Military Tribunals under Control Council Law No. 10: Nuernberg, October 1946-April 1949* (Washington: U.S. Government Printing Office, n.d., vol. 2), 181–82.

anticipated results will justify the performance of the experiment.

4. The experiment should be so conducted as to avoid all unnecessary physical and mental suffering and injury.

5. No experiment should be conducted where there is an *a priori* reason to believe that death or disabling injury will occur; except, perhaps, in those experiments where the experimental physicians also serve as subjects.

6. The degree of risk to be taken should never exceed that determined by the humanitarian importance of the problem to be solved by the experiment.

7. Proper preparations should be made and adequate facilities provided to protect the experimental subject against even remote possibilities of injury, disability, or death.

8. The experiment should be conducted only by scientifically qualified persons. The highest degree of skill and care should be required through all stages of the experiment of those who conduct or engage in the experiment.

9. During the course of the experiment the human subject should be at liberty to bring the experiment to an end if he has reached the physical or mental state where continuation of the experiment seems to him to be impossible.

10. During the course of the experiment the scientist in charge must be prepared to terminate the experiment at any stage, if he has probable cause to believe, in the exercise of the good faith, superior skill and careful judgment required of him that a continuation of the experiment is likely to result in injury, disability, or death to the experimental subject.

Declaration of Helsinki

World Medical Association

1964, revised 1975, 1983, 1989

INTRODUCTION

It is the mission of the physician to safeguard the health of the people. His or her knowledge and conscience are dedicated to the fulfillment of this mission.

The Declaration of Geneva of The World Medical Association binds the physician with the words "The health of my patient will be my first consideration," and the International Code of Medical Ethics declares that, "A physician shall act only in the patient's interest when providing medical care which might have the effect of weakening the physical and mental condition of the patient."

The purpose of biomedical research involving human subjects must be to improve diagnostic,

therapeutic and prophylactic procedures and the understanding of the aetiology and pathogenesis of disease.

In current medical practice most diagnostic, therapeutic or prophylactic procedures involve hazards. This applies especially to biomedical research.

Medical progress is based on research which ultimately must rest in part on experimentation involving human subjects.

In the field of biomedical research a fundamental distinction must be recognized between medical research in which the aim is essentially diagnostic or therapeutic for a patient, and medical research, the essential object of which is purely scientific and without implying direct diagnostic or therapeutic value to the person subjected to the research.

Special caution must be exercised in the conduct of research which may affect the environment, and the welfare of animals used for research must be respected.

The format of this text is that of the *Encyclopedia of Bioethics*, rev. ed. (New York: MacMillan, 1995), 2765-67.

Because it is essential that the results of laboratory experiments be applied to human beings to further scientific knowledge and to help suffering humanity, the World Medical Association has prepared the following recommendations as a guide to every physician in biomedical research involving human subjects. They should be kept under review in the future. It must be stressed that the standards as drafted are only a guide to physicians all over the world. Physicians are not relieved from criminal, civil and ethical responsibilities under the laws of their own countries.

I. BASIC PRINCIPLES

1. Biomedical research involving human subjects must conform to generally accepted scientific principles and should be based on adequately performed laboratory and animal experimentation and a thorough knowledge of the scientific literature.

2. The design and performance of each experimental procedure involving human subjects should be clearly formulated in an experimental protocol which should be transmitted for consideration, comment and guidance to a specially appointed committee independent of the investigator and the sponsor, provided that this independent committee is in conformity with the laws and regulations of the country in which the research experiment is performed.

3. Biomedical research involving human subjects should be conducted only by scientifically qualified persons and under the supervision of a clinically competent medical person. The responsibility for the human subject must always rest with a medically qualified person and never rest on the subject of the research, even though the subject has given his or her consent.

4. Biomedical research involving human subjects cannot legitimately be carried out unless the importance of the objective is in proportion to the inherent risk to the subject.

5. Every biomedical research project involving human subjects should be preceded by careful assessment of predictable risks in comparison with foreseeable benefits to the subject or to others. Concern for the interests of the subject must always prevail over the interests of science and society.

6. The right of the research subject to safeguard his or her integrity must always be respected. Every precaution should be taken to respect the privacy of the subject and to minimize the impact of the study on the subject's physical and mental integrity and on the personality of the subject.

7. Physicians should abstain from engaging in research projects involving human subjects unless they are satisfied that the hazards involved are believed to be predictable. Physicians should cease any investigation if the hazards are found to outweigh the potential benefits.

8. In publication of the results of his or her research, the physician is obliged to preserve the accuracy of the results. Reports of experimentation not in accordance with the principles laid down in this Declaration should not be accepted for publication.

9. In any research on human beings, each potential subject must be adequately informed of the aims, methods, anticipated benefits and potential hazards of the study and the discomfort it may entail. He or she should be informed that he or she is at liberty to abstain from participation in the study and that he or she is free to withdraw his or her consent to participation at any time. The physician should then obtain the subject's freely-given informed consent, preferably in writing.

10. When obtaining informed consent for the research project the physician should be particularly cautious if the subject is in a dependent relationship to him or her or may consent under duress. In that case the informed consent should be obtained by a physician who is not engaged in the investigation and who is completely independent of this official relationship.

11. In the case of legal incompetence, informed consent should be obtained from the legal guardian in accordance with national legislation. Where physical or mental incapacity makes it impossible to obtain informed consent, or when the subject is a minor, permission from the responsible relative replaces that of the subject in accordance with national legislation. Whenever the minor child is in fact able to give consent, the minor's consent must be obtained in addition to the consent of the minor's legal guardian.

12. The research protocol should always contain a statement of the ethical considerations involved and should indicate that the principles enunciated in the present Declaration are complied with.

II. MEDICAL RESEARCH COMBINED WITH PROFESSIONAL CARE (CLINICAL RESEARCH)

1. In the treatment of the sick person, the physician must be free to use a new diagnostic and therapeutic measure, if in his or her judgement, it offers hope of saving life, reestablishing health or alleviating suffering.

2. The potential benefits, hazard and discomfort of a new method should be weighed against the advantages of the best current diagnostic and therapeutic methods.

3. In any medical study, every patient—including those of a control group, if any—should be assured of the best proven diagnostic and therapeutic method.

4. The refusal of the patient to participate in a study must never interfere with the physician-patient relationship.

5. If the physician considers it essential not to obtain informed consent, the specific reasons for this proposal should be stated in the experimental protocol for transmission to the independent committee.

6. The physician can combine medical research with professional care, the objective being the acquisition of new medical knowledge, only to the extent that medical research is justified by its potential diagnostic or therapeutic value for the patient.

III. NON-THERAPEUTIC BIOMEDICAL RESEARCH INVOLVING HUMAN SUBJECTS (NON-CLINICAL BIOMEDICAL RESEARCH)

1. In the purely scientific application of medical research carried out on a human being, it is the duty of the physician to remain the protector of the life and health of that person on whom biomedical research is being carried out.

2. The subjects should be volunteers—either healthy persons or patients for whom the experimental design is not related to the patient's illness.

3. The investigator or the investigating team should discontinue the research if in his/her or their judgement it may, if continued, be harmful to the individual.

4. In research on man, the interest of science and society should never take precedence over considerations related to the well-being of the subject.

SECTION 2

The Ethics of Randomized Clinical Trials

Ethical Difficulties with Randomized Clinical Trials Involving Cancer Patients: Examples from the Field of Gynecologic Oncology

Maurie Markman

In a recent issue of the *New England Journal of Medicine,* two prominent clinical investigators took opposite sides in a debate on the need for and the ethics of randomized clinical trials.[1] The basic argument in support of randomized clinical trials is that in the absence of such studies it is not possible to be certain that a new drug or clinical intervention is actually beneficial to patients with a particular disease or condition, compared either to a "standard" (accepted or approved) therapeutic strategy or to no treatment at all (an untreated control population). The major argument against the performance of randomized clinical trials is that the individual physician's principal ethical responsibility is to the *individual patient* that he or she is treating, and *not* to future patients who may benefit from the potentially important information gained through a well-designed and well-conducted randomized trial. If one accepts this argument, a physician should only recommend that an individual patient participate in a randomized trial if he or she is convinced that neither one of the treatment programs is superior based on previous data available in the medical literature. If it is the *physician's best judgment*—based on his or her interpretation of this data, personal experience, and knowledge of the individual patient's specific medical condition—that one regimen would be preferred over the other(s), then the physician should not recommend that the patient participate in this trial, no matter how important the information gained may be to society.

Physicians working with cancer patients have frequently been able to avoid the difficult ethical dilemma presented above, as experimental (not FDA-approved) antineoplastic agents have traditionally *only* been available to patients who are willing to participate in a clinical trial. Drug development of new agents has followed a logical sequence: toxicity/dose finding studies (phase 1), followed by single-arm efficacy trials in specific disease settings (phase 2), followed by randomized trials to define the "true benefit" of the new therapy (phase 3). In the toxicity studies, the major goal of the treatment is to define the appropriate dose that produces acceptable toxicity, while in the efficacy studies, the aim is to determine if the agent is effective in a particular disease setting. Thus, the physician who believes, based on previously reported clinical data (usually from phase-2 drug trials), that a new drug is potentially superior to the standard therapy would have no choice but to recommend that the patient participate in the trial. In this way, the patient would have a 50 percent chance of receiving the new therapy (and a 50 percent chance of being placed in the control group), compared to a 0 percent chance if he or she does not participate in the study.

We are currently witnessing this process with the new antineoplastic agent, taxol. The drug, which has a unique mechanism of cytotoxic activity, has

Journal of Clinical Ethics, 3, No. 3 (Fall 1992): 193–195. Copyright © 1992 by the Journal of Clinical Ethics. All rights reserved. Reprinted with permission.

recently been demonstrated to cause temporary regression of tumor in approximately 20 to 30 percent of patients with advanced ovarian cancer who have previously failed standard therapy for their disease.[2] At the present time, there is absolutely no evidence that the drug is curative when used in the advanced refractory disease setting, and most responses last less than six to nine months. However, the response rate observed in this particular patient population is superior to what has been demonstrated with other commercially available drugs.

Interest in, and praise for, the effectiveness of taxol has spread far beyond the confines of medical meetings and the peer-reviewed medical literature. This is partly due to the fact that the agent is a natural product, and obtaining sufficient quantities of the drug requires the sacrifice of a large number of endangered trees in the Pacific Northwest. A number of scientists and biomedical companies, as well as the National Cancer Institute, are actively seeking to find new sources of taxol so as to make the drug more widely available to patients with ovarian cancer and other malignancies.

Currently, the Gynecologic Oncology Group, a national multi-institutional cooperative group devoted to the study of cancers involving gynecologic organs, is conducting a randomized trial of a standard chemotherapy regimen (without taxol) compared to a program that includes taxol, in patients with ovarian cancer who have not previously received chemotherapy. This is an important trial, as it should determine what role, if any, taxol should play in the initial management of a patient with advanced ovarian cancer.

A physician hoping to give a patient taxol, in the belief that a regimen that includes this drug may be superior to the current standard regimen, would have to attempt to enter the patient into this randomized trial. But what if the drug, still considered an experimental agent, were made more widely available from the National Cancer Institute? Would a physician who wanted a woman with ovarian cancer to receive taxol be justified in placing the individual on a randomized trial when there were other methods to obtain the drug without randomization? Or, as is frequently asked of cancer specialists when they discuss treatment options with patients, would they recommend this trial to their wife, sister, or mother? This question, perhaps the most difficult

one addressed to oncologists concerning experimental clinical trials, gets to the fundamental core of the issue: Is the physician acting *solely* in the best interest of the patient, or are other considerations (such as the scientific or societal need to know whether one treatment program is superior) playing a role in the doctor's deliberations?

A second example of the physician's dilemma over whether to recommend that a patient participate in a randomized trial—one that is more complex, as it does not involve the use of experimental drugs whose access can be controlled—concerns the current status of chemotherapy for advanced metastatic cancer of the uterus (endometrial cancer). Unfortunately, chemotherapy has only demonstrated limited activity in this disease, with partial responses of short durations being observed in approximately 20 percent of treated patients.

Recently, clinical investigators at the Mayo Clinic reported the results of a nonrandomized trial of a combination chemotherapy regimen in twenty-five patients with advanced cancer of the uterus that employed four commercially available cytotoxic agents.[3] The investigators observed a 60 percent objective response rate, and the authors of the report concluded that the regimen "is highly active in advanced endometrial carcinoma and results in improved survival compared to literature controls."[4] The Mayo Clinic investigators are noted for the quality of their work. In addition, they are generally conservative in the interpretation of their own data. Thus, the results of this trial are quite interesting and encouraging. However, this was a nonrandomized trial, and it is possible that unintentional selection bias may have accounted for the results observed. The only method available to determine definitively if the more toxic, multidrug combination regimen is superior in efficacy to a standard single-agent program would be to conduct a randomized clinical trial.

One can be fairly certain that a randomized trial comparing these two treatment programs will be forthcoming. Should patients be entered into such a trial? Again, the ethical issue for the individual physician comes down to how he or she interprets the results of this investigative program compared to a standard chemotherapy regimen in cancer of the uterus. If the physician cannot accept the results as providing reasonable evidence for superiority of the newer regimen over standard therapy, then he or she is justified in entering patients into such a trial. But if the physician believes that the results suggest increased efficacy with acceptable toxicity, it is difficult to agree with the argument that the physician is acting in the *patient's* best interest if he recommends entry into the randomized trial. The question must be asked again: If this were your wife, mother, or sister, what would you recommend?

A final example illustrates the potential for serious ethical conflict between the importance of obtaining information to define management options for future patients with malignancy, and the critical need to safeguard the patient's best interest. Standard treatment of patients with advanced cancer of the ovary involves an attempt to remove surgically as much tumor as possible from the abdominal cavity (tumor "debulking") prior to the institution of chemotherapy.[5] This is a unique management strategy. In almost all other malignancies, surgery is employed in the initial management of the disease only when it is believed possible that all macroscopic tumor can be removed. However, in patients with ovarian cancer, this surgery is a standard management strategy, even though physicians know that the approach cannot cure patients with disease disseminated throughout the abdominal cavity. What, then, is the justification for this therapeutic strategy?

Multiple retrospective and prospective studies have demonstrated that patients with ovarian cancer who start chemotherapy after surgical resection with small-volume residual disease respond better to the chemotherapy and survive longer than patients with large-volume residual disease.[6] This has led to the conclusion that the surgical removal of tumor increases the effectiveness of chemotherapy, presumably resulting from improved blood supply and delivery of the cytotoxic drug to the remaining tumor, or removal of a large portion of cells that may be resistant to the effects of the anticancer agents. However, this hypothesis has *never* been tested in a randomized trial. It is certainly possible that the surgeon's ability to remove bulky intra-abdominal tumor and leave the patient with small-volume residual disease may simply select patients who would have done well with chemotherapy even if surgery were not performed. Perhaps the factors that permit invasiveness and interfere with a surgeon's

ability to debulk tumor are the same factors that lead to a tumor having an enhanced ability to develop drug-resistant cells rapidly and escape the effects of the antineoplastic agents.

Thus, the only way to answer this important biological and clinical question would be to randomize women with ovarian cancer *who would otherwise be able to undergo debulking surgery* either to have the procedure performed or to start the treatment program with chemotherapy but without surgery. In this way, the role of a major surgical procedure could be evaluated definitively. Unfortunately, the conduct of such a trial leads to serious ethical difficulties. A woman who is randomized to debulking surgery, followed by chemotherapy, will be receiving standard therapy, and her ultimate clinical outcome will be unaffected by the conduct of the trial. However, a woman randomized to receive chemotherapy without surgery cannot be given such a guarantee. While that patient may experience less morbidity by not undergoing the debulking surgery, there is no reason to believe her ultimate outcome will be favorably influenced by participating in this trial. And if it is subsequently determined that surgery does, in fact, play an important role in the management of this condition, *her* survival may have been compromised by participating in the study. Clinical science may have benefitted greatly from the conduct of this study, but individual patients may have paid dearly for their participation. Thus, unless another method can be found to address the question of the role of debulking surgery in patients with cancer of the ovary, this procedure must remain a major part of the management of individuals with the disease.

In this article, I have attempted to present examples of the ethical difficulties with randomized clinical trials experienced by physicians caring for *real* patients with malignant disease. Above all, the physician's responsibility is to the individual patient, and the need to increase knowledge to improve the lot of future patients must always take second place.

NOTES

1. S. Hellman and D. Hellman, "Of Mice but Not Men: Problems of the Randomized Clinical Trial," *New*

England Journal of Medicine 324 (1991): 1585–89; E. Passamani, "Clinical Trials: Are They Ethical?" *New England Journal of Medicine* 324 (1991): 1589–92.

2. W.P. McGuire, E.K. Rowinsky, N.B. Rosenshein, *et al.*, "Taxol: A Unique Antineoplastic Agent with Significant Activity in Advanced Ovarian Epithelial Neoplasms," *Annals of Internal Medicine* 111 (1989): 273–79.

3. H.J. Long, R.M. Langdon, and H.S. Wieand, "Phase II Trial of Methotrexate, Vinblastine, Doxorubicin, and Cisplatin in Women with Advanced Endometrial Carcinoma," *Proceedings of the American Society of Clinical Oncology* 10 (1991): 184.

4. *Ibid.*

5. R.C. Young, Z. Fuks, and W.J. Hoskins, "Cancer of the Ovary," in *Cancer: Principles and Practice of Oncology*, ed. V.T. DeVita, Jr., S. Hellman, and S.A. Rosenberg (Philadelphia: J.B. Lippincott, 1989), 1162–96.

6. *Ibid.*

Of Mice but Not Men: Problems of the Randomized Clinical Trial

Samuel Hellman and Deborah S. Hellman

As medicine has become increasingly scientific and less accepting of unsupported opinion or proof by anecdote, the randomized controlled clinical trial has become the standard technique for changing diagnostic or therapeutic methods. The use of this technique creates an ethical dilemma.[1,2] Researchers participating in such studies are required to modify their ethical commitments to individual patients and do serious damage to the concept of the physician as a practicing, empathetic professional who is primarily concerned with each patient as an individual. Researchers using a randomized clinical trial can be described as physician-scientists, a term that expresses the tension between the two roles. The physician, by entering into a relationship with an individual patient, assumes certain obligations, including the commitment always to act in the patient's best interests. As Leon Kass has rightly maintained, "the physician must produce unswervingly the virtues of loyalty and fidelity to his patient."[3] Though the ethical requirements of this relationship have been modified by legal obligations to report wounds of a suspicious nature and certain infectious diseases, these obligations in no way conflict with the central ethical obligation to act in the best interests of the patient medically. Instead, certain nonmedical interests of the patient are pre-empted by other social concerns.

The role of the scientist is quite different. The clinical scientist is concerned with answering questions—i.e., determining the validity of formally constructed hypotheses. Such scientific information, it is presumed, will benefit humanity in general. The clinical scientist's role has been well described by Dr. Anthony Fauci, director of the National Institute of Allergy and Infectious Diseases, who states the goals of the randomized clinical trial in these words: "It's not to deliver therapy. It's to answer a scientific question so that the drug can be available for everybody once you've established safety and efficacy."[4] The demands of such a study can conflict in a number of ways with the physician's duty to minister to patients. The study may create a false dichotomy in the physician's opinions; according to the premise of the randomized clinical trial, the physician may only know or not know whether a proposed course of treatment represents an improvement; no middle position is permitted. What the physician thinks, suspects, believes, or has a hunch about is assigned to the "not knowing" category, because knowing is defined on the basis of an arbitrary but accepted statistical test performed in a randomized clinical trial. Thus, little credence is given to information gained beforehand in other ways or to information accrued during the trial

New England Journal of Medicine 324, No. 22, May 30, 1991: 1589–1592.

but without the required statistical degree of assurance that a difference is not due to chance. The randomized clinical trial also prevents the treatment technique from being modified on the basis of the growing knowledge of the physicians during their participation in the trial. Moreover, it limits access to the data as they are collected until specific milestones are achieved. This prevents physicians from profiting not only from their individual experience, but also from the collective experience of the other participants.

The randomized clinical trial requires doctors to act simultaneously as physicians and as scientists. This puts them in a difficult and sometimes untenable ethical position. The conflicting moral demands arising from the use of the randomized clinical trial reflect the classic conflict between rights-based moral theories and utilitarian ones. The first of these, which depend on the moral theory of Immanuel Kant (and seen more recently in neo-Kantian philosophers, such as John Rawls[5]), asserts that human beings, by virtue of their unique capacity for rational thought, are bearers of dignity. As such, they ought not to be treated merely as means to an end; rather, they must always be treated as ends in themselves. Utilitarianism, by contrast, defines what is right as the greatest good for the greatest number—that is, as social utility. This view, articulated by Jeremy Bentham and John Stuart Mill, requires that pleasures (understood broadly, to include such pleasures as health and well-being) and pains be added together. The morally correct act is the act that produces the most pleasure and the least pain overall.

A classic objection to the utilitarian position is that according to that theory, the distribution of pleasures and pains is of no moral consequence. This element of the theory severely restricts physicians from being utilitarians, or at least from following the theory's dictates. Physicians must care very deeply about the distribution of pain and pleasure, for they have entered into a relationship with one or a number of individual patients. They cannot be indifferent to whether it is these patients or others that suffer for the general benefit of society. Even though society might gain from the suffering of a few, and even though the doctor might believe that such a benefit is worth a given patient's suffering (i.e., that utilitarianism is right in the particular case), the ethical obligation created by the covenant between doctor and patient requires the doctor to see the interests of the individual patient as primary and compelling. In essence, the doctor-patient relationship requires doctors to see their patients as bearers of rights who cannot be merely used for the greater good of humanity.

As Fauci has suggested,[4] the randomized clinical trial routinely asks physicians to sacrifice the interests of their particular patients for the sake of the study and that of the information that it will make available for the benefit of society. This practice is ethically problematic. Consider first the initial formulation of a trial. In particular, consider the case of a disease for which there is no satisfactory therapy—for example, advanced cancer or the acquired immunodeficiency syndrome (AIDS). A new agent that promises more effectiveness is the subject of the study. The control group must be given either an unsatisfactory treatment or a placebo. Even though the therapeutic value of the new agent is unproved, if physicians think that it has promise, are they acting in the best interests of their patients in allowing them to be randomly assigned to the control group? Is persisting in such an assignment consistent with the specific commitments taken on in the doctor-patient relationship? As a result of interactions with patients with AIDS and their advocates, Merigan[6] recently suggested modifications in the design of clinical trials that attempt to deal with the unsatisfactory treatment given to the control group. The view of such activists has been expressed by Rebecca Pringle Smith of Community Research Initiative in New York: "Even if you have a supply of compliant martyrs, trials must have some ethical validity."[4]

If the physician has no opinion about whether the new treatment is acceptable, then random assignment is ethically acceptable, but such lack of enthusiasm for the new treatment does not augur well for either the patient or the study. Alternatively, the treatment may show promise of beneficial results but also present a risk of undesirable complications. When the physician believes that the severity and likelihood of harm and good are evenly balanced, randomization may be ethically acceptable. If the physician has no preference for either treatment (is in a state of equipoise[7,8]), then randomization is acceptable. If, however, he or she believes that the new treatment may be either more or less successful or more or less toxic, the use of randomization is not consistent with fidelity to the patient.

The argument usually used to justify randomization is that it provides, in essence, a critique of the usefulness of the physician's beliefs and opinions, those that have not yet been validated by a randomized clinical trial. As the argument goes, these not-yet-validated beliefs are as likely to be wrong as right. Although physicians are ethically required to provide their patients with the best available treatment, there simply is no best treatment yet known.

The reply to this argument takes two forms. First, and most important, even if this view of the reliability of a physician's opinions is accurate, the ethical constraints of an individual doctor's relationship with a particular patient require the doctor to provide individual care. Although physicians must take pains to make clear the speculative nature of their views, they cannot withhold these views from the patient. The patient asks from the doctor both knowledge and judgment. The relationship established between them rightfully allows patients to ask for the judgment of their particular physicians, not merely that of the medical profession in general. Second, it may not be true, in fact, that the not-yet-validated beliefs of physicians are as likely to be wrong as right. The greater certainty obtained with a randomized clinical trial is beneficial, but that does not mean that a lesser degree of certainty is without value. Physicians can acquire knowledge through methods other than the randomized clinical trial. Such knowledge, acquired over time and less formally than is required in a randomized clinical trial, may be of great value to a patient.

Even if it is ethically acceptable to begin a study, one often forms an opinion during its course—especially in studies that are impossible to conduct in a truly double-blinded fashion—that makes it ethically problematic to continue. The inability to remain blinded usually occurs in studies of cancer or AIDS, for example, because the therapy is associated by nature with serious side effects. Trials attempt to restrict the physician's access to the data in order to prevent such unblinding. Such restrictions should make physicians eschew the trial, since their ability to act in the patient's best interests will be limited. Even supporters of randomized clinical trials, such as Merigan, agree that

interim findings should be presented to patients to ensure that no one receives what seems an inferior treatment.[6] Once physicians have formed a view about the new treatment, can they continue randomization? If random assignment is stopped, the study may be lost and the participation of the previous patients wasted. However, if physicians continue the randomization when they have a definite opinion about the efficacy of the experimental drug, they are not acting in accordance with the requirements of the doctor-patient relationship. Furthermore, as their opinion becomes more firm, stopping the randomization may not be enough. Physicians may be ethically required to treat the patients formerly placed in the control group with the therapy that now seems probably effective. To do so would be faithful to the obligations created by the doctor-patient relationship, but it would destroy the study.

To resolve this dilemma, one might suggest that the patient has abrogated the rights implicit in a doctor-patient relationship by signing an informed-consent form. We argue that such rights cannot be waived or abrogated. They are inalienable. The right to be treated as an individual deserving the physician's best judgment and care, rather than to be used as a means to determine the best treatment for others, is inherent in every person. This right, based on the concept of dignity, cannot be waived. What of altruism, then? Is it not the patient's right to make a sacrifice for the general good? This question must be considered from both positions—that of the patient and that of the physician. Although patients may decide to waive this right, it is not consistent with the role of a physician to ask that they do so. In asking, the doctor acts as a scientist instead. The physician's role here is to propose what he or she believes is best medically for the specific patient, not to suggest participation in a study from which the patient cannot gain. Because the opportunity to help future patients is of potential value to a patient, some would say physicians should not deny it. Although this point has merit, it offers so many opportunities for abuse that we are extremely uncomfortable about accepting it. The responsibilities of physicians are much clearer; they are to minister to the current patient.

Moreover, even if patients could waive this right, it is questionable whether those with terminal illness would be truly able to give voluntary informed consent. Such patients are extremely dependent on both their physicians and the health care system. Aware of this dependence, physicians must not ask for consent, for in such cases the very asking breaches the doctor-patient relationship. Anxious to please their physicians, patients may have difficulty refusing to participate in the trial the physicians describe. The patients may perceive their refusal as damaging to the relationship, whether or not it is so. Such perceptions of coercion affect the decision. Informed-consent forms are difficult to understand, especially for patients under the stress of serious illness for which there is no satisfactory treatment. The forms are usually lengthy, somewhat legalistic, complicated, and confusing, and they hardly bespeak the compassion expected of the medical profession. It is important to remember that those who have studied the doctor-patient relationship have emphasized its empathetic nature.

> [The] relationship between doctor and patient partakes of a peculiar intimacy. It presupposes on the part of the physician not only knowledge of his fellow men but sympathy. . . . This aspect of the practice of medicine has been designated as the art; yet I wonder whether it should not, most properly, be called the essence.[9]

How is such a view of the relationship consonant with random assignment and informed consent? The Physician's Oath of the World Medical Association affirms the primacy of the deontologic view of patients' rights: "Concern for the interests of the subject must always prevail over the interests of science and society."[10]

Furthermore, a single study is often not considered sufficient. Before a new form of therapy is generally accepted, confirmatory trials must be conducted. How can one conduct such trials ethically unless one is convinced that the first trial was in error? The ethical problems we have discussed are only exacerbated when a completed randomized clinical trial indicates that a given treatment is preferable. Even if the physician believes the initial trial was in error, the physician must indicate to the patient the full results of that trial.

The most common reply to the ethical arguments has been that the alternative is to return to the physician's intuition, to anecdotes, or to both

as the basis of medical opinion. We all accept the dangers of such a practice. The argument states that we must therefore accept randomized, controlled clinical trials regardless of their ethical problems because of the great social benefit they make possible, and we salve our conscience with the knowledge that informed consent has been given. This returns us to the conflict between patients' rights and social utility. Some would argue that this tension can be resolved by placing a relative value on each. If the patient's right that is being compromised is not a fundamental right and the social gain is very great, then the study might be justified. When the right is fundamental, however, no amount of social gain, or almost none, will justify its sacrifice. Consider, for example, the experiments on humans done by physicians under the Nazi regime. All would agree that these are unacceptable regardless of the value of the scientific information gained. Some people go so far as to say that no use should be made of the results of those experiments because of the clearly unethical manner in which the data were collected. This extreme example may not seem relevant, but we believe that in its hyperbole it clarifies the fallacy of a utilitarian approach to the physician's relationship with the patient. To consider the utilitarian gain is consistent neither with the physician's role nor with the patient's rights.

It is fallacious to suggest that only the randomized clinical trial can provide valid information or that all information acquired by this technique is valid. Such experimental methods are intended to reduce error and bias and therefore reduce the uncertainty of the result. Uncertainty cannot be eliminated, however. The scientific method is based on increasing probabilities and increasingly refined approximations of truth.[11] Although the randomized clinical trial contributes to these ends, it is neither unique nor perfect. Other techniques may also be useful.[12]

Randomized trials often place physicians in the ethically intolerable position of choosing between the good of the patient and that of society. We urge that such situations be avoided and that other techniques of acquiring clinical information be adopted. For example, concerning trials of treatments for AIDS, Byar et al.[13] have said that "some traditional approaches to the clinical-trials process may be unnecessarily rigid and unsuitable for this disease." In this case, AIDS is not what is so different; rather, the difference is in the presence of AIDS activists, articulate spokespersons for the ethical problems created by the application of the randomized clinical trial to terminal illnesses. Such arguments are equally applicable to advanced cancer and other serious illnesses. Byar et al. agree that there are even circumstances in which uncontrolled clinical trials may be justified: when there is no effective treatment to use as a control, when the prognosis is uniformly poor, and when there is a reasonable expectation of benefit without excessive toxicity. These conditions are usually found in clinical trials of advanced cancer.

The purpose of the randomized clinical trial is to avoid the problems of observer bias and patient selection. It seems to us that techniques might be developed to deal with these issues in other ways. Randomized clinical trials deal with them in a cumbersome and heavy-handed manner, by requiring large numbers of patients in the hope that random assignment will balance the heterogeneous distribution of patients into the different groups. By observing known characteristics of patients, such as age and sex, and distributing them equally between groups, it is thought that unknown factors important in determining outcomes will also be distributed equally. Surely, other techniques can be developed to deal with both observer bias and patient selection. Prospective studies without randomization, but with the evaluation of patients by uninvolved third parties, should remove observer bias. Similar methods have been suggested by Royall.[12] Prospective matched-pair analysis, in which patients are treated in a manner consistent with their physician's views, ought to help ensure equivalence between the groups and thus mitigate the effect of patient selection, at least with regard to known covariates. With regard to unknown covariates, the security would rest, as in randomized trials, in the enrollment of large numbers of patients and in confirmatory studies. This method would not pose ethical difficulties, since patients would receive the treatment recommended by their physician. They would be included in the study by independent observers matching patients with respect to known characteristics, a process that would not affect patient care and that

could be performed independently any number of times.

This brief discussion of alternatives to randomized clinical trials is sketchy and incomplete. We wish only to point out that there may be satisfactory alternatives, not to describe and evaluate them completely. Even if randomized clinical trials were much better than any alternative, however, the ethical dilemmas they present may put their use at variance with the primary obligations of the physician. In this regard, Angell cautions, "If this commitment to the patient is attenuated, even for so good a cause as benefits to future patients, the implicit assumptions of the doctor-patient relationship are violated."[14] The risk of such attenuation by the randomized trial is great. The AIDS activists have brought this dramatically to the attention of the academic medical community. Techniques appropriate to the laboratory may not be applicable to humans. We must develop and use alternative methods for acquiring clinical knowledge.

NOTES

1. Hellman S. Randomized clinical trials and the doctor-patient relationship: an ethical dilemma. *Cancer Clin Trials* 1979; 2:189–93.
2. *Idem.* A doctor's dilemma: the doctor-patient relationship in clinical investigation. In: Proceedings of the Fourth National Conference on Human Values and Cancer, New York, March 15–17, 1984. New York: American Cancer Society, 1984:144–6.
3. Kass LR. *Toward a more natural science: biology and human affairs.* New York: Free Press, 1985:196.
4. Palca J. AIDS drug trials enter new age. *Science* 1989; 246:19–21.
5. Rawls J. *A theory of justice.* Cambridge, Mass.: Belknap Press of Harvard University Press, 1971:183–92, 446–52.
6. Merigan TC. You *can* teach an old dog new tricks—how AIDS trials are pioneering new strategies. *N Engl J Med* 1990; 323: 1341–3.
7. Freedman B. Equipoise and the ethics of clinical research. *N Engl J Med* 1987; 317:141–5.
8. Singer PA, Lantos JD, Whitington PF, Broelsch CE, Siegler M. Equipoise and the ethics of segmental liver transplantation. *Clin Res* 1988; 36:539–45.
9. Longcope WT. Methods and medicine. *Bull Johns Hopkins Hosp* 1932; 50:4–20.
10. Report on medical ethics. *World Med Assoc Bull* 1949; 1:109, 111.

11. Popper K. The problem of induction. In: Miller D, ed., *Popper selections*. Princeton, N.J.: Princeton University Press, 1985: 101–17.
12. Royall RM. Ethics and statistics in randomized clinical trials. *Stat Sci* 1991; 6(1):52–62.

13. Byar DP, Schoenfeld DA, Green SB, et al. Design considerations for AIDS trials. *N Engl J Med* 1990; 323:1343–8.
14. Angell M. Patients' preferences in randomized clinical trials. *N Engl J Med* 1984; 310:1385–7.

A Response to a Purported Ethical Difficulty with Randomized Clinical Trials Involving Cancer Patients

Benjamin Freedman

In recent years, for a variety of reasons, the mainstay of clinical investigation—the randomized controlled clinical trial (RCT)—has increasingly come under attack. Since Charles Fried's influential monograph,[1] the opponents of controlled trials have claimed the moral high ground. They claim to perceive a conflict between the medical and scientific duties of the physician-investigator, and between the conduct of the trial and a patient's rights. Samuel and Deborah Hellman write, for example, that "the randomized clinical trial routinely asks physicians to sacrifice the interests of their particular patients for the sake of the study and that of the information that it will make available for the benefit of society."[2] Maurie Markman's attraction to this point of view is clear when he writes that "the individual physician's principal ethical responsibility is to the *individual patient* that he or she is treating, and *not* to future patients [emphases in original]." In the interests of returning Markman to the fold, I will concentrate on resolving this central challenge to the ethics of RCTs.

It is unfortunately true that the most common responses from pro-trialists, by revealing fundamental misunderstandings of basic ethical concepts, do not inspire confidence in the ethics of human research as it is currently conducted. Proponents of clinical trials will commonly begin their apologia by citing benefits derived from trials—by validating the safety and efficacy of new treatments, and, at least as important, by discrediting accepted forms of treatment. So far so good. But they often go on to argue that there is a need to balance the rights of subjects against the needs of society. By this tactic, the proponents of clinical trials have implicitly morally surrendered, for to admit that something is a right is to admit that it represents a domain of action protected from the claims or interests of other individuals or of society itself. A liberal society has rightly learned to look askance at claims that rights of individuals need to yield to the demands of the collective. Patients' claims, then, because of their nature as rights, supersede the requirements of the collectivity.

Sometimes, indeed, the surrender is explicit. At the conclusion of a symposium on the ethics of research on human subjects, Sir Colin Dollery, a major figure in clinical trials, complained to the speaker: "You assume a dominant role for ethics—I think to the point of arrogance. Ethical judgments will be of little value unless the scientific innovations about which they are made . . . are useful."[3] But it is the nature of ethical judgments that they are, indeed, "dominant" as normative or accepted guides to action. One may say, "I know that X is the ethical thing to do, but I won't X." That expresses no logical contradiction, but simply weakness of will. But it is, by contrast, plainly contradictory to admit that X is ethical, yet to deny or doubt that one ought to X.

Closer examination and finer distinctions reveal, however, that the conflict between patients' rights

Journal of Clinical Ethics 3, No. 3, Fall 1992: 231–234.

and social interests is not at all at issue in controlled clinical trials. There is no need for proponents of clinical trials to concede the moral high ground.

What is the patient right that is compromised by clinical trials? The fear most common to patients who are hesitant about enrolling is that they would not receive the best care, that their right to treatment would be sacrificed in the interests of science. This presumes, of course, that the patient has a right to treatment. Such a right must in reason be grounded in patient need (a patient who is not ill has no right to treatment) and in medical knowledge and capability (a patient with an incurable illness has rights to be cared for, but no right to be cured).

That granted, we need to specify the kind of treatment to which a patient might reasonably claim a right. It was in this connection that I introduced the concept of *clinical equipoise* as critical to understanding the ethics of clinical trials.[4] Clinical equipoise is a situation in which there exists (or is pending) an honest disagreement in the expert clinical community regarding the comparative merits of two or more forms of treatment for a given condition. To be ethical, a controlled clinical trial must begin and be conducted in a continuing state of clinical equipoise—as between the arms of the study—and must, moreover, offer some reasonable hope that the successful conclusion of the trial will disturb equipoise (that is, resolve the controversy in the expert clinical community).

This theory presumes that a right to a specific medical treatment must be grounded in a professional judgment, which is concretized in the term *clinical equipoise*. A patient who has rights to medical treatment has rights restricted to, though not necessarily exhaustive of, those treatments that are understood by the medical community to be appropriate for his condition. A patient may eccentrically claim some good from a physician that is not recognized by the medical community as appropriate treatment. A physician may even grant this claim; but in so doing, he must realize that he has not provided medical treatment itself. Contrariwise, by failing to fulfill this request, the physician has not failed to satisfy the patient's right to medical treatment.

Provided that a comparative trial is ethical, therefore, it begins in a state of clinical equipoise.

For that reason, by definition, nobody enrolling in the trial is denied his or her right to medical treatment, for no medical consensus for or against the treatment assignment exists.

(The modern climate requires that I introduce two simple caveats. First, I am ignoring economic and political factors that go into the grounding of a right to treatment. This is easy enough for one in Canada to write, but may be difficult for someone in the United States to read. Second, when speaking of treatment that is recognized to be condition-appropriate by the medical community, I mean to include only those judgments grounded in medical knowledge rather than social judgments. I would hope to avoid the current bioethical muddle over "medical futility," but if my claims need to be translated into terms appropriate to that controversy, "physiological futility" is close but not identical to what I mean by "inappropriate." For simplicity's sake, the best model to have in mind is the common patient demand for antibiotic treatment of an illness diagnosed as viral.)

Two errors are commonly committed in connection with the concept of clinical equipoise. The first mistake is in thinking that clinical equipoise (or its disturbance) relates to a single endpoint of a trial—commonly, efficacy. As a function of expert clinical judgment, clinical equipoise must incorporate all of the many factors that go into favoring one regimen over its competitors. Treatment *A* may be favored over *B* because it is more effective; or, because it is almost as effective but considerably less toxic; or, because it is easier to administer, allowing, for example, treatment on an outpatient basis; or, because patients are more compliant with it; and so forth.

Just as equipoise may be based upon any one or a combination of these or other factors, it may be disturbed in the same way. Markman's second example, which discusses the efficacy of a multidrug combination chemotherapy regimen, seems vulnerable to this objection. Even were the results of the Mayo trial convincing with regard to the efficacy of this approach, it has not disturbed clinical equipoise in its favor unless other issues, such as toxicity, have been resolved as well. It is well worth pointing out that the endpoints of trials, particularly in cancer treatment, are far too narrow to disturb clinical equipoise in and of themselves, but they are necessary steps along a seriatim path.

For that matter, in ignoring the compendious judgment involved in ascertaining equipoise, some studies spuriously claim that all of their arms are in equipoise on the basis of one variable (such as five-year survival rates), when they are clearly out of equipoise because of other factors (such as differences in pain and disfigurement).

The second mistake occurs in identifying clinical equipoise with an individual physician's point of indifference between two treatments. Citing the article in which I developed the concept and another article applying it, for example, the Hellmans write, "If the physician has no preference for either treatment (is in a state of equipoise), then randomization is acceptable."[5] But an individual physician is not the arbiter of appropriate or acceptable medical practice.

There are numerous occasions outside of clinical trials where outsiders need to determine whether the treatment provided was appropriate to the patient's condition. Regulators, as well as third-party payers—private or governmental—need to answer the question, as do health planners and administrators of health-care facilities. Disciplinary bodies of professional associations, and, most tellingly, courts judging allegations of malpractice, have to ascertain this as well. It is never the case that the judgment of an individual physician concerning whether a treatment is condition-appropriate (that is, whether it belongs within the therapeutic armamentarium) is sufficient. In all of these instances, however varied might be their rules of investigation and procedure, the ultimate question is: Does the expert professional community accept this treatment as appropriate for this condition? Since clinical equipoise and its disturbance applies to putative medical treatments for given conditions, this is a matter that is determined legally, morally, and reasonably by that medical community with the recognized relevant expertise.

Markman may have fallen into this error, writing repeatedly of the judgment of the treating or enrolling physician (and, in the first page, of the responsibility of "the individual physician") with respect to the clinical trial. There is, however, another way of looking at this. Whereas the status of a putative treatment within the medical armamentarium must be settled by the medical *community*, the application of that judgment *vis-à-vis* a given patient is, of course, the judgment (and the responsibility) of the *individual physician*. This individual clinical judgment must be exercised when enrolling a subject, rather than subjugated to the judgment of those who constructed the trial. Indeed, many studies will list this as a criterion of exclusion: "Those subjects who, in the judgment of the accruing physician, would be put at undue risk by participating."

Another point: the Hellmans write of a physician's duty in treating a patient to employ what he "thinks, suspects, believes, or has a hunch about."[6] This is clearly overstated as a duty: why not add to the list the physician's hopes, fantasies, fond but dotty beliefs, and illusions? Yet patients do choose physicians, in part, because of trust in their tacit knowledge and inchoate judgment, and not merely their sapient grasp of the current medical consensus. It would be a disservice to patients for a physician to see his or her role simply as a vehicle for transmitting the wisdom received from the expert medical community in all cases (though when a departure is made, this is done at the legal peril of the doctor!).

But what follows from this inalienable duty of the treating physician? Not as much as the opponents of trials would have us believe. A physician certainly has the right to refuse to participate in a trial that he believes places some participants at a medical disadvantage. Moreover, if he or she is convinced of that, he or she has a *duty* to abstain from participating. But that only speaks to the physician, and does not necessarily affect the patient. What opponents of trials forget is that the patient—the subject—is the ultimate decision maker—in fact, in law, and in ethics. In at least some cases, the fact that there is an open trial for which a patient meets the eligibility criteria needs to be disclosed as one medical alternative, to satisfy ethical norms of informed consent. A physician with convictions that the trial will put subjects at undue risk should inform the prospective subject of that conviction and the reasons for it, and may well recommend to the subject to decline participation. It will then be up to the patient whether to seek enrollment via another physician.

Most commonly at issue, though, is a physician's preference rather than conviction. In such cases, it is perfectly ethical—and becomingly modest—for a physician to participate in a trial, setting aside private misgivings based upon anecdote as overbalanced by the medical literature.

Finally, something should be said about the underlying philosophical buttress on which anti-trialists rely. Following Kant, the Hellmans argue that the underlying issue is that persons "ought not to be treated merely as means to an end; rather, they must always be treated as ends in themselves."[7] Clinical trials, however, are designed to yield reliable data and to ground scientifically valid inferences. In that sense, the treatments and examinations that a subject of a clinical trial undergoes are means to a scientific end, rather than interventions done solely for the subject's own benefit.

But the Kantian formulation is notoriously rigoristic, and implausible in the form cited. We treat others as means all the time, in order to achieve ends the others do not share, and are so treated in return. When buying a carton of milk or leaving a message, I am treating the cashier or secretary as means to an end they do not share. Were this unvarnished principle to hold, all but purely altruistic transactions would be ethically deficient. Clinical trials would be in very good (and, indeed, very bad) company. Those who follow the Kantian view are not concerned about treating another as a means, but rather about treating someone in a way that contradicts the other's personhood itself—that is, in a way that denies the fact that the person is not simply a means but is also an end. A paradigm case is when I treat someone in a way that serves my ends but, at the same time, is contrary to the other's best interests. It is true that a subject's participation in a clinical trial serves scientific ends, but what has not been shown is that it is contrary to the best interests of the subject. In cases where the two equipoise conditions are satisfied, this cannot be shown.

However, in some cases we are uncertain about whether an intervention will serve the best interests of the other, and so we ask that person. That is one reason for requiring informed consent to studies. There is another. By obtaining the consent of the other party to treat him as an end to one's own means, in effect, an identity of ends between both parties has been created. Applying this amended Kantian dictum, then, we should ask: Is there anything about clinical trials that necessarily implies that subjects are treated contrary to their personhood? And the answer is, of course, no—provided a proper consent has been obtained.

There remain many hard questions to ask about the ethics of controlled clinical studies. Many talents will be needed to address those questions and to reform current practice. Since those questions will only be asked by those who understand that such studies rest upon a sound ethical foundation, I am hopeful that Markman and others will reconsider their misgivings.

NOTES

1. C. Fried, *Medical Experimentation: Personal Integrity and Social Policy* (New York: Elsevier, 1974).
2. S. Hellman and D.S. Hellman, "Of Mice but Not Men," *New England Journal of Medicine* 324 (1991): 1585–89, at 1586.
3. Comment by Sir Colin Dollery in discussion following H.-M. Sass, "Ethics of Drug Research and Drug Development," *Arzneimittel Forschung/Drug Research* 39 (II), Number 8a (1989): 1041–48, at 1048.
4. B. Freedman, "Equipoise and the Ethics of Clinical Research," *New England Journal of Medicine* 317 (1987): 141–45.
5. Hellman and Hellman, "Of Mice," 1586.
6. *Ibid.*
7. *Ibid.*

SECTION 3

Access to Experimental Therapies and Experimentation on "Vulnerable" Populations

Changing Views of Justice after Belmont: AIDS and the Inclusion of "Vulnerable" Subjects

Carol Levine

THE PRINCIPLE OF JUSTICE REVISITED

At the end of the twentieth century, historical time has become compressed. No longer do "eras" last for a century or more. In research ethics, *The Belmont Report* has achieved the status of a historical document already due for re-evaluation. Yet it was published in 1978, just two decades ago. . . .

The Belmont Report represented the culmination of the work of the National Commission for the Protection of Human Subjects of Biomedical and Behavioral Research. In its emphasis on three classic principles of theological and secular ethics—respect for persons, beneficence, and justice—it drew on the centuries-old history of Western thought. In its emphasis on protecting human subjects from harm, coercion, and unconsented experimentation, it reflected the history of the 30 years immediately preceding it.

This emphasis is understandable, given the signal event in the modern history of clinical-research ethics—the cruel and often fatal experiments performed on unconsenting prisoners by Nazi doctors during World War II.[1] American public opinion was shaped by the revelations of unethical experiments such as the Willowbrook hepatitis B studies

at an institution for mentally retarded children;[2] the Jewish Chronic Disease Hospital studies, in which live cancer cells were injected into uninformed elderly patients;[3] and, especially, the Tuskegee Syphilis Study of poor black sharecroppers.[4] The single most influential article was written by Henry Knowles Beecher, a respected anesthesiologist, in the *New England Journal of Medicine*. Beecher described a number of studies at major research institutions that placed subjects at risk and failed to obtain informed consent.[5]

Our basic approach to the ethical conduct of research and approval of investigational drugs was born in scandal and reared in protectionism. Perceived as vulnerable, either because of their membership in groups lacking social power or because of personal characteristics suggesting a lack of autonomy, individuals were the primary focus of this concern.

Today the *Belmont* principles are still firmly in place. But there has been a major shift in emphasis and the beginnings of a shift in practice. Investigators, regulators, and institutional review boards (IRBs) are accustomed to examining the risk-benefit ratio (applying the principle of beneficence) and informed consent (applying the principle of respect for persons). But the selection of subjects as a matter of justice has often been considered last and in only one of its aspects—the protection of vulnerable groups from exploitation as subjects. Making justice an equal partner with respect for persons and beneficence does not reduce the likelihood of conflict among the

From *The Ethics of Research Involving Human Subjects: Facing the 21st Century*, H. Vanderpool, editor, University Publishing Group, 1996, 105–26. Used with permission of the publisher.

EDITORS' NOTE: This article has been edited; notes have been renumbered.

principles or their corollaries; in fact, it adds a layer of complexity.

In *The Belmont Report*, the National Commission stated that justice is relevant to the selection of subjects at two levels—the social and the individual. At the individual level, the National Commission advised that "researchers exhibit fairness: thus, they should not offer potentially beneficial research only to some patients who are in their favor or select only 'undesirable' persons for risky research." At the social level, it said, "distinctions [should] be drawn between classes of subjects that ought, and ought not, to participate in any particular kind of research, based on the ability of members of that class to bear burdens and on the appropriateness of placing further burdens on already burdened persons." Specifically, the National Commission recommended, on the grounds of social justice, that classes of subjects be selected in an order of preference (for example, adults before children), and that some classes of potential subjects (for example, prisoners and the institutionalized mentally infirm) be selected only under certain conditions and perhaps not at all.

AIDS AS A CATALYST

It is ironic that around the same time that *The Belmont Report* was published, the forces of change—in the form of a new disease eventually called AIDS—were already emerging. The first official Centers for Disease Control report from Los Angeles, issued in June 1981, described cases of an unexplained illness in homosexual men who had been treated in the previous 30 months. Although other social, economic, and political forces have contributed to the shift in emphasis in the *Belmont* principles away from protectionism and toward inclusionism, AIDS has been the major catalyst for change.

AIDS took the world by surprise. Disregarding biological and human history, we in the industrialized world had largely come to believe that infectious diseases no longer posed a major threat. Epidemics were, we thought, either relegated to history, curable through one of the miracle drugs of the postwar pharmaceutical armamentarium, or a problem confined to the known diseases of the developing world.

Just as the medical and scientific worlds had to come to terms with the phenomenon of a new and complex retroviral disease, the worlds of law, ethics, and public policy had to grapple with the implications of a communicable disease primarily affecting groups—homosexual men and drug users of both sexes and their children—already stigmatized by mainstream society.

The ethics of research involving human subjects that had developed in the postwar period had focused on individual rights and welfare and on benefits to society through the acquisition of knowledge. It had not been much concerned with threats to public health through communicable diseases, nor with the impotence of medicine to halt or even significantly delay the deaths of large numbers of previously healthy young adults. Some of these young adults and their compatriots refused, in Dylan Thomas's phrase, to "go gently into that good night"; in their "railing against the dying of the light," they accelerated and shaped the deregulation of the drug-approval process that was already underway as a result of pressure from the pharmaceutical industry, legislators, and the public.

The initial demands from people with AIDS and their advocates were based on claims of individual justice and autonomy; that is, sick and dying patients wanted to make their own choices and take their own chances by using unapproved drugs for their lethal condition. The focus was on allowing broader access to ongoing clinical trials by patients who were willing to trade off potentially increased and certainly unknown risk for the possibility, however small, of benefit. Some patients, with the complicity of their physicians, managed to enroll by fudging data or lying outright, a practice well known in cancer trials.[6] Patients who were ineligible for trials because they did not fit the entry criteria or who did not want to be randomized into one of the study groups of a research protocol wanted the option of taking investigational drugs from the trial protocol.

The focus soon broadened, however, to questions of social justice. Groups disproportionately affected by HIV/AIDS—prisoners, drug users, and women (including many members of ethnic minorities)—were excluded from trials, either because of strict protocol entry criteria or because of lack of access to the physicians and healthcare institutions that control research. Interestingly, the initial calls for broadened access often came from those who were included—gay white men—and not just, or possibly not even primarily, from those who were excluded. Many clinicians, desperately seeking therapeutic options, also supported broadened access. . . .

SELECTING THE LEAST VULNERABLE

Underlying the protectionist view of the selection of subjects is the assumption that research is risky or at least burdensome. If this is true, then subjects should be selected in a way that protects those whose social, demographic, or economic characteristics make them particularly vulnerable to coercion and exploitation.

AIDS has been a catalyst for change, and the absence in recent years of the kind of scandal that came to light with depressing regularity in the 1960s and 1970s removed one barrier to change. The view of research as inherently risky and of research subjects as inherently needing protection has changed in the past several years. The actual physical risk in most research studies appears to be quite low. The President's Commission for the Study of Ethical Problems in Biomedical and Behavioral Research asked three large research institutions to summarize their experience with research-related injuries.[7] Each group found a very low incidence of adverse effects. In one institution, out of more than 8,000 subjects involved in 157 protocols, only three adverse effects were reported, including two headaches after spinal taps. Some of these reassuring results may be due to the vigilance of IRBs and investigators in reducing the likelihood of risk in designing and implementing studies. (There are, nonetheless, sporadic reports of serious injury and death to research subjects.)[8] While risk is an element that subjects always should consider when deciding whether to enter a study, it is now often no longer the paramount issue.

OPENING DOORS AT NIH AND FDA

In arguing for wider inclusion criteria in clinical trials, patient advocates and some clinicians have noted that, in the interest of good medical care, drugs should be tested on the populations that will use them. This belief runs counter to the more traditional research view of subject selection, which focuses on testing drugs in a small, homogeneous population in order to detect differences in efficacy and side effects as rapidly as possible.

The conventional view of appeals for broadened access is that they come from advocacy groups, sometimes noisy and disruptive ones. Yet traditional, even conservative, bodies have stated similar views. For example, the Council on Ethical and Judicial Affairs of the American Medical Association (AMA) declared in its 1991 report, "Gender Disparities in Clinical Decision Making," that "results of medical testing done solely on men should not be generalized to women without evidence that results can be applied safely and effectively to both sexes. Research on health problems that affect both sexes should include male and female subjects."[9]

Advocates' efforts have been given additional weight by the Congressional General Accounting Office (GAO). Examining the inclusion of women in clinical trials, the GAO reviewed the practices of the National Institutes of Health and the Food and Drug Administration.[10] In both instances women were found to be underrepresented. In June 1990, the GAO reported that grant applicants and NIH staff were noncompliant with the agency's stated policy of "encouraging" the inclusion of women as research subjects. Although NIH disagreed with some of the GAO's conclusions, in September 1990 it established the Office of Research on Women's Health "to strengthen and enhance the efforts of the NIH to improve the prevention, diagnosis, and treatment of illness in women and to enhance research related to diseases and conditions that affect women."[11]

In a potentially powerful move, because it brings to bear the power of the federal purse, the *NIH Guide for Grants and Contracts* now *requires* the inclusion of women and minorities. The guide states that grant, cooperative-agreement, and contract applicants:

> will be required to include minorities and women in study populations so that research findings can be of benefit to all persons at risk of the disease, disorder or condition under study; special emphasis should be placed on the needs for inclusion of conditions which disproportionately affect them. This policy is intended to apply to males and females of all ages. If women or minorities are excluded or are inadequately represented in clinical research, particularly in

proposed population-based studies, a clear compelling rationale for exclusion or inadequate representation should be provided.

Furthermore, any justification for not including women in such studies will be evaluated by the peer-review group assessing the proposal and factored into the final recommendation. No application or proposal for which the justification for exclusion of women is considered inappropriate will be funded unless such a justification is compelling."[12] To date there has been no official accounting of how this policy is working or whether some projects have not been funded because of lack of representativeness.

In Section 492B of the 1993 NIH Revitalization Act, Congress extended this policy by requiring NIH's director to ensure that "each federally funded research project include women and members of minority groups."[13] The NIH director can authorize exceptions. NIH-funded trials must be analyzed to determine whether women or members of minority groups would respond differently to the intervention or agents being studied. Cost is not a permissible consideration in determining whether inclusion is appropriate. Cost may be considered only when the data regarding women or members of minority groups that would be obtained in the project have been or will be obtained through other means that offer comparable quality. This legislative provision does not answer the question of whether transportation, child care, and other types of financial support that will be necessary to enroll women will be considered legitimate trial costs.

An Institute of Medicine study cautions:

neither adherence to quotas in the composition of a study cohort nor the irrational exclusion of a subgroup of people can be supported scientifically. Determining the number of women to be included in a trial should reflect reasonable hypotheses about the relation of treatment efficacy to sex, not global rules about the composition of study cohorts.[14]

The forces of change have not been limited to the NIH. The GAO's review of FDA policies and practices, issued in October 1992, found that although women were represented in every clinical trial of the 53 drugs approved by the FDA in the previous three and one-half years, for more than 60 percent of the drugs the proportion of women in the trial was less than the proportion of women with the corresponding disease. Women were particularly underrepresented in trials of cardiovascular drugs, even though cardiovascular disease is the leading cause of death in women. The report found that the FDA has not "issued specific guidance or criteria for drug manufacturers to use in determining the extent and sufficiency of female representation in Phase 2 and 3 drug trials." The FDA has not defined "representation" nor provided guidance to drug manufacturers for determining when sufficient numbers of women are included in clinical trials to detect gender-related differences in drug response. As a result, pharmaceutic sponsors are uncertain as to what the FDA expects. The focus of challenges to FDA policies has been the agency's 1977 guidelines for the clinical evaluation of drugs. Until the guidelines were revised in mid-1993, women of child-bearing age were excluded from large-scale clinical trials until the FDA Animal Reproduction Guidelines were completed, except in cases of life-threatening illness. For Phase 1 studies (to determine pharmacokinetics, the safety of a range of doses, or the mechanism of a drug action) the guidelines stated that "in general, women of child-bearing potential should be excluded." For Phase 2 studies (small-scale trials to determine efficacy), women could be included "provided segment II and the female part of segment I of the FDA Animal Reproduction Guidelines have been completed."[15]

Explaining the FDA's decision to revise the guidelines, an FDA working group noted: "In 1993, protecting the fetus from unanticipated exposure to potentially harmful drugs remains critically important, but the ban on women's participation in early clinical trials no longer seems reasonable." The working group cited the scientific benefits of identifying important sex differences in early drug trials, the ethical benefits in terms of enhancing autonomy, and the possibility of reducing the risk of fetal exposure through protocol design (administering a single dose to a woman during or immediately following her menstrual period or after a negative pregnancy-test result).[16]

Even with broadened inclusion criteria, not all patients who want access to promising new agents can be enrolled in clinical trials, either because they fail to meet the inclusion criteria, they live too far away from a research center, or the trials are already closed. Several other mechanisms have been developed, such as the "parallel track," in which qualified patients who cannot enroll in clinical trials may obtain promising drugs through their physicians.[17] Community-based research, especially in cancer and AIDS, has also made clinical trials more accessible to patients. Buyers' clubs make drugs that are on the market in Europe and Asia available to patients, largely without FDA interference.

CHILDREN AS RESEARCH SUBJECTS

Nearly all drugs approved for marketing by the FDA carry a label warning that "this drug is not to be used in children . . ." or "is not recommended for use in infants and young children, since few studies have been carried out in this group. . . ." Pediatricians are forced to extrapolate and estimate dosages for their young patients. As Robert J. Levine has pointed out, "We have a tendency to distribute unsystematically the unknown risks of drugs in children and pregnant women, thus maximizing the frequency of their occurrence and minimizing the probability of their detection."[18]

Protocols involving sick children present particularly difficult choices for investigators, IRBs, primary-care physicians, parents, and foster-care agencies. Investigators typically present information to IRBs to justify the participation of children. Given the ethical imperative to do research, especially on lethal diseases such as HIV/AIDS, an IRB would be hard pressed to justify any delays or significant revisions in a pediatric protocol.

In the past few years, there have been significant advances in pediatric HIV research: notably, studies on AZT, ddI, and ddC. The NIAID now has 15 pediatric AIDS Clinical Treatment Units (ACTUs) within the ACTG. The National Institute of Child Health and Development also has a clinical-trials network, and several other NIH institutes, such as the National Cancer Institute, are also involved in pediatric research. The development of an effective method to prevent maternal-fetal transmission, through the use of anti-retroviral drugs or vaccines, is a high priority nationally and internationally as well.

The public attention on pediatric AIDS has made an impact on pediatric research in other areas. In the fall of 1990, the Pharmaceutical Manufacturers Association published its first survey of drug testing with children. The survey found that 114 pediatric drugs and vaccines were undergoing testing, "although researchers are faced with problems of recruitment, safety and costs for drug testing in children."[19]

The 114 medicines involved 127 research projects, because some of the drugs and vaccines were being tested for more than one use. A quarter of the research projects (32) were for rare diseases; 11 were for genetic disorders, seven each are for HIV/AIDS and growth disorders, and another five were for asthma. Bacterial infections and cancer were the largest categories, with 26 and 24 drugs, respectively. Developing improved DPT vaccines (diphtheria, pertussis, and tetanus) was a high priority. Nine projects dealt with viral infections, including polio, chicken pox, and measles.

Because many of the potential child subjects for HIV/AIDS research are in foster care, their opportunities for participation have been severely limited by the lack of state or agency policies and the reluctance of agency officials to approve the entry of children into trials*. . . .

TOWARD THE 21ST CENTURY

In looking toward the future, we must again he mindful of the past. There still are significant barriers to a full implementation of the principle of justice as exemplified in the selection of research subjects. Two experiences in particular have shaped current attitudes and practices. Two words carry enormous symbolic weight: thalidomide and Tuskegee.

The experience that has most influenced the exclusion of women from research is related to the drug thalidomide: typically it is referred to as the "thalidomide disaster."[20] Thalidomide was synthesized in West Germany in 1954 and approved for marketing in 1958. Its primary use was as a sedative and antidote for nausea in early pregnancy. At least 20 countries approved the over-the-counter sale of thalidomide, including Canada, Great Britain, Australia, and Sweden, but not the United States.

*EDITORS' NOTE: In August 1997 President Clinton proposed that drug companies be required to test their products in children before marketing them for pediatric use. Drug companies oppose the proposal, saying it would put children needlessly at risk and raise costs.

During the same period that thalidomide was being widely distributed, physicians noted an alarming increase in the number of children being born with an unusual and extremely rare set of deformities. The most prominent feature was *phocomelia,* a condition in which the hands are attached to the shoulders and the feet are attached to the hips, superficially resembling the flippers of a seal. By 1962, when sufficient statistical evidence had accumulated to establish thalidomide as the agent causing these deformities, about 8,000 children had been affected. About 35 percent of the women who had received this drug—even a single dose of it—during early pregnancy bore deformed babies. The harm done to women and their infants by thalidomide was not the result of participation in research; it was the result of inadequate research standards (even by contemporary standards), corporate greed, and physicians' uncritical acceptance of promotional claims. The West German firm that developed thalidomide had had to redefine the nature of "sleep" in standard animal tests to prove that the drug had a hypnotic effect; it ignored early and disquieting reports of side effects—including the very serious neurological complication of peripheral neuritis—and it concealed the number of reported cases of this complication. It used money and influence to counter critical reports with favorable ones. Physicians, too, were at fault in succumbing to aggressive promotional efforts to use a new drug when older, more adequately tested drugs were available.

Animal tests that would have proved that thalidomide was teratogenic were not generally performed at the time. However, those that were available would have clearly established the strong possibility of teratogenicity, and it was well known that drugs could cross the placental barrier and affect the fetus. In fact, a British scientist at the firm that held the distribution license for thalidomide discovered that baby rabbits born to mothers given the drug had the same deformities found in children.

In the United States, a cautious FDA official, Dr. Frances Kelsey—suspecting that thalidomide might cause birth defects—delayed marketing approval, thus lessening the impact on American women. Nevertheless, over 1,200 "investigating" doctors did give their patients the thalidomide made available to them by the drug company that was seeking approval (perhaps in an effort to build physicians'

support for the drug). At least 18 thalidomide babies were born in this country as a result, and many more women carrying affected fetuses miscarried.

Dr. Kelsey's caution was well grounded, and the 1962 Kefauver-Harris amendments to the drug-approval laws institutionalized a rigorous preapproval process (Food, Drug, and Cosmetic Act, 1962).[21] Equally important, the powerful emotional impact of the thalidomide experience created an aversion to involving women, especially pregnant women or women of childbearing age, in drug research. Investigators, IRBs, and regulators all approach the inclusion of women of childbearing age in drug trials with considerable caution, if not outright aversion.* Only a few IRBs have developed specific policies in favor of inclusion, and these are in community-based HIV/AIDS research settings. For example, in 1989 the Community Research Initiative (CRI, now the Community Research Initiative on AIDS, or CRIA) in New York City developed the policy statement, "Participants of Reproductive Potential." It states:

> CRI, in recognition of the continuing exclusion of women from clinical trials, will make every effort not to accept a protocol that treats women and men of reproductive potential differently, unless there is solid scientific basis for that difference. In assessing the legitimacy of exclusion criteria regarding the reproductive potential (including pregnancy), CRI will not necessarily place higher value on the potential risk in offspring than on the potential benefit to the trial participant, as in other situations where the potential benefit to the life and health of the patient is considered to justify some increment of risk to the health of the potential offspring. In making this judgment, the CRI will take into account the availability of alternative therapies for the potential parent which present less risk to potential offspring.
>
> CRI will undertake to ensure that all participants in approved trials will receive adequate information about potential adverse reproductive outcomes.

The IRB of the Whitman-Walker Clinic in

---

*EDITORS' NOTE: Thalidomide has made a strong therapeutic comeback and is now being used for patients with leprosy, lupus, HIV infection, and other immune diseases. There are strong warnings against use by pregnant women or women who might become pregnant, but no controls in the open market.

Washington, D.C., has also considered the exclusion of women in HIV-drug studies. Its statement declares: "We call on other IRBs to reject participation in any drug trial that excludes women and to join together to demand systematic drug studies of promising drug treatments for pregnant women and women who decline to use birth control methods. "[22]

In 1975 Bernard L. Mirkin, Professor of Pediatrics and Pharmacology at the University of Minnesota, posed the options available to society bluntly:

> Society may choose to forbid drug evaluation in pregnant women and children. This choice would certainly reduce the risk of damaging individuals through research. However, this would maximize the possibility of random disaster resulting from use of inadequately investigated drugs. In the final analysis it seems safe to predict that more individuals would be damaged; however, the damage would be distributed randomly rather than imposed upon preselected individuals.[23]

The Tuskegee experience presents a barrier of a different sort. This 40-year, Public Health Service sponsored study began in 1932 in rural Macon County, Georgia. Building on both a beneficent motive (using research to replace diminishing funds for syphilis-control programs among poor blacks) and dubious (but then popular) theories about racial differences in disease between blacks and whites, the Tuskegee study enrolled 400 black men with syphilis and 200 members of a control group to study the natural history of the untreated disease. Although the study was originally planned to last only six to nine months, it was extended for 40 years.

The abuses of subjects' rights and welfare during this long period have been well documented: false descriptions of research procedures like spinal taps as treatment; failure to provide currently available therapy and, when it became available, a cure by penicillin; lack of informed consent; the use of burial funds as an inducement to family members to give permission for autopsies.[24] The legacy of Tuskegee is "a trail of distrust and suspicion" that hampers efforts to enroll African Americans in clinical trials as well as to attract them to HIV-prevention and -education programs. Dr. Mark Smith testified to the National Commission on AIDS that the African-American community "is already alienated from the health-care system and the government and . . . somewhat cynical about the motives of those who arrive in their communities to help them."[25] Stephen Thomas and Sandra Crouse Quinn have asserted in a compelling article that the continuing legacy of Tuskegee "has contributed to Blacks' belief that genocide is possible and that public health authorities cannot be trusted."[26]

Although the details of both the thalidomide and Tuskegee stories may have become distorted in the retelling, they easily fit into powerful beliefs about risks to fetuses, on the one hand, and the existence of officially condoned racism to the point of genocide, on the other.

Moreover, important ethical issues in both instances have not been resolved. There is no resolution of the conflict between American society's failure to provide basic healthcare and HIV/AIDS prevention programs to poor communities of color—a matter of social justice—and the potential coerciveness of using research participation as an entry into the healthcare system. "Why," one African-American woman said to me, "am I in such demand as a research subject when nobody wants me as a patient?"

In redressing the imbalance caused by policies that exclude women without scientific or ethical justification, it is important to remember that women, particularly women who are or may become pregnant, have special moral responsibilities to fetuses that they plan to carry to term, as do investigators and IRB members who develop or approve protocols involving women. The ethical obligation not to do harm carries particular force when the recipient of the potential harm is an unconsenting fetus, whose future health and welfare may be unalterably affected. Approval by an IRB of a protocol is not an ethically neutral stance: it is an affirmative statement that the choices to be offered to potential subjects, while perhaps difficult to make, are ethically justifiable. Exposing a fetus to serious risk when there are alternative treatments or when the benefits are modest is not, in my view, an ethically justifiable choice.

The potential of harm to a fetus is a morally relevant factor, not least to the mother herself. The vast majority of women see their own primary interests as identical with those of their fetuses. Women do not lightly undertake any medical intervention that will have an adverse outcome on their fetuses; many women in fact may deny themselves optimal medical care in order to avoid risk. Some, however, may exercise their right to choose medical treatments despite known or unknown risks to the fetus.

Some, perhaps most, protocols may not present any known or foreseeable risks to fetuses; for these protocols, there are (as has already been pointed out) no reasons to exclude women, especially those who are not pregnant or do not plan to become pregnant. Some HIV/AIDS protocols may carry the possibility of minimal or even moderate risk to fetuses, but also offer the possibility of great benefit to women. An obvious example would be a life-saving drug or a cure. Another example might be a study involving a drug to treat a debilitating opportunistic infection for which there are no acceptable alternative therapies. In these cases women should not be excluded automatically but should be given the opportunity to make that calculus for themselves, with careful explanation of the risks and benefits.

There remains, however, the small but worrisome category of studies involving drugs that present high risk to fetuses and minimal or even moderate benefit to women. Some would argue that risks to fetuses, as unconsenting participants, must always outweigh considerations of autonomy. Others would argue that there are never any grounds to override a woman's autonomy and to deny her the choice of whether to participate. In this view, valuing a fetus's welfare more highly than a woman's autonomy is objectionable in principle.

Is there a middle ground? Protocols in other diseases may fail to gain approval on grounds of excessive risk to subjects, even when there are potential benefits. Risks to fetuses cannot simply be dismissed as irrelevant, even if one does not grant them rights. But what would constitute serious or excessive risk? Opinions would differ. . . .

At the extremes, choices about including pregnant women or women of childbearing age are relatively straightforward. Excluding a woman suffering from a life-threatening condition from access to a potentially life-saving drug on the grounds of harm to an unconceived fetus seems not only unjust but harsh. When the woman is pregnant and her life is in danger, her fetus is equally threatened. At the other extreme, to expose women and their actual or potential fetuses

to serious harms when there are alternative therapies or the potential benefits are only trivial honors autonomy at the expense of common sense.

Even if exclusionary barriers related to gender or substance abuse were totally removed, women would still face problems in access to research because of their lack of access to primary healthcare and their special needs for assistance with childcare, transportation, and family responsibilities. Recruitment efforts will have to take into account the multiple roles women play as family caregivers and employees (often in marginal jobs with few opportunities for flexibility). Meeting their own healthcare needs may not be their highest priority; enrolling in research, an alien concept to many, may seem even less important.

The goal is not to convince women to become research subjects, either for their own good or for the good of society, but to make the selection of subjects to undertake the risks and share in the benefits of research more equitable.

Are we headed back to the future? Or can we use the past to create a more just healthcare and research system? As we debate the refining and reinterpretation of the principles of *The Belmont Report*, let us not lose sight of their value as markers of the past and guideposts leading us into the 21st century.

NOTES

1. A.L. Caplan, *When Medicine Went Mad: Bioethics and the Holocaust* (Totawa, N.J.; Humana Press, 1992).
2. D.J. Rothman, "Were Tuskegee and Willowbrook 'Studies in Nature'?" *Hastings Center Report* 12 (April 1982): 5-7.
3. J. Katz, *Experimentation with Human Beings* (New York: Russell Sage Foundation, 1972).
4. J. Jones, *Bad Blood: The Tuskegee Syphilis Experiment*, 2d ed. (New York: Free Press, 1993).
5. H.K. Beecher, "Ethics and Clinical Research," *New England Journal of Medicine* 274 (1966): 1354-60; D.J. Rothman, *Strangers at the Bedside: A History of How Law and Bioethics Transformed Medical Decision Making* (New York: Basic Books, 1991).
6. H.Y. Vanderpool and G.B. Weis, "False Data and Last Hopes: Enrolling Patients in Clinical Trials," *Hastings Center Report* (April 1987): 16-19.
7. The President's Commission for the Study of Ethical Problems in Medicine and Biomedical and Behavioral Research, *Compensating for Research Injuries: The Ethical*

and *Legal Implications of Programs to Redress Injured Subjects* (Washington, D.C.: U.S. Government Printing Office, 1982).

8. See, for example, a report of two deaths in the first days of an NIH trial of a new drug for hepatitis B, and the subsequent cancellation of the study. "Tests of Hepatitis Drug are Stopped as 2 Die," *New York Times,* 9 July 1993, A-10.

9. Council on Ethical and Judicial Affairs, "Gender Disparities in Clinical Decision Making," *Journal of the American Medical Association* 266 (1991): 562.

10. GAO, U.S. Congress, *National Institutes of Health: Problems Implementing Policy on Women in Study Populations,* GAO/T-HRD-90-38, (Washington, D.C.: General Accounting Office, 1990); GAO, U.S. Congress, *Women's Health: FDA Needs to Ensure More Study of Gender Differences in Prescription Drug Testing,* GAO/HRD-93-17, (Washington, D.C.: General Accounting Office, 1992).

11. R.L. Kirschstein, "Research on Women's Health," *American Journal of Public Health* 81(1991): 291-93.

12. NIH, *NIH Instruction and Information Memorandum OER 90-5 (Inclusion of Minorities and Women in Study Population),* 12/11/90 (Bethesda, Md.: U.S. Government Printing Office, 1990).

13. U.S. Public Law 103-43, National Institutes of Health Revitalization Amendment, Cong., 1st sess., (10 June 1993).

14. J.C. Bennett, "Inclusion of Women in Clinical Trials—Policies for Population Subgroups," *New England Journal of Medicine* 329 (1993): 288-92.

15. FDA, *General Considerations for the Clinical Evaluation of Drugs* (Washington, D.C.; U.S. Government Printing Office, 1977).

16. R. Merkatz *et al.,* "Women in Clinical Trials of New Drugs: A Change in Food and Drug Administration Policy," *New England Journal of Medicine* 329 (1993): 271–72.

17. "Expanded Availability of Investigational New Drugs through a Parallel Track Mechanism for People with AIDS and Other HIV-related Disease," 57 *Federal Register* 13250-59.

18. R.J. Levine, *Ethics and Regulation of Clinical Research,* 2nd ed. (Baltimore: Urban & Schwarzenberg, 1986), 240.

19. Pharmaceutical Manufacturers Association, *New Medicines in Development for Children* (Washington, D.C.: Pharmaceutical Manufacturers Association, 1990).

20. The Insight Team of the *Sunday Times* of London, *Suffer the Children: The Study of Thalidomide* (New York; Viking Press, 1979).

21. *Food, Drug, and Cosmetic Act, U.S. Code,* vol. 21, secs. 201-902 (1962, as amended 1980), 321-92.

22. Whitman-Walker Clinic Institutional Review Board, *HIV Drug Studies, Women, and Pregnancy: A Statement from the Whitman-Walker Clinic Institutional Review Board* (Washington, D.C.: Whitman-Walker Clinic IRB, n.d.).

23. B.L. Mirkin, "Drug Therapy and the Developing Human: Who Cares?" *Clinical Research* 23 (1975): 110-11.

24. Jones, *Bad Blood.*

25. National Commission on AIDS, *Hearings on HIV Diseases on African American Communities* (Washington, D.C.: U.S. Government Printing Office, 1990), 19.

26. S.B. Thomas and S. Crouse Quinn. 'The Tuskegee Syphilis Study, 1932-1972: Implications for HIV Education and AIDS Risk Education Programs in the Black Community," *American Journal of Public Health* 81 (1991): 1498-1505.

Unethical Trials of Interventions to Reduce Perinatal Transmission of the Human Immunodeficiency Virus in Developing Countries

Peter Lurie and Sidney M. Wolfe

It has been almost three years since the *Journal*[1] published the results of AIDS Clinical Trials Group (ACTG) Study 076, the first randomized,

New England Journal of Medicine 337, September 18, 1997; 853–856. Copyright © 1997 Massachusetts Medical Society. All rights reserved. Used with permission.

controlled trial in which an intervention was proved to reduce the incidence of human immunodeficiency virus (HIV) infection. The anti-retroviral drug zidovudine, administered orally to HIV-positive pregnant women in the United States and France, administered intravenously during labor and subsequently administered to the newborn infants, reduced the incidence of HIV infection by two thirds.[2] The regimen can save the life of one of every seven infants born to HIV-infected women.

Because of these findings, the study was terminated at the first interim analysis and within two months after the results had been announced, the Public Health Service had convened a meeting and concluded that the ACTG 076 regimen should be recommended for all HIV-positive pregnant women without substantial prior exposure to zidovudine and should be considered for other HIV-positive pregnant women on a case-by-case basis.[3] The standard of care for HIV-positive pregnant women thus became the ACTG 076 regimen.

In the United States, three recent studies of clinical practice report that the use of the ACTG 076 regimen is associated with decreases of 50 percent or more in perinatal HIV transmission.[4-6] But in developing countries, especially in Asia and sub-Saharan Africa, where it is projected that by the year 2000, 6 million pregnant women will be infected with HIV,[7] the potential of the ACTG 076 regimen remains unrealized primarily because of the drug's exorbitant cost in most countries.

Clearly, a regimen that is less expensive than ACTG 076 but as effective is desirable, in both developing and industrialized countries. But there has been uncertainty about what research design to use in the search for a less expensive regimen. In June 1994, the World Health Organization (WHO) convened a group in Geneva to assess the agenda for research on perinatal HIV transmission in the wake of ACTG 076. The group, which included no ethicists, concluded, "Placebo-controlled trials offer the best option for a rapid and scientifically valid assessment of alternative antiretroviral drug regimens to prevent [perinatal] transmission of HIV."[8] This unpublished document has been widely cited as justification for subsequent trials in developing countries. In our view, most of these trials are unethical and will lead to hundreds of preventable HIV infections in infants.

Primarily on the basis of documents obtained from the Centers for Disease Control and Prevention (CDC), we have identified 18 randomized, controlled trials of interventions to prevent perinatal HIV transmission that either began to enroll patients after the ACTG 076 study was completed or have not yet begun to enroll patients. The studies are designed to evaluate a variety of interventions: antiretroviral drugs such as zidovudine (usually in regimens that are less expensive or complex than the ACTG 076 regimen), vitamin A and its derivatives, intrapartum vaginal washing, and HIV immune globulin, a form of immunotherapy. These trials involve a total of more than 17,000 women.

In the two studies being performed in the United States, the patients in all the study groups have unrestricted access to zidovudine or other antiretroviral drugs. In 15 of the 16 trials in developing countries, however, some or all of the patients are not provided with antiretroviral drugs. Nine of the 15 studies being conducted outside the United States are funded by the U.S. government through the CDC or the National Institutes of Health (NIH), 5 are funded by other governments, and 1 is funded by the United Nations AIDS Program. The studies are being conducted in Côte d'Ivoire, Uganda, Tanzania, South Africa, Malawi, Thailand, Ethiopia, Burkina Faso, Zimbabwe, Kenya, and the Dominican Republic. These 15 studies clearly violate recent guidelines designed specifically to address ethical issues pertaining to studies in developing countries. According to these guidelines, "The ethical standards applied should be no less exacting than they would be in the case of research carried out in [the sponsoring] country."[9] In addition, U.S. regulations governing studies performed with federal funds domestically or abroad specify that research procedures must "not unnecessarily expose subjects to risk."[10]

The 16th study is noteworthy both as a model of an ethically conducted study attempting to identify less expensive antiretroviral regimens and as an indication of how strong the placebo-controlled trial orthodoxy is. In 1994, Marc Lallemant, a researcher at the Harvard School of Public Health, applied for NIH funding for an equivalency study in Thailand in which three shorter zidovudine regimens were to be compared with a regimen similar to that used in the ACTG 076 study. An equivalency study is typically conducted when a particular regimen has already been proved effective and one is interested in determining whether a second regimen is about as effective but less toxic or expensive.[11] The NIH study section repeatedly put pressure on Lallemant and the Harvard School of Public Health to conduct a placebo-controlled trial instead, prompting the director of Harvard's human subjects committee to reply, "The conduct of a placebo-controlled trial for [zidovudine] in pregnant women in Thailand would be unethical and unacceptable, since an active-controlled trial is feasible."[12] The NIH eventually relented, and the study is now under way. Since the nine studies of antiretroviral drugs have attracted the most attention, we focus on them in this article.

ASKING THE WRONG RESEARCH QUESTION

There are numerous areas of agreement between those conducting or defending these placebo-controlled studies in developing countries and those opposing such trials. The two sides agree that perinatal HIV transmission is a grave problem meriting concerted international attention; that the ACTG 076 trial was a major breakthrough in perinatal HIV prevention; that there is a role for research on this topic in developing countries; that identifying less expensive, similarly effective interventions would be of enormous benefit, given the limited resources for medical care in most developing countries; and that randomized studies can help identify such interventions.

The sole point of disagreement is the best comparison group to use in assessing the effectiveness of less-expensive interventions once an effective intervention has been identified. The researchers conducting the placebo-controlled trials assert that such trials represent the only appropriate research design, implying that they answer the question, "Is the shorter regimen better than nothing?" We take the more optimistic view that, given the findings of ACTG 076 and other clinical information, researchers are quite capable of designing a shorter antiretroviral regimen that is approximately as effective as the ACTG 076 regimen. The proposal for the Harvard study in Thailand states the research question clearly: "Can we reduce the duration of prophylactic [zidovudine] treatment without increasing the risk of perinatal transmission of HIV, that is, without compromising the demonstrated efficacy of the standard ACTG 076 [zidovudine] regimen?"[13] We believe that such equivalency studies of alternative antiretroviral regimens will provide even more useful results than placebo-controlled trials, without the deaths of hundreds of newborns that are inevitable if placebo groups are used.

At a recent congressional hearing on research ethics, NIH director Harold Varmus was asked how the Department of Health and Human Services could be funding both a placebo-controlled trial (through the CDC) and a non–placebo-controlled equivalency study (through the NIH) in Thailand. Dr. Varmus conceded that placebo-controlled studies are "not the only way to achieve results."[14] If the research can be satisfactorily conducted in more than one way, why not select the approach that minimizes loss of life?

INADEQUATE ANALYSIS OF DATA FROM ACTG 076 AND OTHER SOURCES

The NIH, CDC, WHO, and the researchers conducting the studies we consider unethical argue that differences in the duration and route of administration of antiretroviral agents in the shorter regimens, as compared with the ACTG 076 regimen, justify the use of a placebo group.[15-18] Given that ACTG 076 was a well-conducted, randomized, controlled trial, it is disturbing that the rich data available from the study were not adequately used by the group assembled by WHO in June 1994, which recommended placebo-controlled trials after ACTG 076, or by the investigators of the 15 studies we consider unethical.

In fact, the ACTG 076 investigators conducted a subgroup analysis to identify an appropriate period for prepartum administration of zidovudine. The approximate median duration of prepartum treatment was 12 weeks. In a comparison of treatment for 12 weeks or less (average, 7) with treatment for more than 12 weeks (average, 17), there was no univariate association between the duration of treatment and its effect in reducing perinatal HIV transmission (P = 0.99) (Gelber R: personal communication). This analysis is somewhat limited by the number of infected infants and its post hoc nature. However, when combined with information such as the fact that in non–breast-feeding populations an estimated 65 percent of cases of perinatal HIV infection are transmitted during delivery and 95 percent of the remaining cases are transmitted within two months of delivery,[19] the analysis *suggests* that the shorter regimens may be equally effective. This finding should have been explored in later studies by randomly assigning women to longer or shorter treatment regimens.

What about the argument that the use of the oral route for intrapartum administration of zidovudine in the present trials (as opposed to the intravenous route in ACTG 076) justifies the use of a placebo? In its protocols for its two studies in Thailand and Côte d'Ivoire, the CDC acknowledged that previous "pharmacokinetic modeling data suggest that [zidovudine] serum levels obtained with this [oral] dose will be similar to levels obtained with an intravenous infusion"[20]

Thus, on the basis of the ACTG 076 data, knowledge about the timing of perinatal transmission, and pharmacokinetic data, the researchers should have had every reason to believe that well-designed shorter regimens would be more effective than placebo. These findings seriously disturb the equipoise (uncertainty over the likely study result) necessary to justify a placebo-controlled trial on ethical grounds.[21]

DEFINING PLACEBO AS THE STANDARD OF CARE IN DEVELOPING COUNTRIES

Some officials and researchers have defended the use of placebo-controlled studies in developing countries by arguing that the subjects are treated at least according to the standard of care in these countries, which consists of unproven regimens or no treatment at all. This assertion reveals a fundamental misunderstanding of the concept of the standard of care. In developing countries, the standard of care (in this case, not providing zidovudine to HIV-positive pregnant women) is not based on a consideration of alternative treatments or previous clinical data, but is instead an economically determined policy of governments that cannot afford the prices set by drug companies. We agree with the Council for International Organizations of Medical Sciences that researchers working in developing countries have an ethical responsibility to provide treatment that conforms to the standard of care in the sponsoring country, when possible.[9] An exception would be a standard of care that required an exorbitant expenditure, such as the cost of building a coronary care unit. Since zidovudine is usually made available free of charge by the manufacturer for use in clinical trials, excessive cost is not a factor in this case. Acceptance of a standard of care that does not conform to the standard in the sponsoring country results in a double standard in research. Such a double standard, which permits research designs that are unacceptable in the sponsoring country, creates an incentive to use as research subjects those with the least access to health care.

What are the potential implications of accepting such a double standard? Researchers might inject live malaria parasites into HIV-positive subjects in China in order to study the effect on the progression of HIV infection, even though the study protocol had been rejected in the United States and Mexico. Or researchers might randomly assign malnourished San (bushmen) to receive vitamin-fortified or standard bread. One might also justify trials of HIV vaccines in which the subjects were not provided with condoms or state-of-the-art counseling about safe sex by arguing that they are not customarily provided in the developing countries in question. These are not simply hypothetical worst-case scenarios; the first two studies have already been performed,[22,23] and the third has been proposed and criticized.[24]

Annas and Grodin recently commented on the characterization and justification of placebos as a standard of care: "'Nothing' is a description of what happens; 'standard of care' is a normative standard of effective medical treatment, whether or not it is provided to a particular community."[25]

JUSTIFYING PLACEBO-CONTROLLED TRIALS BY CLAIMING THEY ARE MORE RAPID

Researchers have also sought to justify placebo-controlled trials by arguing that they require fewer subjects than equivalency studies and can therefore be completed more rapidly. Because equivalency studies are simply concerned with excluding alternative interventions that fall below some preestablished level of efficacy (as opposed to establishing which intervention is superior), it is customary to use one-sided statistical testing in such studies.[25] The numbers of women needed for a placebo-controlled trial and an equivalency study are similar.[26] In a placebo-controlled trial of a short course of zidovudine, with rates of perinatal HIV transmission of 25 percent in the placebo group and 15 percent in the zidovudine group, an alpha level of 0.05 (two-sided), and a beta level of 0.2, 500 subjects would be needed. An equivalency study with a transmission rate of 10 percent in the group receiving the ACTG 076 regimen, a difference in efficacy of 6 percent (above the 10 percent), an alpha level of 0.05 (one-sided), and a beta level of 0.2 would require 620 subjects (McCarthy W: personal communication).

TOWARD A SINGLE INTERNATIONAL STANDARD OF ETHICAL RESEARCH

Researchers assume greater ethical responsibilities when they enroll subjects in clinical studies, a precept acknowledged by Varmus recently when he insisted that all subjects in an NIH-sponsored needle-exchange trial be offered hepatitis B vaccine.[27] Residents of impoverished, postcolonial countries, the majority of whom are people of color, must be protected from potential exploitation in research. Otherwise, the abominable state of health care in these countries can be used to justify studies that could never pass ethical muster in the sponsoring country.

With the increasing globalization of trade, government research dollars becoming scarce, and more attention being paid to the hazards posed by "emerging infections" to the residents of industrialized countries, it is likely that studies in developing countries will increase. It is time to develop standards of research that preclude the kinds of double standards evident in these trials. In an editorial published nine years ago in the *Journal*, Marcia Angell stated, "Human subjects in any part of the world should be protected by an irreducible set of ethical standards."[28] Tragically, for the hundreds of infants who have needlessly contracted HIV infection in the perinatal-transmission studies that have already been completed, any such protection will have come too late.

REFERENCES

1. Conner EM, Sperling RS, Gelber R, et al. Reduction of maternal–infant transmission of human immunodeficiency virus type I with zidovudine treatment. N Engl J Med 1994;331:1173-80.
2. Sperling KS, Shapiro DE, Coombs RW, et al. Maternal viral load, zidovudine treatment, and the risk of transmission of human immunodeficiency virus type 1 from mother to infant. N Engl J Med 1996;33i:1621-9.
3. Recommendations of the U.S. Public Health Service Task Force on the use of zidovudine to reduce perinatal transmission of human immunodeficiency virus. MMWR Morb Mortal Wkly Rep 1994; 43(RR-ll):1-20.
4. Fiscus SA, Adimora AA, Schoenbach VJ, et al. Perinatal HIV infection and the effect of zidovudine therapy on transmission in rural and urban counties. JAMA 1996; 275;1483-8.
5. Cooper E, Diaz C, Pitt J, et al. Impact of ACTG 076: use of zidovudine during pregnancy and changes in the rate of HIV vertical transmission. In: Program and abstracts of the Third Conference on Retroviruses and Opportunistic Infections, Washington, D.C., January 28–February 1, 1996. Washington, D.C.: Infectious Diseases Society of America, 1996:57.
6. Simonds RJ, Nesheim S, Matheson P, et al. Declining mother to child HIV transmission following perinatal ZDV recommendations. Presented at the 11th International Conference on AIDS, Vancouver, Canada, July 7–12, 1996. abstract
7. Scarlatti C, Paediatric HIV infection. Lancet 1996; 348: 863-8.
8. Recommendations from the meeting on mother-to-infant transmission of HIV by use of antiretrovirals, Geneva, World Health Organization, June 23–25, 1994.
9. World Health Organization. International ethical guidelines for biomedical research involving human subjects. Geneva: Council for International Organizations of Medical Sciences, 1993.
10. 45 CFR 46.111(a)(1).
11. Testing equivalence of two binomial proportions. In: Machin D, Campbell MJ. Statistical tables for the design of clinical trials. Oxford, England: Blackwell Scientific, 1987:35-53.
12. Brennan TA, Letter to Gilbert Meier. NIH Division of Research Ethics, December 28, 1994.
13. Lallemant M, Vithayasai V. A short ZDV course to prevent perinatal HIV in Thailand. Boston: Harvard School of Public Health, April 28, 1995.
14. Varmus H. Testimony before the Subcommittee on Human Resources, Committee on Government Reform and Oversight, U.S. House of Representatives, May 8, 1997.
15. Draft talking points: responding to Public Citizen press conference. Press release of the National Institutes of Health, April 22, 1997.
16. Questions and answers: CDC studies of AZT to prevent mother-to-child HIV transmission in developing countries. Press release of the Centers for Disease Control and Prevention, Atlanta. (undated document.)
17. Questions and answers on the UNAIDS sponsored trials for the prevention of mother-to-child transmission: background brief to assist in responding to issues raised by the public and the media. Press release of the United Nations AIDS Program. (undated document.)

18. Halsey NA, Meinert CL, Ruff AJ., et al. Letter to Harold Varmus, Director of National Institutes of Health. Baltimore: Johns Hopkins University, May 6, 1997.

19. Wiktor SZ, Ehounou E. A randomized placebo-controlled intervention study to evaluate the safety and effectiveness of oral zidovudine administered in late pregnancy to reduce the incidence of mother-to-child transmission of HIV-1 in Abidjan, Côte D'Ivoire. Atlanta: Centers for Disease Control and Prevention. (undated document.)

20. Rouzioux C, Costagliola D, Burgard M, et al. Timing of mother-to-child HIV-1 transmission depends on maternal status. AIDS 1993; 7: Suppl 2: S49-S52.

21. Freedman B. Equipoise and the ethics of clinical research. N Engl J Med 1987; 317:141-5.

22. Heimlich HJ, Chen XP, Xiao BQ, et al. CD4 response in HIV-positive patients treated with malaria therapy. Presented at the 11th International Conference on AIDS, Vancouver, B.C., July 7–12, 1996. abstract.

23. Bishop WB, Laubscher I, Labadarios D, Rehder P, Louw ME, Fellingham SA. Effect of vitamin-enriched bread on the vitamin status of an isolated rural community—a controlled clinical trial. S Afr Med J 1996;86: Suppl:458-62.

24. Lurie P, Bishaw M, Chesney MA, et al. Ethical, behavioral, and social aspects of HIV vaccine trials in developing countries. JAMA 1994;271:295-301.

25. Annas G, Grodin M. An apology is not enough. Boston Globe. May 18, 1997:C1-C2.

26. Freedman B, Weijer C, Glass KC. Placebo orthodoxy in clinical research. I. Empirical and methodological myths. J Law Med Ethics 1996; 24:243-51.

27. Varmus H. Comments at the meeting of the Advisory Committee to the Director of the National Institutes of Health, December 12, 1996.

28. Angell M. Ethical imperialism? Ethics in international collaborative clinical research. N Engl J Med 1988; 319:1081-3.

Ethical Complexities of Conducting Research in Developing Countries

Harold Varmus and David Satcher

One of the great challenges in medical research is to conduct clinical trials in developing countries that will lead to therapies that benefit the citizens of these countries. Features of many developing countries—poverty, endemic diseases, and a low level of investment in health care systems—affect both the ease of performing trials and the selection of trials that can benefit the populations of the countries. Trials that make use of impoverished populations to test drugs for use solely in developed countries violate our most basic understanding of ethical behavior. Trials that apply scientific knowledge to interventions that can be used to benefit such populations are appropriate but present their own ethical challenges. How do we balance the ethical premises on which our work is based with the calls for public health partnerships from our colleagues in developing countries?

Some commentators have been critical of research performed in developing countries that

might not be found ethically acceptable in developed countries. Specifically, questions have been raised about trials of interventions to prevent maternal–infant transmission of the human immunodeficiency virus (HIV) that have been sponsored by the National Institutes of Health (NIH) and the Centers for Disease Control and Prevention (CDC).[1,2] Although these commentators raise important issues, they have not adequately considered the purpose and complexity of such trials and the needs of the countries involved. They also allude inappropriately to the infamous Tuskegee study, which did not test an intervention. The Tuskegee study ultimately deprived people of a known, effective, affordable intervention. To claim that countries seeking help in stemming the tide of maternal–infant HIV transmission by seeking usable interventions have followed that path trivializes the suffering of the men in the Tuskegee study and shows a serious lack of understanding of today's trials.

After the Tuskegee study was made public in the 1970s, a national commission was established to develop principles and guidelines for the pro-

New England Journal of Medicine 337, October 2, 1997: 1003–1005. Copyright © 1997 Massachusetts Medical Society. All rights reserved. Used with permission.

tection of research subjects. The new system of protection was described in the Belmont report.[3] Although largely compatible with the World Medical Association's Declaration of Helsinki,[4] the Belmont report articulated three principles: respect for persons (the recognition of the right of persons to exercise autonomy), beneficence (the minimization of risk incurred by research subjects and the maximization of benefits to them and to others), and justice (the principle that therapeutic investigations should not unduly involve persons from groups unlikely to benefit from subsequent applications of the research).

There is an inherent tension among these three principles. Over the years, we have seen the focus of debate shift from concern about the burdens of participation in research (beneficence) to equitable access to clinical trials (justice). Furthermore, the right to exercise autonomy was not always fully available to women, who were excluded from participating in clinical trials perceived as jeopardizing their safety; their exclusion clearly limited their ability to benefit from the research. Similarly, persons in developing countries deserve research that addresses their needs.

How should these principles be applied to research conducted in developing countries? How can we—and they—weigh the benefits and risks? Such research must be developed in concert with the developing countries in which it will be conducted. In the case of the NIH and CDC trials, there has been strong and consistent support and involvement of the scientific and public health communities in the host countries, with local as well as United States–based scientific and ethical reviews and the same requirements for informed consent that would exist if the work were performed in the United States. But there is more to this partnership. Interventions that could be expected to be made available in the United States might be well beyond the financial resources of a developing country or exceed the capacity of its health care infrastructure. Might we support a trial in another country that would not be offered in the United States? Yes, because the burden of disease might make such a study more compelling in that country. Even if there were some risks associated with intervention, such a trial might pass the test of beneficence. Might we elect not to support a trial of an intervention that was beyond the reach

of the citizens of the other country? Yes, because that trial would not pass the test of justice.

Trials supported by the NIH and the CDC, which are designed to reduce the transmission of HIV from mothers to infants in developing countries, have been held up by some observers as examples of trials that do not meet ethical standards. We disagree. The debate does not hinge on informed consent, which all the trials have obtained. It hinges instead on whether it is ethical to test interventions against a placebo control when an effective intervention is in use elsewhere in the world. A background paper sets forth our views on this matter more fully.[5] The paper is also available on the World Wide Web (at http://www.nih.gov/news/mathiv/mathiv.htm).

One such effective intervention—known as AIDS Clinical Trials Group protocol 076—was a major breakthrough in the search for a way to interrupt the transmission of HIV from mother to infant. The regimen tested in the original study, however, was quite intensive for pregnant women and the health care system. Although this regimen has been proved effective, it requires that women undergo HIV testing and receive counseling about their HIV status early in pregnancy, comply with a lengthy oral regimen and with intravenous administration of the relatively expensive antiretroviral drug zidovudine, and refrain from breast-feeding. In addition, the newborn infants must receive six weeks of oral zidovudine, and both mothers and infants must be carefully monitored for adverse effects of the drug. Unfortunately, the burden of maternal–infant transmission of HIV is greatest in countries where women present late for prenatal care, have limited access to HIV testing and counseling, typically deliver their infants in settings not conducive to intravenous drug administration, and depend on breast-feeding to protect their babies from many diseases, only one of which is HIV infection. Furthermore, zidovudine is a powerful drug, and its safety in the populations of developing countries, where the incidences of other diseases, anemia, and malnutrition are higher than in developed countries, is unknown. Therefore, even though the 076 protocol has been shown to be effective in some countries, it is unlikely that it can be successfully exported to many others.

In addition to these hurdles, the wholesale cost of zidovudine in the 076 protocol is estimated to be in excess of $800 per mother and infant, an amount far greater than most developing countries can afford to pay for standard care. For example, in Malawi, the cost of zidovudine alone for the 076 regimen for one HIV-infected woman and her child is more than 600 times the annual per capita allocation for health care.

Various representatives of the ministries of health, communities, and scientists in developing countries have joined with other scientists to call for less complex and less expensive interventions to counteract the staggering impact of maternal–infant transmission of HIV in the developing world. The World Health Organization moved promptly after the release of the results of the 076 protocol, convening a panel of researchers and public health practitioners from around the world. This panel recommended the use of the 076 regimen throughout the industrialized world, where it is feasible, but also called for studies of alternative regimens that could be used in developing countries, observing that the logistical issues and costs precluded the widespread application of the 076 regimen.[6] To this end, the World Health Organization asked UNAIDS, the Joint United Nations Programme on HIV/AIDS, to coordinate international research efforts to develop simpler, less costly interventions.

The scientific community is responding by carrying out trials of several promising regimens that developing countries recognize as candidates for widespread delivery. However, these trials are being criticized by some people because of the use of placebo controls. Why not test these new interventions against the 076 regimen? Why not test them against other interventions that might offer some benefit? These questions were carefully considered in the development of these research projects and in their scientific and ethical review.

An obvious response to the ethical objection to placebo-controlled trials in countries where there is no current intervention is that the assignment to a placebo group does not carry a risk beyond that associated with standard practice, but this response is too simple. An additional response is that a placebo-controlled study usually provides a faster answer with fewer subjects, but the same result might be achieved with more sites or more aggressive enrollment. The most compelling reason to use a placebo-controlled study is that it provides definitive answers to questions about the safety and value of an inter-

vention in the setting in which the study is performed, and these answers are the point of the research. Without clear and firm answers to whether and, if so, how well an intervention works, it is impossible for a country to make a sound judgment about the appropriateness and financial feasibility of providing the intervention.

For example, testing two or more interventions of unknown benefit (as some people have suggested) will not necessarily reveal whether either is better than nothing. Even if one surpasses the other, it may be difficult to judge the extent of the benefit conferred, since the interventions may differ markedly in other ways—for example, cost or toxicity. A placebo-controlled study would supply that answer. Similarly, comparing an intervention of unknown benefit—especially one that is affordable in a developing country—with the only intervention with a known benefit (the 076 regimen) may provide information that is not useful for patients. If the affordable intervention is less effective than the 076 regimen—not an unlikely outcome—this information will be of little use in a country where the more effective regimen is unavailable. Equally important, it will still be unclear whether the affordable intervention is better than nothing and worth the investment of scarce health care dollars. Such studies would fail to meet the goal of determining whether a treatment that could be implemented is worth implementing.

A placebo-controlled trial is not the only way to study a new intervention, but as compared with other approaches, it offers more definitive answers and a clearer view of side effects. This is not a case of treating research subjects as a means to an end, nor does it reflect "a callous disregard of their welfare."[7] Instead, a placebo-controlled trial may be the only way to obtain an answer that is ultimately useful to people in similar circumstances. If we enroll subjects in a study that exposes them to unknown risks and is designed in a way that is unlikely to provide results that are useful to the subjects or others in the population, we have failed the test of beneficence.

Finally, the NIH- and CDC-supported trials have undergone a rigorous process of ethical review, including not only the participation of the public health and scientific communities in the developing countries where the trials are being performed but also the application of the U.S. rules for the protection of human research subjects by relevant institutional review boards in the United States and in the developing countries. Support from local governments has been obtained, and each active study has been and will continue to be reviewed by an independent data and safety monitoring board.

To restate our main points: these studies address an urgent need in the countries in which they are being conducted and have been developed with extensive in-country participation. The studies are being conducted according to widely accepted principles and guidelines in bioethics. And our decisions to support these trials rest heavily on local support and approval. In a letter to the NIH dated May 8, 1997, Edward K. Mbidde, chairman of the AIDS Research Committee of the Uganda Cancer Institute, wrote:

> These are Ugandan studies conducted by Ugandan investigators on Ugandans. Due to lack of resources we have been sponsored by organizations like yours. We are grateful that you have been able to do so. . . There is a mix up of issues here which needs to be clarified. It is not NIH conducting the studies in Uganda but Ugandans conducting their study on their people for the good of their people.

The scientific and ethical issues concerning studies in developing countries are complex. It is a healthy sign that we are debating these issues so that we can continue to advance our knowledge and our practice. However, it is essential that the debate take place with a full understanding of the nature of the science, the interventions in question, and the local factors that impede or support research and its benefits.

REFERENCES

1. Lurie P, Wolfe SM. Unethical trials of interventions to reduce perinatal transmission of the human immunodeficiency virus in developing countries. N Engl J Med 1997; 337:853-6.
2. Angell M. The ethics of clinical research in the third world. N Engl J Med 1997; 337:847-9.
3. National Commission for the Protection of Human Subjects of Biomedical and Behavioral Research. Belmont report: ethical principles and guidelines for the protection of human subjects of research. Washington, D.C.: Government Printing Office, 1988. (GPO 887-809.)
4. World Medical Association Declaration of Helsinki. Adopted by the 18th World Medical Assembly, Helsinki, 1964, as revised by the 48th World Medical Assembly, Republic of South Africa, 1996.
5. The conduct of clinical trials of maternal–infant transmission of HIV supported by the United States Department of Health and Human Services in developing countries. Washington, D.C.: Department of Health and Human Services, July 1997.
6. Recommendations from the meeting on mother-to-infant transmission of HIV by use of antiretrovirals, Geneva, World Health Organization, June 23–25, 1994.

International Ethical Guidelines for Biomedical Research Involving Human Subjects

The Council for International Organizations of Medical Sciences (CIOMS) in Collaboration with the World Health Organization (WHO)

Geneva 1993

PREAMBLE

The term "research" refers to a class of activities designed to develop or contribute to generalizable knowledge. Generalizable knowledge consists of theories, principles or relationships, or the accumulation of information on which they are based, that can be corroborated by accepted scientific methods of observation and inference. In the present context "research" includes both medical and behavioural studies pertaining to human health.

Usually "research" is modified by the adjective "biomedical" to indicate that the reference is to health-related research.

Progress in medical care and disease prevention depends upon an understanding of physiological and pathological processes or epidemiological findings, and requires at some time research involving human subjects. The collection, analysis and interpretation of information obtained from research involving human beings contribute significantly to the improvement of human health.

Research involving human subjects includes that undertaken together with patient care (clinical research) and that undertaken on patients or other subjects, or with data pertaining to them, solely to contribute to generalizable knowledge (non-clinical biomedical research). Research is defined as "clinical" if one or more of its components is designed to be diagnostic, prophylactic or therapeutic for the individual subject of the research. Invariably, in clinical research, there are also components designed not to be diagnostic, prophylactic or therapeutic for the subject; examples include the administration of placebos and the performance of laboratory tests in addition to those required to serve the purposes of medical care. Hence the term "clinical research" is used here rather than "therapeutic research".

Research involving human subjects includes:

- studies of a physiological, biochemical or pathological process, or of the response to a specific intervention—whether physical, chemical or psychological—in healthy subjects or patients;
- controlled trials of diagnostic, preventive or therapeutic measures in larger groups of persons, designed to demonstrate a specific generalizable response to these measures against a background of individual biological variation;
- studies designed to determine the consequences for individuals and communities of specific preventive or therapeutic measures; and
- studies concerning human health-related behaviour in a variety of circumstances and environments.

Research involving human subjects may employ either observation or physical, chemical or psychological intervention; it may also either generate records or make use of existing records containing biomedical or other information about individuals who may or may not be identifiable from the records or information. The use of such records and the protection of the confidentiality of data obtained from those records are discussed in *International Guidelines for Ethical Review of Epidemiological Studies* (CIOMS, 1991).

Research involving human subjects includes also research in which environmental factors are manipulated in a way that could affect incidentally-exposed individuals. Research is defined in broad terms in order to embrace field studies of pathogenic organisms and toxic chemicals under investigation for health-related purposes.

Research involving human subjects is to be distinguished from the practice of medicine, public health and other forms of health care, which is designed to contribute directly to the health of individuals or communities. Prospective subjects may find it confusing when research and practice are to be conducted simultaneously, as when research is designed to obtain new information about the efficacy of a drug or other therapeutic, diagnostic or preventive modality.

Research involving human subjects should be carried out only by, or strictly supervised by, suitably qualified and experienced investigation and in accordance with a protocol that clearly states: the aim of the research; the reasons for proposing that it involve human subjects; the nature and degree of any known risks to the subjects; the sources from which it is proposed to recruit subjects; and the means proposed for ensuring that subjects' consent will be adequately informed and voluntary. The protocol should be scientifically and ethically appraised by one or more suitably constituted review bodies, independent of the investigators.

New vaccines and medicinal drugs, before being approved for general use, must be tested on human subjects in clinical trials; such trials, which constitute a substantial part of all research involving human subjects, are described in Annex 2.

THE GUIDELINES

INFORMED CONSENT OF SUBJECTS

Guideline 1: Individual Informed Consent For all biomedical research involving human subjects, the investigator must obtain the informed consent of the prospective subject or, in the case of an individual who is not capable of giving informed consent, the proxy consent of a properly authorized representative.

Guideline 2: Essential Information for Prospective Research Subjects   Before requesting an individual's consent to participate in research, the investigator must provide the individual with the following information, in language that he or she is capable of understanding:

- that each individual is invited to participate as a subject in research, and the aims and methods of the research;
- the expected duration of the subject's participation;
- the benefits that might reasonably be expected to result to the subject or to others as an outcome of the research;
- any foreseeable risks or discomfort to the subject, associated with participation in the research;
- any alternative procedures or courses of treatment that might be as advantageous to the subject as the procedure or treatment being tested;
- the extent to which confidentiality of records in which the subject is identified will be maintained;
- the extent of the investigator's responsibility, if any, to provide medical services to the subject;
- that therapy will be provided free of charge for specified types of research-related injury;
- whether the subject or the subject's family or dependants will be compensated for disability or death resulting from such injury; and
- that the individual is free to refuse to participate and will be free to withdraw from the research at any time without penalty or loss of benefits to which he or she would otherwise he entitled.

Guideline 3: Obligations of Investigators Regarding Informed Consent   The investigator has a duty to:

- communicate to the prospective subject all the information necessary for adequately informed consent;

- give the prospective subject full opportunity and encouragement to ask questions;
- exclude the possibility of unjustified deception, undue influence and intimidation;
- seek consent only after the prospective subject has adequate knowledge of the relevant facts and the consequences of participation, and has had sufficient opportunity to consider whether to participate;
- as a general rule, obtain from each prospective subject a signed form as evidence of informed consent; and
- renew the informed consent of each subject if there are material changes in the conditions or procedures of the research.

Guideline 4: Inducement to Participate   Subjects may be paid for inconvenience and time spent, and should be reimbursed for expenses incurred, in connection with their participation in research; they may also receive free medical services. However, the payments should not be so large or the medical services so extensive as to induce prospective subjects to consent to participate in the research against their better judgment ("undue inducement"). All payments, reimbursements and medical services to be provided to research subjects should be approved by an ethical review committee.

Guideline 5: Research Involving Children   Before undertaking research involving children, the investigator must ensure that:

- children will not be involved in research that might equally well be carried out with adults;
- the purpose of the research is to obtain knowledge relevant to the health needs of children;
- a parent or legal guardian of each child has given proxy consent;
- the consent of each child has been obtained to the extent of the child's capabilities;
- the child's refusal to participate in research must always be respected unless according to the research protocol the child would receive therapy for which there is no medically-acceptable alternative;
- the risk presented by interventions not intended to benefit the individual child-subject is low and commensurate with the importance of the knowledge to be gained; and

- interventions that are intended to provide therapeutic benefit are likely to be at least as advantageous to the individual child-subject as any available alternative.

Guideline 6: Research Involving Persons with Mental or Behavioural Disorders   Before undertaking research involving individuals who by reason of mental or behavioural disorders are not capable of giving adequately informed consent, the investigator must ensure that:

- such persons will not be subjects of research that might equally well be carried out on persons in full possession of their mental faculties;
- the purpose of the research is to obtain knowledge relevant to the particular health needs of persons with mental or behavioural disorders;
- the consent of each subject has been obtained to the extent of that subject's capabilities, and a prospective subject's refusal to participate in non-clinical research is always respected;
- in the case of incompetent subjects, informed consent is obtained from the legal guardian or other duly authorized person;
- the degree of risk attached to interventions that are not intended to benefit the individual subject is low and commensurate with the importance of the knowledge to be gained; and
- interventions that are intended to provide therapeutic benefit are likely to be at least as advantageous to the individual subject as any alternative.

Guideline 7: Research Involving Prisoners   Prisoners with serious illness or at risk of serious illness should not arbitrarily be denied access to investigational drugs, vaccines or other agents that show promise of therapeutic or preventive benefit.

Guideline 8: Research Involving Subjects in Underdeveloped Communities   Before undertaking research involving subjects in underdeveloped communities, whether in developed or developing countries, the investigator must ensure that:

- persons in underdeveloped communities will not ordinarily be involved in research that could be carried out reasonably well in developed communities;

- the research is responsive to the health needs and the priorities of the community in which it is to be carried out;
- every effort will be made to secure the ethical imperative that the consent of individual subjects be informed; and
- the proposals for the research have been reviewed and approved by an ethical review committee that has among its members or consultants persons who are thoroughly familiar with the customs and traditions of the community.

Guideline 9: Informed Consent in Epidemiological Studies   For several types of epidemiological research individual informed consent is either impracticable or inadvisable. In such cases the ethical review committee should determine whether it is ethically acceptable to proceed without individual informed consent and whether the investigator's plans to protect the safety and respect the privacy of research subjects and to maintain the confidentiality of the data are adequate.

SELECTION OF RESEARCH SUBJECTS

Guideline 10: Equitable Distribution of Burdens and Benefits   Individuals or communities to be invited to be subjects of research should be selected in such a way that the burdens and benefits of the research will be equitably distributed. Special justification is required for inviting vulnerable individuals and, if they are selected, the means of protecting their rights and welfare must be particularly strictly applied.

Guideline 11: Selection of Pregnant or Nursing (Breastfeeding) Women as Research Subjects   Pregnant or nursing women should in no circumstances be the subjects of non-clinical research unless the research carries no more than minimal risk to the fetus or nursing infant and the object of the research is to obtain new knowledge about pregnancy or lactation. As a general rule, pregnant or nursing women should not be subjects of any clinical trails except such trials as are designed to protect or advance the health of pregnant or nursing women or fetuses or nursing infants, and for which women who are not pregnant or nursing would not be suitable subjects.

CONFIDENTIALITY OF DATA

Guideline 12: Safeguarding Confidentiality   The investigator must establish secure safeguards of the confidentiality of research data. Subjects should be told of the limits to the investigators' ability to safeguard confidentiality and of the anticipated consequences of breaches of confidentiality. . . .

Drug-Free Research in Schizophrenia: An Overview of the Controversy

Paul S. Appelbaum

The ethics of psychiatric research—in particular drug-free research on schizophrenia—have been the focus of intense interest in the last two years. We have witnessed a proliferation of professional conferences on the topic, often with coverage in the lay press. The American Psychiatric Association has organized a work group to formulate ethical guidelines for psychiatric researchers. At the federal level, the National Institute of Mental Health has indicated its interest in funding research that explores the ethical issues involved in studies of persons with psychiatric disorders.

Why this sudden interest in the ethics of psychiatric research, an area that has been quiescent for nearly a decade and a half? This paper explores the context from which much of this interest has grown: drug-free research on schizophrenia. I consider the roots of the controversy, the nature both of the disorder and of the research that lies at the core of the debate, and the ethical issues that have been raised.

WHY THE CURRENT PROMINENCE OF ISSUES RELATED TO DRUG-FREE RESEARCH IN SCHIZOPHRENIA?

In May 1994, the federal Office of Protection from Research Risks (OPRR) issued a report on its investigation of complaints against a leading group of schizophrenia researchers at the University of California at Los Angeles (UCLA) Medical School. The subjects on whose behalf complaints were filed had participated in a series of studies using Prolixin decanoate, a long-acting, injectable form of a standard antipsychotic agent.

Subjects in the UCLA studies initially went through a one-year, fixed-dose study in which they received injections every two weeks. On the successful completion of the first study, subjects who were willing to continue in the research were enrolled in a second, more controversial protocol. Each subject was assigned, in a randomized, double-blind fashion, to continue the same dose of Prolixin or to receive a placebo injection. After twelve weeks, the groups crossed over, with those subjects who had received active medication now getting placebo, and vice versa. Subjects who were still stable after an additional twelve weeks were then assigned to a withdrawal protocol. The medications were stopped and subjects were followed for at least one year, or until a serious exacerbation or psychotic relapse occurred. The goal of the study was to identify predictors of successful functioning without antipsychotic medication.

Two subjects who had been enrolled in the withdrawal protocol ran into trouble. One subject committed suicide after completion of the formal one-year drug withdrawal study, while continuing to be followed by the research team in a drug-free state. A second person, a young college student, experienced a severe psychotic relapse that began not long after the medication

IRB, Vol. 18, No. 1, 1–5. Copyright © The Hastings Center. Used with permission.

EDITORS' NOTE: All notes have been deleted. Readers who wish to follow up on sources should consult the original article.

was discontinued. During this period, he left school, began to hallucinate, and threatened to kill his parents when he became convinced that they were possessed by the devil. He and his parents alleged that, despite repeated appeals to the research team, it took nine months before he was put back on medication.

In the wake of these episodes, allegations were made to OPRR that the drug withdrawal protocols in which the subjects had been enrolled were unethical because they virtually guaranteed that subjects would relapse; that proper informed consent had not been obtained from the subjects; and that the investigators, who were also the subjects' clinicians, had not monitored their conditions closely enough and had been too slow about pulling them off the protocol and restarting medications.

OPRR's investigation concluded that the design of the research was not unethical, since it comported with current clinical and scientific standards. However, the agency determined that the informed consent obtained from subjects was inadequate, because the consent documents failed to describe clearly the differences between being in the research project and receiving ordinary clinical care. Although UCLA's monitoring of subjects' clinical status was deemed to be acceptable, OPRR also found that subjects should have been informed that their clinicians simultaneously were acting as investigators in the study.

Far from settling the controversy regarding drug-free research in schizophrenia, the OPRR report stimulated renewed consideration of the issues. The controversy was widely covered in the popular media, congressional hearings were held, and a lawsuit was filed against UCLA by the family of one of the subjects. Before considering the ethical issues raised by participants in the debate over drug-free research, however, it may be helpful to know a bit more about schizophrenia and its treatment.

WHAT IS SCHIZOPHRENIA AND HOW IS IT TREATED?

Schizophrenia is a major mental disorder characterized by periods of psychosis or detachment from reality. Patients typically experience hallucinations, delusions, disorganized thinking and behavior, and social withdrawal. Psychiatrists only make a diagnosis of schizophrenia after symptoms have been present for at least six months, but most patients will suffer from the effects of the disorder for the rest of their lives. Periods of relative remission, in which withdrawal and restricted emotions are the most notable characteristics, are frequently punctuated by acute exacerbations, marked by the most florid psychotic symptoms. Persons with schizophrenia experience considerable agony as a result of their disorder; lifetime rates of suicide approximate 10 percent.

Treatment of schizophrenia, once limited to lifetime custodial care, was revolutionized in the mid-1950s by the introduction of the first effective medications for the disorder, the phenothiazine antipsychotics. These drugs—including Thorazine, Mellaril, and Prolixin—appear to have a specific effect on psychotic symptoms, rather than merely "tranquilizing" the patient. Their mechanism of action is believed to involve blockade of brain dopamine receptors, but this continues to be an area of active investigation. Administration of the medications can lead to resolution of acute psychotic episodes and a diminished likelihood of recurrence over time. Eighty percent or more of patients with schizophrenia get some benefit from the medications, and many of those who are resistant to phenothiazines have benefitted from other classes of drugs more recently introduced.

On the other hand, it is clear that currently available antipsychotic medications are a mixed blessing. Though they usually are effective in diminishing symptoms, complete remission is uncommon. Even when maintained on medication, most patients will experience periodic breakthroughs of their psychosis. Moreover, the success achieved by the medications is purchased at the price of substantial side-effects. Acutely, many patients experience drug-induced parkinsonism, muscle spasms called dystonias, feelings of inner restlessness associated with a need to move ("akathisia"), and akinetic states in which the motivation to move and even to think is diminished. Less frequently, patients may experience a potentially fatal hypermetabolic state known as "neuroleptic malignant syndrome"; the most popular of the newer medications, clozapine, can cause dangerous (or life-threatening) suppression of white blood cells (agranulocytosis).

The most profound of the long-term side-effects of the phenothiazine-type medications (and those that act similarly, like Haldol) is tardive dyskinesia. This syndrome is characterized by involuntary muscular movements affecting the face, limbs, and trunk, and sometimes other muscle groups as well. Ranging in intensity from mild to occasionally disabling, tardive dyskinesia occurs in 4 to 5 percent of patients on neuroleptic medication each year. Though it sometimes remits when the medications are stopped, it is often irreversible; patients with tardive dyskinesia may be faced with the choice of continuing the medications, with a possible worsening of the syndrome, or discontinuing them, only to experience an exacerbation of their schizophrenic symptoms. Other delayed neuromuscular syndromes may occur as well.

On balance, though, most patients with schizophrenia tolerate the side-effects of the drugs, both acute and long-term, as a lesser evil compared with untreated schizophrenia.

WHY CONDUCT DRUG-FREE RESEARCH IN SCHIZOPHRENIA?

Given the availability of reasonably effective drugs for the treatment of schizophrenia, and the distress associated with acute episodes of the disorder, one might wonder on what basis researchers perform studies with patients who have been taken off their medication. Three justifications are commonly given.

First, it has been known for many years that some schizophrenic patients can have their medication discontinued without experiencing relapse for a substantial period of time. If such patients could be identified in advance, they would be spared the negative effects of the medication, without undue risk of relapse. At this time, though, there are no good predictors for identifying this patient group. Indeed, developing such markers was the major goal of the UCLA project that stimulated the controversy over drug-free research. To identify patients who do well without medications, the most obvious design is to study subjects in a drug-free state.

Second, the limitations of the current medications point to the desirability of developing new compounds that might be more effective or carry fewer risks. When these new drugs are tested, subjects' current medications are often stopped for a period of several weeks to allow them to wash out of the body, thus minimizing the risk of adverse drug-drug interactions. The medication-free period may also provide a baseline against which the new drug's therapeutic and side-effects can be assessed. Once the trial of the new medication begins, one group of subjects will usually be assigned randomly to receive an inactive placebo, so that their response can be compared with those subjects receiving the new medication.

Third, drug-free research may be helpful in elucidating the pathophysiology of schizophrenia. . . .

WHAT ARE THE RISKS OF DRUG-FREE RESEARCH?

The major risk of taking clinically stable research subjects off their antipsychotic medications is that they will suffer a relapse of their disorder. The most recent analysis of studies involving discontinuation of medication in schizophrenia indicates an overall relapse rate of 54.8 percent during an average follow-up period of 9.7 months. In comparison, 16.6 percent of patients maintained on medication are likely to relapse during the same period of time. Most episodes of relapse occur in the first year after discontinuation. Forty-four percent of subjects off medication will relapse in the first three months, with the total at two years approaching 80 percent.

Efforts to limit the risk of relapse, for example, by eliminating subjects who may be likely to suffer exacerbation of their conditions, are hampered by the absence of reliable predictors. The only significant correlate of likelihood of relapse is the amount of time subjects have been off their medications. Even prolonged stabilization on antipsychotic medications does not seem to reduce the risk of an acute episode once the medications are discontinued. One factor frequently associated with research protocols, however, appears to magnify the risk of relapse: abrupt discontinuation of medication induces a threefold greater risk of relapse than gradual discontinuation over a period of weeks to months.

The effects of a psychotic episode on patients with schizophrenia are not limited to the profound psychic suffering that often accompanies psychosis. Patients may engage in high-risk behaviors, such as assault and suicide attempts. A relapse may destabilize their psychosocial situations, costing them their jobs, housing, and the support of family and friends. Some evidence suggests intermittent use of medications increases the risk of tardive dyskinesia compared with uninterrupted treatment. Most controversially, it has been suggested that psychotic episodes themselves have a "toxic" effect on patients, increasing the likelihood of further episodes in the future and decreasing the long-term effectiveness of existing medications. These claims have been challenged by other researchers, and are by no means generally accepted.

SHOULD WE DO DRUG-FREE STUDIES IN SCHIZOPHRENIA?

Given the risks associated with withdrawal or withholding of medication from patients with schizophrenia, a lively debate is under way about the legitimacy of this form of research. Arguments against drug-free research take a variety of forms. Some advocates for mentally ill persons would ban all studies involving prolonged drug-free periods on the grounds that they threaten subjects with an unacceptable likelihood and level of harm. These critics invoke the provisions of the Nuremberg Code, which demand that researchers avoid unreasonable degrees of risk for research subjects.

Most commentators, however, including the National Alliance for the Mentally Ill, the country's largest advocacy group for persons with mental disorders, have not gone so far as to endorse an absolute ban on drug-free studies. Not only do they fear that progress on the treatment of schizophrenia will be stymied, but they shy away from the implied stigmatization of persons with mental illness. After all, competent persons, even those with major illnesses, generally are allowed to consent to research that induces risk, at times even serious risk. To suggest that persons with mental illness, alone among other competent adults, should not be permitted to participate in risky research labels them as unable to play an equal role in making decisions about their lives.

Thus, most of the criticisms of drug-free research have taken a somewhat narrower approach, looking either to negate some of the justifications for the research or to modify the conditions under which it takes place. Among the suggestions that have been made are that researchers abandon routine use of placebo control groups in clinical trials of new medications; that reasonable precautions be taken to prevent harm to subjects; and that more intensive informed consent procedures be employed.

USE OF PLACEBO IN MEDICATION TRIALS

Drug-free research in schizophrenia has become a lightning rod for discussion of a broader issue in the ethics of experimental design: the legitimacy of using placebo in trials of new medications for serious disorders, when reasonably effective medications are already available. Opponents of placebo use argue that medical ethics, as embodied in the Declaration of Helsinki, require that "[i]n any medical study, every patient—including those of a control group, if any—should be assured of the best proven diagnostic and therapeutic method." This statement, it is claimed, "effectively proscribes the use of a placebo as control when a proven therapeutic method exists." Since the practical question inherent in the development of a new medication is whether it is superior to existing drugs anyway, design of clinical trials should be changed so that new medications are compared with the best current treatments. A more moderate group of critics is willing to permit subjects to consent to participation in placebo-controlled trials, as long as they are aware of the risks of forgoing standard treatment (or even promising experimental treatment). They argue, however, that once potential subjects are well informed about these matters, it is difficult to imagine that many of them would agree to participate in the placebo-controlled study.

Proponents of placebo use, including the U.S. Food and Drug Administration, note that placebos may not be dispensed with quite as easily as some critics suggest. The most problematic situations that arise without the use of placebo controls occur when no differences are detected in the efficacy of the new medication and standard treatment. Such findings might indicate that both medications are equally effective, prompting a search for other advantages of the new drug, perhaps a reduced rate of side effects. Alternatively, however, the results may simply mean that in the circumstances of this particular study, real differences between the medications were obscured, with each appearing to be equally ineffective with this sample.

A variety of methodologic difficulties could underlie the failure to detect real differences between the drugs. Actual differences may have existed, but poor measurement techniques might have precluded them from being detected. Alternatively, each medication may have truly failed to have much effect because of peculiarities of the sample. This is a particular problem in schizophrenia research, where study samples seem to be drawn increasingly from treatment-resistant populations. It is, after all, persons who have not benefitted from existing treatments who are most likely to seek opportunities to try new medications. Whereas the failure to find a difference between new and current treatments in this population could be interpreted as their being equally effective, in fact the results may be due to the selection of an atypical study sample resistant to the effects of all medications. Whether the study's conclusions can be relied upon would only be evident with the inclusion of a placebo control group.

MECHANISMS OF REDUCING RISKS TO SUBJECTS

If drug-free studies are to continue, whether as part of clinical trials or other research, the ethics of research demand that attention be given to means of minimizing the risks faced by subjects. Carpenter and colleagues have suggested several approaches that may be helpful. First, high-risk subjects could be excluded from entry into the study. Although it is impossible at this point to identify those subjects at greatest risk of relapse, individual subjects' histories may help to identify those who are likely to face the greatest risk of harm from psychotic deterioration. This group might include patients with histories of disastrous consequences from deterioration, or those in marginal social situations. Patients who have done exceptionally well on existing treatment might also be excluded, unless the study rationale specifically required their participation, and other safeguards were included.

Who should make these decisions? The National Commission for the Protection of Human Research Subjects suggested that IRBs could require that a "person who is responsible for the health care of a subject" determine that participation will not interfere with that care—a recommendation that could be extended here to insuring that unreasonable risk does not arise. When the potential subject's clinician is also involved in the research, an independent clinical judgment attesting to the appropriateness of including the patient could be required.

In addition, Carpenter and colleagues note that research milieux can be designed with enhanced psychosocial treatments available, since these may mitigate the effects of taking patients off medication. They point to the importance of close monitoring for early signs of relapse, since restarting medication will usually, though not always, prevent the development of a full-fledged psychotic episode. Use of the shortest possible medication-free period, and a study design that offers some benefits to all participants, even those receiving placebo, are also suggested. The latter might be accomplished, for example, by offering subjects in the placebo group the opportunity for an open trial of the new medication at the conclusion of the double-blind study. A final suggestion comes from investigators who have reviewed the literature on relapse after drug withdrawal: slowly tapering medications, rather than stopping them abruptly, appears to reduce the risk of subsequent relapse.

INFORMED CONSENT PROCEDURES IN DRUG-FREE RESEARCH

Much of the criticism of the UCLA studies and similar projects has focused on the procedures they used to get consent from prospective subjects. OPRR's investigation highlighted several inadequacies in the UCLA disclosures. Jay Katz has extended this critique to point to several problems with consent that are particularly likely to arise in research of this sort. He notes that, consistent with physicians' general dislike for discussing adverse consequences with patients, investigators often will be reluctant to describe clearly the probability of relapse and the severity of the symptoms that might be expected. For the same reason, and because it may facilitate recruitment, investigators may blur the distinction between the treatment being provided by the research project and the care patients would otherwise receive.

Katz also points to investigators' reluctance to disabuse subjects of the idea that research procedures are designed primarily to benefit them, rather than for the purpose of generating generalizable research findings. This "therapeutic misconception" appears to be widespread among research subjects. The risk may be especially great when the subjects' treating clinicians are also the investigators in the project. Indeed, one of the subjects turned complainant in the UCLA study was quoted as saying that he was delighted to get into the research program "because I thought I was going to get the premier treatment, while they did a little research on the side." Extra attention from IRBs may be warranted to insure that investigators communicate information targeted specifically at these common problems in investigators' disclosure and subjects' understanding. Persons independent of the research project could be used, for example, to supplement the information potential subjects receive to insure that it is complete and unbiased.

The rationale for allowing patients with schizophrenia to participate in drug-free studies presumes their competence to consent to research. Reassuring data came from a study of a small group of psychiatric patients, most with schizophrenia, showing that their decisions about participation in hypothetical research projects that varied systematically in their risk-benefit ratios were no different from those of a medically ill group. More recent data suggest, however, that hospitalized schizophrenics as a group are at elevated risk of having their capacities to consent impaired, compared with persons with other psychiatric and medical disorders and with matched controls from the general population. Although comparable data from research settings are lacking, there is good reason to believe that similar problems are likely to appear there too. Indeed, some of the information that should be communicated to subjects in drug-free trials may be particularly difficult for persons with schizophrenia to understand. Denial of the presence or seriousness of their illness, for example, is extremely common in schizophrenics, rendering it more difficult for them to accept that

drug withdrawal may result in psychotic relapse. The difficulty that many patients have with abstractions could impair their ability to grasp the negative consequences of decompensation (e.g., "If I become symptomatic again, my family and friends may reject me.")

Given the risks inherent in drug-free studies, and the complexities of the consent process, it may be worth verifying the assumption of subjects' competence by screening potential participants for decision-related capacities. Since capacities exist on a spectrum, higher-risk studies might be limited to patients with better decisionmaking performance. Inclusion of lower-functioning groups, which may be necessary for scientific reasons, may require additional safeguards.

Also of concern is the probability that as subjects in a drug-free condition begin to experience more symptoms, they may lose the decisionmaking capacities they had at the start of the study. One of the UCLA subjects again provides a good example. As he became increasingly delusional, he lied to his caregivers regarding his symptoms, believing "if I told the doctors I was having hallucinations, they would have me arrested or assassinated." Thus, although all subjects at the start of the study may understand the safeguards available, including their right to withdraw at any point, precisely at the time when those safeguards become relevant, subjects may lose the capacity to invoke them. This suggests the desirability of creating mechanisms (e.g., through a durable power of attorney) whereby substitute decisionmakers can act on patients' behalf, if necessary, when they are unable to do so.

CONCLUSION

There are sound reasons to perform drug-free research in schizophrenia. To justify the risk of relapse by subjects in recent studies, however, careful attention must be given to insuring appropriateness of the design, minimization of risks, and adequacy of informed consent.

The UCLA Schizophrenia Relapse Study

Jay Katz

A research study conducted at the Neuro-psychiatric Institute of the University of California, Los Angeles (UCLA), which began in the early 1980s . . . [and was still in progress at the time this article was published in the Fall of 1993—eds.] illustrates the problems I have discussed.* To orient the reader, I briefly summarize three facts about the design of the experiment and two facts about its aftermath that are of concern to me: (1) The study required schizophrenic patients who had recovered from their psychotic disorders to be withdrawn from medication even though "[i]t is generally accepted that maintenance antipsychotic medication will benefit a substantial proportion of chronic schizophrenics."[1] (2) The study expected to produce a relapse (recurrence of symptomatology) in many patient-subjects in order to attain its objective to predict better relapse, particularly of those who would exhibit such severe symptoms as "bizarre behavior, self-neglect, hostility, depressive mood and suicideability."[2] (3) The informed consent form signed by the participants was inadequate in disclosing to the subjects the risks which their participation entailed. (4) The IRB approved the research protocol and informed consent form without asking the investigators for clarifications that might have led the IRB to better protect the subjects of research. (5) The subsequent response to the review of the study by the National Institutes of Health's Office for the Protection of Research Risks (OPRR) did not go far in remedying the problems which came to OPRR's attention.

Saint Louis University Law Journal, Vol. 38:1, pp. 41–51. Used with permission of the publisher.

*EDITORS' NOTE: In a previous section of this article, deleted here, Professor Katz had argued for greater public visibility of the decisions made in the conduct of human experimentation, and had warned against the tendency of local institutional review boards to place the needs of research above the rights and interests of patients.

EDITORS' NOTE: The article has been edited and the notes renumbered.

I also want to emphasize at the outset that my analysis is limited to a review of one of the research protocols, including the informed consent form approved by UCLA's IRB, the action taken by the OPRR, once parents of one of the subjects had lodged a complaint about the study and a perusal of the psychiatric literature pertinent to the research project.[3] I cannot address what might have been disclosed to the subjects in conversations between them and the investigators; about that I have no knowledge. I can only note that the data available from the protocol and the OPRR review hardly suggests that scrupulous attention was paid at any point to full disclosure and consent.

The UCLA experiment was designed to make an important contribution to a better understanding of the need for continuous medication following patients' recovery from a recent onset of schizophrenic disorder. Thus, the research project sought to identify patients who can function without medication because antipsychotic medication can cause tardive dyskinesia, a syndrome consisting of involuntary and potentially irreversible movements for which no known treatment exists.[4]

All potential patient-subjects were being followed in UCLA's After Care Clinic.[5] The study, according to the protocol, consisted of two sequential phases.[6] In the first phase, lasting for twenty-four weeks, the patient-subjects were randomized, in a double-blind design, to one of two groups. The first group received a standardized dose of 12.5 mgm of prolyxin decanoate, an antipsychotic medication, every two weeks, while the second was injected with a placebo, an inert, therapeutically ineffective substance. After twelve weeks, the injections given to members of each group were reversed so that those who had been receiving medication now received a placebo, and vice versa. In the second phase, "all clinically appropriate patients" received no medication, i.e., those who were still on prolyxin were also deprived of the active drug.[7]

The patient-subjects were then followed for at least one year unless "1) the subject withdraws permission for the study or 2) clinical relapse or psychotic exacerbation occurs."[8] Criteria for psychotic relapse included "[high scores on test measures] for hallucinations, unusual thought content, or conceptual disorganization; [for] psychotic exacerbation [fairly severe recurrence of symptomatology; and] for relapse-other type, [high scores] on scales of *bizarre behavior; self-neglect, hostility, depressive mood, and suicidability.*"[9] Apparently the patient-subject's therapist was authorized in the first double-blind phase of the study to break the code for "clinical reasons" but the protocol contained no information, and therefore the IRB could not know, as to when the therapist might take such action. Clearly the intent was to tolerate severe recurrences in symptomatology. Once that had happened "the patient [would] be withdrawn from the study."[10]

The investigators noted in the protocol's section on "Potential Benefits" that since "no study shows 100% relapse in schizophrenics withdrawn from antipsychotics, unquestioned maintenance treatment may for any particular patient involve much risk and little benefit. At present, there is little consistent data regarding predictive factors for patients at low risk of relapse without pharmacotherapy."[11] In that section the investigators also stated

> that clinical relapse or psychotic exacerbation can be expected to occur in at least some of our patient subjects. *However, since most of our patients have been requesting drug withdrawal for months, and since our knowledge as to which acute schizophrenic patients will relapse following drug withdrawal is very meager, we feel this risk is justified, especially in view of the risk of tardive dyskinesia with long-term antipsychotic use.* Withdrawal from antipsychotic medication one year after the psychotic episode is not unusual in standard psychiatric practice for patients with acute, nonchronic schizophrenia, since little clear evidence exists regarding longer-term prophylactic effects for this nonchronic population.[12]

It is true that many schizophrenic patients complain about the side effects of antipsychotic medication. However, therapists who believe that such treatment is clinically indicated generally do their level best to impress on patients the need for remaining on medication or to encourage its resumption as soon as symptoms recur. In the UCLA study, on the other hand, all patients were withdrawn from medication, indeed required to do so, for research purposes until the needs of the study, and not those of the individual patient, had been satisfied.[13] The expectation of relapse was an integral aspect of the research design; it was not an unfortunate consequence of treatment but one which the investigators deliberately induced. This is particularly problematic because of the continuing controversy in psychiatric circles as to whether relapse leads to additional, at times irreversible, injury.[14]

The consent form submitted to the IRB for review and approval informed prospective patient-subjects that "the purpose of this study is to take people like me off medication in a way that will give the most information about the medication, its effects on me, on others and on the way the brain works."[15] It mentioned that an inactive substance (placebo) or an (active) medication would be randomly administered during the first phase and that then "all medication will be stopped and that I will continue to receive regular care at the UCLA After Care Clinic."[16] Stating it in that way could only confuse potential subjects. In the same sentence they were told that medication would be stopped and that they would continue to receive regular care, without alerting them in most explicit language that "regular care" was compromised by the withdrawal of medication.[17]

Moreover, the patient-subjects were not informed at the beginning of the study that already during the first phase they would not necessarily receive optimal individual treatment, but only a *standardized* dose of 12.5 mg of prolyxin. Such a standardized dose can itself lead either to a return of symptomatology or produce unnecessary side effects because it is known that the amount of prolyxin must be tailored to the individual needs of patients with some requiring larger or smaller amounts of medication.[18] The consent form then goes on to describe in considerable detail the psychological tests that would be administered to the patient-subject during the study period. That aspect of the research could have been presented in a more abbreviated fashion and surely, in light of other omissions, did not deserve the space it was given.

With respect to significant risks and benefits the following information was provided:

> I understand that during blood drawing, I may experience pain from the needle prick, a small amount of bleeding, infection or black and blue

marks at the site of the needle mark which will disappear in about 10 days.

I understand that because of the withdrawal of active medication, I may become worse during this study and that either a relapse of my initial symptoms or new symptoms may occur. I understand that I will not be charged for the active medication or the placebo that I am provided during this study. If I do show a significant return of symptoms, I understand the clinic staff will use active medication again to improve my condition. If I would require hospitalization during this study, although this is not likely, I understand that the clinic staff would help to arrange an appropriate hospitalization but the research project would not pay for the hospitalization.

I understand that I may benefit from this study by being taken off medication in a careful way while under close medical supervision. The potential benefits to science in this study are that it will increase my doctor's knowledge of the relationship between the medication, its effect on people such as myself, and on the way the brain functions in certain forms of mental illness.

I understand that my condition may improve, worsen or remain unchanged from participation in this study.[19]

No information was provided as to what constituted a "significant return of symptoms," that it could mean a return of hallucinations, conceptual disorganization, self-neglect, depressive mood, or suicidal ideation. Potential patient-subjects under the care of mental health professionals in an Aftercare Clinic might very well have believed that "significant" did not encompass such dire consequences. Moreover, while it was acknowledged that "I *may* become worse," the consent form of July 1988 did not state that at that time it was known that of those patient-subjects enrolled in the study so far, eighty-eight percent had suffered a relapse.[20]

In light of the high relapse rate it was misleading to aver "that my condition *may* improve, worsen or remain unchanged." The odds favoring relapse were far too great; few subjects would "improve" or "remain the same." Finally, it is not only ironic but also misleading that the risks of a needle prick were discussed in such exquisite detail. Such a forthcoming and honest acknowledgement could only leave patient-subjects with the impression that the investigators would disclose any other risks in similar detail and with similar candor.

The informed consent form should have highlighted in bold face that the primary objective of the study was to advance knowledge for the sake of future patients and, depending on outcome, only of value to some of the subjects' future well-being. The form, further, should have acknowledged that the study was not designed to attend to their *individual* therapeutic needs, and that the subjects exposed themselves to considerable risks. Moreover, the patient-subjects were not presented with any information about the merits of not joining the research project. They were deprived of considering that alternative. To be sure, the informed consent form must be supplemented by the oral informed consent process[21] and the latter may be more important than the former in providing patient-subjects with meaningful disclosures, particularly since the forms are generally written in such incomprehensible language. When, however, as in this instance, the written document provided incomplete information, and with insufficient candor, patient-subjects who are intent on reading it are deprived of crucial information. From a different perspective, the consent form, as written, cannot help but create concerns, though most difficult to substantiate, as to whether the oral informed consent was similarly flawed.[22]

After complaints about the study had come to OPRR's attention[23] and it had discussed the problem with UCLA, a letter from OPRR detailed "the agreed-upon actions" which UCLA would now take:

> [P]rovide (a) more detailed information regarding the risks associated with lengthy withdrawal of antipsychotic medication, including information regarding the likely rates of exacerbation or relapse and the consequences thereof; (b) an indication that, in the event of such exacerbation or relapse, it is likely that antipsychotic medication will need to be resumed; (c) a description of the risks associated with continued fixed dose medication treatment; and (d) a disclosure of alternative courses of treatment . . . .[24]
>
> . . . .
>
> The Continuing Care Brochure will be modified to ensure that it accurately reflects the parameters of the After Care Program's research protocols.[25]

In addition, OPRR required the following additional actions:

> (1) No new subjects should be enrolled in this research until the revised Informed Consent

Documents have been reviewed and approved by the UCLA Institutional Review Board (IRB).

(2) The revised IRB-approved Informed Consent Documents should be used to obtain renewed consent from all subjects currently participating in this research, including subjects for whom clinical monitoring constitutes the only research involvement.

(3) Copies of the revised IRB-approved Informed Consent Documents and of the revised Continuing Care Brochure should be forwarded to OPRR as soon as possible.

(4) UCLA should consider, and OPRR strongly recommends, contacting former research subjects in writing to provide them with the additional information included in the revised Informed Consent Documents. Copies of such communications with former subjects should be forwarded to OPRR as soon as they become available.[26]

OPRR did not insist that UCLA stop the research project immediately, or at least, that the patient-subjects be examined by independent psychiatrists in order to assess their individual treatment needs. In light of what already had transpired, such an opportunity would have made it easier for patient-subjects to decide whether they wished to continue in, or withdraw from, the study. Moreover, in light of the serious deficiencies in the informed consent form,[27] which is one of the prime responsibilities of IRBs to review,[28] OPRR did not institute a thorough investigation of the practices of UCLA's IRB. OPRR's evaluation was sufficiently critical of the IRB process to suggest that the IRB's review of other research proposals may be similarly flawed.[29] Undertaking such an investigation was even more pressing in this case since several subject-patients suffered severe schizophrenic relapses,[30] and one young man allegedly committed suicide.[31]

The revised informed consent form, while an improvement over the previous one, continues to leave patient-subjects uninformed, *inter alia*, about the *specific* severity of relapse which they might suffer, mentioning only "difficulties in relationship with others and problems with work or school"; or what specific "psychotic symptoms or severe symptoms" will lead to providing medication once again. It does not present in any meaningful detail the advantages and disadvantages of participating in the study or receiving customary treatment for their condition. The consent form did not state with sufficient clarity that the primary objective of

the study was to conduct research for the sake of future patients, perhaps of benefit to those enrolled in this study *in the future,* and that it was not therapy for the subject's individual *present* needs. While the consent form now admits that "70-80% of patients who have entered this study in the past have experienced a psychotic exacerbation or relapse within one year" and that "I may become worse during the study," it says nothing about what subjects specifically should consider, and reflect on, before exposing themselves to these risks. On the other hand, with respect to benefits it is noted that withdrawal of medication will keep them from "developing tardive dyskinesia which involves abnormal movements of the face, hands, legs or trunk." And the form goes on to emphasize, "I may benefit from this study by being taken off medication in a careful way while under close medical supervision."[32] The risks deserved at least similar detailed explication and prominence.

What transpired in this study is not unique to UCLA; it is symptomatic of the flawed nature of current regulations and current practices protecting the human rights of research subjects. These flaws, as I have argued throughout this article, extend from the Federal Regulations themselves[33] to the supervision of projects by IRBs and OPRR. Thus, my analysis of UCLA's consent form should not be taken merely as a critique of the nature and depth of the information that was or was not included in the written document, but, more importantly, as a critique of the entire informed consent process. The problems with this study, as with many others, are: (1) subject-patients' consent was manipulated; (2) trivial and non-trivial risks were insufficiently distinguished; (3) the severity of predictable risks was not highlighted nor was the incidence of their likelihood disclosed; and (4) the risks and benefits of non-participation were neither sufficiently disclosed nor satisfactorily discussed. Under these circumstances, patient-subjects were not offered a meaningful choice whether or not to participate in the study.

NOTES

1. Keith H. Nuechterlein & Michael Gitlin, Research Protocol for Developmental Processes in Schizophrenic Disorders Project: Protocol; Double Blind Crossover and Withdrawal of Neuroleptics in Remitted, Recent-Onset Schizophrenia, HSPC #86-07-336 1,6 [hereinafter

Protocol] (on file with author). In a 1988 article the investigators gave a clear account of these research objectives:

> The present study is a prospective examination of prodromal signs and symptoms of schizophrenic relapse, using a systematic and carefully controlled research design. One important improvement over the previous studies is that relapse was defined as the elevation of psychiatric symptoms to the severe or extremely severe level. Thus, minor symptom fluctuations that might often be inconsequential were not considered relapses. In contrast to the studies that defined the period of observation by the necessity to increase medication to avoid a possible relapse, we can be certain that any prodromal changes that we isolated actually did precede a clear relapse.

Kenneth L Subotnik & Keith N. Nuechterlein, *Prodromal Signs and Symptoms in Schizophrenic Relapse*, 97 J. Abnormal Psychology 405, 406 (1988).

2. *Id.*

3. These and all other discussed unpublished documents are in the possession of the author and available upon request.

4. In some patients symptoms of tardive dyskinesia disappear within several months after antipsychotic drugs are withdrawn, but withdrawal of antipsychotic medication does not guarantee that symptoms will vanish. In some patients, symptoms may persist indefinitely. Dorland's Illustrated Medical Dictionary 517-18 (27th ed. 1988).

5. *See infra* note 32 and accompanying text.

6. Protocol, *supra* note.

7. Protocol, *supra* note, at 4.

8. *Id.* at 6.

9. *Id.* (emphasis supplied).

10. *Id.*

11. *Id.* at 7.

12. Protocol, *supra* note, at 8.

13. The protocol does not make clear whether all the patient-subjects had been on medication for at least one year when enrolled in the study, which, according to the investigators, is the time when "in standard psychiatric practice" patients are often taken off medication. *Id.*

14. Although the issue is far from settled, many psychiatrists believe that relapse can be permanently harmful to patients: "[S]ome patients are left with a damaging residual if a psychosis is allowed to proceed unmitigated." Richard J. Wyatt, *Neuroleptics and the Natural Course of Schizophrenia*, 17 Schizophrenia Bulletin 325, 347 (1991). "[N]euroleptic drugs . . . if they fully control all acute episodes, may protect against the otherwise inevitable decline of mental function." R. Miller, *Schizophrenia as a Progressive Disorder: Relations to EEG, CT, Neuropathological and Other Evidence*, 33 Progress Neurobiology 17, 35 (1989).

15. Keith Nuechterlein, Informed Consent Agreement for Patients (Version 1): Double-Blind Drug Crossover and Withdrawal Project 1 (July 1988) [hereinafter Consent Agreement I] (on file with author).

16. *Id.*

17. Being absolutely clear on this point was important since the subjects were recruited from the Continuing Care Program of The Neuropsychiatric Institute UCLA. The brochure, given to patients enrolled in this program, contained the following information:

> THE CONTINUING CARE PROGRAM . . .
>
> . . . is a specialty service combining treatment, research, and training in the care of the individual with psychotic symptoms. Jointly sponsored by NIMH, UCLA, Camarillo-NIP, and the Clinical Research Center, the Program offers continuing care to people who are experiencing their first psychotic episode.
>
> The Program includes inpatient and outpatient treatment as well as an active follow-up evaluation of each person. Fully integrated with these services is a research project aimed at increasing understanding and knowledge of the factors that are related to relapse and remission.
>
> PURPOSE
>
> The goal of the Program is to assist persons in making a successful adaptation to life in the community and to improve their daily living and social skills. An equally important goal is to facilitate the family's coping skills for dealing with mental illness. Where appropriate, consultation with other community agencies and social support networks is provided.
>
> . . . .
>
> AFTERCARE CLINIC
>
> A range of outpatient services are offered through the Aftercare Clinic at the UCLA Neuropsychiatric Institute. Following discharge, patients and their families are provided:
>
> *Group Therapy*: in small groups, patients learn problem-solving skills and interpersonal effectiveness.
>
> *Family Education*: counseling is aimed to upgrade the entire family's coping skills and understanding of the illness, and to facilitate use of resources both within the family and the community.
>
> *Medication* is administered at the lowest optimal dose to maximize coping with symptoms and stressors and to minimize side effects.
>
> . . . .
>
> PARTICIPATION
>
> . . . is voluntary by patients and families in both the research and the clinical services. It is expected that a voluntary agreement to participate for a minimum of two years be made at the point a patient joins the Program.

UCLA Neuropsychiatric Institute, Continuing Care Program of the Mental Health Clinical Center 1-3 (on file with author). Since the Aftercare program serves dual objectives, treatment and research, any experimental interventions needed to be specified and differentiated from therapy with the greatest of care, particularly whenever the research component compromised therapeutic intentions.

18. See *Physician's Desk Reference* 619 (47th ed. 1993) ("Appropriate dosage of Prolyxin Decanoate (Fluphenazine Decanoate Injection) should be individualized for each patient. . . . The optimal amount of the drug and the frequency of administration must be determined for each patient, since dosage requirements have been found to vary with clinical circumstances as well as with individual response to the drug."); *Textbook of Neuropsychiatry* 682 (Stuart C. Yudosky & Robert E. Hales eds., 2d ed. 1991) ("Blood levels vary widely in different patients given the same dose of a neuroleptic. . . . [T]here is no established correlation between serum concentration and clinical response."); Robert F. Asarnow & Stephen R. Marder, *Differential Effect of Low and Conventional Doses of Fluphenazine on Schizophrenic Outpatients with Good or Poor Information-Processing Abilities*, 45 Archive Gen. Psychiatry 822 (1988).

19. Consent Agreement I, *supra* note 15, at 2.

20. Of the 24 patients who entered the drug withdrawal period, 21 have ultimately had psychotic exacerbations or relapses. ranging from 17 to 123 weeks after the last fluphenazine administration. For these 21 exacerbation/relapses plus the 3 psychotic exacerbations during the placebo phase of the crossover, the mean time to exacerbation/relapse is 33 weeks. Of these 24 patients who have developed an exacerbation/relapse after medication discontinuation, 5 exacerbation/relapses occurred after 60 or more weeks (21%), 6 after 40-59 weeks (25%), 7 after 20-39 weeks (29%), 4 after 10-19 weeks (17%), and 2 after less than 10 weeks (8%). Three more remain well after 104, 30 and 23 weeks. Keith H. Nuechterlein, Grant Application: Developmental Processes in Schizophrenic Disorders, RD I MH 37705-07, 1, 84 (Nov. 15, 1988) (on file with author).

21. UCLA claims to have presented much of the information required for informed consent to patient-subject's orally. Department of Health and Human Services (DHHS) regulations at 45 C.F.R. § 46.117 require, however, that the elements of legally effective Informed Consent (specified at 45 C.F.R. § 46.116 (1992)) be embodied in the *written* Informed Consent Document.

22. The special care that, I believe, must be given to the informed consent process whenever the research-therapy distinction is in danger of being compromised, is illustrated by a comment made by my respected colleague and friend Robert J. Levine who read an earlier draft of this paper:

My perception of the investigators' motivation continues to be very different from yours. I see this as an instance of opportunistic research. The physician-investigators did not expose subjects to the risks of withdrawal from medication in order to do research. Rather, in the light of their reading of the results of observations published by others, they decided that it would be in the medical interests of these patients to have their medications withdrawn. Although they knew that some of them would develop symptoms, they could not predict which. What they planned to do was to keep a careful record of their observations of those who developed symptoms. They further made plans to remove patients from the study and treat them if certain specific criteria were met.

Letter from Robert J. Levine to Jay Katz (Sept. 24, 1993) (quoted by permission). Viewing the "motivation" of the investigators as "opportunistic research" in the service of the "medical interests of these patients" co-joins therapy and research. In the UCLA study the patient-subjects' medical interests were subordinated to the inflexibility of the research design. It is this fact that needed to be highlighted in the consent form, notwithstanding any accompanying therapeutic motivations of the investigators. Viewing research also as treatment invites confusion in the minds of all participants as to who they are: physicians or investigators, patients or subjects. In turn, it makes it easier for investigators to take license because of their "benevolent therapeutic intentions." Furthermore, the "specific criteria [for removal from the study]" noted by Levine included relapse to the severest level of psychosis, an unacceptable criterion for clinical practice. Long before that point is reached psychiatrists would urge their patients to resume taking medication. Thus, I would argue that the physician-investigators' conduct was motivated by their research interest, even though they might eventually also bestow benefits on their subjects or future patients. If I am correct, then the patient-subjects' medical interests are in this instance different from, and should not be conflated with, the investigators' research interests.

23. The complaint was lodged by Bob and Gloria Aller, parents of one of the subjects. The story of Greg's participation in, and gradual deterioration during, the study is graphically described in a recent article: Eventually, he not only dropped out of college, but also

took out a carving knife, walked to the door of his mother's kitchen, [and thinking that] "my mom was possessed by the devil," . . . "[m]y plan was to scare the devil out of her literally." The Allers began barricading their bedroom door at night [A few days later] he moved out, [and when he saw Nuechterlein's partner, Dr. Michael Gitlin, Greg kept this information from him, and thus Gitlin]

noted "Moved out from parents. Says no symptoms present. Finishing the semester."
James Willwerth, *Tinkering with Madness*, 42 TIME 41-42 (Aug. 30, 1992). It took five more months, and the article describes what happened during that interval, before he was remedicated at UCLA. *Id.*

24. Letter from J. Thomas Puglisi, Acting Chief, Compliance Oversight Branch of the Office for Protection from Research Risks (OPRR) to Richard Sisson, Senior Vice Chancellor of Academic Affairs at the University of California Los Angeles 1 (Aug. 19, 1992) (on file with author).

25. *Id.* at 2.

26. *Id.*

27. Even after modifying the consent forms initially used, UCLA continues to deny any wrongdoing and contends that the forms and process used to obtain initial consent were appropriate. *See* Letter from Richard Sisson, Senior Vice Chancellor of Academic Affairs at the University of California Los Angeles to J. Thomas Puglisi, Acting Chief, Compliance Oversight Branch of the OPRR 4-5 (Sept. 17, 1992) (on file with author).

28. Federal Regulations instruct IRBs to "determine that all of the following requirements are satisfied: . . . (4) Informed consent will be sought from each prospective subject . . . in accordance with, and to the extent required by § 46.117." 45 C.F.R. § 46.111(4) (1992).

29. The copy of the letter from OPRR to UCLA, made available to me through the Freedom of Information Act, excluded three paragraphs. They may have contained additional criticisms of UCLA'S conduct in this case. See *supra* note 24.

30. Subotnik & Nuechterlein, *supra* note.

31. One participant in the UCLA project committed suicide on March 28, 1992, after being taken off psychotropic medication. Sandy Rovner, *Ethics Concerns Raised in Schizophrenia Study*, WASH. POST, Sept 29, 1992, at H7. The Federal Regulations require that "[w]here appropriate, the research plan makes adequate provision for monitoring the data collected to insure the safety of subjects." 45 C.F.R. § 46.111(6) (1992). The protocol, however, did not describe in sufficient detail the special monitoring that would be provided, even though some of the research subjects could suffer a severe relapse. The protocol only stated that "a member of the clinic staff will meet regularly as needed" with the patient. See *supra* note.

32. Keith Nuechterlein, Informed Consent Agreement for Patients: Double-Blind Drug Crossover and Withdrawal Project 3 (Sept 1992) (on file with author).

33. Shamoo and Irving recently noted that recommendations by various Federal Commissions to consider persons with mental illness as members of a vulnerable group who deserve special protection whenever they participate in research were not implemented. They learned that "[this] outcome was the result in large part of opposition from researchers on mental disorders who claimed that the population in question were no more vulnerable than most persons with severe medical disorders and that the suggested limitations would seriously restrict research on mental disorders." Shamoo and Irving concluded that "the issue of using persons with mental illness as human research subjects has been lost in the shuffle, due in part to the lobbying effort of some researchers on mental disorders." They also raise the important question, "what was the justification for delegating to local IRBs the essential responsibilities for affording protections for persons with mental illness . . . ?" Adil F. Shamoo & Dianne N. Irving, *Accountability in Research Using Persons With Mental Illness* 1, 2(1994) (forthcoming article, on file with author).

RECOMMENDED SUPPLEMENTARY READING

General Works

Brody, Baruch A. *Ethical Issues in Drug Testing, Approval, and Pricing: The Clot-Dissolving Drugs.* New York: Oxford University Press, 1995.

IRB: A Review of Human Subjects Research. Hastings-on-Hudson, NY: Hastings Center, 10 vols. per year.

Katz, Jay; Capron, Alexander M.; and Glass, Eleanor Swift; eds. *Experimentation with Human Beings.* New York: Russell Sage Foundation, 1972.

Levine, Robert J. *Ethics and Regulation of Clinical Research.* 2nd ed. Baltimore, MD: Urban & Schwarzenberg, 1986.

National Commission for the Protection of Human Subjects of Biomedical and Behavioral Research. *The Belmont Report: Ethical Principles and Guidelines for the Protection of Human Subjects of Research.* Washington, DC: U.S. Government Printing Office, 1978.

Rothman, David J. *Strangers at the Bedside: A History of How Law and Bioethics Transformed Medical Decision Making.* New York: Basic Books, 1991.

Vanderpool, Harold Y., ed. *The Ethics of Research Involving Human Subjects: Facing the 21st Century.* Frederick, MD: University Publishing Group, 1996.

Veatch, Robert. *The Patient as Partner: A Theory of Human-Experimentation Ethics.* Bloomington: Indiana University Press, 1987.

Social Welfare and Informed Consent

Annas, George J., and Grodin, Michael A., eds. *The Nazi Doctors and the Nuremberg Code: Human Rights in Human Experimentation.* New York: Oxford University Press, 1992.

Caplan, Arthur L., ed. *When Medicine Went Mad: Bioethics and the Holocaust.* Clifton, NJ: Humana Press, 1992.

Human Radiation Experiments: Final Report of the Advisory Committee on Human Radiation Experiments. New York, Oxford University Press, 1996.

Jonas, Hans. "Philosophical Reflections on Experimenting with Human Subjects." In *Experimentation with Human Subjects,* edited by Paul Freund. New York: Braziller, 1970.

Jones, James. *Bad Blood: The Tuskegee Syphilis Experiment: A Tragedy of Race and Medicine,* rev. ed. New York: Free Press, 1993.

Lasagna, Louis. "Some Ethical Problems in Clinical Investigation." In *Human Aspects of Biomedical Innovation,* edited by E. Mendelsohn, et al. Cambridge, MA: Harvard University Press, 1971.

Lifton, Robert Jay. *The Nazi Doctors: Medical Killing and the Psychology of Genocide.* New York: Basic Books, 1986.

"Trusting Science: Nuremberg and the Human Radiation Experiments." *Hastings Center Report* (symposium, September, October 1996).

The Ethics of Randomized Clinical Trials

Appelbaum, Paul S., et al. "False Hopes and Best Data: Consent to Research and the Therapeutic Misconception." *Hastings Center Report* 17, no. 2 (April 1987): 20–24.

Brody, Baruch A. "Conflicts of Interests and the Validity of Clinical Trials." In *Conflicts of Interest,* edited by D. S. Shim and R. G. Spece. New York: Oxford University Press, 1993.

Christakis, Nicholas. "Ethics Are Local: Engaging Cross-Cultural Variation in the Ethics for Clinical Research." *Social Sciences in Medicine* 35, no. 9 (1992): 1079–1091.

Freedman, Benjamin; Weijer, Charles; and Glass, Kathleen C. "Placebo Orthodoxy in Clinical Research I: Empirical and Methodological Myths," *Journal of Law, Medicine and Ethics* 24 (1996): 243–251.

———. "Placebo Orthodoxy in Clinical Research II: Ethical, Legal, and Regulatory Myths." *Journal of Law, Medicine and Ethics* 24 (1996): 252–259.

Fried, Charles. *Medical Experimentation: Personal Integrity and Social Policy*. New York: American Elsevier, 1974.

Gifford, Fred. "Community-Equipoise and the Ethics of Randomized Clinical Trials." *Bioethics* 9, no. 2 (April 1995): 127–148.

Ijsselmuiden, Carel B., and Faden, Ruth. "Research and Informed Consent in Africa: Another Look." *New England Journal of Medicine* 326, no. 12 (March 19, 1992): 830–834.

Kopelman, Loretta. "Randomized Clinical Trials, Consent, and the Therapeutic Relationship." *Clinical Research* 31(1983): 1–11.

Levine, Carol; Dubler, Nancy N.; and Levine, Robert. "Building a New Consensus: Ethical Principles and Policies for Clinical Research on HIV/AIDS." *IRB: A Review of Human Subjects Research* 13, nos. 1–2 (January–April 1991): 1–17.

Levine, Robert J. "Uncertainty in Clinical Research." *Law, Medicine and Health Care* 16, nos. 3–4 (Winter 1988): 174–182.

Marquis, Don. "Leaving Therapy to Chance." *Hastings Center Report* 13, no. 4 (1983): 40–47.

Miller, Bruce. "Experimentation on Human Subjects: The Ethics of Random Clinical Trials." In *Health Care Ethics*, edited by Donald VanDeVeer and Tom Regan. Philadelphia, PA: Temple University Press, 1987.

Schaffner, Kenneth F., ed. "Ethical Issues in the Use of Clinical Controls." *Journal of Medicine and Philosophy* 1, no. 4 (November 1986).

Tannsjo, Torbjorn. "The Morality of Clinical Research—A Case Study," *Journal of Medicine and Philosophy* 19 (1994): 7–21.

Access to Experimental Therapies and Experimentation on "Vulnerable" Populations

Angell, Marcia. "The Ethics of Clinical Research in the Third World." *New England Journal of Medicine* 337, no. 12 (September 18, 1997): 847–849.

Crouch, Robert, and Arras, John. "AZT Trials and Tribulations," *Hastings Center Report* 28 (forthcoming 1998).

Dubler, Nancy, and Sidel, Victor W. "On Research on HIV Infection and AIDS in Correctional Institutions." *Milbank Quarterly* 67, no. 2 (1989): 171–207.

Grodin, Michael, and Glantz, Leonard E., eds. *Children as Research Subjects: Science, Ethics and Law*. Oxford: Oxford University Press, 1994.

Kass, Nancy E. et al. "Harms of Excluding Pregnant Women from Clinical Research: The Case of HIV-Infected Pregnant Women." *The Journal of Law, Medicine and Ethics* 24, no. 1 (Spring 1996): 36–46.

King, Nancy M. P. "Experimental Treatment: Oxymoron or Aspiration?" *Hastings Center Report* (July–August 1995): 6–15.

Levi, Jeffrey. "Unproven AIDS Therapies: The Food and Drug Administration and ddI." In *Biomedical Politics*. Washington, DC: Institute of Medicine, (1991): 9–42.

Mastroianni, Anna C.; Faden, Ruth; and Federman, Daniel; eds. *Women and Health Research: Ethical and Legal Issues of Including Women in Clinical Studies*. Vols. 1 and 2. Washington, DC: National Academy Press, 1994.

Melnick, Vijaya L., and Dubler, Nancy N., eds. *Alzheimer's Dementia: Dilemmas in Clinical Research*. Clifton, NJ: Humana Press, 1985.

Merton, Vanessa. "The Exclusion of Pregnant, Pregnable, and Once-Pregnable People (a.k.a. Women) from Biomedical Research." *American Journal of Law and Medicine* 19, no. 4 (1993): 369–451.

Miller, Franklin G., and Rosenstein, Donald L. "Psychiatric Symptom-Provoking Studies: An Ethical Appraisal. *Biological Psychiatry* 40 (1997): 403–409.

Shamoo, Adil E., and Keay, Timothy J. "Ethical Concerns about Relapse Studies," *Cambridge Quarterly of Healthcare Ethics* 5 (1996): 373–386.

Thomas, Stephen B., and Quinn, Sandra Crouse. "The Tuskegee Syphilis Study, 1932 to 1972: Implications for HIV Education and AIDS Risk Education Programs in the Black Community." *American Journal of Public Health* 81, no. 11 (November 1991): 1498–1504.

"Twenty Years After: The Legacy of the Tuskegee Syphilis Study." *Hastings Center Report* (November–December 1992): 29 ff.

PART SIX

ALLOCATION,
SOCIAL JUSTICE,
AND HEALTH POLICY

Even if we believe that all men and women are "created equal," it's hard to deny that we are not equal with regard to health. Some of us, the winners in the "natural lottery," are blessed with good health and live to ripe old age without the meddling of physicians and nurses. Others are born with catastrophic diseases requiring massive amounts of high-technology medicine merely in order to survive painfully from day to day.

It is also hard to deny that we are not equal with regard to availability of health care. Some are born into wealthy or middle-class families that can either purchase outright all the health care they want or buy enough insurance to cover their needs. Others come from poor families that cannot afford adequate nutrition, housing, and clothing, let alone insurance for health care. These losers in the "social lottery"—the child in the welfare hotel, the impoverished AIDS patient, the unemployed farm worker—often have desperate needs for care that go unmet.

For those poor enough to meet the definition of poverty stipulated by their state-run Medicaid programs, access to health care is often an entitlement in name only. Since most states reimburse only a small fraction of physicians' usual rates, very few of them are willing to treat Medicaid patients. With the notable exception of some extraordinarily devoted physicians, those who do accept such patients are often poorly qualified and offer substandard care in large, impersonal practices featuring "turnstile" medical attention. Hospitals that deal with a predominantly Medicaid population are notoriously understaffed and undersupplied. Patients are regularly subjected to long waiting periods for necessary treatments during which their conditions may badly deteriorate. And these treatments are often delivered through dangerously antiquated technology. At one Brooklyn hospital, a cancer unit's decrepit radiation unit was nicknamed "the killer" due to its tendency to destroy roughly equal portions of both cancerous and healthy tissue. Yet across the street at the university-affiliated hospital, the insured "paying customers" benefited from state-of-the-art technology and care.

Those who are not poor enough to qualify for Medicaid, yet are too poor to afford private health insurance, pose perhaps the greatest challenge both to our nation's emerging health policy and to our collective moral conscience. Numbering roughly 40 million people, these uninsured individuals must either go without treatment entirely or obtain care from chaotic emergency rooms. Journalist Laurie Kaye Abraham provides us with a compelling and poignant account of the uninsured,

> often in advanced stages of treatable disease, with undiagnosed diabetes attacking their kidneys, or even breast tumors large enough to break through their skin. Their conditions certainly are emergencies now but emergencies that . . . did not necessarily have to be. They got so sick waiting, waiting, waiting, because they had no health insurance and did not think they could afford a doctor until they *really* needed one. And even when things went bad enough that they *really* needed one, they still feared they could not afford it—who knows how expensive a doctor's visit will be?—so they stumbled into the emergency room instead. There, the clerks ask if you have insurance but will not draw in their breath when you say you do not, will not ask you to wait while they confer with someone else, will not, cannot, turn you away. (Abraham 1993, 96)

The first section of Part Six asks how we should think about these inequalities in both the natural and social lotteries. Are they merely instances of misfortune that should elicit pity and perhaps charity, or should we rather view them as injustices calling for rectification? And supposing that health care is a right rather than a privilege, to what kind of health care are we all entitled?

Whereas Section One applies broad questions of political philosophy to health care, Section Two offers a sampler of hard choices forced upon society by the confluence of ever-expanding demands for health care, high-cost technology, and the rise of managed care and other cost-constraining strategies. Section Three is an in-depth study of the various substantive moral principles and procedural devices found in the health care rationer's "toolkit" (Wickler 1992).

JUSTICE AND HEALTH CARE

A crucial and distressing result of the combined natural and social "lotteries" is that roughly 40 million Americans remain uninsured, and millions more remain underinsured. This failure to obtain needed insurance translates into a predictable lack of access to health care. The primary question addressed in Section One is whether this lack of access is unjust or merely unfortunate—a failure of charity or a violation of rights. The President's Commission for the Study of Ethical Problems in Medicine and Biomedical and Behavioral Research confronts this question head-on in its report *An Ethical Framework for Access to Health Care.* According to the Commission, health care is different from other consumer goods in that it is crucially related to our level of well-being, helping us to ward off pain, suffering, and premature death. Like education, health care is necessary to achieve equal opportunity in society. And health care is freighted with "interpersonal significance." As the philosopher Michael Walzer puts it, failure to obtain needed health care in our society is not merely dangerous; it is also degrading, signaling a lack of full citizenship (Walzer 1983). Given the utter unpredictability of many health care needs and the often huge amounts of money necessary to meet them, the President's Commission concluded that the free market alone cannot be counted on to meet these crucial needs and that society therefore has an obligation to help meet them. The Commission insisted, however, that this social obligation is not unlimited; it must be discharged with an eye to the costs and burdens to society in meeting it. Moreover, the fact that society is morally obligated to provide some care does not mean that everyone is entitled to an equal amount of health care or to health care of equal quality. In other words, not all *inequalities* in access to health care constitute *inequities*. So long as everyone is guaranteed access to an "acceptable level" or, as others have put it, a "decent level" of health care, society will have lived up to its moral obligation.

Although the President's Commission's approach lacks the rigor of philosophical analysis, it assembles a broad array of cogent arguments in favor of a right to health care. Interestingly, however, the Commission self-consciously retreated from the vocabulary of rights in attempting to frame its notion of a social duty, a move that has prompted a good deal of criticism from philosophers (Arras 1984; Bayer 1984). If society has a strong duty to ensure every citizen has access to at least a decent level of health care, why not conclude that each citizen has a moral right, as opposed to a legal right, against the government to that level of care?

A more focused and philosophical approach to the question is found in Norman Daniels' work on the connection between equal opportunity and health care. Like the President's Commission, Daniels first attempts to explain what is special about health care needs. As opposed to mere preferences we may have for fine wines or top-of-the-line stereo speakers, our health needs are special in that they relate to our ability to function as normal members of our biological species. If our ability to function normally is impaired—for example, because of a broken arm or cancer cells colonizing our bodies—Daniels observes that we will then be unable to enjoy what he calls the "normal opportunity range" for our society. In other words, illness prevents us from enjoying the range of opportunities—to be, for instance, an athlete, businessperson, or lawyer—that our natural endowment of talents and skills would otherwise entitle us to. Daniels contends this lack of equal opportunity will not be viewed as "merely unfortunate" in any society that is committed to providing equal opportunity to its members. Just as we say that children deprived of a decent education are robbed of their right to equal opportunity, so Daniels concludes that people deprived of adequate health care in our society are treated unjustly.

Although Daniels is firmly committed to viewing access to health care as a matter of justice, he too denies that a right to health care would entitle everyone to all the health care they might want or need. First, our right to health care covers only deviations from normal species functioning, not idiosyncratic desires for, say, nose jobs or "tushy tucks." Second, although health care needs are special compared to goods normally distributed on the free market, they are not so important that society must give them priority over all other needs or go broke trying. Other important interests besides health care—such as needs for good schooling, housing, nutrition, and jobs—must also figure in any robust conception of equal opportunity, so the task for public policy is to weigh and balance all these higher-level interests in fashioning a just *system* that protects equal opportunity. In this view, access to health care is seen as vitally important, but not so uniquely important that making it available to all threatens to break the societal bank.

One important implication of Daniels' position is that the job of health care institutions is to restore our minds and bodies to normal species functioning, that is, to *treat* illness and disability. Although medicine might be usefully deployed to enhance the opportunities of people who are physiologically normal yet lag behind others in terms of various talents and skills, Daniels insists that it is not the proper role of socially guaranteed medicine to *enhance* the abilities and opportunities of otherwise normal individuals. Thus, he would argue, for example, that short children with normal amounts of growth hormone have no right to artificial growth hormone treatments, even if such treatments could enhance their opportunities in a culture that may discriminate against short people. Some might well wonder, however, why medicine should not be used in this way. If we could help such children achieve a more satisfying social life and a more competitive position in society, why not use what medicine has to offer, whether or not we choose to call their condition a disease? (We shall return to this issue in Section Two, where Robert Wright questions whether we should have the right of access to Prozac and other personality-altering drugs.)

This section concludes with philosopher H. Tristram Englehardt, Jr.'s, critique of liberal egalitarian theories of health care justice in "Freedom and Moral Diversity." Engelhardt is a self-described postmodernist and libertarian. His postmodernism derives from his conviction that in the modern world there is no one right, or canonical, answer to the question of what constitutes justice and equality. People from different cultural, religious, or philosophical traditions define these key notions in radically different ways. This is a crucial problem for allocating health care in a pluralistic society, because any scheme for allocating such care must espouse one or another vision of justice and the good life. Engelhardt's libertarianism stems from his conviction that free and equal individuals should not be coerced into accepting, much less paying for, the views of others on such basic but ultimately unresolvable questions as the morality of abortion, physician-assisted suicide, the desirability of organ transplants, and the true nature of equality and social justice. In the face of such important and unresolvable questions, libertarians like Engelhardt insist individuals must remain free from societal or governmental interference to make their own choices. Thus, although it might be perfectly appropriate, even praiseworthy, for many individuals to band together and pool their extra resources to make health care more available to the poor and unfortunate, libertarians insist that no one should be forced to give away his or her resources for the benefit of others. Access to health care thus remains either a matter of buying and selling on the free market or a matter of charity; failure to access adequate amounts of health care is thus viewed by libertarians as unfortunate, but not unjust.

It follows that for Engelhardt the notion of a right to health care is both unfounded and positively dangerous. Unfounded because it must rely on some debatable and not universally endorsed understanding of justice; and dangerous because it necessarily impinges on the rights and lifestyles of those who embrace other visions of the good life. Although Engelhardt concedes that society might possess a moral warrant to tax its citizens for various purposes, including the provision of some level of health care for its needy citizens, he steadfastly resists the notion that this societal choice is demanded by anyone's entitlement.

In addition to engaging liberal egalitarian claims, such as those of Daniels and the President's Commission, on the level of political philosophy, Engelhardt offers some practical suggestions for making health care more widely available without foundering on the prohibitions of his postmodern libertarianism. One way to provide greater health care access for the poor without supporting controversial views of justice and the good life, he contends, would be to establish a voucher system. Given a fund of public monies earmarked for humanitarian purposes, society could distribute health care vouchers to needy individuals who could redeem them at the health system of their choice. Thus, instead of imposing, say, a single view of abortion on all of society, we could leave it up to individuals to cash in their vouchers at avowedly pro-choice or pro-life health plans, as they saw fit. This way, Engelhardt suggests, the poor could obtain expanded access without any accompanying "welfare rights" and without the state imposing a single, official morality on everyone.

Engelhardt's approval of taxation for purposes other than maintaining a so-called "nightwatchman state" consisting solely of police, army, courts and so forth, deviates from orthodox libertarian doctrine, which views all such taxation as forms of theft and forced labor. Likewise, his claim that individual autonomy must be universally respected in a world of moral diversity seems to contradict the thoroughgoing relativism of more robust versions of postmodernism. Still, his critique of welfare rights raises important questions about the legitimacy of state health policies and the wisdom of many practical interventions that the partisans of more egalitarian theories cannot ignore.

Whatever the outcome of the argument between liberal egalitarians such as Daniels and libertarians such as Engelhardt, the notion of a right to health care has only limited usefulness. If we endorsed such a right, what would it mean? And how would it help us answer the tough questions facing health policy experts, legislators, and society today? (Brody 1991)

At most, as Daniels acknowledges, a right to health care would mean that every citizen was entitled to an unspecified amount of health care (a decent minimum) within an overall entitlement to equal opportunity. Since health care needs must ultimately be balanced against other compelling opportunity-related needs, such as nutrition, schooling, and housing, it is impossible to say in the abstract exactly what kind and amount of health care each person is entitled to. Do individuals have a right, for example, to expensive experimental treatments, psychotherapy, organ transplants, AIDS therapies, and so on? Merely stipulating a right to health care does not help us come to grips with these and other crucial questions of health care policy. In each case, we have to ask, How great is the need, how many people will be affected, how likely is the harm, how expensive will the treatment or diagnostic test be, and what alternatives could our scarce public funds support? (See discussion of Section Three.)

In spite of its manifest limitations in resolving some of the most important and pervasive policy debates in health care, the notion of a right to health care is still worth debating. Even though it cannot tell us what level of entitlement is adequate—whether, for example, AIDS patients are entitled to expensive protease inhibitor therapy—it can tell us whether the inability of 40 million people to access health insurance and decent health care is an injustice or merely a large-scale case of bad luck. It might affect the ultimate ability of those millions of people to secure needed health care if we believed society had an obligation based on justice to provide adequate health care for all.

A MISCELLANY OF HARD CHOICES

Section Two surveys several vexing allocation problems confronting health policy experts, legislators, and consumers today. The common focus of these policy case studies is the need to make difficult choices in a context of fiscal scarcity (Morreim 1995). If we had unlimited amounts of money, there would be no need to ration health care; but since money and resources are scarce and health care is expensive, we cannot afford to satisfy everyone's preferences and needs for health care. Even if we can reach consensus that a right to health care exists, we must still learn to assign priorities—a tricky business: Who should be saved when all cannot be saved? Which groups of people and which treatments and diagnostic techniques should have highest priority? The articles in this section give a lively sense of the emerging issues in this area. Because of space limitations, no attempt has been made to present balanced arguments for every issue.

RATIONING HEALTH CARE ACCORDING TO AGE

One important yet highly controversial proposal, based on alarming demographic trends, is to ration health care on the basis of age. The elderly constitute the fastest growing segment of the population and consume a steadily increasing proportion of our nation's health care resources. Demographers estimate, for example, that by the year 2040, those over 65 years of age will represent 21 percent of the total population and account for 45 percent of all health care expenditures. An aging population, coupled with unlimited technological expansion, thus poses a grave threat of "intergenerational conflict," in which the elderly as a class usurp more than their fair share of medical goods and services at the expense of younger persons.

Notwithstanding the disturbing implications of such projections, Americans remain deeply suspicious of targeting the elderly as a class for purposes of rationing. Given the widespread stereotyping of the elderly in a society dedicated to youth and its values, rationing by age strikes many as just another form of invidious discrimination on the order of sexism and racism. Can rationing by age be *ethically* justified?

Two very powerful yet disparate arguments for age-based rationing have recently been developed. In the first, Norman Daniels (1987) suggests that instead of viewing the problem as one of intergenerational conflict, we should view it as a problem of individual prudence. Suppose we could not have all the health care we wanted over our entire lifetime and had to choose, based on a limited amount of dollars, the kind of health care package we would want from cradle to grave. Daniels suggests that it would be rational for individuals to adopt a package emphasizing lifesaving technologies early in life, so as to increase their chances of reaching old age, and adopt low-tech social services and pain relief in their later years. Since all of us, if we are lucky, will eventually become old, this justification for age-based rationing operates *within* individual lives, rather than between competing generations, and thus avoids the sort of stigma attached to racism and sexism. Something very much like this rationing scheme is presently in effect in Great Britain, where the elderly benefit from an impressive array of social and palliative services, but not from life-sustaining technologies like kidney dialysis and total parenteral nutrition.

The second influential argument for age-based rationing comes from Daniel Callahan. In "Aging and the Ends of Medicine," Callahan discerns important "puzzles" about the proper ends of medicine and aging behind the immediate concerns about both financing and demography. Eschewing Daniels's liberal individualistic orientation, which attempts to avoid disputes bearing on the nature of the good life, Callahan argues that we cannot hope to respond adequately and justly to the demographic crisis without first rethinking the meaning of old age and the purposes of health care in our society.

In a nutshell, Callahan claims that the goals of medicine should be twofold: First, to preclude premature death through the deployment of life-sustaining technologies; second, to improve the quality of life, not the length of life, of those who have reached old age. In place of a limitless quest for youthful vigor and longer life in old age, Callahan prescribes a sober vision of a "natural life span," at the end of which death comes not as an outrage or a tragedy, but as a sad and inevitable aspect of the life cycle.

Callahan complements his call for age-based rationing with an appeal for a more supportive context for aging and death in our society—a context that would make our last years better, if not longer. Attentive to critics' warnings of negative symbolism, Callahan argues that the elderly would actually profit both from a rethinking of their place in society and from increased societal support for the humane management of chronic illness.

This agenda for age-based rationing is strenuously challenged by physician-ethicist Christine Cassel, who claims that Callahan's vision is both politically unacceptable and ethically flawed. In "The Limits of *Setting Limits*," Cassel argues, first, that Callahan's communitarian approach sharply conflicts with American traditions of diversity and pluralism. It is not our way, she asserts, to impose a monolithic vision of the meaning of old age, substituting the authority of the state for individuals' rights to self-determination. Second, Cassel points out that the elderly are a highly diverse group—some may be quite intact and vigorous at 90 while others are frail and debilitated at 70—and therefore should be treated on an individual basis rather than according to some "arbitrary" age-based cutoff. Finally, Cassel argues that the imperative of containing health care costs can be addressed in other, less socially damaging ways both by paring waste and excess profit from the system and by basing individualized medical decisions on efficacy rather than age.

RATIONING HEALTH CARE ACCORDING TO ABILITY TO PAY

Another method of rationing is to leave intact both Medicare for the elderly and the largely private system of insurance for the middle and upper classes, while rationing health care to the poor on Medicaid. This is the route taken by the state of Oregon in an ambitious yet highly controversial reform of Medicaid officially enacted as the "Oregon Health Plan" in February 1994. As recounted by Norman Daniels in "Is the Oregon Rationing Plan Fair?" the Oregon plan originated in a "tragic choice" faced by the state legislature in 1987, when it decided to invest its limited remaining health care dollars in prenatal care for thousands of uninsured poor women rather than to fund organ transplants of dubious efficacy for a relative handful of people. It may seem cruel to withhold lifesaving transplants from highly visible poor children, key reformers admitted, but no crueler in reality than allowing the illness and death from lack of prenatal care of largely invisible poor children. And since there were thousands more children who could benefit from prenatal care than children who could benefit from transplants, the state legislators concluded that the money should go where it could do the most good for the most people.

Oregon subsequently envisioned a large-scale reform effort based upon this initial tragic choice. This program simultaneously involved (1) an attempt to guarantee universal access to health care through the expansion of Medicaid benefits to everyone officially defined as poor, (2) a recognition of the necessity of limits in the care that would be provided to everyone in the program, and (3) an open and democratic system for making these difficult decisions. A state Health Services Commission was established to set priorities based in part on cost/benefit calculations and in part on the values of the community. Given the list of priorities, from prenatal care at the top to exotic organ transplants near the bottom, the legislature would determine the exact level of entitlement each year, effectively drawing a line through the list of possible treatments on the basis of how much money the state could afford to spend on health care that year.

Is such a rationing scheme fair to the poor? According to Norman Daniels, the lot of the poor in Oregon may actually be improved overall through the plan's expansion of benefits to more people, in spite of its negative effects on some individual potential organ recipients, though its actual impact will crucially depend upon the amount the legislature devotes to health care each year. Daniels's main objection to the Oregon plan, and to rationing health care to the poor in general, is that it achieves the goal of cost control solely at the expense of poor women and children, who are already a highly vulnerable group. Daniels cogently argues that it is not rationing, per se, that is ethically suspect, but rather rationing care to a small percent of the population that is already disadvantaged, rather than to the vast majority of the population. And while Oregon's attempt to incorporate "community values" into its rationing decisions draws mixed reviews from Daniels, its acceptance of an open and publicly accountable system for making such painful decisions is recognized as an advance over our present system of *covert* rationing to those unable to pay for their care.

RATIONING HEALTH CARE ACCORDING TO MERIT

Suppose we can agree that a right to health care exists based on the notion of equal opportunity—does this mean everyone is entitled to a decent standard of care even if they have squandered their own opportunities for good health? Discussion about rights to health care appears oblivious to any concern for individual responsibility for health. Does each of us have a just claim to medical care against society even when our lack of health is due more to a lack of individual responsibility than to our genetic or social fate? If I am a long-time smoker, is my right to treatment for emphysema or cancer equal to that of my non-smoking neighbor who eats well and jogs daily? In short, should we allocate scarce resources according to the virtue or vice of the recipient?

In "Should Alcoholics Compete Equally for Liver Transplantation?" Alvin Moss and Mark Siegler raise anew the question of whether "personal desert" should ever figure into our allocation

decisions. Ordinarily, our public policies tend not to hold individuals personally responsible for their bad health; life-styles built around cigarettes or Dunkin' Donuts are generally not thought to be punishable by the withholding of medical treatment. But what if the medical commodity is exceptionally scarce, as is the case with transplantable livers, and the disease in question (end-stage liver failure) is eminently preventable by a change in life-style, as is the case (the authors contend) with the disease of alcoholism? Moss and Siegler argue that in the face of extreme scarcity and demonstrable personal responsibility, it is just to give nonalcoholics priority over alcoholics on the list for liver transplants. In short, they argue in this limited context for the principle, "To each according to his or her virtue or vice."

Philosophers Carl Cohen, Martin Benjamin, and others argue in their rebuttal to Moss and Siegler, "Alcoholics and Liver Transplantation," that it is not at all clear that giving livers to reformed alcoholics would be a waste of medical resources. More importantly, they dispute the claim that moral blameworthiness should determine who lives and who dies. If there is no consensus on the true nature of virtue and vice in a pluralistic society, and if such behaviors as smoking and drinking might have some sort of genetic predisposition, we must, they argue, reject the notion that medicine should first inquire into the morality of peoples' habits before deciding whether to treat them.

Any such moralizing of the transplant enterprise would raise interesting questions for policymakers. For example, does the vice in question have to be the cause of the life-threatening condition? If so, why? Further, would we deny a transplant to an alcoholic who had been a documented saint for the greater part of his life? And what about those potential organ recipients who, although not alcoholics, have other problems in the virtue department? For example, should a liver transplant be offered to a teetotaler who also happens to beat his wife, cheat on his taxes, and rape children?

RATIONING EFFECTIVE BUT EXPENSIVE TREATMENT

In contrast to schemes that would ration health care to specific population groups such as the elderly or the poor, managed care organizations

(MCOs) must make difficult allocation decisions that often affect their entire membership, old and young alike. Even when they must choose whether to fund medical interventions that might benefit only a small proportion of their members, such choices will still affect everyone else enrolled in the plan; money spent on one group cannot be spent on other treatments for other members.

A problem common to all health care systems, including MCOs, is deciding whether to provide expensive halfway medical interventions. Modern medicine has served up a vast array of treatments that often do not cure but allow individuals to live their lives with a chronic yet now manageable condition. A good example of such a halfway intervention is chronic kidney dialysis, a technology that saves lives not by curing kidney disease but by periodically cleansing the blood of patients with a dialysis machine. Without dialysis, people with end-stage renal disease would eventually die; with it, they can live productive lives for many years to come. Unlike outright medical cures, however, these halfway interventions often come at a high price both in terms of cost and in terms of lowered quality of life, as with kidney dialysis. In the absence of a genuine cure (such as penicillin for syphilis or a kidney transplant for renal disease), people who depend on halfway interventions often live for a long time, and the cost of their care increases with each passing year.

A pressing example of this problem is discussed in philosopher Leonard Fleck's essay, "Just Caring: Managed Care and Protease Inhibitors." Fleck examines the extraordinarily difficult policy choices facing MCOs in light of the development of some effective new drugs, called protease inhibitors, that help fight AIDS-related infections. Although these drugs certainly do not cure people of their HIV infection, they work remarkably well in limiting the damage to the immune system wrought by the AIDS virus and have thus played a major role in decreasing AIDS-related mortality in the second half of this decade. Protease inhibitors have proven so effective, in fact, that in many cases patients no longer exhibit any signs of viral infection. The virus might well be still embedded in their blood and tissue, but it has often become so well contained as to be virtually undetectable in some patients.

All this is wonderful news. Surely, one might think, if an MCO funds anything, it should pay for drugs that save the lives of AIDS patients and turn this deadly scourge into a manageable chronic illness. It might make sense for MCOs to think twice about paying for relatively ineffective but expensive AIDS drugs, but protease inhibitors really work! (At least for now—their long-range effectiveness is still in dispute.) The bad news, of course, is that these protease inhibitors cost a lot of money—in most cases about $20,000 per year per person. As Fleck notes, considering the possibility that each HIV-infected person might now live for at least another twenty years with the aid of such drugs, the price tag for each long-term survivor would be approximately $400,000—nearly half a million dollars—a daunting sum for the management and membership of any MCO with a substantial number of HIV-infected persons on its roster.

In his policy case study, Fleck would have us imagine we are members of an organizational ethics committee charged with advising the management of an HMO with a small but significant HIV-infected membership. What policy should we recommend: Deny coverage for protease inhibitors, knowing this will mean a premature death for many AIDS patients? Provide full coverage for all HIV-infected individuals, knowing this might endanger the fiscal solvency of the HMO? Or perhaps the best policy lies somewhere in between these extremes. Fleck argues that several intermediate policies might be "just enough," so long as certain procedural requirements are met. How we arrive at collective policy decisions, he observes, can often be just as important as what we substantively decide.

RATIONING EXPERIMENTAL TREATMENTS

When it comes to assigning priorities in health care, we might think we should definitely rank tried and true treatments higher than those that are experimental. Surely, we might say, treatments that have been fully accepted by the medical community, treatments that constitute the standard of care, should be offered to members of MCOs before those that are promising but unproven. Even if we agree that there is a right to health care, there is good reason for thinking that this right should not encompass treatments and diagnostics that have not yet been fully embraced by the medical community. Even though some patients may see a particular experimental drug as their last chance for effective treatment, a right to health care that encompassed any and every untested new drug or device would soon break the bank of any MCO or national health system. Moreover, when we consider that most experimental drugs eventually fail to prove themselves both safe and effective during rigorous controlled trials, such a generous interpretation of the right to health care would lead to results that are not only costly, but also unsafe and ineffective. It is no small wonder, then, that virtually every MCO has an exclusionary clause in its contract with subscribers that rules out coverage for "investigational therapies."

Consider the case of women afflicted with advanced breast cancer for whom standard chemotherapies have failed to effect a remission of the disease. In the absence of any further treatment, these women will likely die in a short time. The only treatment on the horizon, however, is an experimental procedure known as high-dose chemotherapy followed by autologous bone-marrow transplantation (or HDC-ABMT). As philosopher Alex John London explains in "The Story of Christine deMeurers," this treatment holds significant promise for many victims of breast cancer and is currently offered at many hospitals and cancer centers, but it has yet to be fully validated by rigorous scientific studies. The treatment is extremely expensive, costing well over $100,000 per patient. Without this highly invasive and onerous treatment, these women will surely die. Most of them are relatively young, in their 20s and 30s, and many have families who depend on them. In contrast to the deaths of elderly persons, which Daniel Callahan describes as "sad but not tragic," the premature deaths of these young women are tragic. They desperately wish to live, and they view HDC-ABMT not as some far-fetched medical gamble, but as their only remaining shot at continued life. From their point of view, it may seem unfair for their MCOs to foreclose any possibility of potentially helpful treatment. And for those of us witnessing their struggle from the sidelines, it may seem unconscionably hard-hearted of MCOs to deny these women their last remaining chance merely in order to save money. Isn't this, we might well ask, the most egregious possible example of health insurance companies and managed care putting "profits before people?"

Following his narrative of Christine deMeurers, a woman who fought valiant battles against both her MCO and her encroaching terminal breast cancer, Alex John London attempts to put this health policy debate in proper perspective. Rejecting an all-or-nothing perspective on such so-called last-chance therapies, London attempts to focus our attention on the crucial questions we must ask and the procedures we must establish to come to a just and stable resolution of this difficult issue.

RATIONING MEDICAL ENHANCEMENTS

The final health policy debate we highlight here concerns the distinction between medical interventions designed to treat or cure bona fide disease and illness and interventions designed to enhance or optimize otherwise normal individuals. We have just canvassed controversies on treatments that definitely work (protease inhibitors) or might possibly work (HDC-ABMT) for undisputed illnesses such as AIDS and breast cancer. Although the case for such treatments is complicated by their high cost or investigational status, there is no controversy about the appropriateness of medical researchers and physicians targeting these conditions for amelioration. Were researchers to develop relatively inexpensive and effective cures for these conditions, there would be no question about guaranteeing such treatments as essential ingredients in any right to health care. Against this backdrop, the claim to medical interventions designed merely to enhance or optimize otherwise normal human conditions—such as intelligence, height, or personality—might well seem frivolous and preposterous.

Again, however, things may not be so straightforward. Imagine a child (let's call him Jack) of very short stature who happens nevertheless to have the full complement of natural growth hormone in his body. In contrast to children who are short due to a lack of growth hormone, Jack is short because his parents were, not because of any hormonal deficiency. It is well known that children like Jack may face an uphill struggle; short children and adults tend to be discriminated against in our society. With some notable exceptions, taller people tend to get better grades in school, find more attractive dates and mates, and obtain better-paying jobs than short people. As the songwriter, Randy Newman, once put it, albeit somewhat ironically and hyperbolically, in our society "short people got no reason to live."

Consider, then, the response of parents of such short children when they are told that an extended course of artificial human growth hormone injections might add inches to their children's height and opportunities to their lives. Even though they may not regard their children as sick or diseased, they may wish to help them avoid discrimination and reduced opportunities. This, then is an example of a medical intervention designed not to cure disease but to enhance the opportunities of an otherwise completely normal person. If we willingly treat children who are short due to a bona fide disease, that is, lack of growth hormone, because such treatment will open up opportunities to them, why not also treat children who are equally short, face exactly the same sorts of disadvantages in life, and differ only in that their bodies already have natural growth hormone? Why not, in other words, use medicine to advance the cause of equal opportunity even in the absence of a diseased state?

Another example of enhancement is provided by Robert Wright in "The Coverage of Happiness." Although Prozac was originally intended for use as an anti-depressant, many psychiatrists and clinical psychologists have found that the drug also works well for otherwise healthy individuals who are nevertheless unhappy and frustrated due to problems related to their personalities. Some were so attentive to the needs of others that they had lost the capacity for genuine pleasure; others were so weighed down by feelings of inferiority that they found it impossible to take steps to improve their self-esteem, such as asking someone out on a date or asking their boss for a raise. Although most psychiatrists might still regard expensive and protracted psychotherapy to be the best treatment for such conditions, many are now convinced that drugs such as Prozac can produce similar beneficial effects much more quickly and cheaply than therapy. For such patients, Prozac apparently works not like a traditional mood enhancer, but as a personality-altering drug that at best empowers patients to overcome obstacles embedded in their personalities and actually become more as they imagine their "real selves" to be (Kramer 1993).

These claims are obviously controversial, and many physicians and social critics reject them, warning that drugs like Prozac should never be used merely to enhance or optimize the personalities of otherwise normal people (Breggin 1994). But Robert Wright asks us to consider the implications of a genuinely efficacious "cosmetic psychopharmacology." Suppose a drug such as Prozac could effectively make us happier and allow many poor people, perhaps weighed down by low self-esteem, to achieve the same upbeat self-confidence and energy we perceive people nearer the top of the social ladder as possessing. Could not a plausible case be made then for increased access to such a drug on the respectable grounds of providing enhanced opportunity for all?

Norman Daniels thinks not. In "Equal Opportunity and Health Care" (see Section One), Daniels argues against the view that a proper goal of publicly funded medicine is to optimize or enhance otherwise normal human capacities. Instead of advocating that people should be made more equal in their natural talents, skills, and personality structures, Daniels claims only that people should have the opportunity to achieve at the level their natural-born talents, skills, and personalities would have permitted in the absence of disease or disability. In other words, the competition for scarce resources should be fair, but not strictly equal. Although those with more intelligence, height, and bounce in their strides may tend to have better life chances than their less intelligent, shorter, more lethargic peers, Daniels hopes we could find means other than organized medicine—such as Rawls' difference principle (see Introduction)—to aid those who lose out in the natural lottery. But others such as Robert Wright would disagree with Daniels, arguing that if medicine can give people greater happiness or more equal opportunity, then it would be foolish and shortsighted not to deploy all available means toward these laudable goals.

RATIONING FAIRLY: PRINCIPLES AND PROCEDURES

Americans do not like to hear about rationing health care. The term conjures up images of tightwad insurance companies or government bureaucrats deciding that some lives are worth less than others. One of the charges that in 1994 helped scuttle the ill-fated Clinton plan for health care reform was the claim that it would necessitate rationing.

Well aware of the unpopularity of this notion, the Clinton administration actually forbade its 500 consultants to use the word "rationing" in any correspondence or official documents.

But the fact is that we have always rationed health care in one way or another. By far the most widespread method has also been the most morally suspect: rationing care by ability to pay. But we have also rationed organ transplants, intensive care unit beds, and other life-sustaining medical treatments. There are, however, important differences between these traditional forms of rationing and what is happening today under managed care. When the poor and uninsured failed to receive needed care, it was usually not the result of any official policy; their inability to access care was often accepted as if it were a fact of nature. And when patients died of liver or heart failure on a waiting list for an organ transplant, it was usually due to a natural shortage of organs, not to a decision on anyone's part that these lives were simply too expensive to save. So we developed a complicated attitude with regard to rationing: On the one hand, we grew accustomed to the tacit and limited rationing we permitted while fiercely resisting the explicit, publicly imposed rationing, respectively, by doctors on paying customers and by bureaucrats on the poor.

Managed care has changed all this. Operating essentially within closed systems of shared financial resources, MCOs must ration health care on a daily basis. Money spent on expensive but marginally effective treatments cannot be used for other purposes within an MCO, so difficult choices must be made. Under this new dispensation, rationing is explicit; it is implemented by physicians at the bedside; it targets insured populations by restricting potentially beneficial services; and it is justified by fiscal scarcity, rather than by natural shortages (Morreim 1995, Eddy 1996). The notion that rationing would be entirely unnecessary if we would only cut the fat by reorganizing our wasteful health care system has been disproven by history and the fact of scarcity. The question now is not, Shall we ration care? rather, *How* shall we ration, by what principles and processes, and how may we do so without seriously compromising justice and patients' rights?

Section Three examines various proposed methods for rationing health care. We begin with health policy analyst David Eddy, who argues for a form of "cost-effectiveness analysis" in his essay, "The Individual vs Society: Resolving the Conflict." Following a brief explanation of how our health system has traditionally ignored the true costs of health care, Eddy distinguishes two perspectives on the problem. From one angle, which Eddy calls the perspective of society, the imperative is to allocate our resources as efficiently as possible among everyone with a claim to them, thereby getting "the most bang for the buck." But from another angle, the perspective of patient-members who know they are sick and have already paid their health insurance premiums, the imperative is to obtain the desired medical care, no matter what the cost. Eddy then shows the implications of these two different perspectives when applied to the problem discussed by Alex John London in Section Two—experimental bone marrow treatments for women with advanced breast cancer.

Eddy makes two important and controversial claims. First, he asserts that the proper perspective from the vantage point of health policy is that of society. When deciding what treatments to fund, MCOs should, Eddy contends, attempt to quantify the respective benefits of various treatments, divide them by their costs, and then opt for those interventions that provide the greatest good for the greatest number of people. Second, Eddy claims that this perspective, with its emphasis on prevention, will often redound to the benefit of everyone. Instead of paying huge amounts of money, for example, to save a few lives with HDC-ABMT, it will work to everyone's advantage to invest instead in breast cancer screening programs that will save more lives at far less cost. Prior to getting sick, all of us would agree to the prevention strategy because with it we have a better chance of not getting advanced cancer in the first place. Thus, although Eddy embraces a utilitarian mode of rationing, he claims that it is consonant with the idea that rationing can best be justified by the choices of patients themselves.

Another way of stating the utilitarian case for cost-effectiveness analysis is to use the language of "quality-adjusted life years," or QALYs. According to the proponents of QALYs, the goal of health policy should be to increase both the length and quality of people's lives. It isn't enough that people should merely live longer; their lives should also be as high in quality as possible. Like good utilitarian consequentialists, these theorists also hold that a particular health improvement should have the same value no matter who receives it, so it should be provided unless its cost prevents a greater improvement from being offered to someone else. In short, like David Eddy, these theorists contend that we should allocate scarce health care resources so as to do the most good for the most people.

Philosopher John Harris disagrees. Arguing from the widely shared premise that every individual is entitled to equal concern and respect, Harris launches an all-out attack in his essay, "QALYfying the Value of Life." He notes that it is one thing to claim that any given individual might well prefer, say, two years of good health to three years of misery, but another thing entirely to claim that as a matter of health policy "those with more QALYs on offer" should be saved at the expense of those already suffering from lower quality of life. Where *different people* are involved, Harris contends, "it does not follow that treatments yielding more QALYs are preferable to treatments yielding fewer." Indeed, he claims that the QALY approach will necessarily involve unjust discrimination against the elderly, who have fewer QALYs to offer than the young, and also possibly against women and members of minority groups. To endorse QALYs, he contends, is to give free reign to discriminatory judgments of the quality of others' lives. Rather than focusing on some abstract, fungible entity like QALYs, Harris argues that equal weight should be given to concrete, individual persons and their interests, especially to their interest in avoiding premature death. Instead of trying to maximize welfare for the overall aggregate of persons, Harris urges individual health systems as well as national governments to concentrate instead on the avoidance of premature death.

Philosopher Paul Menzel takes this debate over QALYs to a higher level in his essay "Prior Consent to Rationing: Minimizing the Ethical Costs." Menzel agrees with Eddy that the best justification of rationing resides in an appeal to autonomy and individual choice. Rather than viewing rationing as imposed by bureaucrats from on high, Menzel argues that rationing, properly conceived, should represent "people's own hard judgments about the kind of society in which on balance, in the long term, and considering all the realities of cost and scarcity, *they* wish to live." He also agrees with Eddy that the proper time for people to consider what kind and how much health care they should have is *before* they get sick, ideally at the time they enroll in a health plan.

Menzel then deploys this autonomy-based conception of rationing toward the resolution of three important issues. First, he justifies physicians' cooperation in bedside rationing (see Part One, Section Three) on the grounds that such rationing can respect the autonomous choices of individuals regarding their whole lives, rather than merely as sick patients appearing at the physician's doorstep. Second, while noting John Harris' formidable challenge, Menzel mounts a highly qualified and nuanced defense of QALYs, again on the grounds that individuals might consent to this sort of reasoning on the level of health policy. Finally, Menzel draws some interesting and highly controversial implications of his theory for the equitable treatment of the poor. Against the claims of egalitarians like Norman Daniels, Menzel argues that if we take the autonomy and values of poor people seriously, we must conclude that a noticeably lower tier of health care services for the poor can be justified by the likely preferences of poor people for goods such as safety, education, and better nutrition rather than high-quality, high-cost health care. Menzel would thus agree with the result of Oregon's rationing experiment, although he has some serious reservations about the processes through which that two-tiered policy was generated.

The next pair of essays discuss the allocation of scarce, life-saving medical resources in the context of organ transplantation, an area in which explicit rationing is well established. In "Fairness in the Allocation and Delivery of Health Care," religious ethicist and veteran policy analyst James F. Childress examines the criteria for allocating hearts and kidneys developed by the United Network of Organ Sharing (UNOS). Focusing on UNOS' sophisticated point system for assigning priority to recipients—a system based on a number of factors, including patient need, probability of success, time spent on the waiting list, and so on—Childress warns that such quantified and seemingly objective approaches are shot through with value judgments.

Childress then explores the tension between medical need and probability of success. As a religious deontologist, Childress is no friend of unvarnished utilitarianism; he argues, however, that "medical utility"—that is, getting the most use out of each transplanted organ—should figure prominently in the choice of recipients. Focusing on patients with the greatest need—those worst off from a medical point of view—might seem like the most merciful thing to do, but it has a cost in terms of the number and quality of years that might be purchased with our scarce supply of organs. Echoing themes from Eddy and Menzel, Childress argues that patients behind a Rawlsian "veil of ignorance" concerning their own condition and needs would probably opt for a system that used organs to the greatest possible advantage, even if that meant that some of the neediest cases would be passed over. Since reasonable patients would thus give their consent to such a scheme, Childress sees no inherent conflict between stressing both the demands of medical utility and the claims of justice or fairness. Giving organs to those who are most likely to live longer with higher quality of life thus amounts to the just and prudent shepherding of scarce resources.

Robert Veatch, a philosopher and long-time proponent of medical egalitarianism, disagrees with Childress. In "Equality, Justice, and Rightness in Allocating Health Care," Veatch first articulates his egalitarian principle of justice, which states that individuals should have an equal opportunity for well-being. Then Veatch takes issue with both Childress and the UNOS point system on the grounds that they both allot too much weight to medical utility. Claiming the higher ethical ground, Veatch argues it is wrong to balance the claims of utility against the inviolable demands of justice and equality. Thus, rather than giving the highest score to patients who are likely to maximize the usefulness of organs, Veatch would give preference to such factors as length of time on the waiting list or the urgency of medical need. In other words, those who are worst off medically should have the highest priority in the allocation of organs.

Veatch and Childress thus stake out very different positions on the important question of "best outcomes versus equal chances" (Daniels 1993). Childress endorses a strategy that stresses achieving the best outcomes overall, whereas Veatch insists that fairness demands equal chances for all to survive. Why, he asks, should the medically worst off relinquish their claims to a fair chance at life merely because they cannot maximize the usefulness of an available organ?

This disagreement between Childress and Veatch reflects the fact of pervasive value conflicts within a secular, pluralistic society. Should we try to get the most bang for the buck, or salvage the worst-off patients? Should we fund hugely expensive life-saving treatments for the few (such as bone marrow transplants) or cheaper interventions that promise enhanced quality of life for the many (such as hip replacement)? Our inability to reach consensus on such basic but seemingly intractable questions of distributive principles leads Norman Daniels and James Sabin to concentrate on the fairness of our procedures for resolving such knotty questions. In "Last-Chance Therapies and Managed Care," they suggest that if we cannot always agree at the level of principles, then perhaps our best bet is to design various procedural mechanisms that will yield results that are, in the words of Leonard Fleck, "just enough." Keying on the example of HDC-ABMT for advanced breast cancer (discussed in Alex John London's case study in Section Two and in David Eddy's cost-effectiveness analysis in this section), Daniels and Sabin report on a variety of "exemplary practices" recently adopted by managed care plans in the wake of the bad publicity, adverse court decisions, and legislative mandates noted by London. Instead of relying on unilateral denials of care, as in the case of Christine deMeurers, to resolve the tension between the efficient use of resources and the desperate appeals of patients for last-chance therapies, many MCOs are now resorting to such procedural solutions as outside review panels and internal appeals mechanisms that emphasize constructive deliberation and dialogue. By openly experimenting with a variety of such strategies while remaining tolerant of the differing value orientations they represent, Daniels and Sabin hope to "move [us] along a learning curve towards a more patient-centered, cost-effective and ethical health care system." By bringing such tensions and disagreements out into the open where they can be rationally and respectfully discussed among subscribers, patients, physicians, and managers, MCOs will have to acknowledge that such questions are not merely technical and economic, but also deeply political. As London noted, only by dealing with the problems of justly allocating health care through an open and more self-consciously political process can MCOs regain a measure of the trust and legitimacy that they have squandered.

SECTION 1

Justice and Health Care

An Ethical Framework for Access to Health Care

President's Commission for the Study of Ethical Problems in Medicine and Biomedical and Behavioral Research

The prevention of death and disability, the relief of pain and suffering, the restoration of functioning: these are the aims of health care. Beyond its tangible benefits, health care touches on countless important and in some ways mysterious aspects of personal life that invest it with significant value as a thing in itself. In recognition of these special features, the President's Commission was mandated to study the ethical and legal implications of differences in the availability of health services. In this Report to the President and Congress, the Commission sets forth an ethical standard: access for all to an adequate level of care without the imposition of excessive burdens. It believes that this is the standard against which proposals for legislation and regulation in this field ought to be measured. . . .

In both their means and their particular objectives, public programs in health care have varied over the years. Some have been aimed at assuring the productivity of the work force, others at protecting particularly vulnerable or deserving groups, still others at manifesting the country's commitment to equality of opportunity. Nonetheless, most programs have rested on a common rationale: to ensure that care be made accessible to a group whose health needs would otherwise not be adequately met.

The consequence of leaving health care solely to market forces—the mechanism by which most things are allocated in American society—is not

viewed as acceptable when a significant portion of the population lacks access to health services. Of course, government financing programs, such as Medicare and Medicaid as well as public programs that provide care directly to veterans and the military and through local public hospitals, have greatly improved access to health care. These efforts, coupled with the expanded availability of private health insurance, have resulted in almost 90% of Americans having some form of health insurance coverage. Yet the patchwork of government programs and the uneven availability of private health insurance through the workplace have excluded millions of people. The Surgeon General has stated that "with rising unemployment, the numbers are shifting rapidly. We estimate that from 18 to 25 million Americans—8 to 11 percent of the population—have no health insurance coverage at all." Many of these people lack effective access to health care, and many more who have some form of insurance are unprotected from the severe financial burdens of sickness. . . .

Most Americans believe that because health care is special, access to it raises special ethical concerns. In part, this is because good health is by definition important to well-being. Heath care can relieve pain and suffering, restore functioning, and prevent death; it can enhance good health and improve an individual's opportunity to pursue a life plan; and it can provide valuable information about a person's overall health. Beyond its practical importance, the involvement of health care with the most significant and awesome events of life—birth, illness, and death—adds a symbolic aspect to health care: it is special because it signi-

EDITORS' NOTE: Most notes have been deleted. Readers who wish to follow up on sources should consult the original article.

fies not only mutual empathy and caring but the mysterious aspects of curing and healing.

Furthermore, while people have some ability—through choice of life-style and through preventive measures—to influence their health status, many health problems are beyond their control and are therefore undeserved. Besides the burdens of genetics, environment, and chance, individuals become ill because of things they do or fail to do—but it is often difficult for an individual to choose to do otherwise or even to know with enough specificity and confidence what he or she ought to do to remain healthy. Finally, the incidence and severity of ill health is distributed very unevenly among people. Basic needs for housing and food are predictable, but even the most hardworking and prudent person may suddenly be faced with overwhelming needs for health care. Together, these considerations lend weight to the belief that health care is different from most other goods and services. In a society concerned not only with fairness and equality of opportunity but also with the redemptive powers of science, there is a felt obligation to ensure that some level of health services is available to all.

There are many ambiguities, however, about the nature of this societal obligation. What share of health costs should individuals be expected to bear, and what responsibility do they have to use health resources prudently? Is it society's responsibility to ensure that every person receives care or services of as high quality and as great extent as any other individual? Does it require that everyone share opportunities to receive all available care or care of any possible benefit? If not, what level of care is "enough"? And does society's obligation include a responsibility to ensure both that care is available and that its costs will not unduly burden the patient?

The resolution of such issues is made more difficult by the spectre of rising health care costs and expenditures. Americans annually spend over 270 million days in hospitals, make over 550 million visits to physicians' offices, and receive tens of millions of X-rays. Expenditures for health care in 1981 totaled $287 billion—an average of over $1225 for every American. Although the finitude of national resources demands that trade-offs be made between health care and other social goods, there is little agreement about which choices are most acceptable from an ethical standpoint. In this chapter, the Commission attempts to lay an ethical foundation for evaluating both current patterns of access to health care and the policies designed to address remaining problems in the distribution of health care resources. . . .

THE SPECIAL IMPORTANCE OF HEALTH CARE

Although the importance of health care may, at first blush, appear obvious, this assumption is often based on instinct rather than reasoning. Yet it is possible to step back and examine those properties of health care that lead to the ethical conclusion that it ought to be distributed equitably.

WELL-BEING

Ethical concern about the distribution of health care derives from the special importance of health care in promoting personal well-being by preventing or relieving pain, suffering, and disability and by avoiding loss of life. The fundamental importance of the latter is obvious; pain and suffering are also experiences that people have strong desires to avoid, both because of the intrinsic quality of the experience and because of their effects on the capacity to pursue and achieve other goals and purposes. Similarly, untreated disability can prevent people from leading rewarding and fully active lives.

Health, insofar as it is the absence of pain, suffering, or serious disability, is what has been called a primary good, that is, there is no need to know what a particular person's other ends, preferences, and values are in order to know that health is good for that individual. It generally helps people carry out their life plans, whatever they may happen to be. This is not to say that everyone defines good health in the same way or assigns the same weight or importance to different aspects of being healthy, or to health in comparison with the other goods of life. Yet though people may differ over each of these matters, their disagreement takes place within a framework of basic agreement on the importance of health. Likewise, people differ in their beliefs about the value of health and medical care and their use of it as a means of achieving good health, as well as in their attitudes toward the various benefits and risks of different treatments.

OPPORTUNITY

Health care can also broaden a person's range of opportunities, that is, the array of life plans that is reasonable to pursue within the conditions obtaining in society.[1] In the United States equality of opportunity is a widely accepted value that is reflected throughout public policy. The effects that meeting (or failing to meet) people's health needs have on the distribution of opportunity in a society become apparent if diseases are thought of as adverse departures from a normal level of functioning. In this view, health care is that which people need to maintain or restore normal functioning or to compensate for inability to function normally. Health is thus comparable in importance to education in determining the opportunities available to people to pursue different life plans.

INFORMATION

The special importance of health care stems in part from its ability to relieve worry and to enable patients to adjust to their situation by supplying reliable information about their health. Most people do not understand the true nature of a health problem when it first develops. Health professionals can then perform the worthwhile function of informing people about their conditions and about the expected prognoses with or without various treatments. Though information sometimes creates concern, often it reassures patients either by ruling out a feared disease or by revealing the self-limiting nature of a condition and, thus, the lack of need for further treatment. Although health care in many situations may thus not be necessary for good physical health, a great deal of relief from unnecessary concern—and even avoidance of pointless or potentially harmful steps—is achieved by health care in the form of expert information provided to worried patients. Even when a prognosis is unfavorable and health professionals have little treatment to offer, accurate information can help patients plan how to cope with their situation.

THE INTERPERSONAL SIGNIFICANCE OF ILLNESS, BIRTH, AND DEATH

It is no accident that religious organizations have played a major role in the care of the sick and dying and in the process of birth. Since all human beings are vulnerable to disease and all die, health care has a special interpersonal significance: it expresses and nurtures bonds of empathy and compassion. The depth of a society's concern about health care can be seen as a measure of its sense of solidarity in the face of suffering and death. Moreover, health care takes on special meaning because of its role in the beginning of a human being's life as well as the end. In spite of all the advances in the scientific understanding of birth, disease, and death, these profound and universal experiences remain shared mysteries that touch the spiritual side of human nature. For these reasons a society's commitment to health care reflects some of its most basic attitudes about what it is to be a member of the human community.

THE CONCEPT OF EQUITABLE ACCESS TO HEALTH CARE

The special nature of health care helps to explain why it ought to be accessible, in a fair fashion, to all. But if this ethical conclusion is to provide a basis for evaluating current patterns of access to health care and proposed health policies, the meaning of fairness or equity in this context must be clarified. The concept of equitable access needs definition in its two main aspects: the level of care that ought to be available to all and the extent to which burdens can be imposed on those who obtain these services.

ACCESS TO WHAT?

"Equitable access" could be interpreted in a number of ways: equality of access, access to whatever an individual needs or would benefit from, or access to an adequate level of care.

Equity as Equality   It has been suggested that equity is achieved either when everyone is assured of receiving an equal quantity of health care dollars or when people enjoy equal health. The most common characterization of equity as equality, however, is as providing everyone with the same level of health care. In this view, it follows that if a given level of care is available to one individual it must be available to all. If the initial standard is set high, by reference to the highest level of care presently received, an enormous drain would result on the resources needed to provide other goods. Alternatively, if the standard is set low in order to avoid an excessive use of resources, some beneficial services would have to be withheld from people who wished to purchase them. In other words, no one would be allowed access to more services or services of higher quality than those available to everyone else, even if he or she were willing to pay for those services from his or her personal resources.

As long as significant inequalities in income and wealth persist, inequalities in the use of health care can be expected beyond those created by differences in need. Given people with the same pattern of preferences and equal health care needs, those with greater financial resources will purchase more health care. Conversely, given equal financial resources, the different patterns of health care preferences that typically exist in any population will result in a different use of health services by people with equal health care needs. Trying to prevent such inequalities would require interfering with people's liberty to use their income to purchase an important good like health care while leaving them free to use it for frivolous or inessential ends. Prohibiting people with higher incomes or stronger preferences for health care from purchasing more care than everyone else gets would not be feasible, and would probably result in a black market for health care.

Equity as Access Solely According to Benefit or Need Interpreting equitable access to mean that everyone must receive all health care that is of any benefit to them also has unacceptable implications. Unless health is the only good or resources are unlimited, it would be irrational for a society—as for an individual—to make a commitment to provide whatever health care might be beneficial regardless of cost. Although health care is of special importance, it is surely not all that is important to people. Pushed to an extreme, this criterion might swallow up all of society's resources, since there is virtually no end to the funds that could be devoted to possibly beneficial care for diseases and disabilities and to their prevention.

Equitable access to health care must take into account not only the benefits of care but also the cost in comparison with other goods and services to which those resources might be allocated. Society will reasonably devote some resources to health care but reserve most resources for other goals. This, in turn, will mean that some health services (even of a lifesaving sort) will not be developed or employed because they would produce too few benefits in relation to their costs and to the other ways the resources for them might be used.

It might be argued that the notion of "need" provides a way to limit access to only that care that confers especially important benefits. In this view, equity as access according to need would place less severe demands on social resources than equity according to benefit would. There are, however, difficulties with the notion of need in this context. On the one hand, medical need is often not narrowly defined but refers to any condition for which medical treatment might be effective. Thus, "equity as access according to need" collapses into "access according to whatever is of benefit."

On the other hand, "need" could be even more expansive in scope than "benefit." Philosophical and economic writings do not provide any clear distinction between "needs" and "wants" or "preferences." Since the term means different things to different people, "access according to need" could become "access to any health service a person wants." Conversely, need could be interpreted very narrowly to encompass only a very minimal level of services—for example, those "necessary to prevent death."

Equity as an Adequate Level of Health Care Although neither "everything needed" nor "everything beneficial" nor "everything that anyone else is getting" are defensible ways of understanding equitable access, the special nature of health care dictates that everyone have access to *some* level of care: enough care to achieve sufficient welfare, opportunity, information, and evidence of interpersonal concern to facilitate a reasonably full and satisfying life. That level can be termed "an adequate level of health care." The difficulty of sharpening this amorphous notion into a workable foundation for health policy is a major problem in the United States today. This concept is not new; it is implicit in the public debate over health policy and has manifested itself in the history of public policy in this country. In this chapter, the Commission attempts to demonstrate the value of the concept, to clarify its content, and to apply it to the problems facing health policymakers.

Understanding equitable access to health care to mean that everyone should be able to secure an adequate level of care has several strengths. Because an adequate level of care may be less than "all beneficial care" and because it does not require that all needs be satisfied, it acknowledges the need for setting priorities within health care and signals a clear recognition that society's resources are limited and that there are other goods besides health. Thus, interpreting equity as access to adequate care does not generate an open-ended obligation. One of the chief dangers of interpretations of equity that require virtually unlimited resources for health care is that they encourage the view that equitable access is an impossible ideal. Defining equity as an adequate level of care for all avoids an impossible commitment of resources without falling into the opposite error of abandoning the enterprise of seeking to ensure that health care is in fact available for everyone.

In addition, since providing an adequate level of care is a limited moral requirement, this definition also avoids the unacceptable restriction on individual liberty entailed by the view that equity requires equality. Provided that an adequate level is available to all, those who prefer to use their resources to obtain care that exceeds that level do not offend any ethical principle in doing so. Finally, the concept of adequacy, as the Commission understands it, is society-relative. The content of adequate care will depend upon the overall resources available in a given society, and can take into account a consensus of expectations about what is adequate in a particular society at a particular time in its historical development. This permits the definition of adequacy to be altered as societal resources and expectations change.

WITH WHAT BURDENS?

It is not enough to focus on the care that individuals receive; attention must be paid to the burdens they must bear in order to obtain it—waiting and travel time, the cost and availability of transport, the financial cost of the care itself. Equity requires not only that adequate care be available to all, but also that these burdens not be excessive.

If individuals must travel unreasonably long distances, wait for unreasonably long hours, or spend most of their financial resources to obtain care, some will be deterred from obtaining adequate care, with adverse effects on their health and well-being. Others may bear the burdens, but only at the expense of their ability to meet other important needs. If one of the main reasons for providing adequate care is that health care increases welfare and opportunity, then a system that required large numbers of individuals to forego food, shelter, or educational advancement in order to obtain care would be self-defeating and irrational.

The concept of acceptable burdens in obtaining care, as opposed to excessive ones, parallels in some respects the concept of adequacy. Just as equity does not require equal access, neither must the burdens of obtaining adequate care be equal for all persons. What is crucial is that the variations in burdens fall within an acceptable range. As in determining an adequate level of care, there is no simple formula for ascertaining when the burdens of obtaining care fall within such a range. . . .

A SOCIETAL OBLIGATION

Society has a moral obligation to ensure that everyone has access to adequate care without being subject to excessive burdens. In speaking of a societal obligation the Commission makes reference to society in the broadest sense—the collective American community. The community is made up of individuals, who are in turn members of many other, overlapping groups, both public and private: local, state, regional, and national units; professional and workplace organizations; religious, educational, and charitable organizations; and family, kinship, and ethnic groups. All these entities play a role in discharging societal obligations.

The Commission believes it is important to distinguish between society, in this inclusive sense, and government as one institution among others in society. Thus the recognition of a collective or societal obligation does not imply that government should be the only or even the primary institution involved in the complex enterprise of making health care available. It is the Commission's view that the societal obligation to ensure equitable access for everyone may best be fulfilled in this country by a pluralistic approach that relies upon the coordinated contributions of actions by both the private and public sectors.

Securing equitable access is a societal rather than a merely private or individual responsibility for several reasons. First, while health is of special importance for human beings, health care—especially scientific health care—is a social product requiring the skills and efforts of many individuals; it is not something that individuals can provide for themselves solely through their own efforts. Second, because the need for health care is both unevenly distributed among persons and highly unpredictable and because the cost of securing care may be great, few individuals could secure adequate care without relying on some social mechanism for sharing the costs. Third, if persons generally deserved their health conditions or if the need for health care were fully within the individual's control, the fact that some lack adequate care would not be viewed as an inequity. But differences in health status, and hence differences in health care needs, are largely undeserved because they are, for the most part, not within the individual's control.

UNEVEN AND UNPREDICTABLE HEALTH NEEDS

While requirements for other basic necessities, such as adequate food and shelter, vary among people within a relatively limited range, the need for health care is distributed very unevenly and its occurrence at any particular time is highly unpredictable. One study shows 50% of all hospital billings are for only 13% of the patients, the seriously chronically ill.

Moreover, health care needs may be minor or overwhelming, in their personal as well as financial impact. Some people go through their entire lives seldom requiring health care, while others face medical expenses that would exceed the resources of all but the wealthiest. Moreover, because the need for care cannot be predicted, it is difficult to provide for it by personal savings from income. . . .

WHO SHOULD ENSURE THAT SOCIETY'S OBLIGATION IS MET?

In this country, the chief mechanism by which the cost of health care is spread among individuals is through the purchase of insurance. Another method of distributing health care costs is to rely on acts of charity in which individuals, such as relatives and care givers, and institutions assume responsibility for absorbing some or all of a person's health care expenses. These private forces cannot be expected to achieve equitable access for all, however. States and localities have also played important roles in attempting to secure health care for those in need. To the extent that actions of the market, private charity, and lower levels of government are insufficient in achieving equity, the responsibility rests with Federal government. The actual provision of care may be through arrangements in the private sector as well as through public institutions, such as local hospitals.

MARKET MECHANISMS IN HEALTH CARE

One means societies employ for meeting needs for goods and services that individuals cannot produce by themselves is the complex legal and economic mechanism known as a market. When health care is distributed through markets, however, an acceptable distribution is not achieved; indeed, given limitations in the way markets work, this result is practically inevitable.

The Inability to Ensure Adequate Care   First, many people lack the financial resources to obtain access to adequate care. Since American society encompasses a very wide range in income and wealth, distributing goods and services through markets leads to large differences in their consumption. The variations in need for health care do not, however, match variations in ability to purchase care. The market response to variable risk is insurance. Insurance has long existed for certain calamities—such as fire damage to property—and in the past 30 years, a huge market in health insurance has developed that enables people to share some of the financial risk of ill health. The relevant question for determining equity of access thus becomes: Is everyone able to afford access to adequate care through some combination of insurance and direct payment?

Admittedly, "ability to afford" is an ambiguous concept, given different attitudes toward risk and the importance of health care, and, even more important, possibly insufficient information about the likelihood of ill health and about the possible effects of care. For example, people may want an adequate level of care and may be able to afford to pay for it, but they may lack information about the amount of coverage needed to secure adequate care. As a result, the insurance market may not do a good job of providing plans that actually do protect people adequately. And, of course, some people who can afford to pay for their health care (and who would if they knew they would have to go without it otherwise) fail to make sufficient provisions because they rely on others not being willing to let them suffer. Furthermore, the cost of basic health insurance (which does not even guarantee financial access to adequate care in all cases) is high enough to place it beyond the reach of many families by *any* reasonable standard of affordability. Ironically, those who need the most care will find it most difficult to obtain it, both because their disease or disability impairs their opportunities for accumulating financial resources and because insurers will charge them higher rates. . . .

A RIGHT TO HEALTH CARE?

Often the issue of equitable access to health care is framed in the language of rights. Some who view health care from the perspective of distributive justice argue that the considerations discussed in this chapter show not only that society has a moral obligation to provide equitable access, but also that every individual has a moral right to such access. The Commission has chosen not to develop the case for achieving equitable access through the assertion of a right to health care. Instead it has sought to frame the issues in terms of the special nature of health care and of society's moral obligation to achieve equity, without taking a position on whether the term "obligation" should be read as entailing a moral right. The Commission reaches this conclusion for several reasons: first, such a right is not legally or Constitutionally recognized at the present time; second, it is not a logical corollary of an ethical obligation of the type the Commission has enunciated; and third, it is not necessary as a foun-

dation for appropriate governmental actions to secure adequate health care for all.

Legal Rights   Neither the Supreme Court nor any appellate court has found a constitutional right to health or to health care. However, most Federal statutes and many state statutes that fund or regulate health care have been interpreted to provide statutory rights in the form of entitlements for the intended beneficiaries of the program or for members of the group protected by the regulatory authority. . . .

Moral Obligations and Rights   The relationship between the concept of a moral right and that of a moral obligation is complex. To say that a person has a moral right to something is always to say that it is that person's due, that is, he or she is morally entitled to it. In contrast, the term "obligation" is used in two different senses. All moral rights imply corresponding obligations, but, depending on the sense of the term that is being used, moral obligations may or may not imply corresponding rights. In the broad sense, to say that society has a moral obligation to do something is to say that it ought morally to do that thing and that failure to do it makes society liable to serious moral criticism. This does not, however, mean that there is a corresponding right. For example, a person may have a moral obligation to help those in need, even though the needy cannot, strictly speaking, demand that person's aid as something they are due.

The government's responsibility for seeing that the obligation to achieve equity is met is independent of the existence of a corresponding moral right to health care. There are many forms of government involvement, such as enforcement of traffic rules or taxation to support national defense, to protect the environment, or to promote biomedical research, that do not presuppose corresponding moral rights but that are nonetheless legitimate and almost universally recognized as such. In a democracy, at least, the people may assign to government the responsibility for seeing that important collective obligations are met, provided that doing so does not violate important moral rights.

As long as the debate over the ethical assessment of patterns of access to health care is carried on simply by the assertion and refutation of a "right to health care," the debate will be incapable of guiding policy. At the very least, the nature of the right must be made clear and competing accounts of it compared and evaluated. Moreover, if claims of rights are to guide policy they must be supported by sound ethical reasoning and the connections between various rights must be systematically developed, especially where rights are potentially in conflict with one another. At present, however, there is a great deal of dispute among competing theories of rights, with most theories being so abstract and inadequately developed that their implications for health care are not obvious. Rather than attempt to adjudicate among competing theories of rights, the Commission has chosen to concentrate on what it believes to be the more important part of the question: what is the nature of the societal obligation, which exists whether or not people can claim a corresponding right to health care, and how should this societal obligation be fulfilled?[2]

MEETING THE SOCIETAL OBLIGATION

HOW MUCH CARE IS ENOUGH?

Before the concept of an adequate level of care can be used as a tool to evaluate patterns of access and efforts to improve equity, it must be fleshed out. Since there is no objective formula for doing this, reasonable people can disagree about whether particular patterns and policies meet the demands of adequacy. The Commission does not attempt to spell out in detail what adequate care should include. Rather it frames the terms in which those who discuss or critique health care issues can consider ethics as well as economics, medical science, and other dimensions.

Characteristics of Adequacy   First, the Commission considers it clear that health care can only be judged adequate in relation to an individual's health condition. To begin with a list of techniques or procedures, for example, is not sensible: A CT scan for an accident victim with a serious head injury might be the best way to make a diagnosis essential for the appropriate treatment of that patient; a CT scan for a person with headaches might not be considered essential for adequate care. To focus only on the technique, therefore,

rather than on the individual's health and the impact the procedure will have on that individual's welfare and opportunity, would lead to inappropriate policy.

Disagreement will arise about whether the care of some health conditions falls within the demands of adequacy. Most people will agree, however, that some conditions should not be included in the societal obligation to ensure access to adequate care. A relatively uncontroversial example would be changing the shape of a functioning, normal nose or retarding the normal effects of aging (through cosmetic surgery). By the same token, there are some conditions, such as pregnancy, for which care would be regarded as an important component of adequacy. In determining adequacy, it is important to consider how people's welfare, opportunities, and requirements for information and interpersonal caring are affected by their health condition.

Any assessment of adequacy must consider also the types, amounts, and quality of care necessary to respond to each health condition. It is important to emphasize that these questions are implicitly comparative: the standard of adequacy for a condition must reflect the fact that resources used for it will not be available to respond to other conditions. Consequently, the level of care deemed adequate should reflect a reasoned judgment not only about the impact of the condition on the welfare and opportunity of the individual but also about the efficacy and the cost of the care itself in relation to other conditions and the efficacy and cost of the care that is available for them. Since individual cases differ so much, the health care professional and patient must be flexible. Thus adequacy, even in relation to a particular health condition, generally refers to a range of options.

The Relationship of Costs and Benefits   The level of care that is available will be determined by the level of resources devoted to producing it. Such allocation should reflect the benefits and costs of the care provided. It should be emphasized that these "benefits," as well as their "costs," should be interpreted broadly, and not restricted only to effects easily quantifiable in monetary terms. Personal benefits include improvements in individuals' functioning and in their quality of life, and the reassurance from worry and the provision of information that are a product of health care. Broader social benefits should be included as well, such as strengthening the sense of community and the belief that no one in serious need of health care will be left without it. Similarly, costs are not merely the funds spent for a treatment but include other less tangible and quantifiable adverse consequences, such as diverting funds away from other socially desirable endeavors including education, welfare, and other social services.

There is no objectively correct value that these various costs and benefits have or that can be discovered by the tools of cost/benefit analysis. Still, such an analysis, as a recent report of the Office of Technology Assessment noted, "can be very helpful to decisionmakers because the process of analysis gives structure to the problem, allows an open consideration of all relevant effects of a decision, and forces the explicit treatment of key assumptions." But the valuation of the various effects of alternative treatments for different conditions rests on people's values and goals, about which individuals will reasonably disagree. In a democracy, the appropriate values to be assigned to the consequences of policies must ultimately be determined by people expressing their values through social and political processes as well as in the marketplace.

Approximating Adequacy   The intention of the Commission is to provide a frame of reference for policymakers, not to resolve these complex questions. Nevertheless, it is possible to raise some of the specific issues that should be considered in determining what constitutes adequate care. It is important, for example, to gather accurate information about and compare the costs and effects, both favorable and unfavorable, of various treatment or management options. The options that better serve the goals that make health care of special importance should be assigned a higher value. As already noted, the assessment of costs must take two factors into account: the cost of a proposed option in relation to alternative forms of care that would achieve the same goal of enhancing the welfare and opportunities of the patient, and the cost of each proposed option in terms of

foregone opportunities to apply the same resources to social goals other than that of ensuring equitable access.

Furthermore, a reasonable specification of adequate care must reflect an assessment of the relative importance of many different characteristics of a given form of care for a particular condition. Sometimes the problem is posed as: What *amounts* of care and what *quality* of care? Such a formulation reduces a complex problem to only two dimensions, implying that all care can readily be ranked as better or worse. Because two alternative forms of care may vary along a number of dimensions, there may be no consensus among reasonable and informed individuals about which form is of higher overall quality. It is worth bearing in mind that adequacy does not mean the highest possible level of quality or strictly equal quality any more than it requires equal amounts of care; of course, adequacy does require that everyone receive care that meets standards of sound medical practice.

Any combination of arrangements for achieving adequacy will presumably include some health care delivery settings that mainly serve certain groups, such as the poor or those covered by public programs. The fact that patients receive care in different settings or from different providers does not itself show that some are receiving inadequate care. The Commission believes that there is no moral objection to such a system so long as all receive care that is adequate in amount and quality and all patients are treated with concern and respect. . . .

NOTES

1. Norman Daniels, *Health Care Needs and Distributive Justice*, 10 Phil. & Pub. Aff. 146 (1981).
2. Whether the issue of equity is framed in terms of individual rights or societal obligation, it is important to recall that society's moral imperative to achieve equitable access is not an unlimited commitment to provide whatever care, regardless of cost, individuals need or that would be of some benefit to them. Instead, society's obligation is to provide adequate care for everyone. Consequently, if there is a moral right that corresponds to this obligation, it is limited, not open-ended.

Equal Opportunity and Health Care

Norman Daniels

A natural place to seek principles of justice for regulating health-care institutions is by examining different general theories of justice. Libertarian, utilitarian, and contractarian theories, for example, each support more general principles governing the distribution of rights, opportunities, and wealth, and these general principles may bear on the specific issue of health care. But there is a difficulty with this strategy. In order to apply such general theories to health care, we need to know what kind of a social good health care is. An analysis of this problem is not provided by general theories of justice. One way to see the problem is to ask whether health-care services, say personal medical services, should be viewed as we view other commodities in our society. Should we allow inequalities in the access to health-care services to vary with whatever economic inequalities are permissible according to more general principles of distributive justice? Or is health care "special" and not to be assimilated with other commodities, like cars or personal computers, whose distribution we allow to be governed by market exchanges among economic unequals?

Is health care special? To answer this question, we must see that not all preferences individuals have—and express, for example, in the marketplace—are of equal moral importance. When we judge the importance to society of meeting someone's preferences we use a restricted measure of well-being. We do not simply ask, how much does the person want something? Or, how happy an individual will be if he gets it? Rather, we are concerned whether the preference is for something that affects well-being in certain fundamental or important ways (cf. Scanlon 1975). Among the kinds of preferences to which we give special weight are those that meet certain important categories of need. Among these important needs are those necessary for maintaining normal functioning for individuals, viewed as members of a natural species.

Health-care needs fit this characterization of important needs because they are things we need to prevent or cure diseases and disabilities, which are deviations from species-typical functional organization ("normal functioning" for short).

This preference suggests health care may be special in this restricted sense: Health care needs are important to meet because they affect normal functioning. But there is still a gap in our answer: Why give such moral importance to health-care needs merely because they are necessary to preserve normal functioning? Why is preserving normal functioning of special moral importance? The answer lies in the relationship between normal functioning and opportunity, but to make the relationship clear, I must introduce the notion of a normal opportunity range.

The *normal opportunity range* for a given society is the array of life plans reasonable persons in it are likely to construct for themselves. The normal range is thus dependent on key features of the society—its stage of historical development, its level of material wealth and technological development, and even important cultural facts about it. This dependency is one way in which the notion of normal opportunity range is socially relative. Facts about social organization, including the conception of justice regulating its basic institutions, will also determine how that total normal range is distributed in the population. Nevertheless, that issue of distribution aside, normal functioning provides us with one clear parameter affecting the share of the normal range open to a given individual. It is this parameter that the distribution of health care affects.

The share of the normal range open to individuals is also determined in a fundamental way by their talents and skills. Fair equality of opportunity does not require opportunity to be equal for all persons. It requires only that it be equal for persons with similar skills and talents. Thus individual shares of the normal range will not in general be *equal*, even when they are *fair* to the individual. The general principle of fair equality of opportunity does not imply leveling individual differences. Within the general theory of justice, unequal chances of success which derive from unequal talents may be compensated for in other ways. I can now state a fact at the heart of my approach: Impairment of normal functioning through disease and disability restricts individuals' opportunities relative to that portion of the normal range their skills and talents would have made available to them were they healthy. If individuals' fair shares of the normal range are the arrays of life plans they may reasonably choose, given their talents and skills, then disease and disability shrinks their shares from what is fair.

Of course, we also know that skills and talents can be undeveloped or misdeveloped because of social conditions, for example, family background or racist educational practices. So, if we are interested in having individuals enjoy a fair share of the normal opportunity range, we will want to correct for special disadvantages here too, say through compensatory educational or job-training programs. Still, restoring normal functioning through health care has a particular and *limited* effect on an individual's shares of the normal range. It lets them enjoy that portion of the range to which a full array of skills and talents would give them access, assuming that these too are not impaired by special social disadvantages. Again, there is no presumption that we should eliminate or level individual differences: These act as a baseline constraint on the degree to which individuals enjoy the normal range. Only where differences in talents and skills are the results of disease and disability, not merely normal variation, is some effort required to correct for the effects of the "natural lottery."

One conclusion we may draw is that impairment of the normal opportunity range is a (fairly crude) measure of the relative importance of health-care needs, at least at the social or macro level. That is, it will be more important to prevent, cure, or compensate for those disease conditions which involve a greater curtailment of an individual's share of the normal opportunity range. More generally, this relationship between health-care needs and opportunity suggests that the principle that should govern the design of health-care institutions is a principle guaranteeing fair equality of opportunity.

The concept of equality of opportunity is given prominence in Rawls's (1971) theory of justice, and it has also been the subject of extensive critical discussion. I cannot here review the main issues (see Daniels 1985, Chapter 3), nor provide a full justification for the principle of fair equality of opportunity. Instead, I shall settle for a weaker, conditional claim, which suffices for my purposes. Health-care institutions should be among those governed by a principle of fair equality of opportunity, provided two conditions obtain: (1) an acceptable general theory of justice includes a principle that requires basic institutions to guarantee fair equality of opportunity, and (2) the fair equality of opportunity principle acts as a constraint on permissible economic inequalities. In what follows, for the sake of simplicity, I shall ignore these provisos. I urge the fair equality of opportunity principle as an appropriate principle to govern macro decisions about the design of our health-care system. The principle defines, from the perspective of justice, what the moral *function* of the health-care system must be—to help guarantee fair equality of opportunity. This relationship between health care and opportunity is the fundamental insight underlying my approach.

My conditional claim does not depend on the acceptability of any particular general theory of justice, such as Rawls's contractarian theory. A utilitarian theory might suffice, for example, if it were part of an ideal moral code, general compliance with which produced at least as much utility as any alternative code (cf. Brandt 1979). That utilitarian theory could then be extended to health care through the analysis provided by my account. Because Rawls's is the main general theory that has incorporated a fair equality of opportunity principle, I have elsewhere suggested in some detail (Daniels 1985, Chapter 3) how it can be extended, with minor modifications, to incorporate my approach. These details need not distract us here.

The fair equality of opportunity account has several important implications for the issue of access to health care. First, the account is compatible with, though it does not imply, a multitiered health-care system. The basic tier would include health-care services that meet health-care needs, or at least important needs, as judged by their impact on opportunity range. Other tiers might involve the use of health-care services to meet less important needs or other preferences, for example, cosmetic surgery. Second, the basic tier, which we might think of as a "decent basic minimum," is characterized in a principled way, by reference to its impact on opportunity. Third, there should be no obstacles—financial, racial, geographical—to access to the basic tier. (The account is silent about what inequalities are permissible for higher tiers within the system.) Social obligations are focused on the basic tier.

The fair equality of opportunity account also has implications for issues of resource allocation. First, I have already noted that we have a crude criterion—impact on normal opportunity range—for distinguishing the importance of different health-care needs and services. Second, preventive measures that make the distribution of risks of disease more equitable must be given prominence in a just health-care system. Third, the importance of personal medical services, despite what we spend on them, must be weighed against other forms of health care, including preventive and public health measures, personal care and other long-term-care services. A just distribution of health-care services involves weighing the impact of all of these on normal opportunity range. This point has specific implications for the importance of long-term care, but also for the introduction of new high-cost technologies, such as artificial hearts, which deliver a benefit to relatively few individuals at very great cost. We must weigh new technologies against alternatives and judge the overall impact of introducing them on fair equality of opportunity—which gives a slightly new sense to the term "opportunity cost."

This account does not give individuals a basic right to have all of their health-care needs met. Rather, there are social obligations to provide individuals only with those services that are part of the design of a system which, on the whole, protects equal opportunity. If social obligations to provide appropriate health care are not met, then individuals are definitely wronged. Injustice is done to them. Thus, even though decisions have to be made about how best to protect opportunity, these obligations nevertheless are not similar to imperfect duties of beneficence. If I could benefit from your charity, but you instead give charity to someone else, I am not wronged and you have fulfilled your duty of beneficence. But if the just design of a health-care system requires providing a service from which I could benefit, then I am wronged if I do not get it.

The case is similar to individuals who have injustice done to them because they are discriminated against in hiring or promotion practices on a job. In both cases, we can translate the specific sort of injustice done, which involves acts or policies that impair or fail to protect opportunity, into a claim about individual rights. The principle of justice guaranteeing fair equality of opportunity shows that individuals have legitimate claims or rights when their opportunity is impaired in particular ways—against a background of institutions and practices which protect equal opportunity. Health-care rights in this view are thus a species of rights to equal opportunity.

The scope and limits of these rights—the entitlements they actually carry with them—will be relative to certain facts about a given system. For example, a health-care system can protect opportunity only within the limits imposed by resource scarcity and technological development for a given society. We cannot make a direct inference from the fact that an individual has a right to health care to the conclusion that this person is entitled to some specific health-care service, even if the service would meet a health-care need. Rather, the individual is entitled to a specific service only if it is or ought to be part of a system that appropriately protects fair equality of opportunity. . . .

REFERENCES

Brandt, R. 1979. *A Theory of the Good and the Right.* Oxford: Oxford University Press.

Daniels, N. 1985. "Family Responsibility Initiatives and Justice Between Age Groups." *Law, Medicine, and Health Care* 13(4):153–159.

Rawls, J. 1971. *A Theory of Justice.* Cambridge, MA: Harvard University Press.

Scanlon, T. M. 1975. "Preference and Urgency." *Journal of Philosophy* 77(19):655–669.

Freedom and Moral Diversity: The Moral Failures of Health Care in the Welfare State

H. Tristram Engelhardt, Jr.

I.   AN INTRODUCTION: BEYOND EQUALITY

In his 1993 health-care reform proposal, Bill Clinton offered health care as a civil right. If his proposal had been accepted, all Americans would have been guaranteed a basic package of health care. At the same time, they would have been forbidden to provide or purchase better basic health care, as a cost of participating in a national system to which they were compelled to contribute. A welfare entitlement would have been created and an egalitarian ethos enforced.[1] This essay will address why such egalitarian proposals are morally unjustifiable, both in terms of the establishment of a uniform health-care welfare right, and in terms of the egalitarian constraints these proposals impose against the use of private resources in the purchase of better-quality basic health care, not to mention luxury care.

In framing health-care welfare policy, one must address people's fears of being impoverished while at risk of death and suffering when medicine can offer a benefit. Simultaneously, one must confront significantly different understandings of the appropriate use of medicine, the claims of justice, and the meaning of equality. Any approach to providing health care for those who cannot afford it must come to terms with the substantial disagreements that separate individuals and communities regarding provision of health care by the state. In addition, the attempt to frame a uniform policy must confront the nonegalitarian consequences of human freedom. To be free is to make choices that have nonegalitarian results.

I shall argue that our disagreements about equality, fairness, and justice have a depth similar to that of our disagreements about contraception, abortion, third-party-assisted reproduction, and physician-assisted suicide, in that they are not resolvable in general secular moral terms. The lesson of the postmodern era is that there are as many secular accounts of equality, justice, and fairness as there are religious groups, sects, and cults.[2] There is no principled basis for choosing a particular content-full account as canonical. As a consequence, establishing a particular content-full notion of equality, fairness, and justice in health care is the secular equivalent of establishing, for a secular national health-care system, the Roman Catholic proscriptions regarding contraception: it would be morally arbitrary and without secular moral justification. Consequently, there are robust secular moral limitations on the establishment of particular views of equality, limitations resulting from the centrality of human persons as the source of secular moral authority. There are good grounds for holding that current health-care policies, such as those embodied in Medicare, which forbid recipients from paying more for better basic care from participating physicians while coercing them to contribute to this program, are immoral. I argue in this essay that welfare rights in health care, if they are to be established, should be recognized as the creations of limited governmental insurance policies and not as expressions of foundational rights to health care or claims of equality or fairness.[3]

II.   MEDICAL WELFARE: TEMPTATIONS AND DISAGREEMENTS IN THE FACE OF FINITUDE

Health care claims attention because of the dramatic ways in which medicine and the biomedical sciences address our finitude, vulnerability, and mortality. Political support for the governmental provision of

From *Social Philosophy and Policy*, Vol. 14, No. 2, Summer 1997, 180–196. Reprinted with permission from Cambridge University Press.

EDITORS' NOTE: Some notes have been deleted. Readers who wish to follow up on sources should consult the original article.

health care often involves the view that to deny someone health care is to deny him or her protection against suffering, disease, disability, and death. The suppressed premise is that such a denial would be unfair. This view has difficulties. First, one must show how and why needs generate rights. Second, unlike food, clothing, and shelter, which can be provided at relatively minimal costs while still being sufficient for health and life, health care frequently confronts disabilities, diseases, disorders, and threats of death that cannot be overcome even with maximum medical efforts and the costs they involve. Often, illness can be cured only in part, suffering ameliorated only to some extent, disabilities remedied only to some degree, and death postponed only for a short time. In many cases, no matter how much one does, more resources could have been invested with some benefit for some recipients or possible recipients of health care. Just as ever more resources could be invested in avoiding accidental injuries and deaths by improving workplace safety, or invested in diminishing highway deaths by licensing only those cars that have front and side air bags as well as the front-end collision protection available in luxury cars, so, too, in medicine more resources could always be invested in preventive and curative endeavors without ever being fully successful against our finite, vulnerable, and mortal condition. Death and suffering are inescapable, so that we must decide what finite effort we should make to postpone death and avoid some suffering. We must ask whether there is secular moral authority coercively to impose one particular approach and whether it may be an egalitarian one.

The human condition itself conspires against discovering a generally convincing understanding of what should count as a basic adequate package of health-care services. First, there is the problem that medical knowledge is limited and probabilistic. Practicing medicine requires accepting that all life is a gamble, that medicine is a part of life, and that therefore health-care professionals must gamble with the suffering, disability, and death of all whom they treat. Moreover, resources that one might use to improve knowledge and technology are themselves limited. On the one hand, there is not enough money to avoid all suffering, disability, and death. On the other hand, there is not enough knowledge to know with certainty when particular interventions will succeed or fail. As a result, given the fini-

tude of resources and the indefinite range of threats to well-being and life, investments in protection against suffering, disability, and death must take into account probabilities of success and failure. Investments must be limited and one must gamble.

To gamble, one must be willing to lose. Suppose that, as a matter of public policy, one has decided that in order to make good use of resources, one will not provide resources to the poor for a particular intervention—even when it might offer some protection against suffering, disability, and death— because the costs, probability of failure, and/or likely poor quality of results outweigh the possible benefits. In such a case, one must be willing to allow people to experience suffering, disability, and death when the resources are not available. One must also confront the circumstance that those with sufficient resources will purchase protection against death and suffering which is not available to all. In short, since ever more resources could always be invested in health care with some positive benefit, one faces two especially troubling policy questions: (1) May a basic, less-than-optimal package of health care be established for the poor? (2) May individuals, communities, and organizations use their own funds and energies to secure for themselves even better basic protection, as well as supplementary protection, against death and suffering? If secular morality (a) cannot reveal a content-full canonical morality that requires an egalitarian health-care policy, but (b) rather reveals that individuals are the source of secular moral authority, then one will need to endorse a national health-care policy that accepts both moral diversity and inequality.

III.   BAD LUCK, UNFAIRNESS, AND INEQUALITY

If the authority of persons over themselves is morally legitimate, then individuals will, through their free choices, set limits to the realization of government-endorsed visions of the good and of human flourishing. Among the goods with which freedom will collide are those of equality and long life. To be free in any way that allows one to pursue particular goods or goals despite risks of death or disability is to be free to place oneself at risk of needing additional health care. To be free in any way that allows the acquisition of wealth as well as the giving and receiving of funds, valuables, and labor is to be free in ways that produce inequalities in opportunity and outcome. If the authority of governments is derived from the free consent of citizens, then citizens can freely limit governmental authority by withholding consent. Freedom brings into question the plausibility of a uniform and equal basic health-care entitlement. Insofar as people are free and have their own resources, some will take greater risks than others and some will purchase better protection than many can afford. Beyond that, one faces other persistent inequalities and a significant diversity of views about how one should respond to inequalities.

All will die, though some will die in their youth and others will live long lives. Inequality in health is, for many, especially vexing, since it involves significant differences in suffering and length of life. Still, differences in health status are not, on average, dramatically related to the level of access to high-cost health care. Cross-national comparative data concerning health-care investments and life expectancies suggest that differences in access to high-technology medicine pale in importance when compared to differences attributable to gender, income, and genetic luck. Women outlive men, the rich outlive the poor, and high-status individuals tend to outlive low-status individuals. For example, in the United Kingdom men and women in 1991 had life expectancies at birth of 73.2 and 78.8 years, respectively, while those in the United States had life expectancies of 72.0 and 78.9 years, respectively, though the United Kingdom invested $1,151 per person for health care, 7.1 percent of its gross domestic product, in comparison with the United States, which invested $3,094 per person, 13.6 percent of its gross domestic product. At age 80, the life expectancy was 6.3 years for men and 8.3 years for women in the United Kingdom, versus 7.2 years for men and 9.1 years for women in the United States. Though the differences in resource investment for health care likely express themselves in these differences in life expectancies at age 80, in absolute terms the differences due to gender still outweighed the differences between the two systems.

Given these data, a national health-care policy which focused on equality in mortality outcomes would most plausibly direct energies toward developing new ways to address the health needs of men and toward preventing pediatric deaths. Indeed, for egalitarians concerned with equality in life expectancies, a cross-national examination of life-expectancy outcomes by gender would seem to mandate a major commitment to the increased study of diseases of men, an increase in the representation of men in research protocols, and the development of better treatments for life-threatening conditions facing men. Such egalitarians would also favor the prevention of pediatric deaths over improvements in geriatric medicine, because of the robust inequalities in life presented, say, in the comparison between having a life span of twelve years versus one of seventy-two years. If one invokes an expository device such as John Rawls's original position,* one can easily imagine a characterization of the contractors such that they would regard those dying young as the least well-off, and would therefore direct energies against pediatric life-threatening conditions before directing resources to geriatric care, other than perhaps comfort care. A somewhat similar case can be made for directing medical research toward diseases afflicting the poor and persons of low status. In short, a dedicated pursuit of equality in mortality expectations should give priority to medical research and treatment development for men, children, the poor, and persons of low status.

Not all will agree with this approach, either in detail or in its foundations. Since we do not share one concrete morality, the very energies which direct our concerns toward medical issues separate us into disagreeing communities of moral commitment. Disputes regarding bioethics and health-care policy cut to the moral quick regarding equality, not only because individuals and communities differ with respect to the weight assigned to equality interests, but also because of the moral ambiguity of the term itself. If one is to develop an egalitarian policy, one must establish the importance and compelling moral authority of a particular form or understanding of equality. The difficulty is that our understandings of the importance of equality differ substantially.

To appreciate the force of these differences, one might imagine three worlds. The first world has ten people in it, each with six units of goodness or utility. In a second world there are nine people

*EDITORS' NOTE: See the Introduction.

with six units of goodness or utility and one person with ten units. If one is on principle an egalitarian of outcomes, one will regard the second world as worse than the first, even though no one is worse off and the total amount of utility or goodness is greater. If one is morally concerned to rectify the inequalities of the second world, one will incline to what can be characterized as an egalitarianism of envy. That is, one will want all persons to be made equal, even when some have more without dispossessing those who have less. This attitude toward equality can be understood as a form of envy in the sense of an endorsed discontent with the good fortune of others, holding unequalizing good fortune to be unfair, even if it is not at the expense of others. Inequality in and of itself is regarded as a circumstance to be rectified in preference to and in priority over other goods or right-making conditions. Finally, one can consider a third world with nine people with six units of goodness or utility and one person with only one unit. If one wishes to improve the lot of the tenth person as cheaply and efficiently as possible, not because the person's share is unequal, but because that person lacks important goods and satisfactions, one can be characterized as endorsing an egalitarianism of altruism. One is not, in principle, concerned that some have more. Instead, one has sympathy for those who, in having less, lack a good.[4]

How one regards the inequalities presented in the descriptions of these three worlds is important for assessing how one regards inequalities in health care and elsewhere. This is especially significant for health-care policy, given that major differences in per-capita investments in health care across nations do not lead to dramatic differences in mortality expectations, once one has achieved a rather modest level of investment (e.g., Greece does very well with $452 of health care per person).[5] One must look to other considerations for the special place of equality in debates regarding health-care policy. Perhaps the special place given to equality in health care depends on (1) the ways in which medicine is felt to bear on our finitude, in particular, on the postponement of death and the blunting of suffering, as well as (2) the difficulties of steadfastly refusing to commit communal funds to rescue persons with expensive health needs, even when (a) some individuals with disposable

resources may decide to have themselves treated when they have such needs, and (b) individuals without the funds demand such treatment. If one is to set limits on public health-care expenditures when it has been decided that the costs of such interventions on average outweigh the benefits, while recognizing the authority of persons to make choices about themselves and to use their resources as they wish, one must commit oneself to opposing high-cost last-minute state attempts at medical rescue for the poor and one must accept inequalities in access to health care.

Even if one were resolved to set egalitarian limits on health-care expenditures, one would still be confronted with a diversity of equalities. One would need a basis in principle for choosing among: an equality of opportunity in using one's own resources to pursue one's own health-care goals; an equality of opportunity supported by governmental funds in the acquisition of health care; an equality of opportunity supported by governmental funds and by proscriptions against unbalancing this equality by private purchases.[6] If one pursued an equality of outcome rather than an equality of opportunity, one would need to choose among: an equality of outcome supported by research and treatment directed toward avoiding the premature death of men, children, etc.; an equality of outcome directed toward equalizing the likelihood of suffering, including the use of nonvoluntary euthanasia; an equality of outcome directed toward equalizing wealth, etc. One would also need a basis for choosing among conflicting views of governmental authority that could be invoked in the coercive realization of a particular ethos of health-care delivery. Does the government have the moral authority only to ensure that the provision of health care will be honest and nonfraudulent? Does the government also have the moral authority to ensure that everyone receives the health care that the government deems to be appropriate? Does the government have the secular moral authority to forbid the rich from leaving the country in order to purchase better health care abroad?

At stake also are conflicting views of what it is for the state to own the resources which politicians might wish to redistribute for egalitarian purposes, and what it is for individuals and groups to have holdings independently of the state. For example, does one own resources because one has produced them or has been given those resources by those who have produced them? Or does one only own resources if such entitlements conform to a governmentally endorsed understanding of a desirable or right distribution of resources? For that matter, why are communal claims to possess resources advantaged over those made by individuals? In addition, one must decide what counts as just, fair, right, and good. For example, do needs generate rights, so that if resources are not available to meet health-care needs, such a state of affairs is unfair? Or are some outcomes simply unfortunate without being unfair? For instance, if certain screening programs can decrease the risk of developing cancer, does such protection against possible death count as a need that generates a right to a service for which others have a moral obligation to pay? Or is the nonprovision of such a service unfortunate, but not unfair? Or, if one's admission to a critical-care unit will convey a small chance of survival at a very high cost, does one have a need for health care that generates a right to the resources of others in order to purchase such critical care? Or is the nonavailability of such resources, save for the rich, simply unfortunate, not unfair?

There are, in addition, substantive disagreements regarding how to understand the relationship among individuals, communities, societies, and states. These disagreements are functions of different accounts of how one should characterize the communal, societal, and/or political space within which individuals find different kinds of morally authoritative structures. For example, should welfare, in the sense of group-provided insurance against losses in the natural and social lotteries,[7] be provided at the level of the state for all citizens, or instead at the level of particular communities and associations? One might envisage such provision occurring not just through companies, but also through religious and ideological groups. A number of these could transcend national boundaries, such as, perhaps, a worldwide Vaticare health-care welfare system for Roman Catholics, with the payment for care denominated in Vatican lira. Past history indicates that such approaches can succeed quite well even when they are unassociated with a particular religious or moral vision. In our contemporary postmodern

world of deep disagreements regarding appropriate moral understandings of health care, such associations offer the opportunity of maintaining moral and religious integrity within structures committed to a particular vision of health care. Under such an arrangement, one will need to tolerate others' doing evil within their own associations; yet when associations (rather than governments) are the social structures which embody content-full moralities, one can distance oneself as a citizen from such undertakings and avoid immediate collaboration with what one recognizes as wrong.

IV.   HEALTH-CARE WELFARE PROVISION: WHY IT IS SO INTRUSIVE AND PROBLEMATIC

The provision of health care as a basic uniform civil right is more intrusive than any other element of the welfare state: health care dramatically touches all the important passages of life, from reproduction and birth to suffering and death. The commitment to a particular package of services brings with it a particular interpretation of the significance of reproduction, birth, health, suffering, death, and equality (e.g., it involves specific positions regarding artificial insemination by donors, prenatal diagnosis with the possibility of selective abortion, physician-assisted suicide, voluntary active euthanasia, and unequal access to better basic health care). A uniform welfare right to health care involves endorsing and establishing one among a number of competing concrete moralities of life, death, and equality. Because of this tie to morally controversial interventions, the establishment of uniform, universal health-care welfare rights directly or indirectly involves citizens, patients, physicians, nurses, and others in receiving or providing health care in a health-care system which they may find morally opprobrious.

Since all elements of personal behavior have some impact on the likelihood of disease, disability, and death, the establishment of a uniform, encompassing health-care welfare system involves the risk of medically politicizing all elements of personal conduct. For example, how should one regard a person who smokes heavily? Does a smoker irresponsibly expose the nation's health-care system to unnecessary costs? Or is such an individual a super-patriot, supporting the long-term fiscal solvency of the government? That is, should one consider such an individual a cost-saver, taking into account not only the costs of health care for smoking-related illnesses, but also the Social Security obligations (which would increase if the person were to live a more wholesome, longer life), possible long-term Medicare costs (which would be incurred if the individual adopted wholesome, nonsmoking behaviors, and thus lived to be eligible), and possible long-term Medicaid costs (which would rise if the individual adopted wholesome, nonsmoking behaviors, lived longer, and developed Alzheimer's, etc.)? Should one also consider the affluence and therefore increased life expectancies that may result from wealth generated from the tobacco industry? Who burdens whom, and under what circumstances, depends on who pays as well as on the freedom of individuals to agree to engage in certain behaviors and to accept the consequences involved.

An encompassing health-care welfare entitlement does not merely tend to impose a particular vision of morality, human flourishing, and responsible risk-taking; it also tends to constrain the free choice of those with disposable resources. The notion of a guaranteed basic benefit package can take on a coercive character, so that individuals are not allowed to purchase better basic care but may only purchase additional care which is not provided through the guaranteed benefit package. For example, after being compelled by state force to contribute to a Medicare system, so-called beneficiaries may not offer more money for a covered service in order to gain access to a premier physician. Current Medicare law forbids Medicare patients from rewarding their physicians and health-care providers for better basic service. Nor may they legally offer to pay more for a longer, more careful provision of the basic services covered under Medicare. Once covered by Medicare for physician services, for example, they may not volunteer to pay five times the reimbursement schedule (i.e., have Medicare pay its fee and they pay four times that in addition) for a house call by a distinguished internist. In short, their resources are devalued by a system to which they are compelled to contribute and which will then not allow them to benefit from their required

contributions if they wish to purchase better basic care. Substantive, coercively imposed health-care policies come into tension with the free and peaceable choices of individuals (e.g., the patient who might wish to purchase better basic care from a willing physician, while still receiving Medicare benefits which that patient has been compelled to fund).

Health-care welfare rights are, for all these reasons, problematic. The framing of health-care policy requires (1) gambling with human life, (2) accepting unavoidable inequalities in morbidity and mortality, (3) recognizing multiple and competing notions of equality in health care, and (4) acknowledging the intrusiveness of health-care rights if they bring with them particular moral visions of reproduction, suffering, and death. It also requires (5) appreciating the dangers of imposing a particular medicalized view of lifestyles in the service of health policy, and (6) noting the temptation to restrict free choices in order to achieve what is taken to be, on some particular understanding, a suitable level of efficiency or equity, while (7) confronting the diversity of our moral visions.

V. WHY THE MORAL DISPUTES WILL NOT GO AWAY, WHY WE ARE NOT ONE MORAL COMMUNITY WHEN IT COMES TO MATTERS OF HEALTH-CARE WEL-FARE PROVISION, AND WHY A PARTIC-ULAR SUBSTANTIVE MORAL VISION OF FAIRNESS MAY NOT BE IMPOSED ON ALL

It is not merely a matter of fact or of sociological circumstance that we possess diverse understandings of the significance of reproduction, birth, disability, suffering, and death, as well as diverse understandings of how one ought to gamble in the face of finitude or how one ought to take account of our inequalities and disparate misfortunes with respect to death and suffering. The crucial point is that we do not possess the basis for resolving such controversies in terms of a content-full morality. The goal of demonstrating that we are one secular moral community—such that we ought to agree as a matter of justice, fairness, or moral probity regarding an all-encompassing health-care welfare system—is elusive. Rather than uniting citizens in a single moral community, the attempt to develop a uniform, encompassing health-care welfare right, as a matter of principle, and not only as a matter of fact, reveals our moral differences concerning the meaning and importance of equality, as well as our differences concerning the proper understanding of reproduction, suffering, and death.

The difficulty in resolving our moral controversies is foundational: one must already possess particular background moral premises, together with rules of moral evidence and inference, in order to resolve a moral controversy by sound rational argument. One needs a perspective from which one can make a morally authoritative choice among competing visions of the right and the good. An appeal to moral intuitions will not suffice. One's own moral intuitions will conflict with other moral intuitions. An appeal to ever-higher levels of moral intuition will not be decisive either, for further disagreements and appeals can in principle be extended indefinitely. Nor will an appeal to a consensus be any more successful. It will simply raise a number of questions: How does any particular consensus confer moral authority? How extensive must a consensus be to confer such authority? And from whom does such authority derive? (The appeal to consensus appears to invoke a secular version of a claim for the divine authority of majorities: *vox populi, vox Dei.*) In short, how much of a majority authorizes what use of force and why? In order to establish policy, one must know which substantive account of the right and/or the good is authoritative. However, the higher-level perspective from which one would make such a choice must itself be informed by an understanding of the right and/or the good.

Imagine that one agrees that a society—through public policy in general, and in health-care policy in particular—should attempt to maximize liberty, equality, prosperity, and security. To calculate and compare the consequences of alternative approaches, one must already know how to compare liberty, equality, prosperity, and security. The comparative consequences of competing approaches cannot be assessed simply by an appeal to consequences. One must already have an independent morality allowing one to compare the different kinds of outcomes at stake, namely, liber-

ty consequences, equality consequences, prosperity consequences, and security consequences. Nor will attempting to maximize the preferences of citizens determine which health policy has the best consequences. One must first know how to compare impassioned versus rational preferences. One must know how, if at all, one is to revise or correct preferences. In addition, one will need to know God's discount rate for preference satisfaction over time; that is, one must have an absolute standard or must know whether each person's own standard should be used, whatever it might be, in the moment the person attempts the discounting. Nor will it do to appeal to a disinterested observer, a hypothetical chooser, or a set of hypothetical contractors. If such are truly disinterested, they will have no moral sense and will be unable to make a principled choice. To make a principled choice, they must already be informed by a particular moral sense or thin theory of the good. But of course, the choice of the correct moral sense or thin theory of the good is what is at stake. The same difficulty can be recapitulated for any account of moral rationality or of the decision-theoretic resolution of disputes. In order morally to assess behavior or policy, one must appeal to a standard. To use a standard, however, one must know which standard is morally canonical. The result is that a canonical content-full moral vision can be established as binding by sound rational argument only by begging the question. To choose with moral authority, one must already have authoritative normative guidance. The question is: "Which (and whose) guidance?"

Postmodernity as an epistemological predicament, not merely as a sociological fact, is the recognition that, outside of a revelation of a canonical standard, one cannot authoritatively choose among content-full understandings of moral probity, justice, or fairness without begging the question or engaging in an infinite regress. In order to show how a conclusion is warranted, one must always ask whose moral rationality, which sense of justice, is being invoked. At the same time, one must recognize that there are numerous competing moral accounts or narratives. As we have seen, there are numerous and competing understandings of the importance and significance of equality. In such a circumstance, if all do not listen to God, so as to find revealed to them the canonical content-full notion of moral probity, fairness, justice, and equality, and if all attempts by sound rational argument to establish the canonical content-full account of moral probity, justice, and fairness beg the question, then one can arrive at moral authority when individuals meet as moral strangers, not by drawing authority either from God or from reason, but only from the permission of those who participate. Moral authority will not be the authority of God or reason, but of consent, agreement, or permission. General secular moral authority is thus best construed as authorization.[8] The practice of deriving moral authority from permission makes possible a sparse practice of secular morality that does not presume any particular content-full view of the right or the good.

In such circumstances, permission or the authority it provides becomes the source of moral authority without any endorsement of permission as either good or bad. The securing of permission provides authority even when it does not provide motivation (permission does secure secular moral authority for the appropriate, albeit limited, use of state coercion, which can motivate compliance with the practice of deriving authority from permission). The point is that it is possible to secure a justification for state coercion and to determine which instances of coercion carry secular moral authority. The question is not "What will motivate moral action?" (though this issue is important), or "What level of moral disagreement makes governance difficult or impossible?" (or, for that matter, "What strategies by governments support public peace or effective governance?"). The question is, rather, "Under what circumstances can those ruling claim secular moral authority, so that those who disobey laws are not only at risk of being punished, but also at risk of being blameworthy?" Acting with permission offers a sparse, right-making condition for the collaboration of individuals who do not share a common understanding of what God demands or what moral rationality requires, but who claim an authority for their common endeavors.

Secular morality is procedural, and its legitimacy is limited by the consent of those who participate in common endeavors. Consequently, the paradigm moral activities of secular morality are the free market, contract formation, and the establishment of limited democracies.

In particular, democracies will have only that secular moral authority which can be derived either from the actual consent of all their members or from the practice of never using persons without their permission. The result will be that one will at most be able to justify the material equivalent of Robert Nozick's ultraminimal state. The point is that, in the absence of a canonical, content-full secular morality, (1) health-care policy must derive its authority from the consent of the governed, (2) not from a prior understanding of justice, fairness, or equality, and (3) may not be all-encompassing, because the scope of its authority is limited by the limits of the consent of those involved. One will need to create policy instead of attempting to discover guidance in secular morality. One must proceed not by an appeal to a canonical, content-full understanding of the right or the good, but by an appeal to the permission of those involved. There will be no way to discover the correct balance among the various undertakings to which a community could direct its resources (e.g., how one should use common funds when faced with the claims of partisans of whooping cranes versus those of aged humans). As a consequence, limited democracies will be obliged to leave space so that individuals and communities can peaceably pursue their own visions of human flourishing and of appropriate health care. Still, if the state has legitimately acquired common resources, it is at liberty to create limited policy answers. One can explore many of the secular moral limits in health-care policy without attending to the general secular moral limits on state authority, by assuming that the state possesses legitimately acquired funds.[9]

VI. TAKING MORAL DIVERSITY AND LIMITED DEMOCRACY SERIOUSLY

The concern to establish health-care welfare provision is encumbered by a cluster of moral difficulties tied to the inability to establish, by sound rational argument, a canonical morality regarding equality in access, not to mention regarding such important issues as third-party-assisted reproduction, abortion, physician-assisted suicide, and euthanasia. Though there is, on the part of many, a strong desire to establish an encompassing and equal right to health care, there are even stronger grounds for recognizing the morally problematic character of this desire. The substantial and significant differences in moral vision concerning matters of equality—and concerning the appropriate ways to regard reproduction, birth, suffering, and death—make any uniform, governmentally imposed right to health care highly morally problematic. Such an imposition would involve the secular equivalent of establishing a particular religious morality. If we do not share a common understanding of equality, fairness, and justice, and if there is in principle no way through sound rational argument to determine which understanding of justice, fairness, and equality should guide governmental undertakings, and if, in addition, health care is particularly intrusive and morally troubling when it brings with it a content-full moral understanding of reproduction, birth, suffering, and death, then the provision of any general protection against morbidity and mortality is best offered as a limited insurance against losses in the natural and social lotteries.

These considerations argue against any particular universally mandated set of health-care services and in favor of the equivalent of a voucher for the poor, which would allow the purchase of health care from various morally different health-care delivery networks. The limits of secular moral authority require acquiescing in the creation of health-care networks and associations providing morally different forms of basic health care. The only restrictions that may be imposed with secular moral authority will involve the guarantee that participants in the various health-care networks join freely in the particular medical moralities they choose.

In order to establish a limited welfare right to health care without going aground on diverse visions of moral probity and justice, secular health-care provision for the indigent may not be justified in terms of a particular account of equality, fairness, or justice, nor may it establish a particular medical morality regarding reproduction, suffering, and death. The use of vouchers could avoid much of this difficulty if such vouchers could be applied to different alternative, basic menus of service. Different communities or associations with different moral visions could then establish morally competing health-care systems into which individuals could enter for basic services using such vouchers. Better yet would be a policy that avoided even the necessity of establishing basic menus of service and instead allowed the use of health-care purchase accounts to which funds could be provided for the poor to use in purchasing basic medical services.

Under such circumstances, the government would provide basic health-care protection against morbidity and mortality for the indigent without imposing a content-full morality. Medical needs could be both defined and addressed in a range of significantly different terms. In a truly free and limited democracy, competing health-care systems could come into existence to take advantage of the availability of the health-care vouchers (as well as the availability of payments from private insurers and direct payments from patients). For the sake of illustration, one could imagine two systems, one supported by Roman Catholics and another by New Age agnostics. The first would not offer artificial insemination by donors, prenatal diagnosis and abortion, or physician-assisted suicide and euthanasia. It would provide limitations on health-care expenditures in terms of religious understandings of the appropriate line between proportionate and disproportionate care, that is, between ordinary and extraordinary care. This line would vary with the social status of the individual (i.e., it would be *proportionem status*). In addition, religiously attentive hospice and comfort care would be offered to all.

In contrast, the system appealing to agnostic New-Agers would offer artificial insemination for unmarried women, prenatal diagnosis and selective abortion, and specially discounted treatment with an agreement to be euthanatized under certain conditions when health care is unlikely to provide a significant extension of life with an acceptable quality. Hospice care would be tied to effective and painless euthanasia. A voucher system or health-care purchase account that took moral diversity seriously would allow individuals to avoid interventions they recognized as morally inappropriate and to purchase in their stead those they saw as acceptable (or to select care so as to achieve a savings of funds). The result would be a policy that provided basic protection against health-care needs without establishing one view of equality and medical moral probity as dominant over the others.

The data indicate that such a basic welfare package would afford significant mortality protection. If individuals were left free to choose particular packages of basic health care (offered within particular medical moralities and constrained only by the free consent of the participants), then help could be provided for the poor while avoiding the significant moral costs of generally imposing one of the many secular medical moralities at the expense of the others. Such an approach to health-care policy would require accepting our finitude, including the limits of governmental moral authority, while acknowledging our moral diversity.

NOTES

1. The White House Domestic Policy Council, *The President's Health Security Plan* (New York: Times Books, 1993), presents a robustly egalitarian blueprint for health-care policy. In its "Ethical Foundations of Health Reform," the Clinton plan rejects a tiered system: "The system should avoid the creation of a tiered system providing care based only on differences of need, not individual or group characteristics" (p. 11). When the plan recommends that a new federal criminal statute be enacted prohibiting "the payment of bribes, gratuities or other inducements to administrators and employees of health plans, health alliances or state health care agencies" (p. 199), the goal is *inter alia* to proscribe payment to physicians for better basic care. The implications and the stated purpose of the plan are egalitarian.

2. I take it that the postmodern era is characterized by the circumstance, as a matter of sociological fact, (1) that all people do not share the same moral narrative or account, and (2) that this moral diversity is apparent and widely recognized. Moreover, as a matter of our epistemological condition, (3) there is no way to establish in purely secular terms the correct moral narrative or account without begging the question or engaging in an infinite regress, and (4) this is also widely recognized.

3. See also H. Tristram Engelhardt, Jr., *Bioethics and Secular Humanism: The Search for a Common Morality* (Philadelphia: Trinity Press International, 1991), esp. pp. 130–38.

4. One might interpret the so-called Oregon proposal as driven by an egalitarianism of altruism. Oregon proposed limiting the range of health-care resources available to Medicaid recipients so that all the poor could be covered. The proposal was that all the poor should be insured, although (1) Medicaid recipients would not receive the same level of health care as previously, and (2) the affluent would be able to purchase better basic care, as well as luxury care (i. e., there would be a tiered provision of health care with a limited package for the poor and with the affluent left free to purchase whatever they wished and could afford).*

5. Schieber, Poullier, and Greenwald, "Health System Performance."

6. Norman Daniels provides a justification of an egalitarian approach to health care that, in the service of equality of opportunity, advances arguments for proscribing the purchase of better basic diagnostic and therapeutic interventions. See Norman Daniels, *Just Health Care* (New York: Cambridge University Press, 1985). Daniels was among the advisory members of the White House Task Force on National Health Reform, which developed President Clinton's 1993 health-care reform proposal.

7. The term "natural and social lotteries" identifies the natural and social forces that advantage and disadvantage individuals irrespective of their deserts: some live long and healthy lives, while others contract serious diseases and die young (examples of the natural lottery); some inherit fortunes, while others are born destitute (examples of the social lottery).

8. Moral constraints do exist within secular morality; they are derived from the right-making character of appeals to permission as the only source of authority in secular public policy. Even if all do not listen to God, and if reason cannot disclose a canonical content-full moral vision, one can still derive authority from common agreement, that is, from permission. See Engelhardt, *The Foundations of Bioethics,* 2nd ed. (New York: Oxford University Press, 1996), pp. 135–88.

9. I do not here explore the considerable difficulties faced in providing a general secular moral justification for taxation. Instead, attention is directed to how one ought to proceed in using common resources, presuming that they can be acquired legitimately. For my treatment of issues bearing on the legitimacy of taxation, see *The Foundations of Bioethics,* pp. 154–80.

*EDITORS' NOTE: See Part Six, Section Two.

SECTION 2

A Miscellany of Hard Choices
Rationing Health Care According to Age

Aging and the Ends of Medicine

Daniel Callahan

In October of 1986, Dr. Thomas Starzl of the Presbyterian-University Hospital in Pittsburgh successfully transplanted a liver into a 76-year-old woman. The typical cost of such an operation is over $200,000. He thereby accelerated the extension to the elderly of the most expensive and most demanding form of high-technology medicine. Not long after that, Congress brought organ transplantation under Medicare coverage, thus guaranteeing an even greater extension of this form of lifesaving care to older age groups.

This is, on the face of it, the kind of medical progress we have long grown to hail, a triumph of medical technology and a newfound benefit to be provided by an established entitlement program. But now an oddity. At the same time those events were taking place, a parallel government campaign for cost containment was under way, with a special targeting of health care to the aged under the Medicare program.

It was not hard to understand why. In 1980, the 11 percent of the population over age 65 consumed some 29 percent of the total American health care expenditures of $219.4 billion. By 1986, the percentage of consumption by the elderly had increased to 31 percent and total expenditures to $450 billion. Medicare costs are projected to rise from $75 billion in 1986 to $114 billion in the year 2000, and in real, not inflated, dollars.

From *Annals of the New York Academy of Sciences,* Vol. 530: 125–133. Reprinted with permission from The Annals of the New York Academy of Sciences.

There is every incentive for politicians, for those who care for the aged, and for those of us on the way to becoming old, to avert our eyes from figures of that kind. We have tried as a society to see if we can simply muddle our way through. That, however, is no longer sufficient. The time has come, I am convinced, for a full and open reconsideration of our future direction. We can not for much longer continue on our present course. Even if we could find a way to radically increase the proportion of our health care dollar going to the elderly it is not clear that that would be a good social investment.

Is it sensible, in the face of a rapidly increasing burden of health care costs for the elderly, to press forward with new and expensive ways of extending their lives? Is it possible to even hope to control costs while, simultaneously, supporting the innovative research that generates ever-new ways to spend money? These are now unavoidable questions. Medicare costs rise at an extraordinary pace, fueled by an ever-increasing number and proportion of the elderly. The fastest-growing age group in the United States are those over the age of 85, increasing at a rate of about 10 percent every two years. By the year 2040, it has been projected that the elderly will represent 21 percent of the population and consume 45 percent of all health care expenditures. Could costs of that magnitude be borne?

Yet even as this intimidating trend reveals itself, anyone who works closely with the elderly recognizes that the present Medicare and Medicaid programs are grossly inadequate in meeting the real and full needs of the elderly. They fail, most notably, in providing decent long-term care and medical care that does not constitute a heavy out-of-pocket drain. Members of minority groups, and single or widowed women, are particularly disadvantaged. How will it be possible, then, to keep pace with the growing number of elderly in even providing present levels of care, much less in ridding the system of its present inadequacies and inequities—and, at the same time, furiously adding expensive new technologies?

The straight answer is that it will not be possible to do all of those things and that, worse still, it may be harmful to even try. It may be harmful because of the economic burdens it will impose on younger age groups, and because of the skewing of national social priorities too heavily toward health care that it is coming to require. But it may also be harmful because it suggests to both the young and the old that the key to a happy old age is good health care. That may not be true.

It is not pleasant to raise possibilities of that kind. That struggle against what Dr. Robert Butler aptly and brilliantly called "ageism" in 1968 has been a difficult one. It has meant trying to persuade the public that not all the elderly are sick and senile. It has meant trying to convince Congress and state legislatures to provide more help for the old. It has meant trying to educate the elderly themselves to look upon their old age as a time of new, open possibilities. That campaign has met with only partial success. Despite great progress, the elderly are still subject to discrimination and stereotyping. The struggle against ageism is hardly over.

Three major concerns have, nonetheless, surfaced over the past few years. They are symptoms that a new era has arrived. The first is that an increasingly large share of health care is going to the elderly in comparison with benefits for children. The federal government, for instance, spends six times as much on health care for those over 65 as for those under 18. As the demographer Samuel Preston observed in a provocative 1984 presidential address to the Population Association of America:

> There is surely something to be said for a system in which things get better as we pass through life rather than worse. The great leveling off of age curves of psychological distress, suicide and income in the past two decades might simply reflect the fact that we have decided in some fundamental sense that we don't want to face futures that become continually bleaker. But

let's be clear that the transfers from the working-age population to the elderly are also transfers away from children, since the working ages bear far more responsibility for childrearing than do the elderly.[1]

Preston's address had an immediate impact. The mainline aging advocacy groups responded with pained indignation, accusing Preston of fomenting a war between the generations. But led by Dave Durenberger, Republican Senator from Minnesota, it also stimulated the formation of Americans for Generational Equity (AGE), an organization created to promote debate on the burden to future generations, but particularly the Baby Boom generation, of "our major social insurance programs."[2] These two developments signalled the outburst of a struggle over what has come to be called "intergenerational equity," that is only now gaining momentum.

The second concern is that the elderly dying consume a disproportionate share of health care costs. Stanford economist Victor Fuchs has noted:

> At present, the United States spends about 1 percent of the gross national product on health care for elderly persons who are in their last year of life. . . . One of the biggest challenges facing policy makers for the rest of this century will be how to strike an appropriate balance between care of the [elderly] dying and health services for the rest of the population.[3]

The third concern is summed up in an observation by Jerome L. Avorn, M.D., of the Harvard Medical School:

> With the exception of the birth-control pill, each of the medical-technology interventions developed since the 1950s has its most widespread impact on people who are past their fifties—the further past their fifties, the greater the impact.[4]

Many of these interventions were not intended for the elderly. Kidney dialysis, for example, was originally developed for those between the ages of 15 and 45. Now some 30 percent of its recipients are over 65.

These three concerns have not gone unchallenged. They have, on the contrary, been strongly resisted, as has the more general assertion that some form of rationing of health care for the elderly might become necessary. To the charge that the elderly currently receive a disproportionate share of resources, the response has been that what helps the elderly helps every other age group. It both relieves the young of the burden of care for elderly parents they would otherwise have to bear and, since they too will eventually become old, promises them similar care when they come to need it. There is no guarantee, moreover, that any cutback in health care for the elderly would result in a transfer of the savings directly to the young. Our system is not that rational or that organized. And why, others ask, should we contemplate restricting care for the elderly when we wastefully spend hundreds of millions of dollars on an inflated defense budget?

The charge that the elderly dying receive a large share of funds hardly proves that it is an unjust or unreasonable amount. They are, after all, the most in need. As some important studies have shown, moreover, it is exceedingly difficult to know that someone is dying; the most expensive patients, it turns out, are those who are expected to live but who actually die. That most new technologies benefit the old more than the young is perfectly sensible: most of the killer diseases of the young have now been conquered.

These are reasonable responses. It would no doubt be possible to ignore the symptoms that the raising of such concerns represents, and to put off for at least a few more years any full confrontation with the overpowering tide of elderly now on the way. There is little incentive for politicians to think about, much less talk about, limits of any kind on health care for the aged; it is a politically hazardous topic. Perhaps also, as Dean Guido Calabresi of the Yale Law School and his colleague Philip Bobbitt observed in their thoughtful 1978 book *Tragic Choices,* when we are forced to make painful allocation choices, "Evasion, disguise, temporizing . . . [and] averting our eyes enables us to save some lives even when we will not save all."[5]

Yet however slight the incentives to take on this highly troubling issue, I believe it is inevitable that we must. Already, rationing of health care under Medicare is a fact of life, though rarely labeled as such. The requirement that Medicare recipients pay the first $500 of the costs of hospital care, that there is a cutoff of reimbursement of care beyond 60 days and a failure to cover long-term care, are nothing other than allocation and cost-saving devices. As sensitive as it is to the votes of the elderly, the Reagan administration only grudgingly agreed to support catastrophic health care costs of the elderly (a benefit that will not, in any event, help many of the aged). It is bound to be far more resistant to long-term care coverage, as will any administration.

But there are other reasons than economics to think about health care for the elderly. The coming economic crisis provides a much-needed opportunity to ask some deeper questions. Just what is it that we want medicine to do for us as we age? Earlier cultures believed that aging should be accepted, and that it should be, in part, a time of preparation for death. Our culture seems increasingly to reject that view, preferring instead, it often seems, to think of aging as hardly more than another disease, to be fought and rejected. Which view is correct? To ask that question is only to note that disturbing puzzles about the ends of medicine and the ends of aging lie behind the more immediate financing worries. Without some kind of answer to them, there is no hope of finding a reasonable, and possibly even a humane, solution to the growing problem of health care for the elderly.

Let me put my own view directly. The future goal of medicine in the care of the aged should be that of improving the quality of their lives, not in seeking ways to extend their lives. In its long-standing ambition to forestall death, medicine has, in the care of the aged, reached its last frontier. That is hardly because death is absent elsewhere—children and young adults obviously still die of maladies that are open to potential cure—but because the largest number of deaths (some 70 percent) now occur among those over the age of 65, with the highest proportion in those over 85. If death is ever to be humbled, that is where the essentially endless work remains to be done. But however tempting that challenge, medicine should now restrain its ambition at that frontier. To do otherwise will, I believe, be to court harm to the needs of other age groups and to the old themselves.

Yet to ask medicine to restrain itself in the face of aging and death is to ask more than it, or the public that sustains it, is likely to find agreeable. Only a fresh understanding of the ends and meaning of aging, encompassing two conditions, are likely to make that a plausible stance. The first is that we—both young and old—need to understand that it is possible to live out a meaningful old age that is limited in time, one that does not require a compulsive effort to turn to medicine for more life to make it bearable. The second condition is that, as a culture, we need a more supportive context for aging and death, one that cherishes and respects the elderly, while at the same time recognizing that their primary orientation should be to the young and the generations to come, not to their own age group. It will be no less necessary to recognize that in the passing of the generations lies the constant reinvigoration of biological life.

Neither of these conditions will be easy to realize. Our culture has, for one thing, worked hard to redefine old age as a time of liberation, not decline. The terms "modern maturity" or "prime time" have, after all, come to connote a time of travel, new ventures in education and self-discovery, the ever-accessible tennis court or golf course, and delightfully periodic but gratefully brief visits from well-behaved grandchildren.

This is, to be sure, an idealized picture. Its attraction lies not in its literal truth but as a widely accepted utopian reference point. It projects the vision of an old age to which more and more believe they can aspire and which its proponents think an affluent country can afford if it so chooses. That it requires a medicine that is single-minded in its aggressiveness against the infirmities of old age is of a piece with its hopes. But as we have come to discover, the costs of that kind of war are prohibitive. No matter how much is spent, the ultimate problem will still remain: people age and die. Worse still, by pretending that old age can be turned into a kind of endless middle age, we rob it of meaning and significance for the elderly themselves. It is a way of saying that old age can be acceptable only to the extent that it can mimic the vitality of the younger years.

There is a plausible alternative: that of a fresh vision of what it means to live a decently long and adequate life, what might be called a natural life span. Earlier generations accepted the idea that there was a natural life span—the biblical norm of threescore years and ten captures that notion (even though, in fact, that was a much longer life span than was then typically the case). It is an idea well worth reconsidering, and would provide us with a meaningful and realizable goal. Modern medicine and biology have done much, however, to wean us away from that kind of thinking. They have

insinuated the belief that the average life span is not a natural fact at all, but instead, one that is strictly dependent upon the state of medical knowledge and skill. And there is much to that belief as a statistical fact: the average life expectancy continues to increase, with no end in sight.

But that is not what I think we ought to mean by a natural life span. We need a notion of a full life that is based on some deeper understanding of human need and sensible possibility, not the latest state of medical technology or medical possibility. We should instead think of a natural life span as the achievement of a life long enough to accomplish, for the most part, those opportunities that life typically affords people and which we ordinarily take to be the prime benefits of enjoying a life at all—that of loving and living, of raising a family, of finding and carrying out work that is satisfying, of reading and thinking, and of cherishing our friends and families.

If we envisioned a natural life span that way, then we could begin to intensify the devising of ways to get people to that stage of life, and to work to make certain they do so in good health and social dignity. People will differ on what they might count as a natural life span; determining its appropriate range for social policy purposes would need extended thought and debate. My own view is that it can now be achieved by the late 70s or early 80s.

That many of the elderly discover new interests and new facets of themselves late in life—my mother took up painting in her 70s and was selling her paintings up until her death at 86—does not mean that we should necessarily encourage a kind of medicine that would make that the norm. Nor does it mean that we should base social and welfare policy on possibilities of that kind. A more reasonable approach is to ask how medicine can help most people live out a decently long life, and how that life can be enhanced along the way.

A longer life does not guarantee a better life—there is no inherent connection between the two. No matter how long medicine enabled people to live, death at any time—at age 90, or 100, or 110—would frustrate some possibility, some as-yet-unrealized goal. There is sadness in that realization, but not tragedy. An easily preventable death of a young child is an outrage. The death from an incurable disease of someone in the prime of young adulthood is a tragedy. But death at an old age, after a long and full life, is simply sad, a part of life itself.

As it confronts aging, medicine should have as its specific goal that of averting premature death, understood as death prior to a natural life span, and the relief of suffering thereafter. It should pursue those goals in order that the elderly can finish out their years with as little needless pain as possible, and with as much vigor as can be generated in contributing to the welfare of younger age groups and to the community of which they are a part. Above all, the elderly need to have a sense of the meaning and significance of their stage in life, one that is not dependent for its human value on economic productivity or physical vigor.

What would a medicine oriented toward the relief of suffering rather than the deliberate extension of life be like? We do not yet have a clear and ready answer to that question, so long-standing, central, and persistent has been the struggle against death as part of the self-conception of medicine. But the Hospice movement is providing us with much helpful evidence. It knows how to distinguish between the relief of suffering and the extension of life. A greater control by the elderly over their dying— and particularly a more readily respected and enforceable right to deny aggressive life-extending treatment—is a long-sought, minimally necessary goal.

What does this have to do with the rising cost of health care for the elderly? Everything. The indefinite extension of life combined with a never satisfied improvement in the health of the elderly is a recipe for monomania and limitless spending. It fails to put health in its proper place as only one among many human goods. It fails to accept aging and death as part of the human condition. It fails to present to younger generations a model of wise stewardship.

How might we devise a plan to limit health care for the aged, under public entitlement programs, that is fair, humane, and sensitive to their special requirements and dignity? Let me suggest three principles to undergird a quest for limits. First, government has a duty, based on our collective social obligations to each other, to help people live out a natural life span, but not actively to help medically extend life beyond that point. Second, government is obliged to develop under its

research subsidies, and pay for, under its entitlement programs, only that kind and degree of life-extending technology necessary for medicine to achieve and serve the end of a natural life span. The question is not whether a technology is available that can save the life of someone who has lived out a natural life span, but whether there is an obligation for society to provide him or her with that technology. I think not. Third, beyond the point of natural life span, government should provide only the means necessary for the relief of suffering, not life-extending technology. By proposing that we use age as a specific criterion for the limitation of life-extending health care, I am challenging one of the most revered norms of contemporary geriatrics: that medical need and not age should be the standard of care. Yet the use of age as a principle for the allocation of resources can be perfectly valid, both a necessary and legitimate basis for providing health care to the elderly. There is not likely to be any better or less arbitrary criterion for the limiting of resources in the face of the open-ended possibilities of medical advancement in therapy for the aged.

Medical "need," in particular, can no longer work as an allocation principle. It is too elastic a concept, too much a function of the state of medical art. A person of 100 dying from congestive heart failure "needs" a heart transplant no less than someone who is 30. Are we to treat both needs as equal? That is neither economically feasible, nor, I would argue, a sensible way to allocate scarce resources. But it would be required by a strict need-based standard.

Age is also a legitimate basis for allocation because it is a meaningful and universal category. It can be understood at the level of common sense. It is concrete enough to be employed for policy purposes. It can also, most importantly, be of value to the aged themselves if combined with an ideal of old age that focuses on its quality rather than its indefinite extension.

I have become impressed with the philosophy underlying the British health care system and the way it meets the needs of the old and the chronically ill. It has, to begin with, a tacit allocation policy. It emphasizes improving the quality of life through primary care medicine and well-subsidized home care and institutional programs for the elderly rather than through life-extending acute care medicine. The well-known difficulty in getting dialysis after 55 is matched by like restrictions on access to open heart surgery, intensive care units, and other forms of expensive technology. An undergirding skepticism directed toward technology makes that a viable option. That attitude, together with a powerful drive for equity, "explains," as two commentators have noted, "why most British put a higher value on primary care for the population as a whole than on an abundance of sophisticated technology for the few who may benefit from it."[6]

That the British spend a significantly smaller proportion of their GNP (6.2 percent) on health care than Americans (10.8 percent) for an almost identical outcome in health status is itself a good advertisement for its priorities. Life expectancies are, for men, 70.0 years in the United States and 70.4 years in Great Britain; and, for women, 77.8 in the United States and 76.7 in Great Britain. There is, of course, a great difference in the ethos of the United States and Britain, and our individualism and love of technology stand in the way of a quick shift of priorities.

Yet our present American expectations about aging and death, it turns out, may not be all that reassuring. How many of us are really so certain that high-technology American medicine promises us all that much better an aging and death, even if some features appear improved and the process begins later than in earlier times? Between the widespread fear of death in an impersonal ICU, cozened about machines and invaded by tubes, on the one hand, or wasting away in the back ward of a nursing home, on the other, not many of us seem comforted.

Once we have reflected on those fears, it is not impossible that most people could be persuaded that a different, more limited set of expectations for health care could be made tolerable. That would be all the more possible if there was a greater assurance than at present that one could live out a full life span, that one's chronic illnesses would be better supported, and that long-term care and home care would be given a more powerful societal backing than is now the case. Though they would face a denial of life-extending medical care beyond a certain age, the old would not necessarily fear their aging any more than they now do. They would, on the contrary, know that a better balance had been struck between making our later years as good as possible rather than simply trying to add more years.

This direction would not immediately bring down the costs of care of the elderly; it would add new costs. But it would set in place the beginning of a new understanding of old age, one that would admit of eventual stabilization and limits. The time has come to admit we can not go on much longer on the present course of open-ended health care for the elderly. Neither confident assertions about American affluence, nor tinkering with entitlement provisions and cost-containment strategies will work for more than a few more years. It is time for the dream that old age can be an infinite and open frontier to end, and for the unflagging, but self-deceptive, optimism that we can do anything we want with our economic system to be put aside.

The elderly will not be served by a belief that only a lack of resources, or better financing mechanisms, or political power, stand between them and the limitations of their bodies. The good of younger age groups will not be served by inspiring in them a desire to live to an old age that will simply extend the vitality of youth indefinitely, as if old age is nothing but a sign that medicine has failed in its mission. The future of our society will not be served by allowing expenditures on health care for the elderly endlessly and uncontrollably to escalate, fueled by a false altruism that thinks anything less is to deny the elderly their dignity. Nor will it be served by that pervasive kind of self-serving that urges the young to support such a crusade because they will eventually benefit from it also.

We require instead an understanding of the process of aging and death that looks to our obligation to the young and to the future, that recognizes the necessity of limits and the acceptance of decline and death, and that values the old for their age and not for their continuing youthful vitality. In the name of accepting the elderly and repudiating discrimination against them, we have mainly succeeded in pretending that, with enough will and money, the unpleasant part of old age can be abolished. In the name of medical progress we have carried out a relentless war against death and decline, failing to ask in any probing way if that will give us a better society for all age groups.

The proper question is not whether we are succeeding in giving a longer life to the aged. It is whether we are making of old age a decent and honorable time of life. Neither a longer lifetime nor more life-extending technology are the way to that goal. The elderly themselves ask for greater financial security, for as much self-determination and independence as possible, for a decent quality of life and not just more life, and for a respected place in society.

The best way to achieve those goals is not simply to say more money and better programs are needed, however much they have their important place. We would do better to begin with a sense of limits, of the meaning of the human life cycle, and of the necessary coming and going of the generations. From that kind of a starting point, we could devise a new understanding of old age.

NOTES

1. Preston, S. H. 1984. Children and the elderly: divergent paths for America's dependents. *Demography* 21: 491–495.
2. Americans for Generational Equity. *Case Statement.* May 1986.
3. Fuchs, V. R. 1984. Though much is taken: reflections on aging, health, and medical care. *Milbank Mem. Fund Q.* 62: 464–465.
4. Avorn, J. L. 1986. Medicine, health, and the geriatric transformation. *Daedalus* 115: 221–225.
5. Calabresi, G. & P. Bobbitt. 1978. *Tragic Choices.* W. W. Norton. New York, NY.
6. Miller, F. H. & G. A. H. Miller. 1986. The painful prescription: a procrustean perspective. *N. Engl. J. Med.* 314: 1385.

The Limits of *Setting Limits*

Christine K. Cassel

Setting Limits calls for and seeks to defend a new realism about the limits of medical technology, an integral sense of the life span and the ends of medicine appropriate to each part of that life span, a communitarian view of the resources of society, and a principle of fairness in allocation of healthcare resources, especially concerning the needs of different generations. I find this book to be misleading and even dangerous, but not because of the above-mentioned goals. Rather, the policy approaches Callahan maps out to achieve those goals are narrow and incomplete. In addition, some of the premises he accepts are highly questionable—in some cases because of inadequacies in the facts at his disposal, in others because of faulty interpretation of certain data, and most fundamentally because of an antimodernist ideology that does not allow a full appreciation of the radical

demographic, scientific, and cultural changes possible in the society of the future.

Daniel Callahan says explicitly he intends *Setting Limits* to be provocative. This it certainly is. But it is harder to tell just where the author ceases his genuine scholarly appraisal of the problem of limiting medical-care costs of the elderly and begins to play the role of agent provocateur.

Callahan wants to set an age limit for the use of expensive and extensive life-sustaining medical treatment. He urges us to consider death a natural part of life, not to be resisted after a "natural life span." The "natural life span" is defined "biographically" by Callahan to include the range of things one can expect in life in terms of family, work, and personal experiences. The concept of a "natural life span" then becomes the basis for an ostensibly "fair" approach to rationing medical care: He proposes "setting limits" of age (seventy? eighty?) above which no life-prolonging medical care would be provided by public programs.

A longing for community and a sense of fairness between generations in this book strikes part of its antimodernistic tone; Callahan views these undeniably positive goals as achievable only in a world where people don't live so long—a world of the past. Assuring this "fairness" requires across-the-board limits to physicians' freedom to care for their patients. It requires physicians to transfer their primary responsibility from the patient to the community, as represented by some kind of government regulatory function. It gives over to the state the basic function of medical decision-making for an entire group of patients. While I have not before viewed myself as one of the strongest champions of physician autonomy, I find this shift of the object of the physician's responsibility from the patient to the state to be extremely troubling. Indeed, although the "slippery slope" risk is sometimes overstated, we must not forget that medicine working as the arm of the state has always led to major ethical disasters in wartime or in the service of ideologies such as national socialism or Stalinism.

For the individual, to counsel acceptance of death may be sage advice. But such counsel is dangerously misplaced when it is translated into public policy, for the foundation of the American legal system is acceptance and—indeed—protection of diversity and pluralism. The courts, with support from ethicists, have firmly asserted that decisions about life and death, and life-sustaining medical care, must rest on respect for the right of self-determination.

One major premise that must come under question, which prompts and indeed justifies the major conclusion of *Setting Limits*, is that we as a society will not be able to afford to support either unlimited individual choice or unlimited health care as people grow older. This language of crisis, when applied to health-care spending, is widely accepted but rarely examined in detail and outside of any specific rhetorical agenda.

It is not that I view health-care resources as infinite. Nor do I think that we as a society can or should continue to use life-sustaining technology, or any technology for that matter, without a moral context in which its use makes sense, is cost effective, and is in the interest of the community as well as the individual. This is the correct definition of "appropriate"—a term whose complexity must not be underestimated! But looking to an arbitrary age cutoff as a way to achieve these standards is not only politically unrealistic but also ethically flawed.

The first mistake is to assume that at age eighty or eighty-five so little potential benefit can be gained from medical care that few months or years of remaining life would be lost by an arbitrary cutoff of life-sustaining or -extending medical treatment at that point. Callahan chooses the wrong number—somewhere in the seventies or eighties is not the appropriate limit. This is a completely inaccurate interpretation of modern demographic forecasts. While life expectancy has risen to seventy-four for men and seventy-eight for women, this is a statistical projection based on average age at death. Since there are still "premature" deaths, depending on definition—caused by car accidents, hip-fracture complications, suicide, preventable illness such as heart and lung disease—the real limit to natural life of the human species is longer, probably around ninety or ninety-five years.[1] This "biological" natural life expectancy allows for a much greater opportunity range than that defined by Callahan's "biographical" limit. Which shall we use as a standard for letting human beings die—the average life expectancy or the optimal life span? Current demographic studies suggest in fact that not only is life expectancy increasing but life span itself may be increasing.[2] Even if biological life span is limited to ninety-five to one hundred years, there will easily be twenty million people over age eighty by the year 2020. Most of them will be healthy, active people who could contribute to society if our society would allow them to do so. Treatment of a life-threatening illness in an eighty-five-year-old could save ten or fifteen years of life.

A second significant and arguable point of Callahan's analysis is his conclusion that arbitrary cutoffs are fairer and thus have a more positive moral and intergenerational effect on society than will our present course. Five million people currently over eighty would be subject to this rule; under current estimates of life expectancy, in thirty years this number will be twenty million, and if life expectancy continues to increase, that number could be millions more. I suggest that our society will not be able to tolerate such a draconian policy, resulting precipitously in five million deaths. No advanced society could easily accept an across-the-board denial of medical care (which might improve the quality of life as well as extend its duration) to such substantial numbers. The potential for a very negative impact on our society's moral fiber, respect for age, and indeed, respect for people overall, and on the future facing young people growing up in such a society, is profound.

This categorical cutoff is neither the most practical nor the most morally acceptable way to begin cutting health-care costs and rationing health-care spending. There are other ways that lead to a third critique of Callahan's choice of how our nation might save health-care dollars. It has become a truism to point to the amount of waste and excess profit in our health-care system.[3] By combining administrative overhead of $50–$60 billion a year with profits from the range of health-care technologies, an extraordinary savings could then be applied to other worthy purposes such as education, housing, transportation—even long-term care. Furthermore, the clinical influence that these profits and the people who derive benefits from them have on the policy process is as pernicious, if not more so, than the dramatic waste of resources. Because of financial incentives to create and use more technologies, Medicare and other payers continue preferentially to favor high technology interventions over lower technology quality-of-life care or long-term care. Reducing profits to be made would reduce the inappropriate use of such technology and still allow individual decisions.

Two billion dollars per year is spent on renal dialysis; a similar amount on coronary artery bypass grafts. One is clearly a lifesaving treatment; the other is lifesaving only in a minority of cases. Is this too much to spend in either case, in a country that spends $3 billion annually on potato chips?[4] Do we know that dollars spent on dialysis would not be better spent for flu shots in nursing homes? Outcomes of patients with gastrointestinal bleeding are equivalent regardless of whether the patient has endoscopy to determine the source of bleeding, and yet we continue to prescribe and Medicare continues to reimburse endoscopy for that purpose.[5] Physicians are encouraged to request subspecialty consultation at greater cost because of financial incentives established by hospital policies. Geographic variations in rates of surgical procedures—ranging from tonsillectomy and hysterectomy to prostatectomy and lens extraction—suggest surgeons are considering their target incomes rather than demographic needs.[6] There are a number of additional examples of med-

ical situations where efficacy, not age, should be the discriminating factor in utilization decisions.

Change, however, requires political action. Are we so helpless in the face of our own political structure that we are unable to identify more obvious solutions to rising health-care costs than one as extreme and morally treacherous as arbitrary age cutoffs?

Although economists have found that people in the last year of life consume a major part of the Medicare budget, it is not obvious that this is money wasted.[7] All medical care in critical illness is a gamble. People who die may have spent the previous year struggling with illness when death was not predictable. Certainly there are instances of overuse of medical technology at the end of life that prolong dying rather than prolong life. Physicians must learn to deal more directly, reasonably, and compassionately with their dying patients.[8] All of us—health professionals, families, and potential patients—must learn to accept the uncertainty inherent in decisions about the use of high technology. I would prefer to work for social change than accept social engineering—the former seems so much more hopeful and humanistic, the latter so pessimistic and mechanistic. Any arbitrary limit on treatment that excludes the professionals from the agony of uncertainty gives up on the human being as the measure of moral reality.

A fourth problem has to do with "life-prolonging treatments." Medical technologies must be understood in their context. How are we to distinguish between life-extending care and life-improving technologies? For example, a ninety-nine-year-old patient who develops syncope (fainting spells) is admitted to the hospital and found to have periodic interruption of the heart rhythms during which time she passes out. She lives alone, has very severe arthritis, but no other serious illnesses. The treatment of choice for her heart disease (conduction system disorder) is a pacemaker. Without the pacemaker, we will send her home to continue fainting and falling. Either she will fall, break a hip, and lie there until she dies of dehydration, or she will be admitted to the orthopedic service, where at great cost and very poor likely outcome, the broken hip will be tended. The alternative is to give her a pacemaker, which will not only improve the quality of her life by preventing these things from happening but will also extend her life. How are we to make such a decision according to Callahan's proposed scheme?

Manifold other technologies offer the same conundrum to the practicing clinician. Moreover, chronic illness is so complex that any treatment which aims to improve the quality of a person's life may in fact extend that life. Those without terminal illness no doubt will live longer if given meticulous nursing care, good attention to their diabetes, and everything from human interaction to podiatric care. Because these things extend life, should we not use them? The only way to treat the discomfort that would arise would be wholesale anesthesia through morphine or widespread physician-assisted euthanasia. These scenarios would be morally detrimental to our society, no matter how much money they may save or however logically consistent they may be with an abstract idea of a "natural life span."

As life expectancy increases in our society, the variability of health status in old age increases also. A time when many eighty-year-olds can expect to live in good health for fifteen more years is not the time to propose an arbitrary age limit in health-care delivery. "The elderly" are the most diverse, least generalizable group in our society. Physicians need to make more individually tailored decisions, not more arbitrary ones. Urgently needed is better training in geriatric medicine for physicians and a stronger scientific and moral capability to make appropriate decisions on an individual basis.[9] Physicians as a group have been woefully inadequate at assessing individual patients and allowing death to come when that is appropriate. If they understood more about the process of aging—biologically, as well as socially—they would make better decisions. They could better judge the chances of a reasonable outcome of diagnostic or treatment plans if they were more familiar with physiological and clinical studies in aging, and had the clinical skills to differentiate treatable from untreatable disorders. Unfortunate tendencies to generalize about the elderly lead to both overly aggressive and overly nihilistic approaches. Ethics would have a better-defined context with better training in medicine, but better training in ethics is equally important. Callahan is clearly skeptical that physicians will ever be able to claim the moral authority to make appropriate decisions to limit their use of technology and to

respect the life span and the time when death comes. I think he gives up too soon. It is only within the last fifteen or twenty years that the explosion of technology has both seduced the profession of medicine and now in a backlash has begun to force us to learn to confront death.[10] The profession has a long way to go, but must be assigned major responsibility for the moral and social challenges that medical technology poses. An approach to rationing health-care resources which demands that the system treat people as individuals, that efficacy be the major goal of medical treatment, and that the professions and the industry see themselves as serving the public rather than as profit centers, would contribute a great deal more to the quality of our culture, to our society's moral fiber, the beneficence of its intergenerational networks, and its respect for age itself than would an arbitrary age-based cutoff. Better training in how to make these medical and moral judgments needs to be bolstered by better social support for physicians who are able to confront and deal with these shifting grounds. Protection from unjustified liability litigation would go a long way toward improving this decision-making process and making it more individual and more humane, as well as more morally correct.

Setting Limits may have come at exactly the wrong time. Recent studies indicate that, in fact, older and sicker people are now being given less high-technology, life-sustaining treatment, and that what costs money is chronic, long-term care. If we rush too quickly to set limits on aggressive medical treatment, such as treatment of pneumonia, we could play right into an unholy alliance, cutting costs not for any reasoned communitarian motive, but in response to government-directed spending priorities.[11]

If we withhold life-sustaining treatment on an arbitrary basis, we come too near the slippery slope of discrimination or even genocide based on social characteristics which are "undesirable," such as disability, race, religion, class, or sex. This is certainly not Callahan's intention, but the risk is still starkly visible with the hindsight of historical perspective so vivid in the accounts of physician complicity with Nazi anti-Semitism or with psychiatric oppression of dissidents in the Soviet Union, and thus warrants our concern. It is one thing to let people die because their lives have become an inconvenience to them; it is quite another to let them die because their lives have become an inconvenience to us. Some of these people will suffer from chronic illness, which causes them to be dependent and need a great deal of care. Many of those people with chronic illness will want to forgo life-sustaining therapy, and we are obliged to create an ethical system that respects their wishes. But that system will never be created in a society in which a large number of people are fearful that they will not receive appropriate treatment simply because of their age.

In addition, the whole society will suffer. The current aging of society is an unprecedented event, a success of civilization, and we have both an opportunity and a responsibility to shape a society that can appropriately and positively embrace this measure of success.[12] It is the challenge of our success that we create employment, educational and economic structures, and medical care that give all of us as we grow older a positive attitude about the future and about the people with whom we share our society. Callahan's proposal does not allow for medical progress. New treatments for the scourges of old age—Alzheimer's disease, stroke, arthritis—may significantly enhance the quality of life for years before death occurs at the end of a "natural life span," biologically longer than ever before anticipated.[13]

Physicians have been overly strenuous in applying medical technology to some people at the end of life, sometimes even against the patient's expressed wishes. *Setting Limits* is an attempt to take physicians "off the hook," to give them a formulaic approach to these morally and emotionally difficult choices. The attempt fails—it doesn't fix what is broken. We do not need an arbitrary age at which to define someone as socially finished and thus dispensable. Instead, we need a structure for an age-irrelevant society where medical decisions are made on an individual basis. In this latter context, physicians cannot escape their responsibility to understand the biomedical issues of aging and,

equally important, to deal sensitively and responsibly with the ethical issues.

NOTES

1. S. Jay Olshansky, "On Forecasting Mortality," *Milbank Memorial Fund Quarterly* 66 (1988): 482–530.
2. Kenneth G. Manton, "Past and Future Life Expectancy Increases at Later Ages: Their Implications for the Linkage of Chronic Morbidity, Disability and Mortality," *Journal of Gerontology* 5 (September 1986): 672–81.
3. David U. Himmelstein, Steffie Woolhandler, and the Writing Committee of the Working Group on Program Design, "A National Health Program for the United States: A Physicians' Proposal," *New England Journal of Medicine* 320 (January 12, 1989): 102–8.
4. Nancy B. Cummings, "Social, Ethical and Legal Issues Involved in Chronic Maintenance Dialysis," in *Replacement of Renal Function by Dialysis*, ed. John F. Mayer (Boston: Kluwer Academic Publishers, 1988).
5. John M. Eisenberg, *Doctors' Decisions and the Cost of Medical Care* (Ann Arbor: Health Administration Press Perspectives, 1986), pp. 5–27.
6. Uwe E. Reinhardt, "Resource Allocation in Health Care: The Allocation of Lifestyles to Providers," *Milbank Memorial Fund Quarterly* 65 (1987): 153–76.
7. Louise B. Russell, "An Aging Population and the Use of Medical Care," *Medical Care* 19 (June 1981): 633–43.
8. Sidney H. Wanzer et al., "The Physician's Responsibility Toward Hopelessly Ill Patients: A Second Look," *New England Journal of Medicine* 320 (March 30, 1989): 844–49.
9. Robert N. Butler, "The Triumph of Age: Science, Gerontology and Ageism," *Bulletin of the New York Academy of Medicine* 58 (May 1982): 347–61.
10. Christine K. Cassel, "Decisions to Forego Life-Sustaining Therapy: The Limits of Ethics," *Social Service Review* (1987): 552–64.
11. Christine K. Cassel, "Doctors and Allocation Decisions: A New Role in the New Medicare," *Journal of Health Politics, Policy and Law* 10 (Fall 1985): 549–64.
12. Jacob A. Brody, "The Best of Times/The Worst of Times: Aging and Dependency in the 21st Century," in *Ethical Dimensions of Geriatric Care: Value Conflicts for the 21st Century*, ed. Stuart F. Spicker, Stanley R. Ingman, and Ian R. Lawson (Boston: D. Reidel Publishing Company, 1987), pp. 3–21.
13. Jacob A. Brody, "Prospects for an Ageing Population," *Nature* 315 (June 6–12, 1985): 463–66.

Rationing Health Care According to Ability to Pay

Is the Oregon Rationing Plan Fair?

Norman Daniels

The Oregon Basic Health Services Act mandates universal access to basic care, but includes rationing services to those individuals who are Medicaid recipients. If no new resources are added, the plan may make current Medicaid recipients worse-off, but still reduce inequality between the poor and the rest of society. If resources are expanded and benefits given appropriate rankings, no one may be worse-off; though inequality will be reduced, alternative reforms might reduce it even further. Whether the outcome seems fair then depends on how much priority to the well-being of the poor we believe justice requires; it also depends on political judgments about the feasibility of alternative strategies for achieving more egalitarian reforms. Oregon makes rationing public and explicit, as justice requires, but it is not clear how community values influence the ranking of services; ultimately, the rationing process is fair only if we may rely on the voting power of the poor.

EXCLUDING PEOPLE VS. EXCLUDING SERVICES

In 1987, Oregon drew national attention when it stopped Medicaid funding of soft-tissue transplants. Officials justified the action by claiming that there are more effective ways to spend scarce public dollars than to provide high-cost benefits to relatively few people. They insisted that the estimated $1.1 million that would have been spent on such transplants in 1987 would save many more lives per dollar spent if invested in prenatal maternal care.[1] Rather than heartlessly turning its back on children in need of transplants, the state was making a "tragic choice" between two instances of

rationing by ability to pay. The consequences of ignoring "invisible" pregnant women who cannot afford prenatal maternal care are much worse than are those of refusing to fund highly visible children in need of transplants.

The Oregon Basic Health Services Act boldly couples the rationing of health care with a plan to improve access.[2] It expands Medicaid eligibility to 100 percent for those individuals who are at the federal poverty level, creates an Oregon Health Services Commission (OHSC) to establish priorities among health services, requires cutting low-priority services rather than excluding people from coverage when reducing expenditures is necessary, mandates a high-risk insurance pool, and requires employers to provide health insurance or to contribute to a state insurance pool. Oregon must obtain a federal waiver to implement the changes in Medicaid.*

Oregon explicitly rejects the rationing strategy that predominates in the United States: our rationing system excludes whole categories of the poor and near-poor from access to public insurance, denying coverage to *people*, rather than to low-priority *services*. In contrast, the Oregon plan embodies the following principles: (1) there is a social obligation to guarantee universal access to a *basic level* of health care, (2) reasonable or necessary limits on resources mean that not every beneficial service can be included in the basic level of health care, and (3) a public process, involving consideration of social values, is required to determine what services will be included in the basic level of health care.[1,3]

Though these principles are not a complete account of justice for health care, they have considerable plausibility, derive support from theoretical work on justice and health care, and are, to varying degrees, widely believed in by the U.S. popula-

From *Journal of the American Medical Association* 265, No. 17, May 1, 1991:2232–2235. Copyright © 1991 American Medical Association. Reprinted with permission from the publisher.

*EDITORS' NOTE: The Clinton administration approved Oregon's revised application for a Medicaid waiver in 1993; the plan is now in effect.

tion.[4] Nevertheless, these three principles permit rationing care to the poor alone, with serious implications for equality. Thus, critics attack the Oregon plan for making the poor, specifically poor women and children, "bear the burden" of providing universal access.[5]

To evaluate this criticism, we must ask three questions: (1) Does the plan make the indigent groups better-off or worse-off? (2) Are the inequalities the plan accepts justifiable? (3) Is the procedure for determining the basic level of health care a just or fair one? These questions raise issues of distributive justice that go beyond the principles underlying the Oregon legislation.

WHAT DOES THE OREGON PLAN DO TO THE WORSE-OFF GROUPS?

Critics of Oregon's plan appeal to widely held egalitarian concerns when they argue that it makes the poor bear the burden of this effort to close the insurance gap. The strongest sense of "bear the burden" is "being made worse-off." Does the plan, as the critics charge, make the poor worse-off instead of giving priority to improving their well-being?[6,7]

Consider the simplest case first, a zero-sum game with resources. For example, if extrarenal transplants are removed from coverage and no higher-priority services, unavailable before the plan, are added, then current Medicaid recipients will lose some services and the health benefits they produce. They will no doubt then make this complaint: "We bear the burden of the plan. Since we are already the most indigent group, or close to it, we should not have to give up lifesaving or other important medical services so that the currently uninsured can get basic-level health care."

It is important to grasp the moral force of this complaint. Notice that *aggregate* health status for *all* the poor, including current Medicaid recipients and the uninsured, can be improved by the plan, even though current Medicaid recipients are made worse-off. The loss of less-important services by current recipients is more than counterbalanced by the gains of the uninsured. As a result, the plan reduces overall inequality between the poor and the rest of society, albeit at the expense of current Medicaid recipients. Therefore, the complaint cannot be that the plan makes society less equal; instead, it is that even

greater reductions in inequality are possible if other groups sacrifice instead of Medicaid recipients. It is unfair for current Medicaid recipients to bear a burden that others could bear much better, especially since inequality would then be even further reduced.

How stringent is the priority owed the poorest groups when we seek to improve aggregate well-being? Three positions are possible: (1) help the poor as much as possible (*strict priority*); (2) make sure the poor get some benefit (*modified priority*); or (3) allow only modest harms to the poor in return for significant gains to others who are not well-off (*weak priority*). Critics of the Oregon plan insist that we should not settle for weak priority, especially since feasible alternatives help the poor more. The Oregon plan leaves the bulk of the health care system intact. By eliminating the inefficiencies it contains, e.g., by establishing a low-overhead public insurance scheme (as in Canada), or by developing treatment protocols that eliminate unnecessary services, we might be able to avoid making current Medicaid recipients any worse-off. Alternatively, by broadening rationing to cover most of society, as in Canada or Great Britain, we could avoid the criticism that only the poor are being made to bear the burden of improving access.

Proponents of the Oregon plan aim for a more complex case than a zero-sum game with services, however, hoping to add either new services or new revenue sources.[1,3,8] Suppose, for example, the plan makes available "high-priority" services that are currently not adequately provided, such as prenatal maternal care, mental health, and chemical dependency services, while "low-priority" services, e.g., soft-tissue transplants, are not funded. Then current Medicaid recipients will have a *higher* expected payoff from the revised benefits. Since the currently uninsured are also made better-off, and no one is made worse-off (except that taxes may be increased), we have what economists call a *pareto superior* outcome. Of course, those particular Medicaid recipients who need the newly rationed services will be worse-off, but it is reasonable to judge the effects of the system *ex ante*, and the poor as a whole are better-off despite the loss to some individuals who would require soft-tissue transplants.

Thus, with appropriate revisions of Medicaid benefits, the poor will be better-off than they are now. Nevertheless, current Medicaid recipients can object, "We achieve our gain in health status by giving up beneficial services that better-off groups receive; in that sense we 'bear the burden' of the Oregon plan. The poor would improve even more if better-off groups contributed more." The complaint is that social inequality could be reduced in a way that benefits the poor even more.

One version of this complaint appeals to long-term considerations: the Oregon plan makes the poor better-off in the short run but worse-off than they would be in the longer run if a national health insurance scheme were introduced. This claim depends on particular political assumptions about the likelihood of alternative scenarios for reform. In reply, some proponents see the current legislation in Oregon as but the first step in a comprehensive, incremental reform; ultimately, the state would become the major insurer and most powerful purchaser by substituting its basic insurance plan for many private insurance plans as well as for Medicare and long-term care under Medicaid (Sen. John Kitzhaber, verbal communication, January 1991). The debate then focuses on the means to health reform, not its ends; disagreement results from complex political, not moral, judgments.

A second complaint about reducible inequality derives from the Children's Defense Fund's charge that the Oregon plan "exempts" the elderly who are Medicaid recipients from the ranking of services.[5] Poor women and children, who constitute 75 percent of the Medicaid recipients, receive only 30 percent of the benefits in dollars. Much of the rest goes to the elderly who have "spent down" their resources in order to be eligible for long-term care, but these services—as well as all acute care for the elderly who are covered under Medicare—are not included in the prioritization or rationing process. By not establishing priorities among health care services for the elderly, and by financing expansion of Medicaid coverage, primarily by rationing to women and children, the plan seems to suggest that any use of long-term medical services by the elderly is more important than short-term medical services for the young. This would be an irrational ranking on the face of it. If we did not know how old we were and had to allocate resources over our life span, taking our needs at each stage of life into account, we would not consider this ranking a prudent one.[9] A reasonable rationing plan would consider the importance of all health care services, short-term medical as well as long-term care, over an individual's life span, at each stage of life. To avoid what seems to be discrimination by age, rationing should include all age groups. In reply, and as noted, some Oregon proponents intend to expand the plan to cover Medicare and long-term Medicaid care.

Advocates for the Oregon plan argue that additional revenue, which would further reduce inequality, will be easier to obtain when the legislature must visibly cut beneficial services and cannot disguise rationing by raising eligibility requirements for Medicaid. This political judgment ignores evidence from the 1980s, when various states, as well as the federal government, cut important services to the poor, including prenatal maternal care and the Women, Infants, and Children's Program's distribution of food supplements to pregnant women and neighborhood mental health care services. Explicit rationing to the poor made neither politicians nor their constituents so uncomfortable that the cuts were stopped.

In short, we cannot answer the basic question about how the worse-off will fare under the current legislation until we are told what they will get, that is, until the Medicaid benefit package is ranked by OHSC, is funded by the legislature, and is approved for a Medicaid waiver by the Department of Health and Human Services. . . . If the current Medicaid recipients are made worse-off, there is a serious, though not necessarily fatal, objection to the Oregon plan. If we hold only a weak version of the requirement that we give priority to the worse-off, we might still think the plan acceptable even though some of the poor bear the burden of reducing overall inequality. In any case, the Oregon planners hope that rationing will yield a result in which all the poor are better-off than now. Political judgments differ about the likelihood of this preferred outcome.

ARE THE INEQUALITIES THE OREGON PLAN ACCEPTS JUSTIFIABLE?

By rationing lower-priority services to the poor, rather than excluding whole groups of the poor and near-poor from insurance, the Oregon plan reduces inequality in our society, even if current Medicaid recipients are, to some extent, worse-off than they are now. Somewhat paradoxically, even under the scenario in which no one is worse-off, there is still a sense in which the poor bear the burden of the plan, since the plan accepts as official policy an unjustifiable inequality in the health care system.

To see this point, contrast the kind of inequality the Oregon plan accepts with the inequality that arises in the heavily rationed British system.[10] Although about 10 percent of the British public buys private insurance coverage in order to procure various rationed services, the overwhelming majority abides by the consequences of rationing. This produces a more acceptable structure of inequality than would result if the bottom 20 percent of the Oregon population has no access to services that are available to the great majority.[11]

To see why one structure of inequality seems worse than the other, consider how the poor would feel under both. Under the Oregon plan, the poor can complain that society as a whole is content not only to leave them economically badly off, but also to deny them medical services that would protect the range of opportunities that are open to them.[6] There is a basis here for reasonable regrets or resentment, for society as a whole seems content to shut the poor out of mainstream opportunities. They may reasonably feel that the majority is too willing to leave them behind under terms in which the benefits of social cooperation do not reflect their moral status as free and equal agents.[12,13] Alternatively, if health care protects opportunity in a way that is roughly equal for all, except that the most advantaged group has some extra advantages, then this may seem somewhat unfair, but no one group is then singled out for special disadvantages that are viewed as "acceptable" by the economically and medically advantaged majority. Consequently, no group would have a basis for the strong and reasonable regrets that the poor have under the Oregon plan, despite their improvement relative to the current situation.

Thus, even if the poor are better-off under the Oregon plan than now, the plan still accepts an inequality that is not ideally just. It is more just—perhaps much more just—than what we now have, but still not what justice requires. Does this mean we should not implement it? The answer seems to depend on political judgments about the feasibility of alternatives. If one thinks that a uni-

form, universal plan, like Canada's, is a political impossibility in the United States, or if one thinks that introducing the Oregon plan makes further reform in the direction of a uniform plan more likely, then the Oregon plan, even if it is not ideally just, seems reasonable. But if one thinks that introducing the Oregon reform makes more radical reform of the system less likely, then one might well prefer not to make a modest improvement in the justice of the system in order to facilitate a more significant improvement later.

IS THE PUBLIC PROCESS FOR DECIDING WHAT IS "BASIC CARE" FAIR?

The Oregon plan involves public and explicit rationing; it disavows rationing hidden by the covert workings of a market, or buried in the quiet, professional decisions of providers. Its rationing decisions are the result of a two-step process involving separate, publicly accountable bodies. First (step 1), OHSC, which is charged with taking "community values" into consideration, determines priorities among services in a possible benefit package. Second (step 2), the legislature decides how much to spend on Medicaid, given competing demands on state funds. Some lower-priority services may thus not be covered, but the resulting Medicaid benefit package must still be approved by the Department of Health and Human Services. Assessing the fairness of the rationing process requires examining both steps.

Oregon's insistence on publicity is controversial. Calabresi and Bobbitt[14] argue that "tragic choices" are best made out of the public view in order to preserve important symbolic values, such as the sanctity of life. Despite the importance of such symbols, however, justice requires publicity. People who view themselves as free and equal moral agents must have available to them the grounds for all decisions that affect their lives in fundamental ways, as rationing decisions do. Only with publicity can they resolve disputes about whether the decisions conform to the more basic principles of justice that are the accepted basis of their social cooperation.[15]

Actually, going beyond a concern for publicity, Oregon calls for broad public participation in the development of priorities. Public participation is desirable because it may yield agreement about how to resolve disputes among winners and losers in a fair way. It also makes it more likely that outcomes reflect the consent of those individuals who are affected and, since there may not be one uniquely fair or just way to ration services, participation allows the shared values of a community to shape the result. Is the public participation process itself fair, and does it have a real effect on outcomes?

OHSC held public hearings on health services and asked Oregon Health Decisions to hold community meetings throughout the state "to build consensus on the values to be used to guide health resource allocation decisions."[16] At 47 meetings that were held during the early part of 1990, citizens were asked to rank the importance of various categories of treatment and were asked, "Why is this health care service *important to us*?" From these discussions, an unranked list of 13 "values" was distilled. A tally was kept of how often each value was discussed, but we cannot rank the importance of the values on that basis.

One frequent criticism of the community meeting procedure is that it did not involve a representative cross section of Oregonians. Some 50 percent were health professionals; too many were college educated, white, and relatively well-off. Moreover, whereas 16 percent of Oregonians are uninsured, only 9.4 percent of community meeting participants were uninsured, and Medicaid recipients, the only direct representatives of poor children, were underrepresented by half.[5,16] Even if there was no evidence of bias in the meetings, the process is still open to the charge that it consisted of the "haves" deciding what is "important" to give the "have-nots." The charge is twofold. Not only is the composition of the meetings unrepresentative of the interests of those who will be affected, but the task set for the meetings presupposes that rationing will primarily have an impact on an underrepresented minority.

It is difficult to assess the importance of either charge of bias, for we have no way to compare the outcome with an unbiased alternative. Suspicions about the effects of compositional bias would be reduced, however, if there were no bias in the task, that is, if the Oregon plan called for rationing services to the great majority rather than to the poor.

We worry less about who is making a decision if it has an equal impact on everyone, including the decision makers.

The charge of bias is important only if the meetings actually influence the ranking of services (otherwise they are just window dressing). Contrary to public and media understanding, however, the community meetings do not yield a ranking of services, only a general list of community values. Moreover, the list of values cannot be used in any direct way in determining priorities among health services. Some of the "values" are really only categories of services, e.g., mental health and chemical dependency, or prevention. Other values, such as equity (guaranteeing access to all) or respecting personal choice, are things we desire of the system as a whole, not of individual services. And the values relevant to ranking services, such as quality of life or cost-effectiveness or ability to function, are not themselves ranked.

OHSC is well aware of this limitation and views the list of values only as a "qualitative check" on the process of ranking services (Paige Sipes-Metzler, personal communication, June and July 1990). Thus, it believes the community concern for equity is met because the system guarantees universal access to basic care. Community concerns about mental health and chemical dependency, or prevention, are met by making sure that these services are included in the ranking process. Although no weights were assigned to values such as quality of life or cost-effectiveness, they are included as factors in the formal ranking process. The only direct community input into the first attempt at ranking services, however, came from a telephone survey aimed at finding out how Oregonians ranked particular health outcomes that affect their quality of life. By combining this information with expert judgments about the likely outcomes of using particular procedures to treat certain conditions, as well as with information about the costs of treating a population with those procedures, OHSC generated a preliminary cost-benefit ranking of services. Because this ranking drew extensive criticism (*New York Times*, July 9, 1990: A17) and failed to match its own expectations about priorities, OHSC modified its procedure for ranking services. As a result, the OHSC commissioners themselves ranked general categories of services according to their importance to the individual, to society, and to the health plan, and "adjusted" other items.[17] It remains unclear how this process reflects community values, and until we know just how the final rankings were "adjusted," we cannot know what influence public participation has had.

The rationing process involves two decisions, not one. Suppose that we have a fair procedure and a perfect outcome at step 1: the ranking of services captures relevant facts about costs and benefits and represents community values fairly. Unfortunately, fairness at step 1 does not assure it at step 2, because the voting power of the poor is negated in a political process that generally underrepresents them, judging from past voting patterns and outcomes. Therefore, even if there is a consensus at step 1 about what the basic, minimum package should be, there may be well-founded worries that the legislature will not fund it. Indeed, the situation is somewhat worse because OHSC only ranks services, it does not decide what is basic. The funding decision of the legislature determines what basic care is provided.

Clearly, political judgments diverge on how much we can trust the legislature. The crucial issue from the point of view of process, however, is this: because the Oregon plan explicitly involves rationing primarily for the poor and near-poor, funding decisions face constant political pressure from more powerful groups who want to put public resources to other uses. In contrast, if the legislature were deciding how to fund a rationing plan that applied to themselves and to all their constituents, then we might expect a careful and honest weighing of the importance of health care against other goods. The legislature would then have stronger reasons not to concede to political pressures to divert resources, and other groups would be less likely to apply such pressure. If the plan is expanded to include other groups, then the poor may find important allies.

Worries about fairness in the Oregon rationing process thus come from the plan's being aimed at the poor rather than at the population as a whole. Concerns about fairness in the process thus converge with concerns about the kinds of inequality the system tolerates. This does not mean that the Oregon experiment should not be tried; it may produce less overall inequality in health status than we now have. But we should recognize from the start that a system that rations only to the poor

is less equitable and less fair than alternative systems that ration for the great majority of people. To the extent that the inequality ends up troubling many participants in the system, including physicians who will be able to do only certain things for some children and more for others, the strains of commitment to abiding by the rationing will be greater, and rationing may get a worse name than it deserves.

Oregon's plan retains the structure of inequality that it does because states must respond to the problems imposed by a highly inequitable and inefficient national health care system. The plan contains a bizarre irony: the state's Medicaid budget is in crisis because of rapidly increasing costs, largely the result of the burden of long-term care imposed by the elderly, yet the rationing plan focuses on poor children. Oregon did not design a Medicaid system that forces the most vulnerable children and the most vulnerable elderly to compete for scarce public resources. As long as states must respond to problems created by the national system, however, their solutions will inherit its major flaws. Uncoordinated responses by states cannot solve the problems caused by the continuing rapid dissemination of technology, inefficiencies in administering a mixed system, and a growing demand for services in our aging and acquired immunodeficiency syndrome–threatened society.

Oregon offers important lessons for any national effort to address these problems. Nationally, we should embrace Oregon's commitment to provide universal access to basic care and to make rationing a subject of open, political debate, but we should not simply expand the current legislation into a national plan. That would not only reproduce on a larger scale the unjustifiable inequality that the Oregon plan permits. It would also retain at the state level competition for funds between poor children and poor elderly, and it would leave unaddressed the basic problems of inefficiency and rapidly rising costs. In contrast, rationing within a single-payer, public insurance scheme that covered all age groups would more easily address these problems. Whether such a comprehensive scheme is best introduced all at once (on the model of the Canadian system), or is phased in (building on an Oregon-style starting point), is a complex issue. In any case, we have yet to see whether the Oregon plan gives us a clear model for how community values or public participation should influence the design of a national benefit package.

NOTES

1. Golenski J. *A Report on the Oregon Medicaid Priority Setting Project.* Berkeley, Calif: Bioethics Consultation Group; 1990.
2. Senate Bills 27, 534, 935. 65th Oregon Legislative Assembly; 1989 regular sess.
3. Kitzhaber J. *The Oregon Basic Health Services Act.* Salem, Ore: Office of the Senate President; 1990.
4. Blendon RJ, Leitman R, Morrison I, Donelan K. Satisfaction with health systems in ten nations. *Health Aff.* Summer 1990:185–192.
5. *An Analysis of the Impact of the Oregon Medicaid Reduction Waiver Proposal on Women and Children.* Washington, D.C.: Children's Defense Fund; 1990:1–7.
6. Daniels N. *Just Health Care.* New York, NY: Cambridge University Press; 1985.
7. Rawls J. *A Theory of Justice.* Cambridge, Mass: Harvard University Press; 1971.
8. *Preliminary Report.* Salem: Oregon Health Services Commission; 1990.
9. Daniels N. *Am I My Parents' Keeper? An Essay on Justice Between the Young and the Old.* New York, NY: Oxford University Press Inc; 1988.
10. Aaron HJ, Schwartz WB. *The Painful Prescription: Rationing Health Care.* Washington, D.C.: The Brookings Institution; 1984.
11. Temkin L. Inequality. *Philosophy Public Aff.* 1986;15:99–121.
12. Cohen J. Democratic equality. *Ethics* 1989;99:727–751.
13. Scanlon TM. Contractualism and utilitarianism. In: Sen AK, Williams B, eds. *Utilitarianism and Beyond.* New York, NY: Cambridge University Press; 1982:103–128.
14. Calabresi G, Bobbitt P. *Tragic Choices.* New York, NY: WW Norton & Co Inc; 1978.
15. Rawls J. Kantian constructivism in moral theory: the Dewey Lectures. *J Phil.* 1980;77:515–572.
16. Hasnain R, Garland M. *Health Care in Common: Report of the Oregon Health Decisions Community Meetings Process.* Portland: Oregon Health Decisions; 1990.
17. Kitzhaber J. *Summary: The Health Services Prioritization Process.* Salem: Oregon State Senate; 1990.

Rationing Health Care According to Merit

Should Alcoholics Compete Equally for Liver Transplantation?

Alvin H. Moss and Mark Siegler

Until recently, liver transplantation for patients with alcohol-related end-stage liver disease (ARESLD) was not considered a treatment option. Most physicians in the transplant community did not recommend it because of initial poor results in this population and because of a predicted high recidivism rate that would preclude long-term survival. In 1988, however, Starzl and colleagues reported one-year survival rates for patients with

From *Journal of the American Medical Association* Vol. 265, 1296–1298. Copyright © 1991 American Medical Association. Reprinted by permission of the American Medical Association. EDITORS' NOTE: All notes have been deleted. Readers who wish to follow up on sources should consult the original article.

ARESLD comparable to results in patients with other causes of end-stage liver disease (ESLD). Although the patients in the Pittsburgh series may represent a carefully selected population, the question is no longer, Can we perform transplants in patients with alcoholic liver disease and obtain acceptable results? But, Should we? This question is particularly timely since the Health Care Financing Administration (HCFA) has recommended that Medicare coverage for liver transplantation be offered to patients with alcoholic cirrhosis who are abstinent. The HCFA proposes that the same eligibility criteria be used for patients with ARESLD as are used for patients with other causes of ESLD, such as primary biliary cirrhosis and sclerosing cholangitis.

SHOULD PATIENTS WITH ARESLD RECEIVE TRANSPLANTS?

At first glance, this question seems simple to answer. Generally, in medicine, a therapy is used if it works and saves lives. But the circumstances of liver transplantation differ from those of most other lifesaving therapies, including long-term mechanical ventilation and dialysis, in three important respects:

NONRENEWABLE RESOURCE

First, although most lifesaving therapies are expensive, liver transplantation uses a nonrenewable, absolutely scarce resource—a donor liver. In contrast to patients with end-stage renal disease, who may receive either a transplant or dialysis therapy, every patient with ESLD who does not receive a liver transplant will die. This dire, absolute scarcity of donor livers would be greatly exacerbated by including patients with ARESLD as potential candidates for liver transplantation. In 1985, 63,737 deaths due to hepatic disease occurred in the United States, at least 36,000 of which were related to alcoholism, but fewer than 1000 liver transplants were performed. Although patients with ARESLD represent more than 50 percent of the patients with ESLD, patients with ARESLD account for less than 10 percent of those receiving transplants (*New York Times*, April 3, 1990:B6 [col 1]). If patients with ARESLD were accepted for liver transplantation on an equal basis, as suggested by the HCFA, there would potentially be more than 30,000 additional candidates each year. (No data exist to indicate how many patients in the late stages of ARESLD would meet transplantation eligibility criteria.) In 1987, only 1182 liver transplants were performed; in 1989, fewer than 2000 were done. Even if all donor livers available were given to patients with ARESLD, it would not be feasible to provide transplants for even a small fraction of them. Thus, the dire, absolute nature of donor liver scarcity mandates that distribution be based on unusually rigorous standards—standards not required for the allocation of most other resources such as dialysis machines and ventilators, both of which are only *relatively* scarce.

COMPARISON WITH CARDIAC TRANSPLANTATION

Second, although a similar dire, absolute scarcity of donor hearts exists for cardiac transplantation, the allocational decisions for cardiac transplantation differ from those for liver transplantation. In liver transplantation, ARESLD causes more than 50 percent of the cases of ESLD; in cardiac transplantation, however, no one predominant disease or contributory factor is responsible. Even for patients with end-stage ischemic heart disease who smoked or who failed to adhere to dietary regimens, it is rarely clear that one particular behavior caused the disease. Also, unlike our proposed consideration for liver transplantation, a history of alcohol abuse is considered a contraindication and is a common reason for a patient with heart disease to be denied cardiac transplantation. Thus, the allocational decisions for heart transplantation differ from those for liver transplantation in two ways: determining a cause for end-stage heart disease is less certain, and patients with a history of alcoholism are usually rejected from heart transplant programs.

EXPENSIVE TECHNOLOGY

Third, a unique aspect of liver transplantation is that it is an expensive technology that has become a target of cost containment in health care. It is, therefore, essential to maintain the approbation and support of the public so that organs continue to be donated under appropriate clinical circumstances—even in spite of the high cost of transplantation.

GENERAL GUIDELINE PROPOSED

In view of the distinctive circumstances surrounding liver transplantation, we propose as a general guideline that patients with ARESLD should not compete equally with other candidates for liver transplantation. We are *not* suggesting that patients with ARESLD should *never* receive liver transplants. Rather, we propose that a priority ranking be established for the use of this dire, absolutely scarce societal resource and that patients with ARESLD be lower on the list than others with ESLD.

OBJECTIONS TO PROPOSAL

We realize that our proposal may meet with two immediate objections: (1) Some may argue that since alcoholism is a disease, patients with ARESLD should be considered equally for liver transplantation. (2) Some will question why patients with ARESLD should be singled out for discrimination, when the medical profession treats many patients who engage in behavior that causes their diseases. We will discuss these objections in turn.

ALCOHOLISM: HOW IS IT SIMILAR TO AND DIFFERENT FROM OTHER DISEASES?

We do not dispute the reclassification of alcoholism as a disease. Both hereditary and environmental factors contribute to alcoholism, and physiological, biochemical, and genetic markers have been associated with increased susceptibility. Identifying alcoholism as a disease enables physicians to approach it as they do other medical problems and to differentiate it from bad habits, crimes, or moral weaknesses. More important, identifying alcoholism as a disease also legitimizes medical interventions to treat it.

Alcoholism is a chronic disease, for which treatment is available and effective. More than 1.43 million patients were treated in 5586 alcohol treatment units in the 12-month period ending October 30, 1987. One comprehensive review concluded that more than two thirds of patients who accept therapy improve. Another cited four studies in which at least 54 percent of patients were abstinent a minimum of one year after treatment. A recent study of alcohol-impaired physicians reported a 100 percent abstinence rate an average of 33.4 months after therapy was initiated. In this study, physician-patients rated Alcoholics Anonymous, the largest organization of recovering alcoholics in the world, as the most important component of their therapy.

Like other chronic diseases—such as type I diabetes mellitus, which requires the patient to administer insulin over a lifetime—alcoholism requires the patient to assume responsibility for participating in continuous treatment. Two key elements are required to successfully treat alcoholism: the patient must accept his or her diagnosis and must assume responsibility for treatment. The high success rates of some alcoholism treatment programs indicate that many patients can accept responsibility for their treatment. ARESLD, one of the sequelae of alcoholism, results from 10 to 20 years of heavy alcohol consumption. The risk of ARESLD increases with the amount of alcohol consumed and with the duration of heavy consumption. In view of the quantity of alcohol consumed, the years, even decades, required to develop ARESLD, and the availability of effective alcohol treatment, attributing personal responsibility for ARESLD to the patient seems all the more justified. We believe, therefore, that even though alcoholism is a chronic disease, alcoholics should be held responsible for seeking and obtaining treatment that could prevent the development of late-stage complications such as ARESLD. Our view is consistent with that of Alcoholics Anonymous: alcoholics are responsible for undertaking a program for recovery that will keep their disease of alcoholism in remission.

ARE WE DISCRIMINATING AGAINST ALCOHOLICS?

Why should patients with ARESLD be singled out when a large number of patients have health problems that can be attributed to so-called voluntary health-risk behavior? Such patients include smokers with chronic lung disease; obese people who develop type II diabetes; some individuals who test positive for the human immunodeficiency virus; individuals with multiple behavioral risk factors (inattention to blood pressure, cholesterol, diet, and exercise) who develop coronary artery disease; and people such as skiers, motorcyclists, and football players who sustain activity-related injuries. We believe that the health care system should respond based on the actual medical needs of patients rather than on the factors (e.g., genetic, infectious, or behavioral) that cause the problem. We also believe that individuals should bear some responsibility—such as increased insurance premiums—for medical problems associated with voluntary choices. The critical distinguishing factor for treatment of ARESLD is the scarcity of the resource needed to treat it. The resources needed to treat most of these other conditions are only moderately or relatively scarce, and patients with these diseases or injuries can receive a share of the resources (i.e., money, personnel, and medication) roughly equivalent to their need. In contrast, there are insufficient donor livers to sustain the lives of all with ESLD who are in need. This difference permits us to make some discriminating choices— or to establish priorities—in selecting candidates for liver transplantation based on notions of fairness. In addition, this reasoning enables us to offer patients with alcohol-related medical and surgical problems their fair share of relatively scarce resources, such as blood products, surgical care, and intensive care beds, while still maintaining that their claim on donor livers is less compelling than the claims of others.

REASONS PATIENTS WITH ARESLD SHOULD HAVE A LOWER PRIORITY ON TRANSPLANT WAITING LISTS

Two arguments support our proposal. The first argument is a moral one based on considerations of fairness. The second one is based on policy considerations and examines whether public support of liver transplantation can be maintained if, as a result of a first-come, first-served approach, patients with ARESLD receive more than half the available donor livers. Finally, we will consider further research necessary to determine which patients with ARESLD should be candidates for transplantation, albeit with a lower priority.

FAIRNESS

Given a tragic shortage of donor livers, what is the fair or just way to allocate them? We suggest that patients who develop ESLD through no fault of their own (e.g., those with congenital biliary atresia or primary biliary cirrhosis) should have a higher priority in receiving a liver transplant than those whose liver disease results from failure to obtain treatment for alcoholism. In view of the dire, absolute scarcity of donor livers, we believe it is fair to hold people responsible for their choices, including decisions to refuse alcoholism treatment, and to allocate organs on this basis.

It is unfortunate but not unfair to make this distinction. When not enough donor livers are available for all who need one, choices have to be made, and they should be founded on one or more

proposed principles of fairness for distributing scarce resources. We shall consider four that are particularly relevant:

- *To each, an equal share of treatment.*
- *To each, similar treatment for similar cases.*
- *To each, treatment according to personal effort.*
- *To each, treatment according to ability to pay.*

It is not possible to give each patient with ESLD an *equal share*, or, in this case, a functioning liver. The problem created by the absolute scarcity of donor livers is that of inequality; some receive livers while others do not. But what is fair need not be equal. Although a first-come, first-served approach has been suggested to provide each patient with an equal chance, we believe it is fairer to give a child dying of biliary atresia an opportunity for a *first* normal liver than it is to give a patient with ARESLD who was born with a normal liver a *second* one.

Because the goal of providing each person with an equal share of health care sometimes collides with the realities of finite medical resources, the principle of *similar treatment for similar cases* has been found to be helpful. Outka stated it this way: "If we accept the case for equal access, but if we simply cannot, physically cannot, treat all who are in need, it seems more just to discriminate by virtue of categories of illness, rather than between rich ill and poor ill." This principle is derived from the principle of formal justice, which, roughly stated, says that people who are equal in relevant respects should be treated equally and that people who are unequal in relevant respects should be treated differently. We believe that patients with ARESLD are unequal in a relevant respect to others with ESLD, since their liver failure was preventable; therefore, it is acceptable to treat them differently.

Our view also relies on the principle of, *To each, treatment according to personal effort.* Although alcoholics cannot be held responsible for their disease, once their condition has been diagnosed they can be held responsible for seeking treatment and for preventing the complication of ARESLD. The standard of personal effort and responsibility we propose for alcoholics is the same as that held by Alcoholics Anonymous. We are not suggesting that some lives and behaviors have greater value than others—an approach used and appropriately repudiated when dialysis machines were in short supply. But we are holding people responsible for their personal effort.

Health policymakers have predicted that this principle will assume greater importance in the future. In the context of scarce health care resources, Blank foresees a reevaluation of our health care priorities, with a shift toward individual responsibility and a renewed emphasis on the individual's obligation to society to maximize one's health. Similarly, more than a decade ago, Knowles observed that prevention of disease requires effort. He envisioned that the next major advances in the health of the American people would be determined by what individuals are willing to do for themselves.

To each, treatment according to ability to pay has also been used as a principle of distributive justice. Since alcoholism is prevalent in all socioeconomic strata, it is not discrimination against the poor to deny liver transplantation to patients with alcoholic liver disease. In fact, we believe that poor patients with ARESLD have a stronger claim for a donor liver than rich patients, precisely because many alcohol treatment programs are not available to patients lacking in substantial private resources or health insurance. Ironically, it is precisely this group of poor and uninsured patients who are most likely not to be eligible to receive a liver transplant because of their inability to pay. We agree with Outka's view of fairness that would discriminate according to categories of illness rather than according to wealth.

POLICY CONSIDERATIONS REGARDING PUBLIC SUPPORT FOR LIVER TRANSPLANTATION

Today, the main health policy concerns involve issues of financing, distributive justice, and rationing medical care. Because of the many deficiencies in the U.S. health care system—in maternal and child health, in the unmet needs of the elderly, and in the millions of Americans without health insurance—an increasing number of commentators are drawing attention to the trade-offs between basic health care for the many and expensive, albeit lifesaving, care for the few.

Because of its high unit cost, liver transplantation is often at the center of these discussions, as it has been in Oregon, where the legislature voted to eliminate Medicaid reimbursement for all transplants except kidneys and corneas. In this era of health care cost containment, a sense of limits is emerging and allocational choices are being made. Oregon has already shown that elected officials and the public are prepared to face these issues.

In our democracy, it is appropriate that community mores and values be regarded seriously when deciding the most appropriate use of a scarce and nonrenewable organ symbolized as a "Gift of Life." As if to underscore this point, the report of the Task Force on Organ Transplantation recommended that each donated organ be considered a national resource for the public good and that the public must participate in decisions on how to use this resource to best serve the public's interests.

Much of the initial success in securing public and political approval for liver transplantation was achieved by focusing media and political attention not on adults but on children dying of ESLD. The public may not support transplantation for patients with ARESLD in the same way that they have endorsed this procedure for babies born with biliary atresia. This assertion is bolstered not only by the events in Oregon but also by the results of a Louis Harris and Associates national survey, which showed that lifesaving therapy for premature infants or for patients with cancer was given the highest health care priority by the public and that lifesaving therapy for patients with alcoholic liver disease was given the lowest. In this poll, the public's view of health care priorities was shared by leadership groups also polled: physicians, nurses, employers, and politicians.

Just because a majority of the public holds these views does not mean that they are right, but the moral intuition of the public, which is also shared by its leaders, reflects community values that must be seriously considered. Also indicative of community values are organizations such as Mothers Against Drunk Driving, Students Against Drunk Driving, corporate employee assistance programs, and school student assistance programs. Their existence signals that many believe that a person's behavior can be modified so that the consequences of behavior such as alcoholism can be prevented. Thus, giving donor livers to patients with ARESLD on an equal basis with other patients who have ESLD might lead to a decline in public support for liver transplantation.

SHOULD ANY ALCOHOLICS BE CONSIDERED FOR TRANSPLANTATION? NEED FOR FURTHER RESEARCH

Our proposal for giving lower priority for liver transplantation to patients with ARESLD does not completely rule out transplantation for this group. Patients with ARESLD who had not previously been offered therapy and who are now abstinent could be acceptable candidates. In addition, patients lower on the waiting list, such as patients with ARESLD who have been treated and are now abstinent, might be eligible for a donor liver in some regions because of the increased availability of donor organs there. Even if only because of these possible conditions for transplantation, further research is needed to determine which patients with ARESLD would have the best outcomes after liver transplantation.

Transplant programs have been reluctant to provide transplants to alcoholics because of concern about one unfavorable outcome: a high recidivism rate. Although the overall recidivism rate for the Pittsburgh patients was only 11.5 percent, in the group of patients who had been abstinent less than 6 months it was 43 percent. Also, compared with the entire group in which one-year survival was 74 percent, the survival rate in this subgroup was lower, at 64 percent.

In the recently proposed Medicare criteria for coverage of liver transplantation, the HCFA acknowledged that the decision to insure patients with alcoholic cirrhosis "may be considered controversial by some." As if to counter possible objections, the HCFA listed requirements for patients with alcoholic cirrhosis: patients must meet the transplant center's requirement for abstinence prior to liver transplantation and have documented evidence of sufficient social support to ensure both recovery from alcoholism and compli-ance with the regimen of immunosuppressive medication.

Further research should answer lingering questions about liver transplantation for ARESLD patients: Which characteristics of a patient with ARESLD can predict a successful outcome? How long is abstinence necessary to qualify for transplantation? What type of a social support system must a patient have to ensure good results? These questions are being addressed. Until the answers are known, we propose that further transplantation for patients with ARESLD be limited to abstinent patients who had not previously been offered alcoholism treatment and to abstinent treated patients in regions of increased donor liver availability, and that it be carried out as part of prospective research protocols at a few centers skilled in transplantation and alcohol research.

COMMENT

Should patients with ARESLD compete equally for liver transplants? In a setting in which there is a dire, absolute scarcity of donor livers, we believe the answer is no. Considerations of fairness suggest that a first-come, first-served approach for liver transplantation is not the most just approach. Although this decision is difficult, it is only fair that patients who have not assumed equal responsibility for maintaining their health or for accepting treatment for a chronic disease should be treated differently. Considerations of public values and mores suggest that the public may not support liver transplantation if patients with ARESLD routinely receive more than half of the available donor livers. We conclude that since not all can live, priorities must be established and that patients with ARESLD should be given a lower priority for liver transplantation than others with ESLD.

Alcoholics and Liver Transplantation

Carl Cohen, Martin Benjamin, and the Ethics and Social Impact Committee of the Transplant and Health Policy Center, Ann Arbor, Michigan

Alcoholic cirrhosis of the liver—severe scarring due to the heavy use of alcohol—is by far the major cause of end-stage liver disease. For persons so afflicted, life may depend on receiving a new transplanted liver. The number of alcoholics in the United States needing new livers is great, but the supply of available livers for transplantation is small. *Should those whose end-stage liver disease was caused by alcohol abuse be categorically excluded from candidacy for liver transplantation?* This question, partly medical and partly moral, must now be confronted forthrightly. Many lives are at stake.

Reasons of two kinds underlie a widespread unwillingness to transplant livers into alcoholics: First, there is a common conviction—explicit or tacit—that alcoholics are morally blameworthy, their condition the result of their own misconduct, and that such blameworthiness disqualifies alcoholics in unavoidable competition for organs with others equally sick but blameless. Second, there is a common belief that because of their habits, alcoholics will not exhibit satisfactory survival rates after transplantation, and that, therefore, good stewardship of a scarce lifesaving resource requires that alcoholics not be considered for liver transplantation. We examine both of these arguments.

THE MORAL ARGUMENT

A widespread condemnation of drunkenness and a revulsion for drunks lie at the heart of this public policy issue. Alcoholic cirrhosis—unlike other causes of end-stage liver disease—is brought on by a person's conduct, by heavy drinking. Yet if the

From *Journal of the American Medical Association*, Vol. 265, 1299–1301. Copyright © 1991 American Medical Association. Reprinted by permission of the American Medical Association.
EDITORS' NOTE: All notes have been deleted. Readers who wish to follow up on sources should consult the original article.

dispute here were only about whether to treat someone who is seriously ill because of personal conduct, we would not say—as we do not in cases of other serious diseases resulting from personal conduct—that such conduct disqualifies a person from receiving desperately needed medical attention. Accident victims injured because they were not wearing seat belts are treated without hesitation; reformed smokers who become coronary bypass candidates partly because they disregarded their physicians' advice about tobacco, diet, and exercise are not turned away because of their bad habits. But new livers are a scarce resource, and transplanting a liver into an alcoholic may, therefore, result in death for a competing candidate whose liver disease was wholly beyond his or her control. Thus we seem driven, in this case unlike in others, to reflect on the weight given to the patient's personal conduct. And heavy drinking—unlike smoking, or overeating, or failing to wear a seat belt—is widely regarded as morally wrong.

Many contend that alcoholism is not a moral failing but a disease. Some authorities have recently reaffirmed this position, asserting that alcoholism is "best regarded as a chronic disease." But this claim cannot be firmly established and is far from universally believed. Whether alcoholism is indeed a disease, or a moral failing, or both, remains a disputed matter surrounded by intense controversy.

Even if it is true that alcoholics suffer from a somatic disorder, many people will argue that this disorder results in deadly liver disease only when coupled with a weakness of will—a weakness for which part of the blame must fall on the alcoholic. This consideration underlies the conviction that the alcoholic needing a transplanted liver, unlike a nonalcoholic competing for the same liver, is at least partly responsible for his or her need. Therefore, some conclude, the alcoholic's personal failing is rightly considered in deciding upon his or her entitlement to this very scarce resource.

Is this argument sound? We think it is not. Whether alcoholism is a moral failing, in whole or in part, remains uncertain. But even if we suppose that it is, it does not follow that we are justified in categorically denying liver transplants to those alcoholics suffering from endstage cirrhosis. We could rightly preclude alcoholics from transplantation only if we assume that qualification for a new organ requires some level of moral virtue or is canceled by some level of moral vice. But there is absolutely no agreement—and there is likely to be none—about what constitutes moral virtue and vice and what rewards and penalties they deserve. The assumption that undergirds the moral argument for precluding alcoholics is thus unacceptable. Moreover, even if we could agree (which, in fact, we cannot) upon the kind of misconduct we would be looking for, the fair weighting of such a consideration would entail highly intrusive investigations into patients' moral habits—investigations universally thought repugnant. Moral evaluation is wisely and rightly excluded from all deliberations of who should be treated and how.

Indeed, we do exclude it. We do not seek to determine whether a particular transplant candidate is an abusive parent or a dutiful daughter; whether candidates cheat on their income taxes or their spouses; or whether potential recipients pay their parking tickets or routinely lie when they think it is in their best interests. We refrain from considering such judgments for several good reasons: (1) We have genuine and well-grounded doubts about comparative degrees of voluntariness and, therefore, *cannot pass judgment fairly.* (2) Even if we could assess degrees of voluntariness reliably, we *cannot know what penalties different degrees of misconduct deserve.* (3) *Judgments of this kind could not be made consistently in our medical system*—and a fundamental requirement of a fair system in allocating scarce resources is that it treat all in need of certain goods on the same standard, without unfair discrimination by group.

If alcoholics should be penalized because of their moral fault, then all others who are equally at fault in causing their own medical needs should be similarly penalized. To accomplish this, we would have to make vigorous and sustained efforts to find out whose conduct has been morally weak or sinful and to what degree. That inquiry, as a condition for medical care or for the receipt of goods in short supply, we certainly will not and should not undertake.

The unfairness of such moral judgments is compounded by other accidental factors that render moral assessment especially difficult in connection with alcoholism and liver disease. Some drinkers have a greater predisposition for alcohol abuse than others. And for some who drink to excess, the predisposition to cirrhosis is also greater; many grossly intemperate drinkers do not suffer grievously from liver disease. On the other hand, alcohol consumption that might be considered moderate for some may cause serious liver disease in others. It turns out, in fact, that the disastrous consequences of even low levels of alcohol consumption may be much more common in women than in men. Therefore, penalizing cirrhotics by denying them transplant candidacy would have the effect of holding some groups arbitrarily to a higher standard than others and would probably hold women to a higher standard of conduct than men.

Moral judgments that eliminate alcoholics from candidacy thus prove unfair and unacceptable. The alleged (but disputed) moral misconduct of alcoholics with end-stage liver disease does not justify categorically excluding them as candidates for liver transplantation.

MEDICAL ARGUMENT

Reluctance to use available livers in treating alcoholics is due in some part to the conviction that, because alcoholics would do poorly after transplant as a result of their bad habits, good stewardship of organs in short supply requires that alcoholics be excluded from consideration.

This argument also fails, for two reasons: First, it fails because the premise—that the outcome for alcoholics will invariably be poor relative to other groups—is at least doubtful and probably false. Second, it fails because, even if the premise were true, it could serve as a good reason to exclude alcoholics only if it were an equally good reason to exclude other groups having a prognosis equally bad or worse. But equally low survival rates have not excluded other groups; fairness therefore requires that this group not be categorically excluded either.

In fact, the data regarding the post-transplant histories of alcoholics are not yet reliable. Evidence gathered in 1984 indicated that the 1-year survival rate for patients with alcoholic cirrhosis was well below the survival rate for other recipients of liver transplants, excluding those with cancer. But a 1988 report, with a larger (but still small) sample number, shows remarkably good results in alcoholics receiving transplants: 1-year survival is 73.2%—and of 35 carefully selected (and possibly non-representative) alcoholics who received transplants and lived 6 months or longer, only two relapsed into alcohol abuse. Liver transplantation, it would appear, can be a very sobering experience. Whether this group continues to do as well as a comparable group of non-alcoholic liver recipients remains uncertain. But the data, although not supporting the broad inclusion of alcoholics, do suggest that medical considerations do not now justify categorically excluding alcoholics from liver transplantation.

A history of alcoholism is of great concern when considering liver transplantation, not only because of the impact of alcohol abuse upon the entire system of the recipient, but also because the life of an alcoholic tends to be beset by general disorder. Returning to heavy drinking could ruin a new liver, although probably not for years. But relapse into heavy drinking would quite likely entail the inability to maintain the routine of multiple medication, daily or twice-daily, essential for immunosuppression and survival. As a class, alcoholic cirrhotics may therefore prove to have substantially lower survival rates after receiving transplants. All such matters should be weighed, of course. But none of them gives any solid reason to exclude alcoholics from consideration categorically.

Moreover, even if survival rates for alcoholics selected were much lower than normal—a supposition now in substantial doubt—what could fairly be concluded from such data? Do we exclude from transplant candidacy members of other groups known to have low survival rates? In fact we do not. Other things being equal, we may prefer not to transplant organs in short supply into patients afflicted, say, with liver cell cancer, knowing that such cancer recurs not long after a new liver is implanted. Yet in some individual cases we do it. Similarly, some transplant recipients have other malignant neoplasms or other conditions that suggest low survival probability. Such matters are weighed in selecting recipients, but they are insufficient grounds to categorically exclude an entire group. This shows that the argument for excluding

alcoholics based on survival probability rates alone is simply not just.

THE ARGUMENTS DISTINGUISHED

In fact, the exclusion of alcoholics from transplant candidacy probably results from an intermingling, perhaps at times a confusion, of the moral and medical arguments. But if the moral argument indeed does not apply, no combination of it with probable survival rates can make it applicable. Survival data, carefully collected and analyzed, deserve to be weighed in selecting candidates. These data do not come close to precluding alcoholics from consideration. Judgments of blameworthiness, which ought to be excluded generally, certainly should be excluded when weighing the impact of those survival rates. Some people with a strong antipathy to alcohol abuse and abusers may, without realizing it, be relying on assumed unfavorable data to support a fixed moral judgment. The arguments must be untangled. Actual results with transplanted alcoholics must be considered without regard to moral antipathies.

The upshot is inescapable: there are no good grounds at present—moral or medical—to disqualify a patient with end-stage liver disease from consideration for liver transplantation simply because of a history of heavy drinking.

SCREENING AND SELECTION OF LIVER TRANSPLANT CANDIDATES

In the initial evaluation of candidates for any form of transplantation, the central questions are whether patients (1) are sick enough to need a new organ and (2) enjoy a high enough probability of benefiting from this limited resource. At this stage the criteria should be non-comparative. Even the initial screening of patients must, however, be done individually and with great care.

The screening process for those suffering from alcoholic cirrhosis must be especially rigorous—not for moral reasons, but because of factors affecting survival, which are themselves influenced by a history of heavy drinking—and even more by its resumption. Responsible stewardship of scarce organs requires that the screening for candidacy take into consideration the manifold impact of heavy drinking on long-term transplant success. Cardiovascular problems brought on by alcoholism and other systematic contraindications must be looked for. Psychiatric and social evaluation is also in order, to determine whether patients understand and have come to terms with their condition and whether they have the social support essential for continuing immunosuppression and follow-up care.

Precisely which factors should be weighed in this screening process have not been firmly established. Some physicians have proposed a specified period of alcohol abstinence as an "objective" criterion for selection—but the data supporting such a criterion are far from conclusive, and the use of this criterion to exclude a prospective recipient is at present medically and morally arbitrary.

Indeed, one important consequence of overcoming the strong presumption against considering alcoholics for liver transplantation is the research opportunity it presents and the encouragement it gives to the quest for more reliable predictors of medical success. As that search continues, some defensible guidelines for case-by-case determination have been devised, based on factors associated with sustained recovery from alcoholism and other considerations related to liver transplantation success in general. Such guidelines appropriately include (1) refined diagnosis by those trained in the treatment of alcoholism, (2) acknowledgment by the patient of a serious drinking problem, (3) social and familial stability, and (4) other factors experimentally associated with long-term sobriety.

The experimental use of guidelines like these, and their gradual refinement overtime, may lead to more reliable and more generally applicable predictors. But those more refined predictors will never be developed until prejudices against considering alcoholics for liver transplantation are overcome.

Patients who are sick because of alleged self-abuse ought not be grouped for discriminatory treatment—unless we are prepared to develop a detailed calculus of just deserts for health care based on good conduct. Lack of sympathy for those who bring serious disease upon themselves is understandable, but the temptation to institutionalize that emotional response must be tempered by our inability to apply such considerations justly and by our duty *not* to apply them unjustly. In the end, some patients with alcoholic cirrhosis may be judged, after careful evaluation, as good risks for a liver transplant.

OBJECTION AND REPLY

Providing alcoholics with transplants may present a special "political" problem for transplant centers. The public perception of alcoholics is generally negative. The already low rate of organ donation, it may be argued, will fail even lower when it becomes known that donated organs are going to alcoholics. Financial support from legislatures may also suffer. One can imagine the effect on transplantation if the public were to learn that the liver of a teenager killed by a drunken driver had been transplanted into an alcoholic patient. If selecting even a few alcoholics as transplant candidates reduces the number of lives saved overall, might that not be good reason to preclude alcoholics categorically?

No. The fear is understandable, but excluding alcoholics cannot be rationally defended on that basis. Irresponsible conduct attributable to alcohol abuse should not be defended. No excuses should be made for the deplorable consequences of drunken behavior, from highway slaughter to familial neglect and abuse. But alcoholism must be distinguished from those consequences; not all alcoholics are morally irresponsible, vicious, or neglectful drunks. If there is a general failure to make this distinction, we must strive to overcome that failure, not pander to it.

Public confidence in medical practice in general, and in organ transplantation in particular, depends on the scientific validity and moral integrity of the policies adopted. Sound policies will prove publicly defensible. Shaping present health care policy on the basis of distorted public perceptions or prejudices will, in the long run, do more harm than good to the process and to the reputation of all concerned.

Approximately one in every 10 Americans is a heavy drinker, and approximately one family in every three has at least one member at risk for alcoholic cirrhosis. The care of alcoholics and the just treatment of them when their lives are at stake are matters a democratic polity may therefore be expected to act on with concern and reasonable judgment over the long run. The allocation of organs in short supply does present vexing moral problems; if thoughtless or shallow moralizing would cause some to respond very negatively to transplanting livers into alcoholic cirrhotics, that cannot serve as good reason to make such moralizing the measure of public policy.

We have argued that there is now no good reason, either moral or medical, to preclude alcoholics categorically from consideration for liver transplantation. We further conclude that it would therefore be unjust to implement that categorical preclusion simply because others might respond negatively if we do not.

Rationing Effective but Expensive Treatment

Just Caring: Managed Care and Protease Inhibitors

Leonard Fleck

Do HIV-positive patients have any just claims to protease inhibitors? This is really the first issue that needs to be addressed. My short answer to this question is that they have *limited, presumptively just claims*, which is to say the issue is not primarily a matter of social beneficence. There are two sources of the justice presumption, namely, the pronounced effectiveness of these protease inhibitors, and secondly, their ability to protect fair equality of opportunity.

First, the drugs are remarkably effective in about 70% of HIV-positive patients (with some research suggesting that figure might be over 90% for patients who have not used drugs such as AZT). With the most potent of these drugs there are average increases of CD4 counts of 250/mL and reductions in viral burden to undetectable levels.[1] The clinical implications of this are a marked reduction in vulnerability to deadly and debilitating opportunistic infections for these patients. In addition, there have been widespread reports of dramatic improvements in the overall quality of the lives of these patients, i.e., ability to return to work and to enjoy all the other pursuits of normal life.[2] Ordinarily, results like this would warrant inclusion of these drugs in insurance packages as part of the standard of care. That is, it would be presumptively unjust to fail to include coverage for this therapy.

Second, I agree with Norman Daniels that capacity to protect fair equality of opportunity is an essential element of our understanding of the demands of health care justice.[3] It is not the whole of our conception of health care justice, but it is at the core. Given the demonstrated effectiveness of these protease inhibitors, it would seem that affected individuals would have a strong presumptive just claim to them on the grounds that they protect fair equality of opportunity by restoring them to normal species functioning.

We do need to stress the fact that this is a *presumptive* claim: it is defeatable. The primary reason we are having this discussion is that these protease inhibitors are very expensive, not simply on a one-time basis, but repeatedly—for every added year of life we are looking at costs of about $20,000 per person. The mantra of the nineties, with which we are all familiar, is that we have only limited resources to meet virtually unlimited health care needs.[4] Dollars directed to meet some health needs are not available to meet other needs. This, of course, suggests that priorities must be established among health needs.[5] Not all health needs are created equal, morally speaking. Some make stronger claims on limited resources than others. How strong, relatively speaking, are the claims of these protease inhibitors?

No one believes that protease inhibitors represent a cure for AIDS. Therefore, they will not be ranked in the upper tier of health priorities. However, from the perspective of cost-effectiveness, restoration of normal functioning at a reasonable enough cost,

From *Hastings Center Report*. Copyright © The Hastings Center.

they would seem to rank significantly above autologous bone marrow transplants for either breast or testicular cancer. What we might fairly say is that they are squarely in the middle of the mass of halfway medical interventions that define late-twentieth-century medicine. Pessimists might argue that these protease inhibitors will be maximally effective for only two or three years; then they will lose their potency as the HIV virus mutates and defeats them. Optimists, on the other hand, may be inclined to argue that this current generation of inhibitors may have only limited potency, but that the next generation of inhibitors, including integrase inhibitors, may tame the virus so that AIDS becomes a chronic disorder. The "optimal result" expected is that patients would become long-term nonprogressors.

The scare quotes are necessary for the thought that this might be an optimal result, since an outcome like that would be morally scary. If we use cost per quality-adjusted life year saved as a factor in assigning priority to protease inhibitors for health plan funding, then they might be roughly in the same category as major organ transplants where we would have costs of about $20,000 per QALY. As a unit cost, that does not seem to be unreasonable. But the aggregating effects are potentially very troublesome. Apart from kidneys, we do about 8000 major organ transplants each year in the United States. That represents about $1 billion in aggregated costs. The limit we are faced with is the availability of transplantable organs. But there may be as many as one million HIV-positive individuals in the United States. If all of them would have access to protease inhibitors, there would be the potential for adding $20 billion to the cost of health care in the United States per year. Further, we have to assume those numbers would continue to increase for the foreseeable future. Again, if we were successful in achieving "optimal results," say, twenty-year survival with protease inhibitors, then we would be looking at $400,000 costs per life prolonged, plus end-of-life costs, plus the usual range of other health care costs that anyone else in our society might incur. Is it still the case that HIV-positive individuals in our managed care plan have a presumptively just claim to these protease inhibitors at plan expense? And who should have primary moral responsibility for making the relevant policy decisions in these matters within managed care plans, especially in a very competitive cost-conscious health care system?

I will still defend the view that there are just claims to these protease inhibitors, but the claims are *limited*. The responsibility for determining those limits should fall primarily to the board of a managed care plan in conjunction with representatives of the medical staff of that plan and the managed care ethics committee for that plan. The role of the ethics committee is to make "uncontaminated" policy recommendations with respect to cost containment, rationing, and priority-setting within the plan. "Uncontaminated" does not mean that their recommendations are utopian. Almost always, as we shall see below, their recommendations will reflect nonideal judgments of health care justice. What their judgments should not be contaminated by or distorted by are strategic business considerations.

Similarly, plan physicians have at stake their own medical and moral integrity. They will ultimately have responsibility for implementing policies of the board in their practice in the plan. It would be morally irresponsible if physicians were mere tools in the hands of the board. Hence, they must communicate to the board what features of any options being considered would be deeply violative of their medical moral responsibilities as physicians. The analogous responsibility for the ethics committee would be to communicate to the board the features of any option being considered that would be deeply violative of health care justice. The ethics committee should convey to the board their judgment of which option, among several morally permissible options, might be most morally preferable, if in fact the ethics committee can come to something close to consensus on this matter. Beyond that, the board may choose a morally acceptable but sub-optimal option that reflects socially responsible strategic business considerations that seem to be an integral part of our health care system now.

With all that as preface, let us now turn to assessing some specific policy options for our managed care plan with respect to protease inhibitors. We can begin by quickly sweeping some options off the table as badly flawed so far as health care justice is concerned.

Option #1: Postpone making any decision for a year. The main argument that might be deployed in support of this option is that we do not want to waste money on very expensive drugs that might offer no more than short-term false hopes. The fact is that the first protease inhibitors were approved with less than a year of clinical trials. Who knows, the argument goes, what awful surprises might emerge a little later? However, the trials were cut short because the early results were so dramatically positive. Even when we correct for considerable political and commercial pressures associated with these drugs, the results remain morally weighty. The cost of postponing a decision for a year would be the unnecessary loss of some number of relatively young lives within our managed care plan. Speculative fears about side effects cannot be given that much moral weight in these circumstances. Further, if our real concern is costly bad outcomes, then, to give just one example, moral consistency would require that we first put in place a policy of not funding aggressive life-sustaining care in the case of infants born under 750 grams/25 weeks gestation where there is already substantial evidence of very bad outcomes (death or permanent serious disabilities) in a significant majority of cases. In my judgment option #1 fails the minimal justice test.

Option #2: Fund protease inhibitors only to the extent that competing managed care plans fund them. There are clearly corporate self-interest considerations that speak in favor of this option. If there are several very large corporations in an area, and if they all offer options with all the managed care plans in the area (which means the option of switching on an annual basis), then there would be a risk that the first managed care plan to offer coverage of protease inhibitors would attract a disproportionate share of HIV-positive individuals. Further, the argument might be made that an outcome such as this would be unfair; and consequently, managed care plans are not morally obligated to accept such unfair burdens.

But option #2 has some serious, unredeemable moral flaws. First, there are some empirical issues that would have to be addressed. How likely would it be that there would be a large influx of HIV-positive individuals into our plan from competing plans? If there were a very real risk (not just the product of a fevered imagination) of economic failure of the plan as a whole from such an influx, then this might justify reluctantly choosing option #2. If the only morally defensible policy option were unlimited funding for protease inhibitors for all HIV-positive plan members, then, given such

costs, economic failure might be a real-world possibility. But, as I argue below, there are less costly, still "just enough" options, which reduce the plausibility of the economic failure hard moral choice scenario.

Second, there is something morally unsavory about judging what is right and wrong on the basis of what others do. At the very least that would reduce our moral commitments to the lowest common denominator. One might argue that in the world of business that is precisely how moral commitments get defined. However, that assumes that the issue we are faced with is primarily a matter of business ethics (an assumption with which I would strongly disagree), and that business ethics is adequately characterized in terms of lowest common denominator commitments among competitors (also an assumption I reject). On the latter point, there are matters of corporate beneficence where matching what competitors do (and no more) is morally permissible. However, with respect to matters of justice and strong rights claims, that kind of competitive strategy is not morally defensible, unless business ethics is reduced to corporate self-interest. That brings us to our third point.

Some might argue that access to protease inhibitors is only a matter of beneficence. This might be a plausible perspective if protease inhibitors represented marginally beneficial, noncostworthy care. But our earlier arguments showed the benefits are substantial, though fairly costly. Still, there is a presumptive just claim to them. On a priority scale for health care they are somewhere in the middle. That means there will be a substantial number of other medical interventions now covered by our plan that are less beneficial and less costworthy. Fairness would seem to require reducing our commitment to these other interventions before we would be justified in refusing to cover protease inhibitors. At the very least a compelling moral argument would have to be given for refusing to include protease inhibitors as a covered benefit. Competitive economic pressures would not count as such an argument.[6]

Option #3: Let plan members themselves decide what the policy ought to be by something like a direct vote. Readers familiar with my work know that I am a strong advocate of rational democratic deliberation as a fair and reasonable approach to addressing a certain range of rationing decisions.[7]

However, this option, as presented, is outside those bounds. The moral virtue of rational democratic deliberation is that it is supposed to provide a mechanism for a community to make public self-imposed rationing decisions. It is supposed to provide a moral antidote to our typical practice of making rationing decisions invisibly and aresponsibly. It is also supposed to prevent healthy majorities from imposing unjust rationing decisions on sick and vulnerable minorities. The moral space of rational democratic deliberation is delimited by a number of what I refer to metaphorically as constitutional principles of health care justice, one of which would be a principle of non-discrimination. It is that boundary that is violated by option #3. It is much too likely that ongoing patterns of discrimination against HIV-positive individuals would result in an unjust rationing decision in this case, i.e., complete denial of funding or grossly inadequate funding. Further, I would contend that a board that endorsed option #3 would itself be open to the moral criticism that it was abdicating its own moral responsibility. Finally, as we shall see below, there are options available here that would justifiably employ rational democratic deliberation; but the creation of those options will require some responsible decision making by the board first.

Option #4: Let plan physicians make the relevant moral and clinical decisions for individual patients on the basis of their best professional judgment. Like the prior option this one also allows the board to escape responsibility for making these difficult decisions. The basic moral argument in favor of this option is that it is responsive to the complexities of clinical practice.[8] No one doubts the wisdom of a broad measure of respect for clinical autonomy. But unlimited clinical autonomy means the potential for both unlimited costs and unlimited inequities. Individual physicians might be too compassionate or too readily responsive to the demands of patients before them at the expense of the legitimate interests of other patients not before them. Given the widely disseminated hype that protease inhibitors have received, numerous such demands are likely. If enough physicians give in to those demands by patients in the early stages of HIV infection, then there is a good likelihood that plan resources will be squandered on very marginal benefits, which is to say some higher priority, more just health claims might not be met.

An alternative approach is to use economic incentives to shape and constrain clinical autonomy, such as capitation attached to drugs and testing. Here too, however, there is the potential for serious injustices. The first of these would be the problem of invisible rationing. Since there would be no formal rules governing access to protease inhibitors, patients would not know if their physician was being excessively strict in providing access to protease inhibitors, thereby denying them significant and costworthy clinical benefits for reasons of economic self-interest.[9]

Second, under capitation patients with essentially the same clinical status in the same managed care plan might be treated very differently for reasons which are neither their reasons nor for their benefit. The threat of malpractice will protect patients from the most egregious forms of undertreatment, but there is a large enough, gray enough area with respect to protease inhibitors that legal protections will not prevent unjust denials. That gray area exists because of considerable clinical uncertainty regarding optimal initiation of therapy. There are also significant side effects that might give asymptomatic HIV-positive patients pause regarding the initiation of therapy. But under capitation patients are unlikely to be invited to be part of this decision making process. Just rationing protocols ought to be rationally self-imposed, but capitation essentially hands decisional authority to physicians. For these reasons I would reject option #4 as seriously unjust.

Option #5: Let companies that have contracts with our managed care plan decide whether or not they want protease inhibitor coverage for their employees; then price coverage to them experientially. This option is akin in many respects to option #3. It is, for example, primarily a way of shifting moral responsibility away from the board to others whose self-interest is likely to generate a less than just result. Libertarians, of course, will not see it this way. On the contrary, they are likely to see this as the optimal option because each payor decides for themselves what is or is not costworthy care. No one is forced to pay for care he or she does not want. I have addressed elsewhere what I see as the deep moral flaws of libertarianism as a conception of health care justice, so I will not repeat those arguments here.[10] Instead, I will simply point out some of the unseemly consequences specific to this proposal. For one thing, if some companies fund protease inhibitors for their employees but most others do not, then physicians in the same managed care plan will find themselves able to treat some of their HIV-positive patients in a maximally appropriate way while having to allow others to suffer and die prematurely. Outcomes like that can be tolerated as tragic and regrettable when there are absolute shortages of a life-saving drug. Similarly, if a drug is very expensive and yields only marginal benefits, then we find it morally tolerable that only those with personal ability to pay will have access to it. But neither of these conditions obtain with respect to protease inhibitors. At the very least an outcome like this will prove to be morally and psychologically troubling for physicians who find themselves in these circumstances.

Any kind of gatekeeping can be psychologically troubling for physicians, but gatekeeping in the service of a more just distribution of limited resources should not be morally troubling. That, however, is precisely what is not true here. Physicians could initiate appeals on behalf of their unfunded HIV-positive patients. But if the managed care plan responds positively to those appeals, then it sends a signal to the companies who have paid for that coverage that they need not pay for it, which could potentially worsen care for all HIV-positive patients in the plan. Apart from that potential consequence, if the plan responded positively to some appeals on the basis of some moral norm, then the question would be why such a norm did not govern a minimal HIV benefit option that would be part of all their contracts. And, of course, if positive responses were elicited in a rather random or arbitrary non-moral fashion, then those not similarly favored would have cause for just complaint.

Option #6: Fund protease inhibitors for all HIV-positive individuals who believe it is in their best interest that they start on protease inhibitors immediately. This would obviously be the potentially most expensive option our plan could consider with additional annual costs of about $20 million. Is a just and caring managed care plan morally obligated to choose this option? I will argue that this is not a morally obligatory option, but it *may* be a morally permissible option.

The primary consideration that speaks against seeing this option as morally obligatory is that we have little evidence of dramatic medical effective-ness for protease inhibitors in the early stages of infection. Dr. David Ho has been the preeminent medical researcher associated with protease inhibitors. He has a theory that if protease inhibitors are given in the earliest stages of HIV infection they may be able to defeat the virus entirely with three years of protease therapy.[11] But the actual clinical trials were done with patients who were in more advanced stages of AIDS proper. As noted earlier, those trials were aborted after less than a year because of the dramatic results that were achieved. But that provides no evidence for what we might reasonably expect in the way of therapeutic outcomes from earlier administration, say, to patients with CD4 counts above 500/mL. Hence, it would be fair to conclude that in the early stages of HIV infection protease inhibitors are an experimental form of therapy. The moral implication of that is that plan members who were HIV-positive would have no just claim to protease inhibitors at plan expense.

We need to admit that we are in an area of considerable moral uncertainty and moral ambiguity. One of the consequences of my last conclusion is that HIV-positive individuals will have to accept a significant degree of deterioration in their immune systems before they would have access to protease inhibitors at plan expense. There seems to be no medical consensus as to what the medical consequences are of allowing the immune system to deteriorate from CD4 counts of 1100/mL to below 500/mL. There is some evidence suggesting that some such individuals may be vulnerable to some forms of cancer, but the precise causal processes remain mostly a mystery.[12] If our plan had very substantial surplus resources, then a case might be made for providing funding for protease inhibitors in earlier stages of HIV infection. But there are no surplus resources. Those resources would have to be raised from plan members, who might choose to exit the plan rather than pay those higher rates.

Even if those resources could be raised, a significant justice issue would still need to be addressed. Specifically, do individuals in the early stages of HIV infection have stronger just claims to those additional resources than any other patients in the plan with other unfunded health needs? It is very far from obvious that they do. If it is typically the case that deterioration of the immune system occurs over 6–8 years before CD4 counts fall below 500/mL, then we are looking at potential increases in per HIV-positive patient lifetime costs of $120,000–160,000 for benefits that cannot be delineated with any degree of precision. My intuition is that women with advanced stages of breast cancer who had failed conventional chemotherapy would almost certainly have a stronger claim to those resources (so that they could secure ABMT), as well as any number of other patients with other health needs where we are more confident of the likelihood of a significant therapeutic response. It is essentially for this reason that I said earlier that it "*may* be permissible" to fund protease inhibitors for individuals in earlier stages of HIV infection. It *will* be permissible only if substantial medical evidence and moral argument warrant it. For now that evidence and argument are not there.

Option #7: Fund protease inhibitors for those HIV-positive individuals whom best current medical evidence suggests are most likely to benefit significantly. This will involve some set of clinical protocols that will take into account both viral load and CD4 counts below 500/mL. For our plan this will mean about 25 % of our HIV-positive plan members will be eligible for plan funding of protease inhibitors. This will generate costs that ought to be bearable, even in a very competitive health care environment. Some health services may need to be dropped or trimmed in order to control the overall plan budget, but that should not be morally objectionable so long as those are marginally beneficial, low-priority services.

As noted earlier, what option 7 represents is a limited, non-ideal, just-enough option. It is limited and non-ideal because some unknown number of HIV-positive individuals in earlier stages of infection might be faced with serious health problems that might have been averted if they had had access to protease inhibitors earlier in the disease process. But it is still a "just-enough" option because we will be protecting the greatest range of fair equality of opportunity at the lowest feasible cost by choosing this option. That is, "merely" being HIV-positive for the first several years after initial infection does not seem to trigger any diminishment in functional capacities. Individuals can live lives that are quite normal for them from a functional perspective. Later, however, when individuals become vulnerable to serious opportunistic infections there is a real threat of premature death and substantial loss of functional capacity. If protease inhibitors can prevent or forestall that for years, then that generates a strong just claim to those resources *at that point, not before*. It is also significant that individuals who are HIV-positive are generally relatively young, which would also presumptively strengthen their claims to these resources, say, relative to much older patients faced with a terminal illness.

The argument could be made that Dr. Ho's theories will prove to be correct, that protease inhibitors given within months of initial infection defeat the virus entirely so that individuals can look forward to a normal life expectancy, but that delay in therapy will mean very premature death for HIV-positive individuals who will gain only 3–5 years of additional life from them. If this proved to be true, it would be unfortunate that we had committed ourselves to option #7 now, but those premature deaths would not be unjust. We could prevent them only by allocating resources in a way that would almost certainly generate serious and real injustices now on the basis of speculative scientific evidence. Further, that strategy could be justified only if it were generalized. But if it were generalized, that would undermine almost entirely any rational foundation for setting health care priorities in a world of changing and uncertain scientific information.

What I take to be a substantial virtue of option #7 is that it avoids the moral errors associated with our creation of the End Stage Renal Disease program under Medicare. In that program we pay for dialysis and kidney transplants for all who have the relevant need, whether they can benefit very substantially from the therapy or only very marginally, in either case at significant expense to limited public resources. We pay for kidney transplants at public expense but generally not for other major organ transplants. These look like arbitrary distinctions that are seriously unjust. We cannot afford to make that same mistake with AIDS patients, or with others who have comparable serious illnesses. Again, this pertains to another important lesson to be learned from the Oregon approach to health care rationing, namely, that rationing decisions made in an isolated non-systematic fashion are more likely to be unjust, or less likely to be explicable publicly and rationally.

Finally, if option #7 could be rationally and autonomously endorsed by HIV-positive individuals in the plan, as well as by the membership of the plan as a whole, then that would add substantially to the presumptive justness of this option. A mere thought experiment would not be very satisfactory. But there is a real-world option that could be tried within the moral space of rational democratic deliberation. We could permit liberalized and individualized access to protease inhibitors at plan expense. We might permit individuals with CD4 counts below 750/mL the option of accessing protease inhibitors to prevent any further decline in their immune system. This could have very substantial costs to the plan. So they would have to agree to a trade-off. They would have to be willing to give up aggressive and expensive life-prolonging care in the very end stages of disease, when, for example, there was less than a 25% chance they would survive another year. In effect, they decide for themselves which risks are worth taking and which benefits are costworthy enough from their point of view.

In order to protect overall fairness, and in order to make sure such an option did not support any form of invidious discrimination, this option would have to be framed in a way that covered any disease that had a similar enough clinical and cost profile. It may be the case, for example, that some new, very expensive, potentially very effective cancer drugs are being introduced that are not likely to cure a cancer but are likely to yield several good years of remission. They too might need to be taken on a regular basis for years with some uncertainty as to when it would be most cost-effective to begin therapy. They too would have this rationing option, which could be described in most general terms as permission for all patients to trade expensive marginal benefits very late in life for expensive marginal benefits earlier in life. Space does not permit any detailed assessment of what this option might look like in practice, or whether it might prove under close analysis to be seriously morally flawed. But, as a working hypothesis, I would suggest that such an option could be offered for rational democratic deliberation, that some managed care plans could endorse it as being "just enough," and others might reject it as being too morally risky, but both decisions would be "in bounds" morally speaking.

In conclusion, I have argued that a just and caring managed care plan could choose either option

#7 or what I will refer to as #7a. Both are "just enough," whereas I judge the prior options as falling below a minimal standard of justice. Options #7 and #7a are what ought to be recommended to a plan's board. Both options have enough wiggle room (when we really work through the details, such as a 20% co-pay to raise revenue, so long as there is a comparable requirement for comparable drugs for other medical problems) that the requirements of a competitive business environment could be accomodated without threatening the long-term fiscal viability of the plan.

NOTES

1. John Bartlett, "Protease Inhibitors for HIV Infection," *Annals of Internal Medicine* 124 (June, 1996): 1086–88.
2. "The End of AIDS?" *Newsweek* (Dec. 2, 1996): 64-73; David Dunlap, "Hype, Hope, and Hurt on the AIDS Front Lines," *The New York Times* (Feb. 2, 1997), E3.
3. Norman Daniels, *Just Health Care* (Cambridge University Press, 1985), 36–58.
4. Daniel Callahan, *What Kind of Life: The Limits of Medical Progress* (Simon and Schuster, 1990), esp. Chap. 4 "On the Ragged Edge: Needs, Endless Needs," 31–68.
5. This is the primary moral lesson from the Oregon experience with health care rationing. See Leonard M. Fleck, "Just Caring: Oregon, Health Care Rationing, and Informed Democratic Deliberation," *Journal of Medicine and Philosophy* 19 (Aug., 1994): 367–88.
6. For a fuller discussion of these issues see Wendy Mariner, "Business vs. Medical Ethics: Conflicting Standards for Managed Care," *Journal of Law, Medicine. and Ethics*, 23 (1995), 236–46.
7. Leonard M. Fleck, "Just Caring"; see also by Leonard M. Fleck, "Just Health Care Rationing: A Democratic Decisionmaking Approach," *University of Pennsylvania Law Review*, 140 (May, 1992), 1597–1636; and "Just Caring: Rational Democratic Deliberation, Health Care Rationing, and Managed Care," unpublished paper presented at American Bioethics Association meeting in San Francisco Nov., 1996).
8. For this line of argument see David Mechanic, "Professional Judgment and the Rationing of Medical Care," *University of Pennsylvania Law Review*, 140 (May, 1992), 1713–54.
9. For a discussion of the problem of invisible rationing in a managed care context see Leonard M. Fleck, "Justice, HMOs, and the Invisible Rationing of Health Care Resources," *Bioethics*, 4 (April, 1990), 97–120.

10. Tristram Engelhardt's libertarianism is the direct object of my criticisms in my paper "Just Health Care (I): Is Beneficence Enough?" *Theoretical Medicine,* 10 (June, 1989), 167–82.

11. Michael Waldholz, "Dr. Ho's Next Step in AIDS Research is a Remarkable Gamble," *The Wall Street Journal,* (Dec. 17, 1996), Al, A6.

12. Lawrence Altman, "Surviving with AIDS is One Problem; Cancer is Yet Another," *The New York Times* (May 6, 1997), B 10. He writes, "If the cancers are somehow related to problems with the immune system, therapies that prevent HIV damage to the immune system may prevent these cancers as well."

Rationing Experimental Treatments

Bone Marrow Transplants for Advanced Breast Cancer: The Story of Christine deMeurers

Alex John London

It was a frightening discovery.[1] At 32, Christine deMeurers was an active woman with a husband, two children, and a new job as a school teacher. It was 1992 and in the heat of late August the deMeurers were unprepared for the turn their lives were about to take. Christine had been at her new job for less than two months when she found a small lump in her left breast. A visit to her physician and some tests revealed that her worst fears were true; Christine had breast cancer.

The reality of her situation hit like a thunderclap. The speed with which breast cancer is treated can mean the difference between life and death, and the deMeurers knew it. Moving as quickly as possible, Christine underwent a radical mastectomy, radiation therapy, and a course of chemotherapy which ended in March of 1993. By May it was clear that her cancer had spread and Christine was told she had Stage IV metastatic breast cancer.

Like many Americans, the deMeurers received their health insurance through their employer, and like a growing number of people in this country they were members of a managed care plan. Christine had recently been hired to teach at the same school in Elsinore, California, where her husband had been teaching since 1989, and they had each signed up for the least expensive of the three health plans their school offered, Health Net of Woodland Hills, California.

Reprinted with permission from the author.

There is no reason to think that the deMeurers were unhappy with the treatment Christine had received from Health Net by the end of March 1993. Although it had not stopped the spread of her cancer, Christine had received prompt and aggressive treatment for a disease that affects 1 of every 9 American women and is the second leading cause of cancer deaths among women. At the end of these first months of 1993, Christine had exhausted the standard therapies that were available at the time, and it looked as though her cancer would soon overtake her.

Yet Christine's oncologist, Dr. Mahesh Gupta, offered hope. He suggested that Christine might be a candidate for a new procedure known as high-dose chemotherapy with autologous bone marrow transplant, or HDC/ABMT. Although the use of this procedure on women with Stage IV breast cancer was new and its efficacy largely unknown, HDC/ABMT was already accepted as a successful treatment of many non-solid forms of cancer such as Hodgkins disease and leukemia. The theory behind the procedure is simple. There is a direct correlation between the dose of chemotherapy a patient receives and its effect on the targeted cancer. The problem, however, is that there is a natural limit to the amount of these toxic agents the body can endure. In HDC/ABMT physicians remove stem cells from a patient's bone marrow, purify them of cancer cells, and then freeze them for later use. Patients are then exposed to near lethal doses of chemotherapy, up to 10 times the normal level. In addition to killing cancer cells, however, such concentrated amounts of these potent chemicals inevitably kill much of the patient's remaining bone marrow. So after receiving this high dose of chemotherapy the harvested and purified stem cells are transplanted back into the patient. There was, nevertheless, very little information and certainly no consensus among experts as to the efficacy of this procedure on solid tumors like Christine's.

Nevertheless, Dr. Gupta assured Christine that there were still options available, and in a breach of Health Net policy he referred her directly to a colleague at the Scripps Clinic in nearby La Jolla. Dissatisfied with their reception there, the deMeurers flew to Denver where Christine was evaluated by Dr. Roy B. Jones at the University of Colorado. Unlike their reception at Scripps, the deMeurers found a welcome ally in Dr. Jones who examined Christine on June 8, 1993 and told her that she might benefit from the HDC/ABMT procedure. It was a ray of hope in a very dark period of their lives.

On the same day that Christine was being examined by Dr. Jones, however, Health Net formally decided not to pay for the procedure on the grounds that the treatment "is not uniformly accepted as proven and effective for the treatment of metastatic breast cancer." The treatment was excluded under the so-called "investigational clause" in the Health Net contract. The deMeurers were crushed, but undaunted. Together they decided to try to obtain the new procedure any way they could, and they began taking every step possible. Christine secured permission to see a new oncologist who agreed with Dr. Jones' assessment of her situation and agreed to refer her to UCLA medical center. At the same time they began trying to raise the $100,000 it would take to pay for the procedure, and they hired a lawyer to write a formal appeal to Health Net's decision on Christine's behalf.

On June 25, Christine met with Dr. John Glaspy at the UCLA medical center who spelled out the risks involved with the procedure itself, the three months it would take to recover from the severity of the chemotherapy, and the rather steep price tag it entailed. Dr. Glaspy was himself a cautious proponent of the use of HDC/ABMT on women with Stage IV breast cancer, even though a 1992 review article by the respected health policy expert Dr.

David Eddy had concluded that there were no data to support the claim that this procedure was in any way superior to the standard dose of chemotherapy when treating women with metastatic breast cancer.[2] Cautious but optimistic, Dr. Glaspy said that he would perform the procedure if that was what they wanted. The deMeurers readily accepted.

What Dr. Glaspy did not know, what the deMeurers had purposefully made sure he would not know, was that Christine was a member of the Health Net plan. Wary of the influence that they suspected Health Net administrators had already exerted on the course of Christine's care, the deMeurers had decided to present themselves to Dr. Glaspy as paying customers rather than as members of a managed care plan. Ironically, this also prevented the deMeurers from finding out that Dr. Glaspy was a member of the Health Net committee which earlier that year had voted to deny coverage for bone marrow transplants to patients with Stage IV breast cancer.

Soon after their visit to UCLA, the deMeurers learned that Health Net had rejected their appeal. Preliminary tests at UCLA had shown that Christine's cancer had responded to initial doses of chemotherapy, but it was also quickly becoming clear that they would be unable to raise such a substantial amount of money on their own. So the deMeurers authorized their attorney to file for an injunction to force Health Net to pay for treatment and they enlisted Dr. Glaspy's help. The revelation that Christine was a member of Health Net put Dr. Glaspy in a terrible position. As a member of Health Net's transplantation committee, he had advocated covering HDC/ABMT for metastatic breast cancer. But in the end he had agreed with the committee's consensus to exclude it from coverage. Committed to advocating for his patient's interests, on September 13 Dr. Glaspy wrote to Health Net in support of Christine's injunction, "As a physician representing Christine, I have a responsibility to represent her interests and to help her achieve her goals in her health care." Exactly one week later, however, at the request of Health Net lawyers, he submitted a second, much less sanguine statement to Health Net concluding "This procedure is of unproven efficacy in the treatment of metastatic breast cancer, and the results of clinical trials to date are not sufficient to establish beyond doubt that it is superior to standard dose chemotherapy."

The deMeurers felt betrayed and alone. The second letter from Dr. Glaspy only strengthened their resentment of Health Net and their distrust of its doctors. Dr. Glaspy was also painfully aware of the blow he had dealt to the deMeurer's trust. But he was also aware of the dissatisfaction his first letter had caused at Health Net, especially in light of the fact that he was a member of the committee that voted not to cover this procedure. Health Net was upset that a member of its own committee was actively trying to thwart the very regulations he had helped to design, and the phone calls of Health Net officials to Dr. Glaspy's boss, Dr. Dennis Slamon, revealed the depth of the company's dissatisfaction

In an attempt to salvage as much of the medical center's relationship with the deMeurers and with Health Net as possible, Dr. Slamon arrived at a compromise. He decided that UCLA would absorb the costs of Christine's procedure, thus relieving Health Net of any obligation to pay and enabling Christine to receive the healthcare she so desperately wanted. On September 23, 1993 Christine was admitted to UCLA to begin the first phase of treatment. According to her husband, she experienced four disease-free months after recovering from the severe chemotherapy, but by the Spring of 1994 she was ill again and on March 10, 1995 Christine deMeurers succumbed to her cancer.

The story of Christine deMeurers is not typical of most people's experience with managed care, but because it is such an extreme case it casts some of the most serious problems facing the American healthcare system into stark relief. It is the story of a family coping with a terrible disease and unifying around the common cause of exhausting every possible treatment option. It is also the story of a woman who must not only battle cancer, but must also struggle with her insurance company for the treatment she so desperately wants. Similarly, Christine's story illustrates the way physicians have found themselves trapped between two worlds of health care. In Dr. Glaspy we see the old fee-for-service system and the new medicine under managed care clashing in its most palpable form. In these ways, Christine's story is a miniature portrait of the way we think about health care in America and the problems we are facing as the cost of care outstrips our collective ability to pay for it.

After World War II, medical research in the United States flourished, and the marriage of increased research funding with top-flight science gave birth to a formidable array of new therapeutic drugs and devices that enabled physicians to conquer injuries and diseases in a way that would have been unthinkable only years earlier. As amazing as the feats such advances were making possible, however, was the price tag that came with them. The nation's health care expenditures began to climb sharply in the post-war years, and by 1976 General Motors announced that it was spending more money on the health care of its workers than on steel. As the decade drew to a close there was a collective recognition on the part of the corporate sector that something had to be done to keep the cost of health care from hemorrhaging out of control.[3]

Because most Americans receive their health insurance through their employers, the corporate sector was coming to see the high cost of their employees' benefits as a threat to their ability to remain competitive. The choice seemed terrible but unavoidable. How long before industry would have to choose between competitive viability and employee health care? It was in response to this dilemma that managed care companies like Health Net arose with the mandate of stemming the swiftly rising tide of health care costs.

In an important way, the rise of managed care and our reaction to the way it has tried to carry out its mandate illustrates the fundamentally paradoxical relationship that Americans have to medicine in general and to their health care providers in particular. On the one hand, we embrace the values of frugality and fiscal sensibility which lead us to protest against the dizzying rate at which health care costs have been rising. At the same time, we will not tolerate receiving anything less than the latest, most sophisticated health care.[4] We don't want to see restrictions put on our liberty when it comes to being able to seek out and obtain the latest and most advanced medical procedures from the most well-trained providers, yet we also bristle at the restrictions on our liberty that come in the form of the higher taxes, product prices, or insurance premiums that inevitably result from the exercise of this freedom.

In the story of Christine deMeurers we have a concrete and powerful illustration of the way these conflicting values can intersect in the lives of the most vulnerable people. Christine represents the way we have come to look to the frontiers of medicine in the face of the ravages of sickness and disease. Here is a young, productive woman with a life of her own, a family, children, who is also dying from a terrible disease. When the standard modalities of treatment are exhausted, she looks to the frontiers of medical science and places her hopes in a relatively untested procedure of questionable therapeutic value for the chance to live out some portion of her remaining months free of disease. With no other medical options and without the resources to secure this chance for herself, she looks to a third party to cover the expenses and make it possible.

Debate over the benefit that receiving HDC/ABMT had for Christine deMeurers is still mixed. The officials at Health Net stick by their initial decision to deny coverage and Dr. Glaspy admits that Christine would probably have lived longer without the treatment. Clinical trials to test the efficacy of the procedure are under way in a number of cities across the country, but there is still no consensus on whether HDC/ABMT is more effective than standard chemotherapy for women with metastatic breast cancer. For Alan deMeurers, however, the procedure was worth it. It allowed his wife to live a better quality of life for a few short months and to spend one final Christmas with him and their two children. Even if Dr. Glaspy is right, it is the quality of the life Christine led for those four months that matters most to her husband, not simply the length of time she remained alive.

The public reaction to cases like Christine's has mostly been one of outrage. The media was critical of the influence Health Net officials exerted on the medical decisions of the program's physicians, and juries were eager to teach the plan's plutocratic administrators a lesson. In 1993 Health Net lost a lawsuit filed by Jim Fox, the husband of Nelene Fox, a Health Net subscriber who had been denied HDC/ABMT for her Stage IV breast cancer on the grounds that it was experimental and investigational. The jury awarded Nelene's estate $12 million in actual damages and $77 million in punitive damages, although Health Net later agreed to pay only $5 million in exchange for their right to appeal the verdict. Nevertheless, the members of the jury were eager to send a message to health care companies. "You cannot substitute profits for good-quality health care," one juror was quoted as saying.

The Fox verdict precipitated a rash of similar judgments on behalf of women who had been denied coverage for HDC/ABMT for advanced breast cancer, and in 1995 a California arbitration board awarded one million dollars to the estate of Christine deMeurers on the ground that phone calls which Health Net officials had placed to Christine's physicians at various stages in her treatment had exerted undue influence on the doctor-patient relationship. In addition to a fury of litigation, these cases have given rise to legislation in a number of states requiring insurers to pay for HDC/ABMT for women with metastatic breast cancer. The result of these suits and of state congressional action has been to free up patients' access to specialists and to procedures which their insurance providers would otherwise have excluded as investigational or experimental. Yet, amidst the lurid details of some of the questionable activities on the part of officers at Health Net and other HMOs, and in the rush to right what look like injustices that were being perpetrated against the women who were denied access to HDC/ABMT, we seem to have lost sight of the difficult but enduring questions at the very heart of this issue. Should we, should the government or insurance companies, pay for people's access to procedures of this nature? Should we pay for costly medical procedures of unknown therapeutic benefit when there are people struggling to get access to a host of genuinely effective therapies? Are four disease free months in the life of a terminally ill person worth the $100,000 to $200,000 it takes to secure them? Could this money be better spent somewhere else? If we do not draw the line on medical expenses in front of cases like this, then where do we draw it?

In the wake of cases like those of the deMeurers and the Foxs we have struggled with these questions in a very piecemeal and largely inchoate way. On the one hand, the judiciary has consistently sided with plaintiffs in these cases, making it very clear that those with the resources to make themselves heard and with voices articulate enough to make their case compelling can receive access to these sorts of therapies while the less articulate and less well off cannot. On the other hand, as of the end of 1995 at least seven states had mandated coverage for HDC/ABMT for breast cancer although such mandates do not necessarily apply to all forms of insurance providers, and it is rare that such mandates are formulated around a coherent set of health care goals.[5]

The patchwork of judicial and legislative decisions rendered in response to these cases amount to a de facto way of answering the difficult questions posed a moment ago. But surely this is no way to deal with such important and fundamental issues of public policy. The system may provide greater access for some, but in a way that seems arbitrary at best and inequitable or unjust at worst. We may benefit from the psychological comforts of avoiding some very public, "tragic choices," but this is very likely the illusory comfort of the fine new garments the Emperor is wearing.[6] We have to ask ourselves whether we have responded to these cases in such a way as to make the system more just, or whether we haven't simply shifted the burden of injustice off of those who are most capable of defending themselves onto those who are least able to do so.

By acquiescing to the de facto practice that has emerged for dealing with these cases, we have done ourselves, our health care providers, and our third-party payers a terrible disservice. We have left unanswered important questions about which kinds of medical interventions we should be in the business of helping people obtain. We have left the insurance industry without substantive guidelines by which to determine the kinds of interventions they need to cover and the kinds they may need to exclude. This in turn perpetuates a system of disclosure on the part of insurers which keeps subscribers largely in the dark as to the nature of excluded therapies, the methods used for making such determinations, and the process by which the subscriber can influence these guidelines or appeal such decisions. This may have provided litigious subscribers with the power to obtain exotic medical interventions, but the system in which this kind of arbitrary power exists seems to work against our common commitment to reducing health care costs and to spreading the burdens of doing so evenly among the members of society. To

that extent, the maintenance of this piecemeal way of creating public policy works against many of our own explicit and publicly held commitments to fairness and fiscal responsibility.

This leaves subscribers with the unenviable feeling of being trapped in an unfriendly system that has been imposed on them from above. In the absence of some form of communal conversation about these difficult and enduring questions, we will make little headway against the antagonistic and largely adversarial relationship developing between patients, their insurance providers, and the health care workers who are increasingly asked to facilitate the very different aims of these two parties.[7] We need to ask ourselves why so many of these cases wound up in the judicial system. Would subscribers who were given a more active role in the creation of policy guidelines or in the decision-making process of their insurance provider feel the need to take their claims to court? How can we facilitate a more active role for subscribers? Similarly, are there ways we could improve the system so that subscribers whose claims have been denied can appeal their decision and feel that their needs are receiving legitimate and sincere consideration? Would subscribers be as eager to litigate if they felt their claims had received fair consideration in an equitable review process? Would lawsuits have as much merit if insurance companies could point to such a process of appeal?

By giving subscribers a more active role in the formation of the guidelines that govern their care, insurance providers will give their subscribers a stake in making sure such guidelines are both fair and effective. It will also reassure subscribers that they are being treated as ends in themselves and not as mere means. But in order to accomplish these goals we are going to have to improve the way that insurance providers disclose information to their subscribers, and this means that providers and subscribers alike are going to have to deliberate together on how to answer some very important questions. In the case of HDC/ABMT this means that we are going to have to ask whether women with advanced breast cancer should receive coverage for this procedure, and if not, why not.

Health Net, like most managed care companies, denied coverage for HDC/ABMT on the grounds that it was investigational or experimental. The rationale behind this move was simple. First, insurers could make a strong case that there is only an obligation to pay for therapies that are proven to have some therapeutic benefit. The case for this normative claim looks especially strong when we add the premise that there are not even enough resources to cover everyone's access to proven therapies. Second, with this argument on the table the claim that a drug or a procedure is experimental looks more like a straightforward descriptive claim than it does a controversial normative judgment. So excluding an intervention as experimental allowed the insurance provider to maintain the appearance of making coverage decisions without having to make delicate and controversial judgments about the monetary value of the length and quality of human life. Finally, this general attitude toward experimental treatments was perfectly consistent with the public's view of human experimentation in the wake of scandals such as Willowbrook, Tuskegee, and the Jewish Chronic Disease Hospital case.* That is, the denial of access to experimental drugs and procedures fit nicely with the public's view that such things were usually dangerous and to be avoided.

In the 1980s, however, social attitudes towards experimental treatments started to change as patients dying of AIDS began to clamor for access to the experimental drugs and devices which were being held up in what they came to view as a paternalistic system of federal oversight. In the 1980s experimental drugs and procedures came to be seen, not as dangerous things to which no one wanted to be subjected, but rather as the last desperate hope for dying patients. This shift in attitude put pressure on the normative claim that people should not receive access to experimental drugs, but it also brought into question the notion that labeling something as experimental was a purely descriptive and non-normative claim.

Time and again the insurance industry's claim that HDC/ABMT was experimental was challenged by lawyers and physicians. What makes a drug or procedure experimental? Is it the fact that it is not a part of the established medical practice? But medicine is a notoriously recalcitrant social practice and it can take some time for innovative

and effective procedures to be widely adopted. This raises the question of whose medical practice we are talking about. Are we concerned with the standard practices of the larger medical community or only of the most knowledgeable experts? Lawyers had no problem finding expert oncologists to testify about the number of their colleagues who were performing HDC/ABMT on women with advanced breast cancer at some of the most prestigious medical institutions in the world. So if this was the criterion for something's being "experimental," HDC/ABMT didn't seem to fit the bill. Perhaps then something is experimental when it has not received FDA approval. But many of the drugs and procedures involved in HDC/ABMT had received FDA approval for other uses, and there are many drugs and procedures that are used effectively for purposes for which they were not initially approved. Also, FDA approval often requires that a procedure's efficacy be shown in a randomized clinical trial, but there are difficult moral problems associated with conducting this kind of trial on a procedure of this sort.

As a result, in case after case judges and juries told managed care companies that the experimental exclusion clause in their subscriber contract did not apply to HDC/ABMT for advanced breast cancer. But these judgments were based on the inadequate definitions offered by the managed care companies. They should not be taken as speaking to the underlying question of whether this is the sort of treatment third parties should be financing. If policy holders and their providers are going to have an open and productive debate about this question, then they are going to have to ask frank questions about the kinds of health care goals they are willing to support and to what degree. Undoubtedly this is going to require each of us to look at the giant pink elephant standing in the middle of the room: how much money are we willing to spend to improve the quality of a terminally ill patient's life for a few months given the other kinds of health care needs our plan must meet?

The questions raised by cases like that of Christine deMeurers are often perceived as instances of the familiar and intractable conflict between consequentialist concerns about money and utility and deontic concerns for the dignity of

*EDITOR'S NOTE: See Part 5, Section 1.

persons. Although they can easily be understood along these lines, it is important to see that this is not the only or necessarily the best way to think about them. It is true that a careful look at the historical record will show that at the time, many of these cases may have in fact been about a straightforward conflict between money and autonomy. But this might simply be evidence for the inadequacy of this way of structuring the problem rather than for the claim that this is the only way to structure it.

One thing seems clear. To the extent that plan members are forced to submit to policies which they themselves have not either helped to shape or voluntarily chosen, people will continue to feel that someone else has put a price on the length and quality of their lives, and this will continue to foster feelings of antagonism and resentment.[8] To the extent that plan members can actively participate in shaping the policies which govern their treatment or choose their plan based on the policies that best reflect their conception of the value of health care, the restrictions placed on their care will represent an extension of their own autonomy. To that extent they will represent people's considered judgments about the way their needs should be met given the fact of fiscal scarcity and the need to distribute the benefits and burdens of health care fairly amongst the members of the plan. Considerations of costs and benefits may be important factors which shape these decisions, but in the end the moral legitimacy of these decisions will be based on the fact that the resulting policies are the product of the autonomous and considered judgments of the very people they are meant to cover.

In the end, the story of Christine deMeurers confronts us with two basic and interconnected problems. First, how should we answer the difficult questions with which this case confronts us? Second, how can we make sure that there are not more cases like this? How can we ensure that there are structures in place which will facilitate our ability to deliberate about these questions together, and which will reflect the conclusions that such deliberations reach? How can we shape the practices and procedures of our health care system in a way that will facilitate and accommodate this increased interaction between providers, subscribers, and health care workers? We should not shrink from making these difficult decisions together or from the recognition that some of these choices may be tragic, so long as we can maintain the conviction that the decisions we make are fair and that the system we create is more just than the one we have now.

NOTES

1. The details presented here about Christine deMeurers' battle with breast cancer and her HMO have been taken from published accounts by Erik Larson, "The Soul of an HMO," *Time Magazine* (January 22, 1996) and George Anders, *Health Against Wealth* (New York: Houghton Mifflin Company, 1996), chapter seven.

2. David Eddy, "High Dose Chemotherapy with Autologous Bone Marrow Transplantation for the Treatment of Metastatic Breast Cancer," *Journal of Clinical Oncology* 1992, 10(4):657-670.

3. For a more detailed account of the rise of managed care see E. Haavi Morreim, *Balancing Act: The New Medical Ethics of Medicine's New Economics* (Washington, D.C.: Georgetown University Press, 1995) pp.8-17 and George Anders, *Health Against Wealth* op cit.

4. For a trenchant criticism of the conflicting views Americans have about health and health care see Daniel Callahan, *What Kind of Life* (Washington, D.C.: Georgetown University Press, 1994).

5. Reinhard Priester, Karen G. Gervais and Dorthy E. Vawter, *Improving Coverage for Unproven Health Care Interventions* (Minnesota Center for Health Care Ethics, August, 1996), p. 5.

6. For the view that we should avoid the appearance of making tragic choices, even when the choices themselves are unavoidable, see Guido Calabresi and Philip Bobbitt *Tragic Choices* (New York: W. W. Norton and Company, 1978).

7. For an analysis of the way the interests of these three parties can conflict and some suggestions for managing these conflicts see my "Thrasymachus and Managed Care: How Not to Think About the Craft of Medicine" in Ronald Polansky and Mark Kuczewski, eds. *Bioethics: Modern Problems, Classical Solutions* (Pittsburgh: Mathesis Publications, 1998).

8. For a view of the importance of subscriber consent within a managed care plan, see Paul T. Menzel, *Strong Medicine* (New York: Oxford University Press, 1990). For the importance of being able to select a plan that coheres with one's vision of the role of health care in one's life, see Ezekiel J. Emanuel, *The Ends of Human Life* (Cambridge: Harvard University Press, 1991).

Rationing Medical Enhancements

The Coverage of Happiness: When Prozac Meets Universal Coverage

Robert Wright

There are two conversations going on in America right now that might usefully get in touch with each other. One is about President Clinton's health care plan, which includes extensive mental health coverage. The other is about mental health. The second conversation is known as the Prozac debate, though Prozac isn't the issue. This best-selling anti-depressant, said to make people "better than well," is just an emblem for a new age of psychopharmacology in which mental health and mental illness will lose their current meanings. Major depression, minor depression, a dour outlook, occasional moodiness, a short attention span, vocationally costly standoffishness—all these (the scenario goes) will be subject to swift and clean chemical intervention. "Cosmetic pharmacology" will let us custom-build minds and personalities.

The questions raised by cosmetic pharmacology are large, and by no means have they been exhaustively addressed. But also large, and almost entirely unaddressed, is the question of what happens when the government steps in—when Washington becomes the guarantor of this suddenly metamorphosing thing known as mental health. Granted that health care should be an entitlement. Granted even, for the sake of argument, that mental health care, in the traditional sense of the term, should be an entitlement. Should *happiness* be an entitlement?

People have enough trouble with the question of whether psychopharmacology is spiritually legitimate and ultimately beneficial for any one user. Once the government gets involved, the assessment acquires a confounding social dimension. Deciding which productivity-boosting drugs to pay for is a kind of economic policy. Deciding which kinds of patients get them is social policy. When drugs affect

the conscience, or sexual impulses, the government is making moral policy. And all along, in the background, is the question of whether neurochemistry should be a policy lever in the first place.

O.K., O.K.: this is a bit too dramatic. The government already has, via FDA drug approval, a rough kind of control over some of these variables. And even via mental health coverage it won't be able to fine-tune all of them, at least not for now. Prozac is blunt in its effects compared with the anticipated drugs of tomorrow. Still, Prozac is also diverse in its effects, and thus broadly illustrative. Already it is influencing, in small ways, the nation's economy, its moral texture and its social equality, or lack thereof. And in the process, it is suggesting that, oddly, the best way to keep the brave new world grounded in bedrock American values may be to bring cosmetic pharmacology to the masses.

The Prozac-as-policy debate begins with the same question as the Prozac debate: Is psychopharmacology a valid form of self-help? Lately a lot of people have been suggesting not. (See, for example, "Shiny Happy People" by David J. Rothman, TNR, February 14.) The basic argument is that drugs are a palliative; chemicals can address symptoms, but only sustained grappling, through talk therapy or soul-searching, gets at the "real" underlying problem. This argument is usually grounded, implicitly or explicitly, in a kind of dualism that sees mental life as at least partly independent of physiology; there are some places in the mind that molecules just won't take you.

In opposition to this view stand psychological materialists, who insist that all thought and feeling, and all changes therein, are precisely grounded in neurochemistry. Thus, when therapists talk, they emit sound waves that go into their patients' ears and trigger physical signals that go to the brain, which then triggers various other physical things. These things may be as trivial as stimulation of the

From *The New Republic*, March 14, 1994, pp. 24–26, 28–29. Copyright © 1994 The New Republic, Inc. Reprinted by permission of the publisher.

lachrymal glands (crying), which usually makes people feel better at least for a few hours, during which they can schedule another session. Or the change may be more profound, an actual cure. But the materialist's claim has always been that in either case the action is physical; to cure a patient's mental illness is to permanently alter biochemistry. This claim draws only credence from a drug like Prozac, which, by altering brain chemistry, leaves many patients feeling utterly cured, and makes them behaviorally indistinguishable from patients cured by psychotherapy.

The claim also draws credence from what little we know about how Prozac works. A frequent psychological effect of Prozac is to raise self-esteem, and neurologists believe it does this through its primary chemical effect: raising the level of the neurotransmitter serotonin. (Prozac "inhibits re-uptake" of serotonin by the brain cells, as do other less publicized, but similarly effective drugs, such as Paxil and Zoloft.) There is tentative evidence that serotonin levels also rise when self-esteem grows through conventional means—when say, someone gets a promotion or otherwise gains respect at the office. Much research remains to be done, but the best guess for now is that one function of serotonin is to calibrate self-esteem in accordance with social feedback. Thus talk therapists who provide feedback that raises self-esteem may in fact do what Prozac does: raise the serotonin level. Of course, they describe it differently. They say they get the patient to believe in his worth, and that any rise in the serotonin level is incidental. But who knows which comes first—or whether either does?

Even talk therapists who concede that serotonin may be the currency of their influence might still cling to the claim that, by intervening verbally and not chemically, they're raising self-esteem more "authentically" than Prozac does. But in what sense? They don't, after all, actually get their patient a promotion, or otherwise raise the amount of respect he gets. They just convince him that he *deserves* respect—the same thing Prozac does. Of course, in both cases, this belief may then make him more likely to *get* a promotion or more respect. But the initial intervention is in both cases artificial: the objective circumstances of the patient's life haven't changed; his way of looking at life has, along with, apparently, a rise in his serotonin.

Drugs, as chemicals that affect thought and feeling, have always tended to weigh in on the materi-

alist side of the debate. But this century has brought drugs especially forceful in their testimony by virtue of the subtlety of their effects, and the Prozac generation is the latest example. (In *Listening to Prozac*, the book that has framed the Prozac debate, psychiatrist Peter Kramer's former dualism undergoes ongoing, though incomplete, erosion as he describes the psychic make-overs he has witnessed.) No one can be sure about the culmination of this trend—what the final outcome (if any) of the dualism debate will be. My own view is that using the Prozac craze as an occasion to denounce psychological materialism, as many have done, is like choosing D-Day to announce your support of the Axis powers. But for present purposes, the point is more modest: the dualists' basic argument is far from proven and, indeed, has tended to weaken with technological advance. In this light, an intelligent government mental health policy must begin with the assumption that, although any given drug may have bad effects, and thus be undesirable, any good effects are valid—as valid as if earned arduously by lying on a couch and chatting. Pharmacology is not *inherently* suspect.

This is now the operative assumption within the Clinton administration. Last year, as the health care plan was taking shape, mental health coverage drew resistance from the administration's fiscal conservatives, who saw it as a giant dollar-shredder; their nightmare was every American on a therapist's couch, complaining nebulously as the meter ran at a $3-per-minute clip. In reply, mental health advocates, such as Tipper Gore and Ira Magaziner, argued successfully that psychopharmacology was bringing a new age of cheaper and more certain treatment.

This is not to say that the administration's mental health advocates are bullish on "cosmetic pharmacology"—a phrase that doesn't have quite the political resonance of "mental health care." Dr. Bernard Arons, who chaired the administration's mental health advisory group, insists that the line can and will be drawn between the two kinds of intervention. Well, maybe. But the administration has already blurred it a little. In selling mental health coverage, officials have stressed not only pharmacology's cheapness; the very fact that pharmacology works, they have said, is evidence that mental maladies are bona fide, diagnosable diseases, not just vague and elusive discomforts that get mulled over endlessly on the couch. But if successful chemical treatment indeed is the hallmark of a disease, then why aren't all things treated by cosmetic pharmacology considered diseases? And why shouldn't they be? One of the Clinton plan's two prerequisites for mental health treatment is "functional impairment in family, work, school or community activities." Well, those of us who aren't perfect in all our roles are exhibiting some degree of functional impairment. If pharmacology can make us less impaired, and happier, and if there is indeed nothing wrong with chemical intervention in principle, then what's the problem? Why is this not a cure?

The Clinton plan answers this question with its other prerequisite for coverage: the functional impairment must be linked with a "diagnosable mental illness." Here the administration is counting on the American Psychiatric Association's Diagnostic and Statistical Manual (DSM) to distinguish between the merely treatable and the officially pathological. But as Kramer shows in *Listening to Prozac*, what is officially pathological has long depended on what is treatable. For most of this century, people didn't complain of "panic attacks," and doctors didn't know them when they saw them. Freud had deemed panic anxiety unresponsive to psychotherapy, and that was that. But then two drugs, imipramine and Xanax, turned out to stifle panic (though Xanax proved quite addictive). As Kramer puts it, psychiatrists who had "lost touch with panic anxiety" now had to be "educated before they could see the problem." Panic anxiety was "re-created . . . in theoretical terms." Kramer describes such revision as the scholarly "dissection" of mental illness with the scalpel of pharmacology. A more crass (and not really incompatible) view is that it is the market at work. Once something that causes discomfort is treatable, people will pay for the treatment. If you're a psychiatrist, you have to call the discomfort a malady before you can take their money.

There's another dynamic at work, too. As growing numbers of people are thus treated and "cured," the untreated are increasingly conspicuous in their suffering. Mental illness has always been defined somewhat relatively; the more statistically aberrant a condition, the stronger its claim to pathology. Cosmetic pharmacology, by easing various conditions in *some* people, will shore up these claims for the others.

One recent pharmacological "dissection" suggests that some people who exhibit hysterical behavior suffer mainly from oversensitivity to rejection. Some drugs, including Prozac, dull this sensitivity in hysterics and, more to the point, in many nonhysterics. Kramer writes: "Once we focus on rejection-sensitivity apart from hysteria, all sorts of people come to mind to whom the label might apply." Yeah—like everyone. Thus could the concept of pathology grow in lockstep with psychopharmacology. Thus could a government commitment to provide therapy become, willy-nilly, an endlessly growing commitment. Thus could happiness become an entitlement.

Obviously, this won't happen overnight. The DSM evolves slowly. Besides, some analysts, such as Harold Pincus of the APA, argue that the DSM isn't as promiscuous as it is reputed to be. Its growth over the decades, as more things have become treatable, is misleading, Pincus says; new "subcategories" of illness haven't necessarily raised the number of people covered. Cases of panic disorder might just have been shoehorned under a broader label before. Still, as cosmetic pharmacology unfolds, the DSM will have its virtue sorely tested. And I see nothing inherently wrong with extensive surrender (or, alternatively, and perhaps preferably, with dropping the explosive and in many way's unfortunate word "disease," and calling all mental maladies, major, minor and barely noticeable, occasions for welcome intervention).

Anyway, the question of universal health care in the age of Prozac isn't just whether the government will get sucked into the cosmetic pharmacology business. Presumably it can resist if resistance is the right path. The question is whether resistance is the right path. My answer is no.

Just look at what resistance brings—which is to say look at the present situation. For both cultural and economic reasons, Prozac is mainly a drug of the upper and upper-middle classes. (And this is especially true of its "cosmetic" use.) Should the government—should a *Democratic* government—sit idly by when, absent government action, cosmetic pharmacology will be available to some groups, especially the affluent and the white, and not to others?

Of course, lots of things in life are concentrated at the upper end of the income scale. (Money, for example.) What's more, in the realm of health care, this inequity isn't beyond practical justification. Any realistically affordable universal health scheme will reserve "luxuries"—such as nonessential knee surgery diagnosed with expensive nuclear magnetic resonance imaging—for people who can pay more. Still, a robust knee is one thing, and robust self-esteem another. There is something peculiarly obnoxious about denying Prozac to poor people, because what it offers (when it works) is exactly what circumstance has denied many of them. The classic Prozac personality is the personality that so many affluent people absorb during youth, and this absorption is what sustains their affluence. They are upbeat, self-assured, efficient. The Prozac annals contain stories of people who once shirked vocational challenge, or wasted workdays commiserating with themselves—but then, after taking the drug, become human dynamos, wowing the boss, getting that big promotion. Even granting a certain amount of exaggeration, we have to ask: If the drug indeed works in this fashion for any appreciable fraction of people, should it be denied people because they can't afford it? Its absence may be the *reason* they can't afford it.

I am not recommending airdrops of Prozac into Appalachia and South-Central Los Angeles. Though Prozac has clearly helped a lot of people who weren't mentally ill by stringent definition, the evidence that it can improve the life of the *average* person, plucked randomly off the street, is at best sparsely anecdotal, and the anecdotes come from journalists, not psychiatrists. (No one drug will ever be right for everyone; the premise of the Prozac debate is simply that as the future unfolds, more and more people will have a drug that's right for them.) And, though early claims that Prozac can encourage suicide have fallen into question, Prozac's side effects aren't always minor—insomnia, nervousness, sexual dysfunction, etc. Serious pharmacology, cosmetic or otherwise, always calls for clinical discernment. The point is just that whatever degree of discernment is open to the rich should be opened to the poor: the seriously ill, the mildly ill and the not-quite-ill-but-not-beyond-improvement should have access to supervised experimentation if it is likely to help.

Surprisingly, there is some question over how equitably the Clinton plan would help even the undeniably ill. One of the plan's less discussed features is its likely provision of better coverage for the affluent. Each HMO that formed under the plan would, within limits, set its own premium, and if a customer chose a pricey HMO, he—not his employer, not the government—would cover the difference between its cost and the average cost. So lower-income people would cluster in cheaper HMOs. (This is the plan's implicit acknowledgment of the point above: affordable universal care won't be luxurious for everyone.) Though each HMO would cover the same list of maladies, as defined in the DSM, that leaves plenty of wiggle room. Some existing HMOs are said to save money by discouraging treatment for the mentally ill, or by putting them on muddy, paleo-antidepressants, whose patents have expired, rather than pay $2 per pill for the usually cleaner relief of the Prozac generation. Government oversight—which is provided in the Clinton plan—might be needed to ensure equity among the mentally ill.

As for the not-so-ill, the candidates for cosmetic psychopharmacology—their situation would remain in one sense unchanged under the Clinton plan; their chances of getting drugs would vary by income. Liberal prescription might be an unstated benefit of some upscale HMOs—and if it weren't, the affluent could still get wonder drugs by going to a doctor and paying for the visit and the prescription out-of-pocket. In more modest HMOs, cosmetic pharmacology would probably be nil. This shortcoming is not one that any of the alternative health care plans—Cooper, Chafee, etc.—would obviously redress. But that doesn't make it any less of a shortcoming. Our nation has always paid lip service to equality of opportunity. And the stated reason for falling short of that goal has usually been cost. If indeed opportunity can be boosted as markedly, as cheaply, as some Prozac stories suggest, that excuse weakens. (Prozac costs $15 per week at standard prices—plus the occasional half-hour of "maintenance" therapy—and HMOs get bulk deals that cut the price to $8, less than the price of school lunches.)

Redressing the current inequity would of course raise all kinds of fears. Will Prozac simply numb the poor to their harsh world? It is a perfectly good (if slightly patronizing) question. But most people haven't lost much sleep over the other things that numb poor people—alcohol, street drugs, Lotto. At least, we didn't lose much sleep until the drugs started raising our chances of getting shot. It seems odd to have saved all our concern for a drug that, unlike street drugs, may actually help people.

Once the government is paying for drugs, they warrant a special kind of scrutiny. Critics of Prozac have tended to focus on the drug's users, claiming, for example, that inflated self-esteem or indifference to social rejection may hurt them in the long run. Maybe so, but this is a question already being mulled over by the users and their therapists. The more neglected and much harder question is the one that is the government's to ask: What are the larger social effects of the particular kind of happiness brought by a given drug?

People take both cocaine and the designer drug Ecstasy to get happy, yet the effects are in some ways opposite. Cocaine brings a self-centered euphoria, a sense of toughness or smartness or beauty. It inflates the ego. Ecstasy in a sense dilutes the ego, leading people to take an interest, even a joy, in people they might otherwise ignore. Both drugs make people happy, but one makes them happy jerks. Both, also, don't work in the long run. There may be subsequent fits of depression and even a kind of psychosis: and Ecstasy has the added disadvantage of killing brain cells. It may well be that the sorts of euphoria these drugs bring can never become a regular part of the personality. Still, Prozac has shown that more modest elevations needn't be transient; drugs can make people—some people, at least—happier in the long run. There is no reason to doubt that happiness of various stripes can be raised in the long run. Should the government subsidize egocentric as well as empathetic happiness?

This issue is already with us, if in unwieldy form. In *Listening to Prozac*, Kramer describes giving Prozac to "Tess" for a condition that, he somewhat defensively admits, might be described as "heightened awareness of the needs of others." She "heeded the warning of a strong 'superego,' or conscience, that always put work before play." The drug worked. "Where once she had focused on obligations to others, now she was vivacious and fun-loving." But Kramer wonders if Tess will "now give up her work in the projects, as if I had administered her a pill to cure warmheartedness and progressive social beliefs." Then he begins to probe this concern, wondering "whether I was clinging to an arbitrary valuation of temperament, as if the melancholy or saturnine humor were in some way morally superior to the sanguine." A reasonable question for a psychiatrist, given his

role. But surely the government, given its role, isn't exhibiting arbitrary valuation if it chooses not to pay for things that make people less inclined to help others. Where people withhold such help, the government may have to step in and do the job. Why raise taxes to pay for Prozac that creates a need for more taxes?

Tess, in the end, "did not forsake the projects, though she did make more time for herself." This new time, presumably, came marginally at the expense of people in the projects. And, anyway, one can imagine cases in which the patient's peace of mind reaches some critical mass, leaving no time for people she had once helped. Much of the good we do for others is motivated by painful guilt, and often the net social result is good: the happiness we give outweighs the discomfort that prompts the giving.

Tess also moved to another town, the furthest she had lived from her mother; she had overcome "a guilty vigilance over a mother about whom she had strong ambivalent feelings." Kramer (who is utterly aware of the basic moral questions raised by Prozac, notwithstanding the claims of some facile critics) allows that the virtue of this move "depends on one's social values." Yes, and when Tess's Prozac is being paid for by the government, the operative values become clearer. The breakdown of the extended family as a network of social support has cost gobs of tax dollars. (And, back when the extended family functioned better, you can bet that "guilt" and ambivalence" reared their heads more than occasionally.) Does it make sense to spend tax dollars to further decompose the family?

I'm not saying Prozac is inherently an egocentric or socially pathological drug. As Kramer notes, Prozac sometimes frees the self-absorbed to care about others. The anecdotal evidence suggests that the drug has more positive social side effects— externalities, as policy analysts say—than negative ones. The point is simply that happiness is neither a homogeneous nor a socially neutral quality. And there is more logic in subsidizing some kinds of happiness than others. As pharmacology advances, bringing ever more surgical tools of psychic intervention, the government may have the option of choosing between the two, trying to assess the positive and negative externalities embedded in each new miracle molecule.

One can imagine, for example, a divorce antidote. Prozac often dulls the sex drive—especially that great enemy of family values, the male sex drive. Some men say Prozac has saved their marriage, not only by thus stifling extracurricular interests, but by making their marital sexuality more intimate. "My wife was so happy with that side effect, and so am I," says Dr. James Goodwin, the celebrated (and denounced) "pied piper of Prozac," who has single-handedly raised the average serotonin level in the small town of Wenatchee, Washington, and takes the drug himself. Goodwin speaks of male patients who, once on Prozac, look back with dismay at all the time they spent eyeing women lasciviously or buying pornography. (Just think of the careers that could have been saved: Gary Hart and Jim Bakker have both reported taking Prozac since their troubles.) It may be time for Dan Quayle to amend Nancy Reagan's line: Say yes just to Prozac.

On the other hand, some people—often women, by Goodwin's account—say Prozac has given them the courage to leave unhappy marriages. (An interesting question—and an especially valid one once the government is involved—is whether this "courage" suppresses previous worries about the toll divorce would take on children.) Still, one can certainly imagine drugs consistent enough in their effects to, on balance, qualify as a "family values" drug. As pharmacology marches on, Kramer notes, "our accuracy in targeting individual traits will improve." Some of these traits will have moral consequence. It is quite possible that some drugs that pass the psychiatrist's test—they are safe and effective and make the patient better—will fail what should be the government's test; they do more harm than good to society as a whole.

What we have here, clearly, is a mess. The social evaluation of drugs is much too complex to be settled in FDA trials. Seven years after Prozac's debut, we still don't know enough about it, or about other drugs of its generation, to formulate sound policy (beyond my suggested baseline policy that, whatever the degree of access to a drug, it should be socioeconomically equal). And the next generation of drugs may show up before the answers on Prozac are in.

All of which leads to one simple proposal. Let's kill two birds with one stone—make the equitable provision of prescription drugs more affordable and, in the process, *slow things down*. Hillary Rodham Clinton's campaign to cut drug costs met with predictable whining from the pharmaceutical industry: to cut profits, they insisted, is to cut the research incentive. Well, yes. This is exactly the sort of harsh truth that the Clinton administration is so deeply averse to acknowledging. But maybe a slowed pace of research wouldn't be such a harsh truth after all. Maybe having more time to get the answers about Prozac will help us negotiate the next pharmacological wave.

Bear in mind that the tradeoff between affordability and technological advance, as currently calibrated, has no especially compelling logic. Why does Lilly get a fourteen-year monopoly on Prozac? Don't ask me. The answer lies in the distant past, before modern psychopharmacology was on the horizon. Moreover, health insurance has tended to distort the tradeoff in the direction of technological advance. By insulating end-users—the patients—from the actual cost of drugs, insurance leads them to "undervalue" price and "overvalue" progress. That is: it skews the allocation of resources between consumption and investment away from the theoretically "optimal" balance that would result if everyone "voted" with his or her own dollars.

If drug patents were half their current length, the Prozac patent would expire this year, and the cost of a year's supply would drop from around $600 to maybe $50. Providing Prozac to people of all income levels—at least, to those likely to profit from it, who presumably are a minority at all income levels—would change from a stiff, but manageable fiscal challenge to no problem. I can already hear the people at Lilly complaining about how such mindless government meddling slows the march of progress. But in the coming age of psychopharmacology, social progress may—within certain bounds—be inversely related to technological progress.

It is good that the Clinton administration has pushed the government into discussion of mental health just as mental health is getting redefined. "Cosmetic pharmacology" sounds more frivolous than "treatment of mental illness," but it could wind up shaping the nation's character more dramatically. And if the process is left to the marketplace, with no collective guidance, the result may not be pretty.

SECTION 3

Rationing Fairly: Principles and Procedures

The Individual vs. Society: Resolving the Conflict

David M. Eddy

An individual can be in conflict with society whenever the individual uses a disproportionate amount of a health care service without paying for it.[1] This either forces others to cover the cost of replacing the service or, if the cost is not repaid and the service is not replaced, deprives others of the benefits of the service. The first causes others financial harm. The second causes harm to their health. In either case, the "others" are what we call "society."

If the individual is incapable of paying, and if the service is considered essential,[2] then the use of such a service is considered acceptable; it is viewed as part of society's obligation to individuals in need. However, as the individual's ability to pay increases, as the benefit provided by the service decreases, and as the cost of the service increases, the conflict grows.

THE SOURCE OF THE CONFLICT

The potential for conflict arises because in health care, unlike most other sectors of our economy, our country has evolved elaborate mechanisms to spread the high financial costs of medical care. The most obvious mechanism is private health insurance, but Social Security taxes for Medicare, taxes for Medicaid, health maintenance organizations, corporate health plans, and charities are other examples. All these mechanisms have a common feature—the pooling of resources. Individuals pay funds into the pool according to a variety of formulas, and individuals—sometimes the same ones, sometimes others—draw funds from the pool when the need arises.

This pooling of resources has the desirable effects of averaging out what each individual has to pay for health care and greatly reducing the possibility of a disastrous bill. But along with this benefit comes a liability. The pool connects actions of individuals in a way that creates the potential for conflict among them. Ideally, each individual will draw from the pool only his or her "fair share" of resources. In an ideal insurance program, the fair share is determined by Mother Nature; the events that determine which individuals will withdraw from the pool and how much they will withdraw are beyond the individual's control. An example is an earthquake. In health care, however, individuals and their physicians have substantial control over how much individuals withdraw from the pool. If an individual draws more than his or her fair share, then other people will either have to replenish the pool or go without the benefits of the lost services.

WHAT IS A FAIR SHARE?

If the line between a fair share and an unfair share were clear, individuals could be prevented fairly easily from drawing an unfair or inequitable share. Unfortunately, in the context of health care, the concept of fairness or equity is complex and difficult to implement. In health care, "equitable" cannot mean an equal amount of services. Different people have different needs depending on whether they are healthy or sick, the type and severity of

From *Journal of the American Medical Association*, Vol. 265, 2399–2401, 2405–2406. Copyright © 1991 American Medical Association. Reprinted by permission of the American Medical Association.

their disease, and other factors. In the context of health care, a preferable definition of *equitable* is that services should be used in such a way that the services received by each individual should provide them with approximately equal amounts of benefit per unit of resource consumed. Thus, an equitable distribution means equal yield or, more colloquially, equal "bang for the buck." This definition has the desirable property that, if followed, it will use the available resources to yield the greatest total benefit.

The idea is most easily understood through examples. It would not be equitable to use a magnetic resonance imaging test on a person with classic history and symptoms of a stress headache instead of on a person suspected of having a tumor; or to tie up prenatal services by giving a few women monthly ultrasound examinations to keep as mementos, while other women receive no prenatal care at all; or to let a Medicaid budget be drained by a patient who is brain-dead from a gunshot wound and on life support, while scores of other patients with good prognoses go untreated. Put in terms of some measure of effectiveness, such as life expectancy, it would be inequitable to give one person a service that adds 10 days of life expectancy at a cost of $1000 while another person fails to receive a service that would have gained 100 days for the same $1000. Whenever an individual uses services in a way that provides relatively low yield, the potential for conflict exists. Others will either have to pay more money to compensate for the inefficiency or will have to go without the services that went elsewhere.

TWO PERSPECTIVES

If all choices in health care took the form just described, the conflict between an individual and society would probably never arise. When a decision maker faces a limited resource and must determine which of two options yields the greatest benefit from the resource, either the choice will be obvious or it will not make much difference. However, most medical decisions do not take this form. Instead of facing a limited resource and being asked to pick which patient would benefit the most from the resource, most decision makers, especially practitioners, face a patient and must decide which services to provide to that patient. For this type of decision, the connection between

individuals is less obvious, and it is more difficult to appreciate that trying to maximize care for a particular patient will affect the financial or health outcomes of other people.

To understand the conflict between the individual and society, it is helpful to distinguish the two perspectives. In one, which is often called the public health or societal perspective, the decision maker sees a resource and wants to allocate it as efficiently as possible across patients. In the other, which might be called the patients' perspective, the decision maker sees an individual patient and wants to choose resources to optimize that patient's care. Both decision makers have the same goal of providing the best possible health care to the people they serve. However, because they see different people in different settings and make decisions in different directions, the strategies they propose are often in conflict.

TWO POSITIONS

The two perspectives roughly correspond to the two positions each of us can be in with respect to a health care service.[3] We are in one position (the "first position") when we do not yet have a health problem that would need the service and are deciding whether to buy coverage for the service. We are in another position (the "second position") when we have a disease, we know much more about what services we want, and this year's bills have already been paid. With admitted simplification, society is people when they are in the first position, whereas patients are people when they are in the second position. The conflict arises because what is best for us when we are in one position is not necessarily best for us when we are in the other position.[1]

THE CONFLICT

Unfortunately, when decisions are made from the patient's perspective, it is more difficult for the decision maker to determine when an individual is getting a disproportionate share of resources. First, from the patient's perspective, with its narrow focus on one person, it is not obvious that the level of care given to one person will affect the health and economic outcomes of other people. But even when this is appreciated, practitioners and patients can easily depersonalize the other people as "society," an insurance company, or the government, forgetting that these entities are really other patients, premium payers, and taxpayers. Some practitioners even see it as their duty to try to capture a disproportionate share of services for their patients. They perceive themselves as having an ethical responsibility to place the needs of their individual patients above the ill-defined needs of society, to serve as their patients' advocates in a battle with society. Any concern that their patients might receive an unfair share can be rationalized by assuming that if all practitioners look out for other patients with equal vigor, everything will work out fine.

There are several problems with this reasoning. One is that, in fact, we do not maximize the care of all individuals evenly. Some receive large amounts of resources, with little expectation of benefit, while others get far fewer resources even though the yield would have been much greater. The discrepancies affect not only the uninsured who draw from the pool only for urgent care, but also people who ostensibly have full insurance coverage. The discrepancies can occur because of such factors as geography, place of treatment (eg, a research center vs a community hospital), availability of resources, variations in providers' opinions about the outcomes of particular interventions, aggressiveness of the patient, aggressiveness of the physician, recent court cases or news articles, and the strength of a lobby for a particular disease. A second problem is that attempts to maximize every patient's care are likely to drive costs beyond the point that the people who will eventually pay the bill are willing to pay. But an even more impressive problem is that decisions from the perspective of the patients, where the attention is directed toward individuals after they seek care, do not maximize the health of even those individuals.

AN ILLUSTRATION

[I have elsewhere] illustrated these problems with a purposely simplified example of a hypothetical corporation that offered to 1000 of its 50-year-old female employees two options. One option

would cover breast cancer screening from age 50 to 65 years; the other would cover high-dose chemotherapy with autologous bone marrow transplantation (HDC-ABMT) for women who develop metastatic breast cancer. To a woman in the first position (and from the public health perspective), breast cancer screening would reduce her chance of dying of breast cancer by about 0.7 percentage points (from 3.57% to 2.88%), increase her life expectancy by about 44 days, and cost her about $1200. To the same woman, coverage of HDC-ABMT would decrease her chance of dying of breast cancer by about 0.03 percentage points (from 3.57% to 3.54%), increase her life expectancy by about 2.5 days, and cost her about $1500. (The estimates for HDC-ABMT assume that the treatment has a 5% cure rate, which has not actually been demonstrated. The implications of other assumptions can be calculated proportionately. For example, a cure rate of 15% would imply a decrease in probability of dying of 0.09 percentage points and an increase in life expectancy of 7.5 days.) When applied to the 1000 women in the corporation, the first option would prevent about seven breast cancer deaths, add about 120 person-years of life, and cost about $1.2 million. The second option would prevent, at best, one death, would add about 7 person-years of life, and would cost about $1.5 million. Thus, from the first position, the public health perspective, or society's point of view, option 1 provides considerably greater benefit at lower cost and is the preferred program. However, from the perspective of an individual patient who has terminal breast cancer (the second position), a program that covers HDC-ABMT is preferable.

WHY NOT DO BOTH?

How can the conflict be resolved? In addition to highlighting the conflict, this example illustrates several approaches that might be used to try to resolve it. The most obvious question is, "Why not cover both screening and high-dose chemotherapy?"

That is a possibility. Its merits depend on whether women find the additional benefits to be worth the costs. To appreciate the issues, imagine that you are a 50-year-old average-risk woman employed by the corporation. From your point of view, the options appear as shown in Table 1.

Compared with option 1, are you willing to pay about $1100 more to buy option 3 ($2303 − $1195 = $1108), which will reduce your chance of dying of breast cancer by an additional 0.02 percentage points (from 2.88% to 2.86%) and add 2 days of life expectancy? Think hard and understand that if you choose option 3 you will actually have to pay the money; you will not be allowed to pass the cost off to someone else. If you and your coworkers truly prefer option 3, then indeed the solution to the conflict is to cover both screening and HDC-ABMT. This resolves the conflict because although you will be covered for HDC-ABMT, which draws a resource from the pool, you will be paying enough money into the pool to replace the expected cost. Thus, one way to resolve the conflict is to ask people if they are willing to pay for the additional services, and if they are, respect their wishes.

Now suppose you and your coworkers do not think that the benefits of adding HDC-ABMT to screening are worth the cost. Three remaining approaches might be tried to resolve the conflict. One is for the company to give you no choice—it might unilaterally create and bill you for a program that provides coverage for both screening and HDC-ABMT, even though you would rather keep the money than have coverage for HDC-ABMT. This approach, which might be called the "do-it-anyway" approach, does eliminate the health side of the conflict because it covers the ser-

vice and replenishes the fund. However, this approach does not address the financial side of the conflict; you and your colleagues will be forced to pay for something you did not consider to be worth its costs. The do-it-anyway approach only converts the effect of the conflict from a health harm to a financial harm.

A second approach is to make option 3 an employee benefit and pass the costs on to consumers of the corporation's products. Call this the "pass-the-buck" approach. If you are an employee of the corporation, you should like this approach; it gives you a benefit at no cost. The fact that the benefit is not worth the cost is moot as far as you are concerned because you do not have to pay the cost. However, this approach is obviously unfair to the consumers of the product. Not only will they have to pay for a benefit they will never get— the benefit will go to you and your coworkers—but they will be paying for a benefit that the recipients themselves (you) determined was not worth its cost. Consumers might tolerate this for one company and one coverage policy because the costs would be highly diluted. But if this were to become the general method for resolving the conflict between the individual and society, everyone would use it, the costs of all products (and Social Security taxes and income taxes) would be affected, and the total burden on consumers would be huge. Furthermore, this approach boomerangs; you will end up paying for other peoples' health benefits. For example, when you buy a car, about $700 of your money goes to pay for other peoples'

TABLE 1

Health and Economic Outcomes of Three Health Plans From the Perspective of a 50-Year-Old Asymptomatic Average-Risk Woman*

	Baseline	Option 1, Screen	Option 2, HDC-ABMT	Option 3, Both
Probability of getting breast cancer, %	8.22	8.22	8.22	8.22
Probability of dying of breast cancer, %	3.57	2.88	3.54	2.86
Increase in life expectancy, d	0	44	2.5	46
Cost, $†	0	1195	1506	2303

*Calculations performed on CAN*TROL.[4] Screen indicates screening of women between the ages of 50 and 65 years for breast cancer, and HDC-ABMT, high-dose chemotherapy with autologous bone marrow transplantation to age 65 years.

†Present value of costs, discounted to age 50 years at 5%.

health benefits (Walter B. Maher, Chrysler Corporation, written communication, March 4, 1991). Every year, one way or another, every household in the country pays about $7000 for somebody's health care (calculated by dividing the total expenditures for health care by the number of households). Like the previous approach, this one does not solve the conflict between the individual and society; it only hides it better by spreading the financial burden to a larger number of people.

The third approach is to respect your wishes when you say you are not willing to pay for option 3. If you decide that the health benefits of covering HDC-ABMT are not as important to you as the money required to buy that coverage, this approach would take you at your word, not bill you for the cost of HDC-ABMT, and not cover the cost of HDC-ABMT if you should get metastatic breast cancer. This approach, which might be called the "patient choice" approach, is consistent with rationing by patient choice.[5] It resolves the conflict because it does not ask anyone else to pay the cost of a service you yourself were unwilling to pay for. The drawback to this approach is that if you should develop metastatic breast cancer, HDC-ABMT would not be covered. You could change your mind in the sense that you would not be forbidden from getting HDC-ABMT, but you would have to pay for it yourself, in full. You might end up regretting this decision, but that is not a conflict between you and society; it is a choice you made for yourself. You would be in conflict with society only if you tried to demand coverage for the HDC-ABMT, even though you declined to buy it when you had the chance.

An important conclusion of this exercise is that all the approaches that resolved the conflict are based on the same principle—let people decide what they are willing to pay for, respect those decisions, and adhere to those decisions. Notice that this principle would also allow you to choose none of the options. That is, if you look at Table 1 and decide that not even the benefits of option 1 are worth its cost, this principle would say that neither screening nor HDC-ABMT should be covered. This principle is difficult to apply for a variety of practical reasons, such as incomplete information about the relative merits of interventions, variations in peoples' preferences, and the interposition of third-party payment. Nonetheless, the

principle must be understood if practical methods are to be developed to implement it.

The only remaining question is, when should people be asked to make their decisions—when they are in the first position or the second? To determine the guideline for treating breast cancer, should we show Table 1 to women before they get breast cancer, or should we show women who have metastatic breast cancer a modified table that indicates no benefit for screening?

WHICH POSITION IS "CORRECT"?

Both positions are real and have important things to say about the use of health care resources. When resolving the conflict between the individual and society, however, there are several reasons to give precedence to decisions made in the first position. One is that a person in the first position can look into the future to anticipate what he or she would want when he or she reaches the second position. In contrast, once a person reaches the second position, it is too late to fulfill the desires of the first position, at least with respect to that disease. Thus, the first position includes the second, but not vice versa.

But a more impressive reason is that by any aggregate measure of health care quality, such as morbidity rates, mortality rates, life expectancy, measures of health status, or quality-adjusted life-years, and for any specified level of resources, choices made from the first position can always provide as high a quality of care as choices made from the second position and can often provide a higher quality of care. This means that if guidelines are systematically defined from the first position (the public health perspective) more people will live longer, with higher quality, at lower cost than if guidelines are defined from the second position (the patient's perspective). Policies designed from the first position provide greater good for the greater number.

These statements are true because people in the first position always have more options from which to choose. Any option available to the second position is also available to the first position, but there are often options available to the first position that are not available to the second position. To the extent that the additional options available to the first position offer greater benefit and/or lower cost than the options available to the second position, decisions made from the first position will result in a higher quality of care and/or lower cost. In the example, individuals in the first position could choose from any of the options in Table 1. But by the time a person reaches the second position, the only viable option is option 2. Option 1, which would have provided more benefit at lower cost, is no longer available.

One might wonder if guidelines defined from the first position can always provide benefits and costs that are at least as good as guidelines from the second position, are there any advantages to making guidelines from the second position? Choices made from the second position have two main virtues. First, they give the appearance that everything that possibly can be done for an individual patient is being done. I use the word *appearance* because, in fact, while everything will have been done for a patient after he or she gets a disease, everything will not have been done for that person if the person's entire lifetime is considered. Nonetheless, if option 2 or 3 is chosen rather than option 1, neither patients nor physicians will have

to face the emotional anguish of knowing that some potentially beneficial treatment was available but not covered.

The second virtue is closely related to the first. Patients in the second position tend to be much more visible than people in the first position. To the extent that other people who are unrelated to the patient (call them onlookers) place value on attempts to maximize care for an identified individual as opposed to unidentified people, setting policies from the second position can provide the onlookers with vicarious benefit. Memorable examples are a little girl who falls in a well or even whales trapped in Alaskan ice. The vicarious benefit onlookers derive from attempts to save identified individuals offsets at least some of the harm caused by spending large amounts of money that could have yielded greater benefit if used in other ways.

However, both of these virtues can be incorporated in decisions made from the first position. To address the first, add a line to the balance sheet to register the fact that if a woman chooses option 1 but ends up developing breast cancer, she will suffer the anguish of not having HDC-ABMT covered (Table 2). People should think hard about this

TABLE 2

Health and Economic Outcomes of Three Health Plans From the Perspective of a 50-Year-Old Asymptomatic Average-Risk Woman*

	Baseline	Option 1, Screen	Option 2, HDC-ABMT	Option 3, Both
Probability of getting breast cancer, %	8.22	8.22	8.22	8.22
Probability of dying of breast cancer, %	3.57	2.88	3.54	2.86
Increase in life expectance, d	0	44	2.5	46
Probability of suffering the anguish of not having HDC-ABMT covered, %	. . .	3.57	0	0
Cost, $†	0	1195	1506	2303

•Calculations performed on CAN*TROL.4 Screen indicates screening of women between the ages of 50 and 65 years for breast cancer, and HDC-ABMT, high-dose chemotherapy with autologous bone marrow transplantation to age 65 years.

†Present value of costs, discounted to age 50 years at 5%.

additional outcome when making their choices because, under the patient-choice approach, they must live with the decision.

To address the second benefit, the pertinent question is whether the amount of vicarious benefit received by the onlookers is sufficient to outweigh the harm that results from the inefficient use of resources. The amount of such benefit will depend on the nature and visibility of the particular case. Whether right or wrong, live television coverage of attempts to rescue a 5-year-old girl from a well will provide more vicarious benefit than newspaper coverage of a 50-year-old woman fighting with an insurance company for an investigational breast cancer treatment, which in turn will provide more vicarious benefit than hearing about a homeless person who needs better nutrition. To incorporate this feature of a guideline, each option should be studied for the potential of vicarious benefit; a helpful measure is its "newsworthiness."

WHAT HAPPENS NOW?

Our current practices tend to accentuate rather than resolve the conflict. We have little idea of the level of services for which people are willing to pay, we make most decisions from the second position, and we use the pass-the-buck approach to pay for those decisions. The lack of systematic information about the relative benefits and harms of many interventions, and about peoples' preferences for benefits, harms, and costs, deprives us of the anchor we need to determine the total size of the pool, or to determine what constitutes a fair share of services. Most decisions that reflect the second position are not the result of any careful analysis or public debate but simply a consequence of the fact that the great majority of the encounters between individuals and the health care system occur when patients are in the second position. As for paying for services, we have raised the pass-the-buck approach to a fine art. For example, not only do employees get health benefits covered by their employers, who pass them on to consumers, but employees do not have to pay taxes on the benefits as income, the employers can deduct the costs as a business expense, and the government can pass all the lost tax revenues on to

future generations through budget deficits. The fact that most decisions are made from the second position and reflect the patient's perspective produces just what we would expect: most patients want everything possible and expect somebody else to pay for it. Practitioners undoubtedly sense that many of the services they provide are excessive, but their responses vary widely, with some discouraging their use, some staying neutral, and some encouraging them.

Thus, to a great extent the current "solution" to the conflict between the individual and society today is for individuals to try to extract as much from society as possible. We are in a tailspin: individual patients drive up costs, which are passed on to other people, who try to recover their "fair share" by overusing services when their turn comes around.

WHAT IS THE SOLUTION?

Because of the magnitude and complexity of the problem, resolving the conflict will be extremely difficult. To begin, it is helpful to describe what we want to achieve and then try to get closer to that goal than we are now. Ideally, we would have good information about the benefits, harms, and costs of services, about the level of health care for which people are willing to pay, and, correspondingly, about the level of resources that should be made available for health care. Ideally there would be some agreed-on measure of benefit per resource that would serve as a threshold for deciding when coverage of a particular service is fair. When the yield of a service is below the threshold, physicians and patients would voluntarily restrain themselves from seeking coverage for that service from the pool. Conversely, if a particular service has a high yield but is underused, steps would be taken to stimulate that service.

Many problems will prevent us from reaching this ideal. They include lack of good information about the health and economic outcomes of many activities; the fact that the outcomes of a service depend on the specific indications for which it is used (which means there will be few simple guidelines); the lack of a tradition of asking patients their preferences; the fact that preferences are highly personal and variable (which means there will be few single correct answers); and the fact that physicians and patients have strong incentives to maximize services after patients seek care.

Despite these problems, it is certainly possible to improve on our current approach. The first step is to recognize the problem. Physicians and patients must understand that when they attempt to maximize care from the patient's perspective, they might not only be in conflict with society, but they might well be fostering guidelines that are not even in their own long-term interest. Everyone must also understand that behind the abstract label of society are real people; when individuals receive a disproportionate amount of services at the expense of society, they harm the health and finances of other people just like themselves.

The second step is to learn more about the benefits, harms, and costs of the most important interventions and about what people want from the health care system. We should pick two to three dozen representative health problems that span the most important diseases and types of activities, estimate their benefits, harms, and costs, and ask people whether the benefits and harms are worth the costs, using the type of questions described elsewhere.[3] This exercise would provide essential information about whether we are currently spending too much or too little on health care and would provide the threshold that determines the fair share to be covered from pooled resources. The recent programs of the Agency for Health Care Policy and Research are an important step in this direction. The third step is to identify some services that, on the basis of clinical judgment and common sense are suspected to be overused or underused, estimate their health and economic outcomes, and ask people if they are worth their costs. While uncertainty and variability will limit our progress, we can achieve some success by analyzing the extremes. The last steps are to incorporate what we learn into practice policies and then to adhere to those guidelines.

Because it involves human behavior and self-control, the last step will be the most difficult and will require great leadership from practitioners. Medicine has a long tradition of trying to maximize care for individual patients, a tradition not only based on compassion, but strongly reinforced by medical education, pressure from patients, families, the press, the courts, and professional and financial incentives. But the act of pooling resources across individuals requires that that tradition be modified. In return for gaining the benefits derived from sharing costs, individuals must also accept some responsibilities and limitations. A responsibility is to respect others who contribute to the pool. A limitation is to not withdraw from it an unfair share.

NOTES

1. Eddy DM. The individual vs society: is there a conflict? *JAMA.* 1991;265:1446, 1449-1450.
2. Eddy DM. What care is essential? what services are basic? *JAMA.* 1991;265:782, 786-788.
3. Eddy DM. Connecting value and costs: whom do we ask, and what do we ask them? *JAMA.* 1990;264:1737-1739.
4. Eddy DM. A computer-based model for designing cancer control strategies. *NCI Monogr.* 1986;2:75-82.
5. Eddy DM. Rationing by patient choice. *JAMA.* 1991;265:105-108.

QALYfying the Value of Life

John Harris

Against a background of permanently scarce resources it is clearly crucial that such health care resources as are available be not used wastefully. This point is often made in terms of 'efficiency' and

From *Journal of Medical Ethics*, Vol. 13:117. Reprinted with permission from the BMJ Publishing Group.

it is argued, not implausibly, that to talk of efficiency implies that we are able to distinguish between efficient and inefficient use of health care resources, and hence that we are in some sense able to measure the results of treatment. To do so of course we need a standard of measurement. Traditionally, in life-endangering conditions, that standard has been easy to find. Successful treatment removes the danger to life, or at least postpones it, and so the survival rates of treatment have been regarded as a good indicator of success.[1] However, equally clearly, it is also of crucial importance to those treated that the help offered them not only removes the threat to life, but leaves them able to enjoy the remission granted. In short, gives them reasonable quality, as well as extended quantity of life.

A new measure of quality of life which combines length of survival with an attempt to measure the quality of that survival has recently[2] been suggested and is becoming influential. The need for such a measure has been thus described by one of its chief architects: 'We need a simple, versatile, measure of success which incorporates both life expectancy and quality of life, and which reflects the values and ethics of the community served. The "Quality Adjusted Life Year" (QALY) measure fulfills such a role.'[3] This is a large claim and an important one; if it can be sustained its consequences for health care will be profound indeed.

There are, however, substantial theoretical problems in the development of such a measure, and more important by far, grave dangers of its misuse. I shall argue that the dangers of misuse, which partly derive from inadequacies in the theory which generates them, make this measure itself a life-threatening device. In showing why this is so I shall attempt to say something positive about just what is involved in making scrupulous choices between people in situations of scarce resources, and I will end by saying something about the entitlement to claim in particular circumstances, that resources are indeed scarce.

We must first turn to the task of examining the QALY and the possible consequences of its use in resource allocation. A task incidentally which, because it aims at the identification and eradication of a life-threatening condition, itself (surprisingly perhaps for a philosophical paper) counts also as a piece of medical research,[4] which if successful will prove genuinely therapeutic.

THE QALY

I. WHAT ARE QALYS?

It is important to be as clear as possible as to just what a QALY is and what it might be used for. I cannot do better than let Alan Williams, the architect of QALYs referred to above, tell you in his own words:

> The essence of a QALY is that it takes a year of healthy life expectancy to be worth one, but regards a year of unhealthy life expectancy as worth less than 1. Its precise value is lower the worse the quality of life of the unhealthy person (which is what the 'quality adjusted' bit is all about). If being dead is worth zero, it is, in principle, possible for a QALY to be negative, ie for the quality of someone's life to be judged worse than being dead.
>
> The general idea is that a beneficial health care activity is one that generates a positive amount of QALYs, and that an efficient health care activity is one where the cost-per-QALY is as low as it can be. A high priority health care activity is one where the cost-per-QALY is low, and a low priority activity is one where cost-per-QALY is high.[5]

The plausibility of the QALY derives from the idea that 'given the choice, a person would prefer a shorter healthier life to a longer period of survival in a state of severe discomfort and disability'.[6] The idea that any rational person would endorse this preference provides the moral and political force behind the QALY. Its acceptability as a measurement of health then depends upon its doing all the theoretical tasks assigned to it, and on its being what people want, or would want, for themselves.

II. HOW WILL QALYS BE USED?

There are two ways in which QALYs might be used. One is unexceptionable and useful, and fully in line with the assumptions which give QALYs their plausibility. The other is none of these.

QALYs might be used to determine which of rival therapies to give to a particular patient or which procedure to use to treat a particular condition. Clearly the one generating the most QALYs will be the better bet, both for the patient and for a society with scarce resources. However, QALYs might also be used to determine not what treatment to give *these* patients, but which group of patients to treat, or which conditions to give priority in the allocation of health care resources. It is clear that it is this latter use which Williams has in mind, for he specifically cites as one of the rewards of the development of QALYs, their use in 'priority setting in the health care system in general'.[7] It is this use which is likely to be of greatest interest to all those concerned with efficiency in the health service. And it is for this reason that it is likely to be both the most influential and to have the most far-reaching effects. It is this use which is I believe positively dangerous and morally indefensible. Why?

III. WHAT'S WRONG WITH QALYS?

It is crucial to realize that the whole plausibility of QALYs depends upon our accepting that they simply involve the generalization of the 'truth'[8] that 'given the choice a person would prefer a shorter healthier life to a longer period of survival in a state of severe discomfort.' On this view giving priority to treatments which produce more QALYs or for which the cost-per-QALY is low, is both efficient and is also what the community as a whole, and those at risk in particular, actually want. But whereas it follows from the fact that given the choice a person would prefer a shorter healthier life to a longer one of severe discomfort, that the best treatment *for that person* is the one yielding the most QALYs, it does not follow that treatments yielding more QALYs are preferable to treatments yielding fewer where *different people* are to receive the treatments. That is to say, while it follows from the fact (if it is a fact) that I and everyone else would prefer to have, say one year of healthy life rather than three years of severe discomfort, that we value healthy existence more than uncomfortable existence for ourselves, it does not follow that where the choice is between three years of discomfort for *me* or immediate death on the one hand, and one year of health for you, or immediate death on the other, that I am somehow committed to the judgement that you ought to be saved rather than me.

Suppose that Andrew, Brian, Charles, Dorothy, Elizabeth, Fiona and George all have zero life-expectancy without treatment, but with medical care, all but George will get one year's complete remission and George will get seven years' remission. The costs of treating each of the six are equal but George's operation costs five times as much as the cost of the other operations. It does not follow that even if each person, if asked, would prefer

seven years' remission to one for themselves, that they are all committed to the view that George should be treated rather than that they should. Nor does it follow that this is a preference that society should endorse. But it is the preference that QALYs dictate.

Such a policy does not value life or lives at all, for it is individuals who are alive, and individuals who lose their lives. And when they do the loss is principally their loss. The value of someone's life is, primarily and overwhelmingly, its value to him or her; the wrong done when an individual's life is cut short is a wrong to that individual. The victim of a murder or a fatal accident is the person who loses his life. A disaster is the greater the more victims there are, the more lives that are lost. A society which values the lives of its citizens is one which tries to ensure that as few of them die prematurely (that is when their lives could continue) as possible. Giving value to life-years or QALYs, has the effect in this case of sacrificing six lives for one. If each of the seven *wants* to go on living for as long as he or she can, if each values the prospective term of remission available, then to choose between them on the basis of life-years (quality adjusted or not), is in this case to give no value to the lives of six people.

IV. THE ETHICS OF QALYS

Although we might be right to claim that people are not committed to QALYs as a measurement of health simply in virtue of their acceptance of the idea that each would prefer to have more QALYs rather than fewer for themselves, are there good moral reasons why QALYs should none the less be accepted?

The idea, which is at the root of both democratic theory and of most conceptions of justice, that each person is as morally important as any other and hence, that the life and interests of each is to be given equal weight, while apparently referred to and employed by Williams plays no part at all in the theory of QALYs. That which is to be given equal weight is not persons and their interests and preferences, but quality-adjusted life-years. And giving priority to the manufacture of QALYs can mean them all going to a few at the expense of the interests and wishes of the many. It will also mean that all available resources will tend to be deployed to assist those who will thereby gain the maximum QALYs—the young.

. . . There is a general problem for any position which holds that time-spans are of equal value no matter who gets them, and it stems from the practice of valuing life-units (life-years) rather than people's lives.

If what matters most is the number of life-years the world contains, then the best thing we can do is devote our resources to increasing the population. Birth control, abortion and sex education come out very badly on the QALY scale of priorities.

In the face of a problem like this, the QALY advocate must insist that what he wants is to select the therapy that generates the most QALYs for those people who already exist, and not simply to create the maximum number of QALYs. But if it is people and not units of life-span that matter, if the QALY is advocated because it is seen as a moral and efficient way to fulfill our obligation to provide care for our fellows, then it does matter who gets the QALYs— because it matters how people are treated. And this is where the ageism of QALYs and their other discriminatory features become important.

VI. QALYS ARE AGEIST

Maximizing QALYs involves an implicit and comprehensive ageist bias. For saving the lives of younger people is, other things being equal, always likely to be productive of more QALYs than saving older people. Thus on the QALY arithmetic we always have a reason to prefer, for example, neonatal or paediatric care to all 'later' branches of medicine. This is because any calculation of the life-years generated for a particular patient by a particular therapy, must be based on the life expectancy of that patient. The older a patient is when treated, the fewer the life-years that can be achieved by the therapy.

It is true that QALYs dictate that we prefer people, not simply who have *more life expectancy*, but rather people who have *more life expectancy to be gained from treatment*. But wherever treatment saves a life, and this will be frequently, for quite simple treatments, like a timely antibiotic, can be life-saving, it will, other things being equal, be the case that younger people have more life expectancy to gain from the treatment than do older people.

VII. AGEISM AND AID

Another problem with such a view is that it seems to imply, for example, that when looking at societies from the outside, those with a lower average age have somehow a greater claim on our aid. This might have important consequences in looking at questions concerning aid policy on a global scale. Of course it is true that a society's having a low average age might be a good indicator of its need for help, in that it would imply that people were dying prematurely. However, we can imagine a society suffering a disaster which killed off many of its young people (war perhaps) and which was consequently left with a high average age but was equally deserving of aid despite the fact that such aid would inevitably benefit the old. If QALYs were applied to the decision as to whether to provide aid to this society or another much less populous and perhaps with less pressing problems, but with a more normal age distribution, the 'older' society might well be judged 'not worth' helping.

VIII. QALYS CAN BE RACIST AND SEXIST

If a 'high priority health care activity is one where the cost-per-QALY is low, and a low priority activity is one where cost-per-QALY is high' then people who just happen to have conditions which are relatively cheap to treat are always going to be given priority over those who happen to have conditions which are relatively expensive to treat. This will inevitably involve not only a systematic pattern of disadvantage to particular groups of patients, or to people afflicted with particular diseases or conditions, but perhaps also a systematic preference for the survival of some kinds of patients at the expense of others. We usually think that justice requires that we do not allow certain sections of the community or certain types of individual to become the victims of systematic disadvantage and that there are good moral reasons for doing justice, not just when it costs us nothing or when it is convenient or efficient, but also and particularly, when there is a price to be paid. We'll return shortly to this crucial issue of justice, but it is important to be clear about the possible social consequences of adopting QALYs.

Adoption of QALYs as the rationale for the distribution of health care resources may, for the above reasons, involve the creation of a systematic pattern of preference for certain racial groups or for a particular gender or, what is the same thing, a certain pattern of discrimination against such groups. Suppose that medical statistics reveal that say women, or Asian males, do better than others after a particular operation or course of treatment, or, that a particular condition that has a very poor prognosis in terms of QALYs afflicts only Jews, or gay men. Such statistics abound and the adoption of QALYs may well dictate very severe and systematic discrimination against groups identified primarily by race, gender or colour, in the allocation of health resources, where it turns out that such groups are vulnerable to conditions that are not QALY-efficient.[9]

Of course it is just a fact of life and far from sinister that different races and genders are subject to different conditions, but the problem is that QALYs may tend to reinforce and perpetuate these 'structural' disadvantages.

IX. DOUBLE JEOPARDY

Relatedly, suppose a particular terminal condition was treatable, and would, with treatment, give indefinite remission but with a very poor quality of life. Suppose for example that if an accident victim were treated, he would survive, but with paraplegia. This might always cash out at fewer QALYs than a condition which with treatment would give a patient perfect remission for about five years after which the patient would die. Suppose that both candidates wanted to go on living as long as they could and so both wanted, equally fervently, to be given the treatment that would save their lives. Is it clear that the candidate with most QALYs on offer should always and inevitably be the one to have priority? To judge so would be to count the paraplegic's desire to live the life that was available to him as of less value than his rival's—what price equal weight to the preferences of each individual?

This feature of QALYs involves a sort of double jeopardy. QALYs dictate that because an individual is unfortunate, because she has once become a victim of disaster, we are required to visit upon her a second and perhaps graver misfortune. The first disaster leaves her with a poor quality of life, and QALYs then require that in virtue of this she be ruled out as a candidate for life-saving treat-

ment, or at best, that she be given little or no chance of benefiting from what little amelioration her condition admits of. Her first disaster leaves her with a poor quality of life and when she presents herself for help, along come QALYs and finish her off!

X. LIFE-SAVING AND LIFE-ENHANCING

A distinction, consideration of which is long overdue, is that between treatments which are life-saving (or death-postponing) and those which are simply life-enhancing, in the sense that they improve the quality of life without improving life-expectancy. Most people think, and for good as well as for prudential reasons, that life-saving has priority over life-enhancement and that we should first allocate resources to those areas where they are immediately needed to save life and only when this has been done should the remainder be allocated to alleviating non-fatal conditions. Of course there are exceptions even here and some conditions, while not life-threatening, are so painful that to leave someone in a state of suffering while we attend even to the saving of life, would constitute unjustifiable cruelty. But these situations are rare and for the vast majority of cases we judge that life-saving should have priority.

It is important to notice that QALYs make no such distinction between types of treatment. Defenders of QALYs often cite with pride the example of hip-replacement operations which are more QALY-efficient than say kidney dialysis.[10] While the difficulty of choosing between treating very different groups of patients, some of whom need treatment simply to stay alive, while others need it to relieve pain and distress, is clearly very acute, and while it may be that life-saving should not *always* have priority over life-enhancement, the dangers of adopting QALYs which regard only one dimension of the rival claims, and a dubious one at that, as morally relevant, should be clear enough.

There is surely something fishy about QALYs. They can hardly form 'an appropriate basis for health service policy.' Can we give an account of just where they are deficient from the point of view of morality? We can, and indeed we have already started to do so. In addition to their other problems, QALYs and their use for priority setting in health care or for choosing not which treatment to give these patients, but for selecting which patients or conditions to treat, involve profound injustice, and if implemented would constitute a denial of the most basic civil rights. Why is this?

MORAL CONSTRAINTS

One general constraint that is widely accepted and that I think most people would judge should govern life and death decisions, is the idea that many people believe expresses the values animating the health service as a whole. These are the belief that the life and health of each person matters, and matters as much as that of any other and that each person is entitled to be treated with equal concern and respect both in the way health resources are distributed and in the way they are treated generally by health care professionals, however much their personal circumstances may differ from that of others.

This popular belief about the values which animate the health service depends on a more abstract view about the source and structure of such values and it is worth saying just a bit about this now.

I. THE VALUE OF LIFE

One such value is the value of life itself. Our own continued existence as individuals is the *sine qua non* of almost everything. So long as we want to go on living, practically everything we value or want depends upon our continued existence. This is one reason why we generally give priority to life-saving over life-enhancing.

To think that *life is valuable*, that in most circumstances, the worst thing that can happen to an individual is that she lose her life when this need not happen, and that the worst thing we can do is make decisions, a consequence of which, is that others die prematurely, we must think that *each life is valuable*. Each life counts for one and that is why more count for more. For this reason we should give priority to saving as many lives as we can, not as many life-years.[11]

One important point must be emphasized at this stage. We talk of 'life-saving' but of course this must always be understood as 'death-postponing.'

Normally we want to have our death postponed for as long as possible but where what's possible is the gaining of only very short periods of remission, hours or days, these may not be worth having. Even those who are moribund in this sense can usually recognize this fact, particularly if they are aware that the cost of postponing their death for a few hours or days at the most will mean suffering or death for others. However, even brief remission can be valuable in enabling the individual to put her affairs in order, make farewells and so on, and this can be important. It is for the individual to decide whether the remission that she can be granted is worth having. This is a delicate point that needs more discussion than I can give it here. However, inasmuch as QALYs do not help us to understand the features of a short and painful remission that might none the less make that period of vital importance to the individual, perhaps in terms of making something worthwhile out of her life as a whole, the difficulties of these sorts of circumstances, while real enough, do not undermine the case against QALYs.[12]

II. TREATING PEOPLE AS EQUALS

If each life counts for one, then the life of each has the same value as that of any. This is why accepting the value of life generates a principle of equality. This principle does not of course entail that we treat each person equally in the sense of treating each person *the same*. This would be absurd and self-defeating. What it does involve is the idea that we treat each person with the same concern and respect. An illustration provided by Ronald Dworkin, whose work on equality informs this entire discussion, best illustrates this point: 'If I have two children, and one is dying from a disease that is making the other uncomfortable, I do not show equal concern if I flip a coin to decide which should have the remaining dose of a drug.'[13]

It is not surprising then that the pattern of protections for individuals that we think of in terms of civil rights[14] centres on the physical protection of the individual and of her most fundamental interests. One of the prime functions of the State is to protect the lives and fundamental interests of its citizens and to treat each citizen as the equal of any other. This is why the State has a basic obligation, *inter alia*, to treat all citizens as equals in the distribution of benefits and opportunities which affect their civil rights. The State must, in short, treat each citizen with equal concern and respect. The civil rights generated by this principle will of course include rights to the allocation of such things as legal protections and educational and health care resources. And this requirement that the State uphold the civil rights of citizens and deal justly between them, means that it must not choose between individuals, or permit choices to be made between individuals, that abridge their civil rights or in ways that attack their right to treatment as equals.

Whatever else this means, it certainly means that a society, through its public institutions, is not entitled to discriminate between individuals in ways that mean life or death for them on grounds which count the lives or fundamental interests of some as worth less than those of others. If for example some people were given life-saving treatment in preference to others because they had a better quality of life than those others, or more dependents and friends, or because they were considered more useful, this would amount to regarding such people as more valuable than others on that account. Indeed it would be tantamount, literally, to sacrificing the lives of others so that they might continue to live.[15]

Because my own life would be better and even of more value to me if I were healthier, fitter, had more money, more friends, more lovers, more children, more life expectancy, more everything I want, it does not follow that others are entitled to decide that because I lack some or all of these things I am less entitled to health care resources, or less worthy to receive those resources, than are others, or that those resources would somehow be wasted on me.

III. CIVIL RIGHTS

I have spoken in terms of civil rights advisedly. If we think of the parallel with our attitude to the system of criminal justice the reasons will be obvious. We think that the liberty of the subject is of fundamental importance and that no one should be wrongfully detained. This is why there are no financial constraints on society's obligation to attempt to ensure equality before the law. An individual is entitled to a fair trial no matter what the

financial costs to society (and they can be substantial). We don't adopt rubrics for the allocation of justice which dictate that only those for whom justice can be cheaply provided will receive it. And the reason is that something of fundamental importance is at stake—the liberty of the individual.

In health care something of arguably greater importance is often at stake—the very life of the individual. Indeed, since the abolition of capital punishment [in the United Kingdom], the importance of seeing that individuals' civil rights are respected in health care is pre-eminent.

IV. DISCRIMINATION

The only way to deal between individuals in a way which treats them as equals when resources are scarce, is to allocate those resources in a way which exhibits no preference. To discriminate between people on the grounds of quality of life, or QALY, or life-expectancy, is as unwarranted as it would be to discriminate on grounds of race or gender.

So, the problem of choosing how to allocate scarce resources is simple. And by that of course I mean 'theoretically simple,' not that the decisions will be easy to make or that it will be anything but agonisingly difficult actually to determine, however justly, who should live and who should die. Life-saving resources should simply be allocated in ways which do not violate the individual's entitlement to be treated as the equal of any other individual in the society: and that means the individual's entitlement to have his interests and desires weighed at the same value as those of anyone else. The QALY and the other bases of preference we have considered are irrelevant.

If health professionals are forced by the scarcity of resources, to choose, they should avoid unjust discrimination. But how are they to do this?

JUST DISTRIBUTION

If there were a satisfactory principle or theory of just distribution now would be the time to recommend its use.[14] Unfortunately there is not a satisfactory principle available. The task is to allocate resources between competing claimants in a way that does not violate the individual's entitlement to be treated as the equal of any other individual—and that means her entitlement to have her fundamental interests and desires weighed at the same value as those of anyone else. The QALY and other quality-of-life criteria are, as we have seen, both dangerous and irrelevant as are considerations based on life-expectancy or on 'life-years' generated by the proposed treatment. If health professionals are forced by the scarcity of resources to choose, not *whether* to treat but *who* to treat, they must avoid any method that amounts to unjust discrimination.

I do not pretend that the task of achieving this will be an easy one, nor that I have any satisfactory solution. I do have views on how to approach a solution, but the development of those ideas is a task for another occasion.[12] I will be content for the moment if I have shown that QALYs are not the answer and that efforts to find one will have to take a different direction.

I. DEFENSIVE MEDICINE

While it is true that resources will always be limited it is far from clear that resources for health care are justifiably as limited as they are sometimes made to appear. People within health care are too often forced to consider simply the question of the best way of allocating the *health care budget,** and consequently are forced to compete with each other for resources. Where lives are at stake however, the issue is a moral issue which faces the whole community, and in such circumstances, is one which calls for a fundamental reappraisal of priorities. The question should therefore be posed in terms, not of the health care budget alone, but of the *national budget*.[16] If this is done it will be clearer that it is simply not true that the resources necessary to save the lives of citizens are not available. Since the citizens in question are in real and present danger of death, the issue of the allocation of resources to life-saving is naturally one of, among other things, national defense. Clearly then health professionals who require additional resources simply to save the lives of citizens, have a prior and priority claim on the defense budget.

QALYs encourage the idea that the task for health economics is to find more efficient ways of doing the wrong thing—in this case sacrificing the lives of patients who could be saved. All people concerned with health care should have as their priority defensive medicine: defending their patients against unjust and lethal policies, and guarding themselves against devices that tend to disguise the immorality of what they are asked to do.

II. PRIORITY IN LIFE-SAVING

It is implausible to suppose that we cannot deploy vastly greater resources than we do at present to save the lives of all those in immediate mortal danger. It should be only in exceptional circumstances—unforeseen and massive disasters for example—that we cannot achieve this. However, in such circumstances our first duty is to try to save the maximum number of lives possible. This is because, since each person's life is valuable, and since we are committed to treating each person with the same concern and respect that we show to any, we must preserve the lives of as many individuals as we can. To fail to do so would be to value at zero the lives and fundamental interests of those extra people we could, but do not, save. Where we cannot save all, we should select those who are not to be saved in a way that shows no unjust preference.

We should be very clear that the obligation to save as many lives as possible is *not the obligation to save as many lives as we can cheaply or economically save.* Among the sorts of disasters that force us to choose between lives, is not the disaster of overspending a limited health care budget!

There are multifarious examples of what I have in mind here and just a couple must suffice to illustrate the point. Suppose, as is often the case, providing health care in one region of a country[17] is more expensive than doing so in another, or where saving the lives of people with particular conditions, is radically more expensive than other life-saving procedures, and a given health care budget won't run to the saving of all. Then any formula employed to choose priorities should do just that. Instead of attempting to measure the value of people's lives and select which are worth saving, any rubric for resource allocation should *examine the national budget afresh* to see whether

*EDITORS' NOTE: In the United Kingdom, most people receive health care through the publicly financed National Health Service.

there are any headings of expenditure that are more important to the community than rescuing citizens in mortal danger. For only if all other claims on funding are plausibly more important than that, is it true that resources for life-saving are limited.

III. CONCLUSION

The principle of equal access to health care is sustained by the very same reasons that sustain both the principle of equality before the law and the civil rights required to defend the freedom of the individual. These are rightly considered so important that no limit is set on the cost of sustaining them. Equal access to health care is of equal importance and should be accorded the same priority for analogous reasons. Indeed, since the abolition of capital punishment, due process of law is arguably of less vital importance than is access to health care. We have seen that QALYs involve denying that the life and health of each citizen is as important as that of any. If, for example, we applied the QALY principle to the administration of criminal justice we might find that those with little life expectancy would have less to gain from securing their freedom and therefore should not be defended at all, or perhaps given a jury trial only if not in competition for such things with younger or fitter fellow citizens.

A recent BBC television programme calculated[18] that if a health authority had £200,000 to spend it would get 10 QALYs from dialysis of kidney patients, 266 QALYs from hip-replacement operations or 1197 QALYs from anti-smoking propaganda. While this information is undoubtedly useful and while advice to stop smoking is an important part of health care, we should be wary of a formula which seems to dictate that such a health authority would use its resources most efficiently if it abandoned hip replacements and dialysis in favor of advice to stop smoking.

NOTES

1. See the excellent discussion of the recent history of this line of thought in the Office of Health Economics publication *The measurement of health* London, 1985.
2. Williams A. Economics of coronary artery bypass grafting. *British medical journal* 1985; 291; and his contribution to the article, Centre eight—in search of efficiency. *Health and social service journal* 1985. These are by no means the first such attempts. See reference (1).
3. WIlliams A. The value of QALYs. *Health and social service journal* 1985.
4. I mention this in case anyone should think that it is only medical scientists who do medical research.
5. See reference (3): 3.
6. See reference(1): 16.
7. See reference (3): 5, and reference (3).
8. I'll assume this can be described as 'true' for the sake of argument.
9. I am indebted to Dr S G Potts for pointing out to me some of these statistics and for other helpful comments.
10. For examples see reference (I) and reference (2).
11. See Parfit D. Innumerate ethics. *Philosophy and public affairs* 1978; 7, 4. Parfit's arguments provide a detailed defense of the principle that each is to count for one.
12. I consider these problems in more detail in my: eQALYty. In: Byrne P, ed. *King's College studies*. London: King's Fund Press, 1987/8. Forthcoming.
13. Dworkin R. *Taking rights seriously*. London: Duckworth, 1977: 227.
14. I do not of course mean to imply that there are such things as rights, merely that our use of the language of rights captures the special importance we attach to certain freedoms and protections. The term 'civil rights' is used here as a 'term of art' referring to those freedoms and protections that are customarily classed as 'civil rights.'
15. For an interesting attempt to fill this gap see Dworkin R. What is equality? *Philosophy and public affairs* 1981; 4 and 5.
16. And of course the international budget; see my *The value of life*. London: Routledge & Kegan Paul 1985: chapter 3.
17. See Townsend P, Davidson N, eds. *Inequalities in health: the Black Report*. Harmondsworth, Penguin: 1982.
18. BBC 1. *The heart of the matter* 1986, Oct.

Prior Consent to Rationing: Minimizing the Ethical Costs

Paul T. Menzel

The escalating cost of health care has forced people to confront the possibility of rationing—forgoing beneficial care for patients so that the resources might be used either for other current or prospective patients or for entirely different things in life than health care. Rationing of some sort makes eminent sense, not just economically; only those who are fanatics about health and medicine would urge that everything possible be spent on health care for even the slightest marginal benefit. Yet actual rationing of health care is usually thought to exact high, or at least disturbing, ethical costs.

I will examine four of these costs here: (1) the sacrifice of physician loyalty to patients, (2) the substitution of misleading and discriminatory numerical measurements of medicine's human benefit for more sensitive qualitative judgments, (3) the unfair bite that rationing is likely to take first out of poor people's care before it affects wealthier patients, and (4) the general substitution of public, group standards about life and health for the values and decisions of individuals. In my discussion of the second and third costs, especially, I will refer to the state of Oregon's concrete attempt at rationing.

Throughout I will not just elaborate these moral costs but assess them, estimating in particular the extent to which they can be minimized by certain forms of rationing and by certain ways of conceiving of the values that rationing either represents or appears to threaten. Taken together, these four ethical costs portray rationing as preserving or enhancing the welfare of the larger society, at the cost of attending to the needs of each individual patient. Though to some extent these four ethical costs will affect any actual rationing of health care, I will argue that generally they are not as high as is

commonly supposed. To the extent that this claim is correct, rationing's conflict with full respect for individual patients can be significantly diminished.

Another way of stating this general line of argument is to propose a reconception of what rationing represents. Rationing is commonly thought to reflect the "welfare of society"—the needs of people other than the patient whose care gets rationed out. If that indeed is the value that limiting medically beneficial care because of its expense essentially represents, it will (and probably should) be a long time indeed before American society comes to any kind of reasonably secure, ethical satisfaction with rationing. It will be accused, plausibly, of assaulting our most vulnerable citizens, the sick and disabled, so others can retain their desired level of amenities.

As I have argued elsewhere,[1] however, there is a different way of seeing the whole business. Rationing, properly formed, should represent people's own hard judgment about the kind of society in which on balance, in the long term, and considering all the realities of cost and scarcity, *they* wish to live. Concomitantly, commitment to individual patients should involve much more than maximizing their welfare *as patients*. Then respect for individual patients can be reconciled with rationing: if, beforehand, individual patients have consented, or clearly would have consented,[2] to substantive and procedural policies for rationing out care of relatively high expense per benefit, those policies' ethical appeal will rest not merely on the morally controversial goal of increasing aggregate societal welfare but on respect for patients' own values.

I will apply this line of argument, with less success in some cases than in others, to each of the four ethical costs of rationing mentioned above.

Paul Menzel, "Some Ethical Costs of Rationing," *Law, Medicine & Health Care*, 20, nos. 1–2 (1992): 57–66. Reprinted with the permission of the American Society of Law, Medicine & Ethics.

EDITORS' NOTE: This article has been edited and the notes renumbered. Readers who wish to follow up on sources should consult the original article.

PHYSICIAN LOYALTY TO PATIENTS

In some ways this is the easiest case for the reconciliationist line just articulated, but in practical terms it may be one of the hardest.

Superficially the traditional provider ethic of loyalty to each and every individual patient poses an immediate barrier to rationing. A provider's participation in an arrangement in which selected beneficial care is denied because of its excessive cost/benefit ratio seems to be abandonment of a vulnerable person at a time of great need. But the reconciliationist point applies here directly. If (a big if) the very patients whose care is now being rationed out have consented, or clearly would have consented, either to a substantive policy of limiting that sort of care or to a procedural policy for making rationing decisions that has now resulted in limiting their particular care, providers should be able to look patients in the eye with a clean conscience even as they follow through with the rationing process.

The key element in the moral argument here is that patients are more than just patients-at-the-moment. They are people with a dimension I call "integrity"—the ability to manage their lives, and the resources for their lives, over time. Given the structure of a modern health care economy (mainly insurance), controlling the use of even very high cost-per-benefit care is extremely difficult; once patients are insured, whether in private or in public arrangements, both they and providers have strong incentives to overuse care. Determining the outlines of insurance is the most effective point for people to respond to this problem and regain some control over medicine's otherwise virtually endless draw on scarce resources. The problem of controlling the use of care ought to be addressed at an early point in the process, for such a point—insuring—is where the essential trouble starts. To be sure, sometimes there are reasons for not allowing people to precommit themselves to things they might later want to reject. But the best reason, that a later decision is likely to be better, simply does not hold in health care rationing contexts. In their later situation as insured and ill patients, people's capacity to control the resources of their larger lives is sharply diminished. As communities, as individuals, or as both, patients of integrity will want to retrieve that control. . . .

The 1991 Minnesota case of Helga Wanglie provides an interesting illustration of the complex way in which such considerations affect our thinking in a concrete case. Mrs. Wanglie had been in a coma since June, 1990, from which by January, 1991, both physicians and her husband and children agreed she would never regain consciousness. Nevertheless her family wished the life-sustaining ventilator and feeding tubes continued. Her physicians argued that such care was medically futile and that therefore they had no obligation to prescribe it even if the family wanted it for Helga. She had left no clear instructions or any written instructions on the matter, though her husband quoted her as saying that "only He who gives life may take it"; he himself interpreted that to mean that she would want to be given respiratory and nutritional support even if permanently comatose. The cost of her care from November, 1990, when the dispute between the family and physicians began to emerge, until July, 1991, when she died of an infection, exceeded $700,000. Her insurance company never resisted paying; it publicly stated all along that cost should not be a factor in treatment decisions, and that it was willing to pay for her care until a court approved its removal.

Several things are clear about this case. First, it did not really involve the medical futility her physicians claimed; her ventilator and tube feedings really did keep her alive during these months, and as long as she was not in pain (she was comatose), her family's claim that life was still of some value to her (and to them, and perhaps thereby to her) could hardly be denied out of hand by physicians. At the same time, however, it seems equally clear that *if*, before all this happened, Helga Wanglie had been consulted seriously about whether she was willing to devote enough of her accessible resources to insure that even admittedly never-to-recover patients would be kept alive *at the cost of $1 million per year of comatose life*, she would have preferred that the resources be spent on other things. If she could have been questioned beforehand, this would have been the important question, not the much less definitive question of whether she would see some value in a comatose life. If the physicians were going to press to remove life-support, therefore, they should have portrayed it all along as a permissible case of rationing out care that is too expensive for its benefits, not a case where further care had no benefit for the patient (no *medical* benefit, the sort of benefit that they had the expertise to discern).

However, another anomalous factor in the case disturbs this clean argument for physicians rationing out the marginally beneficial ventilator because of its expense. Mrs. Wanglie's insurance company had publicly committed itself to the proposition that cost of care is no object. No doubt that commitment was foolish (not to say, perhaps, dishonest), and more importantly, such an unconditional commitment was undoubtedly out of line with Mrs. Wanglie's and other subscribers' real values despite the short-term public relations value it might have had for the company. Nonetheless, publicly commit itself the company apparently had. That is a good *prima facie* reason why physicians did not have the moral authority to make active rationing judgments in this case.

Other than this mistaken insurance company commitment, Wanglie is a clear case in which substantive rationing judgment could legitimately be made by physicians. Because it is virtually certain that Mrs. Wanglie would not have been willing beforehand to devote the additional resources to her health plan that would be required to sustain a policy of covering life-support at the cost of *$1 million per year of comatose life saved*, it is not crucial that subscriber representatives be integrally involved in developing that rationing guideline.

In summary, then, I would argue that clinicians may participate actively in the rationing process without diminishing their commitment to individual patients if obvious conflicts of financial interest have been removed, if neither the insurers nor clinicians have claimed that cost is no object (and if, ideally, they have positively acknowledged that it *will* be a significant consideration in high cost-per-benefit cases), and if subscribers and patient representatives have had a significant role in giving at least some general normative guidance for rationing. In all cases the crucial test question for justifying rationing is whether as a subscriber beforehand, the patient would in fact have consented to the limitation on care that the provider is now implementing. To the extent that this question can be answered affirmatively with confidence and justification, the requirement of subscriber-patient involvement in setting rationing guidelines diminishes.

QUANTITATIVE MEASUREMENTS OF BENEFIT

Rationing's main target will be high cost-per-benefit care. Its initial attraction is to make our use of health care accountable to what economists call "opportunity costs"—the benefits from an alternate use of the resources that we forgo if we devote those economic resources to a given mode of health care. We want, that is, to use resources well. Obviously, to make any sense of all this, we have to be able to compare the benefits of alternate resource uses. When we draw some limit around health care spending, we make health care resources visibly scarce, and then we need to compare the benefits of alternate health services. We will want to know which benefits are greater, and which we ought to pursue before others.

Having been inevitably launched on this quest, two steps will then become extremely attractive: first, measuring the amount of life we might be saving, and then developing some way of comparing life saved with improvements in the quality of life. For the amount of life saved, an obvious possible unit will be years of life, but how do we compare life saved with improvements in the quality of life? According to one very common-sensical approach, we simply construct a conceptual unit that incorporates both quality and longevity and call it something like a "quality-adjusted life year." ("QALY" for short).[3]

It is hard to overemphasize how helpful such a conceptual unit is in health policy. Should we spend more, for instance, on hip replacements or kidney dialysis? Or save more lives with dialysis or coronary by-pass surgery? With QALYs we at least stand a chance of getting an answer: We can compare quality improvements with life-saving, and saving a life of one quality with saving a life of another.

Given such units' usefulness, it is no surprise, for example, that we find QALYs being used in Oregon's arrangement for rationing Medicaid. The Oregon Health Services Commission, once it took on the task of rank ordering a comprehensive list of health services, quickly found itself considering not only the cost of various services but the quality of life they improved and years of life they saved.[4]

The development and employment of such QALY units, of course, requires some relative numerical ranking of the quality of life (hereafter QOL) in various states of health, as well as a numerical ranking of the value of a given improvement in health status compared to the value of a given life extension. A whole host of skeptical questions can be raised about how to do any of that. Doesn't it discriminate against individuals with longstanding low QOL, since saving their lives would produce fewer QALYs than saving the lives of healthier people? Doesn't the use of a selected sample of persons from whom we elicit the responses that generate the relative values of different health states ignore the perhaps different particular values of the patients affected by the resulting rationing?

Before going further in assessing these criticisms we should note a few basic things about how QALYs work. First a selected group of respondents express their relative valuation of different representative health states. (In Oregon this was 1000 residents through a telephone survey, and in the 1978 York University study that has been used in a number of British National Health Service decisions, it was 70 persons in extended one-to-four hour interviews.) From those responses a "quality index map" of numerical values of QOL from 0.00 (death) to 1.00 (normal health) is constructed for a wide-ranging set of health status categories. Then, for a year of life whose quality is improved by a particular treatment, we multiply the year by the difference between the QOL rankings for the old and new health states to produce the fraction of a QALY which that year of improvement is said to constitute. Similarly, a year of life saved is discounted by the QOL index of the representative health state closest to the health of the person whose life gets extended.

This will give us common numerical units for every benefit produced by a health service. If comparative QALY-production rankings for different procedures are going to serve a more impressive ethical goal than just arithmetically maximizing a cross-personal aggregate of benefits, however, their use will have to be deemed fair to the individuals they end up disadvantaging. The point that then has a chance of saving QALYs will be that people themselves implicitly quality-rank their own lives. We get quality adjustment ratios by consulting the very people who are exposed to the consequences of the rationing decisions that result.

Does this argument work against the major objections to quantitative measurement and maximizing of benefits? Many have mistakenly claimed that use of QALY-production to prioritize health services disadvantages those with low health status to begin with, whose years of life saved constitute

fewer QALYs. Overall, however, QOL adjustment probably does not disadvantage those with low quality of life. With QOL adjustment, *non-lifesaving improvements* from low QOL get more weight in any competition with lifesaving measures than they otherwise would.

Take the example of a patient with kidney failure. Admittedly, QOL adjustment weakens her competitive position in trying to get dialysis. If her QOL is 0.6, she would only gain 6.0 QALYs for her 10 years on $30,000/year lifesaving dialysis, and the resulting $50,000/QALY cost would undoubtedly place her treatment in a relatively low priority position in any rationing. She will be more likely to lose out to hip replacements than if her benefit was counted as 10.0 unadjusted life years.

But in another respect she would gain by quality adjustment. Suppose a kidney transplant would raise her quality of life from 0.6 to 0.8 for 10 years; it would produce 2.0 QALYs above and beyond those produced by dialysis. At a cost, say, of $20,000 for the transplant and $40,000 for subsequent cyclosporin ($4000/year for 10 years), her roughly $7,500/QALY gain[5] puts her claim for a transplant in better stead against other services than if we ignored her jump in QOL. Hip replacements, of course, also gain because of quality adjustment. Though no lifesaving may be involved at all, 15 years at 1.0 instead of 0.9 constitutes a 1.5 QALY gain from just an $8000 operation. This quality adjustment cuts both ways for those with low enough QOL to affect allocations: it benefits such patients in competing for quality enhancing services, though it disadvantages them in competing for lifesaving ones.

Let us explore in further detail the comparison between saving a lower quality life and saving a high quality one. As has been noted, counting QALYs will lead us to save the person with the higher quality life. Indeed you as an individual may prefer a shorter, healthier life to a longer, less healthy one, just as the sample of people whose responses generated the matrix of QOL adjustment indices did. But *both* of those health states are *for yourself.* Have you or they in any way consented to saving the healthier life of one person rather than the lower quality life of *another?*

On the face of it, it's not at all clear. Suppose you later turn out to be an accident victim who could survive, though paraplegic, while someone else could achieve more complete recovery. It could very easily be that each of you "wants to go on living . . . equally fervently" (or maybe even the paraplegic more so), so why should society save the one of you with the "most QALYs on offer"?[6] Your preference for a shorter life of normal health over a lower quality longer life in your own case is not by itself a statement that paraplegic life should someday take second place in a competition between saving two different people. For all we know, *compared to death*, your paraplegic life could still be as valuable to you as anyone else's "better" life is to him or her.

If QALYs are to play a morally acceptable role in prioritizing lifesaving, people simply have to be agreeing to something further when they express those initial quality judgments from which the numerical QOL indices are extrapolated. To see whether that is the case we must look at the precise questions used to establish the numerical rankings. There are four common types:

Time Trade-Off. How much shorter a life in good health would you find preferable to a longer lifetime with the disability or distress you are ranking? (If 10 percent shorter, then QOL is 0.9.)

Standard Gamble. What risk of death would you accept in return for being assured that if you do survive, you will be entirely cured? (If a 10 percent risk, QOL is 0.9.)

Equivalence of Numbers. How many more people with a given chronic, non-fatal illness would have to be saved from death to make saving their lives preferable to saving a smaller number of people in normal good health?[7] (If 10 percent more, QOL is 0.9.)

Direct Ratio. How many times more ill is a person described in one specified state compared with another?

If you turn out to be the paraplegic accident victim with 0.9 QOL, for example, and we could pursue a policy of producing more QALYs by saving someone else, to which of these questions, if any, would your answers that produced the 0.9 QOL rating constitute consent to the policy that now lets you die?

Ambiguity plagues the direct ratio question. Where in "how many times more ill . . . ?" is it

implied that very *lives* themselves, contrasted with death, are more and less worth saving? What is even meant by "how many times more ill"?

The time trade-off question fares no better. In accepting a 10 percent shorter remaining life to avoid a permanent disability, you do not indicate that quality adjusted trade-offs *between* different people's *very lives* are desirable.

Standard gamble suffers from a similar defect. With a 90 percent chance of complete cure from a certain treatment but also a 10 percent chance of dying, you are willing to use the treatment: You are directly expressing only what risks you will take *within your* life.

There is, however, an important conceptual connection between the willingness expressed in the standard gamble and the long-term use of QALYs. Endorsement of QALYs as an allocation method exposes you to a greater risk of being allowed to die should you ever be that paraplegic accident victim, but in return you gain a better chance of either being saved for prospectively normal health or, if you ever are a paraplegic, of receiving greatly quality-enhancing treatment. Let's call this *the QALY bargain.* It is not quite the same as the standard gamble, which concerns the risk of death you would accept to get a cure for your paraplegia. But if, knowing full well what a particular state of illness is like, we would take the gamble of a 10 percent risk of dying in order to restore ourselves to good health, wouldn't we also likely take the QALY bargain?

Generally I think so. To be sure, if one ever does get to the accident victim's paraplegic situation and adjusts in a reasonably normal manner, one will probably want to' live just as fervently as one would if one were the victim with prospective full health. But nonetheless, if people think that should they ever be in that situation, they would in fact take the standard gamble, then why wouldn't they already now be willing to look at their whole unfolding lives as a similar bargain? Past or prospective willingness to take the standard gamble does set some precedent for taking the QALY bargain. Better yet would be "equivalence of numbers" questions, where trade-offs between different people's lives are clear. And best of all would be straightforward QALY-bargain questions themselves.[8] Note that Rosser and Kind's early study used the helpful equivalence-of-numbers question, though it primarily used the relatively worthless direct ratio. It is unclear, however, whether the Oregon telephone survey used any questions from which a person's consent to something like the QALY bargain could legitimately be inferred.

Without some such close connection between the questions used to establish QOL rankings and consent to likely results of counting QALYs, QALYs will remain ethically very suspicious. With the right questions to establish QOL adjustments, however, those links get established. If, but only if, representative people have been asked true QALY-bargain questions in eliciting the resultant numerical QOL adjustments may we presume that similar people who end up being patients would themselves have consented to the use of such QOL adjustments.

Some will still see a major ethical problem with the use of QOL adjustments simply because they are based on interviews with a relatively small sample of the population. Even with the right questions and the right sample of respondents, Harris calls any presumption of people's consent to potential sacrifices on the basis of a small number of other people's responses "truly staggering."[9] He attacks the suggestion that a good reason for presumption is that "it would be impossible to approach everyone who might be affected, certainly not in the detail that can give confidence in the results."[10] The same reasoning, he claims, would justify "abolishing general elections in favor of selecting governments by small sampling along the lines of opinion polls."[11]

Though we may indeed doubt whether sampling should often substitute for general solicitation of opinion, Harris's argument is not persuasive. Undoubtedly people in a democracy want to put many offices up to general election, but it is not at all clear that they wish to tie any health care rationing process as directly to the political process. Oregon, at least for Medicaid services, has placed the debate in at least the legislative arena, but on what basis could we argue that whether the quality of life on kidney dialysis is 0.6 or 0.8 of the quality of normal, healthy life is better settled directly by an electorate? We have legislatures precisely because we think it best not to decide everything by initiative or referendum, and legislatures in turn rely on other registrations of value because they think it best not to make all the decisions necessary for government policy on the legislative floor.

There is one point, however, where QALYs face a much more difficult problem of extrapolating values from the expressed preferences of a few: people with congenital illnesses and handicaps. One critic, O'Donnell, throws an appropriate rhetorical question in QALYs' face: "What about that Dublin boy confined to a wheelchair since birth?"[12] Should we really discount the value of saving his life because of its relatively low quality? Here (not often elsewhere in his attack on QALYs) O'Donnell is correct. There is no point in time at which such a boy can even be conceived or presumed to agree to any QALY bargains that make saving his life less urgent than saving the life of someone in normal health. The extrapolated prior consent argument for QALYs does not apply to him or other cases of congenital impairments.

In summary, the use of QALYs is not as objectionable ethically as many critics claim. Such quantitative measurements of value are, however, morally problematic. The questions used to elicit QOL adjustment indices must be explicit about the use of the responses to make trade-offs, and it is doubtful whether QALY-production assessments can ever be fairly used to allocate resources among patients with non-congenital illnesses and those with illnesses that identifiably began before any plausible age of consent.

RATIONING POOR PEOPLE'S CARE

The fundamental drive behind rationing is the competition of other things in life besides health care for our finite resources. Once that elementary point is acknowledged, it should be expected that the fewer the resources to which people have access, the more attractive rationing health care becomes. Thus, poor people, if they can control the use of their resources (their own private resources plus any societally assisted ones to which they have access), would naturally ration care before wealthier people would.

In that respect, there is nothing suspicious or surprising about the fact that one of the first openly acknowledged instances of rationing in the U.S. is Oregon's recent plan for Medicaid. Oregon's decision to replace restrictions on eligibility for state-assisted health care with restrictions on the more expensive-per-benefit care in the plan is particularly laudable. Disturbing, however, is the fact that the floor of covered care that finally emerges from the process of prioritizing different health services is a direct function of whatever aggregate of money the Oregon legislature happens to authorize for the system. If that total is very low, even services relatively high on the priority list could be rationed out; conversely, if the state is having a good year financially and the legislature is acting very generously, all but the very lowest priority items might be funded when the resources would better be used for other needs in the lives of poor people. What seems missing is any independent sense of the level of minimally decent care to which poor people ought to have access.

Some would attack the Oregon arrangement more frontally than this: any rationing of poor people's health care without equivalent rationing of others' care is unjust. Elsewhere I have argued against any such "medical egalitarianism regarded as a matter of moral principle."[13]

My rejection of medical egalitarianism takes both a positive and negative form. Positively, what must be said is that permitting a noticeably lower tier of services for the poor can be based on respect for poor persons' own preferences. If poor, I will rationally and knowledgeably prefer to spend less on preserving health and saving life than if I am well off. Especially in choosing whether to cover and pay for statistically expensive, marginally beneficial procedures, lower income people will properly choose differently. To flatten out these differences through uniform health services *without* changing the basic distribution of income rides roughshod over poor people's preferences for the only lives they have to live. If wider injustice is the problem, it should be attacked by redistributing economic resources generally, not by restricting the choices of the poor when those choices are plausibly rational within their real life context.

Negatively, we should note the failure of various arguments for medical egalitarianism.[14] Take the argument based on the caring for others in need said to provide the basic glue of social solidarity. It fails because a truly caring non-poor person should not choose for a poor person what she (the non-poor person) wants for herself. Instead she should put herself in the poor person's shoes. I may want liver transplants covered in my health plan even if I could convert the savings from excluding them to other uses I value, but if I really were the poor person I would almost certainly not include such an expensive service in preference to devoting the resources to other (to me then) more urgent things. Caring benevolence that takes the initial feelings of the contributor as unquestioned, without critical adjustment for the situation of the recipient, is surely superficial.

Another argument for medical egalitarianism focuses on equal opportunity. Though stronger, it, too, fails. The essential argument is that people ought to have roughly equal opportunities to achieve the more universally desired goods in life. Since illness and disability are major, unequal barriers to such opportunity, health care ought to be distributed straightforwardly according to medical need.[15]

To see how problematic this argument is, we need to note that the concept of opportunity involves three sorts of reference: some goal or set of goals toward which we are striving, a particular obstacle or set of obstacles to that goal from which we are free, and the absence of all insurmountable obstacles to that goal. Equal opportunity in particular then refers to people's mutual freedom from the same set of particular obstacles to the same set of goals. The argument for the special importance of health care based on equal opportunity omits one of these elements: a set of goals to which illnesses are impediments.

The argument is then caught on the horns of an impossible dilemma. If its point is just that the opportunity to pursue *any* set of goals is set back by disease and disability, then, though that may in fact be largely true, it would certainly seem appropriate for a rational poor person to adjust his level of medical care downward from what the middle class selects in order to balance out his health care needs with other important goals. The set of *all* goals, after all, is the point of the project. On the other hand, if the implicit goals of the opportunities which health care helps to equalize exclude or downgrade the competing goals which might lead a rational poor person to adjust his preferred level of health downward, we get locked in an argument about why health care's particular ultimate goals are so important. The concept of "opportunity" performs no magic here at all in abstraction from the real lives of preferring individuals.

It might be replied that neither any and all goals nor any particular, question-begging, restricted set of goals is presupposed by health care's connection with "equal opportunity." Health care instead gets its importance by preserving or restoring opportunity in a very simple, neutral, straightforward sense: a person's entire future potential.

This argument may work well in classic arguments for paternalism: we keep the child (or the child in us) from mortgaging its future. In the context of our current discussion, however, the argument is unpersuasive. The departure from medical egalitarianism does not feature an irrational child but focuses on a rational poor person who selects a leaner package of health care. Moreover, major parts of health care do not represent "future potential" any more than a whole variety of other preferences do. For example, additional insurance that covers lifesaving transplants at 60 looks like a potential-preserving use of resources to a 50- or 60-year-old (compared, say, to lengthy vacations in Hawaii), but for a poor person at 40 that item in a life-long health care package may not represent "potential" nearly as much as better housing for her family.

In the last analysis, the attraction we have to the proposition that a decent minimum of health care for the poor is roughly equal to the care others obtain reflects at best only practical considerations, not sound moral principle. Perhaps, for example, providers just inevitably fall into the routine of using a uniform conception of "good," "basic" care, so there is no way other than complete exclusion of specific services to distinguish a decent minimum from the common care for the middle class. (Note, though, that this provides only a highly qualified and partial argument for equal care. It does not allow us to see equal care for equal medical needs as ideal, nor, of course, does it help when we get to making policy decisions about reimbursing for discrete, separable items, as Oregon was doing.)

Or in particular historical circumstances, lumping the poor in with the middle class under a unitary standard of required care may seem to be the only politically feasible way of getting additional resources to the poor. In a sense, then, the public is justified in giving resources to poor people as medical care even when they would benefit more from devoting some of those resources to other things. (But then note: the attitudes that politically restrict government to that form of provision are themselves the problem. They are public attitudes, for which the public is still on the hook.)

We should thus reject any *principle* of equal care for equal medical needs. Therefore the Oregon arrangement, for example, is not morally objectionable on its face simply because its rationing pertains to poorer persons without touching the middle class. There are some other reasons, however, for objecting to Oregon's singling out of poor people for special rationing treatment.

What rational recipients themselves would choose in shaping a system of care for their larger lives is the preferable framework for conceiving of a decent minimum of care, and that can justify a lower level of health services for lower income people. Yet in Oregon's case it is not poor people who by and large are making the fundamental choices from which rationing and the final floor of accessible care emerge. The problem is not just that people other than the poor themselves are doing both the final prioritizing and the funding which determines the final cut-off line; that may be understandable, and virtually inevitable politically. But there are further unnecessary problems. Oregon's telephone survey to elicit the QOL rankings that influence the final priority list of health services did not focus on lower income people especially at all. More importantly, the legislature is working with a rather stacked deck in funding Medicaid: otherwise non-poor elderly, covered by Medicare but not for normal nursing home care, spend more than half the Medicaid budget on nursing home care after spending themselves down into medical indigence.

Most objectionably, the total situation in Oregon cannot be accurately described as simply an attempt of the state to bite the rationing bullet for state-assisted citizens while others have not had similar courage to ration their privately paid medical resources. Another major group assisted by the state, the elderly on Medicare, have not had their care nearly as significantly and explicitly rationed as have the poor. Meanwhile, persons privately insured through employer-paid premiums receive a roughly 40 percent subsidy from the government in the form of a tax break on their insurance.[16] Middle and upper class citizens have their care heavily subsidized by the government with little attempt by the state to ration their care. Rationing care may indeed be mandatory for a health care system truly responsible to prior consumer choices, and Oregon's attempt to ration care for the poor may even benefit its poor.* Moreover, there may be nothing wrong with rationing the care of public assistance recipients while leaving privately insured individuals free to pay for their own fatter, unrationed plans. But what is actually in place in Oregon today as a result of state and federal policies combined is different, and not nearly so unobjectionable. Non-poor citizens supported by the government face little if any explicit rationing, while poor citizens, receiving much smaller aggregate government support, face rationing.

It is logical that health care rationing bite first on services for the poor before it affects the care of others, but it is hardly conscionable for a society to ration poor people's care explicitly and then turn around and not only fail to ration, but highly subsidize, the care of others who are much better off. *Oregon's* rationing plan may not be ethically objectionable by itself, but the full picture—its plan together with federal Medicare and tax subsidy policy—is.

PUBLIC VS. INDIVIDUAL STANDARDS OF VALUE

One of the apparent costs of rationing arrangements seems to be the use of large group policies that ride roughshod over individual differences in what people value. Oregon, for example, draws up one ranked list of services despite the many differences about the preferred order of that list that undoubtedly exist among its Medicaid recipients. Morally this has to be a source of concern if the basic justification of rationing is that it reflects the prior refusal of informed, forward-looking subscribers to pay more to include the rationed-out items in their coverage. How serious a moral problem, though, is this apparent dominance of group over individual values?

Undoubtedly communities can be very irrational in collective decisions that they make. One

of the worst instances of this on the current rationing scene is the apparent confusion about expense in relation to the incidence of health problems in Oregon. Certain treatments for relatively common diseases that ranked low in Oregon's initial cost/QALY list got raised much higher on the list after later public discussion.[17] While it is politically understandable how services for "popular" diseases will get raised on the list, it is completely irrational: Of the treatments for a rare and a common disease that were initially ranked equal, the treatment for the rare disease costs less in the aggregate because there are fewer cases to absorb expense. A typical person stands just as much to gain from including treatments for ten equally rare diseases as from including treatments for one disease that is ten times more common than each of the rare ones, so that if the costs for all the treatments are the same *per case*, then the rare diseases come out equal to the ten times more common disease in cost/benefit effect. The rareness of a disease should make no difference in treatment priority if expense per case is no higher.

At a higher level, however, there may be equal confusion in the complaint that group rationing decisions will swamp out individual preferences. If all care is covered and none rationed, we get the impression that all individual choices are being satisfied; the individual patient who does not wish the care can still exercise her right of informed refusal. By contrast, it seems that if by a collective process a group of citizens that is not a voluntary association restricts certain care, the choices of individual dissenters who are willing to pay to have that care covered are being slighted.

The alleged contrast between these two cases in their respect for individual values and preferences is misleading, however. It is admittedly unfortunate, and a certain diminution of their liberty, that dissenters in the rationing case do not have their choices reflected in the final shape of their health plan. Yet equally, if no care is rationed, individuals who would prefer not to pay for coverage of some of the care that is then provided do not have their choices accommodated. We ought to see the failure to ration when people's considered prior preferences demand rationing as also a disparity between larger group choices and individual values. To be sure, the denial of care to an individual who would have preferred coverage can have

---

*EDITORS' NOTE: See Part Six, Section Two, "Is the Oregon Rationing Plan Fair?" by Norman Daniels.

more individually tragic results at a later stage (e.g., death), but not rationing can be just as much the failure of a group to accommodate individual choice as rationing is when good-faith dissenters prefer to pay more.

We must remember that autonomy, not just aggregate efficiency, is one of the values that supports selective rationing. Some dimensions of rationing will always remain morally suspect, but rationing's fundamental conflict with respect for the individual patient-subscriber is not as severe or intractable as most people assume.

NOTES

1. P. Menzel, *Strong Medicine: The Ethical Rationing of Health Care* (Oxford University Press, New York, N.Y., 1990), Chapters 1 and 2, especially pp. 10-15.
2. On the conditional moral legitimacy of presuming a person's consent, see Menzel, supra note 1, pp 22-36.
3. QALY is pronounced to rhyme with "holly." Such a unit has also been referred to as "well-years" or "health state utilities."
4. D. Hadorn, "The Oregon Priority-Setting Exercise: Quality of Life and Public Policy," *Hastings Center Report* 21 (3): 11 suppl. (May-June, 1991). . . .
5. 8.0 QALYs for $60,000: 2.0 QALYs more than 6.0 produced by dialysis.
6. J. Harris, "QALYfying the Value of Life, "*Journal of Medical Ethics* 13: 117 (1987). . . .

7. Or how many people in a better state of illness would have to be cured for one to think the situation better than curing a smaller number of patients in a worse-off condition? . . .
8. I now think that this QALY bargain is not what we are confined to if we use the Equivalence of Numbers questions (now in the literature called Person Trade-Off questions) to elicit numerical rankings.
9. J. Harris, "More and Better Justice," in J. Bell and S. Mendus, eds. *Philosophy and Medical Welfare* (Cambridge University Press, Cambridge, England, 1988), at p. 87.
10. Menzel, supra note 1, p. 89
11. Harris, . . . ibid.
12. M. O'Donnell, "One Man's Burden," *British Medical Journal* 293 (6538): 59 (July 5, 1986). . . .
13. Menzel, supra note 1, pp. 116-128. . . .
14. Menzel, supra note 1, pp. 119-126. . . .
15. A sophisticated version of this argument has been articulated by N. Daniels, *Just Health Care* (Cambridge University Press, Cambridge, 1985). . . .
16. The larger point here about rationing care for the poor in the light of our government's larger Medicare and tax subsidy support for the non-poor is made by C. Dougherty, "Setting Health Care Priorities: Oregon's Next Steps," *Hastings Center Report* 21 (3): 1 supp. (May-June, 1991). As to the 40 percent figure, note that employer-paid premiums are excluded entirely from taxable income: from the employee's 15-33 percent federal income tax and 7.8 percent Social Security tax, from the employer's 7.8 percent Social Security match, and from any state and local income taxes.
17. Hadorn, supra note 8, p. 11 suppl.

Fairness in the Allocation and Delivery of Health Care: A Case Study in Organ Transplantation

James F. Childress

Several cases in the last few years have stirred rumblings of distrust in the process of selecting recipients of scarce organs for transplantation. Mickey Mantle's rapid liver transplant, which came shortly after he was put on the waiting list in June 1995,

James F. Childress, "Ethical Criteria for Procuring and Distributing Organs for Transplantation," in *Practical Reasoning in Bioethics* by James Childress, Indiana University Press, 19??. Reprinted with permission from the publisher.

because of end-stage liver failure secondary to cirrhosis and cancer, was only the most recent. In 1993 Governor Robert P. Casey of Pennsylvania, age sixty-one, received an experimental and risky heart-liver transplant at the University of Pittsburgh Medical Center because his hereditary disease, amyloidosis, had caused his liver to produce an abnormal protein that then accumulated in the walls of his heart. Even though his medical team had expected a wait of four to six weeks, the thirteen-hour operation commenced just hours after his name had been entered onto the waiting list at the United Network for Organ Sharing (UNOS), the national organ transplantation and procurement network. . . .

SELECTION OF RECIPIENTS OF SCARCE ORGANS FOR TRANSPLANTATION

The scarcity of organs for transplantation will probably remain a problem for the indefinite future; indeed, it is probable that the demand will always exceed the supply, unless animal organs can be used or artificial organs can be developed. Under these circumstances, there will be difficult questions regarding the procedural and substantive standards for patient selection. Who should choose recipients of donated organs and by what criteria?

DONATED ORGANS AS PUBLIC RESOURCES

Why not simply let the physicians, nurses, and others involved in transplantation select patients? Why shouldn't selection be viewed as a medical decision to be made by the appropriate professionals? There are some important reasons for developing general public criteria of patient selection—criteria that are developed with input from the public and publicly stated and defended. Apart from special cases—for example, when living donors of kidneys designate a recipient or beneficiary—it can be argued that, from a moral standpoint, donated organs belong to the public, to the community. This fundamental conviction undergirded the Task Force's deliberations and recommendations regarding fair access to organ transplantation: Donated organs should be viewed as scarce public resources to be used for the welfare of the community. Organ procurement and transplant teams receive donated organs as trustees and stewards for the community. Their dispositional authority over those organs should be limited and constrained.

There is increasing demand that the public participate in formulating the criteria for patient selection in order to ensure that they are fair. In general, the evidence presented to the Task Force and published since then indicates that organ procurement and transplantation teams usually make morally responsible decisions in allocating and distributing organs. However, some widely publicized exceptions have

generated public controversy and perhaps even reduced organ donations—some of these appeared to the public to reflect favoritism to wealthy foreign nationals. The demand for public participation in the formulation of criteria for the allocation and distribution of organs stems in part from the nature of the organ procurement system—it depends on voluntary gifts by the public, that is, by individuals and their families, to the community. Indeed, there are important moral connections between policies of organ procurement and policies of organ distribution. On the one hand, it is obvious that the success of policies of organ procurement may reduce scarcity and hence obviate some of the difficulties of patient selection. On the other hand, distrust is a major reason for public reluctance to donate organs, and policies of procurement may be ineffective if policies of distribution are perceived by the public to be unfair and thus untrustworthy. Hence public participation—for example, in UNOS—is important. "Organ allocation falls into the region of public decision-making," as Jeffrey M. Prottas insists, "not medical ethics and much less medical tradition."[1] . . .

JUSTICE AND MORALLY RELEVANT AND IRRELEVANT CHARACTERISTICS

Justice not only involves public participation—a matter of fair process—but also substantive standards. "Justice" may be defined as rendering each person his or her due, and it includes both formal and material criteria. The formal criterion of justice is similar treatment for similar cases, while material criteria specify relevant similarities and dissimilarities among patients and thus determine how particular benefits and burdens will be distributed.[2] There is debate about the *moral relevance* and *moral weight* of various material criteria, such as need, merit, societal contribution, status, and ability to pay. Different theories of justice tend to accent different material criteria; however, some criteria may be acceptable in some areas of life but not in others.

A fundamental issue for organ transplantation is determining which material criteria are justifiable for the allocation and distribution of donated organs. Standards of justice permit rationing under conditions of scarcity, but they rule out selection criteria that are based on morally irrelevant characteristics, such as race or gender. The major debates focus on which characteristics of patients are morally relevant and which are morally irrelevant in the two stages of selection for organ transplantation: (1) formation of a waiting list, and (2) distribution of available organs to patients on the waiting list.

WAITING LISTS: PROBLEMS IN ADMISSION

There is general agreement that the waiting list of candidates for transplantation should be set largely according to medical criteria, i.e., the need for and the probability of benefiting from an organ transplant. There is, of course, debate about whether these medical criteria should be defined broadly or narrowly (for example, how high should we set the standard for minimal efficacy?), about how to specify these criteria, about the relevance of several different factors to the determination of need and efficacy, and about which criteria should have priority in case of conflict.

Why are both need and probability of success important? They reflect *medical utility* which requires the maximization of welfare among patients suffering from end-stage organ failure. Medical utility should not be confused with *social utility*.[3] While social utility focuses on the value of salvageable patients for society, medical utility requires that organs be used as effectively and as efficiently as possible to benefit as many patients as possible. For example, if there is no reasonable chance that a transplant will be successful for a particular patient, it could even be unethical to put the patient in line to receive a scarce organ.

Efforts are made through UNOS and elsewhere to develop fair policies for allocating and distributing organs to patients on waiting lists, but it is more difficult to ensure equitable access to waiting lists for organ transplants. There is evidence that women, minorities, and low-income patients do not receive transplants at the same rates as white men with high incomes.[4] For example, in one study, females were approximately 30 percent less likely than males to receive a kidney transplant, black dialysis patients were only 55 percent as likely as white dialysis patients to receive a cadaver transplant, and patients receiving dialysis in units in higher income areas had higher transplant rates. A primary source of unequal access appears to be in the decisions about who will be admitted to the waiting list rather than in the decisions about who will receive donated organs (although the waiting times may be quite

unequal). Serious questions were raised, for instance, about the admission of Mickey Mantle to the liver transplant waiting list, even though there is no reason to believe that his selection from the waiting list was unfair. However, more research will be required to determine the extent to which unequal access to kidney transplantation, for example, hinges on patient choices and legitimate medical factors rather than on physician sequestration of patients in dialysis units, physician failure to inform and refer some groups of patients, or physician bias in the selection of patients seeking admission to waiting lists. . . .

UNOS POINT SYSTEM FOR CADAVERIC KIDNEYS

Although UNOS has developed computerized point systems for the allocation of hearts, livers, and kidneys, I will use the point system for kidneys as the primary example because it has received the most attention and has undergone major alterations in light of conflicting values. In October 1987, UNOS implemented a point system for cadaveric kidneys, based on a proposal by Thomas E. Starzl and colleagues.[5] This system required that cadaveric kidneys be offered to patients on the local waiting list (defined as either the individual transplant center recipient list or a shared list of recipients within a defined procurement area) in descending order, with the patient with the highest number of points receiving the highest priority. The original point system consisted of three major parameters: the degree of sensitization, reflected in panel reactive antibodies (PRA, ten points maximum), time on the waiting list (ten points maximum), and HLA matching (twelve points maximum), with some attention to logistics and urgency. Critics noted that the point values for time waiting and high PRA overrode all other point allocations so that the first patient to appear on the print-out had high PRA levels but poor HLA matches. And most of the requests for area variances involved PRA and antigen match.

After much discussion, UNOS in 1989 adopted a revised point system that stressed HLA matching because of evidence about its long-term impact on graft survival. This revised point system accorded less weight to sensitization and to time on the waiting list, as well as to logistics and urgency.

According to the UNOS policy statement, "for the national pool, the new allocation system will ensure optimal use of every cadaver kidney offered, since it will identify very well matched recipients. Highly sensitized patients will be chosen when excellent matches emerge. Kidneys will be shipped to highly sensitized patients generally only when negative crossmatches had [sic] been obtained at the donor center. Within each match category fractions of a point acquired for waiting time will determine the order in which patients with the same match score would be listed.[6] Medical urgency status could be requested under some circumstances, but it is rare because dialysis is usually possible as a backup. The policy of mandatory sharing of zero antigen mismatches continued, and a payback policy was adopted for centers receiving organs that had to be shared. ABO blood-group matching remained the same— blood group "O" kidneys could be transplanted only into blood group "O" patients except in the case of kidneys that were mandatorily shared because of HLA match; otherwise "O" patients would be greatly disadvantaged because "O" organs are usable in other blood groups, whereas "O" patients can only use "O" organs.

Another major change occurred in 1995 when the point system for kidney transplants was revised to increase the number of kidneys allocated by waiting time alone, thereby reducing the reliance upon certain HLA matches. Research had indicated that zero ABDR mismatched kidneys have a graft survival as high as kidneys with a six-antigen match, while the graft survival of kidneys with zero AB and three BDR mismatch levels are not significantly better than unmatched grafts. Thus, the UNOS board decided to mandate sharing of all zero mismatched kidneys but to eliminate points at the zero AB and three BDR mismatch levels and to assign seven points for zero BDR mismatches, five points for one BDR mismatch, and two points for two BDR mismatches. As a result of this shift in the point system, UNOS projected that the number of kidneys allocated by waiting time alone would increase from approximately 10 percent to approximately 40 percent. The remainder would be allocated according to a mix of HLA matching, waiting time, PRA, and age (with additional points given for young people, in a policy that will be discussed below).

ASSESSMENT OF POINT SYSTEMS FOR ALLOCATING ORGANS

How are such point systems to be assessed? I will first consider the value of computerized point systems in general and then the value of particular point systems. Many of the supposed advantages and disadvantages of point systems for the allocation of organs hinge on their alleged *objectivity*. Even though a point system does not eliminate the individual physician's judgment—the art of medicine—regarding, for example, the final decision about the use of an organ for any particular patient, it does reduce the physician's discretion. For example, Thomas Starzl contends that "the effect of [his original] point system was to diminish judgmental factors in case selection, which in the past probably had operated to the disadvantage of 'undesirable' potential recipients, including older ones and possibly ethnic minorities.[7] Even though many concede that some decisions have certainly been affected by physicians' subjective biases—for example, in admission to waiting lists— many also stress that it is important for physicians to be able to practice the art of medicine in view of the individual features of particular cases, such as predicting efficacy for a particular patient. According to Daniel Wikler, a computerized point system can systematize decision making by focusing on a full range of data and "can convince patients and the public that a routine, sound plan is in place," perhaps enhancing perception of fairness in distribution or at least stimulating public discussion.[8] However, in focusing on objectivity, we must not forget that the selection and assignment of weights (points) to these factors rest on values.

With the exception of time on the waiting list, the criteria used in the different point systems for kidneys are medical in the sense that they involve medical techniques used by medical personnel and arguably influence the likely success or failure of the transplant. However, while medical in these senses, these criteria are not value free or value neutral. The vigorous debate about how much weight each criterion should have is only in part technical and scientific (e.g., the impact of HLA matching); it is to a great extent ethical. In kidney transplantation, some factors, such as quality of antigen match and logistical score, focus on the chance of a successful outcome; in different ways both medical urgency and panel-reactive antibody focus on patient need; and time on the waiting list introduces a nonmedical factor, even though it may overlap with panel-reactive antibody because sensitized patients tend to wait longer for transplants. The points assigned to these various factors thus reflect value judgments about the relative importance of patient need, probability of success, and time of waiting—all factors stressed by the federal Task Force on Organ Transplantation.

MEDICAL UTILITY IN PATIENT SELECTION

Both patient need for a transplant and the probability of a successful transplant reflect medical utility. Medical utility is not necessarily at odds with fairness, even though they sometimes come into conflict. It is a fundamental mistake to suppose that "medical utility" and "fairness" are necessarily in tension so that if one is met the other is infringed, and it is a fundamental mistake to suppose that "fairness" always dictates priority to queuing or randomization over "medical utility." Indeed, in some contexts determination of "medical utility" may be required by the principle of fairness. It may be "unfortunate" when one patient receives an organ over another because of "medical utility," but it is not necessarily "unfair." Appeals to "medical utility" in the distribution of organs do not necessarily violate the principle of equal concern and respect; judgments based on "medical utility" do not necessarily show disrespect and contempt, which, by contrast, are inevitable in judgments based on patients' comparative "social utility." Furthermore, acceptance of "medical utility" does not commit one to utilitarianism as a foundational or substantive moral doctrine; "medical utility" can (and should) be accepted in any defensible deontological framework as well. Holding that a lexical or serial order of these criteria is impossible also does not entail utilitarianism. In addition, using a Rawlsian contract metaphor, we can argue that in a fair set of decision-making circumstances behind the veil of ignorance, patients not knowing their own medical conditions would choose criteria of "medical utility." Such a hypothetical contract allegedly makes the distribution fair to potential recipients. Finally, others also argue that fairness to donors requires that organs be used effectively and efficiently.

Judgments about medical need and probability of success, as already noted, are value-laden. Consider, for example, the debates about what will count as *success*—such as length of graft survival, length of patient survival, quality of life, rehabilitation—and about which factors influence the *probability of success*. Some contraindications are well established, such as mismatched blood group or positive donor-recipient crossmatch. Over time the UNOS point system for kidneys has stressed, to varying degrees, tissue matching on medical utility grounds. It is also not unfair to use tissue matching, not only because of medical utility, but because tissue matching functions as a kind of natural lottery, which involves the randomness of the HLA match between available donors and recipients. However, there is vigorous debate about the relative importance of tissue matching now that cyclosporine and other immunosuppressive medications are available, and this technical debate influences judgments about the conditions under which kidneys should be shared outside the location where they are retrieved. For example, since cyclosporine is nephrotoxic, a retrieved kidney needs to be transplanted sooner than usual in order to increase the chances of successful transplantation when that immunosuppressive medication is used. Furthermore, studies also indicate that the length of cold ischemic time prior to the kidney's transplantation has an impact on graft survival.

Tissue matching needs ongoing scrutiny. First, in view of the scientific controversy, it is essential to see if certain levels of tissue match or mismatch really make significant differences in the outcome of transplantation over time. Second, it is morally imperative to monitor the operation of the point systems to make sure that tissue matching does not have unjustified discriminatory effects, for example, against blacks and other minorities. As noted, discrimination may already occur against blacks and other minorities in admission to waiting lists, and tissue matching may have discriminatory effects for some patients on the waiting list. For example, most organ donors are white, certain HLA phenotypes are different in white, black, and Hispanic populations, the identification of HLA phenotypes is less complete for blacks and Hispanics, nonwhites have a higher rate of end-stage renal disease, and nonwhite populations are disproportionately represented on dialysis lists. In this context, Robert Veatch argues that "if organs are to be allocated on the basis of degree of tissue match, the policy is, de facto, a whites-first policy."[9] Monitoring the operation of each point system will provide evidence regarding discriminatory effects. If such discriminatory effects emerge, then it may be necessary to sacrifice some probability of success in order to take affirmative action to protect blacks and other minorities. Indeed, such considerations figured significantly in the UNOS decision to alter, in 1995, the point system for the allocation of cadaveric kidneys to eliminate points given from some levels of match and to increase the role of time on the waiting lists.

Sometimes there is a tension between urgency of need and probability of success. Robert M. Veatch contends that "a justice-based allocation . . . would demand that highest priority be given to medical need and length of time the patient has been in need."[10] Apparently some potential recipients would choose such criteria. For example, in determining who will receive a heart, members of a Canadian transplant team note, "it becomes a difficult ethical issue as to whether the patient with the better outcome or the individual with the greatest urgency should receive the heart. The patients themselves would opt for the patient with the greatest urgency and by and large that is the decision taken by the team. However, one is conscious of the fact that one may be affecting the overall success rate by making choices in favor of individual patient urgency rather than making them on the basis of success."

Tensions between medical urgency and probability of success may vary greatly depending on the organ in question. For instance, there is debate in heart transplantation about the use of artificial hearts and other assist devices, in part because they have sometimes given patients priority for scarce donor hearts on the basis of medical need, even though their chances for success may have been minimal. Critics such as George Annas charge that using the total artificial heart as a temporary bridge to transplantation does not save lives; it only changes the identities of those receiving heart transplants by giving very sick patients priority.[11] And UNOS revised its criteria for the allocation of hearts so that patients on mechanical assist devices would no longer receive priority

over all other candidates in their area; under the revised allocation system, patients who require inotropic agents and are in intensive care units would also appear in the top priority group. One goal of this revision was to remove any incentive for a physician to put a patient on an assist device in order to improve his or her chances of getting a heart transplant.

In liver transplantation, to take another example, the dominant practice has been to give the sickest patient the highest priority, but "medical utility" (and some would include cost-effectiveness) would often dictate placing the liver in the fittest patient and realizing the greatest medical benefit (at the lowest cost). Another reason for priority to those with a higher probability of benefit is that "as time goes on . . . the fitter patients become increasingly ill, their survivability on the waiting list declines, and their operative risk soars." Nevertheless, as Olga Jonasson notes, there is clearly one case in which the sickest of all patients awaiting liver transplants is also the best candidate for successful transplantation—the young, previously healthy patient with fulminant acute liver failure.

The category of medical urgency may not be as important when an artificial organ can be used as a backup (for example, dialysis for end-stage renal failure). However, some argue that medical urgency should include not only the immediate threat of death but also the likelihood of not receiving another organ because of presensitization particularly because sensitized patients now constitute a hard core of the waiting lists for kidney transplants. The Task Force recommended that a highly sensitized patient who is predicted on the basis of either a computer antibody analysis or an actual crossmatch to accept the transplant should be given priority over equivalently matched nonsensitized patients. And yet the success rates may be lower for sensitized patients than for nonsensitized patients.

Another problem is that medical urgency is a manipulable category. It is reportedly abused at times by physicians eager to protect their patients by declaring them medically urgent in order to increase their chances for a transplant. These reports are not implausible in light of studies indicating that physicians are willing to lie in order to promote their patients' welfare in the health care system, such as using a misleading category in order to enable the patient to have a diagnostic procedure covered by health insurance.

In short, it is not at all clear that a general, a priori formulation of the appropriate relation between medical need and probability of success within medical utility is defensible, in part because of the variations in organ systems. Thus, the proposals may have to be organ specific, and variations can be expected in policies from one organ to another. Ongoing monitoring and assessment of current policies, with public input and with special attention to the proper use of the category of medical urgency, appears to be the most appropriate action. As the federal Task Force recommended,

> A decision on how to apply the criterion of urgency must be developed by a thoughtful and broadly representative group, which must struggle with the concept of [the] best use of organs in the context of compassion and humanitarianism. Because donated organs are a scarce resource, policies to resolve conflicts between equity and efficiency that arise in the distribution of organs should be determined by a broadly representative group that includes patient, community and ethical perspectives, as well as those of the medical professionals involved.[12]

TIME ON THE WAITING LIST

Many including this writer have argued that randomization or time on the waiting list is a fair way to allocate scarce lifesaving resources under some circumstances. I developed my argument to this effect in 1970 when the debate was mainly about kidney dialysis.[13]. . . At that time I argued that once the pool of medically eligible candidates has been determined, it is then fair to make the final selection by randomization or queuing. However, I believe that matters are somewhat different when the scarce medical resource is an organ, which cannot be reused. Now I would argue that medical utility should also be used to determine which candidate should receive the organ, after the eligible candidates have been identified on grounds of medical utility. A major reason is not wasting the gift of life; the organ has been donated for effective use. Giving an organ to a patient who has a very limited chance of success, perhaps because of poor tissue match, increases the probability that he or she will then need another transplant for survival,

further reducing the chances for others as well as for his or her own successful transplantation.

Nevertheless, it is important to reject positions that rule out queuing or time on the waiting list as morally irrelevant or even morally pernicious. For example, Olga Jonasson argues that "length of time on the waiting list is the least fair, most easily manipulated, and most mindless of all methods of organ allocation," and Ruth Macklin argues that the principle of "first come, first served" is inapplicable and even inequitable in the allocation of scarce medical resources because it ignores different medical needs and prognoses.

By contrast to those positions, if two or more patients are equally good candidates for a particular organ according to the medical criteria of need and probability of success, their time on the waiting list may be the fairest way to make the final selection. This approach is similar to that recommended by the federal Task Force.[14] The original UNOS point system for kidneys gave more weight to time on the waiting list and also to sensitization, but since highly sensitized patients are likely to spend more time on the waiting list they were, in effect, counted twice. Some argued that such double counting is justifiable because of their difficulty of obtaining organs, while others noted that such patients might then receive priority over much better matched patients. In the revised point system in 1989, time on the waiting list functioned more as a tiebreaker in the allocation of kidneys in the UNOS point system, while in the revised point system in 1995, it again received greater weight (the point value was raised from 0.5 to one point for each full year of waiting time).

Queuing is often favored because it appears to be objective and impersonal, but the justification of its use in patient selection depends on certain values (or principles), such as fair opportunity. And there are both ethical and practical problems. It is not always easy to determine when a patient entered the waiting list; one way is the accession time on the UNOS list. But, as Jonasson notes, it is easy to manipulate this criterion, for example, by putting patients on the list before they become dialysis dependent. In addition, it is important to note that the fairness of queuing (as well as of randomization) depends in part on background conditions. For example, some people may not seek care early because of limited financial resources and insurance; others may receive inadequate medical advice about how early to seek transplantation; and so forth.

There are clear differences in orientation between two approaches to time on the waiting list—use time on the waiting list unless there are substantial differences in medical utility, or follow medical utility unless there are no substantial differences and then use time on the waiting list. However, they should, practically speaking, end up at the same place, *if* there is a consensus on what constitutes "substantial differences in medical utility. . . .

THE ACCESS OF FOREIGN NATIONALS TO ORGANS DONATED IN THE UNITED STATES

Another major question arises from the Task Force's recommendation that "donated organs be considered a national resource": Should foreign nationals have access to organs donated in the United States? The issue of geographical boundaries, or "accidents of geography," is international as well as intranational. Of the approximately 6,000 cadaveric kidneys transplanted in the United States in 1985, 300 went to nonresident aliens who had come to the United States for medical care, and 200 to 250 additional kidneys were shipped abroad for use in other countries.

The debate about transplanting organs obtained in the United States into foreign nationals and about exporting those organs invokes various moral principles as well as diverse convictions about the ownership of donated organs. Some who propose physician discretion in the selection of patients insist that the ideal of medical humanitarianism precludes the use of criteria such as national residence. By contrast, critics of physician discretion contend that the distribution of donated organs is not merely or even primarily a matter of medical humanitarianism but of social humanitarianism. I agree that donated organs belong to the community, that procurement and transplantation teams only serve as trustees and stewards of donated organs, and that the debate essentially concerns social rather than medical humanitarianism.

It should not be surprising that the most vigorous and divisive debate on the federal Task Force centered on the access of foreign nationals to cadaveric organs donated in the United States. Members of the Task Force sought to balance principles of fairness, beneficence (expressed as compassion and generosity), and utility and efficiency, particularly in the avoidance of kidney wastage. There was little or no interest in excluding foreign nationals altogether, for instance, when organs would otherwise go to waste. Rather, the debate focused on whether to adopt (1) a policy of U.S. citizens and residents first—sometimes called "Americans first"—which would allow some nonresident aliens on waiting lists but would not allow them to receive any particular donated organ unless no U.S. citizen or resident could benefit from it, or (2) a policy that would set a ceiling on the number of nonresident aliens on the waiting list, but would accord equal treatment to everyone on the list, regardless of national residence. The Task Force recommended the first policy for hearts and livers and the second policy for kidneys, recommending a ceiling of 10 percent until the matter could be reviewed by the OPTN (which became UNOS).

The majority of the Task Force distinguished between these two policies on the grounds that kidneys are not as scarce as extrarenal organs, and dialysis is usually available and feasible as a backup or an alternative to transplantation in the treatment of end-stage renal failure. However, eight of the twenty-five members of the Task Force dissented from the recommendation for renal organs. These dissenters argued that it is unfair to members of the national community to deny or to delay their access to organs donated in the United States and unfair to use taxpayers' money to obtain kidneys that would be distributed to nonresident aliens. . . .

After reviewing various arguments, UNOS adopted a policy that established some limits and directions but relied mainly on a procedure of accountability in the transplantation of nonresident aliens. It required UNOS members to charge the same fees for nonresident aliens as for domestic patients, to treat all patients accepted on transplant waiting lists according to UNOS policies for the equitable distribution of donated organs, and to arrange any exportation of organs through UNOS and then only after no suitable recipient could be located in the United States or Canada (included because of sharing arrangements). Accountability was established in several ways. On the local level, centers that accept nonresident aliens on their waiting lists should establish a mechanism for community participation and review. On the national level, the UNOS committee on foreign relations has a right to audit all transplant center activities relating to nonresident aliens and will automatically review any center that has more than 10 percent of its transplant recipients from foreign nationals.

ABILITY TO PAY

So far I have examined issues of patient selection for organs for transplantation—both formation of the waiting list and selection to receive a particular organ—apart from questions of costs. Yet organ transplants are notoriously very expensive. Our society has responded very differently to different organ transplant procedures. Through Medicare's End-Stage Renal Disease (ESRD) program, virtually everyone who needs a kidney transplant (or dialysis) is covered, while coverage for heart and liver transplantation is at best spotty. Should ability to pay function as a criterion for admission to waiting lists? Should there be a "green screen" for access to waiting lists for organ transplantation? These questions cannot be directly addressed by UNOS; they emerge on other levels for other social institutions, particularly for the federal and state governments.

As part of its efforts to propose policies to ensure equitable access to organ transplantation, the federal Task Force on Organ Transplantation offered several arguments in favor of increasing societal funding for organ transplants—on the one hand, for immunosuppressive medications for organ transplants already funded (mainly kidneys), and, on the other hand, for extrarenal organ transplants not currently funded.

The Task Force concluded that coverage for immunosuppressive medications was important because, for example, wealth discrimination had reentered the ESRD program, which had been designed to eliminate distribution of artificial and transplanted kidneys according to ability to pay. Noting that approximately 25 percent of the transplant population (for all organs) lacked state or private coverage for immunosuppressive medications, especially cyclosporine, which was then estimated to cost approximately $5,000 to $7,000 a year, the Task Force "found evidence that inability to pay for immunosuppressive medications had been a factor in the initial selection of patients for transplantation" and that some transplant recipients had undergone nonmedically indicated—and potentially risky—changes in their medications because of the costs. The Medicare coverage that was subsequently approved, in part in response to the Task Force report, was limited to one year after the transplant. Further study is needed to determine the extent to which limited coverage of immunosuppressive medications limits access to transplants. (The coverage is now being gradually extended to a full three-year period.)

Much of the Task Force's concern about fair access focused on extrarenal organs—hearts and livers—in view of the limited and uneven provision of funds for them. And, according to the Task Force, there are several arguments for a societal obligation, to be discharged by the federal government as a last resort, to provide funds for extrarenal transplants in order to ensure fair access. One argument focuses on the *continuity* between extrarenal organ transplants and other medical procedures that are already covered, such as kidney transplants and dialysis. Appealing to the principle of consistency or universalizability, this argument accepts the precedent value of prior and current policy decisions. Still another premise in the argument is empirical—extrarenal transplants are comparable in efficacy and costs to procedures that are routinely covered. In response to worries about cost containment, defenders of public funding for organ transplantation hold that it is unfair to impose the major burden of cost containment on patients with end-stage organ failure who need transplants. The burdens of cost containment should themselves be distributed equitably across categories of patients needing health care.

A second argument focuses on the *distinctiveness* or *uniqueness* of organ transplantation, particularly the social practices of procurement that provide the organs for transplantation. This argument identifies an important moral connection between organ procurement, including organ donation, and organ distribution and allocation. In its efforts to increase the supply of organs, our society requests donations of organs from people of all socioeconomic classes—for example, through presidential appeals for organ donations or through state "required request" and "routine inquiry" statues, which mandate that institutions inquire about an individual's or family's willingness to donate, or even request such a donation. However, it is unfair and even exploitative for society to ask people, rich and poor alike, to donate organs if access to donated organs will be determined by ability to pay rather than by medical need, probability of success, and time on the waiting list.[15]

A third and related argument builds on societal opposition to commercialization and commodification of human body parts, as expressed in various laws and policies. . . . Federal legislation—as well as legislation in some states—prohibits individuals from transferring organs over which they have dispositional authority for valuable consideration.[16] In addition, various professional organizations involved in organ transplantation have taken a stand against the sale of organs for transplantation. It is difficult, according to this third argument, to distinguish (1) buying an organ for transplantation and then hiring a surgeon to perform the procedure from (2) purchasing an organ transplantation procedure that includes a (donated) organ as well as the surgeon's (and others') services.

These last two principled arguments may be combined with consequentialist arguments. There are legitimate worries about the impact of unequal access to organ transplants, based on inability to pay, on the system of organ procurement that includes gifts of organs from individuals and their families. As I noted earlier, there is substantial evidence that attitudes of distrust limit organ donation; this distrust appears to be directed at both organ procurement (e.g., the fear the potential donors will be declared dead prematurely) and organ distribution (e.g., the concern that potential transplant recipients from higher socioeconomic classes will receive priority). Thus, it is not at all surprising that after Oregon decided to stop providing Medicaid funds for most organ transplants, "a boycott of organ donations was organized by some low-income people." And cynical comments about how rapidly famous people, such as Mickey Mantle, receive scarce organ transplants reflect public suspicion of organ allocation policies.

A final argument is closely related to the first one, but instead of building on what the society has already decided to do regarding other health care, it focuses on the federal government's obligation, at least as a last resort, to ensure fair access to health care, including organ transplantation, by removing financial barriers, if necessary. For example, this argument might appeal to what the President's Commission for the Study of Ethical Problems in Medicine and Biomedical and Behavioral Research construed as society's obligation to provide equitable access to an adequate level of health care without excessive burdens.* (Even though this argument may appear to be independent of social practices, it may—and should—nevertheless appeal to principles and values embedded in those practices.) Whatever the foundation of the obligation, there will still be vigorous debate about what counts as an adequate level of health care and whether organ transplants qualify. And this debate moves us to questions of *macroallocation*. It is now standard to distinguish microallocation from macroallocation. For example, Engelhardt uses the term "macroallocation" to refer to "allocations among general categories of expenditures," and the term "microallocation" to refer to "choices among particular individuals as to whether they will be recipients of resources and in what amount. "[17]

The question of microallocation is *who* will receive a particular scarce good; the questions of macroallocation focus on *how much* of a good will be made available, where financial resources can alter the availability of that good, such as organ transplants or AZT for AIDS patients. It is important to note that while macroallocation and microallocation are analytically distinct, they are significantly related. Obviously macroallocation decisions determine the extent of scarcity and the difficulty of patient selection by in part determining how much of a good will be made available in a society. If a particular technology or mode of health care is in limited supply, as is often the case, then there may be difficult microallocation decisions about who will receive this particular scarce good. But problems in microallocation may also have an impact on macroallocation decisions. For instance, it has been argued that the federal

*EDITORS' NOTE: See Part Six, Section One.

government decided to provide virtually universal funding for treatments for end-stage renal disease in part to eliminate the problem of patient selection for kidney dialysis and transplantation, that is, the problem of having health care professionals and committees explicitly determine who would live and who would die. . . .

CONCLUSION

In conclusion, I want to draw together several points and mention a few others that grow out of this analysis and properly set the context for discussion of a political-legal right to health care. First, I have stressed the principle of fairness (equity or justice). This principle is not easy to specify or to apply, for there are vigorous disputes about its meaning (e.g., whether it excludes medical utility) and about its weight (e.g., when it comes into conflict with other principles).

Second, fairness is not the only principle; there are others, including utility and respect for personal autonomy. Fairness does not always oppose such principles as medical utility, as I argued in my proposals for a fair use of medical utility (medical need and probability of success) in the allocation and distribution of organs for transplantation. Even when there are conflicts it is not possible to indicate in advance exactly which principle should have priority. Seeking to balance these various principles is a worthy process and goal, but sometimes trade-offs are inevitable in policies of allocation and distribution.[18]

Third, if we ask about the fairness of providing or not providing funds for extrarenal transplants, it may be difficult to answer that question in an unfair system. If, as Norman Daniels argues, "our system is, in general, unjust,"[19] then it may be difficult to determine whether it would be just or unjust to press for and obtain funds for organ transplants or AZT or some other treatment. Which policy of allocation would be more likely to lead to a more just system? And, if neither would, which should be adopted as the morally preferable—perhaps because more just—policy within an unjust system? I will provide a context for such judgments in the next chapter, when I consider a general political-legal right to health care, which is currently missing from U.S. health policy.

Fourth, not only do our reflections about policies of allocation and distribution occur within a particular sociopolitical context, but that context itself often changes over time. Thus, it may be appropriate to develop policies to reaffirm some principles or values that have been neglected, or even overridden, in order to maintain their significance for the society over time.[20] There is no reason to suppose that within the range of ethically acceptable policies only one should be implemented over time.

Finally, ethical theories, including theories of justice and fairness, may have only limited applicability, partly in view of conditions that limit their feasibility. The phrase "applied ethics"—the application of ethical principles, rules, and theories—is not the most appropriate, for the task for ethics is more that of illuminating the ethical presuppositions and implications of the choices we have to make in the real world, in response to such questions as how organs should be distributed and allocated and whether organ transplants should receive societal funds. Those questions arise in a complex mix of social, political, scientific, medical, and other factors. "Illumination" rather than "resolution" is the main contribution of ethical theory, and it properly takes the form of "practical ethics" rather than "applied ethics."

NOTES

1. Jeffrey M Prottas, "Nonresident Aliens and Access to Organ Transplant," *Transplantation Proceedings* 21 (June 1989) 3428.
2. For a discussion of criteria of justice, see Beauchamp and Childress, *Principles of Biomedical Ethics*, 4th ed. (New York: Oxford University Press, 1994), chap. 6.
3. For the distinction between "medical utility" and "social utility," see James F. Childress, "Triage in Neonatal Intensive Care: The Limitations of a Metaphor," *Virginia Law Review* 69 (April 1983): 547-61.
4. See P. W. Eggers, "Effect of Transplantation on the Medicare End Stage Renal Disease Program," *New England Journal of Medicine* 318 (1989): 223-29.
5. See T. E. Starzl, T. R. Hakala, A. Tzakis et al., "A Multifactorial System for Equitable Selection of Cadaver Kidney Recipients," *Journal of the American Medical Association* 257 (1987): 3073-75.
6. UNOS, *Final Statement of Policy: UNOS Policy Regarding Utilization of the Point System for Cadaveric Kidney Allocation* (Richmond, VA: UNOS, April 4, 1989), which

gives the history of the policy development to that point, as as well as an overview of the different stages and arguments involved in the policy formation.

7. T. E. Starzl, R. Shaprio, and L. Teperman, "The Point System for Organ Distribution," *Transplantation Proceedings* 21 (June 1989): 3434.

8. Daniel Wikler, "Equity, Efficacy, and the Point System for Transplant Recipient Selection," *Transplantation Proceedings* 21 (June 1989): 3437.

9. Robert M. Veatch, "Allocating Organs by Utilitarianism Is Seen as Favoring Whites over Blacks," *Kennedy Institute of Ethics Newsletter* 3 (July 1989):1 and 3.

10. Robert M. Veatch, *Death, Dying and the Biological Revolution*, rev ed. (New Haven: Yale University Press, 1989), p. 210.

11. George J. Annas, "No Cheers for Temporary Artificial Hearts," *Hastings Center Report* 15 (October 1985).

12. Task Force, *Organ Transplantation*, pp. 88-89.

13. James F. Childress, "Who Shall Live When Not All Can Live?" *Soundings* 53 (1970): 339-55.

14. See Task Force, *Organ Transplantation,* chap. 5.

15. Contrast Norman Daniels, "Comment: Ability to Pay and Access to Transplantation," *Transplantation Proceedings* 21 (June 1989): 3434. For a sharp criticism see F. M. Kamm, "The Report of the U.S. Task Force on Organ Transplantation: Criticisms and Alternatives," *Mount Sinai Journal of Medicine* 56 (May 1989): 207-20.

16. See PL 98-507.

17. H. Tristram Engelhardt, Jr., *Foundations of Bioethics* (New York: Oxford University Press, 1986), p. 369, n. 7.

18. For a sketch of a model of balancing, which is, however, not fully consistent, see "The UNOS Statement of Principles and Objectives of Equitable Organ Allocation," *UNOS Update* (August 1994), pp. 20-38. For a strong argument against balancing medical utility against justice, with justice interpreted as requiring "opportunities for equality of health," see Robert M. Veatch's response to an earlier version of this chapter.* My reasons for rejecting much of Veatch's position appear in the argument for medical utility in the previous chapter as well as in the overall argument of this chapter, even though I do not directly address his arguments.

19. Norman Daniels, *Just Health Care* (Cambridge: Cambridge University Press, 1985), which has greatly influenced these concluding remarks.

20. Guido Calabresi and Philip Bobbitt, *Tragic Choices* (New York: Norton, 1977).

*EDITORS' NOTE: See this section.

Equality, Justice, and Rightness in Allocating Health Care: A Response to James Childress

Robert M. Veatch

James Childress has given us a carefully reasoned and generally plausible account of an ethics of allocating resources and its implications for organ transplantation, one that reflects a moral theory far more subtle than a simple strategy of maximizing good consequences from the scarce health care resources we have available. He shows that the decisions made about ethical theory make a difference in how people will get treated by the health care system. Rather modest changes in the theory, however, can have important implications for decisions such as who should get scarce organs for transplantation.

I would like to suggest some places where some of these small changes in the general theory would be plausible and then comment on how that has forced me in my role as a member of the Washington Regional Transplant consortium to vote for a different kidney allocation formula.

Childress and I agree that justice or fairness is one among several right-making principles for moral action. This implies that it is theoretically possible that, depending on one's formula for resolving conflict among ethical principles, a policy that is just or fair may turn out not to be exactly the policy that is ethically right, all things considered. Before tackling the question of the correct formula for resolving

From *A Time To Be Born and A Time To Die: The Ethics of Choice,* Barry S. Kogan, editor, Aldine de Gruyter, 1991. Copyright © 1991 Walter de Gruyter, Inc., New York. Reprinted with permission from the publisher and the author.

such conflict among principles, about which Childress and I differ on certain particulars, it is going to be necessary to clarify exactly what we mean by justice. Then I will try to reveal why this makes me opt for a somewhat different strategy for allocating kidneys than Childress appears to favor. I will close with some comments on how justice ought to relate to the other moral principles for allocating kidneys or any other scarce health resource.

THE PRINCIPLE OF JUSTICE

Deciding what is just or fair entails understanding whether there is a moral right-making characteristic of actions or polices or practices that is independent of the other usual considerations we take into account in deciding about right conduct. In particular, is the right allocation simply a matter of spreading resources around so that they produce the greatest amount of good in aggregate or so that people are free to act autonomously in using their private property; or is there some unique and independent consideration separate from these factors that pulls on us in deciding who should get a kidney or a scarce hospital bed or Medicare dollar?

Many ethical traditions have recognized that there is a moral principle independent of utility that bears on how resources should be distributed. They variously hold that there is a natural law, a law created by God, or that reason requires that one thing to consider in allocating resources is that they be distributed justly. One approach that permits some convergence of these disparate views is to ask what reasonable people would recognize as just if they had general knowledge of the facts of nature and human psychology, but no knowledge of their particular interests or needs. This approach does not necessarily require us to agree on why people under such circumstances would agree. Some might say they would agree because there is a preexisting moral law, others because reason would require it, or because it is a prudent way to protect self-interest. Regardless, there seems to be considerable convergence that, at least in certain circumstances, justice has something to do with an allocation that is not based solely on getting as much total or average utility out of the resources being allocated. Our sense of justice has something to do with recognizing the fundamental equality of persons. Although

the argument cannot here be developed in detail, virtually all the ethical traditions participating in the current discussion recognize that the principle of justice creates a presumption in favor of equality. In my view, people under the circumstances I have described would agree that one right-making characteristic of an allocation practice would be that it gives people an opportunity for equality of well-being. This is what I shall refer to as the egalitarian principle of justice. Recall that whether it is right, on balance, to give people such an opportunity for equality of well-being will have to be settled later . . . .

JUSTICE IN ALLOCATING ORGANS FOR TRANSPLANT

This brings us to the question of what would count as a just practice for allocation of kidneys or other organs for transplant. We should realize at this point that the just allocation is not necessarily the allocation that will produce the most benefit. In some cases, because of decreasing marginal utility, we find ourselves in the fortunate position that arranging resources so as to produce greater equality will also maximize the aggregate amount of good that is done. Transplantation, however, is one of many areas in health care where often a policy of giving resources to the worst-off group will be terribly inefficient in producing good because the worst off are so sick that large resource commitments do relatively little good. Thus we will have to decide not only what is just, but also whether the right course is based on producing justice, good health outcomes, or some combination thereof.

Childress is surely correct in dissociating justice from social utility. Even if considering the social usefulness of potential transplant recipients is a reasonable way of figuring out how to do the most good with organs, it is not the way to promote justice. He is also on the right track when he warns that medical criteria are not value free. Not only that, medical criteria may turn out to be surrogates for social criteria. Persons of lower social classes do more poorly medically. They lack the education, social support network, and resources to follow regimens necessary for the complex care following transplant. Physicians have correctly argued that patients were poor medical risks for transplant because of their fragile social environments.

Appeals to medical criteria may simply be social criteria in disguise.

Childress goes on, however, to a dangerously confusing claim. He says that "both patient need. . . and probability of successful transplantation reflect medical utility." It is particularly misleading, if not wrong, to say that "'medical utility' may be a criterion of fairness." I am not sure what this means, but, if I understand, I think this is simply wrong.

I take the criterion of medical utility to be that an individual has a moral claim to a transplant to the extent that it is predictable that a medical good will come from transplanting the organ to that individual. There is a great deal of room for dispute about what counts as a medical good, but that will not be critical here. We are talking about the prediction of the goods of years of life added or suffering and incapacity alleviated.

It should be conceded that allocating organs on the basis of medical utility may also happen to contribute to opportunities for equality of medical well-being, but that is surely an accident, not the result of striving for maximizing medical utility. Contrary to Childress, appeals to "medical utility" in the distribution of organs do necessarily violate the principle of equal concern and respect. The least well-off are not given equal respect; it is only luck if they happen to get the most medical utility from an organ. Often that will not be the case. Childress is correct that medical utility might be accepted in a deontological framework, but only to the extent that it incorporates some ethical principle other than justice. Some deontological frameworks do this. But it is a mistake not to recognize that, in such cases, the incorporation or medical utility takes place in spite of its prima facie violation of the justice principle. Only when we go on to examine the relation between justice and rightness will we be able to know if this is acceptable.

The UNOS point systems for allocating kidneys provide a perfect test case for practical application of one's understanding of justice in health resource allocation. As Childress describes, the original UNOS point system gave points for various factors including HLA matching, waiting time, panel reactive antibodies (PRA), logistics, and urgency. Although what follows will be somewhat of an oversimplification, it is within reason to attribute the various points in the formula to either medical utility or justice considerations. The 12-point maximum assigned to HLA were clearly points for the purpose of promoting medical utility. The degree of HLA match predicts the likelihood of a successful graft. On the other hand, the other points seem to be included as a way of giving transplant candidates a more equal chance of getting an organ even though the factors represented by the points generally have nothing to do with predicting medically good result. For example, the 10 points that could have been assigned for urgency surely have nothing to do with whether the transplant candidate would do well; to the contrary, the more urgent the transplant, the worse off the patient and the greater likelihood of a poor outcome. Likewise, points were included for PRA because persons with high PRA are more unlikely to have another chance to get an organ that is usable. Time on the waiting list is an indirect measure of how difficult it is for a person to be matched successfully. Thus persons with O blood group, high PRA, and antigens that are difficult to match are likely to be on the list a longer time and, if a suitable organ becomes available, they can be said to have greater need, not only because they have been waiting longer, but because they are less likely to get another chance.[1]

Still oversimplifying, one can say that the original Starzl formula used about one-fourth of its points (12 of 48) as a measure of medical utility and three-fourths as a measure of fairness or justice. It was thus not perfectly just, but gave justice considerable weight.

It should be pointed out how arbitrary this allocation was. Based on the original example in the Starzl proposal, if only antigen matching had been considered half as important, urgency twice as important, and waiting time scores calculated in proportion to length of wait, then the patient who scored the lowest would have moved to the top of the list. Nevertheless, the Starzl formula can be said to be approximately three-fourths committed to justice. Would that the same could be said for other governmental programs.

The real problem has arisen with the recently revised point system. Clinicians, typically being committed to medical efficiency even at the expense of justice, had protested that the Starzl formula was paying too much attention to need and not enough to medical utility. The result was a radical shift in the direction of antigen matching, the measure that is included because of the widespread belief that antigen matching increases probability of successful grafts. Now points included for medical utility have risen to approximately two-thirds of the total. Those whose need is great and who have a substantial chance to benefit from an organ will have a much harder time getting the organ. This is thought acceptable because they have somewhat less chance of benefit than others who get a large number of points for antigen matching.

One problem with this is that, contrary to Childress's claim, likelihood of a good antigen match is far from random. Members of certain social groups are known to be statistically harder to match with an organ with a good chance of success. The losing groups strikingly are often those who are oppressed in other social allocations. Blacks and Hispanics, for example, are more likely to have antigens that are hard to match. Unidentifiable antigens are more frequent in these populations. For those for whom all six antigens cannot be identified, it is impossible to have a perfect match with a donor.[2]

Thus the point system is rigged so that blacks and Hispanics are known in advance to be at risk for not being able to get points. Likewise, women are known to have higher risk for panel-reactive antibodies. Although those with high PRA levels get points when they are matched with a suitable organ, those points can still be offset by the points assigned to others for a good tissue match, leaving the high PRA patient waiting in line even though possibly another suitable organ may never come along. Other groups known to be in need because they are difficult to match are those in the O blood group. If justice requires arranging social practices such as organ allocation systems so as to give people an equal opportunity, then the new (Terasaki) point system is far more unjust even than the original Starzl system. It is two-thirds rigged against justice, while the Starzl system is three-fourths justice-oriented.

Let me be very clear that I am not objecting in principle to the use of point systems for making allocation decisions. I agree that they provide at least some semblance of objectivity. Moreover, they give us a concrete formula for understanding how we are relating utility and justice. In the case of the new formula for kidneys, however, we are purposely demoting concerns for justice. We are making decisions that are known to work (statisti-

cally) against blacks, Hispanics, women, and others who are hard to match. Although to my knowledge the data are not available, it seems reasonable that the system will work against any who are in genetic groups distant from those that dominate the donor pool. It is likely, for example, that Jews, to the extent they reflect an atypical genetic endowment, will be hard to match. At the very least we should say of such an arrangement that we are sacrificing justice for medical utility. Whether that is ethically acceptable will have to be determined when we decide what the relation of justice to other ethical principles, such as utility or social beneficence, should be. . . .

JUSTICE AND RIGHT ALLOCATION

This leads me to the conclusion that justice requires allocating health resources so as to produce opportunity for equality of health insofar as possible. To the extent that Childress incorporates other considerations, such as medical utility, we are in disagreement. I am particularly distressed when he says, apparently conveying what is just or fair, that "macroallocation decision[s] should be subject to resolution in part through scientific and medical information about effectiveness and efficiency in reducing morbidity and premature mortality." That is a formula that invites sacrificing fairness to the altar of aggregate efficient production of utility.

Still, I have admitted, as he has, that justice or fairness is not the only ethical consideration. There are other principles that could come into play in deciding what is the right allocation of scarce health resources. Some of these considerations are based on other principles that are deontological in character, that is, they do not focus directly on the production of good consequences. For example, it is conceivable that some scarce resources have been promised to individuals who do not have claims of justice to them. I am open, as apparently Childress is, to the necessity of balancing such competing moral principles as justice or autonomy or the duty to avoid killing.

The real controversy, however, is not over these principles, but rather over the conflict between justice and utility or social beneficence.[3] Childress says that "It is not possible to indicate in advance exactly which principle should have priority." Elsewhere, he has supported an approach that would balance competing claims. I want to go on record that I oppose this strategy as being terribly dangerous and contrary to our common moral sense.

First, note a double danger. Childress has already incorporated considerations of medical utility into his formulation of what is just or fair. He now tells us that justice or fairness will have to be further diluted by being balanced or prioritized with other principles, including utility or benefi- cence. If utility counts for half (or two-thirds in the new kidney formula) of what it means to be just or fair and then on top of that one must balance the fair course of action with the one that is called for by the principle of utility or beneficence, there is very little left of a commitment to equality of well- being. It is doubly diluted.

Even if Childress were to follow me in limiting justice to opportunity for equality of well-being, his approach of reconciling the claims of justice with those of utility would still be dangerous. It is a position that commits one logically to the view that in some cases if there is enough utility, the rights of individuals can always be sacrificed. In this case the right being sacrificed is an entitlement right, the right to the resources needed to have an opportunity for equality of well-being insofar as possible. In other cases the right may be a liberty right, such as the right to refuse medical treatment or refuse to be an unwilling subject of medical research. If justice and autonomy can be traded off against utility, one is logically committed to the position that, if enough good would be done, an individual can be sacrificed against his will to the aggregate good. That is a view I reject. It is a view the Judeo-Christian tradition rejects. It is a view that a liberal democratic society rejects. In particu- lar, we are committed to the view that no amount of social good would justify coercing individuals to be subjects to Nazi-like medical experiments against their will. The only way one can remain committed in principle to that position is to acknowledge that no amount of beneficence or social utility can override the moral claims grounded in the nonconsequentialist principles such as autonomy or justice. In the example we are pursuing, no amount of medical utility should per- mit one to override the claim of justice that would

lead to a policy of allocating scarce medical resources such as kidneys on the basis of who is worst-off.

This position is probably viewed by many, including Chidress, as extreme. It is often chal- lenged by what I call the infinite demand (or bot- tomless pit) argument. It is said that as soon as we come up against someone with an incurable med- ical need serious enough to classify the individual as among the worst-off, that person will command in the name of justice all society's resources. That would leave others destitute, which seems absurd.

The infinite demand problem is a serious one for an egalitarian, but there is a plausible response. First, all that is called for is opportunity for equali- ty as far as possible. The principle does not call for using resources that will do no good for the least well-off. We do not need to give a kidney to some- one dying of cancer. Assuming someone in a per- manent vegetative state gets no objective benefit from medical treatment, we do not need to give a PVS patient a kidney.

Second, under the principle of autonomy, per- sons retain the right to refuse treatment. A person with a terrible incurable illness may find it appro- priate to refuse treatment to let the dying process continue. He would not find the use of resources on his behalf beneficial.

Third, if literally all the world's resources went to someone medically incurable, eventually others would be even worse-off. They would become the ones with claims of justice. Although this is a limit at the extreme, it is a limit.

Fourth, I have acknowledged that other noncon- sequentialist principles legitimately conflict with justice. If resources have been promised to others, they do not necessarily go to those who have claims of justice. Likewise, persons who are legiti- mate owners of resources may have autonomy rights that limit the use of resources for the least well-off. Also, the autonomy of the least well-off may lead them to yielding their claims of justice either because they are altruistic or because, as in the Rawlsian maximin case, they find it is in their interests to surrender their claims to equality. Contrary to Rawls, however, I describe this as waiving justice, not allocating in the name of jus- tice. Moreover, in my formula it is only the least well-off who have the authority to waive the claims of justice. It is not something that rationality requires and therefore can be argued by anyone in the social system.

All of these taken together lead me to the confident conclusion that the bottomless pit problem is not an insurmountable one. If others, including Childress, do not agree, then they are forced to retreat to the dangerous territory where justice gets balanced against utility. That, however, is a terrible position to be in. I prefer to avoid it by never permitting mere utility to offset nonconsequentialist ethical considerations such as justice.

Even if such a balancing gamble is taken, however, it is still crucial to keep it separate from our conclusions about what is fair or just. If we have to incorporate points for HLA matching in our kidney allocation formula, let us at the very least state as clearly as possible that we are not doing it in the name of what is just or fair. Rather we are sacrificing justice in order to make the system more efficient or utility maximizing.

NOTES

1. It is probably fair to point out that since high PRA also contributes to length of time on the waiting list, it may be double-counted in the formula.
2. Technically, the points are assigned on the basis of mismatches. Still, if the donor organ has six identified antigens, then a recipient for whom only five antigens can be identified is said to have a mismatch for at least one of the donor's antigens. The maximum number of points is thus reduced accordingly.
3. I will use the two interchangeably. Some would attempt to distinguish between beneficence and nonmaleficence and then determine a formula for relating the two. That is an interesting issue, about which Childress and I may disagree, but it is not crucial in this context.

Last-Chance Therapies and Managed Care: Pluralism, Fair Procedures, and Legitimacy

Norman Daniels and James Sabin

I. COVERAGE FOR UNPROVEN LAST-CHANCE THERAPIES

The most difficult and explosive responsibility for any health care system is deciding whether patients with life-threatening illnesses will receive insurance coverage for unproven treatments they believe may make the difference between life and death.

Potentially life-saving treatments with proven efficacy and safety (proven net benefit) and quack treatments for which there is no scientific rationale, rarely pose major problems about insurance coverage. In a country as wealthy as the United States, effective last-chance treatments without alternatives generally are and should be covered virtually all the time. When shared resources from cooperative schemes are involved, as in public or private insur-

ance, rather than individuals paying with their own resources, quack treatments will and should virtually never be covered, even if the patient or doctor passionately believe in the purported cure.

The difficult practical and ethical challenges come from promising but unproven last-chance treatments, for which we use high-dose chemotherapy with autologous bone marrow transplant (ABMT) for advanced breast cancer as our key example.[1] Not covering treatments that ultimately prove to be effective lets curable patients die prematurely, and even if a treatment ultimately proves to be ineffective, not covering it may create the impression that critically ill patients are being abandoned in their moment of need. Covering treatments that ultimately prove to be ineffective or harmful reduces the quantity and quality of the patient's remaining life, wastes substantial resources, and undermines clinical research. These are the moral stakes in the decision.

There are also other costs and risks in these decisions. Denials of coverage for seriously ill people are highly visible. Even health plans that use impeccable science and patient-centered deliberation while trying to hold the traditional, contractually-specified line against unproven therapies risk horrendous publicity, expensive litigation, and legislative mandates requiring coverage.

We shall later see (in Section II) that there is room for reasonable people to disagree about how to weigh the conflicting values and principles in these cases. There is no convincing, principled argument or social consensus for determining the relative importance of (1) giving some (how much?) priority to meeting the *urgent claims* of patients in last-chance situations, (2) providing *stewardship* of collective resources, (3) producing the public good of *scientific knowledge* about the effectiveness of unproven therapies, and (4) respecting *patient autonomy* through collaborative decision making about risks and benefits.

We can try to gloss over the ethical uncertainties in these cases by pretending that terms like "investigational," "experimental," and "medical necessity" tell us what to do. These terms, however, explain little and dodge the genuine ethical dilemmas. Without extensive explanation of the reasoning process they will not—and should not—satisfy the public or the courts. The ethical challenges posed by unproven but promising last-chance technologies are not helped at all by the language of current medical insurance benefit contracts. They are also made harder to solve by the climate of distrust that surrounds insurers, including managed care organizations (MCOs) of all types. Why should the public accept as *legitimate* decisions made by MCOs that limit access to "unproven" last-chance therapies, especially if some responsible clinicians and their patients believe them to be effective?

In a three-year research project involving collaboration with a number of leading managed care organizations, we have been investigating, through a series of policy case studies, how insurers and health plans make coverage decisions about the adoption and application of new technologies.[2] In this policy discussion, we report on some very promising "exemplary practices" we have observed for managing last-chance therapies. We believe it would be premature to try to choose among these "exemplary practices." Because of the deep moral disagreement about the underlying issues, it would be wise for society to experiment with several promising strategies in order to learn more over time about how well they work and how morally acceptable they seem in light of actual practice.

Before describing the moral disagreement in more detail in Section III, we shall begin with some background about the scientific and societal context in which the practices we describe have been developed. In Section IV, we describe the "exemplary practices" in more detail, showing how the differences among them might be mapped onto different moral views about the weight we should assign various relevant considerations. In Section V, we return to the issue of the legitimacy of MCO decisions, suggesting how some of these practices could meet more general conditions for establishing legitimacy. In Section VI, we discuss a consequence of our view that we should experiment with a variety of fair procedures, namely that we may have to learn to tolerate what looks like violations of a formal requirement of justice. Finally, in the concluding section, we suggest ways in which the different "exemplary practices" can provide valuable lessons about coming to grips with limits in the domain of health care.

II.   A BRIEF SOCIAL HISTORY

By 1989, and definitely by 1990, patients with advanced breast cancer, with the support of some clinicians, began to seek coverage for admittedly experimental use of ABMT from MCOs, including our collaborating sites. Analogues to this treatment had proven effective for some lymphatic cancers, and there was some scientific rationale for extending the treatment to solid tumors. Despite the enthusiasm of the clinicians, and the desperate belief of the breast cancer patients, many of whom were well-organized and informed, there was at the time no hard clinical evidence, and especially no controlled trials, that showed an advantage to the risky treatment over standard treatments.

During this period in the early 1990s, technology assessment of the therapy was undertaken at a number of our collaborating MCOs and by the Medical Advisory Panel (MAP) of the BC/BS Technology Evaluation Center (TEC).[3] The

National Cancer Institute authorized four randomized clinical trials for ABMT in advanced breast cancer in 1991 (with support from TEC), but these results would not be available for some time. There were no published controlled clinical trials until the Bezwoda et al. study in 1995.[4] Early evaluations of this technology had to be based on weaker forms of evidence. Between 1991 and 1994, several MCOs (as well as the Oregon Health Services Commission) decided that the technology was not ready for standard coverage, based on this early evidence regarding safety and efficacy. (As early as 1990, one of our collaborating sites, Health Partners, provided coverage under "alternative funding" for participation in clinical trials.) Similarly, early evaluations by the MAP found that there was inadequate evidence of efficacy or net benefit for ABMT for advanced breast cancer.

It was not until February 1996 that the BC/BS Medical Advisory Panel (MAP) finally decided that the therapy did meet its criteria for status as a noninvestigational technology. At its February 1996 meeting, the MAP evaluated evidence from the only published study of a randomized clinical trial (Bezwoda et. al. 1995), as well as evidence from ongoing studies. The discussion suggested that the published study could not support conclusions about the greater efficacy of the therapy over standard treatments used in the U.S., but the MAP voted that its criteria were met.[5] A consideration of the identical evidence in June 1996 by California State Blue Shield led to the decision that the MAP criteria were not yet satisfied.[6] Several MCOs that had undertaken similar technology assessments also continued to believe, as of mid-1996, that there was insufficient evidence to show that the therapy met reasonable criteria of safety and efficacy for advanced breast cancer in comparison to standard treatments—even if it had by then become nearly "standard" therapy.

Like HIV patients desperate to try "promising" drugs prior to full FDA testing, however, breast cancer patients in the early 1990s demanded that they be allowed to decide whether the risks were worth taking.[7] The "gatekeeper" here, however, was not the FDA, charged with keeping unsafe pharmaceuticals off the market, but insurers, who, by contract, had no obligation to provide coverage for "investigational" treatments. When some MCOs, with adequate, evidence-based reason on

their side, insisted the therapy was still "investigational" and "unproven," and might even prove worse than standard therapies, patients pursued both litigation and legislation, and the media "exposed" the denials. As early as 1991, *60 Minutes* featured a story about Aetna declining coverage for ABMT for breast cancer. In California in 1993, the estate of Neline Fox won an $89 million suit against Healthnet, which had originally denied coverage, then provided it. The suit charged the delay cost Fox her life. This suit cast a pall over traditional procedures for assessing the status of last chance therapies.

Throughout the early 1990s, many insurers were providing coverage for patients participating in approved clinical trials. Unfortunately, this coverage seemed "arbitrary and capricious" according to an important study in the *New England Journal of Medicine*, which said coverage was not correlated with pretreatment clinical characteristics of the patients, the design or phase of the study, or the response to induction therapy.[8] That study showed that as many as three out of four patients seeking coverage for participation in a trial were granted it, and another half of those who threatened legal action when initially denied also received coverage. Activism clearly paid off for patients seeking treatment.

Responding to well-organized and highly visible advocates for these women, some state legislatures mandated coverage as early as 1994 and 1995, despite protests, for example in Minnesota and Massachusetts, that the mandates would make it impossible to continue proper clinical trials aimed at finding out if the procedure was truly superior to standard therapy. In other states, though legislative mandates were not passed, lawsuits in effect compelled coverage, since large punitive damages were imposed where coverage was denied or delayed. The resulting legal climate made it too risky and costly to deny what was still an unproven therapy.

Some insurers responded earlier than others to the handwriting on the wall, reading the message that traditional efforts to manage last chance therapies by "holding the line" against investigational treatments were not working. Following the *60 Minutes* expose in 1991, Aetna, under the initiative of William McGivney, introduced a procedure in which an independent panel would be invoked when patients wanted a last-chance treatment that internal review denied coverage for (see Section IV for more detailed discussion). The same approach was adopted by Kaiser of Northern California in 1993. Other approaches were introduced in the same period, including Oregon Blue Cross Blue Shield's (1994) use of a transplant coordinator to manage the coverage of clinical trials for unproven last-chance therapies. In 1996, Health Partners introduced a special process for evaluating "promising therapies" that fall in the space between clearly investigational and standard treatment. It is this "new wave" of approaches that is the focus of our discussion in subsequent sections.

Before turning to the details of these newer approaches, we want to make three points. First, the social climate—including well-organized women's groups, a crusading media, committed practitioners, suspicious courts, and opportunistic legislators—clearly made the standard "technology assessment" approach to holding the line against coverage for last-chance "investigational" therapies untenable. Second, the legal and political interventions also had the effect of making it more difficult to find out if high-dose chemotherapy with stem cell support actually worked for advanced breast cancer. Although some MCOs decided to provide coverage for clinical trials, others (for example Harvard Community Health Plan, in an evaluation just before the Massachusetts mandate in 1994) were ethically uneasy about insisting on participation in trials, where patients would not always get the experimental regimen. The effect of compelling coverage meant that enrollment in NIH sponsored clinical trials was slowed. The public intervention through the courts and legislatures thus had the effect of frustrating another publicly supported goal in health care, namely, to make the system more efficient by pushing it to adopt "outcomes-based" medicine.

Third, the challenge to limit-setting by MCOs has its international analogues in publicly administered and financed health care systems that offer universal coverage. Even where public agencies might be thought to be a more "legitimate" locus for limit-setting decisions, a similar moral challenge is made. The suggestion is that "bureaucratic" decisions driven too much by "budget limitations" ignore the fact of urgent need in these cases, that is, that the moral priorities of decision makers

are inappropriate. It would take us too far afield to discuss the similarities and differences between these cases (e.g., in England, Norway, and New Zealand) and those in the U.S., but it is important to see that the moral dimension of these issues arises across differences in institutional design, financing, national culture, and even incentives. We return to this issue briefly in Section V.

III. MORAL DISAGREEMENT AND ACCESS TO LAST-CHANCE THERAPIES

Reasonable people disagree about the best way to manage access to last-chance therapies because they disagree about the relative importance of several values or principles that come into conflict in these cases. In a pluralist society, where the underlying disagreement may involve conflicts among more comprehensive and systematic moral views, this means there is no one way of managing last-chance therapies that all agree is morally superior. In effect, we may have to learn to live with alternative best practices, not agreement on one approach, even if, as we shall see in Section V, this raises a challenge to one aspect of our traditional thinking about fairness and justice.

The general and difficult moral problem that all health plans must solve is how to meet the diverse needs of the insured population under reasonable resource constraints. This problem involves balancing population-centered concerns against patient-centered ones. Promising but unproven last-chance treatments evoke the general problem especially sharply since so much is at stake for the individual patients while at the same time the proposed treatments are often quite costly.

The major population-centered concerns are the prudent use of shared resources ("stewardship") and the promotion of public goods, such as knowledge about safety and efficacy produced through clinical trials. Those who emphasize these concerns will prefer policies under which collective resources would only be used for last-chance treatments that meet a threshold of established net benefit, and unproven therapies, if paid for at all, would only be covered in the context of controlled clinical trials, including randomized controlled trials in which a patient might receive a placebo or the standard treatment.

The key patient-centered concerns include: giving proper attention to patient needs, especially urgent needs as in the last-chance situations; avoiding harm, including the psychological harm that can arise from adversarialism; and managing uncertainties and risks through collaborative treatment planning. Those who emphasize these concerns will prefer policies for last-chance treatments that create a much lower standard of evidence that must be met for a treatment to be offered to a patient and that allow patients and their clinicians more leeway in judging the relative weight of risks and benefits. They are less likely to promote policies that would require patients to enter controlled trials, since they have no assurance in those trials of receiving the desired treatment.

Reasonable people will differ, however, in the degree to which they want to trade population-centered values in favor of patient-centered ones because of the urgency of the situation. There is no higher-level agreement on how much weight to give to the competing values or principles. Careful deliberation may resolve some of the conflicts, for often our views are not systematically considered, but it is unlikely to eliminate all of them. In many cases, the disagreement about weights may reflect significant differences in comprehensive moral views that people hold. For example, some "communitarians" will give more weight to guardianship of collective resources and the maximization of health benefits for a community that is cooperating to share resources. Classic liberals will give more weight to respect for individual autonomy. "Communitarians" and "liberals" will recognize the relevance of the reasons to which the other gives priority, since in other contexts, these factors also count as reasons for them in their thinking about how to solve the general problem of meeting needs under resource constraints. But the disagreement about weights or priorities will probably persist.

This disagreement about weights will then lead people to have different views about the acceptability of different ways of managing last-chance therapies. In the next section, we draw on our empirical study of decision making about coverage in MCOs to describe in more detail a set of "exemplary practices" regarding promising but unproven last-chance therapies. Our point is to show how they can be thought to reflect these dif-ferent judgments about how to weigh competing values. We do not try to show that any one is best, since we know of no persuasive argument to that conclusion. Rather, we present each as a reasonable, good-faith effort to solve the problem.

IV.   SOME EXEMPLARY PRACTICES IN MANAGING LAST-CHANCE THERAPIES

We begin with the earliest approach to managing last-chance therapies, the terminal illness program William McGivney started at Aetna in 1991. This program, used primarily in an indemnity insurance context, served as Aetna's *modus operandi* until the end of 1996 after Aetna purchased and merged with U.S. Healthcare. It was later adapted for use in an MCO setting by Northern California Kaiser Permanente and eventually became the model for the 1996 Friedman-Knowles legislation in California.

In the Aetna program, when medical directors in the field received a request for an unproven but promising last-chance cancer treatment that was not covered under established company policy, they referred the request to the home office at Hartford, where a consulting oncologist reviewed the clinical situation. A key feature of the program was that the home-office oncologist was only empowered to *approve* requests. If the consulting oncologist believed the request did not represent reasonable clinical practice for the particular patient, the case was automatically referred outside the company for independent review by the Medical Care Ombudsman Program in Bethesda, Maryland.

The Ombudsman Program, which was founded by Grace Monaco in 1991, provides independent expert opinion about appropriate treatment in serious but ambiguous clinical situations. On a timetable which can be as short as 24 hours, the Ombudsman Program will put together a panel of 2–3 experts with no affiliation to the insurer or the provider of the proposed treatment, to assess whether the proposed treatment has any scientific rationale for the particular patient. This is not a technology assessment of the new technology but an expert clinical assessment of the *potential value of the technology for a particular patient*. Typically, at least one of the experts is prepared to testify in court if the case should come to litigation.

Aetna did not restrict its own consulting oncologist from rendering negative coverage decisions because the consultant lacked competence. Any time that specialized technical expertise was needed, Aetna could have hired additional consultants at less cost to itself than using the Ombudsman Program. The problem Aetna was trying to solve with its terminal illness program was one of *trust*, not lack of technical expertise. The fact and appearance of "conflict of interest" was removed: if Aetna would say no only if an independent consultant said no, then the "no" should not be construed as a cost-driven decision. In circumstances of life-threatening illness and ambiguous information, the patient's trust in the decision-making process can be the difference between peace and outrage, or acceptance versus litigation.

In 1993, the Northern California region of Kaiser Permanente took the program that Aetna had developed in a primarily *indemnity* insurance context and adapted it for its own 3600 physician *prepaid group practice HMO*. Kaiser's experience helps us understand the mechanism through which Aetna's innovative way of addressing the patient's concern about the insurer's potential conflict of interest helps the decision-making process.[9]

Like Aetna, Northern California Kaiser Permanente decided to let patients in last-chance situations know that they could go outside of Kaiser for an independent opinion from the Ombudsman Program if they were not satisfied with the internal decision-making process. This was a controversial step for Kaiser to take. Some Kaiser doctors worried that allowing automatic appeal outside the HMO would diminish the group's ability to manage care rationally and feared that the program itself might be very costly.

What actually happened was exactly the opposite of what was feared. From 1994–1996, only 6 of the 2.5 million northern California members asked for referral to the Ombudsman program. When the patients' concerns about insurer trustworthiness and potential conflict of interest were addressed in advance by the option of going outside of Kaiser for independent consultation, patients and families were much readier to enter into a reflective dialogue with their Kaiser physicians about what treatment approach really made sense for them.

The Aetna-Kaiser "last-chance" policy might simply be dismissed as a cost-benefit calculation

made by the MCO. Put cynically, it is better to pay for a few treatments than face lawsuits, any one of which would be more costly than a bunch of treatments. But it also can be defended—and is by some MCOs that adopt it—on more explicitly moral grounds that connect its adoption with our earlier discussion.

The policy can be defended morally in this way. It recognizes the fundamental importance in a medical system of "shared decision making" between patients and clinicians about risk taking. If an unproven last-chance therapy is viewed by some acknowledged experts as the most appropriate treatment for the patient, and if the patient understands the risks as presented by parties on all sides, then organizations have no better option than to rely on the informed decision of the patient and her clinician. This is not the same as saying that a patient can be granted just any last wish regarding treatment: there must be some basis in evidence and expert view that the therapy is not quackery. In the external review model, that expert view is provided by the independent panel. Under those conditions, simply refusing to provide coverage fails to acknowledge the obligation not to impose paternalistically a plan's own judgment about acceptable risks and benefits on the choices of desperately ill patients with few options. To be sure, the role of the MCO as a guardian of shared resources is reduced, but this is defensible in light of both the urgency of the patients' needs, and the special importance, in light of the uncertainty and the severity of need, of promoting a climate of shared decision making. Indeed, a proponent of this view might even say that the decision to hold to a hard-line denial is so likely to lead to a waste of resources in the legal and political climate that actually surrounds MCOs that the more efficient way to respect resources is to adopt the more lenient strategy toward last-chance therapies.

The Aetna-Kaiser approach has been embodied in new legislation. Under the Friedman-Knowles Experimental Treatment Act, passed by the California legislature in 1996, the kind of independent consultation process that Aetna and Kaiser Northern California have piloted will become mandatory for all California insurers starting July 1, 1998. The provisions of the bill are quite detailed, but the basic concept is simple. If a patient with a condition that has no effective therapy and is likely to cause death within two years is denied coverage for a new treatment that has some scientific promise, an independent expert review of the decision must be offered.

What is so important about the Friedman-Knowles bill is the effort to use legislation to influence the quality of the decision-making process without making any attempt to mandate what the decisions themselves should be. The bill does not mandate any specific treatments as so many states have done and continue to do. Rather, it mandates an organizational decision-making process designed to reduce fears about conflict of interest and increase deliberative reflection and clarity about the reasons for coverage decisions. (We note that in August 1997, the California Legislature considered legislation that takes a step backwards—toward mandating coverage for ABMT for breast cancer. Some proponents of the legislation say it eliminates "inequities" in coverage, since state employee benefits mandate ABMT but other insurers do not, an issue we return to in Section VI; critics say the state should not be making these disease-specific sorts of coverage decisions.)

Oregon Blue Cross Blue Shield has developed an approach to unproven bone marrow transplant regimens that reflects a slightly different moral framework. In 1993, in the aftermath of the *Fox* v. *Healthnet* case, Oregon Blue Cross Blue Shield created a new, full-time role of transplant coordinator. The transplant coordinator is a clinically experienced nurse whose job is to work directly with patients and families, transplant programs, employers, and the Oregon Blue Cross Blue Shield benefit systems to create mutually satisfactory individualized treatment plans.

Whereas Aetna and Kaiser use the option for independent review outside of the organization to allay patient concerns about conflict of interest and promote collaboration, Oregon Blue Cross Blue Shield's distinctive approach is an unusually open and accountable process of deliberation and reason-giving and an especially strong emphasis on supporting scientific treatment evaluation. Instead of the infamous "gag rule," the Oregon program has developed what might be called a "let's talk it over openly and at great length rule!"

In ethics classes at medical, nursing, and business schools we try to teach students to identify the key facts and values in a situation and to develop options to advance the most important values that apply. This is what the Blue Cross transplant coordinator does every day, except she does it in circumstances of time pressure and high emotion, not in a classroom. When we interviewed her for our research project, we told her that her role seemed to be $^1/_3$ nurse clinician, $^1/_3$ nurse manager, and $^1/_3$ ethics professor.

Here are the kinds of things the transplant coordinator says in dealing with the multiple stakeholders in the decision-making process:

• To a confused and frightened patient: "Do you have this article about the treatment? Have you read this other one? I'm going to be at the library this afternoon—why don't you come and meet me there and we can go over the information together?"

• To explain the importance of consistency to a wealthy patient: "Just because you're a VIP who lives in the West Hills, you don't really want to make me treat you any differently than the person who comes to clean your house, do you?"

• To an employer who wants Blue Cross to cover an employee for a treatment that has no scientific justification: "But it's not based on sound science. Do you want to do the same thing for all the other women in your employee group? And even if you do, what will you tell their sisters who can't have the treatment? We want to be able to support scientific research that's going to answer the question."

• And, to a provider who is asking the insurer to cover an unproven treatment: "Then build your case to us, make your proposal so that when we make this decision, we can have sound rationale for a similar case on the next patient that you or someone else may send to us."

These comments illustrate the kind of deliberative dialogue that will have to happen hundreds of thousands and perhaps millions of times for doctors, patients, health plans, and society to move along a learning curve towards a more patient-centered, cost-effective, and ethical health care system.

The Oregon Blue Cross process, like the Aetna-Kaiser, places its ultimate emphasis on encouraging open deliberation between patient, clinician, and, in this case, coordinator. When we asked the coordinator how she was able to achieve trust with patients without the promise of an external, independent review, as in the Aetna-Kaiser approach, she said that she would view an instance of a patient going to external review as a failure on her part to have engaged the patient in the kind of deliberative give and take that her approach requires. The promise of external review, she feared, could lure patients away from the need to engage in deliberation with her.

Although deliberation and shared decision making were the key goals, Oregon Blue Cross Blue Shield has another priority as well—supporting clinically important research. If a promising but unproven last-chance treatment is available in a scientifically valid clinical trial, the plan will cover it. The coordinator claimed that as of our visit in June, 1996, no patients had resorted to litigation, and a significant number decided that the unproven treatments they initially requested were, after careful thinking, not really what they wanted.

In contrast to the Aetna-Kaiser approach, Oregon Blue Cross Blue Shield appears to put more emphasis on redirecting its stewardship responsibility toward supporting research. At the same time, since outright denial of unproven therapies was much less likely than in a traditional "hold the line" approach, it became possible to involve the patient in shared decision making.

In 1996, Health Partners, a prominent HMO in Minnesota, began to develop a special policy regarding "promising" but still unproven therapies. For selected "promising treatments," Health Partners will provide coverage even though the technology still falls into the category of "investigational" and would traditionally be excluded from coverage by contract language. The rationale for singling out the category of "promising treatments" is to introduce consistent policy about a particular technology, thereby avoiding case-by-case responses to individual requests.

Although this approach clearly relaxes the traditional hard line about stewardship, it keeps the health plan in control of what counts as "promising." Compared to the case-by-case decision-making by Aetna, Kaiser of Northern California, and Oregon Blue Cross Blue Shield, the Health Partners approach appears to place more emphasis on the organization's stewardship role. It remains to be seen whether the approach of offering greater consistency technology-by-technology at the cost of less flexibility in deciding individual cases leads to more or less conflict and litigation.

V. LEGITIMACY AND FAIRNESS

MCOs operate in a social climate of distrust. The vigorous effort at cost containment initiated by large employers (and the government) has largely been invisible to the public. Instead, managed care organizations have taken the heat for cost containment and system change. In this climate of distrust, the issue of legitimacy arises in a sharp form: why should patients or clinicians who think they are being denied medically appropriate treatments, even unproven last-chance therapies, accept as legitimate the decisions of MCOs? More to the point, under what conditions should the public come to view these decisions as legitimate?

Elsewhere,[10] we have argued that if the following four conditions were met, MCOs would take a large step toward earning legitimacy, at least over time:

1. Decisions regarding coverage for new technologies (and other limit-setting decisions) and their rationales must be publicly accessible.
2. The rationales for coverage decisions should aim to provide a *reasonable* construal of how the organization should provide "value for money" in meeting the varied health needs of a defined population under reasonable resource constraints. Specifically, a construal will be "reasonable" if it appeals to reasons and principles that are accepted as relevant by people who are disposed to finding terms of cooperation that are mutually justifiable.
3. There is a mechanism for challenge and dispute resolution regarding limit-setting decisions, including the opportunity for revising decisions in light of further evidence or arguments.
4. There is either voluntary or public regulation of the process to ensure that conditions 1–3 are met.

These four conditions capture at least the central necessary elements of a solution to the legitimacy and fairness problems for coverage decisions about new treatments. Condition 1 requires openness or publicity, that is, clarity about the reasons for decisions. Condition 2 involves some constraints on the kinds of reasons that can play a role in the rationale: it recognizes the fundamental interest all parties have to finding a justification all can accept as reasonable. Conditions 3 and 4 provide mechanisms for connecting deliberation and decisions within MCOs to a broader deliberative process, that is, for making them accountable to the results of a wider deliberation about what fairness requires.[11]

The procedures for managing last-chance therapies discussed in the previous section can meet these conditions. The first point to note is that the rationale for a plan's adopting one procedure rather than another should itself be made public, as Condition 1 requires. In such a rationale, giving more weight to responsibility for stewardship (as perhaps in the "promising-therapy" strategy) than another strategy does is the type of reason that meets Condition 2; so does the opposite weighting. Our main point in the discussion in the previous section is that each of the exemplary strategies could be defended publicly with reasons that meet these legitimacy conditions. What varies among these procedures is not the appeal to inappropriate reasons but the different weights reasonable people might give to relevant reasons.

In their implementation, any of these procedures should meet the conditions as well. For example, in the procedure followed by Oregon Blue Cross Blue Shield in managing patients who may be left out of available clinical trials, there is an effort to engage the patient in reason-giving of exactly the sort required by Condition 2. Similarly, the results of previous deliberations about particular cases could be made publicly available (still respecting confidentiality), so they were accessible to other patients seeking to develop claims about coverage in their cases. In effect, a kind of case law should emerge that governs the operation of the MCO and is accessible to patients and clinicians. Similarly, the kind of deliberation engaged in by the external ombudsman program used by Aetna and Kaiser, and now mandated by California law, could also meet the publicity conditions and the restrictions on types of reason-giving.

We noted earlier that the legitimacy problem in the U.S. has its analogue in publicly administered systems. In other countries, even where public commissions have been established to approve "principles" for priority-setting and limit-setting in those systems, the agencies that make actual decisions often keep their results quiet, perhaps implicit in quietly made budget decisions, and fail to meet the conditions we articulate. We believe compliance with these conditions would contribute to establishing greater legitimacy for hard choices made in those systems as well.

VI.   FORMAL VS PROCEDURAL JUSTICE

There may not be just one best or fairest way to manage last-chance therapies. At least, reasonable people may not agree on what the best procedure is, and in light of that disagreement, we should experiment with a family of "best practices," or so we have argued. There is a troubling implication of this view that some may view as a fatal objection. We see it not as a flaw in our approach but as a manifestation of an unavoidable moral uncertainty, which we must learn to respect and to live with.

Here is the problem. Suppose we have two patients, Groucho and Harpo, who are indistinguishable with regard to the relevant features of their cases. Both make the same claim that they need a particular high-dose chemotherapy with stem cell support for their advanced cancers. Let us suppose that this treatment has not yet been shown to provide a net benefit for the condition, which is in any case fatal on standard treatments. Groucho belongs to BestHealth and Harpo to GreatCare, two responsible MCOs that manage last-chance therapies in different ways. For the sake of specificity, suppose BestHealth uses a version of the external appeal procedure (like Aetna or Kaiser) and that GreatCare covers people in clinical trials if they meet the protocols or can make a reasonable case that they should be so covered (like Oregon Blue Cross Blue Shield). Suppose finally that Groucho is denied the transplant but that Harpo is given it. When Groucho hears about Harpo, should we agree if he complains that one of them has been treated unfairly?

Groucho claims that a fundamental principle of justice has been violated, the *formal* principle that like cases be treated similarly. If his case is just like Harpo's in all relevant ways, then they should either both get the treatment or neither should. The formal principle does not tell us how both should be treated, only that they should be treated similarly. Specifically, if there are *reasons* why Harpo should get the treatment, Groucho insists, then they apply equally to him, and he should receive it as well.

Groucho's complaint that a formal principle of justice is violated actually turns on there being a substantive reason or principle that grounds the decision to treat Harpo. To see this point, consider this variation on the case: in both MCOs, a coin is flipped about whether to give the treatment. Groucho loses and Harpo wins. When Groucho complains that like cases are being treated dissimilarly, we can now say to him, "The cases are unlike: there was a coin toss, and you lost and he won." There is no violation of the formal principle if there is a non-reason-based procedure used to distinguish the cases, as there is in the case of a coin toss. Alternatively, we can construe this as a case in which a principle is appealed to and uniformly applied, namely the principle that winners but not losers of coin-tosses (or other random processes) will get the treatment.

Neither BestHealth nor GreatCare flips coins, however. Within their different procedures, each encourages the giving of reasons and the deliberation about cases in light of reasons. We presuppose that the difference in their procedures for managing these cases rests on a difference in the ways the two organizations weight certain values, i.e., the values of urgency, stewardship, and shared decision-making with patients. Suppose further that we are right to claim there is no argument we all can accept that shows that one weighting (and thus one procedure) is clearly morally more justifiable than the other. That weighting, and thus the choice of fair procedure, is itself the focus of reasonable disagreement.

Generally, when there is a violation of the formal principle of justice, we are challenged to evaluate the weight attributed to a reason or principle that was applied in one case but not the other. We are asked to find a difference in the cases, that is, to show that they were not really similar in all relevant ways, or to affirm the uniform application of that reason or principle or of some alternative principle. But in the condition of moral pluralism we face, we have no candidate principle that purports to enjoy "our" endorsement independently of the fair procedure we are employing. A reason that may seem compelling or decisive in one process may not have that force in another. To be sure, we are not flipping coins in either case. We are deliberating carefully in a reason-driven and reason-giving way. But the weight given reasons in each setting is a reasonable reflection of other moral disagreements and moral uncertainty—the very uncertainty about what counts as a just outcome that compels us to adopt a procedural approach to fair outcomes. Groucho can be told this: Harpo was given the treatment because his plan reasoned about his case differently than your plan, and both ways of reasoning are relevant and arguably fair.

How tolerable would a system be if it produced situations in which a Groucho and Harpo were treated differently? We might think it makes a difference how centralized or decentralized a system is. In a decentralized system such as ours, for example, it may be difficult to require that insurance schemes use one rather than another procedurally fair way of deliberating about cases (though legislation such as the Friedman-Knowles Experimental Treatment Act imposes uniformity, at least at one stage of decision making). On what basis should the choice between procedures and weightings be made? Can we show a superior outcome to insisting on one such process rather than another? Without such a compelling regulatory reason, we might have trouble justifying public regulation requiring just one form of managing last-chance cases.

Despite the decentralization in our health care system, however, our courts arguably can impose a kind of unifying framework. Groucho might sue BestHealth, saying that not only does he want the treatment, and not only does some clinician he prefers say it is appropriate, but GreatCare has given the treatment to someone just like him. In practice, the courts could make unworkable an effort to experiment with different fair procedures to see what their advantages and disadvantages really are. On the other hand, what has often carried the day in actual suits on these matters is a demonstration of a lack of fair process and a kind of arbitrariness within an organization. If each of the fair procedures constitutes a reasonable defense against that sort of claim, then the courts might welcome an effort to rely more directly on fair procedures applied within plans. An analogy here would be the way in which the courts have welcomed decision making by ethics committees in hospitals as a preferable route to having these kinds of cases continuously adjudicated in the courts.

Would it be a compelling regulatory reason that we find differential treatment unacceptable and have to avoid it, if only by insisting on uniform process by convention? That might be true in a decentralized system, but it seems even more likely to be true in a national health care system. In the U.K., for example, it might seem more troubling that Groucho did not get his transplant in London but Harpo got his in Manchester. Here too, however, there might be disagreements among *meaningful political units*, the districts, about what constituted the "best" procedure. If that is true, then there might be even more reason to tolerate variation than there is in the U.S., where people are grouped into insurance schemes, not meaningful political units that have ways of selecting their procedures in a democratic fashion.

How acceptable differential treatment would be seems to depend, then, on whether a persuasive political rationale for uniformity can be developed. In a decentralized system, the political rationale would have to be sufficient to override the presumption that "private" insurers have the authority to select from among a set of comparably fair procedures. Of course, the political rationale might simply be that the legal system would not allow differential treatment; but that too remains to be seen.

In a national health care system, the political rationale for uniformity would have to show that differential treatment among districts was less acceptable than giving them the autonomy to select their own procedures. If meaningful political units, like districts, felt strongly enough about their choices of procedures, the costs of uniformity might be too high. For the problem we are facing, then, it remains unclear how unacceptable it would be for Harpo to get a last chance when Groucho does not.

VII.   CONCLUSIONS

Making decisions and policies about payment for promising but unproven last-chance therapies presents the most difficult moral and clinical policy challenge a health care system can face. Important values, all of which command respect and attention, inevitably come into conflict in these difficult situations, especially (1) giving some (how much?) priority to meeting the *urgent claims* of patients in

last-chance situations, (2) providing *stewardship* of collective resources, (3) producing the public good of *scientific knowledge* about the effectiveness of unproven therapies, and (4) respecting *patient autonomy* through collaborative decision making about risks and benefits.

General principles of distributive justice do not tell us how to weigh the relative claims of these competing considerations. Nevertheless, the insurers and MCOs whose programs we describe have developed procedures for making decisions and policies that can be defended on the basis of justifiable—although different—weights they give to the different values. In our decentralized, competitive system—largely in response to political and legal pressures patients and clinicians have focused on these plans—an important social experiment has emerged. Different procedural "solutions" to the problem of limit setting in the case of new technologies are being developed and honed in practice. What can we learn from the experiment?

If we as a society can tolerate the inevitable differences in decisions and policies that the different configurations of values will create, we will have an opportunity to learn from the dialectic between principles and practice. We will see more clearly through a legacy of specific decisions and their outcomes just what the moral and nonmoral benefits and costs of the different approaches are. What we learn will help us refine our notions of fair procedure and in turn help us produce better solutions to the general problem of limit-setting in health care that all societies are struggling with. In the last 20–30 years, we have learned much and seen important changes in how individual clinicians and patients negotiate the difficult issues of clinical planning in the context of threats to life itself. If we have enough societal fortitude, and a modicum of strong political leadership, close study of the experiences generated by the kinds of programs we have described can help us do the same at the level of social policy.

NOTES

1. We distinguish the case of promising but unproven last-chance therapies from the case of treatments that professionals decide are futile. In futility cases, the judgment of the professional is that there will be harm to the patient, or there is at least clear evidence that there will

be no benefit. The patient or family might disagree, perhaps because they seek miracles or perhaps because they view mere physiological functioning as a benefit. Here there is a conflict between stewardship and the somewhat confusing notion of patient "autonomy." The conflict eases if we restrict the plausible core of patient autonomy to a (positive) right to participate in decisions about treatment and a (negative) right to refuse treatment, and we distinguish that core from an (implausible) "entitlement" to have whatever treatment one desires, which involves unrestricted claims on resources held by others. There is also a conflict between paternalism (in the form of a legitimate concern to avoid doing harm) and a patient's or family's judgment about what counts as a benefit. These are interesting issues, but this kind of case is marked by clear professional judgment rooted in considerable *certainty about the evidence*. In the last-chance cases we are concerned with, it is professional *uncertainty*, not certainty, that is key.

2. Case studies completed to date include, Sabin, J., Daniels, N., 1997a. "How MCOs deliberated about coverage for lung volume reduction surgery: A Focal Case Study," (unpublished manuscript), and Wilkinson, S., Sabin, J., and Daniels, N. 1997. "How MCOs decided to cover pallidotomy for advanced Parkinson's Disease: A Focal Case Study," (unpublished manuscript). See also Daniels, N. and Sabin, J. 1997. "Limits to Health Care: Fair Procedures. Democratic Deliberation, and the Legitimacy Problem for Insurers," *Philosophy and Public Affairs* 26, no. 4 (Fall 1997): 303–350.

3. Other technology assessment centers not affiliated with MCOs, such as ECRI, also undertook evaluations.

4. Bezwoda, W.R., Seymour, L., Dansey, R.D., "High-dose Chemotherapy with Hematopoietic Rescue as Primary Treatment for Metastatic Breast Cancer: A Randomized Trial." 1995. *J Clin Oncol* 13:2483-89.

5. The MAP criteria are as follows:

   1. The technology must have final approval from the appropriate government regulatory body.
   2. The scientific evidence must permit conclusions concerning the effect of the technology on health outcomes.
   3. The technology must improve the net health outcome.

4. The technology must be as beneficial as any established alternative.
5. The improvement must be attainable outside the investigational settings.

The South African study (Bezwoda et. al. 1995) used as its control a regimen of standard chemotherapy that was inferior in outcomes to the conventional therapy that would standardly be available in the U.S. and elsewhere. Showing that high-dose chemotherapy was superior to a conventional regimen that itself was far inferior to conventional therapy commonly in use should not persuade us of the superior efficacy of the high-dose regimen.

6. The California Blue Shield evaluation took place in a public setting, the only such open technology assessment process that we know of aside from Oregon Health Resources Commission. At its discussion, the panel seemed comfortable supporting its conclusion only after it was assured that no one actually wanting the high-dose chemotherapy was unable to get it, despite its investigational status.

7. See Norman Daniels, *Seeking Fair Treatment: From the AIDS Epidemic to National Health Care Reform*, New York: Oxford University Press, 1995, Chapter 6.

8. Peters, W.P., and Rogers, M.C. 1994. "Variation in Approval by Insurance Companies for Coverage of Autologous Bone Marrow Transplantion for Breast Cancer," *NEJM* 330:7:473-7.

9. Beebe, D.B., Rosenfeld, A.B., Collins, N.: "An Approach to Decisions about Coverage of Investigational Treatments." *HMO Practice* 11(2): 65-67, 1997 (June).

10. See Daniels and Sabin, "Limits to Health Care: Fair Procedures, Democratic Deliberation, and the Legitimacy Problem for Insurers," *Philosophy and Public Affairs* 26, no. 4 (Fall 1997): 303–350.

11. These conditions were developed independently but fit reasonably well with the principles of publicity, reciprocity, and accountability governing democratic deliberation cited by Amy Gutmann and Dennis Thompson, *Democracy and Disagreement* (Cambridge: Harvard University Press, 1996). For reservations about their account, see Norman Daniels, "Enabling Democratic Deliberation," Pacific Division of the American Philosophical Association, March, 1997.

RECOMMENDED SUPPLEMENTARY READING

General Works

Abraham, Laurie K. *Mama Might Be Better Off Dead: The Failure of Health Care in Urban America.* Chicago: University of Chicago Press, 1993.

Agich, George J., and Begley, Charles E., eds. *The Price of Health.* Boston, MA: D. Reidel Publishing Co., 1986.

Annas, George J. *Standard of Care: The Law of American Bioethics.* Oxford: Oxford University Press, 1993.

Beauchamp, Dan E. *The Health of the Republic: Epidemics, Medicine, and Moralism as Challenges to Democracy.* Philadelphia, PA: Temple University Press, 1988.

Brock, Dan W. *Life and Death: Philosophical Essays in Biomedical Ethics.* New York: Cambridge University Press, 1993.

Daniels, Norman. *Just Health Care.* Cambridge: Cambridge University Press, 1985.

———. *Seeking Fair Treatment: From the AIDS Epidemic to National Health Care Reform.* New York: Oxford University Press, 1995.

Daniels, Norman; Light, Donald W.; Caplan, Ronald L. *Benchmarks of Fairness for Health Care Reform.* New York: Oxford University Press, 1996.

Dougherty, Charles. *Back to Reform: Values, Markets, and the Health Care System.* New York: Oxford University Press, 1996.

Emanuel, Ezekiel. *The Ends of Human Life: Medical Ethics in a Liberal Polity.* Cambridge, MA: Harvard University Press, 1991.

Hall, Mark A. *Making Medical Spending Decisions: The Law, Ethics, and Economics of Rationing Mechanisms.* New York: Oxford University Press, 1996.

Morreim, E. Haavi. *Balancing Act: The New Medical Ethics of Medicine's New Economics.* Washington, DC: Georgetown University Press, 1995.

President's Commission for the Study of Ethical Problems in Medicine and Biomedical and Behavioral Research. *Securing Access to Health Care.* Washington, D.C.: U.S. Government Printing Office, 1983.

Justice and Health Care

Arras, John. "Retreat from the Right to Health Care: The President's Commission and Access to Health Care." *Cardozo Law Review,* 6 (1984): 321–345.

Bayer, Ronald. "Ethics, Politics, and Access to Health Care: A Critical Analysis of the President's Commission." *Cardozo Law Review,* 6 (1984): 303–320.

Brock, Dan; Buchanan, Allan; Daniels, Norman; Wikler, Daniel. *Genes and the Just Society: Genetic Intervention in the Shadow of Eugenics.* (forthcoming).

Brody, Baruch. "Why the Right to Health Care is Not a Useful Concept for Policy Debates." In *Rights to Health Care,* edited by T. J. Bole III and W. B. Bondeson. Netherlands: Kluwer Academic Publishers, 1991.

Buchanan, Allen. "Equal Opportunity and Genetic Intervention," *Social Philosophy and Policy,* 12, no. 2 (Summer 1995): 105–135.

Callahan, Daniel. *What Kind of Life: The Limits of Medical Progress.* New York: Simon & Schuster, 1990.

———. *Seeking Fair Treatment: The Lesson of AIDS for National Health Care.* New York: Oxford University Press, 1995.

Gutmann, Amy. "For and Against Equal Access to Health Care." *Milbank Quarterly* 59 (Fall 1981): 542–560.

Murphy, Timothy F., and Lappé, Marc A., eds. *Justice and the Human Genome Project.* Berkeley: University of California Press, 1994.

Shelp, Earl E., ed. *Justice and Health Care.* Dordrecht, Holland: D. Reidel Publishing Co., 1981.

Veatch, Robert M. *The Foundations of Justice: Why the Retarded and the Rest of Us Have Claims to Equality.* New York: Oxford University Press, 1986.

Walzer, Michael. *Spheres of Justice: A Defense of Pluralism and Equality.* New York: Basic Books, 1983.

A Miscellany of Hard Choices

Rationing Health Care According to Age

Binstock, Robert H., and Post, Stephen G., eds. *Too Old for Health Care? Controversies in Medicine, Law, Economics and Ethics.* Baltimore, MD: Johns Hopkins University Press, 1991.

Callahan, Daniel. *Setting Limits.* New York: Simon & Schuster, 1987.

Daniels, Norman. *Am I My Parents' Keeper?* New York: Oxford University Press, 1987.

Homer, Paul, and Holstein, Martha, eds. *A Good Old Age? The Paradox of Setting Limits.* New York: Simon & Schuster, 1990.

Jecker, Nancy S. "Age-Based Rationing and Women." *Journal of the American Medical Association* 266, no. 21 (December 4, 1991): 3012–3015.

———. ed. *Aging and Ethics: Philosophical Problems in Gerontology.* Clifton, NJ: Humana Press, 1991.

Rationing Health Care According to Ability to Pay

Arras, John. "Health Care Vouchers and the Rhetoric of Equity." *Hastings Center Report* 11 (August 1981): 29–39.

Bodhenheimer, T. "The Oregon Health Plan—Lessons for the Nation." *The New England Journal of Medicine.* Part One—337, no. 9 (August 28, 1997): 651; Part Two—337, no. 10 (September 4, 1997): 720.

Fleck, Leonard M. "Just Caring: Oregon, Health Care Rationing, and Informed Democratic Deliberation." *Journal of Medicine and Philosophy* 19 (1994): 367–388.

Garland, Michael J. "Justice, Politics, and Community: Expanding Access and Rationing Health Services in Oregon." *Law, Medicine and Health Care* 20 nos. 1–2 (Spring–Summer 1992): 67–81.

Lomasky, Loren. "The Small but Crucial Role of Health Care Vouchers." *Hastings Center Report* 11 (August, 1981): 40–42.

Menzel, Paul. "The Poor and the Puzzle of Equality." In *Strong Medicine,* by Paul Menzel. New York: Oxford University Press, 1990.

Rationing Experimental Treatments

Daniels, Norman, and Sabin, James. "Limits to Health Care: Fair Procedures, Democratic Deliberation, and the Legitimacy Problem for Insurers." *Philosophy and Public Affairs* 26, no. 4 (Fall 1997): 303–350.

Eddy, David. "High-Dose Chemotherapy with Autologous Bone Marrow Transplantation for the Treatment of Metastatic Breast Cancer." *Journal of Clinical Oncology* 10, no. 4 (1992): 657–670.

Pongrace, Paul Earl, III. "HDC/ABMT Experimental Treatment or Cure All? (Ask the Insurance Companies)." *The Journal of Pharmacy & Law* 2, no. 2, (1994) 329–356.

Priester, Reinhard; Gervais, Karen G.; Vawter, Dorthy E. *Improving Coverage for Unproven Health Care Interventions.* Minneapolis: Minnesota Center for Health Care Ethics, 1996.

Rationing Medical Enhancements

Allen, David, and Fost, Norman, eds. "Access to Treatment with Human Growth Hormone: Medical, Ethical, and Social Issues." *Growth, Genetics and Hormones* 8 (May 1992): 1–77.

Breggin, P. *Talking Back to Prozac.* New York: St. Martin's Press, 1994.

Canterbury, R J., and Lloyd, E. "Smart Drugs: Implications of Student Use." *Journal of Primary Prevention* 14 (1994): 197–207.

Davis, Kathy. *Reshaping the Female Body: The Dilemma of Cosmetic Surgery.* New York: Routledge, 1995.

Dean, W; Morgenthaler, J.; and Fawkes, S. *Smart Drugs II: The Next Generation.* Menlo Park: Health Freedom Publications, 1993.

Elliott, C. "Hedgehogs and Hermaphrodites: Toward a More Anthropological Bioethics." In *Philosophy of Medicine and Bioethics: A Twenty-Year Retrospective and Critical Appraisal,* edited by R. Carson and C. Burns. Dordrecht, The Netherlands: Kluwer Academic Publishers, 1997.

Gardner, William. "Can Human Genetic Enhancement Be Prohibited?" *Journal of Medicine and Philosophy* 20 (1995):

65–84.

Jorgensen, O. L., and Christiansen, Jens L. "Growth Hormone Therapy—Brave New Senescence: GH in Adults." *Lancet* 341 (1993): 1247–1248.

Kramer, Peter D. *Listening to Prozac.* New York: Viking, 1993.

Parens, Erik, ed. *Enhancing Human Traits: Conceptual Complexities and Ethical Implications.* Washington, D. C.: Georgetown University Press, 1998.

White, Gladys. "Human Growth Hormone: The Dilemma of Expanded Use in Children." *Kennedy Institute of Ethics Journal* 3, no. 4 (December 1993): 401.

Rationing Fairly: Principles and Prodedures

Aaron, Henry J., and Schwartz, William B. *The Painful Prescription: Rationing Health Care.* Washington, D. C.: Brookings Institution, 1984.

Anders, George. *Health against Wealth.* New York: Houghton Mifflin Company, 1996.

Blank, Robert H. *Rationing Medicine.* New York: Columbia University Press, 1988.

Blustein, Jan, and Marmor, Theodore R. "Cutting Waste by Making Rules: Promises, Pitfalls, and Realistic Prospects." *University of Pennsylvania Law Review* 140, no. 5 (May 1992): 1543-1572.

Churchill, Larry R. *Rationing Health Care in America: Perceptions and Principles of Justice.* Notre Dame, IN: University of Notre Dame Press, 1987.

Daniels, Norman. "Rationing Fairly: Programmatic Considerations." *Bioethics* 7, nos. 2–3 (1993): 224–233.

Daniels, Norman, et al. "Meeting the Challenges of Justice and Rationing." *Hastings Center Report* 24, no. 4 (July–August 1994): 27–42.

Eddy, David M. *Clinical Decision Making: From Theory to Practice.* Sudbury, MA: Jones and Bartlett, 1996.

Kamm, Frances M. *Morality, Mortality: Death and Whom to Save from It.* Oxford: Oxford University Press, 1993.

"The Law and Policy of Health Care Rationing: Models and Accountability." *University of Pennsylvania Law Review* 140, no. 5 (May 1992): 1505–1998.

"Managed Care Systems: Emerging Health Issues from an Ethics Perspective." *Journal of Law, Medicine and Ethics* 23, no. 3 (symposium 1995).

Menzel, Paul T. *Medical Costs, Moral Choices.* New Haven, CT: Yale University Press, 1983.

———. *Strong Medicine: The Ethical Rationing of Medical Care.* New York: Oxford University Press, 1990.

Nelson, James Lindemann. "Measured Fairness, Situated Justice: Feminist Reflections on Health Care Rationing." *Kennedy Institute of Ethics Journal* 6 (1996): 53–68.

Wikler, Daniel. "Ethics and Rationing: 'Whether,' 'How,' or 'How Much'?" *Journal of the American Geriatrics Society* 40, no. 4 (1992): 398–403.

APPENDIX

RESOURCES IN BIOETHICS

Bibliographies

Goldstein, Doris Mueller. *Bioethics: A Guide to Information Sources*. Detroit, MI: Gale Research Company, 1982.

Hastings Center. *Hastings Center's Bibliography of Ethics, Biomedicine, and Professional Responsibility*. Frederick, MD: University Publications of America, 1984.

Lineback, Richard H., ed. *Philosophers' Index*. Bowling Green, OH: Bowling Green State University, Philosophy Documentation Center. Issued quarterly.

Walters, LeRoy, and Kahn, Tamar Joy, eds. *Bibliography of Bioethics*. Washington, D.C.: Kennedy Institute of Ethics, Georgetown University. Published annually.

Yesley, Michael S. *ELSI Bibliography: Ethical, Legal and Social Implications of the Human Genome Project*. Washington, D.C.: U.S. Department of Energy, Office of Energy Research, 1993.

Bibliographical Services

Childress, James F., and Gaare, Ruth D., eds. *Bio-Law: A Legal and Ethical Report on Medicine, Health Care, and Bioengineering*. Frederick, MD: University Publications of America. Monthly updates of cases on 14 different topics in bioethics.

Hastings Center. "In the Literature." Annotated bibliography of recent titles in bioethics, published as a regular feature of the *Hastings Center Report*.

Reading Packets are available at $3 each through the Center for Biomedical Ethics, University of Minnesota, Suite N504 Boynton, 10 Church St. SE, Minneapolis, MN 55455-0346, or call 612-624-9440. Subjects include Artificial Nutrition and Hydration, Transplantation, Termination of Treatment of Adults, Distributing Limited Health Care Resources, Resuscitation Decisions, The Determination of Death, Individual Responsibility for Health, and New Frontiers in Genetic Testing and Screening: The Human Genome Project.

Scope Notes Series. Washington, D.C.: National Reference Center for Bioethics Literature, Kennedy Institute of Ethics, Georgetown University. A series of review essays and annotated bibliographies on a wide variety of topics in bioethics. Subjects include Living Wills and Durable Powers of Attorney (no. 2), Surrogate Mothers (no. 6), In Vitro Fertilization (no. 10), Anencephalic Infants as Potential Organ Sources (no. 12), Maternal-Fetal Conflicts (no. 14), Basic Resources in Bioethics (no. 15), The Human Genome Project (no. 17), Active Euthanasia and Assisted Suicide (no. 18), Nursing Ethics (no. 19), A Right to Health Care (no. 20), Genetic Testing and Screening (no. 22), and Human Gene Therapy (no. 24). Beginning with no. 15, all Scope Notes can also be found in the *Kennedy Institute of Ethics Journal*. To order reprints at $5 each, call 800-638-8480 or write the National Reference Center for Bioethics Literature, Kennedy Institute of Ethics, Georgetown University, Washington, D.C. 20057.

Data Bases

Bioethicsline. A National Library of Medicine on-line bibliographical data base covering the literature of the health sciences, law, religion, philosophy, the social sciences, and the popular media. Produced by the Information Retrieval Project at the Kennedy Institute of Ethics, Georgetown University, and supplied to the NLM MEDLARS system at the National Institutes of Health. Updated bi-monthly.

To order *free* bibliographical computer searches, call the National Reference Center for Bioethics Literature, Kennedy Institute of Ethics, Georgetown University, at 800-633-3849.

Dialog. Dialog Information Services, Inc., 3460 Hillview Ave., Palo Alto, CA 94304.

Lexis / Nexus. Mead Data Central, 9443 Springboro Pike—DM, P.O. Box 933, Dayton, OH 94501.

Bioethics Centers and Organizations

*Denotes recommended internet sites.

American Society for Bioethics and Humanities
4700 W. Lake Ave.,
Glenview, IL 60025-1485
847-375-4745
http://www.asbh.org

American Society of Law, Medicine, & Ethics
765 Commonwealth Ave., 16th Floor
Boston, MA 02215
617-262-4990
http://lawlib.slu.edu/aslme

Bioethics Center
University of Virginia
Box 348, UVA Health Sciences Center
Charlottesville, VA 22908
http://www.med.virginia.edu/inter-dis/bio-ethics/
Undergraduate Program in Bioethics
512 Cabell Hall
Charlottesville, VA 22903
http://minerva.acc.Virginia.EDU/~bioethic/

Bioethics Program
Howard University College of Medicine
520 W St. NW
Washington DC, 20059
202-806-6300

*Biomedical Ethics Unit
McGill University

3690 Peel St.
Montreal PQ, H3A 1W9 Canada
514-398-6980
http://www.mcgill.ca/bioethics

*Center for Bioethics
University of Pennsylvania
3401 Market St. #320
Philadelphia, PA 19104-3308
215-898-7136
http://www.med.upenn.edu/~bioethic/

Center for BioMedical Ethics
Case-Western Reserve University
School of Medicine
2119 Abington
Cleveleand, OH 44106
216-368-6196
http://www.cwru.edu/med/bioethics/bioethics.html

Center for Ethics and Humanities
Michigan State University
C-201 E. Fee Hall, East
Lansing, MI 48824
517-355-7550
http://www.med.umich.edu/psm/psm.html

Center for Ethics, Medicine, and Public Issues
Baylor College of Medicine
Houston, TX 77030
713-798-5678
http://www.bcm.tmc.edu/ethics/

Center for Health Care Ethics
St. Louis University Medical Center
1402 S. Grand Blvd.
St. Louis, MO 63104

The Centre for Applied Ethics
University of British Columbia
227-6356 Agricultural Rd.
Vancouver, B.C.
http://www.ethics.ubc.ca/resources/biomed/

Hastings Center
Garrison, NY 10524-5555
914-424-4040
http://www.ats.edu/spons/H0000089.HTM

Hastings Center West
324 Holyoke St.
San Francisco, CA 94134
415-468-6459

Institute for Jewish Medical Ethics
645 14th Ave.
San Francisco, CA 94118
800-258-4427
http://www.hia.com/hia/medethic/

Kennedy Institute of Ethics
Georgetown University
Washington D.C., 20057
800-MED-ETHX
http://guweb.georgetown.edu/kennedy/

*MacLean Center for Clinical Medical Ethics
University of Chicago
MC6098
5841 S. Maryland
Chicago, IL 60637
312-702-1453
http://ccme-mac4.bsd.uchicago.edu/CCME.html

Medical History and Ethics
A-204 Health Sciences, SB-20
University of Washington
Seattle, WA 98195
206-543-4802

National Bioethics Advisory Commission
6100 Executive Boulevard, Suite 5B01
Rockville, MD 20892-7508
301-402-4242
http://bioethics.gov/cgi-bin/bioeth_counter.pl

NIH Clinical Center
BioEthics Program
Bldg. 10, Rm. 1C116
Bethesda, MD 20892
301-496-2429
http://www1.od.nih.gov/ogcethics/home.html

Pacific Center for Health Policy and Ethics
USC Law Center 444
University Park, CA 90089-0071

Pope John Center for the Study of Ethics in Health Care
186 Forbes Rd.
Braintree, MA 02184
http://www.pjcenter.org/pjc/

Poynter Center for the Study of Ethics and American Institutions
Association for Practical and Professional Ethics
Indiana University
410 N. Park Ave.
Bloomington, IN 47405
812-855-0261
http://www.indiana.edu/poynter/index.html

University of Minnesota Center for Bioethics
Suite N504 Boynton
410 Church St. SE
Minneapolis, MN 55455-0346
612-624-9440
http://www.med.umn.edu/bioethics/

University of Pittsburg Center for Medical Ethics
Medical Arts Building Suite 300
3708 Fifth Ave.
Pittsburg, PA 15213-3405
412-647-5700
http://www.law.pitt.edu/mdethics/

Encyclopedias

Becker, Lawrence C. and Charlotte B., eds. *Encyclopedia of Ethics*. New York: Garland,
     1992. 2 vols.

Edwards, Paul, ed. *Encyclopedia of Philosophy*. New York: Macmillan, 1967.

Reich, Warren T., ed. *Encyclopedia of Bioethics*. 2nd ed. New York: Free Press, 1995.
     5 vols.

Journals

Journals that focus primarily on bioethics:

Bioethics

Cambridge Quarterly of Healthcare Ethics

Hastings Center Report

IRB: A Review of Human Subjects Research

Journal of Clinical Ethics

Journal of Law, Medicine & Ethics

Journal of Medical Ethics

Journal of Medical Humanities and Bioethics

Journal of Medicine and Philosophy

Kennedy Institute of Ethics Journal

Theoretical Medicine

Philosophical journals that regularly feature articles on bioethics:

Canadian Journal of Philosophy

Ethics

Philosophy and Public Affairs

Social Theory and Practice

Legal journals often contain bioethics-related essays, and their voluminous footnotes
are an excellent source of further bibliographical data. An indispensable guide to this
literature is the *Index of Legal Periodicals*. The following journals regularly feature useful
articles:

American Journal of Law and Medicine

Harvard Law Review

Yale Law Journal

Medical and nursing journals with significant bioethical contributions:

American Journal of Nursing

Annals of Internal Medicine

Archives of Internal Medicine

Journal of the American Medical Association (JAMA)

Lancet (British)
New England Journal of Medicine
Nursing Research
Pediatrics
Perspectives in Biology and Medicine

Religious and theological journals:
Journal of Religious Ethics
Linacre Quarterly
Theological Studies

Health policy journals:
Health Affairs
Journal of Health Politics, Policy and Law
Milbank Quarterly (often publishes excellent supplementary issues devoted to such topics as decision making for the elderly and AIDS)

Instructional Aids

Clouser, K. Danner. *Teaching Bioethics: Strategies, Problems, and Resources*. Hastings-on-Hudson, NY: Hastings Center, 1980.

Dax's Case: Who Should Decide? An hour-long film about the burn patient discussed in the case study in Part Two, Section Two of this text. Produced by Concern for Dying and available from Filmakers Library, 124 E. 40th St., New York, NY 10016, 212-808-4980, or from Choice in Dying, 200 Varick St., New York, NY 10014.

Scope Note Number 9: *Bioethics Audiovisuals: 1982–1988*, 12 pp. Available through National Reference Center for Bioethics Literature (see under Bibliographical Services above).

Scope Note Number 16: *Teaching Ethics in the Health Care Setting: Survey of the Literature and Sample Syllabus*. Parts I and II. In *Journal of the Kennedy Institute of Ethics* 1, nos. 2–3 (June/September 1991): 171–185, 263–273.

Graduate Programs in Bioethics

"Graduate Programs in Bioethics and the Medical Humanities," revised February 1994. A report listing bioethics programs in the United States, available on-line from the University of Pennsylvania Bioethics Internet Project at http://www.med.upenn.edu/bioethics.